THE BASIC EMT

Comprehensive Prehospital Patient Care

Dan Schott

CONGRATULATIONS

You now have access to MERLIN for
The Basic EMT: Comprehensive Prehospital Patient Care,
second edition,
by **Norman E. McSwain, Jr., and James L. Paturas!**

sign on at: http://www.mosby.com/MERLIN/McSwain

A website just for you as you learn prehospital emergency care with the new
second edition of The Basic EMT: Comprehensive Prehospital Patient Care

what you will receive:

Whether you are a student, an instructor, or a clinician, you'll find information just for you. Things like:
- Content Updates
- Links to Related Products
- Author Information, Answers to Frequently Asked Questions, and more

plus:

WebLinks

An exciting new program that allows you to directly access hundreds of active websites keyed specifically to the content of this book. The WebLinks are continually updated, with new ones added as they develop. **Peel the top layer only from the sticker on this page and register with the listed passcode.**

Free access to Mosby's Virtual Classroom with NEW textbook purchase.

Talk to your instructor about Mosby's Virtual Classroom! This instructor-driven, online learning environment allows your instructor to provide you with convenient access to course syllabuses, additional activities and review exercises, and a whole lot more. When your instructor chooses to take advantage of this powerful tool, your access to Mosby's Virtual Classroom is FREE for one year with the purchase of a NEW textbook. Purchase a NEW print workbook and you will receive FREE access to the interactive online workbook for an entire year! Find out more at MERLIN.

MERLIN

Mosby's **E**lectronic **R**esource **L**inks & **I**nformation **N**etwork

Mosby
A Harcourt Health Sciences Company

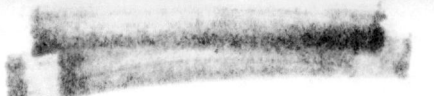

SECOND EDITION

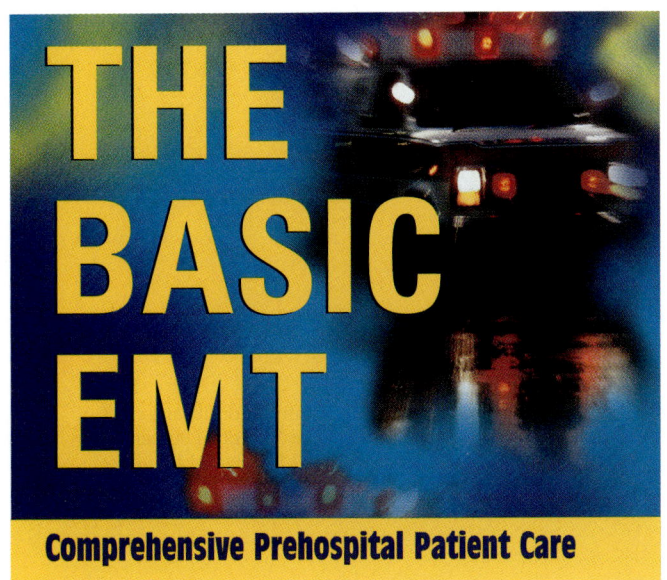

THE BASIC EMT
Comprehensive Prehospital Patient Care

NORMAN E. McSWAIN, Jr., MD, FACS, NREMT-P
Professor of Surgery
Tulane University School of Medicine
New Orleans, LA

JAMES L. PATURAS, EMT-P
Director, Emergency Medical Services
Bridgeport Hospital
Bridgeport, CT

with 783 illustrations

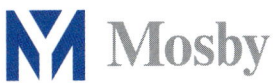

A Harcourt Health Sciences Company
St. Louis   London   Philadelphia   Sydney   Toronto

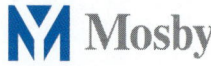

A Harcourt Health Sciences Company

Publisher: Andrew Allen
Executive Editor: Claire Merrick
Developmental Editor: Laura Bayless
Editorial Assistant: Lisa Brightwell
Project Manager: Catherine Jackson
Project Specialist: Jeff Patterson
Design Manager: Judi Lang
Cover Designer: Teresa Breckwoldt

SECOND EDITION

Copyright © 2001 by Mosby, Inc.

Previous edition copyrighted 1997

All rights reserved. No part of this publication may be reproduced or transmitted in any form or by any means, electronic or mechanical, including photocopy, recording, or any information storage and retrieval system, without permission in writing from the publisher.

Permission to photocopy or reproduce solely for internal or personal use is permitted for libraries or other users registered with the Copyright Clearance Center, provided that the base fee of $4.00 per chapter plus $.10 per page is paid directly to the Copyright Clearance Center, 222 Rosewood Drive, Danvers, Massachusetts 01923. This consent does not extend to other kinds of copying, such as copying for general distribution, for advertising or promotional purposes, for creating new collected works, or for resale.

Mosby, Inc.
A Harcourt Health Sciences Company
11830 Westline Industrial Drive
St. Louis, Missouri 63146

Printed in the United States of America

Library of Congress Cataloging-in-Publication Data
The basic EMT: comprehensive prehospital patient care.—2nd ed./[edited by] Norman E. McSwain, Jr., James L. Paturas.
   p. cm.
  Includes index.
  ISBN 0-323-01116-0 (hardcover)—ISBN 0-323-01110-1 (softcover)
  1. Medical emergencies. 2. Emergency medical technicians. I. McSwain, Norman E., 1937-
    II. Paturas, James L.

RC86.7 .B376 2001
616.02′5—dc21

                                                                                       00-069943

Dedication

Forty-five years ago, no training program was available to educate prehospital personnel in the management of trauma patients. J.D. 'Deke' Farrington, MD, felt that trauma victims deserved better than an unattended ride to the hospital in the back of a hearse. In 1958 he convinced the Chicago Fire Department that firefighters should be trained to manage emergency patients. Along with Dr. Sam Banks, Deke started the Trauma Training program in Chicago. More than three million people have been trained according to the guidelines they developed. Still, no standards for ambulance design and equipment existed, communication systems between physicians and EMTs were missing, and national standards for training and certification had yet to be written.

Deke was involved in every aspect of the origins of EMS; nothing happened without his hand or his influence.

"Training of ambulance personnel and others responsible for the emergency care of the sick and injured on the scene and during transport" (March 1968) Task force chairman JD Farrington (basis for the 81-hour course)

"The advanced training for emergency medical technicians/ambulance" (September 1970 Subcommittee on Ambulance services) JD Farrington, Chairman (basis for the 480-hour course)

"Medical requirements for Ambulance Design & Equipment" (1967) Subcommittee for ambulance services; JD Farrington, Chairman (basis for the essential equipment list)

"EMS design and criteria" (May 1971) Committee on AMBULANCE design and criteria; JD Farrington, committee member (basis for the KKK standards for vehicles)

As a member of the National Academy of Sciences/National Research Council committee, Farrington helped write the famous paper, "Accidental Death and Disability, The Neglected Disease of Modern Society." His ideas and support launched the National Association of EMTs, and he was one of the major players in the National Registry of EMTs for more than 15 years.

This "Moses" of EMS was the son of a Baptist minister in the deep South. His nickname was short for Deacon.

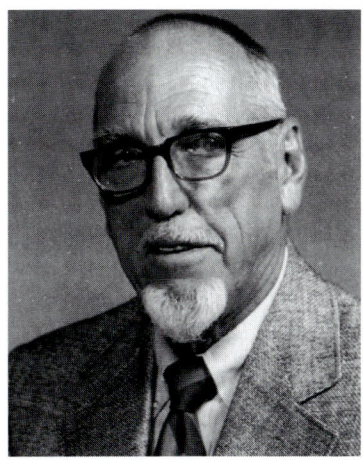

Joseph D. "Deke" Farrington, MD, FACS
Father of EMS
January 16, 1909–January 20, 1982

Born in Richmond, Virginia, he lived in every state in the impoverished South. He attended the University of Alabama when it was only a 2-year medical school in Birmingham, before obtaining his MD degree at Rush Medical School in Chicago. He lost his mother at an early age due to a lack of proper medical care. This experience, along with his love for people and his religious training, was most likely the source of his zeal to improve the care of the injured patient.

Twenty-nine years before the publication of this textbook, "Deke" Farrington published the article that was the focal point for the beginning of EMS. "Death in a Ditch" is the landmark paper most often identified as the point of change in prehospital care. Most people in EMS have heard of it, but many have not read it. In the first few paragraphs it is easy to grasp the state of prehospital care in the 1960s and Deke's vision of what it should be. We have come a long way in doing what he asked. Don't stop now. Continue to improve yourself and the care that you provide.

Contributors to the Second Edition

FOREWORD
Richard C. Hunt, MD, FACEP
Professor and Chair
Department of Emergency Medicine
SUNY Upstate Medical University
Syracuse, New York

CHAPTER 2
Jeff G. deGraffenreid, Paramedic, M.Ed.
Paramedic Team Leader
Johnson County Medical Action Emergency Medical Services
Olathe, Kansas

CHAPTER 3
Jorge A. Martinez
Chair, Emergency Medicine
Louisiana State University Medical Center
New Orleans, Louisiana

Larry D. Weiss, MD, JD
Clinical Associate Professor of Medicine
Louisiana State University
New Orleans, Louisiana

CHAPTERS 5 AND 36
J. Mark Lockhart, NREMTP
Maryland Heights Fire Protection District
Maryland Heights, Missouri

CHAPTER 7
John Chamberlain
EMS Specialist-Educator
PreHospital Care Office
University of Pittsburgh Medical Center
Pittsburgh, Pennsylvania

Stephen R. Carden, EMT-P
JHPC Program Coordinator
Bridgeport, Connecticut

CHAPTERS 8, 12, 13, 16, AND 41
Larry Hatfield, REMT-P
Creighton University EMS Education
Omaha, Nebraska

CHAPTER 9
Dawne W. Orgeron, RN, EMT-P
EMS Administrator
New Orleans Health Department
New Orleans, Louisiana

CHAPTERS 17 AND 19
Will Chapleau, RN, EMT-P
Good Samaritan Hospital
Downer Grove, Illinois

CHAPTERS 18 AND 31
Michael Werdmann, MD, FACEP
Chairman, Department of Emergency Medicine
Bridgeport Hospital
Bridgeport, Connecticut

CHAPTERS 20 AND 30
Richard L. Judd, PhD, EMSI
Central Connecticut State University
New Britain, Connecticut

CHAPTER 21
John Pelazza, EMT-P
American Medical Response of CT
Bridgeport, Connecticut

CHAPTER 23
Scott B. Frame, MD, FACS, FCC
Department of Surgery
University of Cincinnati Medical Center
Cincinnati, Ohio

CHAPTERS 24, 27, AND 28
Merry J. McSwain, BSN, RN, NREMT-P
Masters Candidate in Trauma/Critical Care
University of Alabama—Birmingham
School of Nursing
Birmingham, Alabama

CHAPTER 25
Jeffrey Salomone, MD, FACS, NREMT-P
Assistant Professor of Surgery
Emory University School of Medicine
Atlanta, Georgia

CHAPTER 29
Steve Mercer, NREMT-P
Iowa Department of Health
EMS Bureau
Des Moines, Iowa

CHAPTER 32
Elizabeth M. Wertz, RN, BSN, PhRN, EMT-P
Pediatric Alliance, PC
Carnegie, Pennsylvania

CHAPTERS 33 AND 38
Greg Chapman, EMT-P
Hudson Valley Community College
Troy, New York

CHAPTER 34
William R. Metcalf, EMT-B
Division Chief, EMS and Special Services
North Lake Tahoe Fire Protection District
Incline Village, Nevada

Jim Linardos, EMT-I
Fire Chief
North Lake Tahoe Fire Protection District
Incline Village, Nevada

CHAPTERS 35 AND 40
Augie Bamonti, EMTP, RN
Chicago Heights Fire Department
Chicago Heights, Illinois

CHAPTER 37
Ben Blankenship, EMT
Emergency Response Supervisor
Great Lakes Chemical Corporation
South Arkansas Operations
El Dorado, Arkansas

CHAPTER 39
Steve Kidd
Company Officer
Orange County Fire/Rescue Division
Orange County, Florida

John Czajkowski
Company Officer
Orange County Fire/Rescue Division
Orange County, Florida

CHAPTER 41
Bret C. Gilliam, Captain
Ocean Tech
Bath, Maine

CHAPTER 42
G. H. Adkisson, MC, USN, Captain
Commanding Officer
Medical Corps, U.S. Navy
Fort Sam Houston, Texas

APPENDIX A
Catherine A. Parvensky Barwell, RN, MED, PHRN, EMT-IT
MCP Hahnemann University
Philadelphia, Pennsylvania

Merry J. McSwain, BSN, RN, NREMT-P
Masters Candidate in Trauma/Critical Care
University of Alabama—Birmingham School of Nursing
Birmingham, Alabama

Contributors to the First Edition

We want to thank the contributors to the first edition:

Michael Armacost, NREMT-P, BS
Brent R. Asplin, MD, NREMT-P
Christopher M. Cannon, MSN, MPH, MBA, CHE
Stephen R. Carden, EMT-P
Vincent P. Cezus, RN, MBA, NREMT-P
Drew E. Dawson, EMT-B
Scott B. Frame, MD, FACS, FCC
Mike Hartzog, MD
Donna Hastings, EMT-P
Lawrence M. Hatfield, Jr., REMT-P
Leah J. Heimbach, JD, RN, NREMT-P
David R. Johnson, MD, FACEP
Richard L. Judd, PhD, EMSI

Mark Lockhart, NREMT-P
Steven A. McLaughlin, MD
Stuart D. McNicol, NREMT-P
Merry J. McSwain, NREMT-P
Steve Mercer, NREMT-P
Patrick F. Moore, REMT-I, I/C
Chris Neal, EMT-P
Earl H. Neal, EMT-P
F.R. Fritz Nordengren, EMT-P
Dawne W. Orgeron, RN, EMT-P
Rick Petrie, EMT-P
Michael J. Werdmann, MD, FACEP
Elizabeth M. Wertz, RN, BSN, PHRN, EMT-P

We would also like to especially acknowledge Roger Dean White, MD, and William R. Metcalf, EMT-B, for their contribution as co-authors of the first edition.

Acknowledgments

Anyone who reads this textbook knows that it is not a product of the editors or the authors. It is far more than that. This particular text has been very complex because of the style and the concern that all of the users' needs are met by including all of the objectives of the National Standard Curriculum in a readable fashion while adding the enhancement information that will make the EMT-B more well rounded.

The book that you are about to read is an output of a team. The team is like any sports team that you have been a part of or watched. We are very pleased to have been pushed, prodded, pulled, and helped along each step by what must be the finest team in the publication business. The developmental editor, Peg Waltner, spent many hours going over the text material to make sure that there was consistency from chapter to chapter in style, language, illustrations, and other aspects. She took over in the middle of the project at a difficult time and made it a success. Enough cannot be said of the endless contributions and the frustrations managed by those in the St. Louis Production Department, including Catherine Jackson and Jeff Patterson. Production folks spend many hours looking at the minutia of photos, illustrations, text, and the layout. Without them, their patience, their outstanding knowledge, and their leadership, this book would have never become a reality. Any writing is done with flaws, missed concepts, oversights, and lost thoughts. The reviewers, Catherine Parvensky Barwell and Merry McSwain, have spent long hours into the night and on off weekends looking for these details. Perhaps most importantly for the EMT-B student who reads the text, the instructor who teaches with it, and the ultimate user, the patient, they have made sure that every concept and every objective was covered completely. Anyone who has seen the photographic work of Rick Brady knows of his skill and understanding of EMS photography. Many of the readers have seen and used his work in other books for a long time. We are very pleased to have had the benefit of his experience with this book.

Finally, and most importantly, is the executive editor for the publisher, who is the big brother, the mother, the disciplinarian, the godfather, the leader, the whip holder (and user), who makes the entire process work. We have worked with Claire Merrick on a number of products. We hope to do so again. There is no question that she is the quarterback, the coach, and the captain of this team. Without her leadership this book would have never be finished. She is the very best in the business.

I do not exist day to day without the other half of my personal team. Vanessa Lee and I have been together almost 15 years. She is my maker, my companion, and my friend. Without her I could not survive in academic medicine.

Norman E. McSwain, Jr.

On a similar note, I could not get through a day without the support of Liz Butcher. Since titles do not mean much to me, the important part is that Liz is an equal member of the team who keeps me on the straight and narrow at the hospital. For that I thank her and will be forever in her debt.

James L. Paturas

Publisher's Acknowledgments

The publisher would like to thank the following reviewers who read, commented on, and helped fine-tune the manuscript.

Linda M. Abrahamson, EMT-P, RN
EMS Education Coordinator
Silver Cross Hospital
Joliet, Illinois

Joe Acker, AHT, EMT-P
Coordinator, EMT-I Program
Northern Alberta Institute of Technology
Edmonton, Alberta, Canada

Brenda Beasley
EMS Program Director
Calhoun Community College
Wedowee, Alabama

Sharon "Skipper" Boyko, RN, CEN, CFRN, EMT-P, TNCC (I)
Flight Nurse
Aero Med of Spectrum Health
Grand Rapids, Michigan

Robert Carter, NREMT-P
Affiliate Faculty, Hopkins Outreach for Pediatric Education
The Johns Hopkins Children's Center
Baltimore, Maryland

Robert Cook, NREMT-P
Paramedic Supervisor
Hamilton Hospital
Webster City, Iowa

Jeff G. DeGraffenreid, Paramedic, M.Ed.
Paramedic Team Leader
Johnson County Medical Action Emergency Medical Services
Olathe, Kansas

Bob Elling, MPA, NREMT-P
Program Director
Hudson Valley Community College
Institute of Prehospital Emergency Medicine
Troy, New York

Richard Ellis, NREMT-P
Instructor
United States Air Force EMT Program Manager
Sheppard Air Force Base
Texas

Marie Godspodareck
University of Alabama
School of Health Related Professions
Birmingham, Alabama

Larry Hatfield, NREMT-P
EMS Education
Creighton University
Omaha, Nebraska

Victor Hernandez, EMT-P
Sierra College
Rocklin, California
Emergency Training and Consultations
Truckee, California

David LaCombe, NREMT-P
EMS Educational Programs Coordinator
University of Miami School of Medicine
Center for Research in Medical Education
Miami, Florida

Jeffrey Lindsey, Paramedic
Education Specialist
VFIS and St. Petersburg Junior College
Largo, Florida

Andrew McDonell
Director of Paramedic Education
Victoria University
Melbourne City, Australia

Merry McSwain, RN, NREMT-P, BSN
Masters Student in Trauma/Critical Care
University of Alabama in Birmingham
School of Nursing
Birmingham, Alabama

William R. Metcalf
Division Chief, EMS and Special Services
North Lake Tahoe Fire Protection District
Incline Village, Nevada

James B. Miller, EMT-P
U.S. Army EMT Program Manager
91W Branch

Debra O'Callaghan, EMT
BLS Coordinator
Thomas Jefferson University Hospital
Philadelphia, Pennsylvania

John Eric Powell, MS, NREMT-P
Flight Paramedic
University of Tennessee Medical Center—Knoxville
Knoxville, Tennessee

Severo A. Rodriguez, NREMT-P
Instructor
Emergency Medical Technology
University of Texas Health Science Center
San Antonio, Texas

Judith Ruple, PhD
EMT Instructor
The University of Toledo
Toledo, Ohio

Jose Salazar
Jose Salazar & Associates
EMS Consulting & Education
Sterling, Virginia

Karen Snyder, RN, CEN, EMT-P
EMS Educator
Cincinnati State Technical and Community College
Cincinnati, Ohio

Andrew William Stern, NREMT-P, MPA, MA
Town of Colonie Emergency Medical Services
Colonie, New York

Gail Stewart, EMT-P
Emergency Medical Services Programs Director
Santa Fe Community College
Gainesville, Florida

A. Keith Wesley, MD, FACEP
Director, EMS Education
Sacred Heart Hospital
Eau Claire, Wisconsin

Cindy Wojton, PA, EMT-P
BLS Coordinator
Thomas Jefferson University Hospital
Philadelphia, Pennsylvania

Matthew Zavarella, BSAS, NREMT-P, EMT-P
University of Mississippi Medical Center
Department of Emergency Medical Technology
Jackson, Mississippi

History of EMS

During the late 1700s, Napoleon Bonaparte appointed Baron Dominique-Jean Larrey to develop the medical patient care system for the French army. One of findings was that leaving wounded soldiers on the field for several days increased the complications and suffering. He felt that this delay in treatment resulted in needless deaths. "The remoteness of our ambulances deprived the wounded of the requisite attention," he wrote. In 1797, Larrey developed a method to send trained medical personnel into the field to provide medical care to the wounded soldiers and to provide medical care en route to the field hospital. This action increased their chances of survival and benefited Napoleon's conquest efforts. He designed a special carriage staffed with medical personnel to access all parts of the battlefield. The carriage became known as the *ambulance volante*, or *flying ambulance*.

Baron Larrey developed all of the precepts of emergency medical care used today: 1) rapid access to the patient by trained personnel, 2) field treatment and stabilization, and 3) rapid transportation back to the medical facility, while 4) providing medical care en route. Although removal of the wounded and dead from the battlefields has existed in some form since early Greek and Roman times, Larrey can still be considered the "father of emergency medical services."

During the War between the States, both sides attempted to emulate the medical practices of the Napoleonic wars with little success. Lack of funding, government support, and dedicated personnel prevented the development of an effective system. During the Second Battle of Bull Run in August of 1862, on the Yankee side alone 3000 wounded lay in the field for 3 days and 600 wounded lay for 1 week. James Brady and Walt Whitman reported that facilities were primitive and many wounded died in agony. At that time the ambulance service was run by the Quartermaster Corps. It was transferred to surgeon general Jonathan Letterman, MD, to organize. He reinstated Larrey's concepts.

At the Geneva Convention of 1864 an agreement was developed among the European countries to recognize the neutrality of hospitals, the sick and wounded, all persons involved in medical care, and ambulances. It provided safe passage across battle lines for all medical and injured personnel. On August 22, 1864, the organization adopted for its logo the reverse of the Swiss flag. The logo was a red cross on a white background. The name that they adopted was the International Red Cross.

In 1867 Major General Rucker won the "best of kind" for an ambulance that was adopted as the regulation ambulance. It had extra springs on the floor, more elasticity to the stretchers, and improved ventilation.

The first ambulance service in the United States was created in Cincinnati in 1865 at Cincinnati General Hospital. This service still operated in the fire department. Other services followed at Grady Hospital in Atlanta, Charity Hospital in New Orleans, and several hospitals in New York City and other major cities. In December of 1869 the first month of operation of the ambulance service of the Free Hospital of New York (Bellevue) ran 74 calls. A total of 1466 calls were run in 1870. The dispatch system was different from that used today. The hospital ran a bess, which triggered a weight to fall, lighting the gas lamp to wake the physician and the driver. It also caused the harness, saddle, and collar to drop on the horse and opened the stable doors. However, this improved care was mostly limited to the larger cities.

During World War I and especially during World War II, the military medical corps proved their worth in field assessment and early management of injured personnel. Although the military system of emergency care became well developed, the development of a civilian system lagged far behind.

In the mid-1950s, J.D. "Deke" Farrington, MD, FACS (the Father of modern EMS), and others, questioned why the lessons learned by the military medical corps during World War II and the Korean War could not be brought into the civilian community to improve the standard of civilian care. At that time, emergency medicine and EMS were not what we know today. In San Francisco, New York, New Orleans, and other American cities, interns were assigned to ambulances to provide care for the victims of trauma and other conditions outside of the hospital. Most hospitals did not have a place to manage emergencies. Some hospitals had set up an unstaffed "emergency room" at the back of the hospital. The "ambulance driver" had to ring the doorbell beside the emergency room door so that the nurse could come down from the ward to unlock the door. The nurse then checked the patient and called a physician from home if she thought that the patient was really sick. (Did you ever wonder why modern emergency departments are in the rear of the hospital and not out front? Tradition.) All the physicians on staff had to take turns "covering the emergency room." A patient involved in a major wreck with multiple fractures, and perhaps a ruptured spleen or a head injury, might be seen by an ophthalmologist or a dermatologist. Many physicians knew that they were ill prepared to handle trauma or a major myocardial infarction, but there was no alternative.

Until the concept arose that nonphysicians could be trained to provide this kind of emergency care, the majority of the prehospital care was merely transportation provided by the local mortuary. The victim was driven to the hospital in a hearse with no one in the "patient compartment" except the patient and perhaps a family member.

Many people began to question the efficacy and even ethics of this transportation. When the paper titled "Accidental Death and Disability: The Neglected Disease of Modern Society" was written by the National Academy of Sciences and the National Research Council in 1966, it became apparent that much improvement could be made by changing the emergency vehicles themselves and improving the training of EMTs, communications, record keeping, and the care provided upon arrival to the facility.

At the Airlie House conference (May 1969) sponsored by the Committee on Trauma, American College of Surgeons and Committee on Injuries, American Academy of Orthopaedic Surgeons, "Recommendations for an Approach to an Urgent National Problem" was written. This conference indicated that immediate attention and control were needed in the areas of transportation and communication. Developing standards for ambulance design and equipment was recognized as "painfully slow."

Dr. Farrington and Dr. Sam Banks developed a trauma training school for the Chicago Fire Department that served as the prototype of what later became the first EMT-Ambulance (EMT-A) training program. The task force involved in the design of the program for the United States Department of Transportation (USDOT) included Deke Farrington, Rocco Morando, Oscar Hampton, Walter Hoyt, Walter Hunt, Robert Oswald, Peter Safar, and Joseph Territo.

At the same time that the EMT-A training program was evolving, Eugene Nagle in Miami; Ron Stewart and Jim Page in Los Angeles; John Waters in Jacksonville, Florida; Costas Lambrew in New York; Mark Vasu in Grand Rapids, Michigan; Jim Warren in Columbus, Ohio; and others began to provide "paramedic care." Originally designed for cardiac patients, all types of patients soon received the type of prehospital cardiac care developed by Pantridge and Geddes in Belfast, Ireland. Small communities, such as Newton, Kansas, under the direction of Jim Werries, had developed a cardiac care EMS service by the early 1970s, but these were isolated situations. Kansas was like many of the states during the period that worked in isolation to develop a method of providing prehospital care for its citizens. It was not until 1974 to 1975 that Kansas had the statewide program going at the basic level and partially evolved at the EMT-Paramedic (EMT-P) level.

The initial training program was called the Advanced Training Program of EMT. The USDOT organized a subcommittee on ambulance services, which developed the standards on which this course was based. Many of those leaders who have been identified were active in the development of this curriculum. Nancy Caroline and her team at the University of Pittsburgh was awarded the contract from the USDOT to write the National Standard Curriculum for the EMT-P. This modular training program included sections that then became the basis for the EMT-Intermediate (EMT-I).

Up until the late 1970s, most of the federal involvement came through the USDOT under the leadership of Leo Schwartz and Robert Motley. A new EMS act was passed in 1976 that gave money and responsibility to the U.S. Department of Health, Education, and Welfare. Chicago trauma surgeon David Boyd led this enactment, which resulted in the development of state and local EMS regions throughout the United States.

The National Registry of EMTs (NREMT) was created shortly after the Airlie Conference. This organization was responsible for registering and reregistering EMTs based on completion of the USDOT standard EMT-A curriculum (and later the EMT-I and EMT-P training). The NREMT developed written and practical examinations based on the objectives of these courses to examine and register those who satisfactorily completed the examination process. Most states use the NREMT's process in whole or in part as the basis for licensure.

The "Star of Life" is a logo patented by the American Medical Association in 1967. It represents the three rivers of life and the staff of Aesculapius. It was given to the NREMT as the EMT logo. When Dawson Mills of the USDOT asked the American Red Cross to use the red cross as the EMS logo for ambulances and was refused, he asked "Deke" Farrington if the USDOT could use the Star of Life on all ambulances in the United States, and Farrington approved it. The six points of the star were named by Leo Schwartz.

The National Association of EMTs (NAEMT), founded in 1975, was developed to represent EMTs at all levels. The state EMS directors formed the National Association of State EMS Directors (NASEMSD) to share ideas and develop strategies for EMS development across state lines. Another organization, the National Council of EMS Training Coordinators (NASEMSTC), is also charged with sharing educational ideas across state lines.

The National Association of EMS Physicians (NAEMSP) was formed to provide leadership in medical direction of EMS services. This association is the focus of activities, discussion, and meetings for physicians involved either full- or part-time in EMS.

This brief overview can only mention a few highlights in the development of EMS in the United States. However, even this history underscores how far EMS has evolved from its roots in European battlefields.

Table of Important Events in EMS

Year	Event
1899	First motorized ambulance operated out of the Micheal Reese Hospital in Chicago; reached a speed of 16 miles per hour
1901	President McKinley shot in Buffalo and transported in a motorized ambulance
1922	Committee on Treatment of Fractures formed
1931	Outline of Treatment of Injuries, American College of Surgeons
1939	Committee on Fractures and Other Injuries formed
1954	Survey of EMS systems performed by ACS/COT chairman Alan Dimick, MD; 64 cities, 5 years of data (1/4 excellent, 1/3 unacceptable)
1955	Saturday Evening Post article, "Let Those Crash Victims Lie—Ambulance Attendants are Trained to Handle Them," published
1959	Symposium on Medical Aspects of Traffic Safety formed
1960	"Management of Fractures and Soft Tissue" published by Committee on Trauma, American College of Surgeons
1957	Chicago Fire Department training program developed by "Deke" Farrington, MD
1960	Cardiopulmonary resuscitation (CPR) successful (Kouwenhoven)
1960	"CPR"—*Journal of the American Medical Association* article published by Jude
1962	AMBU bag developed
1962	"Thumper," developed by Michigan Instruments
1962	"Resusci-Anne," developed by Laerdal
1965	Life Pack 33 developed
1966	"Accidental Death and Disability—The Neglected Disease of Modern Society" published by NRC-NAS
1966	Presidents Commission on Highway Safety formed
1966	Highway Safety Act enacted
1967	"Death in a Ditch" published by "Deke" Farrington, MD
1967	Mobile Coronary Care Units developed by Pantridge
1967	Traction splint developed by Glenn Hare
1967	"Star of Life" patented by American Medical Association
1967	Jaws of Life developed by George Hurst
1969	Ohio Heartmobile developed
1969	Arlie House Conference formed
1969	American Medical Association Commission on EMS formed
1969	Helicopter used for civilian medical transportation
1969	EMT-A published by Dunlap and Associates
1970	National Registry of EMTs (NREMT) founded
1970	"Emergency" television series with Johnny and Roy
1973	Emergency Medical Services Act enacted
1975	National Association of EMTs (NAEMT) founded
1975	ACLS developed by American Heart Association
1978	ATLS pilot course developed in Auburn, Nebraska
1979	ATLS approved by ACS/COT
1979	Joint Review Committee for EMT-Paramedic accreditation formed
1981	Prehospital Trauma Life Support (PHTLS) approved by NAEMT and ACS/COT
1981	BTLS developed by Alabama Chapter of ACEP
1983	PHTLS pilot courses run in Iowa, Connecticut, and Louisiana

EMS grew exponentially after the early 1980s. So many people contributed so much that an attempt to list all of these contributions would leave out many of the major players. This does not detract from all of the work done by each of them. It only points out the growth of EMS in the United States and the world. A small example is all of those who made possible the spread of PHTLS to 25 countries and greater than 300,000 providers trained by the year 2000 and a similar spread of BTLS by its contributors.

Norman E. McSwain, Jr.

Introduction

by **Norman E. McSwain, Jr.** MD

The chance to help a fellow human being happens only occasionally to most people. To have this chance every day comes only to a few. However, with that opportunity falls the obligation to provide this service as completely and flawlessly as possible. An imperfectly or partially performed task is not acceptable to a sick or injured patient, nor should it be to the EMT. The EMT must have a basic bank of knowledge, the observational power to gather information, the analytical insight to balance actions and their outcomes, the clinical understanding to arrive at decisions, the strength to carry them out, and the composure to do so quickly and efficiently.

To achieve this, the EMT must dedicate himself or herself to the acquisition and maintenance of the knowledge required to make these judgments. This is a lifelong obligation. Learning must not stop when the initial training period is over. Every week new information becomes available that changes the approach to patient care. Each day the EMT must dedicate himself or herself to acquiring new knowledge and perfecting current knowledge and skills. Patients expect no less, and EMTs must do the same.

At the scene of an emergency, once scene safety is secured, the patient becomes the most important person present. Patients do not choose to be in their current condition. Yes, they may have made foolish decisions that got them into their present predicament, but nonetheless they did not choose specifically to be there. Also, they did not choose the EMT who will provide them with care. On the other hand, the EMT did choose to be an EMT, did choose to provide patient care, and in one way or another did choose to be on that particular call. Since the patient did not choose us and we chose him or her, it is our responsibility to give 100% of our time, knowledge, and effort to the patient. All of us should strive to have all the knowledge possible, provide the best care possible, and achieve the best outcome on each of our patients. We must treat each of our patients as we would wish to be treated or as we would wish a member of our family to be treated. The patient expects that of us, and we should expect it of ourselves. The patient cannot afford for the EMT to have a "bad day."

The goal of the prehospital provider has always been to get the patient safely to the hospital. It has never been the goal to completely treat the patient in the field. Some conditions are field-manageable; others are not. Providing definitive care for the patient's condition is the goal of each individual involved in patient care, regardless of their background and training. One of the most important factors in the survival of any patient is the time from the onset of the emergency to the provision of definitive care.

Definitive care has various levels depending on the skill, knowledge, and equipment at hand and patient condition. The more complex levels of care do not minimize that provided by the EMT in the field; each level is critically important to the survival of the patient.

Consider a patient with cardiac arrest. Definitive care for this patient is to reestablish cardiac rhythm, cardiac output, and perfusion to vital organs. The first step of definitive care is returning the patient's cardiac output to normal, and at a minimum, maintaining the perfusion to the brain, heart, lung, and other vital organs. This first step is frequently achievable in the field through cardiopulmonary resuscitation (CPR), adequate ventilation, and defibrillation. However, CPR is only a holding pattern.

The next level of definitive care is to find the cause of the cardiac arrest and take steps to prevent its recurrence. This step is usually not achievable in the field; it must be done in the hospital. Perhaps coronary bypass or even a heart transplant will be required to treat the patient. The care of this patient begins in the field but does not end until the patient is fully rehabilitated and returned to normal activity. As you can see, each level of definitive care is necessary for recovery. The sooner each level of definitive care is reached, the greater the patient's chance for survival.

Definitive care of trauma patients usually cannot be provided in the field. The definitive care of the severely injured is hemorrhage control, decompression of an intracranial hematoma, or other procedures that can only be done in the operating room (OR). However, this does not mean that the pneumatic antishock garment (PASG) plays no role in the management of trauma patients. Several types of "holding patterns" can be carried out to transport the patient quickly and safely to the OR: adequate ventilation to provide oxygenation of the red blood cells in the lungs, assistance in achieving perfusion of tissues, immobilization of fractures so that the patient is not further harmed en route to the hospital, and expedient transportation to the appropriate facility.

The "appropriate facility" is also important in trauma management. The patient should be taken quickly to the hospital most capable of delivering the level of care required. If a community has two hospitals and only one of the hospitals is committed to managing trauma patients (an OR staff is available and in-house), the trauma patient should be taken to the hospital committed to the care of trauma patients.

The important part the EMT-Basic plays in the management of the emergency patient is to initially recognize the patient's problem. It is not necessary to make a diagnosis (although cardiac arrest is certainly a diagnosis), but it is important to recognize the problem for the patient. In a cardiac arrest, the problem is that the patient's heart is no longer beating and that the patient is no longer breathing; therefore vital organs are no longer being perfused. It is not the EMT-Basic's responsibility to identify the causes of the problem; this determination will be made later at the hospital. The EMT-Basic's responsibility is to recognize and solve the problem by getting the patient to the hospital with the heart and brain in an oxygenated condition.

The care that you as an EMT-Basic provide for your patients is basic but important. The final goal is a surviving patient who returns to a productive life after discharge from the hospital. To achieve this goal, you must (1) "do no harm" and (2) provide the best definitive care for the patient's condition based on your training and knowledge. This care will be based on your "best guess" as to the patient's problem. Quick access to the scene, knowledge of the needs of the patient, swift application of definitive care, and rapid delivery of the patient to the hospital are the skills that you provide.

Norman E. McSwain, Jr.

Preface

This textbook follows the EMT-Basic curriculum, which helps EMTs form a foundation in assessing and treating their patients. The philosophy behind this curriculum is twofold:

- To direct the EMT toward a symptom-based rather than the previously disease-based management system to provide patient care
- To reduce the complexity of the language of the course to make it easier for the individual taking an EMT course to understand the terminology

Symptom-based assessment is one of the quickest and simplest ways to approach prehospital care. When the EMT arrives on the scene, he or she will rapidly assess the patient, focusing on the new assessment techniques, and determine the treatment based on the signs and symptoms. There may be several different causes as to why the patient may have cold and clammy skin, have a weak pulse, and be short of breath, but the cause is not as important right now as medications with which the EMT-Basic can assist the patient.

A simplistic language (nonmedical) is the second goal of the new EMT-Basic curriculum. This textbook uses this simple, nonmedical terminology in addition to the accepted terminology used in the medical field.

The editors of this textbook share the opinion that EMTs should be taught to think and should have enough knowledge to be able to make correct patient decisions. This will increase the chance of an improved EMT/patient encounter. This textbook meets the needs of the instructor as well as the student. The basic approach is there for the instructor, medical director, and EMT to use, but if a more in-depth approach is needed, the material is in this book to help achieve this goal. The editors have also tried to provide a textbook for quick and easy reference to the necessary information. The chapters follow the guidelines set forth in the EMT-Basic curriculum. The chapters are set up to "stand alone" so that instructors can use them in the designated order or develop their own order.

This textbook is a collaboration of the work of the many contributors and editors from the first and second editions as well as the two editors whose names appear on the cover. In addition, this text could not have been written without the support of all of the physicians and EMS personnel who started EMS, as well as the hundreds of surgeons, emergency physicians, internists, anesthesiologists, and EMTs who have followed in their footsteps.

In terms of years of experience, the contributors and editors have amassed more than a millennium of experience in both prehospital and inhospital patient care. As with the first edition the contributors and editors bring to this text their continued experiences and knowledge to provide you with the most up-to-date and time-honored information available.

Foreword

It is an honor and privilege to write the foreword for this important contribution toward the education of out-of-hospital providers. The text's authors are leaders in the EMS, and I can think of no better combination for educating EMTs than an EMS physician and a paramedic. The authors' passion for excellence in EMS education is unequaled.

Throughout the text the authors address the value of medical direction. Through the interaction EMS physicians have with EMTs, we learn from each other. We learn together in classrooms, on the radio, and most importantly at the patient's bedside. From that important foundation we care for patients together better. This text is not regurgitation of old material in a new format. It is dynamic and includes new essential material on patient presentations that we see every day, including altered mental status, substance abuse, head trauma, and abdominal emergencies. Important new content areas include use of AEDs, diving emergencies, and military EMS.

When I was an EMT, we didn't have algorithms, step-by-step procedures, chapter review questions, and summaries. We surely did not have student workbooks, test generators, and slide sets on CD-ROMs. The editors and authors have incorporated state-of-the-art adult education tools with the ultimate goal for you to have the knowledge and skills to care for patients better.

The text parallels the new U.S. Department of Transportation EMT-Basic National Standard curriculum, but the text goes way beyond the objectives of that curriculum. "Passing the test" is one goal of any student taking a course. This book and its associated materials will certainly help you achieve that goal. However, the additional content affords you the opportunity to become a "thinking man's EMT," expanding your horizons beyond what you have to know for the text. This philosophical approach of the text moves you beyond a "technician" to a true "professional."

As an EMT you probably spend more time with a patient in the street, in the house, and in the ambulance than any other health care professional during that patient's illness or injury. You have an enormous impact on the patient's care and have the opportunity to care for the patient for a longer period of time than most of us in health care. This exemplifies how important you have become to the rapidly changing health care environment.

Today, patients wait days or weeks for an appointment with a health care provider. EMS is different. You are there within minutes of a patient's call for help to 911. You have become far more than an "ambulance technician." EMS providers have become the ultimate safety net for the public's health. Increasingly we have become recognized as medicine's front line. EMS systems have captured the attention of all major health organizations and federal agencies concerned for the public's health, including the American College of Emergency Physicians, American Heart Association, American Public Health Association, American College of Surgeons, National Association of EMS Physicians, and others.

We see society's failures and successes at caring for the public's health. Our success is in providing quality patient care and caring for our patients. Our future success will be from research that will guide us in taking care of patients better and by continuing to integrate ourselves within the entire health care community.

As you become a "thinking man's EMT," this text will prompt you to want to discover and learn more. This text will become the anchor for your career in Emergency Medical Services—the ultimate safety net for American's health care.

Richard C. Hunt, MD, FACEP

Contents

Section One
Introduction to EMS 1

1 Introduction to EMS 3
Emergency Medical Provider 5
Emergency Medical Service System 6
Health Care Delivery System 7
Common EMS System Variables 9
Future of EMS 15
Future of the EMT 15
EMS System Challenges 15

2 Roles/Responsibilities of the EMT 20
Emergency Medical Services System 21
Communication 22
Roles and Responsibilities 24
Professional Attributes 26
Professional Ethics 27
Certification and Licensure 27
Professional Organizations 28

3 Medical/Legal Principles 31
Medical Control 32
Prehospital Medical Record Documentation 33
Consent for Medical Care and Transportation 33
Consent in the Incompetent Adult Patient 35
Surrogate Consent 36
Providing Treatment at a Possible Crime Scene 37
EMT's Scope of Practice 37
Right to Receive Care Without Interruption 38
Right to Receive Appropriate Care 38
Organ Donation 39

4 EMS Medical Director 42
EMS Medical Director 44
Medical Direction 45

5 Well-Being of the EMT 53
Assess Scene for Hazards 54
Body Substance Isolation 55
Overview of Special Scenes 55

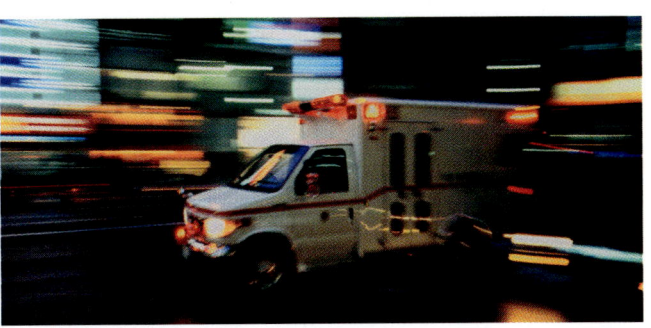

Death and Dying 60
Dealing with the Dying Patient and Family Members 61
EMT's Reaction to Emergencies 63
EMT's Family and Friends 64
Understanding Stress 65

6 Infection Control 74
Importance of Body Substance Isolation 76
Common Infectious Diseases 77
Guidelines for Bloodborne Pathogen Protection 78
Methods for Personal Protection for the EMT 80

7 The Human Body 86
Medical Terminology 87
Musculoskeletal System 88
Body Systems 95
Body Cavities 105

8 Assessment 113
Patient Assessment 117
General Impression and Plan of Action 117
Scene Survey 118
Initial Patient Assessment 120
Rapid Focused History and Physical Examination 126
Baseline Vital Signs 137
Signs Versus Symptoms 137
Pulse 138
Ventilations 140
Blood Pressure 141
Skin Color and Temperature 142

Level of Consciousness 142
Pupil Reaction 144
SAMPLE History 144
Vital Signs Review 145

9 Management of Shock 150
Anatomy and Physiology 153
Pathophysiology 159
Assessment 165
Management 167

10 Airway Management and Ventilation 177
Anatomy and Physiology 180
Assessment 184
Management 186

11 Advanced Airway Management Skills 212
Anatomy and Physiology 215
Pathophysiology of Airway Compromise 216
Assessment: Indications for Endotracheal Intubation 216
Management 217
Advance Directives 231

12 Scene Size-up and the EMS Call 235
Types of EMS Calls 238
Citizen Access and Communication 240
Dispatching the Ambulance 241
En Route to the Scene 241
At the Scene 243
Bioethical Considerations 247
Transportation Considerations 249
Emergency Department 249
Continuum of In-hospital Care 251

Section Two
Nontraumatic Emergencies 255

13 General Pharmacology 257
Overview of the Use of Medications by the EMT 258
Medication Names 259
Forms of Medications 259
Drug Dynamics 261
Reading Labels and Prescriptions 263

Specific Medications 264
Assessment and Management 264

14 Respiratory Emergencies 272
Respiratory System 275
Pathophysiology 275
Management 282

15 Cardiovascular Emergencies 288
Anatomy 291
Physiology 292
Pathophysiology 296
Assessment 297
Management 298
Automated External Defibrillation 300

16 Early Defibrillation 306
Sudden Cardiac Death 307
Automated External Defibrillator 310
Postresuscitation Care 315
Maintenance of the AED 315
Maintaining AED Skills 315

17 Altered Mental Status 323
Causes of Altered Mental Status 324
Assessment of the Patient with Altered Mental Status 330

18 Allergies 335
Anatomy and Physiology 336
Pathophysiology 337
Assessment 338
Management 339

19 Toxic Emergencies: Poisoning and Overdose 343
Poison Control Centers 344
Anatomy and Physiology 345
Assessment 346
Management 348
Substance Abuse 350

20 Behavioral Emergencies 355
Behavior 356
Behavioral Emergencies 357
Magnitude of Mental Health Problems 357

Assessment of Behavioral Emergencies 358
Primary and Secondary Psychologic Crises 361
Medicolegal Considerations 368
Management and Emergency Medical Treatment 369

21 **Obstetric and Gynecologic Emergencies 372**
Anatomy and Physiology 373
Pathophysiology 379
Assessment 381
Management 382
Alleged Sexual Assault 391

Section Three
Trauma 401

22 **Kinematics of Trauma 403**
Definitions 405
Precrash, Crash, Postcrash 405
Physics of Energy Exchange 406
Blunt Trauma 410
Motorcycle Collisions 425
Pedestrian Injury 427
Falls 429
Sports Injuries 430
Blast Injuries 431
Penetrating Injuries 432

23 **Soft Tissue Injury and Bleeding Control 442**
Anatomy and Physiology 445
Pathophysiology 447
Assessment 451
Management 452
Controlling Bleeding 456

24 **Head Trauma 460**
Anatomy of the Head 462
Pathophysiology of the Head 467
Assessment of Head Injuries 471
Management of Head Injuries 476

25 **Chest Trauma 476**
Anatomy 477
Physiology 481
Pathophysiology 483
Heart 486

Assessment 486
Management 487

26 **Abdominal Emergencies 493**
Anatomy 494
Physiology and Pathophysiology 497
Assessment 500
Management 501

27 **Spinal Trauma 504**
Nervous System 507
Anatomy of the Spine 508
Pathophysiology of the Spine 510
Assessment of Spinal Injuries 511
Management if Spinal Injuries 513
Skills 514

28 **Musculoskeletal Trauma 529**
Anatomy and Physiology 531
Muscle and Bone Interaction to Produce Motion 532
Pathophysiology 536
Assessment 542
Management 545
Practical Skills: Splinting 546

29 **Environmental Emergencies 560**
Anatomy and Physiology of Temperature Regulation 561
Pathophysiology: Environmental Factors Affecting Body Temperature 564
Assessment of Environmental Emergencies 565
Management of Environmental Emergencies 566
Generalized Cold Exposure 566
Localized Cold Exposure 569
Heat Exposure 571
Burns 573
Water-Related Emergencies 577
Bites and Stings 578

Section Four
Special Patient Populations 583

30 **Geriatric Patients 585**
Aging 586
Anatomy and Physiology 587

Dementia and Alzheimer's Disease 591
Assessment: General Considerations 592
Medications and the Elderly 594
Initial Assessment 595
Assessment and Emergency Medical Care of Acute Illness 595
Assessment and Emergency Medical Care of Trauma 596
Environmental Problems 597
Geriatric Cases 598
Suicide 599
Elder Abuse 599

31 Infants and Children 604
Pediatric Patients 605
Pathophysiology 612
Pediatric Basic Life Support 614
Pediatric Basic Airway and Respiratory Adjuncts 615
Pediatric Resuscitation 617
Assessment and Management of Common Pediatric Medical Emergencies 618
Pediatric Trauma 622
Other Pediatric Problems 630
Children with Special Needs 632
Pain Control in Infants and Children 633
General Considerations 633

32 The Patient with Special Needs 638
Pathophysiology 640
Assessment 648
Management 652
Family Considerations 655
EMT-B Considerations 655
Guidelines for Disability Awareness 656

Section Five
EMS Operations 659

33 Lifting and Moving Patients 661
Time-Dependent Medical Problems 662
Minimization of Risk 663
Mechanics of Lifting 664
General Guidelines for Safe Lifting 664

Guidelines for Safe Lifting of Cots and Stretchers 665
Guidelines for Carrying Patients and Equipment 666
Guidelines for Safe Carrying Procedures on Stairs 666
Guidelines for Reaching 668
Guidelines for Pushing and Pulling 668
Principles for Moving Patients 668
Equipment for Moving Patients 672
Equipment Maintenance 678
Patient Positioning 679
Transportation Considerations 680

34 Communications 686
Components of an EMS Communication System 687
Public Access 691
Emergency Medical Dispatch 692
General Guidelines for Radio Communication 693
Communication with Medical Direction or Destination Facility 694
Communication en Route to the Hospital 695
In-Person Communication with Facility Staff 696
Essential Principles of Interpersonal Communication 697
Communication with Special Patients 697
Legal Concerns 698

35 Documentation 701
Patient Care Report 702
Special Situations 711

36 Quality Improvement 715
Quality Assurance 717
Quality Assessment Methods 718
Quality Improvement Loop 719
The Emergency Medical Technician's Role in Quality Assurance 722

37 Ambulance Operation 724
Ambulance 725
Medical Equipment 726
Portable Kits 730
Nonmedical Equipment 731

Daily Inspections   731
Dispatch   734
En Route   734
Positioning the Unit   736
Arrival at the Scene   738
Transferring the Patient to the Ambulance   738
En Route to the Receiving Facility   739
At the Receiving Facility   739
En Route to the Station   739
Post-run   740

38 Interagency Interface 742
Dispatcher   743
First Responders   744
Advanced Life Support Paramedics   744
Other Levels of Advanced Life Support   745
Aeromedical Services   745
Child Protective Services   751
Elder Abuse Services   752
Managed Care Organizations   752
Interacting with Law Enforcement Agencies   752
Search and Rescue   754
Conflict Resolution   755

Section Six
Special Topics   759

39 Gaining Access   761
Types of Rescue Operations   762
Rescue Action Plan   764
Vehicle Rescue Incidents   765

40 Emergency Preparedness   774
Disaster and Multiple-Casualty Response   776
Hazardous Materials Response   782

41 Diving Emergencies   791
The Physics of Air   793
Pressure, Volume, and Density   794
Barotrauma Injuries Occurring During Descent   794
Barotrauma Injuries Occurring During Ascent   795
Pathophysiology   797
Assessment   799
Management   801

42 Military EMS   806
Military Echelons of Care   808
Emergent Care in the Tactical Environment   809
Weapons of Mass Destruction   815
Triage   820
Comparison of Civilian Versus Military Casualty Management   821

Appendix A: CPR Review   825
Appendix B: National Registry of Emergency Medical Technicians (NREMT) Skill Sheets   842
Appendix C: National Highway Traffic Safety Administration (NHTSA) Technical Advisory Panel (TAP) Standards   862
Answers to Review Questions   865
Glossary   871
Illustration Credits   895
Index   899

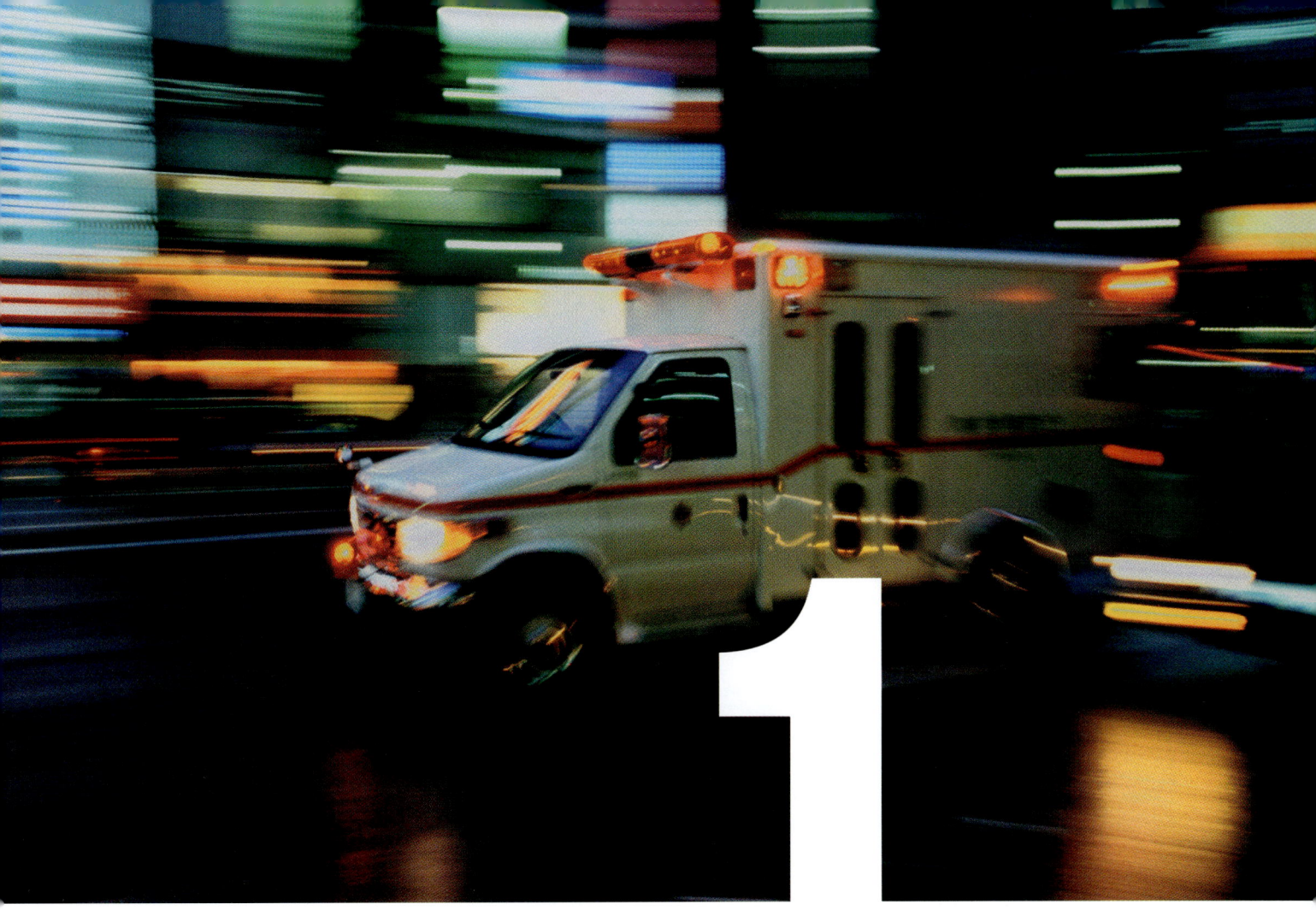

Section One

Introduction to EMS

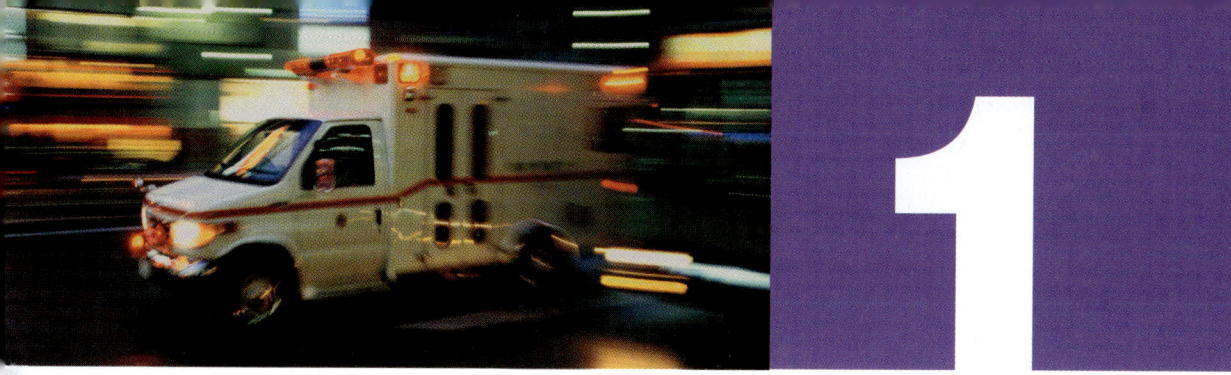

Introduction to EMS

Lesson Goal

The goal of this chapter is to provide the EMT-Basic with an introduction to emergency care by defining the history of the emergency medical services system and the role that the EMT-Basic plays in that system and the overall health care system.

Scenario

It is a cold, snowy evening in northeastern Connecticut in March 1974. Traffic is light and moving very slowly. A station wagon carrying a family returning home from a movie is approaching a sharp curve in the road. As they round the curve they suddenly see a car up on a jack missing a tire. The cars hazard lights are barely visible through the haze of the snow. The driver of the station wagon reflexively swerves to avoid the disabled car and begins to slide sideways on the snow-covered road. The station wagon is broadsided by a coal truck that was following too closely, is pushed into a ravine, and finally comes to rest upside down. An eerie silence descends over the scene. Several cars pull up, and people stare at the sight of the demolished car below them. The truck driver descends into the ravine and approaches the station wagon. He sees that two of the children were thrown from the vehicle and the remaining passengers are unconscious and bleeding. He turns and shouts at a car on the road, "Call for help! Go down the mountain and call Casey's Funeral Home. Tell them that we need their ambulance in a hurry! A lot of people are hurt!" The driver speeds off in search of a phone to call the funeral home.

 When the call for help is made, who will respond to this collision? What kind of training will they have? Where will they come from? Will the victims in this collision receive the same kind of care that someone would receive in a different part of the country?

Key Terms to Know

Acute care
Assessment
Chronic care

Curriculum
Definitive care
Diagnosis

Emergency medical services
  (EMS) system
EMT-Basic (EMT-B)

EMT-Intermediate (EMT-I)
EMT-Paramedic (EMT-P)
Extended care facility

Key Terms to Know (cont'd)

Fee-for-service
Health care delivery system
Home care
Managed care
Prehospital care
Prehospital provider
Stabilization
Tiered response system

Learning Objectives

As an EMT-Basic, you should be able to do the following:

DOT

- Define emergency medical services (EMS) system.
- Differentiate the roles and responsibilities of the EMT-Basic from those of other prehospital care providers.

Supplemental

- Define *emergency medical care*.
- Define the role that emergency medical services play in the public health community and the public safety community.
- Define *emergency medical technician* (EMT).
- Describe pertinent history, current events, and the future outlook for the EMT.
- Explain how emergency medical care relates to other components of the health care delivery system.
- Identify the role played by the United States Department of Transportation (DOT) in the training of the EMT.
- Identify common EMS system models.
- Describe the difference between an assessment-based approach to emergency care and a diagnosis-based approach.
- Explain the differing goals of initial and continuing education for the EMT.
- Identify the various components of EMT training.
- Identify the various certifying bodies for the EMT.
- Demonstrate a basic understanding of the types of health care that are available in the United States.
- Describe how changes in the health care system will affect the EMS system.
- Describe current challenges facing EMS systems.
- Identify current trends and likely future changes in EMS systems.

The emergency medical technician-Basic (EMT-B) who is the focus of this book is the foundation of the emergency medical service system (Figure 1.1). More EMT-Bs participate in the prehospital health care system than any other provider, and they are an essential part of almost every emergency medical service system.

An **emergency medical services (EMS) system** is one in which medical care is provided to people who suddenly become seriously ill or injured. It involves rapid response, **assessment** (determining what is wrong), **stabilization** (treating life-threatening conditions and packaging for transportation), transportation, and **definitive care** (the final medical treatment provided to correct the initial illness or injury). One of the most important elements in the EMS system is the EMT. No matter where an emergency occurs, how the patient is transported, or to what type of facility the patient is transported, the person who provides the initial prehospital emergency medical care (the EMT) is the constant factor that always remains the same.

This chapter provides an introduction to EMS and explores its relationship with the health care system. It describes the individual components of an EMS system and how they interact, as well as some of the most common system organizational models. It defines and briefly explores the history of EMS and the EMT and the role they play in the health care system. The components of the EMS system, as well as highlighting the general training, certification requirements, and EMT educational programs found throughout the country, are reviewed. This chapter explores challenges facing EMS systems and speculates about future changes.

 EMS is an essential component of the health care delivery system

✓ EMS occupies a position between a public safety service and a public health service. It is not one or the other; it is a little bit of both.

Emergency Medical Provider

The heart of the EMS system is the EMT. *EMT* is a general term used to describe the majority of personnel involved in the provision of emergency medical care outside of the hospital. There are several different levels of emergency care providers throughout the country.

1. *First responder.* In many cases, one of the first individuals to respond to the scene of an emergency is the "first responder." Historically in the public safety sector, many first responders have come from the ranks of fire and police departments. There are also many industries who have developed first responder programs, such as chemical and oil companies, forestry services, and telecommunications companies. The United States Department of Transportation (DOT) has developed a 40-hour training program for the first responder, which incorporates basic emergency care and interface with EMTs.
2. **EMT-Basic (EMT-B).** This term describes the basic level of emergency medical technician identified by the DOT. The EMT-B provides basic emergency medical care and is the cornerstone of the EMS workforce. By some estimates, as many as 500,000 EMT-Bs are currently certified in the United States alone.
3. **EMT-Intermediate (EMT-I).** The EMT-I has additional training in assessment beyond the EMT-B level. In addition, the EMT-I will be trained to use intravenous therapy and a limited selection of medications.
4. **EMT-Paramedic (EMT-P).** The most advanced level of EMT identified by the DOT is the EMT-P, or paramedic. The EMT-P has advanced assessment skills and is trained in a variety of invasive interventions, administration of medications, intravenous solutions, and other advanced treatment techniques.

✓ The EMT-B represents the cornerstone of the EMS system. Most prehospital providers start their education in EMS with the EMT-B course, which is also a prerequisite for the other two training courses, EMT-I and EMT-P.

History of the EMT

As with the modern EMS model, the birth of the EMT can be traced back to *Accidental Death and Disability: The Ne-*

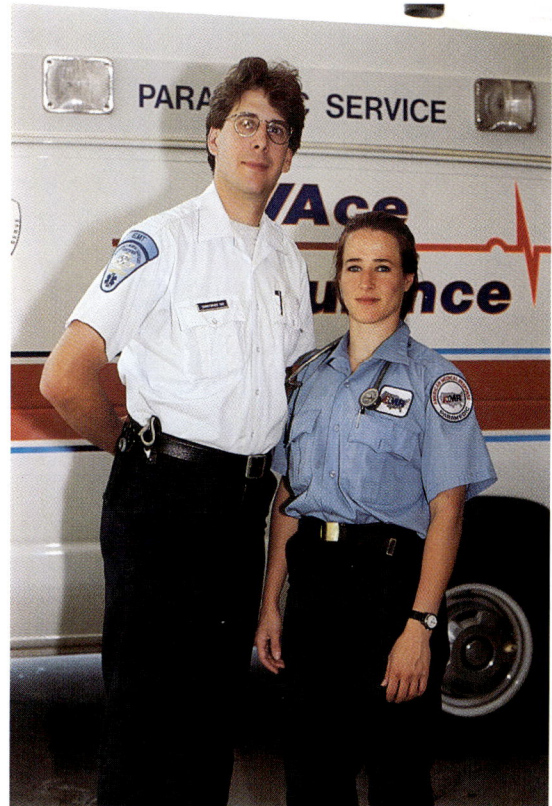

FIGURE 1.1 The EMT is the foundation of the EMS system.

glected Disease of Modern Society, a research paper published in 1966 by the National Academy of Sciences. The authors cited the large number of preventable deaths and disabilities that were occurring in the United States and identified the contributing factors for this trend. One of the key factors focused directly on the people who provided emergency medical care. Although the authors did not question the intentions of these providers, they strongly recommended that a standard minimum level of training be developed and implemented. Decisions were made concerning the basic knowledge and skills that would be necessary to improve **prehospital care.** This information was then transformed into a training curriculum (a standardized course description and outline), and the initial course introduced in 1969 was called EMT-Ambulance (EMT-A).

Based on the 1966 research paper, the federal government passed legislation in 1973 (the Emergency Medical Services Systems [EMSS] Act of 1973) and specifically identified standardized training for prehospital personnel as an essential goal of the EMS system. The initial legislation that prompted the DOT to create the EMT-A training course also created federal grant programs for states to develop EMS systems. This requirement

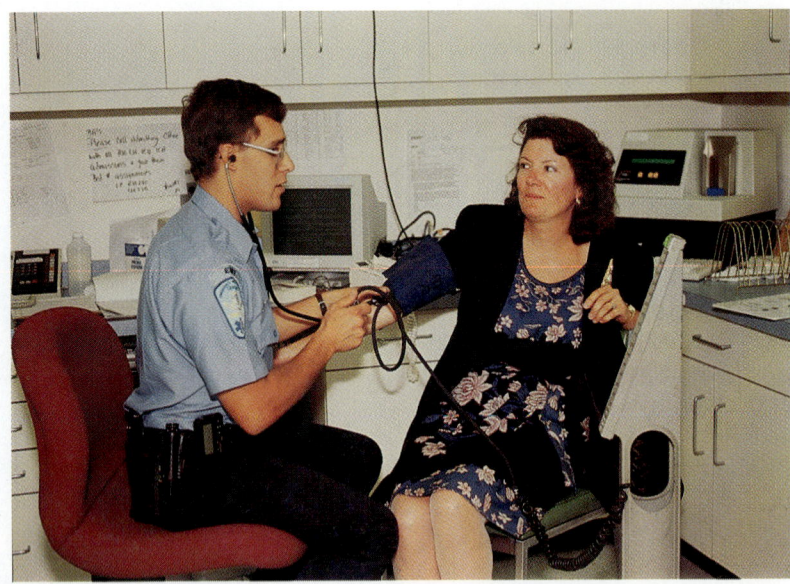

FIGURE 1.2 Some communities use EMS personnel to deliver basic public health services.

prompted most states to adopt the DOT national standard EMT curriculum and to reference the DOT curriculum in most state statutes or regulations.

Responsibility for developing the training programs was assigned to the DOT because of the emphasis on highway-related injuries. Within the DOT, the National Highway Traffic Safety Administration (NHTSA) Office of Occupant Protection and EMS have evolved into the agency with principle responsibility for continuing to develop and revise the EMT programs.

> ✓ The federal government developed the original national training standards for EMS personnel. States adopted the federal standards as a requirement for receiving federal grant funds.

Emergency Medical Service System

The EMS system is a large and complicated network of people, vehicles, equipment, and facilities that is organized to respond in a rapid, organized fashion to emergency medical incidents. The EMS system occupies an interesting and important place in the health care industry, which is a system constructed to meet all of the health care needs of the public (Figure 1.2). This position of the EMS between public safety and public health often leads to interesting conflicts. It is clearly a public safety service, much like police and fire services, that society provides to meet the basic needs of the population (Figure 1.3). It is also clearly a part of the public health care system, an essential component that provides early out-of-hospital care and transportation.

History of EMS

The history of the EMT and EMS are intricately linked. Although emergency medical care has been provided in the out-of-hospital environment for hundreds of years, the idea of linking the various components into organized systems is a relatively new concept. During the late 1960s and early 1970s, several research projects were initiated to explore the possible alternatives to improving the state of emergency medical care in the field. By the early 1970s, it was clear that a large number of components were necessary to work together as a system for patients to receive the most benefit.

As previously discussed, the U.S. Congress passed the EMSS Act of 1973, which identified 15 "essential" components of an EMS system. To provide both the means and an incentive for states and local communities to develop comprehensive EMS systems, the government made millions of dollars of grant funding available to states and communities that developed EMS systems.

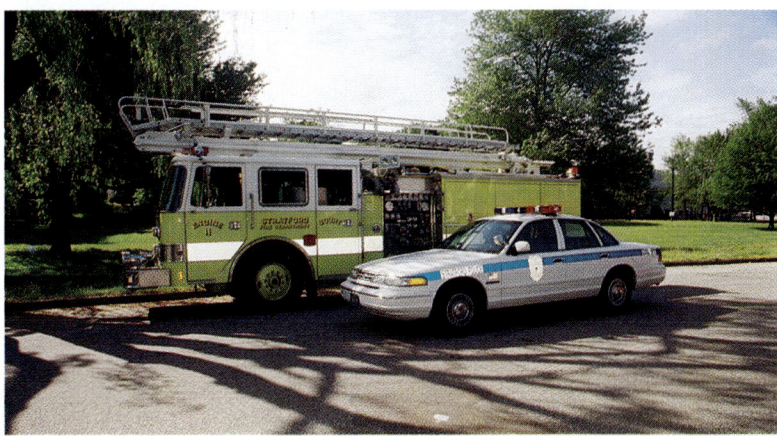

FIGURE 1.3 EMS is often considered a public safety service like police and fire departments.

Although the federal EMS programs of the 1970s were ahead of the times, there were also limits. For example, in the list of "essential" components, there is no mention of statutes (laws) or regulations to create or empower EMS systems. The issue of appropriate funding for EMS was not addressed, and physician medical direction also was conspicuously absent.

As EMS systems continued to evolve, so has systems thinking. In 1988 an attempt to redefine the components of an EMS system was initiated through the Technical Assistance Program (TAP) offered by the NHTSA (Box 1.1). TAP evaluates state EMS systems using 10 standard components. In addition to evaluating the presence and quality of each of the components, the TAP process also gives significant consideration to the interaction between the components.

> ✓ The role of the EMT-B within the health care system is undergoing dramatic change. The DOT continually revises the training course, and the health care system is always looking for new ways to use the EMS workforce.

> **Box 1.1** **10 Standard Components of an EMS System as Identified in the NHTSA Technical Assistance Program (1988)**
>
> 1. Regulation and policy
> 2. Resource management
> 3. Human resources and training
> 4. Transportation
> 5. Facilities
> 6. Communication
> 7. Public information and education
> 8. Medical direction
> 9. Trauma systems
> 10. Evaluation

Health Care Delivery System

It is essential to understand types of care and how the EMS system integrates and supports the **health care delivery system.** The overall health care system is a network of people, facilities, support services, and equipment that meets the general health care needs of the population (Figure 1.4). Overlaying the delivery of health care is the financing or payment for care, which is most often discussed in terms of insurance. It is the insuring, or payment, of health care that determines how and by whom health care is provided.

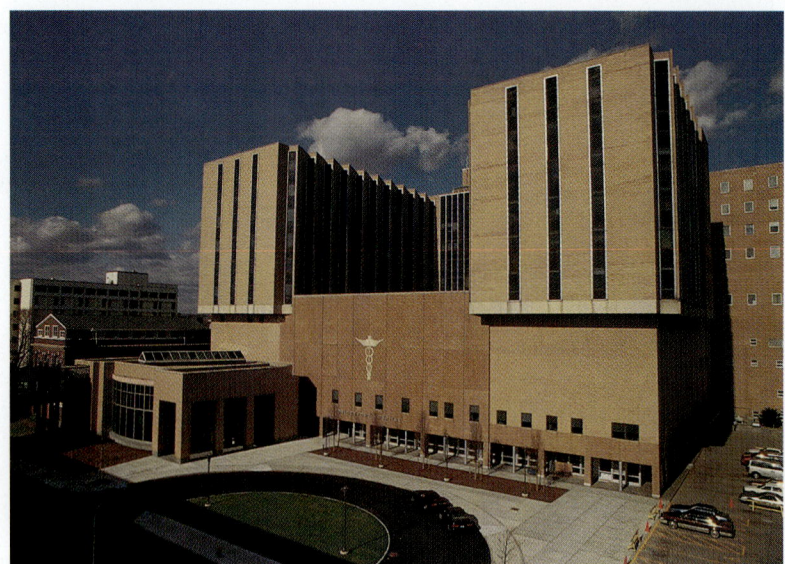

FIGURE 1.4 EMS is an integral component of the health care delivery system.

The health care delivery system is in a state of constant change. However, the rate of change has accelerated dramatically in recent years with the dramatic advances in technology, reimbursement, and medical science.

Acute Care

A major component in the health care delivery system is **acute care.** Access to the acute care setting often begins with an emergency call for prehospital emergency medical care and transportation of the patient to the hospital. Once a patient receives acute intervention and definitive treatment, he or she may need additional ongoing health services outside of the acute facility. Acute care generally is provided by a hospital, with the most intensive medical interventions on a 24-hour-a-day basis. The hospital provides emergency and trauma care, critical intensive care, surgical intervention, and a broad spectrum of diagnostic testing services such as radiology, cardiology, and laboratory services.

Restorative Care

Restorative care involves the treatment and therapy necessary to return the patient to a "normal" condition or function. The restorative care facility provides the patient with intensive rehabilitation to assist with walking and functional independence. The EMT-B is essential in the support of care to the patient requiring restorative care since these patients often will require ambulance transportation to and from the restorative care facility and the various treatment centers that may be used during their rehabilitation.

Chronic Care

When a patient continues to require health care intervention and does not improve, **chronic care** is required. In the United States, chronic care is provided in facilities such an **extended care facility,** a nursing home, or the patient's own home.

Home Care

Home care is provided to patients in need of less intensive care after intervention in an acute care facility. Home care typically provides nursing and other therapy interventions in the home as ordered by the physician. The EMT-B may be called upon to help support theses types of care with either direct intervention or transportation services.

Health Care System Changes

The health care system is in the process of significant evolution. Many reasons exist for these changes, including the ever increasing cost of health care and access to care. Pressure from businesses and government, largely driven by concerns about cost, have fostered these changes. Health care costs have continued to escalate at a rapid rate.

The most global change in the health care system is the shift from **fee-for-service** financing to **managed care.** As the health care system continues to move toward a managed care model with increasing reductions in payments, the entire health care community is going to be challenged to maintain quality in the face of shrinking resources. Policy makers and providers will need to proceed cautiously to avoid unnecessary and unfortunate sacrifices in quality for the sake of saving money.

 The EMS system and prehospital providers play a key role in the shift to managed care.

Common EMS System Variables

For all of the variability in EMS systems in the United States, several common attributes characterize EMS systems (e.g., level of service, type of personnel, where the service is housed). No evidence shows that any one of these characteristics or models is better than another. It is how they work together in the system that is the critical aspect.

Level of Service

Before the early 1970s, only a single level of emergency care was available in the United States, which was very basic and not standardized in any way. However, several different "levels" have been developed since 1973. Communities are able to pick and choose, mix and match, depending on the will of the community and the available dollar resources.

Basic Life Support

The term *basic life support* (BLS) is used to describe a level of service that provides noninvasive emergency care. BLS involves cardiopulmonary resuscitation (CPR), basic control of external bleeding, splinting, spinal immobilization, normal childbirth, and other uncomplicated forms of emergency care. A BLS system focuses on the critical aspects of life (e.g., maintain breathing and circulation and transport the patient without doing additional harm). The most common type of provider in BLS systems is the EMT-B, but other BLS providers might include first responders.

Advanced Life Support

Advanced life support (ALS) is a general term used to describe any form of emergency care that is above the BLS level. It usually involves the use of invasive techniques (e.g., intravenous therapy and drug administration) and often includes the use of more sophisticated equipment such as cardiac monitors. The principle behind ALS systems is to take more advanced therapy to the patient rather than waiting for the patient to reach the hospital. ALS systems often have impressive results, particularly with patients experiencing cardiac problems, but they also involve a high cost and put a lot of demands on the workforce for education and maintenance of skill proficiency. Two nationally recognized levels of ALS providers are the EMT-I and the EMT-P. In addition to these three national standard levels of EMT (EMT-B, EMT-I, and EMT-P), dozens of other intermediate levels of provider exist throughout the United States.

Tiered Response System

A variation on the model of the all-BLS or all-ALS system is called a **tiered response system,** which involves layers of care. As previously discussed, the first level of care is usually BLS provided by first responders or EMTs. The next layer is the ALS layer, which backs up the BLS providers by responding to those patients who will benefit from ALS care. Chapter 38 deals with the interface between BLS and ALS. In some systems, a third tier, air medical transportation, is available.

Types of Service Delivery Models

Another set of common attributes among EMS systems is how or where the providers are housed or the kind of agency for which they work.

Fire Department

Many of the earliest examples of prehospital care in the United States can be traced to the community fire department. Today, many fire departments are actively involved in the delivery of EMS, either as the emergency care and transportation agency or as the first responder agency in a tiered system (Figure 1.5).

Private Ambulance

The private ambulance industry also has a long history in EMS in the United States. The private ambulance industry has grown from the funeral home ambulance services of the 1940s and 1950s to those communities where they were used to transport nonemergency patients and those EMS systems where a contract for the provision of 911 EMS exists. Regardless of their origin, the private ambulance industry is a vital part of the modern EMS system (Figure 1.6).

Hospital-Based Service
Hospital-based services range from simple transportation services for the hospital's patients to sophisticated ALS services that provide primary EMS response to the surrounding community. For the **prehospital provider**, one unique aspect of the hospital-based service is that it often offers the opportunity to gain more experience through work in the emergency department or other hospital areas when not working on the ambulance (Figure 1.7). The hospital-based model also offers the opportunity for enhanced relationships between the emergency department personnel and prehospital personnel.

Public Third Service
An additional type of EMS provider agency is a third public safety service offered by government agencies other than police and fire protection agencies, hence the term *third service*. An example of this type of model can be found in Denver, Colorado. The EMTs that work for these agencies are state or local municipal government employees, just as police officers and fire fighters are in the city.

Industrial
Another common EMS system model is the industrial EMS system. Large industries in the United States often have their own EMS system set up within the confines of the building or operation. The industry will often provide everything from first response through transportation using company personnel, equipment, and vehicles. Examples of this type of EMS system can be found in such industries as mining and off-shore oil refineries.

Military
EMS is also in the military. Although titles and ranks vary among the military services, each service (Army, Navy, Air Force, etc.) operates their own complete EMS system (Figure 1.8). The first responders are soldiers with basic first-aid training. The ALS back-up comes in the form of corpsmen with more sophisticated tools and techniques.

> ✔ As noted, EMS may be provided by a variety of organizational entities, including the government and private industry. All models have advantages and disadvantages.

EMS System Financing

How individual EMS agencies handle their system financing (revenues and expenses) is one of the key characteristics that will help to ensure future success and growth. EMS financing includes fundraising, capital expenditures, payroll, and general operating expenses. A brief description of examples for EMS system financing models follows.

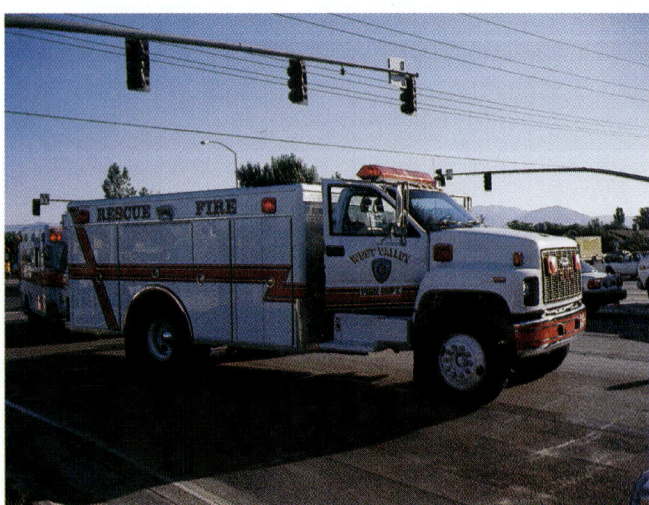

FIGURE 1.5 The fire service is actively involved in EMS delivery.

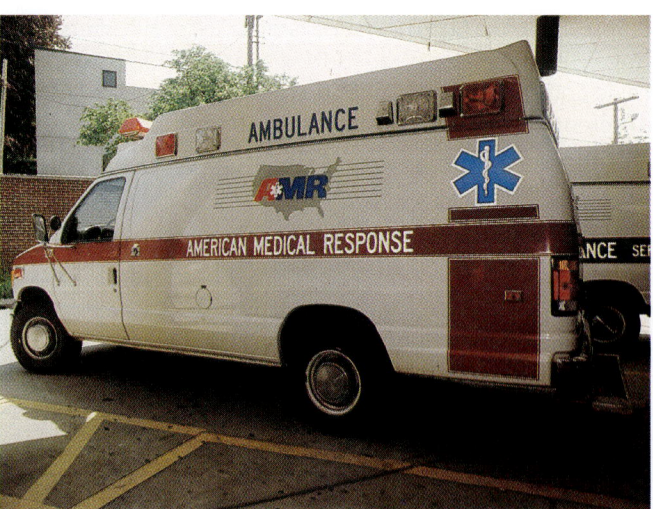

FIGURE 1.6 The private ambulance industry has expanded far beyond basic transportation services.

Payroll Considerations

The terms *volunteer* and *paid* often are used to differentiate between those EMTs who are compensated and those who are not. In recent years, however, this distinction has blurred considerably. Large portions of the United States receive EMS and fire protection from dedicated volunteer professionals within their community. At the other end of the scale are the systems that use EMT-Bs who are full-time employees. In many cases, those systems with paid personnel also operate at the ALS level.

Driven largely by a desire to attract and keep dedicated volunteers, many of the EMS agencies that formerly relied on the nonpaid volunteer are now offering some sort of compensation. The pay status of EMS providers has nothing to do with their level of dedication, commitment to quality community service, skills, or knowledge level.

EMS System Revenue Sources

Adequate revenue to support an EMS operation continues to be a tremendous challenge for EMS systems. In an effort to generate revenue to offset capital and operating expenses, several different models have been instituted across the country. These methods include fee-for-service, subscription, government subsidy.

Fee-for-service. A fee-for-service system charges a fee for the services that it provides. Payment comes from the patient, private insurers, and government insurers (Medicare and Medicaid). This type of model is found in the hospital-based and private ambulance industry and is becoming an increasingly common finance model for volunteer, fire, and third services ambulance agencies.

Subscription. Several EMS systems are funded solely through donations. Much like the volunteer fire departments, they earn their revenue from a variety of fund-raising activities in the community. A variation on this theme is the subscription form of funding. In this case the EMS agency sells a "subscription" to individuals or families in the service area. This financing model is not limited to volunteer services. One of the largest private companies in the country, the Acadian Ambulance Service in Louisiana, operates almost exclusively on a subscription basis.

Subsidized. This model includes the fire service–based EMS system that does not bill for services, the private systems that bill patients but also receive a government payment to make the business profitable, and volunteer services that receive a subsidy to cover nonpersonnel operating expenses.

EMT-B Training Curriculum

In 1989, 20 years after the introduction of the initial EMT-A training program, the DOT began its most comprehensive revision of the EMT training program **curriculum,** which was then published in 1994. The most significant change included a renewed emphasis on science as the foundation for deciding which medical interventions would be used. A change in the approach to training the EMT also resulted from this initiative. In addition, EMT-A

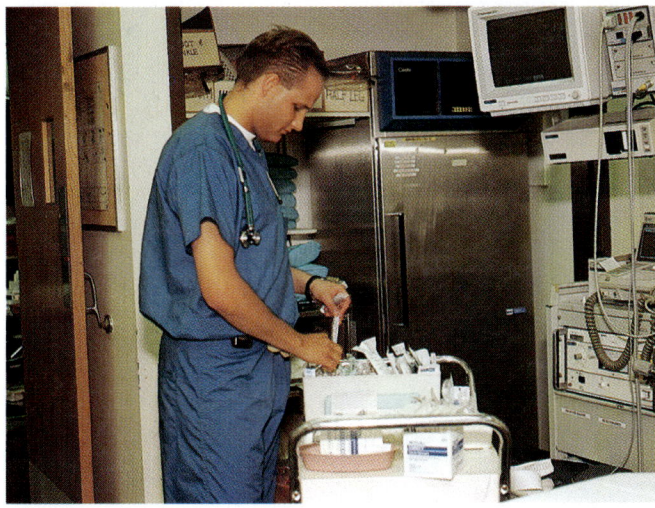

FIGURE 1.7 Hospital-based ambulance services offer staff a variety of opportunities to gain experience.

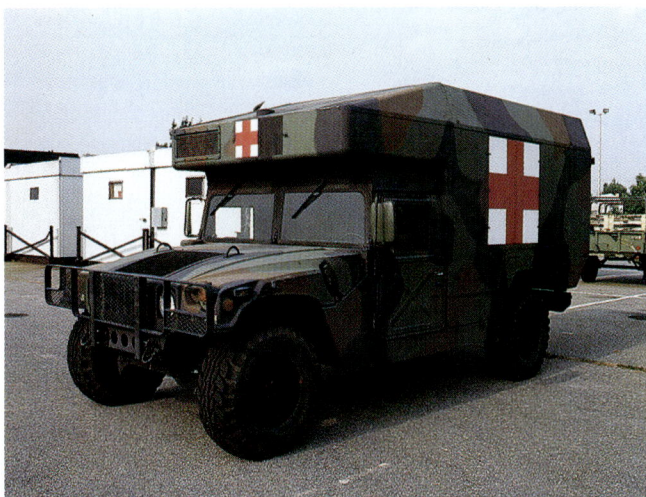

FIGURE 1.8 Each branch of the military operates its own EMS system.

was changed to EMT-B in recognition of the fact that many EMTs work in settings other than ambulances.

At the same time that the DOT initiated this comprehensive revision of the training curriculum for the EMT-B, the health care delivery system in the United States was undergoing change that continues today. Based on an urgent need to control cost and increase efficiency in the health care system, one of the major new directions being considered is an expansion or change in the way that nonphysician and nonnurse health care providers, such as the EMT, are used in the health care delivery system.

The EMT-B is often the first contact that the patient has with the health care system and plays a role in determining how and where the patient will receive definitive care. Preparing the EMT-B for this critical role begins with an educational process that attempts to focus on the crucial information needed to expedite care and transportation to a hospital.

As with any broadly used standard, the EMT-B national standard curriculum is a compromise between medicine, politics, and reality. If the EMT-B were trained purely from the medical perspective, the course would be extremely long in duration and comprehensive. However, considering that many EMTs are volunteers with limited time for training or with dual-role responsibilities like fire fighters, the other reality is a cost-benefit analysis, which is where politics enters the scenario. When all three of these factors come together in one place, compromise results.

For EMS, compromise means that all providers are not equal. The EMT-B is the classic example of the compromise discussed here. The EMT-B is an educated, thinking individual who brings knowledge, experience, intuition, and common sense to the emergency scene. Nevertheless, the EMT-B training course, which provides the student with knowledge and practical skills, has undergone many philosophic changes and compromises over the years. The most recent revision of the curriculum represents perhaps the most dramatic of these compromises in its approach to basic prehospital care.

> ✓ Because every state in the United States uses the national standard DOT curriculum as a minimum standard, the EMT student will learn all of the required material included in the national program.

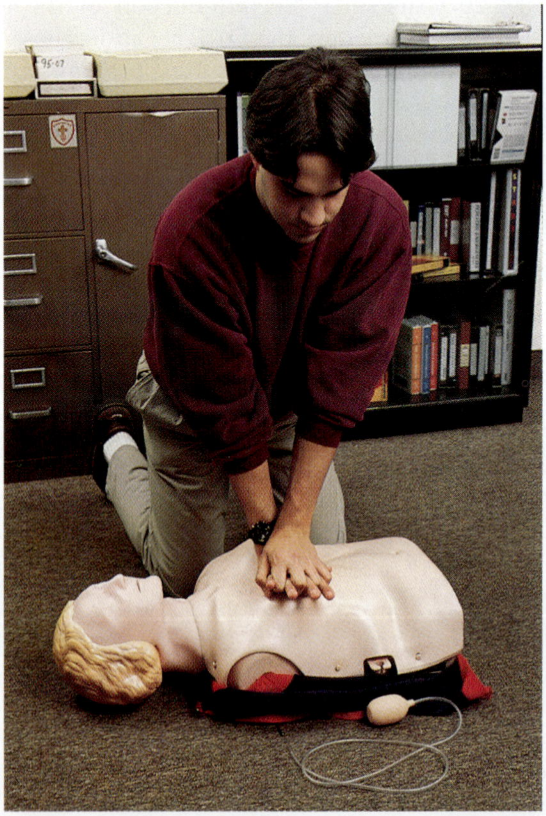

Prerequisites

The national standard curriculum requires that the EMT-B student complete a course of study in Basic Car-

FIGURE 1.9 CPR training is a prerequisite for entering the EMT-B training program.

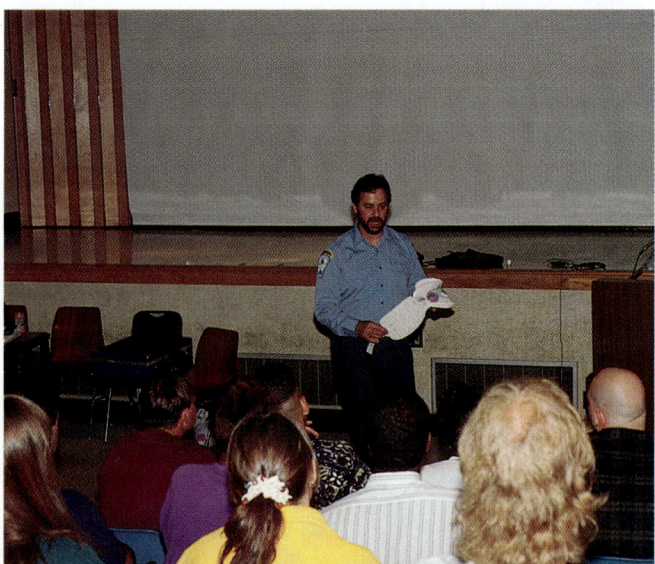

FIGURE 1.10 The EMT-B course will include classroom lectures.

diac Life Support before entering the EMT course. This course teaches students to deliver CPR and is offered in many communities under the auspices of the local EMS agency, the American Heart Association, or the American Red Cross (Figure 1.9). In addition, since EMS is a physically and mentally demanding profession, individuals seeking to complete an EMT-B training course will need to possess the physical and mental characteristics necessary to deal with the demands of emergency medical care.

Educational Experience

The EMT-B training course involves several types of educational experiences. The national standard curriculum requires that the EMT-B student participate in at least 110 hours of instruction. This instruction includes lectures and participation in practical skill sessions. The student must also make a commitment to independent study (Figures 1.10 to 1.12) and read this and other texts to supplement the classroom instruction.

Clinical Experience

In addition to the time spent in the classroom, the national standard curriculum requires that EMT students have the opportunity to see and work with patients in a clinical setting (Figure 1.13). This requirement may be accomplished by riding on EMS units, or it may involve observation in an emergency department or physician office. The objective of these clinical exercises is to give the student the opportunity to have interactions with actual patients under the supervision of experienced health care professionals before he or she is faced with the first patient in an emergency situation. The national standard curriculum requires that the EMT-B student interact with at least five patients as a part of the training program.

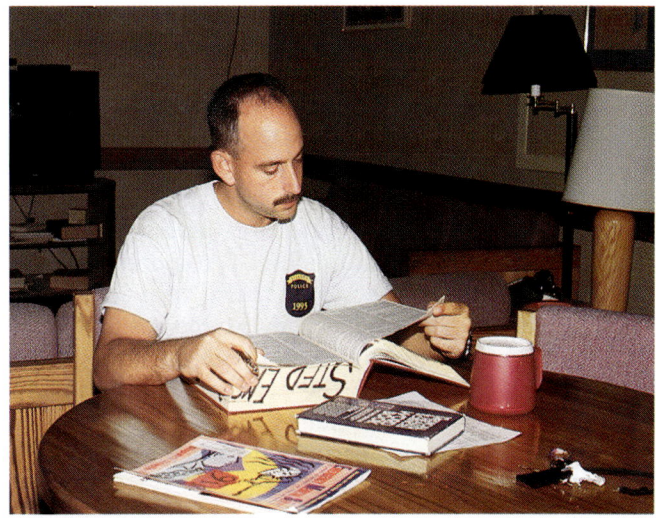

FIGURE 1.12 The EMT-B course requires a commitment to study outside of the classroom.

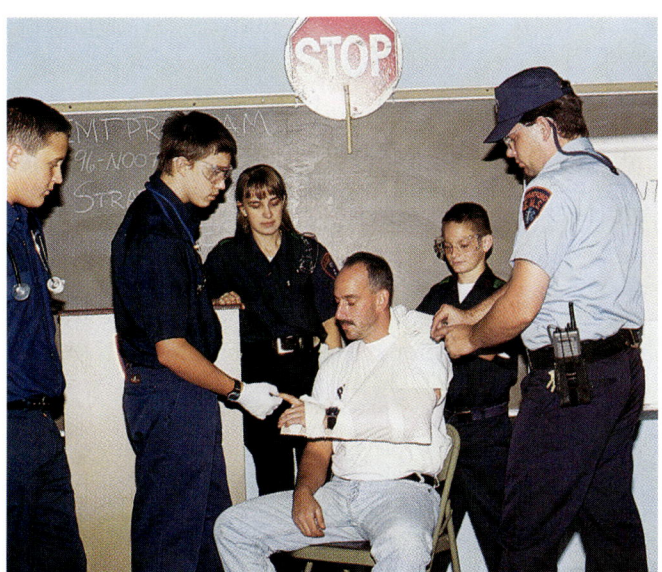

FIGURE 1.11 Practical skill sessions allow the student to actually perform the EMT skills.

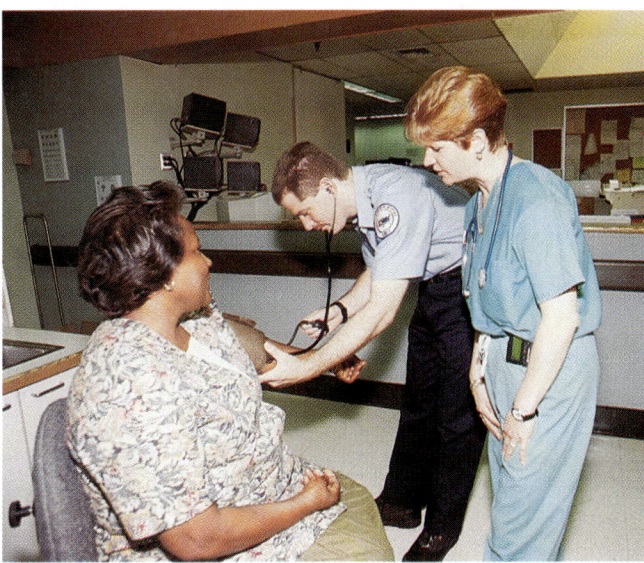

FIGURE 1.13 The EMT student will have the opportunity to practice assessment skills in the clinical setting.

Approach to Teaching EMTs

Assessment-Based Versus Diagnosis-Based Emergency Care

During the last revision of the national standard EMT curriculum, experts faced a challenging system-imposed limit. The knowledge required by the EMT-B was continuing to grow at the same time that politics and reality dictated that the minimum number of hours in the course could not be increased. More information had to fit into the same time frame that was used before. The decision was made to go back to an assessment-based approach, which is based on a simple recognition of the patient's signs and symptoms. This is contrary to the diagnosis-based approach, which takes the results of patient assessment and matches them with known injuries or diseases to arrive at a **diagnosis.**

An example that illustrates this assessment-based approach is one in which the EMT-B responds to a patient with chest pain. The treatment will be to administer oxygen, place the patient in a comfortable position, reassure the patient, assist the patient with his or her medications, and transport to the hospital. This treatment will be exactly the same whether the patients condition is muscular pain, angina pectoris, or an acute myocardial infarction.

The assessment-based approach does not imply that the EMT-B is not capable of learning the difference. On the contrary, it acknowledges the reality that the EMT-B does not always need to know the difference between different diagnoses but needs to know how to manage the problems or conditions that the patient has.

✓ The EMT-B training program takes an **assessment-based approach** to emergency medical care. The EMT-B is taught to quickly recognize important signs and symptoms and rapidly respond with appropriate emergency medical care

Initial Training Versus Continuing Education

EMS education has two distinct components: initial and continuing education. The EMT-B course is not intended to create a prehospital emergency care expert on the first day out of the classroom but rather to provide the basic knowledge and skills necessary to be fully functional on that first day. However, EMS education is a continuous process, and it requires that individuals commit themselves to the constant process of upgrading and maintaining knowledge and skills through continuing education (CE).

CE is accomplished in a variety of ways from a formal classroom setting to something as simple as reading professional journals, reviewing videotapes, or listening to audiotapes. Case review sessions, in which a particular case is discussed and critiqued by a group of EMTs and perhaps a physician, is another form of CE. The common thread through all of these forms of CE is that the EMT-B will be building on the basic information received in the initial EMT-B course.

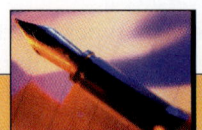

Tips from the Pros

Many EMT-B students turn to an experienced EMT-B, EMT-I, or EMT-P to help them through the course. Although experienced prehospital providers can be a lot of help, a risk is involved. Although veteran EMS providers are excellent resources and mentors for EMTs who have completed the course, they are not the only help for completing the course and achieving initial certification.

Another approach to successful completion of the EMT-B course is for the students to help one another by forming study groups, practicing together, and spending extra time with the instructor. All of these things will better prepare the student for successful course completion. Once the new EMT completes the course and accomplishes certification, he or she should actively seek experienced EMTs and draw on their valuable experience to build on the lessons learned in the EMT training course.

Licensure and Certification

Initial certification. After successful completion of the initial EMT-B training course, the student has the opportunity to achieve state and/or national certification. In general, certification involves a written examination and a demonstration of skill competency. However, states vary in the details of their certification processes. Many states use a national certification process administered by the National Registry of EMTs (NREMT) (Figure 1.14).

Recertification. The EMT-B is required to demonstrate periodically that he or she still possesses the basic knowledge and skills necessary to function as an EMT-B. Most states and the NREMT require CE as a component of the recertification process. In addition, many states require a written and/or practical examination during the recertification process.

> ✓ The EMT-B training program involves classroom lecture and practical skill sessions. A clinical experience, which provides the opportunity to practice assessment skills on live patients, is also required. The course concludes before the student takes the state or national certification examination

Future of EMS

EMS in the future likely will be very different than it is now. More emphasis may be placed on transportation services, the scope of practice may expand beyond simple emergency care, and based on the lack of definitive research, the amount of ALS that is provided in the field may be reduced. The most significant issues will continue to be system financing, enhancing research opportunities, rapid changes in technology, and workforce issues.

Many futurists have indicated that unless major research initiatives are carried out soon that conclude continuing or enhancing ALS interventions, there may be a reduction in the number of ALS services. In addition, reimbursement for performing ALS interventions will continue to be evaluated by the federal government. A new EMS model, based on an broader BLS approach, may very well be the EMS model of the future. As the health care delivery system changes and as different societal needs and priorities arise, the EMS system will need to change at the same time to remain relevant in the changing world.

The NHTSA EMS division produced a document titled *EMS Agenda for the Future*, which serves as a guide for EMS providers, health care organizations and institutions, government agencies, and policy makers. This document is a strategic plan and needs assessment, which has been developed to help guide EMS into the next millenium. It examines what has been learned in the past 30 years and creates a vision for the future.

Future of the EMT

During the next millenium it is likely that more dramatic changes will develop within the health care system. EMS and the EMT-B, which are now 30 years old, will also undergo dramatic change in the future. There will be a greater emphasis on research in the EMS system of the future (Figure 1.15).

In addition to an increased role in research, the EMT-B of the future probably will be much more involved in the transportation business than in the emergency medical business. Advancements in technology will continue to affect the EMT-B in the areas of education, cost, access to the equipment, and its approved use (based on science). Another major trend is the changing demographics in the United States and a population that is aging. The EMT-B will spend more time dealing with this older patient population and will need a greater emphasis on recognition and treatment of geriatric diseases (Figure 1.16).

EMS System Challenges

Although tremendous change and controversy have occurred from the beginnings of EMS to the present, there seems to be no slowing of this change. As EMS embraces the new millenium, the challenges it faces will continue to escalate.

Financing

EMS continues to be a high-cost service. In the early years of explosive growth, the cost-effectiveness of the system was never questioned. Health care consumers have come

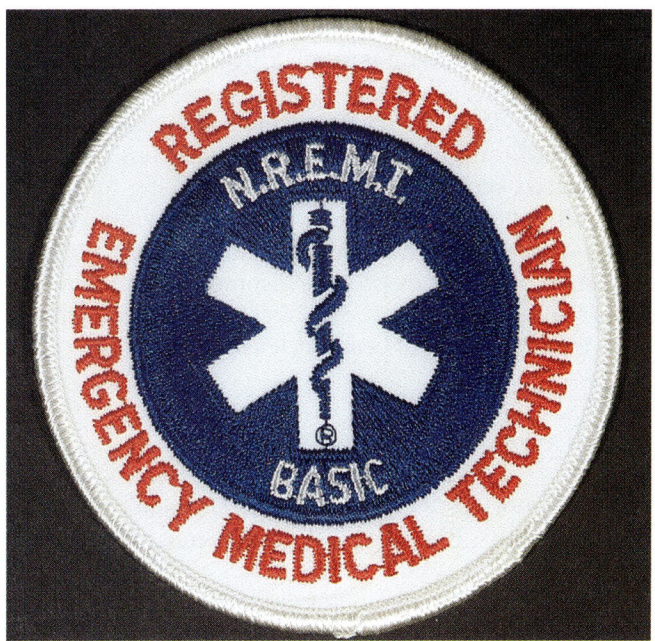

FIGURE 1.14 After completion of the EMT-B training course, the EMT-B student will have the opportunity to achieve certification. Many states use a national certification process administered by the National Registry of EMTs, which is a nonprofit, national certifying body.

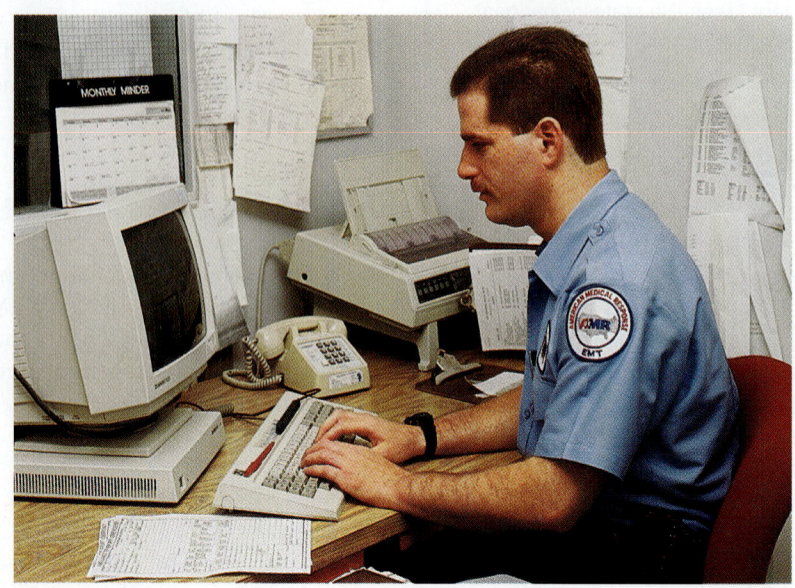

FIGURE 1.15 The EMT of the future will be actively involved in research, including data entry and analysis.

to appreciate that health care is also costly. In this new area of cost-consciousness in health care, EMS systems everywhere are finding it more difficult to find adequate funding.

Fee-for-service revenues are being squeezed by contract health care (managed care). Government subsidies are reduced because of the tax squeeze being felt by almost all governments, large or small. Individual donations, subscriptions, and payments are severely reduced as people have less disposable income to share. Finding ways to adequately finance health care in general, and in EMS in particular, will be an increasing challenge.

Workforce

The EMS workforce continues to be an issue of concern for the industry. EMS at times is considered a young person's occupation with 5 years considered a long time to stay in the field. As with other industries that depend on a young workforce, the workforce pool of young people is not as big as it once was. For the first time, EMS agencies are beginning to focus seriously on keeping people rather than simply replacing them. This approach toward improving working conditions, compensation, and benefits is paying off with people staying in the field for a longer time. Careers of 10 to 15 years (or longer) are now common; however, maintaining a workforce sufficient to meet community needs will continue to challenge EMS systems.

Research

One of the first priorities for spending money is to use it on things that definitely work or return a benefit. Unfortunately, EMS has just begun to effectively conduct formal research that can prove that what is done in the field works. For those things that do work, it is difficult to establish their value or cost-effectiveness. For example, it is clear that a sophisticated and well-integrated EMS system reduces deaths from cardiac arrest. However, the cost of developing the system measured against the number of lives saved indicates an extremely small benefit received for the dollars expended.

EMS systems at the local, regional, state, and national levels need to continue to invest significant time, effort, and dollars into research that is aimed at evaluating the effectiveness of EMS systems based on patient outcomes. Without basic, fundamental research and justification,

EMS stands to lose more financial resources, especially at the ALS level, and may see a gradual move toward BLS as the most common level of service.

Technology

Another challenge is technology and the demands it places on personnel. The rate of change in technology today is phenomenal. Even the experts in the computer and telecommunications industries are hard-pressed to keep up with these changes. As more technology becomes available at an increasing rate of speed, EMS systems will need to be careful of the effect that it has on the workforce. Along with technology comes training requirements. The importance of operator skill and efficiency go up, and the cost of developing and maintaining the necessary technical expertise escalates. EMS systems will be challenged to evaluate and implement new technology in ways that achieve maximum patient benefit without the costs exceeding the benefits.

> ✓ Although more than 30 years old, EMS systems are still faced with a number of challenges. In particular, challenges in the workforce, research, technology, and finance areas will test EMS systems and EMS personnel as they have never been tested in the past.

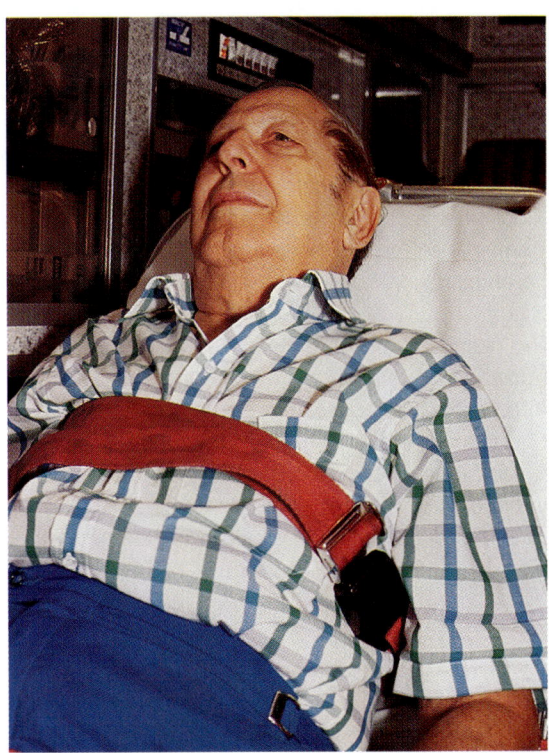

FIGURE 1.16 In the future, the EMT-B will spend more time dealing with the older patient population and will need a greater emphasis on recognition and treatment of geriatric diseases.

Summary

- The EMS system is a critical part of the overall health care delivery system. It has a dual role as a public safety service and a public health service.
- The EMT-B is the foundation level of prehospital provider. The EMT-B course provides all of the basic knowledge and skills necessary to provide emergency medical care outside of the hospital. All other levels of prehospital provider training and certification originate from the EMT-B program.
- The EMT-B program is based on a national standard training curriculum developed by the United States Department of Transportation (DOT) and adopted by individual states. The national standard program is intended to be a minimum standard, and many states and local jurisdictions have developed enhancements to the basic EMT-B course.
- The EMT-B program has been in existence for 30 years. It has undergone continuous revision and improvement over the years. The most recent revision involved a change in philosophic approach to the training course. Specifically, the course has shifted from a diagnosis-based approach to an assessment-based approach to training the EMT-B.
- The EMT-B training program involves at least 110 hours of instruction plus clinical experience. The student must make a personal commitment to additional study outside the classroom to be successful in the program.
- After completion of the EMT-B program, the student is required to participate in a certification process administered by the state EMS agency or the National Registry of EMTs (NREMT) before he or she is recognized as a certified EMT-B.

Scenario Solution

Less than 10 minutes after the collision occurs, a large vehicle with flashing lights quickly pulls up to the scene. It looks like a van with a large box on the back. It has the word "Ambulance" on the sides and hood, but it does not look like the combination hearse and ambulance that people were expecting.

The occupants of the ambulance jump out and efficiently move down to the station wagon with their boxes of supplies. They quickly begin to assess the patients, and they ask a number of bystanders to help with simple tasks because there are so many victims hurt. They quickly stop the patients' bleeding, splint broken bones, and move the patients to the ambulance. In less than 10 minutes, the ambulance pulls away toward the hospital.

As the bystanders begin to move back toward their cars, one long-time area resident says to another, "Say, where did that ambulance come from and who were those people in it? It sure didn't look like Casey's Funeral Home hearse and ambulance!"

The second resident says, "Haven't you heard? That was the brand-new town ambulance, and those people are emergency medical technicians. They've been trained according to new government standards. They sure looked like they knew what they were doing, didn't they?"

The first bystander responds, "We've seen many people die on this mountain road in the past. It's nice to know that with improved training and equipment these new EMTs will be able to offer better care to their patients."

Key Terms

Acute care Short-term medical treatment for an injury or disease with rapid onset, severe symptoms, and short duration, such as injuries resulting from an automobile collision.

Assessment Process that includes an oral interview and a physical examination. Assessment allows the EMT to gather information or clues that are useful in deciding which emergency medical interventions will be used. The results of the assessment also are communicated to the medical personnel at the receiving hospital.

Chronic care Health care provided for a persistent injury or disease with little change or slow progression, such as Alzheimer's disease; typically, this care is provided in an extended-care facility.

Curriculum Description of an educational program; usually includes learning objectives for the students as well as guidelines or rules for conducting the program (e.g., number of hours, number of lessons, etc.).

Definitive care Treatment provided to cure or resolve a patient's current illness or injury (e.g., surgery to repair a badly fractured bone or to reattach an amputated limb).

Diagnosis Identification of a disease or condition. The results of the assessment are compared with known injury or illness patterns to identify a disease or condition.

Emergency medical services (EMS) system Complex organization composed of people, equipment, and facilities designed to respond to the emergency health care needs of the community.

EMT-Basic (EMT-B) Basic level of emergency medical technician education identified by the United States Department of Transportation; provides basic emergency medical care.

EMT-Intermediate (EMT-I) Level of emergency medical technician between the level of EMT-Basic and EMT-Paramedic. The EMT-I has additional education in assessment over the EMT-B level. In addition, the EMT-I will be educated to use intravenous therapy and a limited selection of medications.

EMT-Paramedic (EMT-P) The most advanced level of prehospital emergency care provider identified by the United States Department of Transportation. The paramedic has advanced assessment skills and is trained in a variety of invasive medications, intravenous solutions, and other advanced treatment techniques.

Extended care facility Facility providing inpatient chronic or restorative patient care; often referred to as a *nursing home*.

Fee-for-service In a fee-for-service model, the patient accesses a health service and pays a fee for such care. In this approach, no limits are placed on the patient in selection of medical providers or access to the health care system.

Health care delivery system Large, complex network of people, equipment, and facilities designed to meet the general health care needs of the population.

Home care Health care provided to the patient outside of a licensed health care facility, such as in the patient's home or the home of a relative.

Managed care Form of health care insurance. Managed care plans control costs by monitoring how medical professionals treat patients, limiting referrals to specialists, and requiring preauthorization before care is rendered. Managed care also usually includes negotiated payment rates with providers that are discounted below the normal fee-for-service rates.

Key Terms (cont'd)

Prehospital care Health-related services provided to the patient outside of the hospital, generally at home, work, or in the field.

Prehospital provider A generic term for an individual who provides clinical prehospital care (e.g., EMT-B, EMT-I, EMT-P).

Primary care provider Physician who oversees the medical care for a patient in the managed care system; also called a *gatekeeper*.

Stabilization Process of bringing a patient's emergency medical condition under control.

Tiered response system Level of service at which multiple response of first responders, EMT-Basics, and EMT-Paramedics work together at the scene of an emergency. The type of care will determine the level of care to be provided.

Review Questions

1. Which federal agency developed the initial standards and continues to be responsible for development and revisions of the national standard EMT curricula?
2. Describe the role that EMS plays in the overall health care system. Explain.
3. The national standard EMT-B curriculum teaches an _____ approach to emergency medical care.
4. Describe the various types of roles that the EMT-B can be found working in.
5. Describe the difference between fee-for service and managed care.
6. The primary role of a tiered system is to provide _____.

Answers to these Review Questions can be found at the end of the book on page 865.

Roles and Responsibilities of the EMT

Lesson Goal

The goal of this chapter is to help the EMT-Basic understand the primary functions of being an EMT, including skills, knowledge, ethical behavior, and empathy.

Scenario

While picking up a late dinner at a local eatery, your emergency medical services (EMS) crew has been dispatched to a call from an elderly lady in need of assistance. As your partner drives to the address, you both notice that the house has no lights on outside. As you leave the ambulance you quickly glance in the mirror to check for oncoming traffic. You also make sure that the portable radio is in your possession. The unknown call nature and absence of lighting have heightened your awareness.

As you approach the residence, your partner stands beside the front door, knocks from the side, and announces "ambulance." You are greeted by a kind, frail-appearing, elderly lady who invites your EMS crew to come inside. When you ask her how you can assist, she replies with a long list of problems. "My health is failing. My diabetes is much worse since my insurance has changed. My prescriptions are all different with my new doctor, and I just can't drive to the store as easily as I used too. I haven't eaten well for days, and my trash can just tipped over. Can you please help me."

As you pick up the scattered garbage and place it back into the trash can, your partner inquires if the patient has any physical complaints. "No. I feel pretty good today. My blood sugar tested fine, and I certainly don't need to go to the hospital."

? Being an emergency medical technician (EMT) involves working with human beings in need. Some will need every assessment and skill you learned in class, and others will just require an open heart. The roles and responsibilities of the EMT vary as much as the situations that EMTs encounter. What actions during the call revealed your professionalism? What actions during the call displayed your concern for safety? What actions during the call displayed your understanding of the EMS system and medical direction?

Key Terms to Know

Certification
Emergency medical services (EMS) system
Emergency medical technician (EMT)
Licensure
Patient advocacy
Quality improvement

Learning Objectives

As an EMT-Basic, you should be able to do the following:

DOT

- Define *emergency medical services (EMS) systems*.
- Differentiate among the roles and responsibilities of the emergency medical technician-basic (EMT-B) from other prehospital care providers.
- Describe the roles and responsibilities related to personal safety.
- Discuss the roles and responsibilities of the EMT-B toward the safety of the crew, patient, and bystanders.
- Define *quality improvement* and discuss the EMT-B's role in the process.
- Define *medical direction* and discuss the EMT-B's role in the process.

Supplemental

- Explain the various methods used to access the EMS system in differing communities.

Prehospital emergency medical care is a field like no other. It is an ever evolving and changing profession in which the reality of life and death is confronted at a moment's notice. The responsibility of assisting people in their greatest time of need is monumental. The **emergency medical technician (EMT)** should acquire the knowledge, skills, and attitude necessary to fulfill the role of prehospital care provider. To give patients their greatest opportunity for survival and recovery, the EMT must know what his or her roles and responsibilities are in the EMS system. Society expects the EMS industry to provide not only emergent medical care but also emotional support for the patient and family members.

EMTs must always remember that personal safety is of the highest priority. The EMT must learn to assess the scene to ensure the safety of the crew and the patient. This chapter discusses the EMS system and the roles and responsibilities of the EMT. Safety, quality improvement, medical direction, and state statutes and regulations are also explored.

Emergency Medical Services System

The **emergency medical services (EMS) system** is a health care system that has many components. The system approach requires a large commitment of teamwork to achieve the best service using existing resources. Not every EMS system will look the same, but most will include the following components:

- An administrative agency will be responsible to govern the activities of the EMS. This can be in the form of a city or county government, a private corporation, a fire service, or a combination. The administrative agency will develop the policies and procedures for the service.
- The EMS system will have a medical director who leads the service's clinical patient care.
- The EMS system will also make a provision for medical control. Medical control is direct communication between the EMT in the field to a physician (Figure 2.1). This physician will consult directly with the EMT in determining the best patient care plan.
- Protocols are a set of guidelines that provide a standardized approach to the delivery of patient care in the system. Some of the procedures will be emergent interventions and may be standing orders. Other less emergent procedures will be done after consultation with medical control.
- Public education is another important component in the EMS system. This component educates the public about recognizing an emergency, accessing the system, and teaching citizens what to do before the ambulance arrives.
- A communications center is a crucial aspect of an EMS system. The center dispatches ambulances

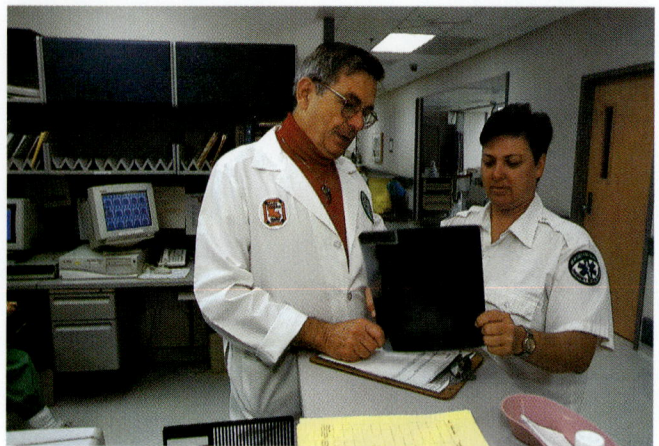

FIGURE 2.1 The medical director and EMT-B work together to ensure the best possible patient care.

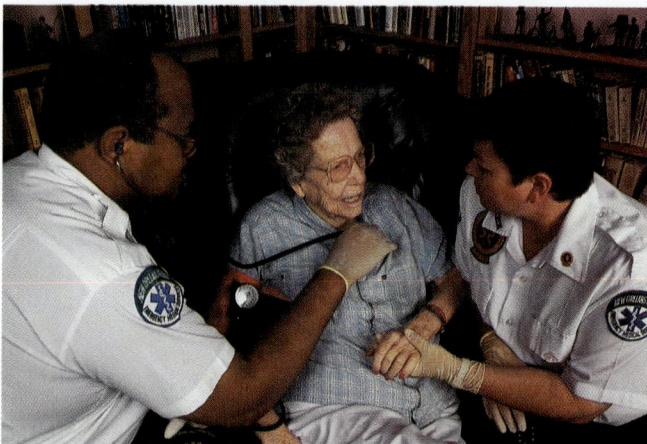

FIGURE 2.2 The EMT-B should always remember to use both verbal and nonverbal cues to reassure patients.

and makes sure that the system's resources are appropriately disseminated. Many communication centers use specially trained emergency medical dispatchers to deliver pre-arrival instructions and correctly prioritize calls.
- The EMS system will also make a provision for continuing education. The goal of continuing education should be to keep the EMT on the cutting edge of prehospital medicine.
- The quality of an EMS system needs to be measured. This ongoing process is known as quality assurance. The information gathered would then be used to improve the system in an attempt to deliver the highest level of service possible.
- Many systems have a formal plan to address situations when existing resources are overwhelmed. A mutual aid agreement with neighboring areas ensures that help will be available when needed.

A systems approach with these components increases an EMS agency's ability to provide superior patient care.

Access to the System

The EMS system is unique in that it can be accessed by anyone at any time. The means of access can vary from community to community. Some use a special 7-digit phone number for access, whereas others use the universal access number 911 because of its ease of memory. Many 911 systems are enhanced to give the dispatcher other specific information. For the EMS system to be of value to the community, it must be easily accessible.

Quality Assurance and Quality Improvement

For an EMS system to be its best, it must also have a means to continuously monitor and measure the quality of care delivered. A quality assurance program evaluates data (such as response times, scene times, adherence to protocols, and other indicators of quality) to identify trends. This helps a system to know what it does well and what it needs to work on based on a uniform set of data. After a system has identified a weakness, through education, it can improve.

EMS systems may also use a **quality improvement** program for evaluating system performance that is usually based on the perceptions of the customer. It is also an ongoing effort to refine and enhance the system. Its focus may be on clinical issues or different aspects such as billing, unit maintenance, or other support functions. Quality improvement relies on the customer as the ultimate indicator of quality.

Communication

Personal Communication

The EMT must strive to become a master at communication. The EMT will communicate verbally and nonverbally with every patient that he or she encounters. The spoken word is verbal communication, and the actions of the EMT are nonverbal communication. While the EMT is assessing the scene, the patient is also assessing the EMT. The actions of the EMT will often be

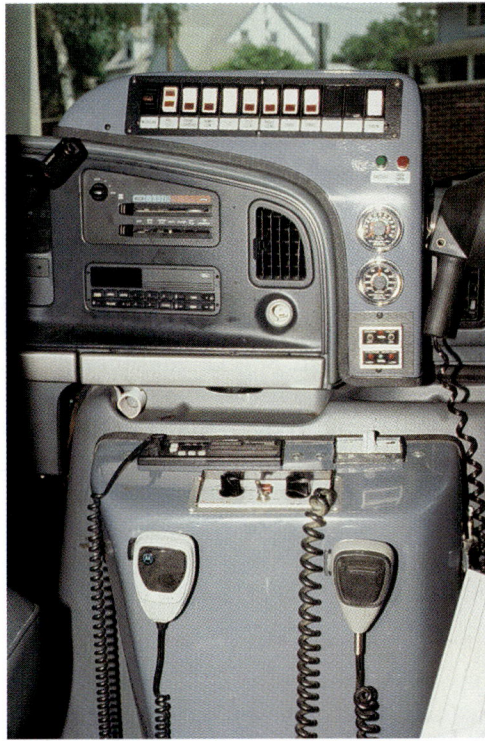
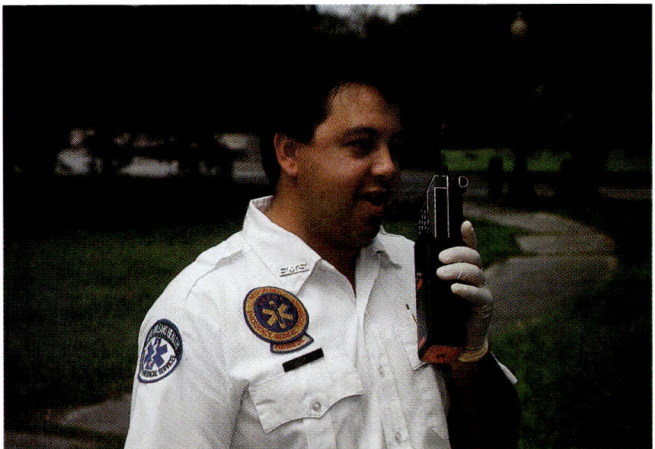

FIGURE 2.3 The EMT-B will need to master radio communications.

the first communication between the parties. The EMT should strive to display a calming demeanor in all situations (Figure 2.2). A patient who perceives a nervous, anxious, or excited care giver may have a decreased level of confidence in the EMT. Actions such as running to a patient and yelling are alarming and may increase the patient's anxiety. Patient's who are anxious are more challenging to treat. The EMT must remember that part of the care and treatment for all situations is reassurance and acting in a calm and professional manner.

Radio Communication

Radio communication is an important component of most EMS systems. The EMT needs to be proficient in radio operations. Nearly every call will require the EMT to talk on a radio to communications centers and hospitals (Figure 2.3). The radio is also a safety device for EMTs who find themselves in danger. It is important to have the ability to call for police assistance when needed. The general principles of radio communications, as well as specific guidelines for EMS communications, are discussed in detail in the Chapter 34.

Patient Communication

Communicating with patients is an essential skill for the EMT. As discussed previously, communication is verbal and nonverbal. This section focuses on verbal communication.

The EMT should identify himself or herself by name, title, and name of the service (e.g., "Hello, my name is Brian. I'm an EMT with LaSalle Ambulance."). The EMT must also receive consent from the patient to begin treatment (e.g., an EMT could ask, "May I help you?"). After receiving consent to treat the patient, the EMT must also inform the patient of the treatment plan, its anticipated results, and the potential problems of following and not following the plan.

Establishing good rapport with the patient during the initial assessment will aid in compliance of the patient during treatment. Patients trust that the EMT will be honest and provide quality care for them. The EMT should never lie or be disrespectful to the patient. A commitment to responsive communication between the EMT and the patient will facilitate smooth interaction.

Team Building and Leadership

Quality communication between ambulance team members is important. The EMS personnel must be working toward a common goal. Communication is the cornerstone for a good team relationship. The EMT's employer may designate a specific role for each employee. One team member may be designated the lead EMT, or Team Leader, but the roles will frequently overlap and require a team effort. The EMT crew must use the strengths of one another to provide the highest quality of care to the patient. This will also strengthen the working relationship.

Roles and Responsibilities

The role of the EMT is diverse and includes a variety of duties outside of patient care, including many before and after a call (Figure 2.4). Preparation is the goal of precall operations. The EMT will need to be mentally, physically, and emotionally prepared. Maintaining medical knowledge and keeping current with trends outside of the hospital is also important.

After a response, the EMT will need to restock the ambulance in preparation for future calls. The EMT will also be involved with documentation of the call events on the patient care report. The EMT may also need to seek help in dealing with critical-incident stress from allied mental health professionals after disturbing calls. The role of the EMT will also include many noncall activities that may include public relations, community education, station duties, and more.

Safety and the EMT-B

Personal Safety

The EMT needs to realize that a solid foundation regarding personal safety and self-preservation are paramount to career longevity. Emergency call scenes can be hazardous whether the EMT works in an urban, suburban, or rural setting. Arriving at work well rested, having an appropriate fitness level, and being confident about EMT skills are important aspects of personal safety. The EMT must also have an excellent working knowledge of all equipment and its location on the ambulance. The EMT must understand the policies and procedures that define the EMS agency and the EMS system of which he or she is a part. For further discussion on personal safety issues, refer to Chapter 5.

Safety of Crew, Patient, and Bystanders

The EMT has a family-like responsibility for the safety of other crew members. A cooperative team approach to crew safety is beneficial during hazardous call scenes. The crew must respond to all calls in a safe and appropriate manner. Not every EMS call will require a "lights and siren" response. EMTs must be knowledgeable of the geographic area, traffic patterns, and all traffic laws by which they must abide. Special educational courses are available to prepare the EMTs who have the responsibility of driving the emergency vehicle. EMTs also have the responsibility of providing a safe environment for patients in their care and for bystanders.

Responsible Patient Care

Patient Assessment

Before any emergency medical treatment can begin, the EMT must begin the process of identifying what is wrong with the patient. Patient assessment is the systematic collection of information about the patient and includes both historical information and information related to the current illness or injury. This information can be obtained through observation, physical assessment, examination, and response to interventions. Frequent reassessment of the patient is necessary. Chapter 8 provides additional information on this subject.

Patient Care Based on Assessment Findings

EMTs have the knowledge to recognize life-threatening conditions, evaluate the status of patients, and provide appropriate treatments. The EMT should be a critical thinking provider who initiates treatments based on assessment findings. No single treatment plan will fit every problem that is encountered. Prompt and effective treatment may include emergency airway control, traumatic injury management, or cardiopulmonary resuscitation.

Transportation and Transfer of Patients

Lifting and Moving Patients Safely

In most instances the EMT will be involved in shifting the patient from the site where he or she was found to a medical facility. This relocation may involve the simple task of moving a patient from the bed to the ambulance cot and then carrying the patient to the ambulance, or it may involve the use of other lifting and moving devices

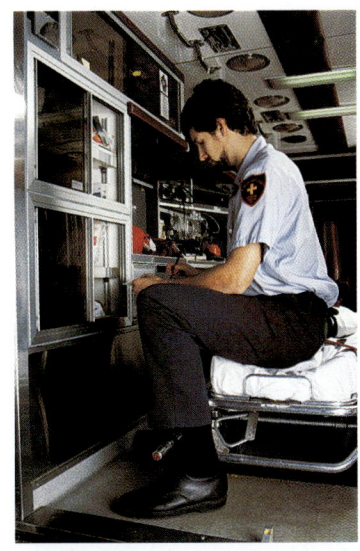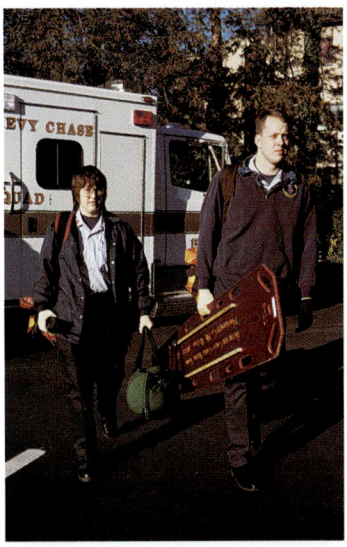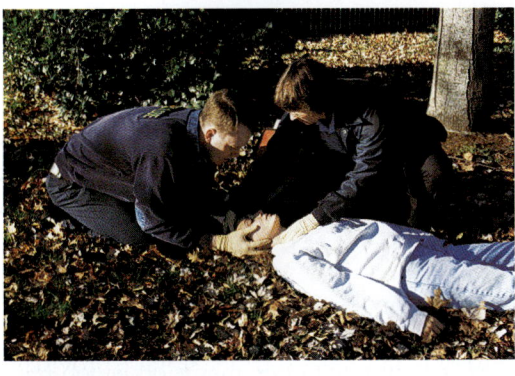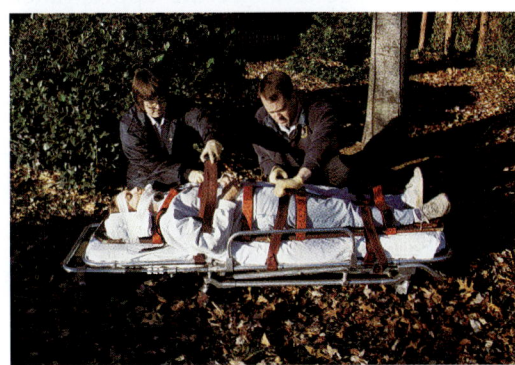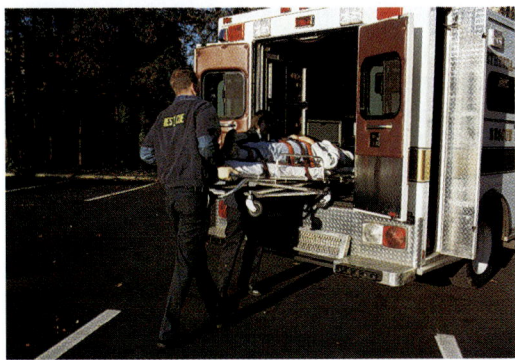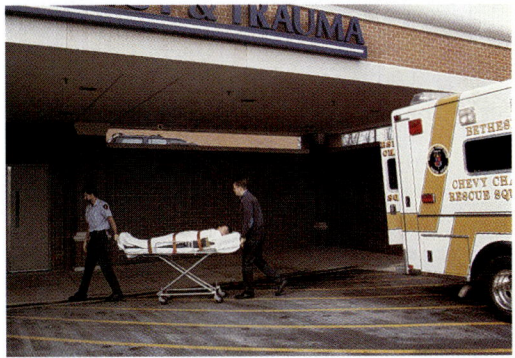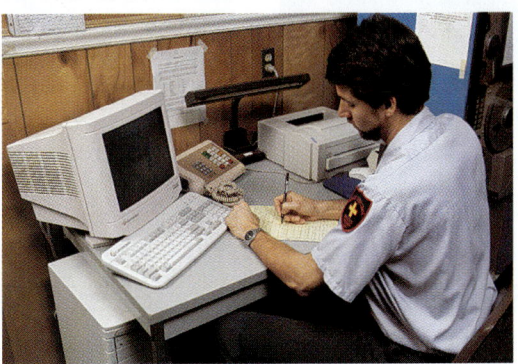

FIGURE 2.4 The job of an EMT is important and requires knowledge of many skills.

(Figure 2.5). Chapter 33 provides additional information on this subject.

Safe Transportation

Efficiently deciding the correct time to move from the call scene to a transportation mode is an important skill for the EMT. This is especially evident with the critical trauma patient. Respecting the role that EMTs play with quick assessment and rapid transport may greatly affect patient outcome. Providing a smooth and comfortable ride to the hospital will greatly increase the perception of the patient that they have been cared for well. Conversely, a rough ride will leave an unpleasant lasting memory. Drivers and passengers should always be secured with seat belts. Securing the patient to the ambulance cot and securing the cot into the back of the ambulance is an important safety step. EMTs should use car seats for children when age and size are appropriate. Safely and efficiently delivering the patient to his or her destination is a major portion of the EMTs responsibility.

Transfer of Care

Selecting the most appropriate medical facility is accomplished by an evaluation of the illness or injury that the patient is experiencing, as well as the location and availability of hospital resources. Correctly choosing specialty hospitals like trauma centers or chest pain centers may greatly affect a patient's risk of morbidity and mortality. The EMT often is responsible for communicating verbally with the receiving hospital or its designee before arriving. A written prehospital care report is also an essential tool for communicating information to the receiving hospital. Once the EMT has arrived at the receiving facility, it is important for the EMT to transfer the care of the patient face to face with another provider. At this meeting all pertinent information about the patient should be relayed.

Record Keeping and Data Collection

Every time an EMT encounters a patient, he or she is responsible for accurately recording the events and findings in a patient care report. This legal medical record usually includes details about the circumstances of the call, the findings of the patient assessment, and a description of care rendered and its results. Chapter 35 discusses this process in detail.

Patient Advocacy

In addition to the specific responsibilities described previously, the EMT also has a responsibility to be a patient advocate. **Patient advocacy** means that a person has placed his or her medical care in the EMT's hands when requesting emergency medical assistance. The EMT must represent the patient and act in the patient's best interest until that responsibility can be passed on to another provider in the health care system.

Other Related Functions

EMTs may encounter many other job-related functions depending on the setting in which they work. Not all EMTs work on ambulances. For example, some EMTs work as community educators, some in industry, and others in sports medicine. The EMT's ability to perform the various functions and tasks required by the job provides stimulation and rewards. The EMT should be a well-rounded individual willing to accept challenge.

Professional Attributes

The EMT is a respected individual who is dedicated to helping others. The EMT is also a human being whose attitude and professionalism help establish credibility and rapport with patients, allied health care providers, and other professional responders. EMTs must be conscious of the way they present themselves to others. Most emergency services require EMTs to wear a uniform that is clean and orderly to display a professional image (Figure 2.6). The combination of appearance and actions by the EMT leaves a lasting impression. Successful EMTs are leaders who are skilled, compassionate, honest, and physically and emotionally stable. The nature of prehospital medicine will test these qualities frequently.

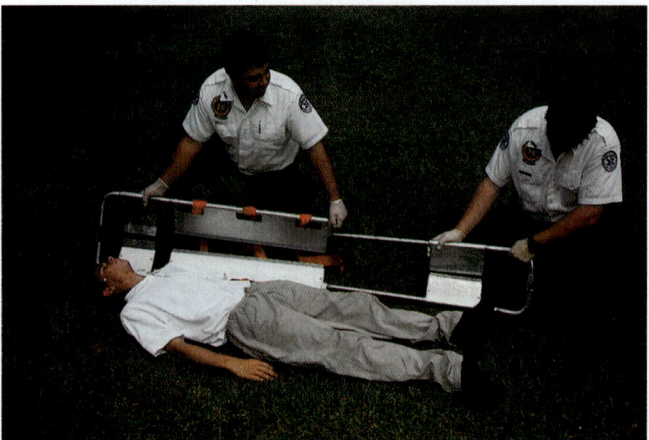

FIGURE 2.5 Sometimes moving the patient may require use of specialized lifting and moving devices.

Professional Ethics

Ethics are moral principles or standards that govern the conduct of a group of people. In the medical profession, ethics deals with the relationship between the provider and the patient, the patient's families, and fellow allied health care providers. The EMT will be involved in decisions concerning ethics and must uphold the highest standards of ethics.

The EMT is required to maintain patient confidentiality at all times. The information that the EMT receives from or about a patient is confidential. EMTs have an obligation to protect a patient's privacy. This information may not be released to a third party without the patient's consent. Delivering a verbal and written report of the patients condition to the person at the receiving facility who will be providing direct patient care is not considered a third-party release. For example, the EMT giving a report to the hospital nurse or physician to provide a continuum of care is not a violation of confidentiality.

In 1948, the World Medical Association adopted the *Oath of Geneva*. In 1978, the National Association of Emergency Medical Technicians (NAEMT) adopted the *EMT Oath* and a *Code of Ethics* (Boxes 2.1 to 2.3). These three documents detail the guiding principles for professional EMT service, and all EMTs should be familiar with them.

Legal Considerations

A variety of external factors govern the way in which an EMT functions. These factors may be formal, such as laws, regulations, and local ordinances. They may vary significantly between states and communities. The external factors may also be informal, such as ethics, morals, or standard of care.

EMTs are responsible for knowing and complying with the laws and regulations that govern their practice. They are also responsible for understanding and applying appropriate ethics, morals, and standards of care with each patient they encounter. All EMTs should strive to provide and ensure the highest level of EMS in an effective, caring, and professional manner while fulfilling their legal obligations.

Certification and Licensure

Licensure, certification, recertification, and continuing education policies and procedures vary from state to state. It is the EMT's responsibility to understand the laws and requirement of his or her state. EMTs must continually update and broaden their knowledge (Figure 2.7). The responsibility for continuing education is upon the EMT, whether they are paid or are a volunteer. Most states recognize EMTs by either licensure or certification. **Licensure** means that a governing body has granted permission for the individual to perform certain acts. **Certification** means that an agency or association has granted a certificate that attests to the accomplishments of a set of requirements by an individual.

Box 2.1   The Oath of Geneva

I solemnly pledge myself to consecrate my life to the service of humanity; I will give to my teachers the respect and gratitude which is their due; I will practice my profession with conscience and dignity; the health of my patient will be my first consideration; I will respect the secrets which are confided in me; I will maintain by all the means in my power the honor and noble traditions of the medical profession; my colleagues will be my brothers; I will not permit considerations of religion, nationality, race, party, politics, or social standing to intervene between my duty and my patient; I will maintain the utmost respect for human life from the time of conception; even under threat, I will not make use of my medical knowledge contrary to the laws of humanity. I make these promises solemnly, freely and upon my honor.

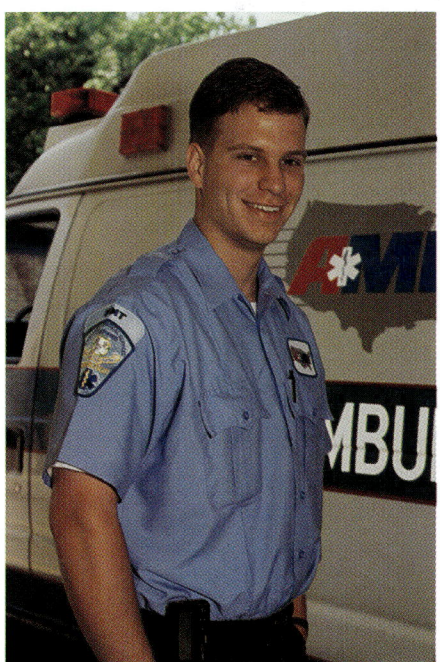

FIGURE 2.6 The EMT-B must look and act professional at all times.

Box 2.2 The EMT Code of Ethics

Professional status as an Emergency Medical Technician and Emergency Medical Technician–Paramedic is maintained and enriched by the willingness of the individual practitioner to accept and fulfill obligations to society, other medical professionals, and the profession of Emergency Medical Technician. As an Emergency Medical Technician at the basic level or an Emergency Medical Technician–Paramedic, I solemnly pledge myself to the following code of professional ethics:

A fundamental responsibility of the Emergency Medical Technician is to conserve life, to alleviate suffering, to promote health, to do no harm, and to encourage the quality and equal availability of emergency medical care.

The Emergency Medical Technician provides services based on human need, with respect for human dignity, unrestricted by consideration of nationality, race, creed, color, or status.

The Emergency Medical Technician does not use professional knowledge and skills in any enterprise detrimental to the public well-being.

The Emergency Medical Technician respects and holds in confidence all information of a confidential nature obtained in the course of professional work unless required by law to divulge such information.

The Emergency Medical Technician, as a citizen, understands and upholds the law and performs the duties of citizenship; as a professional, the Emergency Medical Technician has the never-ending responsibility to work with concerned citizens and other health care professionals in promoting a high standard of emergency medical care to all people.

The Emergency Medical Technician shall maintain professional competence and demonstrate concern for the competence of other members of the Emergency Medical Services health care team.

An Emergency Medical Technician assumes responsibility in defining and upholding standards of professional practice and education.

The Emergency Medical Technician assumes responsibility for individual professional actions and judgment, both in dependent and independent emergency functions, and knows and upholds the laws which affect the practice of the Emergency Medical Technician.

An Emergency Medical Technician has the responsibility to be aware of and participate in matters of legislation affecting the Emergency Medical Technician and the Emergency Medical Services System.

The Emergency Medical Technician adheres to standards of personal ethics which reflect credit upon the profession.

Emergency Medical Technicians, or groups of Emergency Medical Technicians, who advertise professional services, do so in conformity with the dignity of the profession.

The Emergency Medical Technician has an obligation to protect the public by not delegating to a person less qualified any service which requires the professional competence of an Emergency Medical Technician.

The Medical Technician will work harmoniously with, and sustain confidence in, Emergency Medical Technician associates, the nurse, the physician, and other members of the emergency medical services health care team.

The Emergency Medical Technician refuses to participate in unethical procedures and assumes the responsibility to expose incompetence or unethical conduct of others to the appropriate authority in a proper and professional manner.

Continuing Education

Licensure and certification are only the beginning of the EMT's education. EMTs have a responsibility to keep up-to-date on issues affecting the out-of-hospital medical field. This is accomplished through continuing education. Every EMT, no matter how busy the system in which they work, will experience a decay of knowledge and skills over time. EMTs can stay informed about the rapidly changing field of EMS through many different types of continuing education, including case reviews, lectures, hospital setting rotations, and self-study. The goal of continuing education should not be just to meet a state requirement for recertification but rather to increase and refresh the medical knowledge that a provider has.

Professional Organizations

Several national and state organizations are available for EMTs. The common goal of these organizations is to promote continuity and professionalism within EMS occupations. Organizations serve an important role in ad-

> **Box 2.3 The EMT Oath**
>
> Be it pledged as an Emergency Medical Technician, I will honor the physical and judicial laws of God and man. I will follow that regimen which, according to my ability and judgment, I consider for the benefit of patients and abstain from whatever is deleterious and mischievous, nor shall I suggest any such counsel. Into whatever homes I enter, I will go into them for the benefit of only the sick and injured, never revealing what I see or hear in the lives of men unless required by law.
>
> I shall also share my medical knowledge with those who may benefit from what I have learned. I will serve unselfishly and continuously in order to help make a better world for mankind.
>
> While I continue to keep this oath unviolated, may it be granted to me to enjoy life and the practice of the art, respected by all men, in all times. Should I trespass or violate this oath, may the reverse be my lot. So help me God.

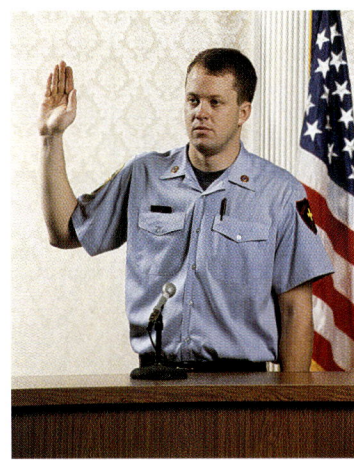

FIGURE 2.7 Keeping licensure and certifications current is an important part of the EMT-B's responsibilities.

vancing the profession of emergency services in many areas, including education, leadership, legislation, and standards. These organizations can be contacted for additional information.

National Association of Emergency Medical Technicians

The NAEMT was formed in 1975 by a group of nationally registered EMTs from existing state EMT organizations, national EMT leaders, and the National Registry of Emergency Medical Technicians (NREMT) to serve the needs of EMTs throughout the country. The association's goals are to promote the professional status of the EMT. Other national EMS organizations include the following:

- National Association of Search and Rescue
- National Association of State EMS Directors
- National Association of EMS Physicians
- National Flight Paramedics Association
- National Association of EMS Educators
- American Academy of Medical Administrators

These are just some examples of organizations through which EMTs and other EMS professionals can enrich themselves and pursue their specific interest. Belonging to a professional organization is a good way to be on the leading edge of prehospital medicine.

National Registry of Emergency Medical Technicians

The NREMT, founded in 1970, is a nonprofit organization that prepares and administers standardized testing materials for the EMT-B, EMT-I, and EMT-P. This agency documents the EMT's level of ability according to recommended standards by the administration of validated testing. The NREMT's goal is to promote and improve the delivery of EMS. Many states use the NREMT as the state certifying process.

Professional Journals

The EMT has several journals and trade magazines available to keep themselves aware of the latest changes and advancements in an ever-changing industry. These journals also offer a national forum for discussions about topics that face the industry.

Summary

- An EMT is viewed as a leader in the prehospital phase of the health care system and frequently interacts with many people of differing levels of training.
- The EMT's responsibilities include on-the-scene duties and precall preparation.
- The EMT will need to make a commitment to quality communication, be dedicated to excellence, portray a professional appearance, and exhibit a professional attitude.
- Most of an EMT's time will not be spent in emergency situations, but when the time arrives, he or she must be prepared to respond.
- The EMT will most likely have the opportunity at some point to make a monumental difference in someone's life.

Scenario Solution

Your intuition leads you to ask the patient if she has any food in the house. She embarrassingly shakes her head no. Your partner returns from the kitchen with the patient's medications, and your EMS crew spends a few minutes helping the elderly lady understand the order and amounts of medications that are to be taken tomorrow. You and your partner make eye contact, and it is obvious that you have the same thought. Your partner leaves and quickly returns with the meal that was to be dinner.

The elderly lady is amazed at your kindness and begins to cry. "This is the nicest thing that anybody has done for me in a long time!" The patient then agrees to let your partner call the local agency that assists elderly persons with independent living. As your partner arranges for an agency visit, you make radio contact with the base hospital physician to discuss the situation and your plan. The physician commends you for your actions and agrees that it would be fine to leave the patient at home.

Key Terms

Certification The act of certifying or state of being certified. In the legal sense, certification is analogous to licensure.

Emergency medical services (EMS) system Complex organization composed of people, equipment, and facilities designed to respond to emergency health care needs of the community.

Emergency medical technician (EMT) A person trained in and responsible for the administration of specialized emergency care and the transportation to a medical facility of victims of acute illness or injury. The Department of Transportation training guidelines for EMTs include a 110-hour course of instruction and clinical time.

Licensure The process by which the EMT-B is issued a license or certification by the state government agent. The licensure process implies compliance with federal and state guidelines.

Patient advocacy A process by which the patient places responsibility for his or her care and well-being in the hands of others.

Quality improvement A term used interchangeably with *quality assurance*. However, in quality improvement the emphasis is placed on improving performance at individual and system levels with less punitive means.

Review Questions

1. As an EMT, what documents will guide your ethical approach to prehospital medicine?
2. In your own words, what is an EMT?
3. Besides working on an ambulance, what other occupations use the EMT's training?
4. Other than the "lights and sirens" types of calls, what will be your attitude in dealing with patients with less critical needs who have accessed your care?
5. What is the importance of quality improvement in an EMS system?

Answers to these Review Questions can be found at the end of the book on page 865.

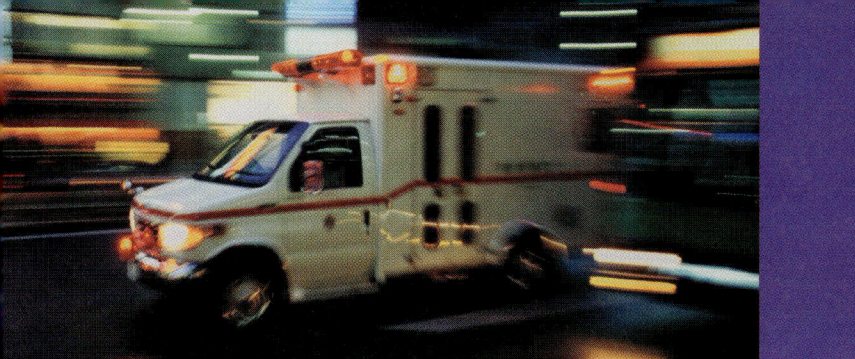

3

Medical/Legal Principles

Lesson Goal

This is a unique chapter from the National Standard Curriculum (NSC). It includes NSC objectives but expands upon and explains them with cases. The goal is to emphasize to the student that, in the current litigious climate in the United States, the EMT must be aware of the potential of legal suit. The EMT must carefully document each step of patient care and the indications for performing that measure. Patient rights must be a primary concern.

Scenario

You and your partner arrive at the scene of a two-vehicle collision involving four people. The first car contains two restrained teenage boys, both of whom respond to your questions but have slurred speech. Both boys are 16 years of age and have blood coming from their mouths. On the dashboard of the car you notice a crack pipe and a bag of white crystals. You also notice two empty vodka bottles in the back seat of the automobile. As you begin extricating the two boys from the automobile, they scream at you and refuse transportation to a medical facility. One of the boys tells you that his father is an attorney and will file a lawsuit if you tell anyone about the crack pipe and empty vodka bottles.

In the second car, an adult male and female, both unrestrained, appear intoxicated and have the smell of alcohol on their breath. The man, seated at the steering wheel, does not appear injured except for an abrasion on his forehead. He complains of numbness in his arms. The woman is in the back seat, although she was sitting in the front seat before the accident. She appears pale and only moans unintelligible words. She has erratic breathing and an open laceration to her scalp that bleeds profusely. You also note that she has a deformed right forearm and an open fracture of her lower leg.

When you approach the vehicle, the man identifies the woman in the car as his wife. He does not want you to take him or his wife to the hospital. He tells you that if you remove either him or his wife from the car, he will contact his lawyer and sue you and your ambulance company. Upon further questioning, you note that the man cannot tell you the date and has trouble remembering his name.

? How do you approach the teenage boy's protests about being transported to a medical facility? How do you address the male driver's refusal to accept transportation to the hospital? How do you manage the female passenger? How should you deal with the crack pipe, bag of crystals, and alcohol bottles in the boys' automobile? How should you deal with the evidence that suggests intoxication of the adult male driver?

Throughout this chapter, the term *emergency medical technician (EMT)* refers to all prehospital care providers.

Key Terms to Know

Abandonment
Assault
Battery
Crime scene
Confidentiality
Confusion

Consent
Durable power of attorney
Duty to act
Emancipation
Expressed consent
Head injury

Implied consent
Incompetent patient
Informed consent
Intoxication
Minor
Negligence

Refusal of care
Restraint
Right to Refusal
Scope of practice
Standard of practice
Surrogate consent

Learning Objectives

As an EMT-Basic, you should be able to do the following:

DOT

- Describe how an emergency medical technician (EMT) allows refusal of medical care and the interactions that must occur between the medical control physician and the EMT.
- Compare the functions of an EMT with those of a law enforcement officer at a crime scene.
- Define the EMT-Basic scope of practice.
- Discuss the importance of do not resuscitate (DNR) (advance directives) and local or state provisions regarding EMS application (Chapter 4).
- Define *consent* and discuss the methods of obtaining consent.
- Differentiate between expressed and implied consent.
- Explain the role of consent of minors in providing care.
- Discuss the implications for the EMT-Basic in patient refusal of transportation.
- Discuss the issues of abandonment, negligence, and battery and their implications to the EMT-Basic.
- State the conditions necessary for the EMT-Basic to have a duty to act.
- Explain the importance, necessity, and legality of patient confidentiality.
- Discuss the considerations of the EMT-Basic in issues of organ retrieval.
- Differentiate among the actions that an EMT-Basic should take to assist in the preservation of a crime scene.
- State the conditions that require and EMT-Basic to notify local law enforcement officials.

Supplemental

- Describe the rights of patients to make decisions regarding their medical care.
- Describe when a patient may not refuse medical care.
- Be able to correctly document the forensic aspects of a scene.

The emergency medical technician (EMT) often deals with situations that have medicolegal implications when providing prehospital care. This chapter discusses the legal issues that most often occur at the scene: the importance of documentation, questions regarding consent, and treatment at the scene of a crime. When consent issues arise, EMTs must understand the rights of the patient to accept or reject treatment and/or transportation. In addition, the EMT sometimes faces situations in which, despite the protests of the patient and/or family members or bystanders, the standard of practice requires the provision of prehospital care. In general, when the EMT arrives at the scene, he or she should understand that the patient must consent before the EMT performs interventions. The patient may express consent directly by requesting intervention or imply consent by cooperating with the EMTs.

Occasionally, the EMT will arrive at the scene of an apparent crime. In these situations, the EMT has an obligation to initiate prehospital protocols while disturbing as little of the crime scene as possible. In emergency situations, EMTs must initiate appropriate prehospital care. However, EMTs must conduct all interventions with the awareness that they should disturb the physical evidence as little as possible.

Medical Control

The EMT should maintain contact with medical control when managing cases with medicolegal implications. Most medical control physicians have dealt with medicolegal issues that commonly arise in emergency situations. Therefore the physician may assist the EMT in analyzing the emergency scene and determining the obligations of the EMT to treat the patient versus the patient's right to refuse treatment and transportation. Two-way communication between the physician and EMT allows the physician to give step-by-step guidance regarding the medicolegal issues. Depending on the situation, two-way communication allows the physician to speak with the patient, family member, or bystander and discuss the apparent or perceived problem resulting in a refusal to accept prehospital care.

Contact between a medical control physician and EMTs should always occur on a recorded channel. Assuming that most prehospital providers act reasonably, such documentation will usually help defend providers when a party questions their actions. In some cases, EMTs may want to contact medical control just to record and document legal information. In addition, contact with medical control allows the EMT to inform the physician of a potential crime scene. In some systems, medical control can then notify law enforcement authorities. In addition, medical control can assist the EMT in providing prehospital care while minimizing the disturbance of physical evidence at the scene.

Prehospital Medical Record Documentation

The three most important words in medicine when completing a prehospital medical record form are "Document, document, document." The EMT should record all essential and relevant information pertaining to the prehospital scene. Complicated situations require additional detail. The Scenario provides an example of a prehospital scene becoming progressively more complicated. In the scenario, the occupants of the vehicles suffer severe injuries. Medicolegal issues developed after the EMTs initiated prehospital interventions. In such a situation, the EMT should devote more attention to proper documentation. For example, the EMT should document the mental and physical status of all four patients. The EMT should carefully record his or her interaction with the patients and the physical description of the environment in which the dialogue took place.

Thus by documenting in detail the facts as they occur, the EMT can demonstrate a logical step-by-step basis for the actions taken at the scene. By documenting this information the EMT creates a document that a third party can review to resolve the legal issues of the case. Also, a contemporaneous record provides the most reliable means of recollection when courts resolve the legal issues of the case.

Editor's Note

The saying "If it is not written down, it did not happen" applies in a court of law. An example of this application is an EMT-Paramedic (EMT-P) who gets sued because he or she places an endotracheal (ET) tube in the patient's esophagus instead of the trachea.* The EMT-P had vivid recollection (as did his partner who was also in the patient compartment during the transportation) that the breath sounds in both lungs, lack of sounds in the epigastrium, improved electrocardiograph (ECG) strips, moisture in the tube, and the pulse oxygen percentage indicated throughout the transportation that the ET tube was in the correct position in this patient who is suffering from severe asthma. This assumption was further emphasized by the fact that the EMTs carried out three intubation attempts and correctly determined that the ET tube was in the esophagus on the first two attempts. The ET tube most likely became dislodged when the patient was transferred from the gurney to the emergency department bed. There would be no question that the EMTs did their job correctly if they had documented their actions.

In the court room, the run report revealed that the only documented vital signs, patient condition, and care rendered was on initial arrival on the scene. Throughout the 37 minutes that the EMTs were on the scene and transporting the patient, there were no other notations in the records and none of the ECG records were attached to the run report. The EMTs stated that they did not have time to document in the runs of patient care. However, with two EMTs, some notation could have been done and later transferred to the run report. Even an EMT working alone can jot down some information to later jog his or her memory as to the details. The two EMTs remained in the emergency department for 1 hour before the completion of the run and did not spend any of that time doing the paperwork correctly.

In court it was the word of a frightened EMT-P against that of the aggressive plaintiff's attorney that the ET tube was not placed in the esophagus initially and the EMT-P had not correctly evaluated that patient. A complete record would have prevented the entire case.

*This is based on an actual case. Some of the details have been changed to disguise and protect the EMTs, but the facts are correct.

Consent for Medical Care and Transportation

General Consent Issues

Informed consent refers to the basic doctrine concerning the provision of medical treatment by health care providers. This doctrine states that before a health care provider may render medical treatment to a patient, the patient must express consent directly by requesting intervention or imply consent by cooperating with the EMTs. Patients directly consent to treatment by stating orally or in writing that they request medical treatment or by signing a form authorizing medical treatment. Implied consent is when a patient acts in a manner that suggests that he or she accepts the treatment offered. For example, if an

EMT begins to insert an intravenous line and the patient puts his or her arm out to comply with the EMT, the EMT can infer that the patient consents to have the intravenous line started. **Expressed consent** is when the patient gives consent either in writing or orally for EMTs to provide treatment.

The **emergency consent doctrine** is another exception to the general rules regarding consent. Despite the EMT's duty to properly inform the patient about his or her injury, situations exist in which the patient lacks the ability to understand the nature and severity of the medical condition and the consequences of refusing treatment. The emergency consent doctrine allows a health care provider to give medical care to a patient in an emergent situation if the patient lacks the ability to understand the situation. Examples of situations that may affect the patient's ability to understand include unconsciousness, severe intoxication, or head injury. In these situations, the health care provider may provide emergency care despite the absence of formal consent by the patient. In the Scenario, the boys suffered potential life-threatening injuries. They have blood oozing from their mouths, suggesting that they may have sustained head injuries. Based on the crack pipe and the empty bottles of vodka in the automobile, they may have an altered sensorium as a result of severe intoxication. Thus they may not have the capability of providing an informed refusal. Therefore the EMT should contact medical control to discuss potential injuries and how they may affect the boys' mentation. The EMT should prudently transfer the boys to the hospital, under the auspices of medical control, rather than honoring the boys' demands to refuse transportation.

Refusal of Care

The informed consent doctrine includes an inherent right for **refusal of care**. Just as a patient has the right to accept medical care, he or she also has the right to refuse medical care. In *Cruzan v. Director, Missouri Department of Health*, the U.S. Supreme Court affirmed an individual's right to refuse medical treatment. However, the Court did not specifically grant minors the unconditional right to accept or refuse treatment. Before an individual may refuse medical care, the health care provider has the duty to inform the patient of his or her condition. The health care provider must determine whether the patient has the mental capability to understand the nature of his or her medical problem and the consequences of refusing treatment. Therefore the EMT is responsible for communicating with his or her patient to determine the mental capacity of the patient and explain the nature of the medical condition, the treatment required, and the consequences of refusing treatment. EMTs should not allow mentally incompetent or suicidal patients to refuse medical care.

Minor Consent

Laws define a **minor** as a person younger than either 18 or 21 years of age. Each state has rules defining the age at which an adolescent becomes an adult under the law. Adults, or majors, may legally contract, vote, drink alcohol, and consent or refuse medical treatment. Most states also have laws allowing minors to consent for medical care without approval or authorization of their parents. For example, states typically allow minors to give consent for treatment of sexually transmitted diseases, drug rehabilitation, and mental illness. Allowing minors to consent for these specific illnesses promotes treatment without fear of involving their parents. However, most states have not specifically authorized the right of a minor to refuse medical care. The EMT is responsible for knowing and understanding his or her state's laws regarding this matter.

Fortunately, parents or guardians in most emergency situations accompany minors. Consequently, health care providers obtain consent to treat a minor from the person or persons who have legal custody of the child. In most cases, the minor's parent provides consent. Competent parents have a near absolute right to give consent for treatment of their child; however, parents do not have an absolute right to refuse medical care for their child. For example, a parent does not have an absolute right to refuse medical care in an emergency situation in which the lack of medical treatment would result in serious bodily injury or death of the minor. In such cases the parent's right to refuse treatment does not override the state's compelling interest in preventing unnecessary injury or death of the minor. EMTs should call for support from law enforcement personnel when parents do not allow EMTs to provide urgent or emergent medical care to their children or when parents otherwise act unreasonably and jeopardize the health of their children.

The Scenario involves two boys who sustained injuries in a motor vehicle accident. A rapid assessment of the boys demonstrates obvious bleeding from the mouth. This finding suggests possible injuries to the head and cervical spine and compromised airway. Hypoxia can complicate any of these injuries and affect the boys' mentation. Therefore they may not have the ability to comprehend their potential injuries. Their stated refusal to allow transportation to the hospital may be a result from cerebral hypoxia, which adversely affects their ability to make informed decisions regarding the treatment of their injuries. More importantly, the crack pipe and empty vodka bottles may reflect potential **intoxication**. Like cerebral hypoxia, alcohol or drug intoxication may affect the boys' appreciation of the severity of their potential injuries and their ability to make rational and informed decisions regarding medical treatment.

At 16 years of age, the law considers both boys as minors. In emergencies, they usually have the right, based on state statute, to consent to medical treatment. However, minors may not have the right to refuse medical care in some states. The "mature minor doctrine" allows minors to consent to medical care. This doctrine states that before a minor may enter into any legally binding agreement, he or she must have the capacity to understand. Health care providers should not allow a minor to refuse medical care when the minor lacks the ability to understand.

EMTs should also consider whether their patient qualifies as an emancipated minor. **Emancipation** allows minors to have certain legal rights normally endowed to adults, including the right to contract and the right to administer business affairs. Emancipation usually results from a court order in which the court provides the minor with papers certifying emancipation. Certain situations automatically give rise to emancipation, including marriage, military service, and in some states, pregnancy. Nonetheless, without evidence that overtly demonstrates emancipation, the EMT may make a good-faith appraisal of the scenario and treat an underage patient as a minor.

Consent in the Incompetent Adult Patient

Competent patients have a general legal right to refuse prehospital medical treatment and transportation to the hospital. However, this right applies when several factors exist:

1. The patient appears awake, alert, and oriented.
2. The patient has the capability of understanding the nature and severity of the medical condition or injury.
3. The patient does not pose a suicidal risk.
4. The patient does not appear under the influence of intoxicants or has not suffered a medical problem or injury that affects his or her ability to understand the condition or injury.

Thus if the patient appears stuporous, unconscious, or severely intoxicated or suffered an injury or acute medical condition that affects his or her ability to understand the situation, then the patient lacks the capacity to refuse medical care.

When confronted with a possibly **incompetent patient**, the EMT should perform a mental status examination. The patient's medical condition and mental status may both interfere with his ability to understand. If a patient cannot understand the nature and severity of his or her injury and the consequences of accepting or rejecting treatment for his or her condition, then the patient cannot provide informed consent.

Before honoring a refusal, the EMT should document the information in detail and discuss the refusal with medical control. If medical control grants the refusal, the EMT should again advise the patient of the risks of refusal. Ultimately the decision to allow a patient to refuse medical care depends on the mental competency of the patient. Generally, EMTs should not allow clinically incompetent patients to refuse medical care. However, EMTs should not fight with patients who physically resist treatment. In these situations, the EMT should call for assistance from law enforcement personnel. EMTs may restrain patients who pose an immediate risk to themselves or others despite direct observation. However, the EMT should contact medical control as soon as possible to discuss the situation and get a verbal order for the **restraint**.

Providing emergency care when the patient does not consent to the treatment can result in charges against the EMT for assault and/or battery. EMTs are subject to liability for (1) **assault** if their actions put the patient in immediate fear of harm and (2) **battery** if they touch a person without his or her consent, even if the EMT justifiably believes that the action is necessary to save the patient's life. These laws are grounded in the fundamental concept that all adult human beings of sound mind have a right to determine what is to be done with their bodies. Laws governing when the EMT can begin treatment vary among the states.

In the Scenario, the unrestrained driver has evidence of a head injury in a high-impact motor vehicle accident. He also smells of alcohol and appears intoxicated. Upon questioning, he does not know the date and has difficulty remembering his own name. This information suggests that the driver may have suffered a **head injury**. The driver's complaint of arm numbness suggests that he may have a cervical spine injury. A strong possibility exists of a concurrent closed-head injury and cervical spine injury. The potential closed-head injury may affect the driver's ability to understand his potential injuries, specifically the potential severity of his injuries and the need for timely intervention to minimize his injuries. Furthermore, the potential closed-head injury may affect the driver's capability of understanding any information relayed to him by the EMT. The driver's questionable orientation supports this conclusion.

In addition to the potential closed-head injury, the patient appears intoxicated and smells of alcohol. Both the alcohol and the blunt head trauma may alter the patient's sensorium. Therefore the EMT should suspect that the driver lacks the ability to appreciate the severity of his potential injuries. The EMTs may not properly obtain informed consent from the patient because of his questionable mental competency; however, the EMT should make an attempt to do so. As the EMT discusses the situation with the driver, he or she should evaluate the driver's overall physical status, including the nature, extent, and severity of his injuries; his level of consciousness; his mental status; his ability to comprehend his injuries and environment; and his ability to carry on a coherent conversation regarding the situation.

The EMT should document this information in the record. In addition, the EMT should contact the medical control physician and convey this information. The EMT should specifically state that the patient refused treatment and transportation. The EMT and physician should discuss the facts and determine whether the driver can understand the situation in its entirety and whether he may legitimately refuse prehospital emergency medical care.

If the physician and EMT determine that the driver lacks the capability of understanding his medical condition and injuries, they may provide care if an exception to the informed consent doctrine exists. The exceptions discussed previously include mental incompetency, suicidal risk, and the emergency consent doctrine. Health care providers should do several things when deciding to treat a patient without consent:

1. The EMT should attempt to discuss the situation again with the patient and, if he or she is competent, obtain consent for treatment and transportation.
2. The EMT should explain to the patient the reasons that he or she will receive treatment and the risks of not providing treatment.
3. Medical control should try to locate the patient's closest relatives and inform them of the decision to treat and transport the driver despite his or her refusal.
4. The EMT should document the entire encounter in the record, including the facts of the situation, the patient's refusal, the discussion with medical control, reasons behind the decision to treat, and the fact that the EMT discussed this information with the driver after making the decision to treat.

Courts formally make the determination of mental competency. However, while health care providers do not determine legal competency, they routinely determine clinical competency through a mental status examination. A patient may lack clinical competency as a result of intoxication, injury, or a mental illness and may lack the capability of understanding the nature and severity of his or her medical condition. Therefore the patient may not have the ability of truly consenting to or refusing treatment.

Surrogate Consent

In the prehospital setting, EMTs experience situations in which family members, or surrogates, make decisions for a patient with an emergency medical condition or acute injury. Most of these cases involve uncomplicated situations. The classic example of **surrogate consent** occurs when parents consent for treatment of their children. Other situations include spouses who consent for treatment of the other spouse or adult children who consent for treatment of an ill parent. Most states have laws describing who may act as a surrogate decision maker regarding heath care.

The *power of attorney for health care matters* is an example of a legally sanctioned surrogate. The court grants an individual the right to make health care decisions for a patient in case he or she becomes ill and mentally incompetent. The court grants the power of attorney expressly through a document that details the authority of the surrogate. Before the surrogate begins to make decisions regarding health care matters for the patient, he or she should display the document to the health care provider. The power of attorney activates only if the ill patient loses mental competency and cannot understand information regarding the disease, injury, or illness that is affecting his or her ability to make informed decisions regarding medical treatment. Thus the power of attorney for health care matters does not give the surrogate the right to override decisions related to health care matters as long as the ill patient maintains his or her capacity to understand and act. Therefore a competent patient maintains the right to make decisions regarding treatment.

Other situations exist where the closeness of a relationship allows a surrogate to make health care decisions. Parents have such rights with regard to their children. Depending on state law, spouses may consent for treatment of the other spouse but only when the spouse loses the capability of understanding. However, most states limit surrogate authority regarding refusal of medical treatment. Typically, husbands may refuse medical care for their wives, and vice versa, when the spouse has a chronic or protracted terminal disease and the ill spouse no longer has the capability of understanding or making rational decisions. However, courts often do not recognize a spouse's right to refuse emergency medical care for the other spouse who has a treatable illness.

In the Scenario, the EMTs have no readily apparent proof that a marital relationship exists between the man and woman. However, the EMT should approach this situation in good faith. EMTs may rely on reasonable representations of the parties and the physical evidence, although the facts of a situation may negate that reliance. In this case, because both the man and woman appear intoxicated, the man may claim that the woman is his wife to prevent further evidence of his driving while intoxicated since a wife cannot be forced to testify against her husband. In addition, the man may make the claim because of **confusion** related to his head injury. The lack of orientation provides evidence of confusion. Moreover, based on his confusional state, the man may not understand the severity of the woman's injury. On the other hand, if he had awareness of the severity of her injuries, he would certainly not refuse medical care for his wife.

In this complicated situation, faced with the man's claim that he is the woman's husband, which is associated with the man's confusional state as a result of possible intoxication and head injury, the EMT should contact medical control and discuss the situation. Based on this conversation the EMT and physician can determine whether to honor the man's refusal or proceed with medical treatment and transportation despite his protests.

Providing Treatment at a Possible Crime Scene

EMTs often respond to an emergency at a **crime scene**. The EMT primarily has a responsibility to treat patients at the scene. Nonetheless, when the EMTs arrive at a possible crime scene, they have a duty not to disturb the crime scene any more than necessary when providing medical care. Activities like extrication, physical examination, intubation, splinting extremities, and cardiopulmonary resuscitation (CPR) may require the EMT to move the patient and disturb the emergency scene to render necessary and proper emergency medical care. The EMT should make a concerted effort to remember the environment as it existed at the time that he or she arrived. In the Scenario, the EMT should note the location of the four victims when he or she first arrived at the scene of the accident. The EMT should also note the location of potential evidence, including the crack pipe, bag of crystals, and empty vodka bottles.

If possible, the EMT should not disturb the evidence at all. In this situation, the EMTs may not have to move the crack pipe and bag of crystals located on the dashboard while evaluating and removing the boys from the car. However, if extrication or treatment of the patients required movement of the crack pipe, bag of crystals, or empty vodka bottles, the EMT should mentally note the initial location of the evidence. In addition, he or she should document this information in the record.

The public often mistakes EMS personnel for law enforcement officers at an emergency scene. Therefore victims and bystanders may react toward them in a cooperative or adversarial manner. They may tell the EMT information more appropriate for law enforcement. In those situations, the EMT should identify himself or herself to the victims or bystanders and encourage them to provide forensic information to the police. Nevertheless, EMTs should make a concerted effort to remember the information offered by victims or bystanders. Such information, whether verbal or physical, may have value in a subsequent criminal investigation.

If someone identifies evidence to the EMT, the EMT should note the type of evidence, its presentation, its location, and what happened to the evidence after its presentation or discovery. The EMT may point out the evidence to law enforcement officers when they arrive on the scene. EMTs should document in the record all pertinent information regarding the environment of the emergency or crime scene and the type and location of potential evidence. They should document the information in an objective manner, without personal opinions about the nature of the evidence. If possible, they should document the name and address of the person providing the information.

EMTs, like other health care providers, have a general duty of **confidentiality** toward their patients. The EMT should not disclose details of medical problems or details about the patient's medical history. However, most states have laws dealing with the discovery of contraband or other evidence of unlawful conduct. EMTs must generally disclose this evidence to the appropriate authorities.

For example, most states require that witnesses report elder abuse and child abuse. Therefore if the emergency scene suggests such abuse, the EMT has a heightened responsibility to note the condition of the elder or child, including bodily evidence that suggests abuse. For example, if EMTs find a child alone in a house with multiple bruises to the face, arms, and legs, they should consider the possibility of child abuse. They should then record in detail the environment, finding the child alone, and the physical condition of the child. If they find a belt next to the child, they should appropriately document this in the record. However, they should not remove the belt from the scene, nor should they move the belt unless necessary to treat the child. In addition, the EMTs should notify the police regarding the potential for child abuse. The police will then evaluate the scene for evidence of a crime.

Depending on state law, the EMT may have a responsibility to report that the drivers of the automobiles appeared intoxicated. Police often detect this information directly because they often arrive at the scene of the accident before or during the presence of EMTs. Regardless of the presence of police, EMTs should not disturb the emergency scene in search for evidence to prove intoxication. That lies within the purview of law enforcement.

EMT's Scope of Practice

EMTs have acquired special skills and knowledge that enable them to render basic emergency care. With this knowledge comes significant legal responsibility. EMTs have legal responsibilities to the patient, the medical director, and the public. EMTs should be familiar with their **scope of practice.** The EMT's practice includes providing for the well-being of the patient by rendering necessary interventions. Interventions are limited to the skills taught in EMT classes based on the United States Department of Transportation National Standard Curriculum, and any additional skills defined in state legislation regulating the practice of EMTs. Additional skills may be incorporated into the EMT's practice by medical direction through the use of protocols and standing orders. EMTs should never attempt to perform additional skills that they have not been certified to perform in accordance with state law—even if they believe that they will help the patient.

The EMT's ability to function is contingent on medical direction. Medical direction can be accomplished through a number of mechanisms. On-line medical direction is provided through telephone and radio communications to the EMT during the course of providing prehospital care to the patient. The EMT may also provide care with off-line medical direction in accordance with approved standing orders or protocols. The EMT is responsible to the medical director for any treatment that is provided or omitted in the prehospital care setting.

> ✓ The EMT is allowed to practice a limited form of medical care under the authority of a state's medical practices act and its related regulations. The law or regulations spell out the EMT's scope of practice. Typically, the EMT functions under the supervision of a physician medical director.

Right to Receive Care Without Interruption

Abandonment is failure to provide care for the patient once it has been initiated. Abandonment can result in the EMT being subject to liability for negligence. Abandonment can take many forms. Each of the following examples can result in a charge of abandonment:

1. The EMT initiates care and leaves the patient or turns him or her over to someone who has less training.
2. The EMT leaves the patient unattended for a brief period of time and his or her condition worsens or additional injury is sustained.
3. The EMT fails to transfer information to the receiving facility regarding the patient's history, treatment, or current condition.
4. The EMT fails to respond to or complete an ambulance call.
5. Once the EMT has responded, something happens that stops the response, such as equipment failure or a change in the EMT's own health status, and the incident is not immediately reported.

> ✓ Patients have the right to receive care in an uninterrupted fashion until they are stable or no longer need assistance. EMTs have the duty to provide this care.

Right to Receive Appropriate Care

The EMT is expected to provide the same level of care that any other competent EMT with equivalent training would provide. Failure to provide this standard of care is defined as **negligence**. To prove negligence, the complaining party must prove four elements:

1. *The EMT had a duty to act.* A duty to act implies a contractual or legal obligation to provide patient care. The duty may be formal, such as when the ambulance service has contracted to provide emergency care to the citizens of the community; or implied, such as when the EMT initiates treatment of the patient. A duty can also be implied when the patient calls for an ambulance and the dispatcher confirms that an ambulance will be sent.
2. *A breach of the duty to act occurred.* A breach of the duty to act can be shown by offering evidence that the EMT did not conform to the standard of care (the level of care that would have been provided by any other EMT in the same situation) by rendering inappropriate care, failing to act at all, or acting beyond the scope of practice. The EMT must act as a reasonable, prudent EMT would in the same or similar circumstances.
3. *The patient experienced a physical or psychological injury as a result of the breach of duty.*
4. *The EMT's action or failure to act was the proximate (or immediate) cause of the patient's injury.* A patient being transported in an ambulance that crashes would have little difficulty proving that the crash was the proximate cause of some of his or her injuries. However, a patient who sustains a ruptured appendix while riding in an ambulance is not as likely to be successful in asserting that the injuries were proximately caused by the ambulance transportation.

On occasion, the EMT may not actually have a legal duty to act but may have moral or ethical obligations to consider. In many states, while off duty, the EMT is not legally obligated to stop at the scene of a car crash. How-

> ✓ Failure to provide appropriate medical care is defined as *negligence* and may result in significant legal liability for the EMT.

ever, ethical obligations may demand the EMT do so. These obligations may be even more pronounced if the EMT is driving the ambulance outside his or her service area and observes a car crash.

Organ Donation

Whenever possible, the EMT should tactfully inquire whether the patient is an organ donor. To be an organ donor, the patient must have signed a document granting legal permission to procure organs from him or her. The EMT can obtain this information by interviewing the family members, having them look in the patient's wallet for an organ donor card, or having them look at the driver's license, which, in some states, lists the intent to be an organ donor. An organ donor should not be treated differently than other patients requesting treatment. The EMT's role in organ donation is to identify the patient as a potential donor, establish communication with medical direction to relay this information, and provide appropriate care to maintain organ viability.

Summary

- Most patients should provide express consent for treatment. In general, EMTs may presume implied consent when a patient calls them to a scene, and the law generally presumes implied consent in emergency situations and for unconscious or confused patients.
- Most states allow minors to consent for treatment, especially if they are old enough to have the capacity to understand. In an emergency, the EMT may proceed to treat minors under a presumption of implied consent. EMTs should obtain consent from parents when they are present. If a parent refuses life-saving interventions for a child, EMTs should contact law enforcement officials and proceed with urgent interventions. Many states do not allow minors to refuse emergency medical care.
- All states have laws and regulations allowing for surrogate decision making for incompetent patients. EMTs should not allow the surrogate to act unreasonably.
- EMTs should provide urgent and emergent care at the site of a possible crime, as they would in any other situation. They must balance their general duty of confidentiality toward their patient with a duty to report criminal behavior or evidence to the police.

Scenario Solution

Health care providers may optimally procure consent to treat a minor from the minor's parents or guardian. However, in the absence of parents or a guardian, the EMT should evaluate the seriousness of the situation and understand the general rule of erring on the side of treatment. A decision to provide treatment despite the refusal of a minor should occur after discussion with medical control. The conversation between the physician and the EMT will verify the discussion of the boys' medical condition and the absence of a parent or guardian. Furthermore, in some states minors may not refuse medical treatment, especially in an emergency situation.

In this scenario it appears that the male driver lacks the capability of understanding his situation because of his potential head injury and/or his intoxicated state. This suggests that the EMTs should treat and transport the driver despite his protests. The information that supports the invocation of this exception must appear in detail in the record. Similar to invoking the emergency exception, the EMTs must discuss the situation with medical control before treating an incompetent patient without appropriate consent. The EMT should revisit the driver and discuss the situation. The EMT should reevaluate the driver's capability to understand. If the driver still lacks the ability to understand, the EMT should inform the driver that he will not honor his refusal to treat and transport.

The facts of this scenario fulfill the criteria to invoke the emergency consent doctrine. The woman, involved in a high-impact motor vehicle accident, did not use a seat belt, had blunt head trauma, and ended up in the back seat of the car. She lost consciousness and had irregular breathing. She had profuse bleeding from a scalp laceration, a broken forearm, and an open fracture of the lower leg. Based on the description, she suffered a potential head injury, cervical spine injury, blunt trauma to the chest and abdomen, and hemorrhagic shock from the blunt trauma and scalp lacerations, which are all life-threatening injuries. She could not understand because of confusion and probably presented in shock.

In this situation, the EMT should infer that this patient would want prehospital medical treatment and transportation to a hospital for definitive therapy. Because she has a severe life-threatening injury and lacks the ability understand, she would meet the emergency exception and not have to expressly consent to treatment and transportation. The EMTs should contact

Scenario Solution (cont'd)

medical control immediately and explain to the physician the seriousness of the woman's injuries. Through the dialogue with medical control, the EMTs should document that the woman's situation requires emergency medical treatment and that she cannot provide informed consent. The EMTs should begin medical treatment, arrange extrication, and provide transportation to the hospital as soon as possible despite the objections of the male patient.

Key Terms

Abandonment Failure to provide continuing care for the patient once it has been initiated.

Assault Creation of immediate fear of harm in another individual.

Battery Touching a person without the person's permission; includes treating a patient without the patient's permission.

Confidentiality Privacy that is afforded to patient-related information.

Confusion Inability to understand the situation.

Consent Doctrine that states that before a health care provider may render medical treatment to a patient, the patient must express consent directly by requesting intervention or imply consent by cooperating with the EMTs.

Crime scene Location where the crime occurred. Everything present in and around the scene is a potential clue or evidence and should not be disturbed.

Durable power of attorney (for health care matters) The court grants an individual the right to make health care decisions for a patient in case he or she becomes ill and mentally incompetent.

Duty to act Responsibility to provide appropriate medical care.

Emancipation Legal doctrine that allows a person to make legal decisions regarding his or her health.

Expressed consent Patient states consent either in writing or orally for EMTs to provide treatment.

Head injury Damage to the brain (see Chapter 24).

Implied consent Patient implies that he or she wants care by his or her actions, or if the patient is unconscious or impaired, he or she would consent to care if able.

Incompetent patient Patient who is unable to make legal decisions. Usually an act of the court may be judged to be in such a state because of a medical or mental condition.

Informed consent Doctrine that allows a patient to accept or refuse treatment based on disclosure of information about the medical condition and the risks, benefits, complications, potential outcome, and alternatives of the suggested treatment.

Intoxication Above the legal limit of alcohol or drugs.

Minor Below the age to make a legal decision.

Negligence Failure to exercise the degree of care that a reasonable person would exercise under the same circumstances.

Refusal of care Decline treatment based on an informed consent.

Restraint Physical "restraints" to prevent a patient from injuring himself, herself, or others.

Right to refusal A court-granted right of a competent person to refuse medical care.

Scope of practice Usually defined by the state law that authorizes the EMT to function to provide patient care under the supervision of a physician.

Standard of practice The level of care that a reasonable EMT would provide for the patient in a similar situation.

Surrogate consent Informed consent provided by another.

Review Questions

1. An adult patient may refuse life-saving medical care if he or she:
    i. Is awake, alert, and oriented
    ii. Is capable of understanding the medical situation
    iii. Does not pose a suicidal risk
    iv. Does not appear under the influence of alcohol or drugs
    v. Has not suffered a mental problem or injury that affects understanding
    a. All of the above must be present.
    b. None of the above must be present.

Review Questions (cont'd)

    c. Only (i) must be present.
    d. Only (iii) must be present.
2. A patient may refuse medical care if he or she has consumed alcohol or suffered a head injury provided that:
    a. The patient is not too impaired to walk away from the scene under his or her own power
    b. The EMT has discussed the situation in detail with medical control and received permission to release the patient
    c. The patient will sign a refusal form
    d. The patient or another family member is an attorney
3. What should an EMT do if a parent refuses emergency care for his or her child or if a surrogate refuses emergency care for an incompetent adult?
    a. The EMT should request assistance from law enforcement and restrain the patient for transportation if necessary.
    b. The EMT should use leather restraints on the patient to prevent harm to the patient's wrists
    c. The EMT should carry handcuffs and use them in this situation and should perform a citizen's arrest and notify medical control of his or her actions.
    d. The EMT should leave the patient on the scene as the patient has requested (patient's rights).
4. What is the most important fact for the EMT to document when a patient refuses care?
    a. That the patient signed a refusal form
    b. That the patient's attorney is present or has been called
    c. The patient's mental state and medical condition
    d. That others on the scene have witnessed the patient's signature on the refusal form
5. Should an EMT collect evidence at a crime scene?
    a. The EMT should collect all possible evidence and document its location, time of collection, and description of the material.
    b. The EMT should touch nothing except what is absolutely required for proper patient care.
    c. The EMT should proceed immediately to the patient and start providing care while the other EMT should photograph the scene with a Polaroid camera immediately on arriving to record the scene.
    d. In the event of a major crime, the EMT should touch nothing, including the patients (except to give oxygen) until law enforcement has arrived.

Answers to these Review Questions can be found at the end of the book on page 865.

Suggested Readings

Ayers RJ: Legal considerations in prehospital care, *Emerg Med Clin North Am* 11(4):853, 1993.

Canterbury v. Spence, 464 F 2d 772, (DC Cir), cert denied, 409 US 1046 (1972).

Cruzan v. Director, Missouri Department of Health, 497 US 261, 110 Sct 2841, 111 L Ed 2d 224 (1990).

Hartman KM, Liang BA: Exceptions to informed consent in emergency medicine, *Hosp Physician* 35(3):53, 1999.

Informed consent and the impaired patient: an emergency medicine case study, *Emergency Physician Legal Bulletin* 9(2):1, 1998.

Mallon WK, Russell MA, editors: Forensic emergency medicine: Part I, *Top Emerg Med* 21(2), 1999.

Merz JF: On a decision-making paradigm of medical informed consent, *J Leg Med* 14(2):231, 1993.

Nyman DJ, Sprung CL: Informed consent: essentials and specific exceptions, *J Crit Illn* 6(9):891, 1991.

Ochs MA, Binder J, editors: Emergency medical services, *Top Emerg Med* 21(1), 1999.

Rosoff AJ: *Informed consent: a guide for health care providers*, Rockville, Md, 1981, Aspen.

Russell MA, Mallon WK, editors: Forensic emergency medicine. Part II, *Top Emerg Med* 21(3), 1999.

Schloendorff v. Society of NY Hospital, 211 NY 125, 105 NE 92 (1914).

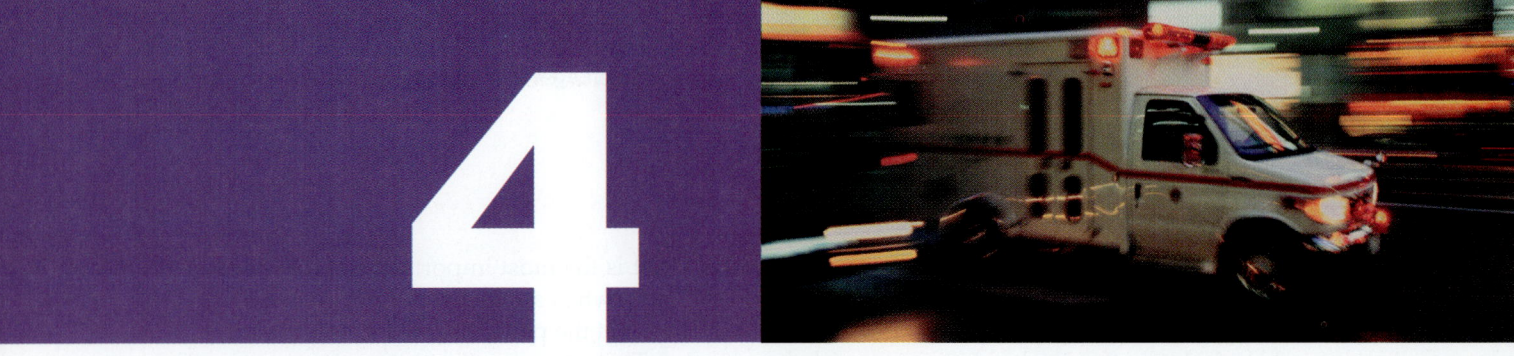

4

EMS Medical Director

Lesson Goal

EMTs at all levels do not have a license to practice medicine and therefore must work under the license of a physician. The goal of this chapter is to define the relationship between the EMT and the medical director and the roles and responsibilities of the EMS medical director.

Scenario

A call is received by the dispatch center regarding a two-car collision. One of the occupants is trapped, and another is up and walking. No other information is available.

On arrival at the scene, two cars are noted close to each other. Major damage is present to the door of one vehicle and to the front end of the other. A victim is trapped in the vehicle with the crushed door. An individual dressed in civilian clothes is reaching through the window with his hands on the patient. As you get out of your unit, he tells you that he is an EMT-B from the next state, that the man is not breathing, and that he needs to insert an endotracheal tube.

The man walking around smells strongly of alcohol. He has several lacerations on his face, and a bulls-eye fracture is seen in windshield of the car that he was apparently driving. He refuses to get into the ambulance. He tells you belligerently that he is going to get into his car despite the damage and go home. He then opens his car door.

 How are you going to handle this situation?

Key Terms to Know

Direct medical direction
Immediate medical direction
Medical direction

Medical director
Off-line medical direction
On-line medical direction

Physician extenders
Prospective medical direction
Protocols

Standing orders

42

Learning Objectives

As an EMT-Basic, you should be able to do the following:

Supplemental

- Describe the roles and responsibilities of the emergency medical services (EMS) medical director.
- Identify three approaches to EMS medical direction.
- List the components of prospective medical direction.
- Identify the components of immediate medical direction.
- List the components of retrospective medical direction.
- Explain the importance of the relationship between the EMT and the medical director.
- Define the difference between protocols and standing orders.

Health care delivery requires the participation, cooperation, and coordination of several different types of providers. This is particularly true in emergency medical services (EMS). One of the most important relationships between prehospital providers in EMS is the relationship between the physician and the EMTs, which should be cooperative because they are fighting against the same enemies—death and illness.

When the concepts that led to the creation of the modern EMS model were being developed in the 1960s and 1970s, the intent was to provide improved emergency care before the patient's arrival at the emergency department. This was to be done by using well-trained, nonphysician personnel working under the direction of a physician. The physician would take full medical and legal responsibility of the EMTs by being actively involved in their training, setting up the EMS system, reviewing the care that was provided in the field, and making necessary changes to ensure that the care meets national standards. This type of care has been provided by physicians riding in ambulances since as early as 1865 in Cleveland, Ohio and in 1867 in New York City, but it caught on only in major cities. In the smaller cities and towns the transportation service was provided frequently by the local funeral home, without emphasis on patient care. A benchmark article written by the father of EMS in the United States, Dr. Deke Farrington, identified that prehospital care in small towns was usually poor. Farrington embarked on methods of providing good patient care by **physician extenders** in the field to deliver the patient to the emergency department in the same or better condition than when he or she was found and to reduce the amount of time between onset of the illness or injury and the beginning of emergency care.

These prehospital physician extenders were specially trained individuals who were prepared to act as the physician's eyes, ears, and hands in the prehospital evaluation and management of the emergency patient. They became known as emergency medical technicians (EMTs) and thus began the vital connection between the physician, the prehospital provider, and the patient. The EMT, as part of the medical care team, is the link that was missing in the early days of EMS in the United States. This team would not work if the EMT and the EMS medical director did not work together and respect each other.

The delivery of health care in every state in the United States is governed in part by a law commonly known as a *medical practice act*. This law typically spells out who can provide medical care and under what circumstances. To implement the physician extender concept, EMTs had to be given authority to deliver health care through appropriate state laws or regulations. In almost every instance, the medical practice laws and regulations place the responsibility for EMT practice on a physician who agrees to supervise the prehospital providers. This supervision is particularly true of EMTs (Intermediate [EMT-I] and Paramedic [EMT-P]) who perform advanced life-support skills. In most cases, these individuals may not even practice without the specific authorization of a physician. Today, even most emergency medical technician-basics (EMT-Bs) function under the broad supervision of a physician.

Many terms have been associated with this relationship between the physician and EMS providers, such as *medical control*, **medical direction,** and *medical oversight*. The term *medical direction* is used to describe the role of the physician who is responsible for the emergency care provided in an EMS system. There have also been various titles assigned to the physician who fills this role, such as medical director and medical advisor. However, this text also uses use the term **medical director** to describe the physician who provides medical direction to an EMS system. Instead of focusing on titles, however, the EMT needs to focus on the function that the physician has in the EMS system, how the physician will affect his or her practice as an EMT, and how the EMT can work with and become friends with the medical director to provide better care to the patient.

The relationship between the physician and the prehospital provider has its foundation in history, theory, law, and the common health care delivery principle that the best patient care results from the cooperative efforts of many different types of providers. Because the EMT will have a great deal of exposure to physicians and will likely work under the guidance of an EMS medical director, it will be useful for the EMT to develop a basic understanding about EMS medical direction. This chapter discusses EMS medical direction, explores the roles and responsibilities of the physician in the EMS system, and describes the relationship between the medical director and the EMT (Figure 4.1).

> ✓ One of the most important relationships in an EMS system is the relationship between the EMT and the physician who serves as the EMS medical director. They need each other to carry out their responsibilities and the patient benefits when they understand each other and work well together.

EMS Medical Director

At the beginning of EMS development, no specific medical specialty or training program prepared physicians to take on EMS medical direction responsibilities. Early EMS medical directors came from many different medical specialties such as surgery, cardiology, orthopedics, primary care, and emergency medicine. They had little or no formal training in EMS and learned as they went along. Those early medical directors did an excellent job, but EMS medical direction suffered from a lack of consistency and a lack of standards.

As EMS has evolved, medicine has evolved with it, and EMS medical direction is now recognized as a specialized area requiring a standard set of knowledge and skills. As evidence of the evolution of EMS medical direction, EMS is now either a requirement or an elective in many medical school curricula. EMS is also part of the core curriculum in emergency medicine residency programs, and EMS fellowships are offered at several residencies throughout the country. Several postgraduate training programs have been developed specifically to train EMS medical directors, and a group of interested medical directors formed an organization to address prehospital issues. This organization, known as the National Association of EMS Physicians (NAEMSP), has now become a very well-respected national organization with several hundred members. Membership is open to emergency physicians, surgeons, family physicians, internists, or any physician interested and involved in prehospital care. EMS personnel are permitted to join as affiliate members. The NAEMSP has written protocols, position papers, and an outstanding textbook on medical direction. The material in this chapter is in general or specific compliance with their philosophy, goals, and written position papers.

Regardless of formal education or training, the physician who provides medical direction to an EMS system should have the following interests and background:

1. Familiarity with the design and operation of prehospital EMS systems
2. Experience in prehospital emergency care of the acutely ill or injured patient
3. Routine participation in base-station radio direction of prehospital emergency units
4. Experience in emergency department management of the acutely ill or injured patient
5. Routine active participation in emergency department management of the acutely ill or injured patient
6. Active involvement in the training of basic and advanced life-support prehospital personnel
7. Active involvement in the medical audit, review, and critique of basic and advanced life-support prehospital personnel
8. Participation in the administrative and legislative process affecting the regional and/or state prehospital EMS system
9. Active involvement in field patient care

Types of Physician Involvement

The EMS medical director must be involved in two different types of activities to accomplish the components of medical direction. The first is administrative in nature and is known as **off-line medical direction** or *indirect*

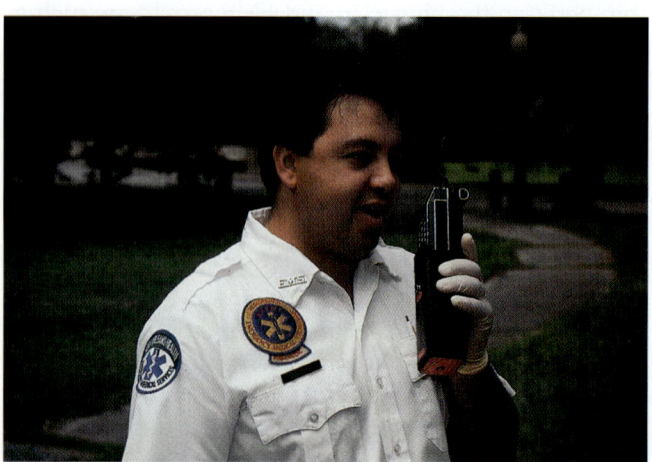

FIGURE 4.1 The EMT-B and the medical director work together as part of the health care team.

medical control. It includes activities such as writing protocols and reviewing EMT performance. The amount of time and effort required by the medical director to accomplish these administrative duties will vary depending on the size and complexity of the EMS system.

The second component of the EMS medical director is clinical in nature and is known as **on-line medical direction** or **direct medical direction**. This activity includes providing radio or telephone instructions to prehospital providers; direct observation of the system; and individual performance by responding to the scene, teaching in primary and ongoing EMS education, and providing prehospital patient care.

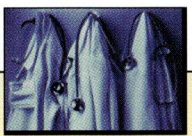

Physician Notes

There are two philosophies in the training of EMS personnel:

- The EMT should be trained to strictly follow memorized rules as a ritual. The EMS roll will require that the EMT think little and carry out care according to a set plan.
- The EMT should be provided with the knowledge, through initial training and continuing education, to make judgments based on a fund of knowledge and the situation as it presents at the scene.

It is the philosophy of the editors of this text that the latter method provides that best and most complete patient care.

Early in EMS system development, there was a greater emphasis on real-time physician involvement in emergency care delivery, so direct medical direction seemed to be the more important role. The EMS role has evolved, and as prehospital providers have demonstrated their competence, emphasis has shifted to the indirect form of medical direction. The theory is that a well-organized system with well-trained personnel who have been empowered to use their knowledge to perform judgment decisions while following good protocols and with good equipment should need little intervention by the physician as the emergency is taking place. This excludes the teaching and on-site supervision of the medical director of the EMS service.

> ✓ EMS is the delivery of prehospital medical care. In this United States and in the U.S. health care system, the physician is the responsible authority for health care delivery. However, EMS seems to work best when physicians and EMTs cooperate to deliver high-quality patient care.

Medical Direction

Medical direction of EMS systems is provided in many different ways that vary at the state, region, and local levels. Medical direction may be provided (1) by a single physician who makes all the decisions and carries out all of the responsibilities at the state or local level or (2) by a group of physicians who act collectively through a consensus process to provide medical direction to the system. It does not matter which system is used, as long as a working system is in place. The EMT will need to learn which medical direction model is used in his or her EMS system.

Three Components of Medical Direction

Whether by one or by a group of physicians, medical direction at its most basic level means that physicians determine what emergency medical care will be provided in an EMS system and exactly how the care will be provided. This standard setting and definition of process occurs through three components.

Prospective Medical Direction

Prospective medical direction includes the range of activities with which a medical director may be involved that occur *before* the emergency occurs. For example, the medical director should have a major influence on the care provided in a system by being actively involved with the training of the providers in the system, identifying the equipment that will be used to treat patients, assisting with selection of personnel, and developing the

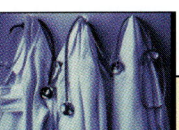

Physician Notes

The care of the patient in the field is different from the care of the patient in the hospital. Although the same method of patient care is used (initial assessment, resuscitation, focused assessment, and definitive care), the end points of each step and the way that some of the procedures are carried out are different because of the unique setting that the out-of-hospital environment presents. Therefore for the medical director to understand what the field situation is like, to be able to design the system, and to be able to judge the quality of the care provided by the EMT, the medical director must spend time in the field. This may be once a week or every day depending on the activity of the service. The medical director cannot stay in the hospital and expect to understand what goes on at the scene of an emergency.

protocols used for patient care, ambulance dispatch, and the ambulance placement strategy.

The prospective phase of EMS medical direction begins when a community first makes the decision to provide EMS service. After each run and periodically, the various aspects of how the service is set up and run should undergo an insightful evaluation by the medical director and prospective changes should be made in the protocols for the ensuing runs.

The community identifies the type of EMS that it wants and the resources and limitations on system design (budgets, response times, etc.). Once the community has identified the system goals, the EMS medical directors, the EMS agency, and the EMS providers begin to develop a system that will meet the public's needs.

The initial action is identification of the level of prehospital service that is required to provide the desired patient care for the community. After this decision is made, protocols are written, training programs are designed, ambulance equipment and supplies are purchased, mechanisms for retrospective review are implemented, and appropriate patient care report forms are produced. All of these activities must be compatible with local, state, and federal laws and regulations. In a well-designed EMS system, the medical directors will be directly involved in each of these decisions. They may not be the actual decision makers in each case, but they should have the opportunity for significant input. Although the administrative entity that provides the financial support for the service also has concerns and responsibilities, the factors that affect the quality of medical care ultimately must be the responsibility of the physician. Inevitably, a conflict will arise between the medical and administrative aspects of the system. Although both sides can argue that they should have the ultimate authority, the best solution likely will be found through compromise because both aspects are important. A system cannot exist without appropriate budget and administrative support, and it cannot exist without medical input and oversight.

Protocols. Protocols are the overall steps in patient care management that are to be undertaken by the EMT at every patient contact. A protocol is the instruction sheet or plan that is followed to have a successful patient outcome. Protocols are usually created for the emergency medical conditions that are most likely to be encountered in an EMS system, and they will address each step of prehospital care to be provided. There are national protocols (e.g., the protocols for management of the trauma patient developed by the American College of Surgeons/Committee on Trauma [ACS/COT] and the American College of Emergency Physicians [ACEP]), and there are state and local protocols. Some medical directors and EMS systems elect to develop their own protocols, whereas others may share protocols or use a generic source of protocols with modifications for the special needs of the local community.

A protocol can be symptom-based (e.g., coma, chest pain, seizure, and impending delivery) or diagnosis-based (e.g., diabetes, myocardial infarction, epilepsy, and pregnancy). The symptom-based approach is more common in prehospital protocols, especially at the EMT-B level, because it is often difficult to establish a prehospital diagnosis. Because the usual prehospital patient presents with specific complaints or symptoms, a protocol for reacting to the symptoms or complaint is easier to develop and easier for the EMT to learn because he or she is not required to make a diagnosis before beginning treatment. The EMT may only have time to address and treat the initial complaint or the most serious condition before getting to the hospital. For longer transport times, developing an in-depth fund of knowledge is beneficial for patient care.

Once protocols are developed by the medical director or EMS committee, they are usually put through an approval process within the local medical community. Even if a system medical director has the authority to act independently, it is often wise to seek outside input. Protocol approval may come from a state or local government agency, or it may come from a state or local medical organization. The goals of this approval process are to ensure that (1) the medical community agrees with the proposed level of prehospital care, (2) the proposed level of care and protocols accurately reflect the standard of care in the community, and (3) the protocols provide community-wide medical support for the prehospital system.

Once the protocols are approved, prehospital personnel need to be oriented to the protocols. Specific emphasis should be placed on any differences between the generic EMT curriculum and the skills and knowledge necessary to implement the protocols.

✓ EMS system design and function have both an administrative perspective and a medical perspective. Systems work best when decisions are made through cooperation and consensus building. Systems and patients suffer when one side or the other attempts to exert inappropriate power.

As discussed previously in this chapter, prospective medical direction involves several different aspects. The prospective medical direction is used to start up the EMS service; then all components are monitored daily just as patient's vital signs and initial survey are monitored every few minutes. Changes are made as appropriate

The EMS system will also need to put a process in place to review system performance to ensure that the protocols are used appropriately and that the protocols are having the desired effect.

> ✓ Protocols are the tool used by the medical director to clearly spell out how each patient should be evaluated and managed.

Standing orders. Standing orders are those components of prehospital care that the EMT may perform before contacting the physician by radio or telephone for further instructions. Protocols are often confused with standing orders, but they are actually two very different concepts. Protocols describe the big picture and total treatment, whereas standing orders refer to a much more limited range of actions.

At the beginning of advanced EMS in the United States, voice communication was thought to be absolutely necessary and to be desirable at the basic level. It was believed by most physicians involved in medical direction that voice communication should always be established after initiation of the standing orders; only radio failure should prevent such communication. Research in the mid to late 1980s proved that this is not necessary. The research showed that (1) there is no difference in survival with or without on-line medical direction, (2) less time is spent in the field without the requirement to call the hospital, and (3) prehospital providers are capable of making decisions without "reporting in" before providing patient care. This outcome was true not only for voice communication but also for electrocardiograms that were sent to the hospital via telemetry.

With information now available about the effectiveness of standing orders, many EMS systems are shifting away from requirements for direct, on-line medical direction and instead are focusing more on the use of standing orders. As experience continues to build, it is becoming clear that the key to success of a standing orders-based system is the presence of an effective indirect medical direction review process to ensure that the standing orders are being used safely and effectively when EMTs have a solid fund of knowledge. The EMT is not left alone with this process. When problems arise or there is a question, the good EMT will call medical control for help. It is inevitable that patients and conditions will be encountered that do not exactly fit the standing orders no matter how extensive that they are.

> ✓ Standing orders define those assessments and treatments that can be done before contacting a physician.

Training. Prospective medical direction also includes participation in the education of prehospital personnel. All states require that the objectives set forth in the National Standard Curriculum as developed by the U.S. Department of Transportation (DOT) are the minimal educational requirement. Some states, local communities, or instructors decide that a more in-depth level of knowledge is needed by the EMT to provide the best level of patient care. Because of the variance, this textbook includes the material set forth by the National Standard Curriculum and enhances information for a more well-rounded fund of knowledge that the instructor can use as he or she sees fit. Even if it is not included as part of the training program that is being used, the additional information is available as needed to add to the EMT-B's fund of knowledge.

At the most basic level, the medical director will be included in discussions and decisions about content and format of the training programs that will be used to prepare system personnel for their duties. If a decision is to be made to exceed or vary from the National Standard Curriculum, then the medical director should have input into the decision.

Special skills or knowledge, required or approved by the medical director, also influence EMT training in the system. For example, the National Standard Curriculum identifies intubation as an optional skill. A medical director's decision about whether EMTs in the system will use this skill will have significant educational implications.

As discussed previously, protocols developed by the medical director will also have an influence on training in the system. The length and complexity of the protocols will have training implications. Also, the frequency with which the protocols need to be revised will have an influence on the training program.

In addition to providing input into the training issues in an EMS system, the medical director should be frequently involved in the presentation of training. Many physicians are an excellent resource for some aspects of the EMT training program. Having them present in the classroom provides an excellent opportunity for EMTs and the medical director to get to know one another. When the training is over, the medical director and the EMTs are well acquainted.

In addition to the provision of input into initial training, the medical director will also have a great deal of information to feed to the continuing education program for the EMS system. Protocol revisions, changes in medical science, and the output of the system's quality assurance program (discussed in detail in Chapter 36) will provide a great deal of material for the continuing education process.

> ✔ The medical director should be involved in all aspects of the EMT's training, including decisions about what will be taught and how it will be taught. The medical director should also actively participate in teaching EMTs.

Ambulance equipment and supplies. At first glance, it might seem that decisions about what types and brands of equipment and supplies will be used in the system would not be a medical decision. After all, a bandage is a bandage. However, all prehospital equipment is not the same, and the medical director should be involved in decisions about the equipment and supplies so that the clinical perspectives can be added to the purchase decision.

In many instances, state or local government will dictate the minimum equipment and supplies that must be carried on an ambulance to be eligible for a license. In addition, the basic equipment and supplies needed for an ambulance has been defined in a list jointly developed by the ACS/COT and the ACEP. This list specifies the minimal equipment necessary to provide adequate patient care at the basic, intermediate, and advanced levels. Deviations from the essential (minimal) equipment and supplies can be by need of the local community or by changes in prehospital care standards. However, when making such changes the EMS service must take into consideration that most state statues include this essential list in their licensing process. The ACEP also has a position paper defining the optimal prehospital advanced life-support skills and medication. These and other ACS/COT and ACEP papers on medical control may be useful resources for the EMS medical director. The NAEMSP provides a text book and a course on how to be a medical director.

Local variations in response time, transport time, and vehicle use will influence the inventory of equipment and supplies that must be available. Although it is the responsibility of the administrative entity to keep supplies available on the unit, it is the responsibility of the medical director to work with the providers to identify what is required and how many of each are necessary to fulfill the mission.

> ✔ Because EMS equipment and supplies have varying results from a medical perspective, the medical director should be involved in making purchase and inventory decisions.

Ambulance placement strategy. How many ambulances are needed in a system and where they are positioned is a subject that is very important both in the design and the daily management of an EMS system. The medical director has an important role based on the patient care to be given and the access that patients have to patient care in this process.

The demand for EMS services is not steady in any geographic area. Instead, the frequency of medical emergencies and the locations change based on many factors, including time of day, day of week, weather, special events, etc. Sophisticated computer modeling systems are available to determine the optimal placement of vehicles. These sophisticated systems also move vehicles depending on demand variations. Such systems work well in large systems, but in the smaller systems with only a few calls each day, a more improvisational strategy will work just as well.

There is a medical component to the decision about where to place vehicles and how to use them. The medical characteristics of a community will dictate demand variations and the priority of the medical emergencies that may occur. The medical director provides valuable input to system administrators since there are many variables that apply only to the local system. Final decisions about placement should not be made without input from the medical director.

Communication. As discussed in Chapter 34, the communication function assumes a variety of important roles in EMS systems. Perhaps the most surprising function is that the communications center is a place where emergency medical care is delivered. More and more dispatch centers are adopting the principles of prearrival medical instruction and priority (basic life support [BLS] versus advanced life support [ALS]) dispatching. These two concepts involve dispatchers giving emergency care instructions to callers over the telephone until emergency units arrive on the scene, as well as sorting and prioritizing calls so that the patient with the greatest need gets help first.

> ✔ The EMS medical director needs to be involved in the planning, development, and implementation of the dispatch function, including medical priority dispatch and the delivery of prearrival instructions.

Immediate Medical Direction

The **immediate medical direction** includes the range of activities that the medical director and his or her designees provide while the emergency is taking place. For example, many EMS systems provide the capability for the EMT to speak directly with a physician by phone or radio to receive instructions about how to take care of a particular patient (direct [on-line] medical control). Physicians should ride along with EMTs and observe their job performance, providing coaching and assistance as needed, as part of the educational process (indirect [off-line] medical control) (Figure 4.2).

Direct. Direct (on-line) medical control of the EMS call is provided by a physician conferring by radio or telephone about patient care strategies. Although this method of providing medical control is not used as frequently as it was in the past, it is still an essential component in any EMS system. In the past, physician-to-EMT communication was a routine occurrence. Now EMTs function most often under protocols that may include standing orders and only contact the physician for direct medical decision making when an unusual occurrence or situation does not fit an established protocol or to report that a patient is being transported to the hospital.

The physician who provides direct medical control usually is not the same physician who has responsibility for the administrative, prospective, or retrospective aspects of an EMS system's medical direction. More often than not, the direct medical control is provided by the physician on duty in the receiving hospital or base station. On arrival at the hospital, the immediate phase continues when the physician provides personal feedback to the EMTs about the patient and the care given.

Indirect. To maintain a level of knowledge and proficiency in the EMS system, the medical director needs to observe the system in action (indirect [off-line] medical control). This should include observation in the dispatch center and ride-alongs with crews in the system. The EMT who has the opportunity to "host" the medical director has a tremendous opportunity to learn and to teach.

Retrospective Medical Direction

Retrospective medical direction describes the activities conducted by the physician *after* the call is complete. This should involve review of the emergency call by the medical director from a medical perspective. The medical director will use this case-review approach to identify system issues and individual performance issues with EMTs (Figure 4.3). The retrospective medical direction is also known as *quality assurance* or by some other quality-related term. Quality assurance is discussed in Chapter 36; however, the basics are covered here.

Case review. The EMS medical director should be involved in the routine review of the emergency medical calls handled by the EMS system. In large systems, (1) the medical director might review a percentage of the calls, or (2) all calls can be reviewed by the supervisor or training officer and "fall outs" or "outliers" only are reviewed by the medical director. In smaller systems, the medical director may review all of the runs. The purpose of this review is to identify system-wide issues such as

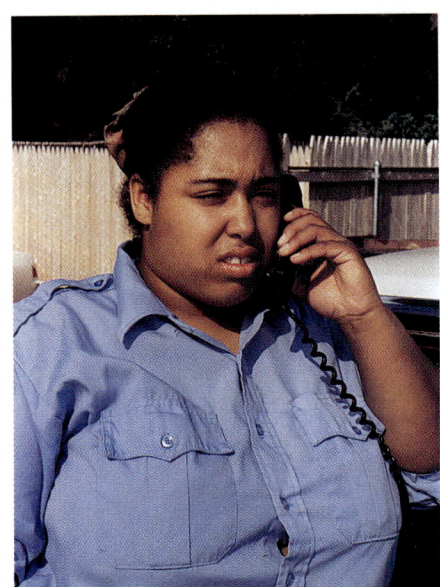
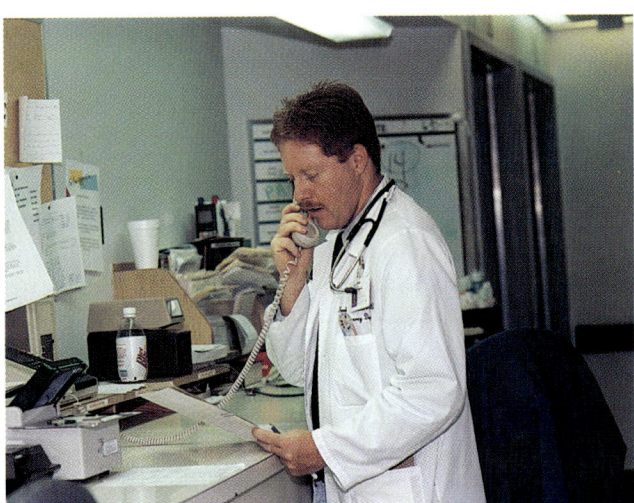

FIGURE 4.2 Immediate medical direction.

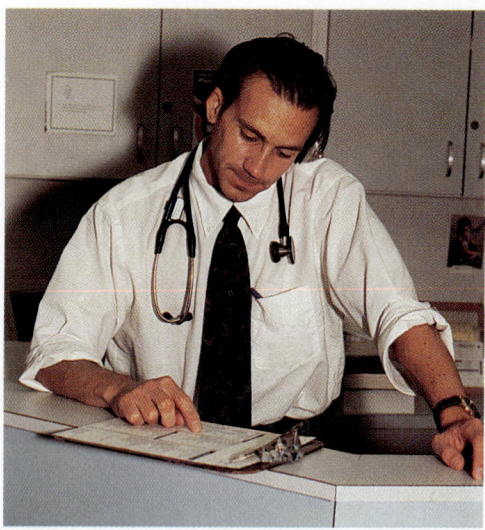

FIGURE 4.3 One aspect of retrospective medical direction is the review of patient care reports by the medical director.

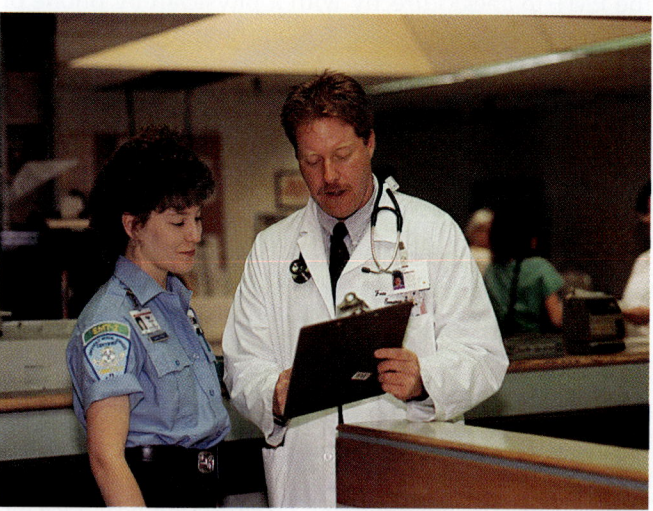

FIGURE 4.4 Individual EMT counseling is another part of retrospective medical direction.

response-time problems or skill problems that affect everyone. It also serves to identify individual providers who may have specific educational needs.

The case review will typically involve the physician looking at the patient care report that was prepared by the EMT, as well as the hospital records for the patient if they are available. An individual case review will usually focus on five questions:

1. Was the prehospital field diagnosis the same as the emergency department diagnosis?
2. Was anything done in the field that should not have been done?
3. Was anything not done in the field that should have been done?
4. Was there inappropriate delay in transporting the patient to the hospital?
5. Was the patient transported to the appropriate hospital?

> ✓ The EMT will have many of his or her patient care reports reviewed by the medical director and may have the opportunity to talk with the medical director about specific patient encounters.

EMT counseling. Another aspect of retrospective medical direction is the medical director's role in dealing with performance issues with individual EMTs (Figure 4.4). When inappropriate care is rendered by a specific EMT or if a question arises about the care provided, the medical director should have the opportunity to talk to the EMT. If the issue is an educational problem, the medical director can provide instruction to correct the situation. As described in Chapter 36, this interaction with individual EMTs should take place on a one-on-one basis with the individual EMT and should be approached as a positive and constructive learning situation.

Education. The medical director should also be involved in EMT educational programming as a component of retrospective medical direction. Using trends and performance information obtained from the case review process, the medical director should design and participate in the presentation of continuing education sessions for the EMTs in the system. The medical director should also identify and participate in the delivery of formal training programs that may be useful to system personnel, such as Emergency Medical Dispatch, Pre-Hospital Trauma Life Support, and Basic Trauma Life Support.

System review and revision. Another significant aspect of retrospective medical direction is the constant focus on system efficiency and medical effectiveness. The medical director must constantly monitor the state of the EMS system, through available data sources, and work aggressively with system administration to keep the system at a maximum level of effectiveness. An ongoing mechanism must be in place to allow the medical director to have access to system administrators and to participate in strategic planning for the system.

> ✓ EMS systems are not static, and the EMS medical director must constantly evaluate and provide input as the system evolves and changes.

Summary

- One of the most important relationships in an EMS system is between the EMT and the physician who serves as the EMS medical director. They need each other to carry out their responsibilities, and the patient benefits when they understand each other and work well together.
- EMS is the delivery of prehospital medical care. In the United States and in the U.S. health care system, the physician is the responsible authority for health care delivery. However, EMS seems to work best when physicians and EMTs cooperate to deliver high-quality patient care.
- EMS medical direction is emerging and evolving as a sophisticated specialty. However, the medical education process is still sorting out how to prepare physicians for this role. In the interim, EMS medical directors come from broad and diverse backgrounds.
- EMS system design and function have both administrative and medical perspectives. Systems work best when decisions are made through cooperation and consensus-building between the EMS medical director and system administrators. Systems and patients suffer when one side or the other attempts to exert inappropriate power.
- Protocols are the tool used by the medical director to clearly spell out how each patient should be evaluated and managed.
- Standing orders define what medical care can be provided to the patient before physician contact is made.
- The medical director should be involved in all aspects of the EMT's training, including decisions about what will be taught and how it will be taught. The medical director should also actively participate in teaching EMTs.
- Because EMS equipment and supplies have varying results from a medical perspective, the medical director should be involved in making purchase and inventory decisions.
- The EMS medical director needs to be involved in the planning, development, and implementation of the dispatch function, including medical priority dispatch and the delivery of prearrival instructions.
- The EMT will have many of his or her patient care reports reviewed by the medical director and should have the opportunity to talk with the medical director about specific patient encounters.
- EMS systems are not static, and the EMS medical director must constantly evaluate and provide input as the system evolves and changes.

Scenario Solution

The best friend that the EMT has in this and many other situations is the physician at the medical command authority handling direct medical control or the EMS medical director. The EMT wanting to intubate the patient may or may not be legal in your state. This is certainly outside of their own medical control and protocols. The "drunk" who is trying to drive away probably should not be able to sign out.

You need help. Your help is your medical director. He or she will give you immediate advice as to how to handle this situation via radio, will protect you if you get sued by any of those involved, will comfort you in your frustration, and will develop for you a CME program that will address these issues.

If any one of the system participants fails to deliver, the system fails. When they all work together, the system excels.

Key Terms

Direct medical direction Clinical type of medical direction that involves real-time direction of prehospital providers in the delivery of emergency care; also known as *on-line medical direction*.

Immediate medical control Range of activities that a medical director provides while the emergency is taking place (e.g., giving instructions to EMTs via radio or telephone).

Key Terms (cont'd)

Medical direction Various duties that a physician supplies in support of an EMS system; includes protocols, case reviews, educational programming, etc.

Medical director Physician who supplies medical direction to an EMS system.

Off-line medical direction Administrative duties carried out by the EMS medical director (e.g., writing protocols, negotiating destination policies, retrospective review of EMT performance); also known as *indirect medical direction*.

On-line medical direction Clinical type of medical direction that involves real-time direction of prehospital providers in the delivery of emergency care; also known as *direct medical direction*.

Physician extenders Specially trained individuals who are prepared to act as the physician's eyes, ears, and hands in the prehospital evaluation and management of the emergency patient.

Prospective medical direction Range of activities with which a medical director may be involved before the emergency occurs (e.g., training of EMTs).

Protocols Written or printed instructions or plans for carrying out an activity. In EMS, a protocol is a document that describes, usually in a step-by-step manner, the method that is used to deal with a set of symptoms or conditions.

Standing orders Patient care instructions in writing that authorize specific steps in patient assessment and intervention without the requirement of direct medical contact by radio or telephone; usually very specific in what can be done and contained within the patient care protocols.

Review Questions

1. The responsibilities of the medical director are to:
   i. Oversee the clinical activities of the EMS
   ii. Oversee the operational activities of the EMS
   iii. Ensure that all employees report to work on time
   iv. Review the patient care provided by the EMTs
   v. Develop protocols for patient care
   vi. Critique individual prehospital calls
   vii. Order supplies for patient care
   viii. Assist with ambulance placement strategy
   a. i, ii, iii, vi, and viii
   b. i, iii, iv, v, and viii
   c. i, iv, v, vi, and vii
   d. All of the above

2. The three components of medical direction are:
   a. Prehospital supervision, immediate radio control, run report review
   b. Prospective, immediate, retrospective
   c. Protocol development, scene supervision, ambulance purchase
   d. System development, field supervision, run report review

3. Which of the follow statements is true:
   a. Prehospital care by the EMT-Basic is done under the license of physicians.
   b. EMT-Bs are licensed to provide patient care independently.
   c. EMT-B protocols need not have physician review.
   d. Patient care provided by EMT-Bs is NOT subject to review by the medical director of the service.

4. Standing orders and protocols are as follows:
   a. They describe the same process.
   b. Standing orders are part of the protocols of a service.
   c. Protocols are part of the standing orders of a service.
   d. Standing orders do NOT require the approval of the medical director.

5. While the call is in progress, immediate medical supervision of the EMT-B's care means that:
   a. The medical director must monitor all medical radio communication
   b. The medical director should review only those calls when he or she provides orders
   c. Standing orders before notification of the physician or nurse at the hospital is acceptable
   d. Only a physician is allowed to communicate with the EMT-B via radio for medical orders

6. The medical director of an EMS:
   a. Should frequently ride the ambulance with the working EMT-B
   b. Has no role in the back of an ambulance
   c. Has no role on the scene
   d. Should ONLY monitor calls and be involved with patient care after the patient arrives at the hospital

Answers to these Review Questions can be found at the end of the book on page 865.

5

Well-Being of the EMT

Lesson Goal

The goal of this chapter is to provide information that will help the EMT-Basic take care of himself or herself, provide skills for dealing with death, and identify support systems for dealing with stress.

Scenario

You respond to a call for an accidental injury at a local park. En route, dispatch advises that the caller had no patient information, only that someone was hurt at the playground and an ambulance was needed. As you arrive on the scene, you notice a small crowd gathered in the grassy area around the playground. You and your partner don your body substance isolation (BSI) gear as required by your infection control policy, grab your equipment, and head for the crowd. The bystanders part to let you through, and you observe a teenage male patient supine on the ground with a visibly upset female subject cradling his head in her lap. The patient is clutching his right chest. The female explains that her boyfriend was stabbed by a male with a large knife about 5 minutes ago. You immediately request law enforcement assistance and begin your assessment of the patient. He is conscious and alert with increasing difficulty breathing. He has a 1-inch stab wound to the right anterior chest, mid-clavicular region, just above the nipple. You hear a sucking sound from the wound and immediately cover it with an occlusive dressing and tape it on three sides. As you continue your assessment, the girlfriend lets out a blood-curdling scream. You look up to see the crowd running and a male subject standing about 15 feet away with a boot knife in his right hand. He tells you to "leave him alone and let him die."

 How did you get into this situation? How could it have been avoided? Now that it has happened, how should you proceed to resolve the situation?

Key Terms to Know

Body substance isolation (BSI)
Critical incident
Critical incident stress debriefing (CISD)
Environmental stressors
Hazardous materials
Personal stressors
Psychosocial stressors
Stress

Learning Objectives

As an EMT-Basic, you should be able to do the following:

DOT

- Explain the importance of surveying the scene and determining scene safety.
- Discuss the importance of body substance isolation (BSI).
- List personal protective equipment and considerations necessary for special situations, including:
  - Hazardous materials
  - Crime scenes
  - Rescue operations
  - Exposure to bloodborne pathogens
  - Exposure to airborne pathogens
  - Violent scenes
- Discuss the possible reactions that the patient and family may exhibit when confronted with death and dying.
- List the steps that the emergency medical technician-basic (EMT-B) will take to approach a family confronted with death and dying.
- List the possible reactions that the EMT-B may experience when faced with trauma, illness, death, and dying.
- List the possible reactions that the family of the EMT-B may exhibit because of their indirect involvement with EMS.
- Recognize the signs and symptoms of critical incident stress, and discuss the benefits of debriefing.
- List the steps that the EMT-B should take to prevent, reduce, and alleviate stress.

Of all the helping professions, the emergency medical services (EMS) system is one of the most challenging and fulfilling. Emergency medical technicians (EMTs) begin their careers filled with new knowledge, new skills, and new opportunities. EMTs are special people with special training. They are excited, challenged, and long to discover all that EMS has to offer.

The fast-paced, action-oriented world of EMS heightens the enthusiasm of the new EMT (Figure 5.1). Many new EMTs think that they are invincible, but before long, this sense of invincibility fades as the stresses of EMS begin to take their toll. All EMTs must learn to recognize the signs of stress and know how to alleviate it.

Regardless of the classes attended or hours spent studying, there is nothing that can completely prepare EMTs for what is before them. Few stop to consider the risks and demands that will be placed on them. It is up to all EMTs to heed the instruction, guidance, and direction of those who are training and orienting them. EMTs must appreciate their technical training (Figure 5.2) and the need to prepare for the risky, demanding, and emotionally draining part of their day-to-day work. The EMT must actively choose to be safety conscious, to take precautions, and to maintain a balanced, healthy lifestyle. This chapter should be read carefully. More than any other chapter, this one is written especially for the EMT.

Assess Scene for Hazards

A scene is not safe until the EMT determines it to be safe (Figure 5.3). Although a scene such as the one in the opening scenario initially may appear to be safe, that does not mean that it will continue to be safe. EMTs constantly must be cautious to ensure that the scene remains safe. Several factors must be checked:

- Is the ambulance or rescue vehicle parked in the nearest safe location?
- Does the unit need to be moved because of danger of fire, explosion, or escaping gases?
- Is it safe to approach the patient? If the scene is not safe, make it safe or do not enter. Police officers or fire fighters may be required to secure some scenes (Figure 5.4).
- Does the patient need to be moved immediately because of hazards?
- Is specialized equipment, such as turnout gear or breathing apparatus, needed to approach the patient?

It is important to survey the scene thoroughly. Even in an emergency, with people screaming and calling for help, surveying the scene for safety is an essential step. The lives of the EMT, his or her partner, and the patient may depend on it. For information on completely surveying the scene, see Chapter 12.

> ✓ Do not endanger yourself by rushing into a scene. Think before you act. It is important to understand that the hazards you face may not always be obvious. A butcher knife, a liquor bottle, an ash tray, or even a broom stick are all common household items that could become a weapon. Be aware of your surroundings, stay alert, and be cautious!

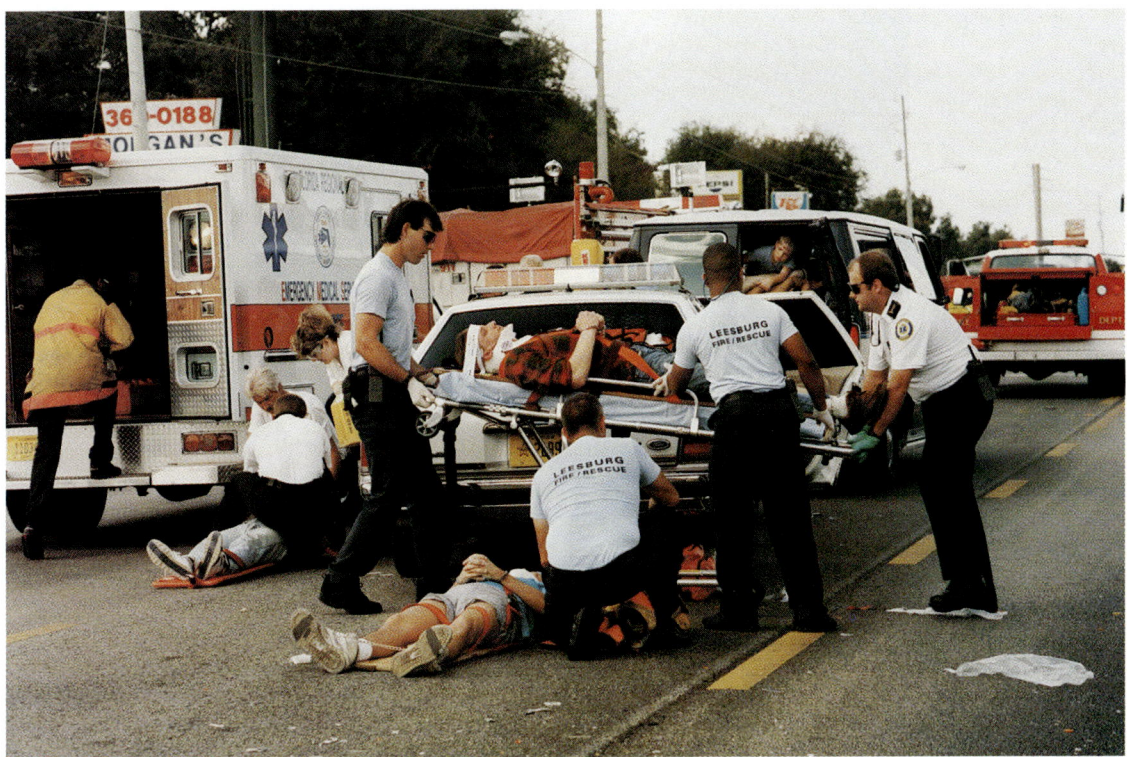

FIGURE 5.1 The EMS world is exciting and fast-paced.

Body Substance Isolation

The Centers for Disease Control and Prevention (CDC) provides guidelines for **body substance isolation (BSI)** based on the most current information and research (Figures 5.5 to 5.9). These guidelines, previously called *universal precautions*, are updated on a regular basis. The term *universal* means that the guidelines are to be followed consistently for all patients everywhere, not just those who raise suspicion. These precautions are especially important in the prehospital care setting because the risk of being exposed to blood is increased and the infection status of the patient is usually unknown. The guidelines are established for the protection of the health care provider and the patient. Chapter 6 discusses the use of BSI in greater detail.

Overview of Special Scenes

The EMT is exposed to many situations that require personal protection, special equipment, and special procedures. An overview is provided for each of the most commonly encountered special scenes. More details are provided throughout the text.

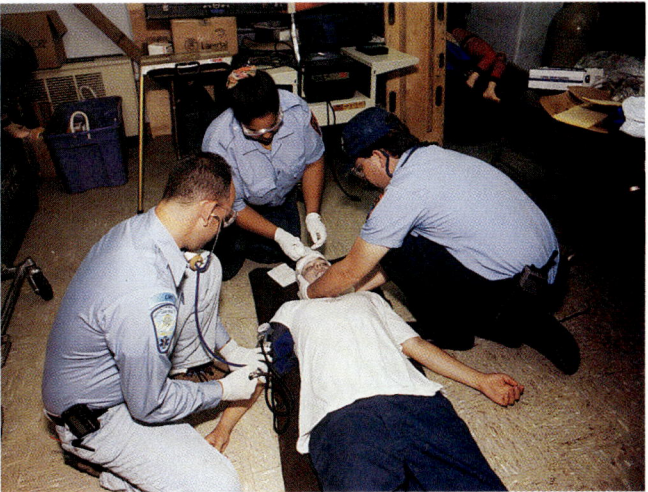

FIGURE 5.2 EMTs practicing simulated scenarios in class.

Hazardous Materials Scene

Hazardous materials (HAZMAT) teams are usually dispatched when dangerous materials require special handling. EMS often arrives at the scene before the HAZMAT team.

- Ambulances should be equipped with binoculars to allow EMTs to view the scene from a distance.

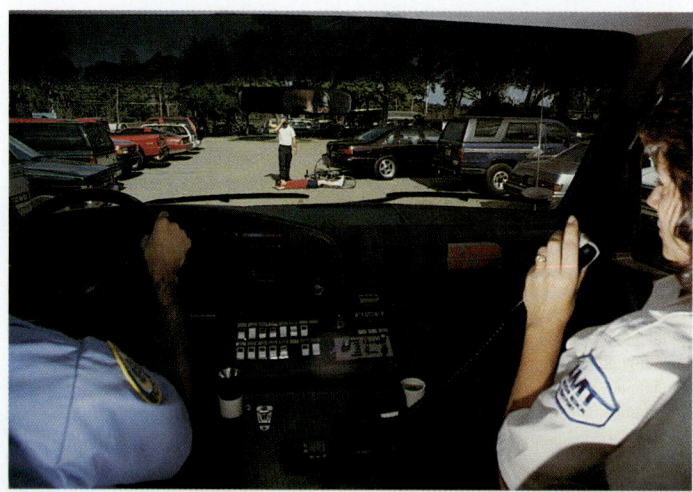

FIGURE 5.3 Survey the scene for hazards, the number of patients, the mechanism of injury, and the need for extrication.

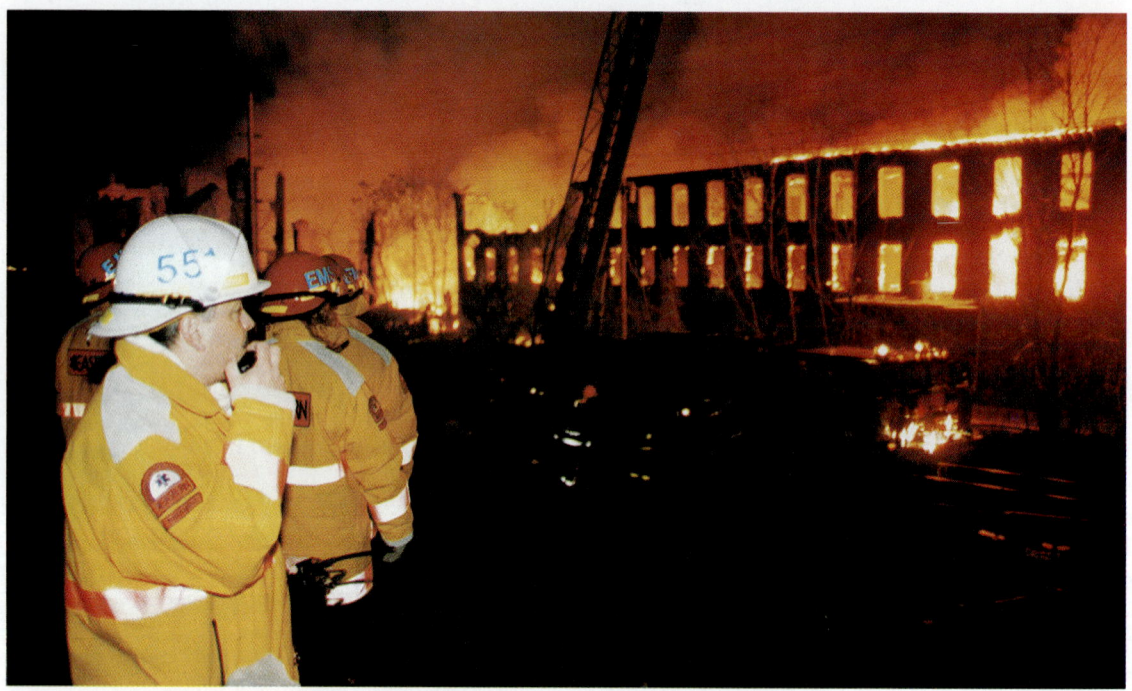

FIGURE 5.4 Do not endanger yourself by rushing into a scene. Think before you act.

- Placards on transport vehicles and containers provide clues and information about the contents (Figure 5.10).
- A copy of the *Emergency Response Guidebook (ERG)*, published by the United States Department of Transportation (DOT), should be available in all emergency service vehicles, including ambulances.[1] A full version of the *ERG2000* is available for download at the DOT website, www.dot.gov, and is updated periodically.

- The EMT should remain a safe distance from the scene. EMTs provide emergency care only after the scene is safe and the patient has been decontaminated. When responding to a known hazardous materials incident or when it is suspected that a hazardous material is involved, the ambulance should be parked at a safe distance *upwind* from the scene as recommended in the *Emergency Response Handbook*.
- Hazardous materials scenes are controlled by special HAZMAT teams. If the EMT has completed specialized HAZMAT training and is going to operate in

---
[1] Transport Canada, U.S. Department of Transportation, Transport and Communications of Mexico: *2000 emergency response guidebook (ERG2000)*, Washington, DC, 2000, DOT.

Well-Being of the EMT | Chapter 5   **57**

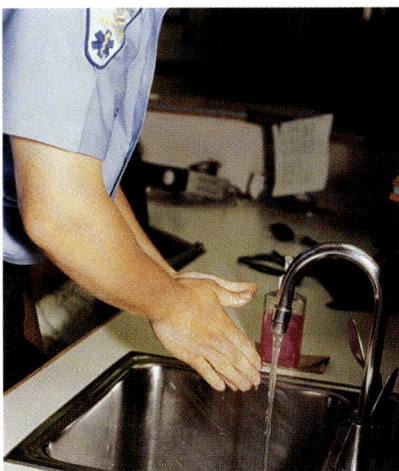

FIGURE 5.5 Handwashing is the most important procedure in preventing the spread of infection.

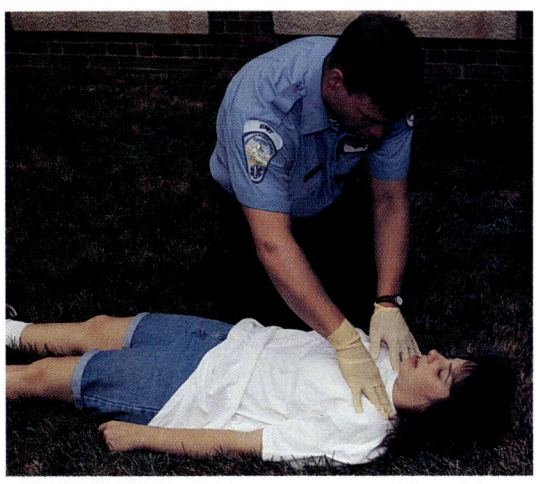

FIGURE 5.7 Gloves should be put on before arriving at the scene and before touching any patient.

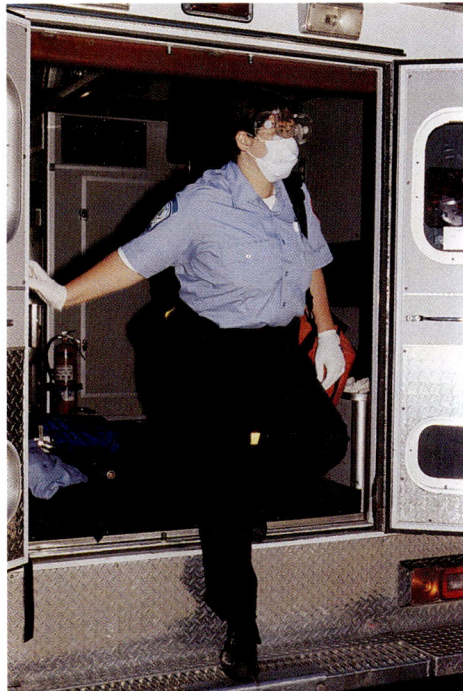

FIGURE 5.6 Personal protective equipment should be worn in situations that are likely to generate drops or sprays of blood or other bodily fluids.

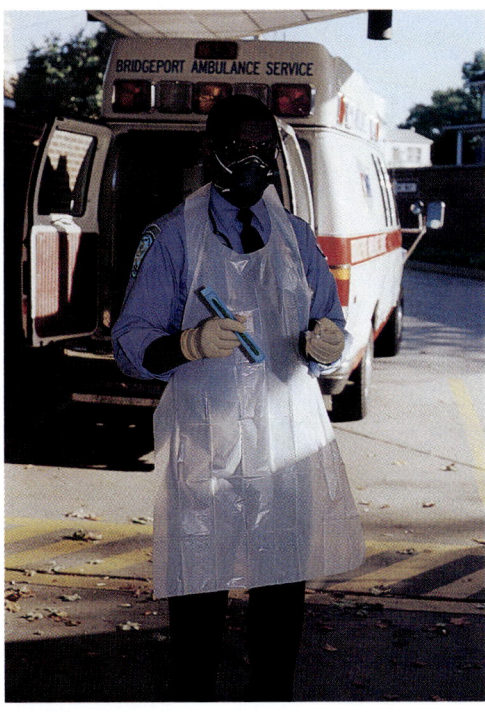

FIGURE 5.8 When you suspect that blood or fluids may be splashed, put on a gown as well as gloves, mask, and eye protection.

close proximity to the hazardous substance, he or she will need to wear protective clothing and respiratory protection up to and including a hazardous materials suit and self-contained breathing apparatus. Specialized training for EMTs is required in some locations.

> ✓ Incidents involving hazardous materials require special training and special equipment to be safely and effectively managed. The EMT should recognize the unique nature of these situations and call for the necessary specialized equipment and personnel to deal with them. Chapter 40 discusses this subject in more detail.

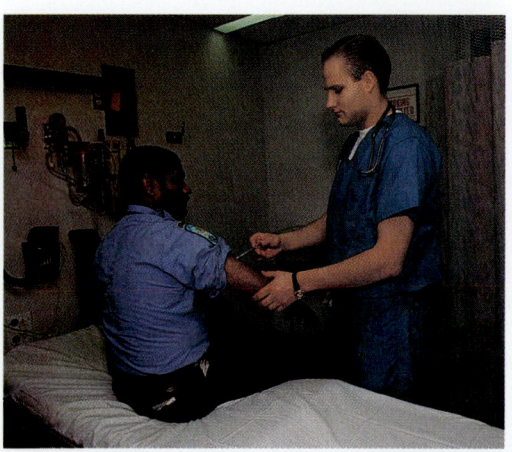

FIGURE 5.9 Immunizations preferably should be completed before the EMT comes in contact with patients.

Rescue Scene

A rescue scene requires additional time, equipment, personnel, and cooperation with other emergency services.

- After ensuring that the scene is safe, the EMT's primary responsibility is providing medical care to the patient.
- EMTs must be alert to potential threats to life such as electricity, fire, explosion, and hazardous materials.
- Protective clothing usually will need to be worn, including turnout gear, puncture-proof gloves, a helmet, and safety glasses or goggles.
- Rescue teams must be requested for extensive or heavy rescue (Figure 5.11).

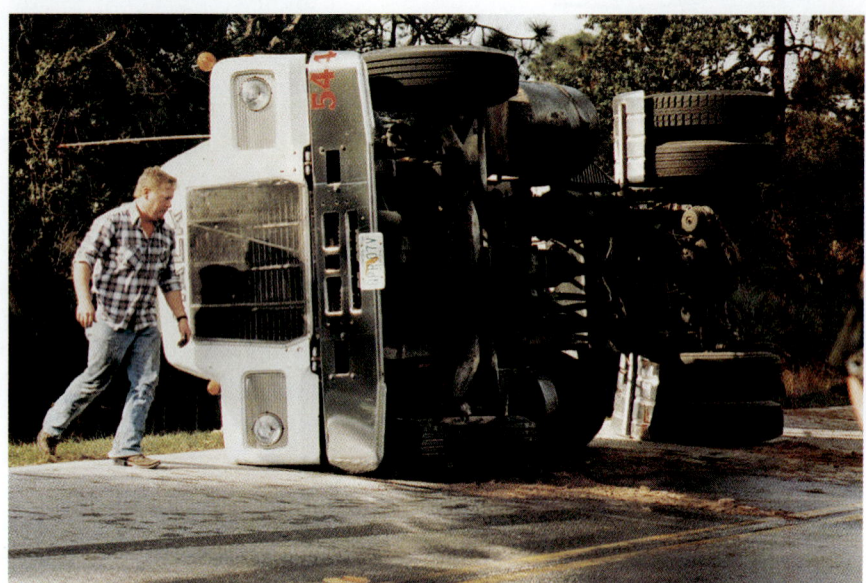

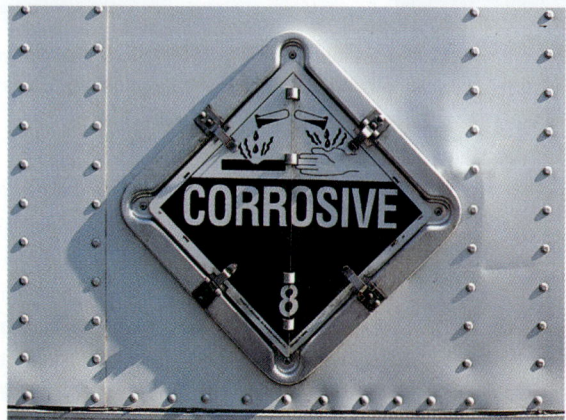

FIGURE 5.10 Look for placards on transportation vehicles and containers that provide clues and information about the contents.

- A number of specialized training programs are available for EMTs to further their understanding and rescue skills.

> ✓ Like hazardous materials incidents, extrication requires special training, experience, and equipment. The EMT should be able to recognize the need for extrication and know where to access the specialized personnel and equipment to complete the rescue.

Violent Scene

EMTs are too frequently faced with violent scenes. The violence may be targeted at the EMTs for "interfering" or may be aimed at others. The EMT should not take any unnecessary chances.

- Violent scenes should always be controlled by law enforcement personnel before the EMT provides patient care (Figure 5.12).
- Most EMTs are not prepared to intervene in violent situations. It is not the EMT's responsibility to provide law enforcement.
- The EMT should be especially cautious if the perpetrator of the crime is still on the scene.
- The EMT should be observant for blood on people's clothing, hidden weapons, and potential weapons.
- The EMT should be alert to bystander or family reactions. Watch for indicators of retaliation and revenge attempts.
- The EMT should never hesitate to request that a police officer ride in the ambulance with the violent patient to the hospital.

> ✓ Scenes in which a violent act has been committed are among the most dangerous that the EMT will face. The EMT should be able to recognize dangerous situations and request assistance from law enforcement personnel when necessary.

Crime Scene

On occasion, EMTs may be called to a scene that is criminal in nature. Whether or not patient care is delivered, the EMTs have an additional responsibility to preserve the crime scene and act as witnesses.

- Many crime scenes are also violent, so the EMT should keep the guidelines pertaining to violent scenes in mind.

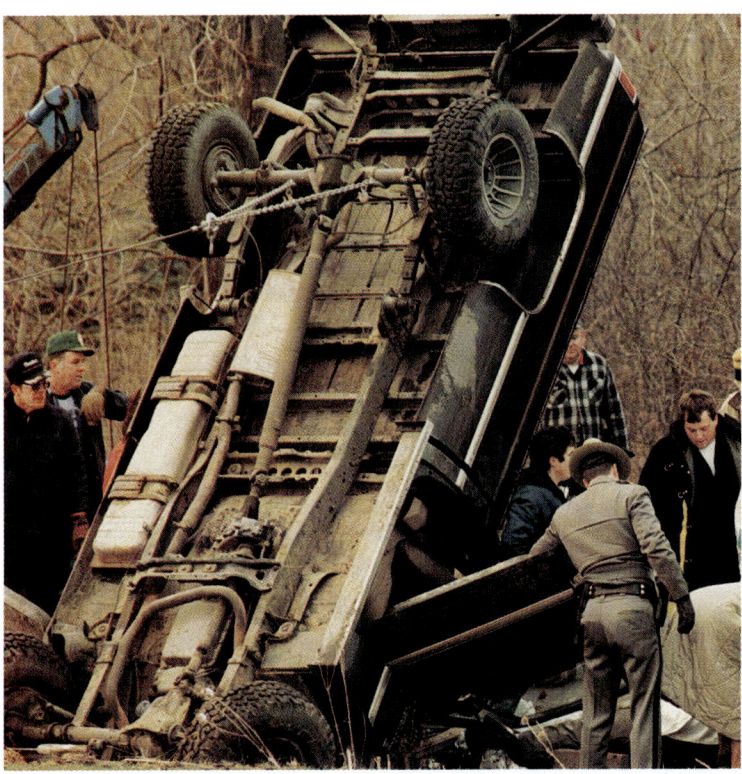

FIGURE 5.11 Special equipment and skills are needed to handle certain incidents.

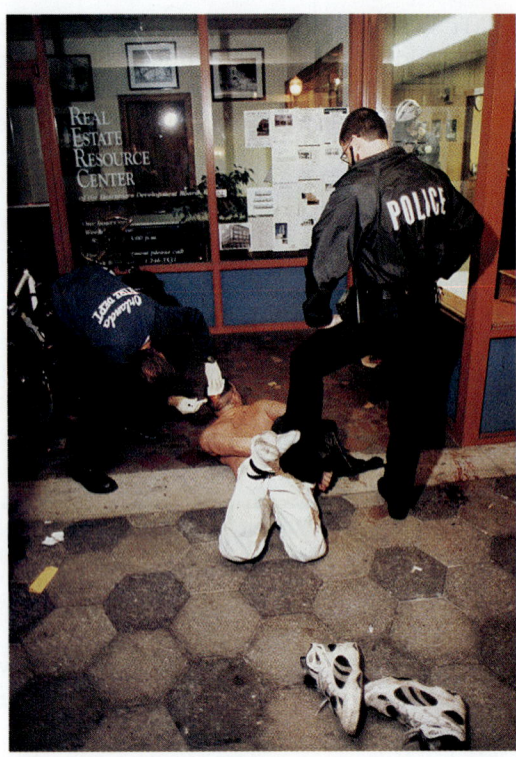

FIGURE 5.12 Violent scenes should always be controlled by law enforcement personnel before the EMT provides patient care.

- The EMT must not disturb the scene unless required for medical care.
- The EMT must take the same path in and out of the scene to avoid disturbing evidence.
- The EMT must not touch anything or remove anything.
- The EMT must save all clothing that is removed during patient care and avoid damaging bullet or knife holes in clothes by cutting through the holes when removing clothing.
- The EMT must assist the police officer when a statement is requested or if called as a witness for court. Professional courtesy prevails, as does the EMT's responsibility to society.

✓ Although the EMT's primary responsibility is patient care, he or she should do everything possible to preserve a crime scene and avoid disturbing or removing evidence unless it is absolutely necessary. If something must be moved, a mental note should be made of its original location and law enforcement should be informed of the item being moved and the original location.

Death and Dying

The scene of a sudden death or of a dying patient is almost always an emotionally charged setting. If the patient was ill or died because of a medical cause, death may or may not have been expected. Death resulting from injury and trauma to the body is never expected.

Terminally ill people go through stages in thinking about what is happening to them. These stages have been described by Dr. Elisabeth Kübler-Ross in her book *On Death and Dying*[2] (Figure 5.13):

- *Denial*: "Not me!" A mental defense mechanism creates a buffer between the reality of the present condition of those who are dying and the reality that they are actually dying from that condition.
- *Anger*: "Why me?" Anger is expressed because they do not feel that they deserve to die now.
- *Bargaining*: "OK, but first let me . . ." People who are dying may bargain with God, themselves, their family, or the medical professionals around them to let them do something in particular before dying. They may have a strong sense that they need to see someone, do something, or take care of important arrangements before their death.
- *Depression*: "OK, but I haven't . . ." People who are dying are filled with self-pity, regrets, and a lack of fulfillment at thoughts of their life ending. They usually become silent and retreat into their own world of sadness and despair.
- *Acceptance*: "OK, I'm not afraid." Dying patients eventually accept that their death is inevitable. It does not mean that they are happy or have completely resolved the matter of dying, but at this stage they are able to accept it.

Some patients experience these marked stages, whereas others do not experience the stages in a clear-cut manner. Some patients go through these stages slowly, whereas others progress relatively quickly. Some patients experience more than one stage at the same time or return to previous stages. The EMT should not expect to see a pattern repeated in all dying patients. Much depends on the person, the circumstances, and the time frame involved. In emergency response situations, EMTs often witness a mixture of stages, responses, and emotions.

Family and close friends at the scene may also respond in a range of ways and emotions. They are almost always anxious. This anxiousness may escalate to complete panic and loss of personal control. They may express anger at themselves out of guilt, or they may lash out at others, such as EMTs. They may be demanding of the

---
[2] Kübler-Ross E: *On death and dying*, New York, 1997, Simon & Schuster.

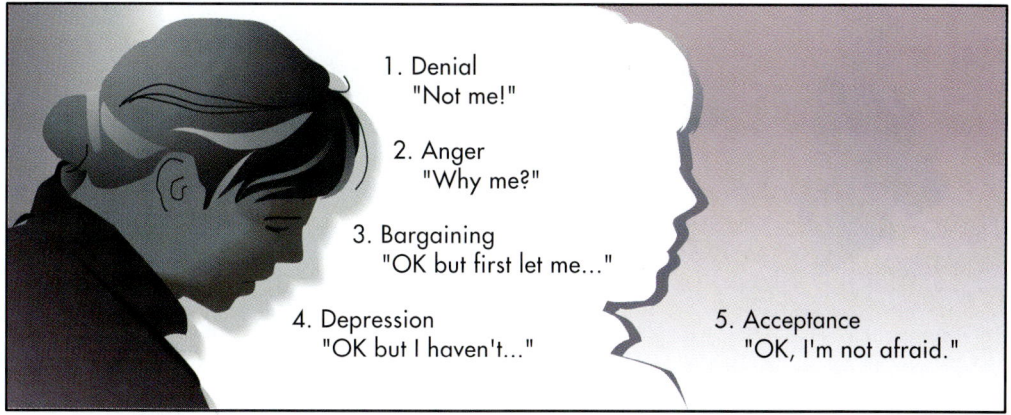

FIGURE 5.13 Stages of the grief process.

EMTs and say things like, "Just hurry and get him to the hospital." Family members may cry uncontrollably and experience dizziness, vomiting, or fainting. Others may want to help so much that they grab onto the EMTs, move equipment, or get in the way. Still others become silent and withdrawn, perhaps even leaving the room or scene.

> ✓ The phases of death and dying are experienced by patients and their families. The EMT may be faced with a patient or family member in any of these stages. Recognition of the normal psychologic process that is at work will help the EMT deal with the situation.

Dealing with the Dying Patient and Family Members

The EMT must remain calm, professional, and in control when other people and circumstances are out of control (Figure 5.14).

- EMTs must identify themselves and clearly communicate what they are doing and where they are transporting the patient.
- EMTs should allow family members, unless they are young children, to remain with their loved ones if they insist. Otherwise, they should be encouraged to provide information to another EMT in another room and should be kept informed about what is happening.
- Local protocols will determine if family is allowed to ride in the ambulance, and if so, whether in the patient compartment or up front with the driver. Quick arrangements may be made for relatives to ride to the hospital with other emergency personnel, such as a police officer. If family members are going alone to

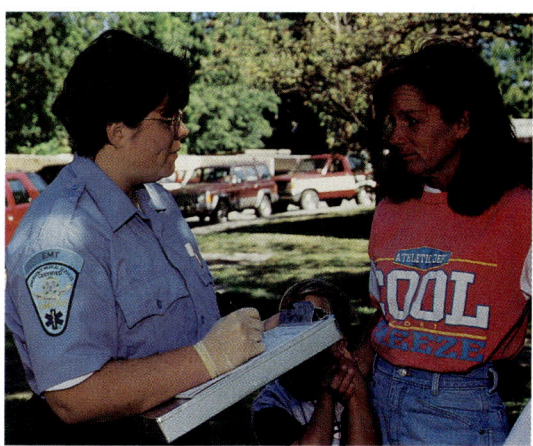

FIGURE 5.14 The EMT must remain calm, professional, and in control when other people and circumstances are out of control.

the hospital, encourage them to have a friend or neighbor drive or to call a taxi.
- If the patient is alone, the patient should be assured that his or her family will be located and notified. Notification is usually done by hospital staff. The EMT should provide reassurance and pass on information about relatives to the hospital personnel.
- EMTs should avoid negative or confidential statements about the patient's condition. These comments could easily be overheard by the patient, family members, or bystanders. The patient may hear the EMT, even if he or she appears to be unresponsive. Hearing is the last sense to be lost.
- EMTs should be honest with the patient and the family. The facts should be stated using a gentle tone of voice and a reassuring touch, if appropriate.
- The patient and family should not be falsely reassured, but they can be given some hope. The EMT should let the patient know that everything that can be done to help will be done.

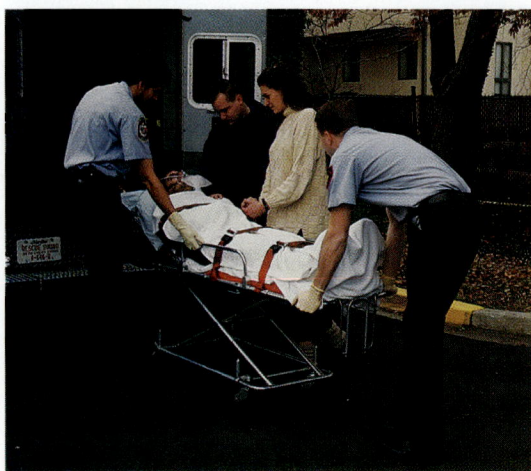

FIGURE 5.15 If family arrives at the scene before the patient dies, arrange for them to see the patient. If immediate transportation is required, allow them to say a quick goodbye.

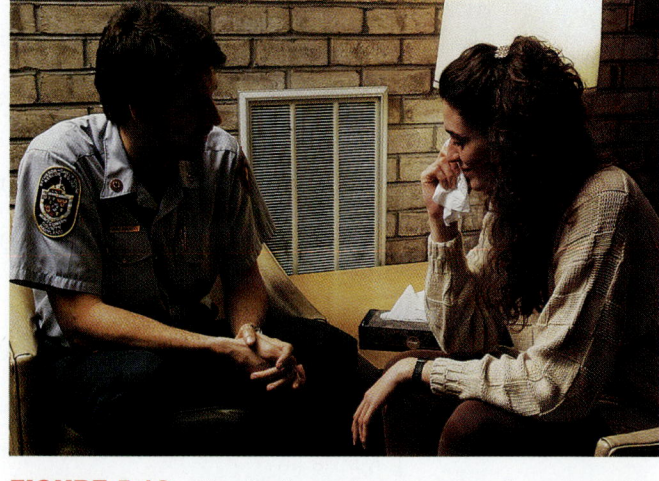

FIGURE 5.16 Allow family members to express themselves without judgment.

- Privacy should be ensured for the patient from onlookers and bystanders.
- EMTs should offer comfort and help to family members. The first priority is the dying patient. Family members, however, also may be injured or in emotional shock from witnessing their loved one's injury or illness.
- If other family members are involved and are seriously injured, they should be protected temporarily from the reality of a dying or dead loved one. If they themselves are unstable, knowledge of the other person's death may deprive them of their will to survive. The EMT should not volunteer information unless asked, and the circumstances should be weighed carefully before providing an answer.
- Those close to the patient may express anger or rage. Their anger or insults should not be taken personally. The EMT should be tolerant and should not be defensive or retaliate. The EMT should try to understand their feelings and communicate that he or she will do everything possible to help them and their loved one.
- If family arrives at the scene before the patient dies, arrangements should be made for them to see the patient. If immediate transportation is required, they should be allowed to say a quick good-bye. It is important to allow them to express their love, address unfinished business, or say good-bye as their needs dictate. The EMT should explain that the patient may still be able to hear and understand even though he or she appears unresponsive (Figure 5.15).
- The patient should be treated with dignity and respect, especially as death is near. Families will watch closely to see how their dying relative is treated. The EMT should be gentle and aware of how his or her attitudes and actions may be perceived at the time and later during their grieving process. The greatest possible respect should be shown. The EMT should talk to the patient, touch him or her as if they were responsive, and explain what is going to be done before any movement or change is initiated.
- The EMT should listen closely and empathetically and allow family members to express themselves without judgement. The EMT should let them know that it is all right to react to how they feel. Everyone's grief response is different.
- The EMT should help the family in any way possible. They may want an item of special meaning from another room or simply may ask for a tissue. They may want to be held or to pray. They may want the EMT to just stay with them and remain silent (Figure 5.16).
- Some people want to touch or hold the body after death. This request should not be denied unless it is a crime scene or it compromises the EMT's care and local protocol.
- If possible, the EMT should stay with the body and family until police, the medical examiner, or the coroner arrives. Local protocol should be followed.

Remember that the physical care given to the dying patient by the EMT must be equaled by the emotional care and support that is provided to the patient and the family.

> ✓ The EMT is not only responsible for care of the patient. In almost every situation, the EMT will be faced with family members or other individuals who are close to the patient. These people also need careful attention and treatment.

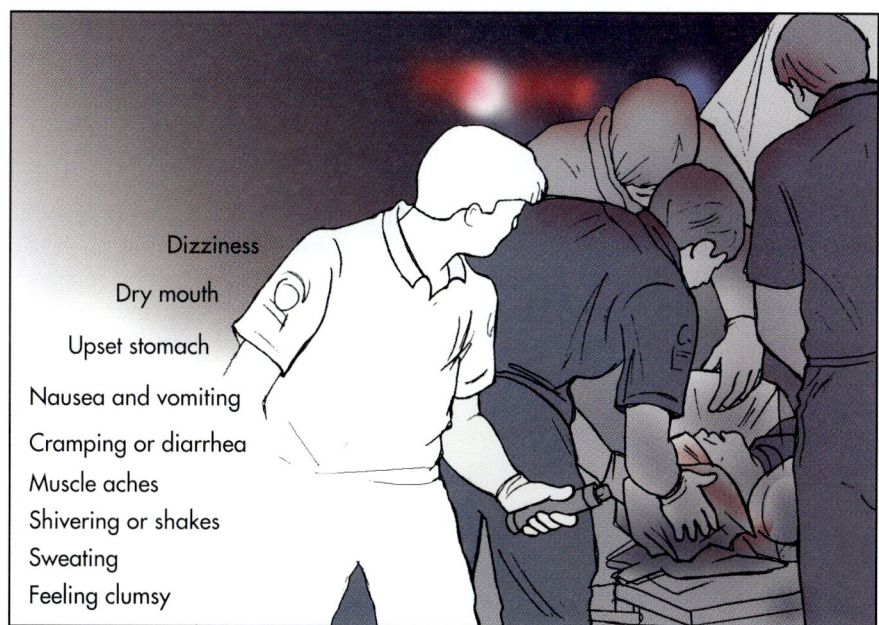

FIGURE 5.17 Signs and symptoms that an EMT may experience while responding to an emergency call or while on a scene.

EMT's Reaction to Emergencies

EMTs regularly face serious illness, traumatic injury, dying patients, and death. Once the alarm sounds or the call is dispatched, all attention is focused on the emergency response. It is not uncommon for EMTs en route to a scene to notice themselves shaking or shivering. Once at the scene, most emergency care providers function on automatic control as they rely on their technical training.

Emergency response causes a number of physical and emotional effects on EMTs. They should be aware of their own response to situations rather than forcing thoughts out of their mind or denying the feelings within them.

Physiologic Response

When EMTs are responding to an emergency or are faced with a stressful scene, information is relayed to the brain through their senses. What do they see, hear, smell, or touch on arrival? All of the gathered information is processed by the outer layer, or cortex, of the brain. The cortex interprets the significance of the information based on memories from past circumstances and logic. If the cortex and sympathetic nervous system determine that a challenge must be met, a situation must be overcome, or a threat exists, a physiologic reaction occurs. Physiologic reaction simply means that the normally functioning human body will respond in a physical way. Epinephrine (adrenaline) and other chemicals are released to prepare the body to deal with the situation. Respirations, heart rate, and blood pressure increase. Muscles tighten, pupils dilate, and glucose is released into the blood for immediate energy.

The type of response described in the previous paragraph is often referred to as *fight or flight*. The body and mind are hyperalert and ready to fight or run away. This response is normal and healthy. It allows for self-protection and self-defense, accomplishment of more than usual, or quick retreat from a situation that may be life threatening.

One of the most difficult factors for an EMT to deal with is the element of surprise. It is more difficult to respond quickly and appropriately after arriving at a scene that is surprising. The fight-or-flight response is almost guaranteed to start. The EMT should try to find out all that he or she can while en route. Gathering information before arrival at the scene allows for mental preparation, and the EMT will less likely be caught off guard. Back-up crews should be warned if they are about to face an unpleasant scene, such as badly mutilated bodies. EMTs can more readily and easily deal with something with which they are mentally prepared.

While responding to an emergency or on the scene, an EMT may experience some of the following signs and symptoms of the normal response to a stressful situation (Figure 5.17):

- Upset stomach
- Dry mouth
- Nausea and vomiting
- Pounding heart
- Shivering or shakes
- Sweating

- Feeling clumsy
- Stomach cramping
- Diarrhea
- Muscle aches
- Dizziness

The EMT should acknowledge that his or her body and mind are reacting to the stressful situation. New EMTs may be faced with scenes that they could never have imagined. They have no frame of reference or experience to reassure them about what they are seeing, hearing, smelling, and touching. New EMTs can expect a range of physical reactions to stressful situations.

> ✓ In addition to the psychologic reaction to EMS work, the EMT will experience a physical response to the stresses and pressures of this occupation. Understanding this physical reaction is the first step in the process of managing the response.

Disciplining the EMT's Reaction

After the EMT acknowledges that his or her body and mind are reacting normally to the circumstances, he or she should take a few slow, deep breaths. The EMT has been trained to respond to emergency situations and is there to help others. The EMT's mind should be focused on what he or she should be "doing," and "thoughts and feelings" should be considered after the call. The EMT should remember that he or she has at least one partner and possibly others on the scene to assist.

Tips from the Pros

Most EMTs are very curious, wanting to see all that they can see and know all that there is to know at a scene. There are, however, times when this drive can be a personal disadvantage. At the scene of a particularly gruesome event, such as some kinds of suicides or homicides, stop yourself. You should be observant in the event that you later are called as a witness, but even though you are drawn to focus on the facial expression or eyes of the deceased or some other detail, stop yourself. It does no good to memorize and implant these visual images in your mind.

Working as an EMT exposes you to significant suffering and pain. Focus on caring and helping people, not on compiling an inventory of memories of their pain and suffering. It will only keep you from sleeping at night.

EMTs who are feeling extremely shaky, upset, or physically ill should let their partner know so they can help the affected EMT through the situation. If after taking all these steps the EMT finds his or her reactions interfering with patient care, the EMT should inform his or her partner and return to the ambulance. Although exiting the scene is the least ideal way of coping, it is better than vomiting or fainting at the scene. Back-up can be called or other emergency responders on site can assist the affected EMT's partner. If the inability to deal with emergency scenes happens repeatedly, the EMT will need to seek counseling.

For most new EMTs, this extreme reaction never happens. They will go through a process of recognizing how they react to calls and situations. As time goes by, their comfort zone increases. They are able to gain experience and refer to past outcomes. EMTs should never strive to become "hardened." EMTs who brag, "I've seen it all, and nothing bothers me," are not being honest or fair to themselves or those around them.

Healthy and well-adjusted EMTs acknowledge that facing human suffering is an unpleasant and potentially stressful part of their job. They recognize that some calls stimulate thoughts and feelings within them. They do not deny or suppress those thoughts and feelings but consider them after the call. They know that they are free to discuss the call with their partner or peers. They know that opportunities are available to further deal with things that really bother them.

> ✓ The EMT must learn to deal with the emotions and physical reactions that are prompted by certain situations. Very often, physical and emotional reactions must be controlled so that patient care can be continued.

EMT'S Family and Friends

EMTs work long hours and rotate shifts. They are exposed to danger and are required to take certain risks. EMTs face a greater chance of being injured or killed at work than many other professions. EMTs may have carefully weighed the risks involved with their work and have come to terms with what the risks mean to them, but have their family and friends done the same? Significant strain can be placed on the EMT whose spouse, significant other, or family does not understand or accept what he or she does.

If the family and friends of the EMT are willing to listen, the EMT should share thoughts and feelings with them (Figure 5.18). The worst thing an EMT can do is isolate work from personal life, thinking that no one outside of EMS can understand. The family and friends are a valuable resource. It may be true that they cannot understand completely, but they do need to know when the EMT is upset or stressed by things at work. The EMT can tell them about calls or situations without breaking patient confidentiality, and they also need to know why the EMT finds the work challenging and fulfilling. If they understand that the EMT is happy in his or her work, they will be more understanding of the inconvenience that is caused. They may be less likely to complain about shifts or being on call and how that interferes with plans and activities.

The EMT should be cautious that he or she does not give the impression of "living for being an EMT." It is true that EMS is exciting and rewarding. It is also true that most EMTs are very dedicated, action-oriented individuals who have a tendency to become obsessed with doing a good job and continually improving. However, personal and professional lives must be balanced. It is no wonder that family members get upset at the EMT who stops by the ambulance base regularly on their time off to "see what's happening" rather than spending time with them.

For some EMTs, their work becomes the most important thing in life. Some EMTs "can't get enough," so they join volunteer emergency response units in addition to their regular duties. Other aspects of their life begin to suffer, such as family, friends, hobbies, interests, parenting, home responsibilities, and their health. The result is that these EMTs may end up alone, without family or friends to support them. These EMTs may realize too late that they should have devoted more time and energy to their relationships and friendships.

If work is overwhelming personal and family life, some adjustments should be considered:

- Trading shifts or duty time with other EMTs to accommodate special times or events with family and friends
- Requesting a rotation, location, or duty assignment in an area that is not as busy
- Choosing or requesting shifts that better coincide with the schedule of family and friends
- Requesting shift hours and rotations that allow for more time to relax with family and friends

Fortunately, most EMS systems today are aware of the importance of an EMT's support system. Programs and seminars are available that address emergency services personnel and their families. Topics include the personality profiles of emergency personnel, orientation to EMS stress, communication, the family as a support system, problem solving, and building strong relationships.

EMTs who have long and fulfilling careers in EMS realize that a life exists beyond their work. They understand the importance of their family, friends, and other interests. A balanced personal and professional life offers them support, security, and safety.

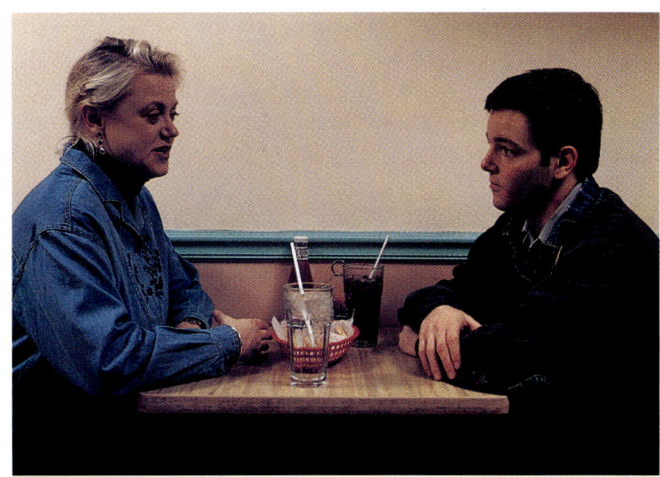

FIGURE 5.18 If your family and friends are willing to listen, make certain to share your thoughts and feelings with them. Your family and friends are part of your support system.

> ✓ EMS can easily consume those individuals who commit to a career in it. It is essential that an EMT have a balanced life, both inside and outside of EMS, to maintain his or her mental and physical health.

Understanding Stress

Stress is an internal response to external factors. The word *stress* comes from a Latin term meaning 'strain, pressure, or force.' Originally, stress described a mechanical force that was placed on an object. Gradually, stress has come to mean emotional strains that are placed on individuals because of work, family responsibilities, or lifestyle changes.

In general terms, an EMT experiences the following:

- A physical or psychologic response to demands placed on them
- A response to a perceived change, challenge, or threat

Stress is a common occurrence. Some stress is helpful and necessary to motivate and satisfy. Positive or beneficial stress is usually referred to as *eustress*. Stress that gets out of control or has negative aspects is usually referred to as *distress*. Stress is often grouped into three main categories or causes:

1. Environmental
2. Personal
3. Psychosocial

Environmental Stressors

The EMT experiences numerous **environmental stressors** on a regular basis. The following are examples of environmental stressors:

- Demanding physical labor
- Lights, sirens, alarms, and noise
- Weather conditions and temperature extremes
- Angry, impatient bystanders and family
- Emergency driving and response (Figure 5.19)
- Sharing quarters with other EMTs
- Long hours and shifts
- Overwork from high call volume

Personal Stressors

EMTs often place stress on themselves. **Personal stressors** form from the way a person thinks and feels. This type of stress is usually influenced by experiences and memories. The following are examples of personal stressors:

- Anxiety about being responsible for a person's life
- Making life-and-death decisions
- Fear of making a serious error
- Dealing with dying patients and grieving family members
- Anxiety about being competent as an EMT or about passing local, state, and national EMT examinations
- Guilt or anger about mistakes or criticism

Psychosocial Stressors

Psychosocial stressors are initiated by contact with other people. EMTs interact with many people each day in their personal and professional lives, and therefore the risk of encountering psychosocial stressors is high. The following are examples of psychosocial stressors:

- Agitated and combative patients
- Abusive parents of a young patient
- Patients under the influence of alcohol or drugs
- Patients from a violent domestic situation
- Death of a child or infant
- Hospital staff who do not listen to or respect the EMT (Figure 5.20)
- Conflicts with supervisors, dispatchers, or medical directors
- Incompatibility with a partner

Chronic or Cumulative Stress

A common misconception among EMS personnel is that a stressful response or distress is always caused by a significant event. Major calls involving disaster, destruction, and multiple deaths often evoke distress in EMS personnel. However, a significant toll is taken on the EMT emotionally, mentally, and physically because of frequent ongoing stressors such as those just listed. This type of stress is referred to as *chronic stress* or *cumulative stress*.

Chronic stress can become overwhelming if ignored. Unchecked chronic stress is also a set-up for "the straw that

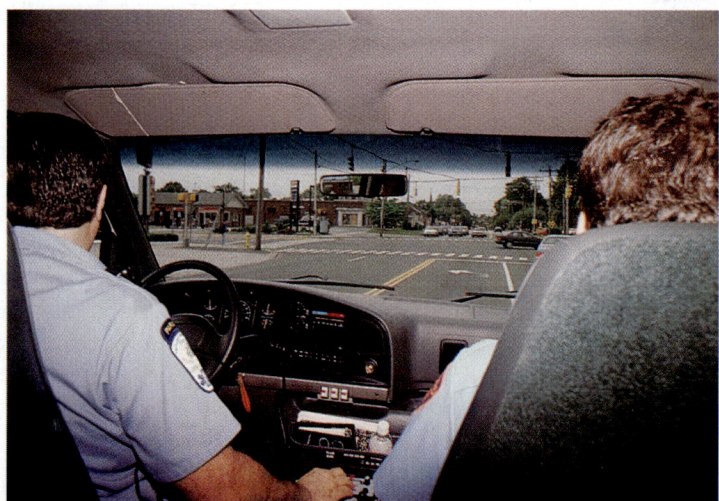

FIGURE 5.19 An EMT regularly experiences numerous environmental stressors.

broke the camel's back" syndrome. An EMT experiencing chronic stress does not have the energy reserve to cope with a significant or even moderately stressful single event.

Acute Stress

Significantly difficult calls or critical incidents may cause an acute stress reaction. EMTs may be overpowered or overwhelmed by an emergency call, scene, or situation in which they are placed. The following are examples of circumstances that may cause an acute reaction:

- Responding to a serious illness or injury and the patient is known to the EMT
- Serious injury or death of a coworker
- Disaster or mass casualty situation
- Threat or attack on the EMT's life
- Involvement in a fatal collision while responding to another emergency call
- Witnessing child abuse or homicide
- Facing a scene with multiple mutilated bodies
- Infant or child trauma or amputation
- Infant, child, elder, or spousal abuse

A **critical incident** is any event or circumstance that overwhelms the EMT's usual coping skills. Some critical incidents affect only one EMT, whereas others are of such magnitude that they affect everyone at the scene.

Posttraumatic Stress Disorder

Some EMTs suppress their emotions and refuse to talk about them or participate in debriefing after a critical incident or traumatic event. This kind of unnatural and unhealthy suppression of emotions and thoughts may lead to posttraumatic stress disorder (PTSD).

PTSD is a serious condition involving illness, personality changes, and self-destructive behavior. Unfortunately, some EMTs have taken their own lives in suicide. PTSD should not be ignored. PTSD interferes with every aspect of an EMT's life, including relationships, work, rest, sleep, and most importantly, the EMT's health. PTSD cannot be self-diagnosed or diagnosed by a peer. PTSD is a diagnosis made only by psychiatrists and psychologists. However, EMTs should recognize the characteristics of PTSD:

1. The EMT has been exposed to a critical incident or disturbing event.
2. The EMT avoids and blocks thinking about, talking about, or being reminded about the incident.
3. Despite these attempts at avoidance, the EMT re-lives the incident in his or her thoughts, dreams, or real life.
4. Signs and symptoms of emotional, behavioral, mental, or physical change are noted that were not present before the incident.
5. The signs and symptoms of dramatic change last longer than 1 month.

Warning Signals of Stress

Various degrees of distress affect people differently. The four categories for noting change include physical, emotional, behavioral, and cognitive. *Cognitive* refers to thoughts or thinking capacity. Although one may experience one or more of these signals for various reasons, it is important to understand that a stress reaction may be occurring. For example, chills, upset stomach, and diarrhea are signs and symptoms of the flu, but they may also be indicative of stress.

Although there are infinite examples and combinations of change that stem from distress, Tables 5.1 and 5.2 provide a summary of examples. The EMT should learn to watch for and recognize indicators of stress in himself or herself and in others.

Burnout

A catch phrase during the 1980s and early 1990s was, "He or she is burned out." *Burnout* is roughly defined as the

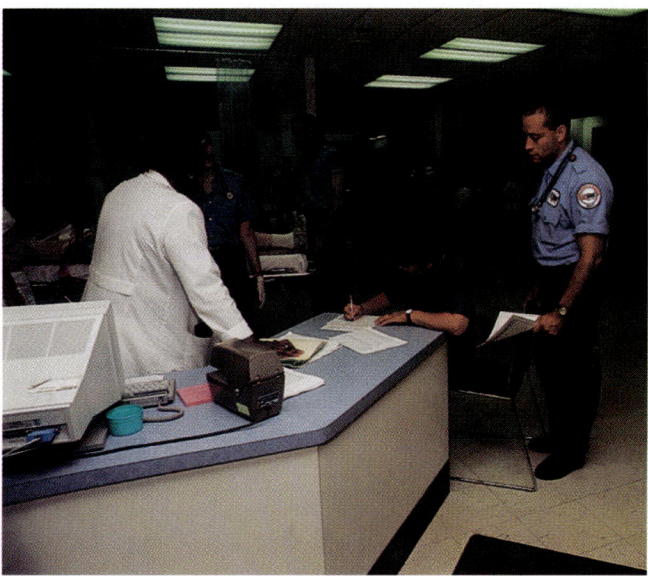

FIGURE 5.20 Psychosocial stressors are initiated by contact with other people.

TABLE 5.1 Distress Signals Requiring Immediate Corrective Action

Physical*	Cognitive	Emotional	Behavioral
Chest pain	Decreased alertness to surroundings	Panic reactions	Significant change in speech patterns
Difficulty breathing	Difficulty making decisions	Signs and symptoms of shock	Excessively angry outbursts
Excessive blood pressure	Hyperalertness	Phobic reaction	Crying spells
Collapse from exhaustion	Generalized mental confusion	General loss of control	Antisocial acts (e.g., violence)
Cardiac arrhythmias	Disorientation to person, place, time	Inappropriate emotions	Extreme hyperactivity
	Serious disruption in thinking	Wishing to die	Irritability to coworkers, family members, and friends
Excessive dehydration	Seriously slowed thinking		
Dizziness	Problems in naming familiar items		
Excessive vomiting	Problems recognizing familiar people		
Blood in stool	Difficulty sleeping/nightmares		

*These indicate a need for medical evaluation.

TABLE 5.2 Common Signs and Symptoms of Distress Not Requiring Immediate Action

Physical	Cognitive	Emotional	Behavioral
Nausea	Confusion	Anticipatory anxiety	Change in activity
Upset stomach	Lowered attention span	Denial	Withdrawal
Tremors (lips, hands)	Calculation difficulties	Fear	Suspicion
Feeling uncoordinated	Memory problems	Survivor guilt	Change in communications
Profuse sweating	Poor concentration	Uncertainty of feelings	Change in interactions with others
Chills	Seeing an event over and over	Depression	Increased or decreased food intake
Diarrhea	Distressing dreams	Grief	Increased smoking
Rapid heart rate	Disruption in logical thinking	Feeling hopeless	Overly vigilant to environment
Muscle aches	Blaming someone	Feeling overwhelmed	Excessive humor
Sleep disturbance	Inability to concentrate	Feeling lost	Excessive silence
Dry mouth		Feeling abandoned	Unusual behavior
Shakes		Worried	
Vision problems		Wishing to hide	
Fatigue		Anger	
Loss of appetite		Feeling numb	
		Identifying with victim	

build-up of distress until the individual is no longer productive. Burnout is almost always used with negative meaning, sometimes as an excuse for taking sick time, but it might be a symptom of a deeper dissatisfaction. For instance, an EMT who is burned out might be expressing dissatisfaction with the way his or her career has turned out. The reason for this career dissatisfaction is often because the EMT ignores his or her own needs while caring for others. Burnout is a process that can often be traced to a lack of self-care.

Critical Incident Stress Debriefing

As discussed previously, a critical incident is any event or situation that overwhelms the EMT's usual coping skills.

In recent years, a process known as **critical incident stress debriefing** (CISD) has been introduced to EMS with great success. Dr. Jeff Mitchell, author and advocate of CISD, is paraphrased as saying the following:

> Defusing and debriefings can be powerful processes that prevent serious stress reactions from becoming extremely damaging to emergency personnel. They have frequently accelerated the recovery process. If they are overused for routine events, defusing and debriefing can be diluted and their power substantially reduced. They should be reserved for events that have extraordinary power to negatively affect emergency personnel.

The process of CISD involves a team approach, including mental health professionals and peer support personnel from police, fire, EMS disaster management, and other emergency-oriented organizations. Clergy may also be asked to be on the team. Four or five team members hold a debriefing led by a mental health professional. Interagency and interjurisdictional cooperation is encouraged (Figure 5.21). A formal CISD should be conducted between 24 to 72 hours after a major incident.

Criteria for considering and holding a CISD are as follows:

- Many individuals within a group appear to be distressed after a call.
- The signals of distress appear to be severe.
- Personnel demonstrate numerous behavioral changes.
- Personnel make significant errors on calls occurring after the critical incident.
- Personnel request help.
- The event is extraordinary.
- Various agencies are showing the same reactions.
- Signals of distress continue beyond 3 weeks.

The CISD process is confidential and is not an investigation or an interrogation. It is designed to open discussions about feelings, fears, and reactions to the incident. The CISD leaders and mental health personnel evaluate the information, provide feedback, and offer suggestions about overcoming the stress.

CISD accelerates the normal recovery process of emergency personnel after the experience of a critical incident. The process works well because thoughts and feelings are vented quickly and the environment is supportive and nonthreatening.

A comprehensive system for managing critical incident stress includes the following:

1. Preincident stress education
2. On-scene peer support

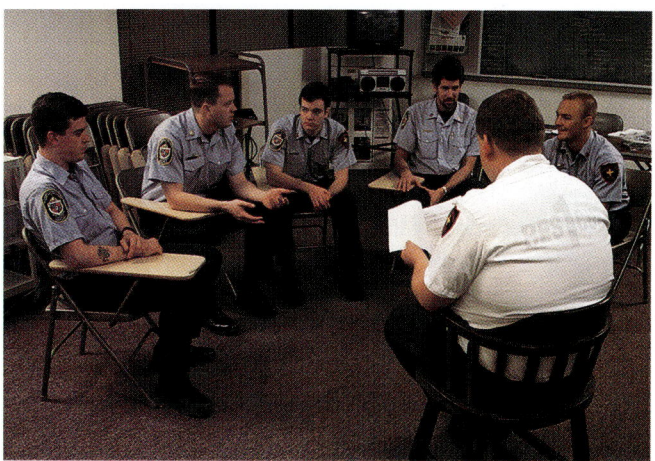

FIGURE 5.21 The process of critical incident stress debriefing involves a team approach.

3. One-on-one support
4. Disaster support services
5. Defusing
6. Critical incident stress debriefings
7. Follow-up services
8. Spouse and family support
9. Communication outreach programs
10. Other health and welfare programs, such as wellness programs

Stopping Stress from Becoming Distress

It is possible to prevent, reduce, and alleviate stress that leads to distress. Managing the stress level of one's profession is 100% his or her responsibility. Some of the following 12 suggestions are general and could apply to almost anyone, whereas others are targeted specifically for the EMT.

1. Balance life, including work, recreation, family, friends, etc.
2. Recognize that personality includes physical, mental, emotional, and spiritual needs. Self-care is important in each of these areas
3. Maintain a positive attitude at all times
4. Maintain a healthy diet. Diet can compromise performance, stamina, and the ability to manage stress. A poor diet can cause stress to increase and health to decline, putting EMTs and their patients at risk. The following dietary guidelines are edited from *Emergency Services Stress* by Jeff Mitchell, PhD, and Grady Bray, PhD.[3]

---

[3] Mitchell JT, Bray GP: *Emergency services stress: guidelines for preserving the health and careers of emergency services personnel,* Englewood Cliffs, 1990, Prentice-Hall.

> **Attitudes**
>
> *by Charles R. Swindoll*
>
> Words can never adequately convey the incredible impact of our attitude toward life. The longer I live the more convinced I become that life is 10 percent what happens to us and 90 percent how we respond to it.
>
> I believe the single most significant decision I can make on a day-to-day basis is my choice of attitude. It is more important than my past, my education, my bankroll, my successes or failures, fame or pain, what other people think of me or say about me, my circumstances, or my position. Attitude keeps me going or cripples my progress. It alone fuels my fire or assaults my hope. When my attitudes are right, there's no barrier too high, no valley too deep, no dream too extreme, no challenge too great for me.
>
> From Swindoll CR: *Strengthening your grip*, Dallas, 1982, Word Inc. Used by permission of Insight for Living.

> **Dietary Guidelines for Emergency Personnel**
>
> - Avoid sugar, salt, white bread, alcohol, and caffeine as much as possible.
> - Increase the consumption of complex carbohydrates, such as whole grain breads, granola, and bran, so that the total calories from carbohydrates in the diet is closer to 48% than its current average of 28%.
> - Dramatically reduce the intake of fatty foods. Avoid or reduce consumption of fried foods, nuts, fatty meats, chips, and other foods high in fat.
> - Watch especially the intake of foods that are known to be loaded with cholesterol, such as eggs, cheese, shrimp, crab, and butter.
> - Use polyunsaturated and monosaturated fats instead of saturated fats.
> - Aim at a 50% reduction of refined sugars.
> - Reduce salt intake by 15% to 70%, depending on current consumption.
> - Try to eat only as many calories as are expended in a day.
> - If overweight, decrease food intake and increase exercise.
> - Increase the consumption of fruits, vegetables, and whole grains.
> - Substitute low-fat and nonfat milk for whole milk. Also use low-fat dairy products.
> - Consume more fish and poultry.
> - Become a label reader and watch out for foods that have a high hidden salt or sugar content.
> - Use multivitamin supplements, but do not overdo it.
> - Avoid crash diets.
> - Check with your physician before dieting.
> - Once you lose weight you have to be careful not to revert to poor eating habits. It will be necessary to maintain proper nutrition and proper exercise to keep the weight off.

5. Develop an exercise plan and follow it (Figure 5.22). Working as an EMT is a physically demanding career. EMS requires physically fit people with stamina. To be less than physically fit invites injury and premature death. A popular opinion that remains to be studied is that many deaths of emergency services personnel could be prevented if the responders had been physically fit.

    Most studies agree about the benefits of regular exercise. Some of the benefits are as follows:
    a. Better self-image and self-esteem
    b. Reduced risk of injury
    c. Weight management
    d. Better sleep
    e. Increased lung and heart capacity
    f. Decreased heart rate and blood pressure
    g. Increased muscle mass, strength, and stamina
    h. Higher energy levels and reduced feeling of tiredness

6. Do not smoke. Smoking is the number one cause of preventable death in North America. Smoking leads to heart disease, lung cancer, and other respiratory ailments. Smoking in spite of all the evidence literally is deadly.

7. Limit or avoid substance abuse, including alcohol and other drugs. Alcohol should never be consumed while on duty. Alcohol undeniably affects a person's coordination, performance, judgment, and behavior. Alcohol depletes the body of vitamins B and C, leaving it more vulnerable to stress and disease. The use of alcohol or drugs as a coping mechanism is a danger sign.

    Do not believe the myth that emergency responders always drink because it goes with the job. Police, fire, and EMS personnel should be examples because they see the results that alcohol can have on people. Emergency responders should lead the campaigns in their communities for drinking and driving awareness. If you or someone you know cannot stop drinking, seek professional help.

    Abuse (misuse) of other drugs (whether legal or illegal) is equally damaging to the EMT, both mentally and physically. Substance abuse of any type cannot be tolerated in EMS.

8. Get 7 to 8 hours of sleep every 24 hours.

9. Be sure to get enough rest and relaxation. Getting enough rest and relaxation is good advice for anyone but is particularly important for the EMT. The fast-paced, strenuous, demanding world of EMS

must be balanced with adequate recovery time for the body and mind.
10. Develop hobbies. Enjoying hobbies ties in with balancing your life. The EMT must foster other interests and activities. Be creative, do what comes naturally, do what interests you, and have fun while you do it.
11. Have a healthy sense of humor. Use tasteful humor to break the tension and provide relief at work and at home. A certain degree of morbid or dark humor is inevitable within EMS; the key is "within EMS." Family and friends may become offended or misunderstand an EMS joke that your partner laughed about. Another precaution is to make sure that patients do not feel that they are the target of your humor.
12. Learn more about the human aspect of being an EMT. Challenge yourself to read books, attend seminars, and take classes that focus on the human aspects of being an EMT. Even though the literature or session may not be targeted to EMS, ask yourself, "Could it help me do my job better?"

Some possible topics for additional study include the following:
a. Dealing with grief and the grieving process
b. Stress management skills
c. Crisis intervention skills
d. Understanding and preventing suicide
e. Dealing with alcohol and drug abuse
f. Disaster psychology and preparedness
g. Dealing with violent patients

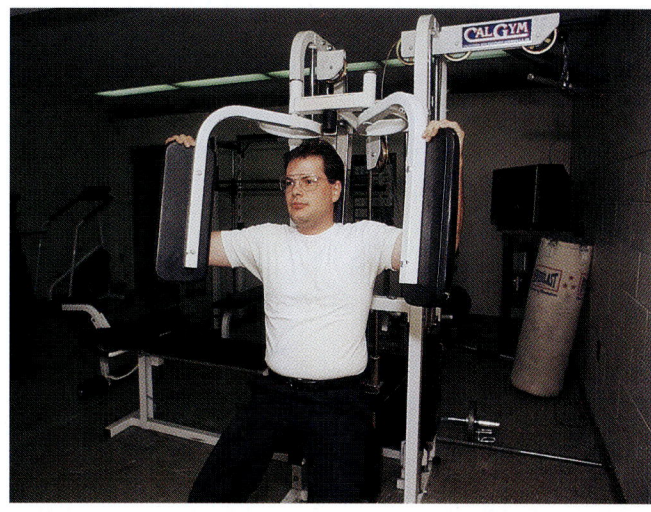

FIGURE 5.22 Develop an exercise plan and discipline yourself to follow it.

h. Problem-solving skills
i. Human interactions and communications
j. Behavioral and psychiatric emergencies
k. Helping victims of abuse
l. Understanding the helping professions

Make the decision now to begin developing safe and healthy habits that will pave the way for a long and productive career in EMS.

Summary

- Taking care of yourself is a prerequisite to taking care of others. The way you take care of yourself and others at a scene begins by noting anything special about the scene. Certain scenes, such as those with hazardous materials, rescue needs, violence, and crime, require the EMT to respond differently. Decisions must be made to address other factors in addition to patient care.
- EMTs regularly face death. Dying patients may go through stages in their thinking, including denial, anger, bargaining, depression, and acceptance. The EMT must remain calm, professional, and in control when other people, such as family and friends, and circumstances are out of control. The physical care given to the dying patient must be equaled by the emotional care and support provided to the patient and family.
- EMTs experience internal changes and feelings relating to emergencies. They should be aware of their own response to situations rather than forcing thoughts out of their mind or denying the feelings within them. EMTs who have long and fulfilling careers in EMS realize that life exists beyond their work. They understand the importance of their family, friends, and other interests. A balanced personal and professional life offers them support, security, and safety.
- Stress is an internal response to external factors, including environmental, personal, and psychosocial. EMTs may feel emotional strain because of their work, family responsibilities, or lifestyle changes. Stress may be chronic, or cumulative, meaning it is ongoing and accumulates over a period of time. Stress may also be acute as a result of an overwhelming situation.
- Posttraumatic stress disorder (PTSD) occurs from the unnatural and unhealthy suppression of emotions and thoughts after a critical incident or traumatic event. PTSD is a very serious condition involving illness, personality changes, and self-destructive behavior. Critical incident stress debriefing (CISD) is defusing and debriefing that may prevent serious stress reactions from damaging emergency personnel.

Summary (cont'd)

- EMTs must learn how to prevent and reduce stress that leads to distress. Twelve suggestions are provided with the most important ones including the following:
    - Balancing you life
    - Caring for yourself physically, mentally, emotionally, and spiritually
- Maintaining a positive attitude
- Maintaining a healthy diet
- Disciplining yourself to follow an exercise plan
- Managing your stress level is one area of your life that is completely your responsibility.

Scenario Solution

In the scenario, the EMTs were at a distinct disadvantage because the first indication they had of a problem was when they discovered that the patient was a victim of violence. They found themselves in a dangerous situation because they did not have good information regarding the nature of the call or the patient's problem. Unfortunately, not having the best or most reliable information when responding to a call is a fact of EMS life. In calls dispatched as assaults, domestic disturbances, or otherwise potentially violent natures, you must exercise extreme caution when responding and on the scene. On all other calls, you must maintain a heightened sense of awareness about the potential for violence or danger to you and your partner until you are ensured that a threat does not exist.

The EMTs in this scenario now find themselves in the unenviable position of having a potentially critical patient while being threatened by a man with a knife. What do you do?

Do not make any sudden moves. Communication is almost always the key to the outcome of situations such as this one. Immediately identify yourselves as "ambulance personnel." Now is not the time to be specific about your title or level of training. People who are upset may mistake EMS personnel for law enforcement officers.

Next, indicate that you will leave immediately. Ask the man to put down the knife so that you and your partner are able to leave. As the patient is in need of immediate care, ask if you can take him with you to the hospital. Abide by the answer you receive, whether yes or no, and leave immediately.

Return to the ambulance and drive away *without* lights or sirens. Radio immediately for the estimated time of arrival of the police and provide an update of the situation, including the intended use of a knife. Remember the guidelines for a violent scene:

- Violent scenes should always be controlled by law enforcement personnel before the EMT provides patient care.
- EMTs are not sufficiently trained, equipped, or paid to intervene in violent situations. It is not the EMT's responsibility to provide law enforcement. Do not play cop.
- Be especially cautious if the perpetrator of the crime is still on scene.
- Be observant for blood on people's clothing, hidden weapons, and potential weapons.
- Be alert to bystanders or family reactions. Watch for indicators of retaliation and revenge attempts.

Turn off the lights and siren as you near the address to which you have been dispatched. Stop at least half a block away from the address and check if the police have arrived yet. If the police have arrived, cautiously proceed to park at the scene. If the police have not arrived yet, radio your arrival on scene and communicate that you are waiting in the ambulance for the police. As you wait, be observant for any signs of activity in or around the house.

Following the guidelines for a violent scene will minimize the risk of being trapped and becoming a target of violence.

Key Terms

Body substance isolation (BSI) Isolation of substances that are excreted from the body to prevent the spread of communicable diseases.

Critical incident An event or circumstance that overwhelms one or more of the people present.

Critical incident stress debriefing (CISD) A confidential meeting in which a team consisting of mental health professionals, police, fire, and EMS disaster management personnel meet with prehospital providers to

Key Terms (cont'd)

discuss a critical incident for the purpose of debriefing and alleviating stress.

Environmental stressors Strains and pressures from factors in the environment that can affect the EMT (e.g., weather conditions, noise levels, and shift work).

Hazardous materials Chemical substances (solid, gas, or liquid) that are toxic to humans; unprotected exposure to these chemicals may result in severe illness or death.

Personal stressors Strains and pressures caused by the stress a person places on himself or herself from factors such as expectations, anxiety, and guilt.

Psychosocial stressors Stressors that are initiated by contact with other people.

Stress An internal response to an external factor such as work, family responsibilities, or lifestyle changes.

Review Questions

1. Body substance isolation (BSI) is important to the EMT because:
   a. The EMT may be contagious and expose the patient to communicable diseases from other patients
   b. The risk of exposure to body fluids is increased and the infection status of the patient is usually unknown
   c. The EMT is not exposed to patients with communicable diseases on a regular basis
   d. Federal regulations require EMS personnel to wear BSI gear when caring for some patients

2. You respond to a call for a shooting. As you arrive and exit the ambulance, the police officer on the scene advises you that the patient is critical and this is a crime scene. Your actions would include all of the following EXCEPT:
   a. Not disturbing the scene unless required for medical care
   b. Taking the same path in and out of the scene to avoid disturbing evidence
   c. Saving all clothing removed during patient care
   d. Waiting for police approval before moving or transporting the patient

3. You and your partner respond to a call for a possible sudden death. Upon arrival, the patient has obvious signs of lividity and rigor. The patient's husband becomes very upset when he is told that his wife is dead. He is crying and begins to pound his fists on the kitchen table. He is in what stage of dealing with his wife's death?
   a. Anger
   b. Denial
   c. Bargaining
   d. Depression
   e. Acceptance

4. True or False: When dealing with the family of a dying patient, it is best for the EMT to be honest without creating false hope.

5. During your last shift, your unit responded to a multicar accident in which two teenagers died. Their car left the roadway at a high rate of speed and was wrapped around a utility pole upon your arrival. Both patients had open head injuries, open fractures, and were obviously dead. In the 2 days since the accident, you have not slept well and your stomach has been upset. You are most likely experiencing:
   a. A bad case of influenza
   b. Stress as a result of the accident
   c. Food poisoning
   d. Hepatitis A

6. Signs and symptoms of critical incident stress in an individual or organization include all of the following EXCEPT:
   a. The signals of distress appear to be severe
   b. Personnel demonstrate numerous behavioral changes
   c. The signals of distress continue beyond 3 weeks
   d. Personnel visit the patients involved in the hospital

7. To reduce job-related stress, an EMT should recognize personal limits, have a positive attitude, exercise regularly, get plenty of rest, and:
   a. Participate in as many work-related activities as possible
   b. Maintain a balanced, healthy diet and lifestyle
   c. Work overtime on weekends and holidays
   d. Drink alcoholic beverages on a regular basis

Answers to these Review Questions can be found at the end of the book on page 865.

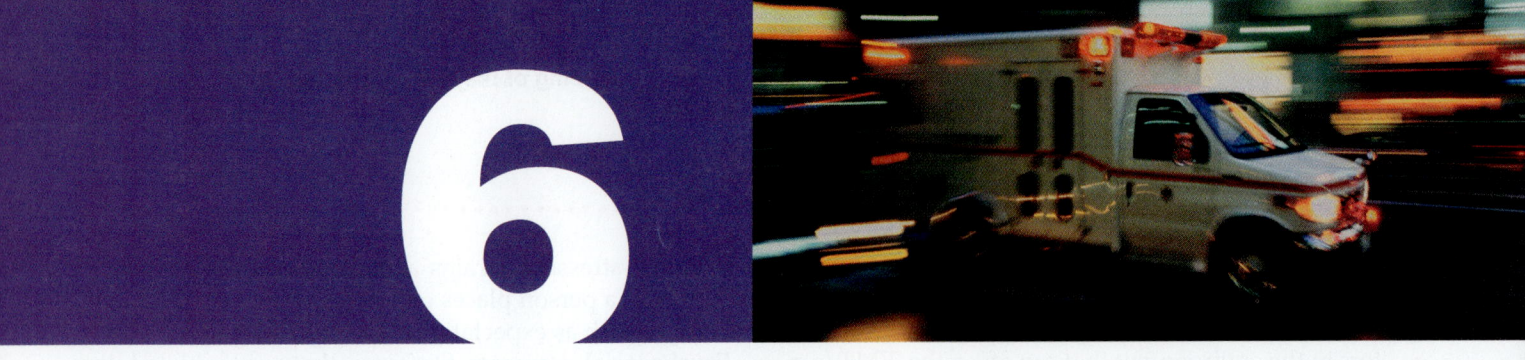

6

Infection Control

Lesson Goal

Thirty years ago it was macho for the EMT to arrive at the hospital covered with blood from the scene of a major trauma. In the latter part of the twentieth century and into the twenty first, medical knowledge has proved that this is a poor practice, risking disease to the EMT, other patients, and the EMT's family and friends. This chapter discusses this problem and how to prevent it.

Scenario

You are responding to an ambulance call for "general illness." The patient is a middle-age man who is vomiting a large quanity of bright red blood. The floor and walls of the bathroom are covered with the blood vomitus as is the patient. Members of his family tell you that he was released from the hospital last week with the same problem. They state that he has had the "alcohol liver" for several years and that the doctor told him that the "blood spiders" on his skin are from his alcohol abuse. They also state that he drinks two bottles of grocery store wine a day.

You note that the patient is thin with almost glassy yellow skin with telangectasis throughout his skin. His abdomen is large and blotted as if it may burst. He has needle track marks on his arms. He is coughing up a small amount of white mucus when he is not vomiting. He also reports a recent hospital admission for pneumonia.

 This situation contains many warning signs for the EMT. What are they? What steps should the EMTs take to protect themselves and others from the danger in this situation?

Key Terms to Know

Airborne pathogens
Bloodborne pathogens
Body fluid or substance
Body substance isolation (BSI)
Centers for Disease Control and Prevention (CDC)
Communicable disease
Exposure control plan
High-efficiency particulate air (HEPA) respirator
Infectious disease
Microorganisms
Occupational Safety and Health Administration (OSHA)
Personal protection
Protective equipment
Vaccination

74

Learning Objectives

As an EMT-Basic, you should be able to do the following:

DOT

- Discuss the importance of body substance isolation (BSI).
- Describe the steps that the EMT should take for personal protection from airborne and bloodborne pathogens.
- List the personal protective equipment necessary for exposure to airborne and bloodborne pathogens.

Supplemental

- Discuss common infectious diseases to which the EMT may be exposed.
- Discuss the Occupational Safety and Health Administration (OSHA) and Centers for Disease Control and Prevention (CDC) guidelines for bloodborne pathogens.

In the prehospital setting, the emergency medical technician (EMT) frequently comes into contact with patients who have a communicable disease. A **communicable disease** can be passed or communicated from one organism to another. The term **infectious disease** also is frequently used to describe these diseases. These two terms are used interchangeably in this chapter because they have essentially the same meaning for the prehospital provider. Communicable diseases are generally classified as children's diseases (minimal risk for the EMT), those that are

Patient Care Algorithm

Scene Assessment

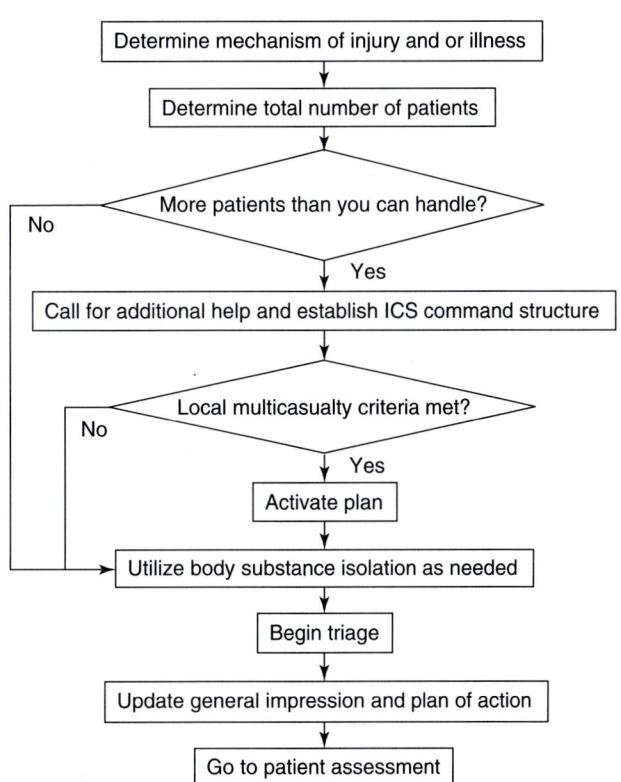

TABLE 6.1 Recommendations for Protective Equipment in the Prehospital Setting

Task	Disposable Gloves	Gown	Mask	Protective Eyewear
Controlling spurting blood	Yes	Yes	Yes	Yes
Controlling minimal bleeding	Yes	No	No	No
Emergency childbirth	Yes	Yes	Yes, if splashing is likely	Yes, if splashing is likely
Oral/nasal suctioning, manually clearing airway	Yes	No	Only if splashing is likely	Only if splashing is likely
Handling and cleaning contaminated equipment	Yes	Only if splashing is likely	No	No
Taking blood pressure	No	No	No	No
Taking temperature	No	No	No	No

spread by air (moderate risk for the EMT), and those that are spread by body fluids (major risk for the EMT).

Often there is no indication that a disease is communicable. When the EMT either is told or suspects that a patient has a communicable disease, the management of the patient and the treatment priorities remain unchanged. However, the EMT may need to take additional steps to protect the emergency medical services (EMS) crew members and to ensure that the disease is not spread to family members, other patients, or healthcare workers. These steps include understanding the importance of body substance isolation (BSI; also known as universal or standard precautions), understanding how the common infectious diseases are spread, knowing the risk associated with each disease, knowing the basic pathophysiology of each disease as it applies to the prehospital environment and **Occupational Safety and Health Administration (OSHA)** and **Centers for Disease Control and Prevention (CDC)** guidelines for dealing with bloodborne pathogens, and knowing the methods for personal protection from bloodborne and airborne pathogens.

In a disaster situation in which bodies have been lying on the scene, a different type of protection is required. The EMT should know how to access this special information if the situation should ever arise in his or her community.

Importance of Body Substance Isolation (Universal or Standard Precautions)

On December 6, 1991, OSHA published the standard designed to protect employees who are at risk for exposure to bloodborne pathogens. **Bloodborne pathogens** are **microorganisms,** present in blood and body fluids, that can cause disease. EMTs are especially susceptible to bloodborne pathogen exposure because they usually work in high-risk environments. However, blood is not the only form of **body fluid or substance** that can carry the organisms that result in communicable diseases. The simplest approach for the EMT is to consider any substance from the body (e.g., blood, urine, feces, tears, saliva, spinal fluid) as being highly dangerous. EMTs should wear protective devices while performing patient care in situations in which the chances of being exposed to body substances are high, such as with cardiopulmonary resuscitation (CPR), intravenous (IV) life-line insertion, trauma, and

Editor's Note

Many terms are used in different regions of the United States that mean the same thing. Three of these terms relate specifically to this chapter: standard precautions (SP), universal precautions (UP), and body substance isolation (BSI). The most descriptive of these terms is BSI since it describes exactly what is being done. However, it is impossible to change well-used terms in a community when the change is no more than a name change. Therefore these three terms are used interchangably throughout this text.

✓ Bloodborne pathogens are microorganisms, such as viruses and bacteria, that can cause disease. EMTs must protect themselves from exposure to these microorganisms. The EMT should wear protective equipment when performing any procedures in the prehospital setting that may result in exposure to blood or other body fluid that can transmit communicable diseases.

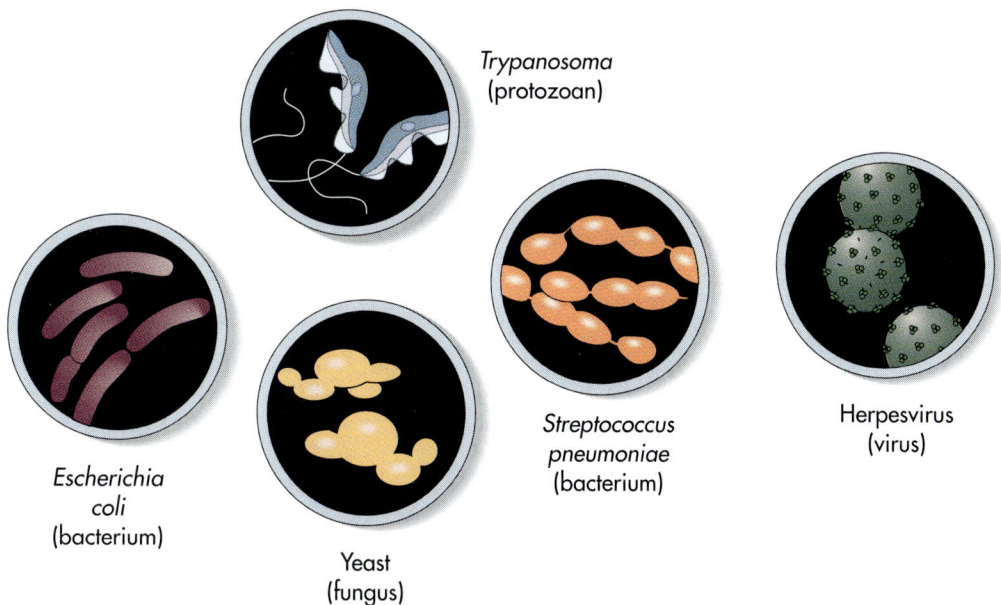

FIGURE 6.1 An infectious disease is caused by the presence of microorganisms in the body, including bacteria, viruses, protozoa, and fungi.

childbirth. Table 6.1 lists tasks that the EMT commonly performs in the prehospital setting along with the CDC recommendations for the type of **protective equipment** that EMTs should wear when completing these tasks.

Common Infectious Diseases

An infectious disease is caused by the presence of microorganisms in the body. These microorganisms are usually bacteria, viruses, or fungi (Figure 6.1). Most communicable diseases are not life threatening, but some are, such as hepatitis, new strains of tuberculosis, and acquired immunodeficiency syndrome (AIDS). The EMT can be exposed to these diseases when coming into contact with a patient who is infected. Communicable diseases are transmitted through various ways, including the following:

1. *Direct contact.* Direct contact is made by touching an infected patient or infected body fluid, such as kissing, sexual intercourse, and introducing contaminated fluid to an open wound. Simply shaking the hand of an AIDS patient does not transmit the infection.
2. *Droplet inhalation.* Droplet inhalation occurs when the EMT breathes in the infected moisture that the patient exhales or coughs out.
3. *Contaminated needle puncture.* This occurs when the EMT works with another health care professional who administers an injection to a patient, when the EMT searches a patient and is stuck with the needle that the patients uses for IV drug use, or when contaminated sharps are not placed in the proper disposal containers.
4. *Bites.* Bite injuries occur when the EMT is bitten by either an animal or a human. The most severe infections are associated with human bites if the skin is broken.
5. *Blood transfusions.* Blood transfusions that are administered in the prehospital setting may put the EMT at risk for infection either by blood from the patient coming into contact with an open wound on the EMT or by a needle puncture during preparation of the transfusion. Although transfusions are carefully checked for contaminations at the time of preparation, not all infectious diseases can be detected.
6. *Contaminated materials.* Contaminated materials are a source of infection for the EMT when they contain body substances or fluids from the patient. These materials include handkerchiefs, washcloths, towels, sheets, or used wound-dressing material.

> ✓ Communicable diseases are transmitted through various ways, such as direct contact, droplet inhalation, contaminated needle puncture, bites, blood transfusions, and contaminated materials.

The EMT should be familiar with communicable diseases. Many diseases are contagious for only a portion of the time that the person is ill. This is most common with

TABLE 6.2 Communicable Diseases Encountered in the Prehospital Setting

Disease	Mode of Transmission	Communicable Period
Common Childhood Diseases		
Measles (rubeola)*	Airborne droplets or secretions from the mouth, nose, and eyes	At symptom onset (about 4 days before the rash appears) and for about 2 more days
Rubella (German measles)*	Airborne droplets or contaminated materials	A week before the rash appears and for about 4 more days
Mumps*	Airborne droplets or contaminated materials	At symptom onset and as long as 9 days after the salivary glands swell up
Chickenpox*	Airborne droplets or direct contact with secretions from the nose and mouth	A few days before the rash appears and for about 6 days after the vesicles become apparent; moist scabs are still infectious
Other Serious Communicable Diseases		
Meningitis	Airborne droplets or direct contact with secretions from the nose and mouth	Variable—lasts as long as the bacteria are present in the nasal and oral secretions
Tuberculosis	Airborne droplets	Variable—lasts as long as the bacteria are present
Hepatitis (viral) type A	Ingestion of food or water that has been contaminated by infected feces	Towards the end of the incubation period (which is about 4 weeks) and for a few more days
Hepatitis (viral) type B (serum)*	Sexual contact or puncture with a contaminated needle	Weeks before the first symptoms appear and can last for years
AIDS	Sexual contact, being punctured with a contaminated needle, and across the placenta to a fetus	High-risk periods from exposure until the blood test is positive (weeks to months), and from positive blood test until the disease develops
Sexually Transmitted Diseases		
Gonorrhea	Direct contact with pus drainage from the mucous membranes of the infected person	On contact and until treated
Syphilis	Direct contact with the infectious drainage from the lesions; can be transmitted from a mother to the infant across the placenta; and rarely by contact with contaminated materials.	Upon contact and until treated
Genital herpes	Sexual contact; also infants can become infected if delivered to a woman with an active outbreak	At symptom onset and for 4 to 7 days

*Vaccinations exist for the disease.

the childhood diseases (e.g., measles, chicken pox, mumps). Others, such as hepatitis C, last for the life of the patient. This contagious time is called the *communicable period*. The communicable diseases that the EMT is likely to encounter in the prehospital setting, the means by which they are transmitted, and their communicable period are listed in Table 6.2.

Guidelines for Bloodborne Pathogen Protection

Under federal law, the director of the CDC has developed standards for health workers, which include emergency response personnel to reduce the risk of becoming infected with a communicable disease through exposure to bloodborne pathogens and to identify circumstances in which exposure is likely to occur. These standards are enforced by OSHA and apply to emergency response personnel, whether paid or volunteer. The standards require that the employer develop an **exposure control plan,** which must contain certain elements that describe how the employer will protect its employees. For the purposes of this chapter, *employer* is defined as the organization that is responsible for the paid or volunteer EMS provider. Box 6.1 lists the specific items required for inclusion in the plan.

✓ OSHA regulations to reduce the risk of exposure to communicable diseases apply to emergency response personnel.

Box 6.1 Exposure Control Plan Requirements

- A list of the jobs and the procedures in which exposure to bloodborne pathogens may occur
- A timeline and method by which the plan is to be implemented
- A plan outlining how exposure incidents will be handled
- A plan for annual review and update to include any changes in the workplace that may result in bloodborne pathogen exposure

Box 6.2 OSHA Bloodborne Pathogen Training Session Topics

- Overview of the modes of transmission of bloodborne pathogens
- Principles regarding the control of risk
- Medical management of those who have been exposed
- Appropriate equipment cleaning techniques
- Appropriate packaging techniques for specimens
- Methods of using personal protective equipment

Box 6.3 Additional Required Employer Action

- Provide personal protective equipment, hepatitis B vaccination, and a confidential medical evaluation and follow-up visit to the employee at no cost.
- Develop a written schedule to clean and decontaminate equipment and the work area after blood or other potentially infectious material has been exposed to the area.
- Devise procedures to handle regulated waste.
- Ensure that warning labels are secured to containers that are used to store or transport blood or other wastes that are potentially infectious.
- Maintain records on each employee who may be at risk of exposure and records that training has occurred as prescribed.

In addition to the exposure control plan, the employer must also provide training for its personnel, as soon as they are retained, at least annually. This training is to be free of charge and conducted during normal work hours. Box 6.2 outlines the required topics for inclusion in the training session. On completion of the training session, the personnel must be provided with access to a copy of the OSHA standard, an explanation of the employer's exposure control plan, and an opportunity to ask questions.

> ✓ Employers are required to have an exposure control plan, provide free training, and provide free protective equipment.

The employer must also take actions to comply with the OSHA standard (Box 6.3). The employer must keep the medical and training records identified in Box 6.3 for a specified period of time. The employer must maintain the medical records for the duration of employment plus 30 years and keep the training records for 3 years from the date that the training occurred.

In addition to the employer requirements, the EMT has important responsibilities to ensure a safe working environment:

- The EMT must remove gloves and jewelry and wash his or her hands thoroughly for at least 30 seconds after each patient contact.
- If the gloves have been punctured during the client contact, the EMT must clean his or her hands and all areas potentially touched by the body fluids with hydrogen peroxide, Clorox, alcohol, or other strong disinfectant that is effective against viruses. The EMT should consider using antiviral medication in the event of needle puncture or laceration from the client's teeth. The local emergency department will have a protocol to follow.
- The EMT must wipe down the floor, walls, and stretcher at least once a day with a 1:10 mixture of household bleach and water or an appropriate commercial cleaning solution.
- The EMT must wipe down frequently used items such as radios, stethoscopes, monitors, and oxygen tanks.
- The EMT must place contaminated trash and linen in the appropriate containers (Figure 6.2).

> ✓ The EMT has important responsibilities to ensure a safe working environment.

When body fluids have spilled on ambulance surfaces or equipment, the EMT should wear disposable

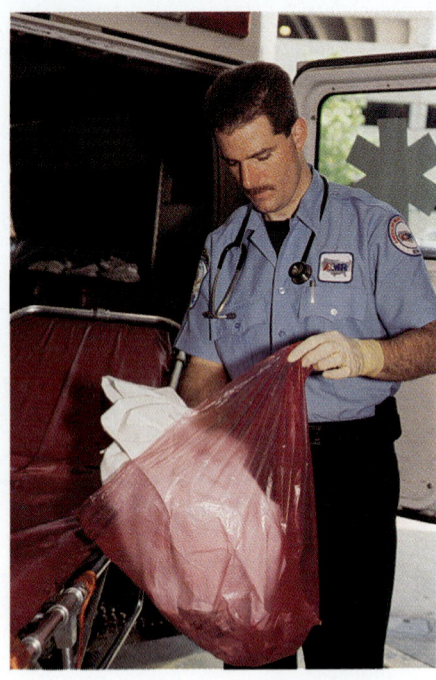

FIGURE 6.2 Properly disposing of contaminated linens and dressings is one way EMTs can protect themselves from exposure to disease-causing organisms.

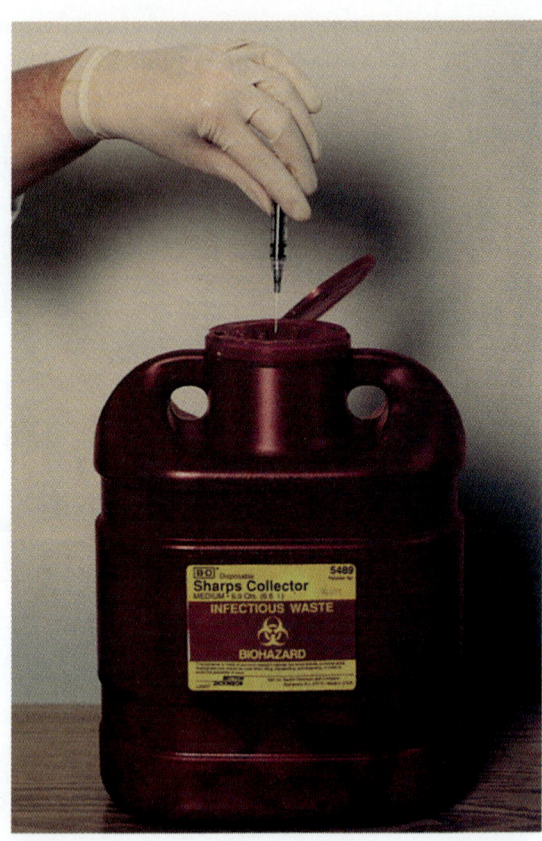

FIGURE 6.3 Contaminated needles must be disposed of in proper containers.

gloves and eye protection. The EMT must also do the following:

- Clean up blood spillage by absorbing the spill with disposable paper towels or linen, and clean the area with the 1:10 mixture of bleach and water or an appropriate commercial cleaning solution.
- Dispose of sharp items such as needles in approved containers (Figure 6.3).
- Thoroughly clean suction equipment that has been used following the manufacturer's recommendations.
- Discard disposable respiratory equipment and thoroughly clean the nondisposable parts (such as laryngoscopes).
- Scrub backboards, straps, and cervical spine immobilization devices with hot, soapy water, rinse well with plain water, and let them thoroughly dry.
- The pneumatic antishock garment (PASG) should be cleaned according to manufacturer's recommendations, which usually includes scrubbing the garment with warm, soapy water and thoroughly rinsing and drying.

Methods for Personal Protection for the EMT

To minimize the risk of exposure to a communicable disease process, the EMT must be familiar with methods of **personal protection. Body substance isolation** (BSI) is a process that health care providers use to separate or isolate themselves from potentially dangerous body substances. BSI is accomplished through several means. Handwashing is an easy and effective method of preventing disease transmission. After transporting any patient, the EMS crew members should always wash their hands thoroughly on arrival at the health care facility. Ideally, and for the patient's safety, EMTs should wash their hands before and after coming into contact with each patient. The EMT can accomplish handwashing using soap and hot water or one of the commercial water-free cleaning solutions that are available (Figure 6.4).

BSI also can be accomplished with the use of basic personal protection equipment (Figure 6.5):

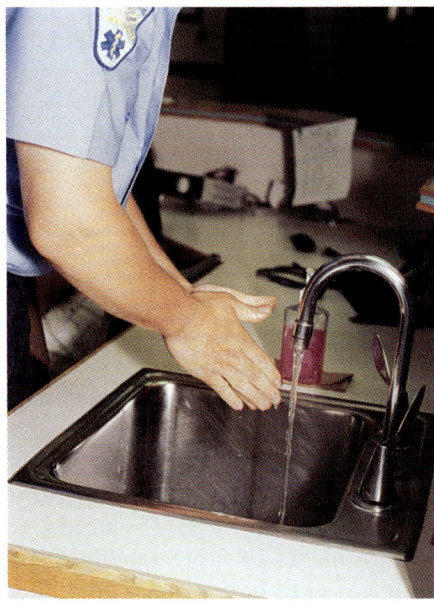
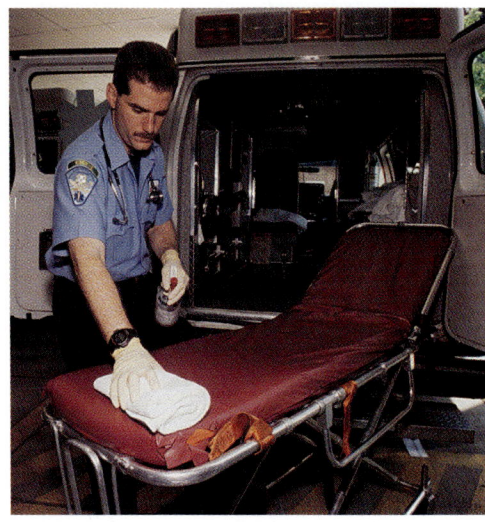

A **B**

FIGURE 6.4 Handwashing **(A)** and washing equipment **(B)** after each patient contact removes disease-causing organisms and lessens the risk of infection.

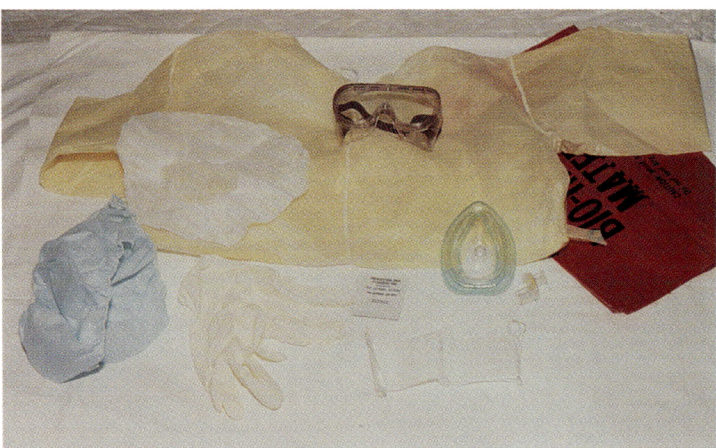

FIGURE 6.5 Various protective devices that the EMT should wear while rendering patient care, including eye protection, gloves, gown, and face mask.

1. *Eye protection.* Health care workers can use prescription eyeglasses to protect their eyes from the splashing of body substances that are emitted from the patient. However, eyeglasses should be equipped with removable side shields, which prevent substances from getting into the eyes from the side. Several eye protection devices are also available, such as goggles, for people who do not wear glasses. They usually cover the area surrounding the eyes. Goggles effectively protect the eyes from exposure to body substances. Protective eyewear or face shields are required when contamination of the eyes is likely; however, they are not required for routine care. The EMT should carry eye protection in an easily accessible place so that he or she does not lose valuable time when the protection is needed.

2. *Gloves.* All EMS personnel should don disposable gloves before initiating emergency care. Vinyl or latex disposable gloves are especially appropriate when the EMT may come into contact with body fluids, especially blood or bloody body fluids. The gloves should fit tightly at the wrists. The EMT should put on a new pair of gloves between contact with different patients. General purpose utility

> **Editor's Note**
>
> OSHA rules that apply to the EMS situation have been developed with the protection of the EMT, his or her family, and the other patients as the major objective. However, the rules are strict with heavy fines of thousands of dollars for each offense to the individual EMT and to the EMS service. These include no food in the patient compartment of an ambulance, no application of lipstick or lip balm while in the patient compartment, and a change of clothes after certain patient contact. Like many government regulations, the rules apply to the private industry and not necessarily to the government-run EMS services. Each EMT must understand these regulations and whether they apply to the EMS service for which he or she works. Situations exist when the EMT must follow these regulation when inside a private ambulance but not in a government vehicle, even on the same call. The EMT must understand the rules as they apply to his or her own EMS service and the community in which he or she works.

> **Tips from the Pros**
>
> The most important aspect of protecting the EMT from communicable diseases is handwashing. Gloves alone are not effective to prevent transmission.

gloves are needed for cleaning vehicles and equipment. The best type to use are those with extended cuffs, which may be cleaned and reused. However, the EMT should not use utility gloves if they are peeling, cracked, or discolored or if they have punctures, tears, or other evidence of deterioration. While wearing gloves, the EMT should avoid handling personal items, such as pens and combs, that may become contaminated with body fluids.

> **Tips from the Pros**
>
> EMTs who develop a rash when using disposable gloves can often find relief by using allergen-free vinyl or nitrile gloves, which are available through various medical supply companies. Handwashing solutions, such as Betadine or other idoine-containing fluids, frequently produce allergies.

> **Tips from the Pros**
>
> All EMS personnel should become accustomed to putting gloves on before they leave the unit to ensure that it becomes second nature.

3. *Gowns.* The EMT should wear a gown when splashing to the skin or clothing is likely to occur, such as during field delivery of an infant and after major trauma. Once the work is complete, in addition to discarding the gown in an appropriate fashion, the EMT should change his or her uniform.
4. *Face masks.* The EMT should wear surgical-type face masks to protect against possible blood splatter or with patient who are known or suspected to have a disease that is transmitted through the air. Masks are required when contamination of the mucosal membranes, mouth, or nose is likely; however, they are not required for routine care. If a patient is known or suspected to have tuberculosis, the EMT should wear a **high-efficiency particulate air (HEPA) respirator.** If possible, the EMT should transport the patient in an ambulance that is well-ventilated to the outside. These precautions are necessary because tuberculosis may stay in the air for an extended period. The EMT should strongly consider having the patient wear an HEPA respirator or a surgical mask as well.

> **Tips from the Pros**
>
> When developing specifications for ambulance purchase, be sure to include an exhaust fan and windows that can be opened in the patient compartment.

5. *Resuscitation equipment.* Pocket masks, bag-valve-masks, and other ventilation devices should be available immediately to all EMS personnel to minimize the need for mouth-to-mouth resuscitation. If the EMT uses disposable items, they should be used once and then discarded. If they are not disposable, the EMT must clean them thoroughly and disinfect them in accordance with the manufacturer's recommendations.

Should body fluid contact occur, the rights of the EMT and the patient may be at odds. When communicable diseases are involved, some states have determined that the EMT's right to know supersedes the patient's right to privacy. Other states require that patient consent be obtained before information is released. The EMT is responsible for determining, in advance of an exposure, what their state law requires.

> ✓ The EMT can accomplish adequate BSI by using basic precautionary equipment such as eye protection, gloves, gowns, face masks, and resuscitation equipment.

Use of protective devices on a regular basis will ensure that the risk of exposure to a communicable disease is minimized. Wearing protective devices should be so common that it becomes second nature and does not require a delay in initiating patient care. The EMT is responsible for knowing state laws regarding exposure. Before starting work in the prehospital setting, EMTs should ensure that they are up to date on all of the recommended immunizations. These include *Haemophilus influenzae* B (HIB); diphtheria-pertussis-tetanus (DPT); measles, mumps, and rubella (MMR); polio; and hepatitis B vaccinations, and a tetanus booster every 10 years. This process of **vaccination** involves the introduction of examples of the target organisms into the body so that the body can develop its defenses against the agent.

There is an upswing in the occurrence of tuberculosis (TB or Tbc) in the United States. Part of this problem is due to new strains that are resistant to the usual TB medications. EMTs exposed to patients with potential Tbc should be evaluated for potential exposure and appropriate treatment. EMTs should be tested for TB annually with the use of tuberculin purified protein derivatives (PPDs).

> ✓ The EMT should obtain all of the recommended immunizations, including HIB, DPT, MMR, polio, and hepatitis B vaccinations, and a tetanus booster every 10 years.

Summary

- Protection of the EMT, the EMT's family, and other patients is a priority in the management of all patients. The amount of protection needed varies according to the situation. At the very least the EMT should wear gloves for every patient contact. If body fluids come into contact with the skin, these areas should be cleaned throughly with strong disinfectants. This process is called *body substance isolation* (BSI), *standard precautions* (SP), or *universal precautions* (UP).
- EMTs are especially susceptible to bloodborne pathogen exposure because they usually work in high-risk environments.
- The EMT should wear protective equipment while initiating patient care in situations in which the chances of being exposed to pathogens are high, such as CPR, intravenous insertion, trauma, and childbirth.
- Infectious diseases can be transmitted by direct contact, inhalation of droplets, contaminated needle puncture, bites, blood transfusions, and contaminated materials.
- The EMT can be exposed to communicable diseases in the prehospital setting, including:
    - Common childhood diseases, such as measles, rubella, mumps, and chickenpox
    - Other serious diseases, such as meningitis, tuberculosis, hepatitis, and AIDS
    - Sexually transmitted diseases, such as gonorrhea, syphilis, and genital herpes
- The Occupational Safety and Health Administration (OSHA) enforces standards to protect emergency response personnel from becoming infected through exposure to bloodborne pathogens.
- Employers are required to have an exposure control plan in place, provide training for their personnel, and provide personal protective equipment for employees.
- Body substance isolation (BSI) can be accomplished by using basic precautionary equipment such as eye protection, gloves, gowns, face masks, and resuscitation equipment (i.e., bag-valve-masks and pocket masks).

Scenario Solution

This patient has signs and symptoms of severe liver disease, a respiratory problem, and possible immune system suppression. The signs and symptoms of liver disease are vomiting bright red blood, yellow skin, and a protruding abdomen. Severe liver disease can be secondary to a history of alcohol abuse or any of the viral hepatitis diseases. The cause of his liver disease is unknown. He may have been exposed to hepatitis B or C or AIDS from sharing needles or from blood transfusions before such testing was available. The needle tracks may indicate a risk of HIV infection, which can compromise his immune system and make him susceptible to tuberculosis or several other contagious pulmonary diseases.

In managing this patient, the entire crew should observe strict BSI by taking the following actions:

1. Ensure that the patient is treated in a professional manner (not condescending or demeaning).
2. Explain to the patient that the precautions are medically necessary.
3. Provide appropriate emergency care of the patient, including management of airway, breathing, and circulation.
4. Avoid contact with any of the patient's bodily fluids.
5. Wear gloves.
6. Wear eye protection.
7. Wear a gown.
8. Wear an HEPA respirator (having the patient wear an HEPA respirator is not recommended because he or she is actively vomiting and the mask may compromise his or her airway).
9. Calmly reassure the patient during treatment and transportation.
10. Open the windows in the ambulance to facilitate airflow and ventilation in the patient compartment.
11. Thoroughly disinfect the inside of the ambulance, any equipment used in treating the patient, and the cot, and dispose of bed linen appropriately.

Observing the precautions discussed in this section will protect the EMT in the workplace and ensure appropriate patient care. Although most of the OSHA standard requirements for compliance are placed on the employer, most of the specific tasks will be delegated to the EMT who provides direct patient care.

Key Terms

Airborne pathogens Microorganisms, present in the air, that cause disease.

Bloodborne pathogens Microorganisms, present in the blood, that cause disease.

Body fluid or substance Any matter excreted or emitted by the body that may contain infectious microorganisms.

Body substance isolation (BSI) Isolation of substances that are excreted from the body to prevent the spread of communicable diseases.

Centers for Disease Control and Prevention (CDC) A division of the United States Public Health Service that is responsible for activities related to control and prevention of disease processes.

Communicable disease A disease that can be transmitted from one person to another through body fluids, air ingestion, or skin contact.

Exposure control plan The plan that an employer is required to develop in compliance with the Occupational Safety and Health Administration standard, to minimize the risk that employees will become exposed to a communicable disease.

High-efficiency particulate air (HEPA) respirator A mask worn over the mouth and nose that decreases the spread of infection of airborne pathogens such as tuberculosis.

Infectious disease A disease that can be transmitted from one organism to another; an active state of infection.

Microorganism A microscopic organism (plant or animal).

Occupational Safety and Health Administration (OSHA) Division of the United States Department of Labor that is responsible for establishing and enforcing safety and health standards in the workplace.

Personal protection Steps taken to decrease the risk that the rescuer will become exposed to a communicable disease.

Protective equipment Equipment that is used to decrease the risk that the rescuer will become infected with a communicable disease.

Vaccination Introduction of a vaccine (a mixture of weakened or dead microorganisms) into the body to produce immunity to a specific disease.

Review Questions

1. Situations in which the chance of being exposed to pathogens is high are:
   a. Talking to and shaking hands with an AIDS patient
   b. Eating food after dressing an open wound using no gloves
   c. Driving the EMS unit with a patient in the patient care compartment who has hepatitis C
   d. Eating at the same table as a patient who has AIDS
2. Important types of protection for the EMT from communicable disease exposure are:
   a. Gloves, mask, and Kevlar vest
   b. Mask, cap, gown, and antibiotics
   c. Mask, glove, and hepatitis vaccination
   d. Gown, mask, air pack, and gloves
3. Methods of transmission of communicable diseases are:
   i. Examining patients without gloves
   ii. Poor or no handwashing after patient care
   iii. Being inside the patient's house
   iv. Breathing the same air as the patient
   v. Patient body fluids on open skin lesions
   vi. Improper patient care compartment after each patient transportation
   vii. Shaking hands with the patients
   a. ii, iii, v and vii
   b. i, ii, iv, and vi
   c i, ii, v, and vi
   d. All of the above
4. Common childhood diseases that can present a risk of exposure to the EMT are:
   i. Measles
   ii. Mumps
   iii. Chicken pox
   iv. Pink eye
   v. Pneumonia
   vi. Gastroenteritis
   vii. Scarlet fever
   a. i, ii, iii, iv, and vii
   b. i, ii, iii, iv, v
   c. ii, iii, iv, v, and vi
   d. All of the above

The statements in questions 5-8 have two parts. The parts are:
   a. True, true and related
   b. True, false
   c. True, true and unrelated
   d. False, true

5. OSHA bloodborne pathogen training sessions are important because patients frequently spit on patients.
6. Masks should be worn for ALL patient encounters because they prevent airborne infection exchange.
7. Hand contamination is a problem when dressing wounds because the blood of all patients may have communicable diseases.
8. The failure to carry out proper protection is a risk to the family of the EMT because the failure to follow OSHA rules can result in a large fine to the EMT.

Answers to these Review Questions can be found at the end of the book on page 865.

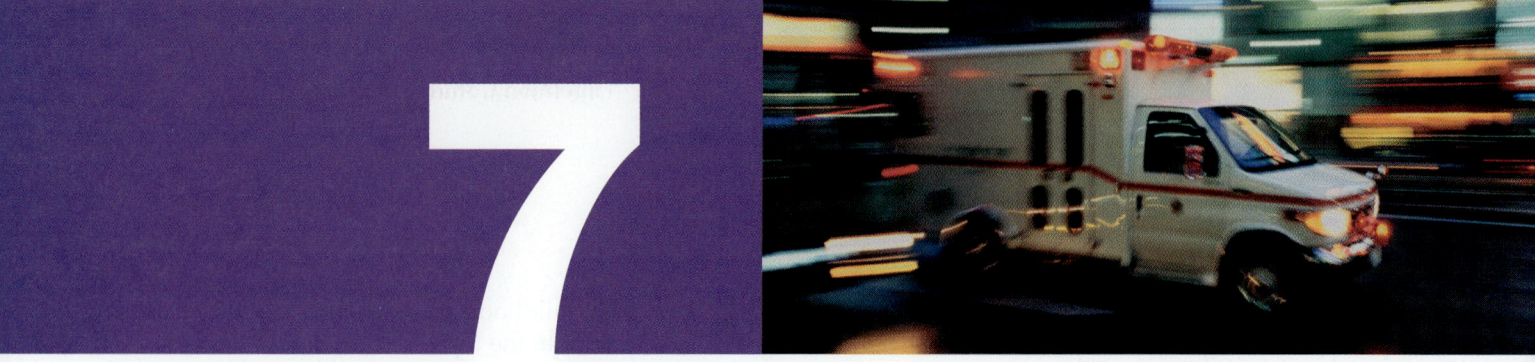

7

The Human Body

Lesson Goal

The goal of this chapter is to help the EMT-Basic understand the primary structure of the human body and its relationship with illness and injury and the care rendered by the EMT-basic.

Scenario

You are called to respond to a hunting accident. You arrive on the scene to find a 35-year-old male patient lying on his back in heavy brush at the base of a tree. The patient was shot from his tree stand by another hunter and fell 15 feet to the ground. He is responsive and alert. After assessing the patient, you find that he has a small cut on his chin and shot-gun pellets under his chin, on his right chest, on his right buttock, and on the outside of his right thigh. He also has an obvious open deformity of his right thigh and multiple pellet wounds just above his knee.

 Using directional medical terminology, describe the specific location of the upper leg deformity and pellet injuries. Which human system may be compromised as a result of the deformity in the right upper leg? When communicating with the hospital, how will the EMT describe these injuries?

Key Terms to Know

Abdominal quadrants	Brachial artery	Clavicle	Face
Acromion	Brain stem	Colon	Femoral arteries
Alveoli	Bronchi	Coronary arteries	Femur
Aorta	Capillaries	Dermis	Fibula
Arteries	Cardiac muscle	Diaphragm	Frontal
Atria	Carina	Diastolic pressure	Heart
Automaticity	Carotid arteries	Endocardium	Hemoglobin
Autonomic nervous system	Carpals	Epicardium	Hinged joint
Ball-and-socket joint	Cartilage	Epidermis	Hip joint
Blood	Central nervous system	Epiglottis	Hormones
Blood pressure	Cerebellum	Erythrocytes	Humerus
Blood vessels	Cerebrum	Esophagus	Iliac crest

Key Terms to Know (cont'd)

- Integumentary system
- Intercostal muscles
- Involuntary muscles
- Ischium
- Joints
- Kidney
- Large intestine
- Larynx
- Leukocytes
- Ligaments
- Lungs
- Mandible
- Manubrium
- Maxilla
- Medical terminology
- Metabolism
- Metacarpals
- Metatarsals
- Muscles
- Musculoskeletal system
- Myocardium
- Nasal bone
- Occipital
- Olecranon
- Orbit
- Ovaries
- Parasympathetic nervous system
- Parietal
- Parietal pleura
- Patella
- Perfusion
- Pericardium
- Peripheral nervous system
- Peritoneum
- Phalanges
- Pharynx
- Plasma
- Platelets
- Prefix
- Pubis
- Pulmonary arteries
- Pulmonary veins
- Radial artery
- Radius
- Respiratory depth (tidal volume)
- Respiratory quality
- Respiratory rhythm
- Retroperitoneal space
- Ribs
- Root word
- Scapula
- Skeleton
- Skull
- Small intestine
- Sternum
- Subcutaneous tissue
- Suffix
- Sympathetic nervous system
- Systolic pressure
- Tarsals
- Temporal
- Tendons
- Testes
- Thorax
- Tibia
- Trachea
- Ulna
- Ureter
- Urethra
- Veins
- Venae cavae
- Ventilatory rate
- Ventricles
- Vertebrae
- Visceral pleura
- Vocal cords
- Voluntary muscles
- Xiphoid process
- Zygomatic bones

Learning Objectives

As an EMT-Basic, you should be able to do the following:

DOT

- Identify the following directional terms: medial, lateral, proximal, distal, superior, inferior, anterior, posterior, midline, right and left, apices, midclavicular, bilateral, and midaxillary.
- Describe the structure and function of the following major body systems: respiratory, circulatory, musculoskeletal, integumentary, nervous, and endocrine.

Supplemental

- Describe the various components of medical terminology, including medical abbreviations.

The goals of prehospital emergency medicine are to provide proper care and transportation to an appropriate facility for each patient. To reach these goals, prehospital care focuses on "assessment-based" patient management. The foundation of patient assessment is a working knowledge of the anatomy (structure) and physiology (function) of the human body. Patient assessment and appropriate use of appropriate medical terminology allow the emergency medical technician–basic (EMT-B) to communicate effectively with other health care professionals.

This chapter reviews anatomic terms, the skeletal system, and body systems. Medical terms are also introduced. This information will enable the EMT-B to begin building the foundation for quality patient assessment and management.

Medical Terminology

Medical terminology is the language unique to the medical profession. Medical terminology is useful to know because it allows health care providers to communicate in a precise and effective manner with other medical personnel. Many medical terms come from Greek or Latin. Terms are based on a **root word** combined with a prefix, suffix, and/or another root. Translating a medical term into "normal" English often requires several words to communicate the same thought. For example, the medical term *appendectomy* means "surgical excision or removal of the appendix." The root word *append*, meaning appendix, is combined with the suffix *ectomy*, meaning surgical excision or removal, to form the medical term. Medical terminology is a code that allows for precise meanings to be expressed with few words. Table 7.1 contains some common root words and their meanings.

A **prefix** is made up of one or more syllables and is located at the beginning of the word. Prefixes usually indicate direction, how, or how much. Table 7.2 contains some common prefixes and their meanings. A **suffix** is located at the end of the word. Table 7.3 contains some common suffixes and their meanings.

Abbreviations are common in the medical field, and it is helpful for the EMT-B to be able to recognize and use them when appropriate. However, some abbreviations may mean different things to different people. Their use should be avoided whenever the potential exists for confusion or when communicating with the general public. Table 7.4 contains some of the more common abbreviations and their meanings.

> ✓ Medical terms are composed of prefixes, root words, and suffixes. It is important for the EMT-B to understand medical terminology to communicate effectively with other health care professionals.

Directional Terminology

When assessing a patient, understanding the terminology associated with the external features of the human body is crucial. Terms used to describe directional anatomy are based on the assumption that the body is in the anatomic position. In this position, the patient stands upright and faces forward. The arms are down at the sides, and the palms face forward (Figure 7.1). When the terms *right* and *left* are used, they refer to the patient's right and left. Table 7.5 contains terms and their definitions are helpful when assessing a patient's condition and reporting assessment results (Figure 7.2).

> ✓ Use of the correct directional anatomy terms ensures that accurate patient information will be conveyed in a concise, professional manner to the receiving health care facility.

Musculoskeletal System

The **musculoskeletal system** is the framework for the body, protects vital internal organs, and provides for body movement. The two major components of the musculoskeletal system are the bones that make up the skeleton and the muscles.

Skeletal System

The **skeleton** is made up of 206 bones that give the body structure and work with the muscles to provide for movement (Figure 7.3). The skeleton is divided into eight components: joints, skull, bones of the face, spinal column, thorax, pelvis, upper extremities, and lower extremities. The skeletal system provides the framework for the human body, thus visual deformity of an extremity will most likely indicate a skeletal injury.

TABLE 7.1 Root Words and Meanings

Root	Meaning
Cardi	Heart
Oste	Bone
Gastr	Stomach
Nephr	Kidney
Phleb	Vein
Trache	Trachea
Thorac	Chest

TABLE 7.2 Prefixes and Meanings

Prefix	Meaning	Example
Ambi-	Both, both sides	*Ambi*dextrous
Pre-	Before, in front of	*Pre*operative
Hypo-	Under, below	*Hypo*thermia
Epi-	Upon	*Epi*gastric
Inter-	Between	*Inter*costal
Post-	After, behind	*Post*natal

TABLE 7.3 Suffixes and Meanings

Suffix	Meaning	Example
-ectomy	Excision	Append*ectomy*
-itis	Inflammation	Periton*itis*
-centesis	Surgical puncture	Pericardio*centesis*
-meter	Instrument to measure	Thermo*meter*
-scopy	Visual examination	Broncho*scopy*
-paresis	Partial paralysis	Hemi*paresis*

TABLE 7.4 Abbreviations and Meanings

Abbreviation	Meaning
AMI	Acute myocardial infarction
ASHD	Ateriosclerotic heart disease
BP	Blood pressure
C	Centigrade
CA	Cancer
CCU	Cardiac care unit
CHF	Congestive heart failure
COPD	Chronic obstructive pulmonary disease
CSF	Cerebrospinal fluid
CVA	Cerebrovascular accident
Dx	Diagnosis
ECG	Electrocardiogram
F	Fahrenheit
Fx	Fracture
GI	Gastrointestinal
Gm	Gram
ICU	Intensive care unit
IV	Intravenous
O_2	Oxygen
RN	Registered nurse
Rx	Treatment

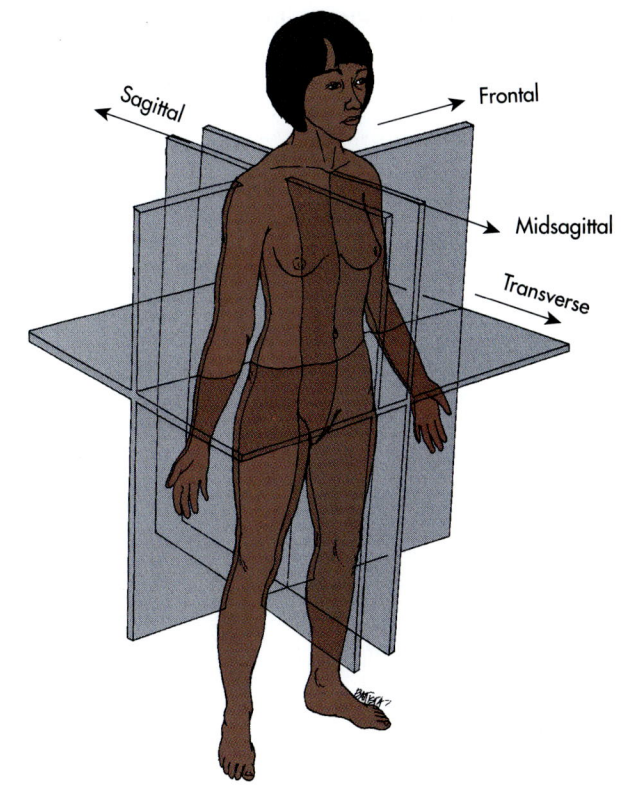

FIGURE 7.1 Anatomic position.

TABLE 7.5 Common Directional Terminology

Torso	Trunk of the body	The chest is located in the torso.
Midline	Imaginary line running vertically down the middle of the body, dividing it in half	The nose is located in the midline.
Medial	Toward the midline	The heart is medial to the right arm.
Lateral	Away from the midline	The ears are located laterally on the head.
Proximal	Closer to the trunk	The elbow is proximal to the wrist.
Distal	Farther from the trunk	The wrist is distal to the elbow.
Superior	Above	The head is superior to the shoulders.
Inferior	Below	The feet are inferior to the knees.
Midaxillary	Imaginary line running vertically from the middle of the armpit to the ankle	The midaxillary line divides the body into anterior and posterior.
Anterior	Toward the front	The abdomen is located anterior to the spine.
Posterior	Toward the rear	The spinal column is located posterior to the heart.
Midclavicular	Imaginary line drawn vertically from the middle of the clavicle to the pelvis	The nipples are located in the midclavicular line.
Bilateral	Pertaining to both sides	The patient had bilateral wrist deformities.
Dorsal	Toward the back	The buttocks are located on the dorsal side of the body.
Ventral	Toward the front	The abdomen is located on the ventral side of the body.
Palmar	Relating to the palm	The patient had a palmar wart.
Plantar	Relating to the sole of the foot	The patient had a plantar wart.
Prone	Lying face down	The patient was found prone.
Supine	Lying face up	The patient was found supine.
Fowler position	Sitting up	The patient was placed in the Fowler position on the stretcher.
Trendelenburg position	Feet up, head down	The patient was placed in the Trendelenburg position.
Apices	Plural of apex, which is the uppermost section of a structure	The uppermost portion of the liver is the apex.

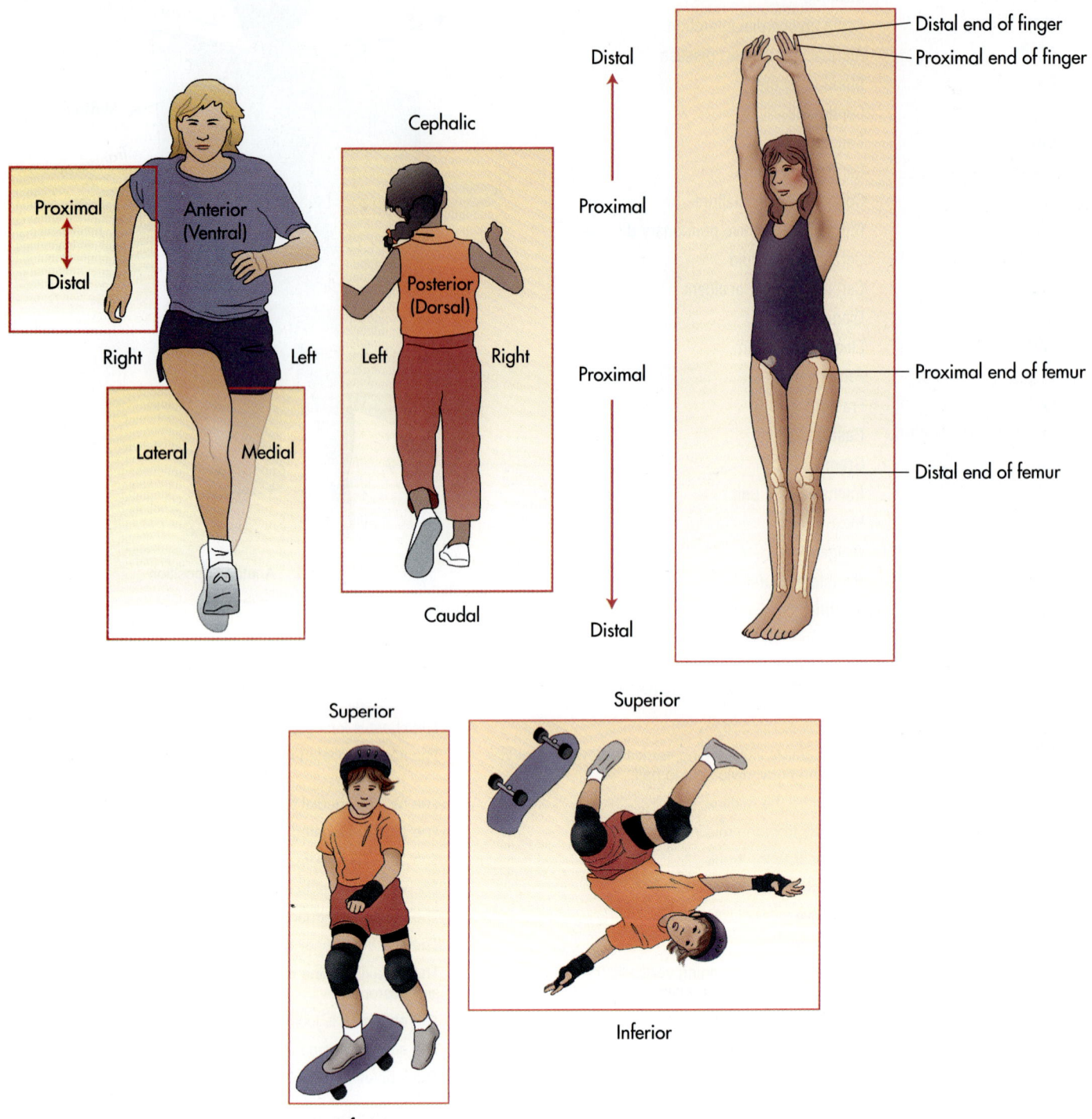

FIGURE 7.2 Common directional terms.

Joints

Joints are the points at which bones connect to other bones. **Cartilage** is located between the bones where they come together to lubricate and cushion the joint. **Ligaments** hold the bones together. There are various types of joints: ball-and-socket joint; hinged joint; pivot joint, and fused, or sutured, joint (Figure 7.4). The **ball-and-socket joint** moves freely in all directions (e.g., hip and shoulder), whereas the **hinged joint** moves in only one direction (e.g., elbow and knee). A pivot joint rotates but only on one axis (e.g., first cervical and second cervical vertebrate). A sutured joint contains bones that have minimal movement for expansion and contraction only (e.g., bones of the skull).

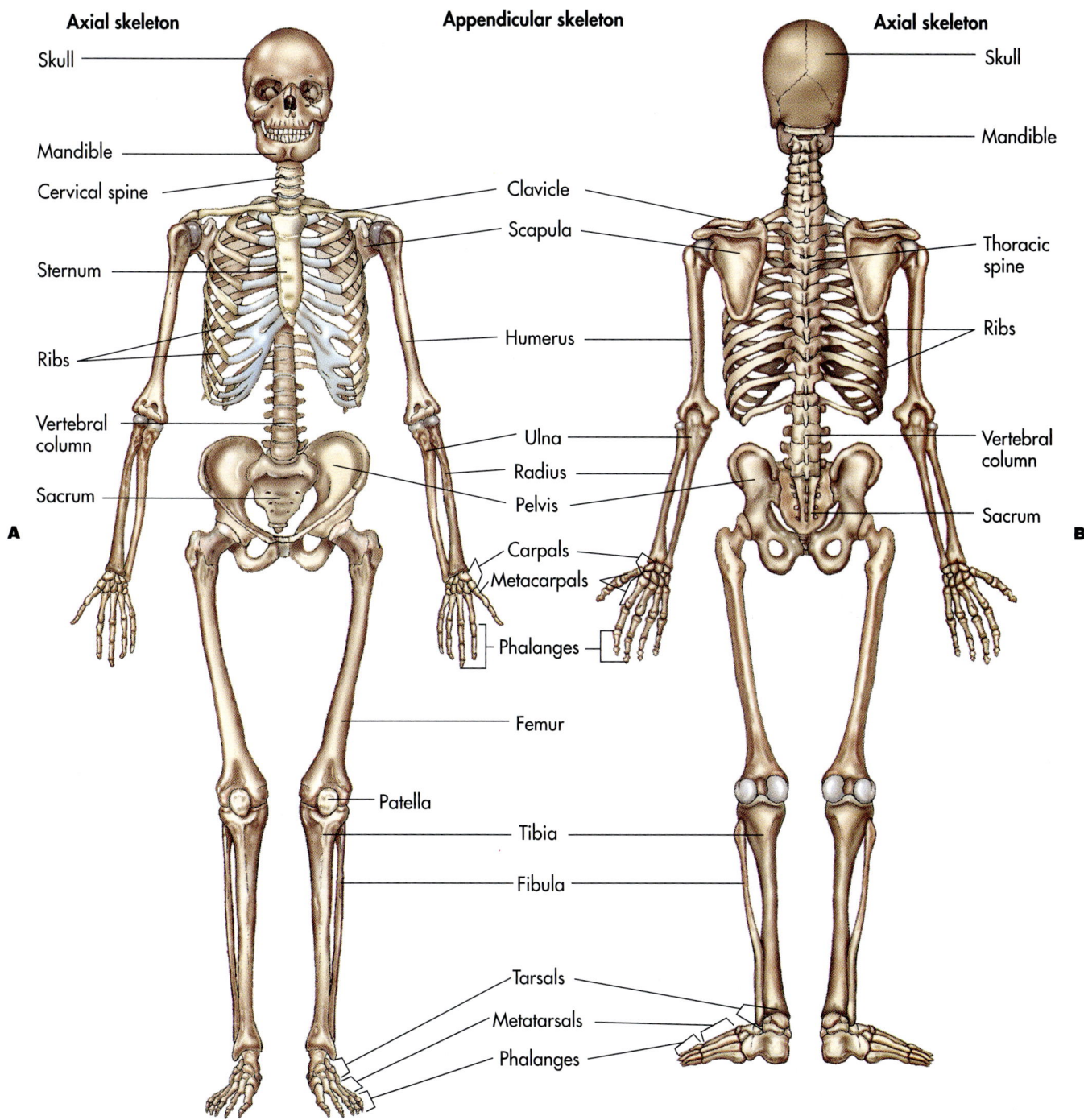

FIGURE 7.3 The skeleton. **A,** Anterior view. **B,** Posterior view.

Skull

The **skull** houses and protects the brain and is divided into four major areas (Figure 7.5):

1. **Frontal** (anterior section)
2. **Occipital** (posterior section)
3. **Temporal** (sides)
4. **Parietal** (top)

Bones of the Face

The **face** is made up of five major bones. The **nasal bone** forms the nose. Only the proximal one third of the nasal bone is actually bone; the distal two thirds are cartilage. Two **maxilla** form the upper jaw, and two **zygomatic bones** make up the cheeks. The **mandible**, or lower jaw, is the only moveable face bone. The **orbit** (eye socket) is made up of the edges of the frontal, nasal, zygoma, and maxilla bones.

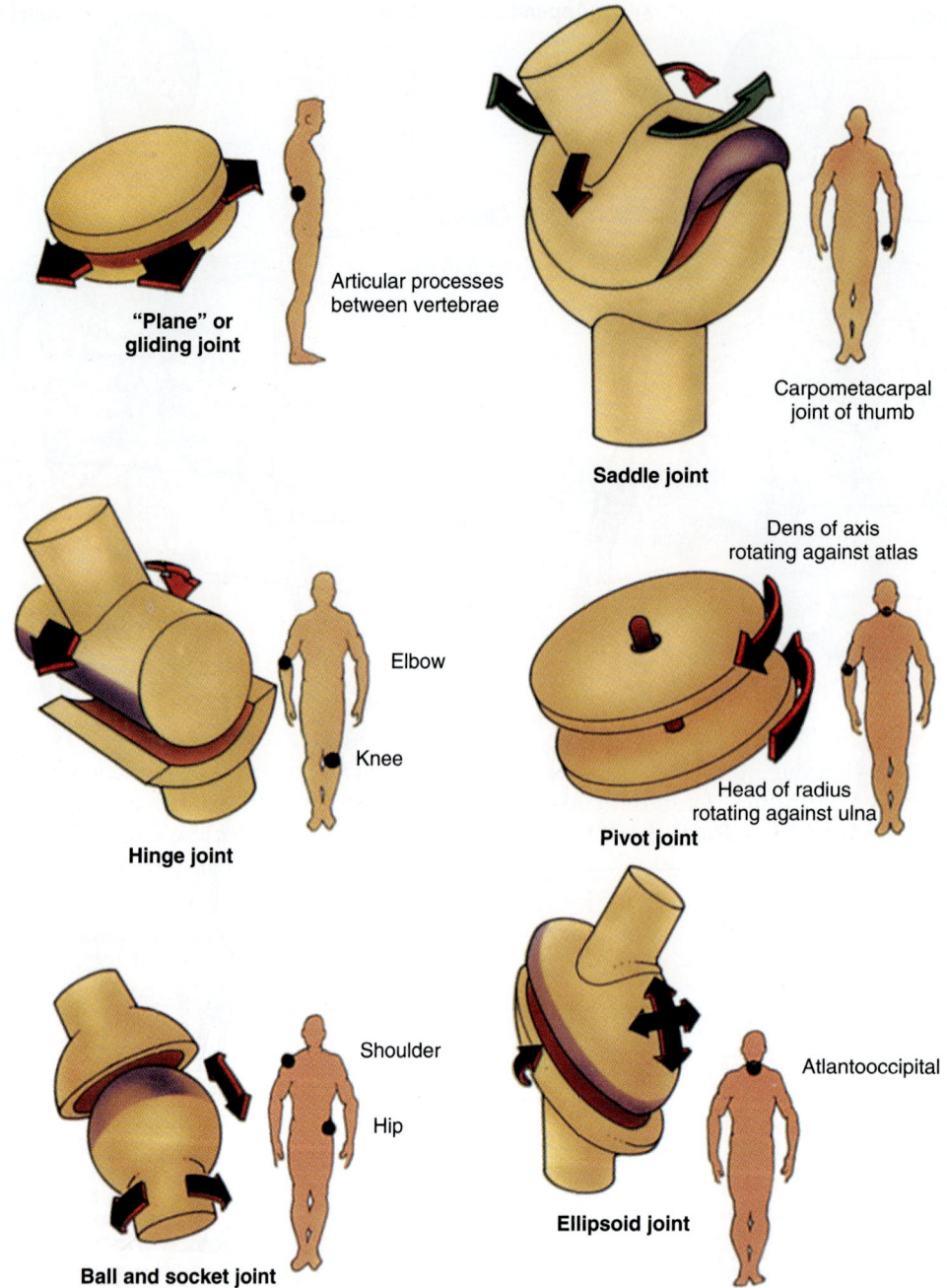

FIGURE 7.4 Different types of joints and their locations throughout the body.

Spinal Column

The spinal (vertebral) column is composed of 33 individual bones called **vertebrae** (Figure 7.6). Beginning at the proximal end of the spinal column, the first seven vertebrae are called the *cervical vertebrae*, the next 12 are called the *thoracic vertebrae*, followed by five lumbar vertebrae, five sacral vertebrae, and ending with four coccyx vertebrae. The spinal column forms the flexible backbone that supports the torso and head. It also protects the spinal cord, which is contained within a central canal created by the vertebral column. The vertebrae are separated by cartilage that cushions the vertebrae and allows the spine to move freely.

Thorax

The **thorax** consists of the **ribs**, sternum, and 12 thoracic vertebrae (Figure 7.7). Twelve pairs of ribs are attached posteriorly to the thoracic vertebrae. Of these 12 pairs,

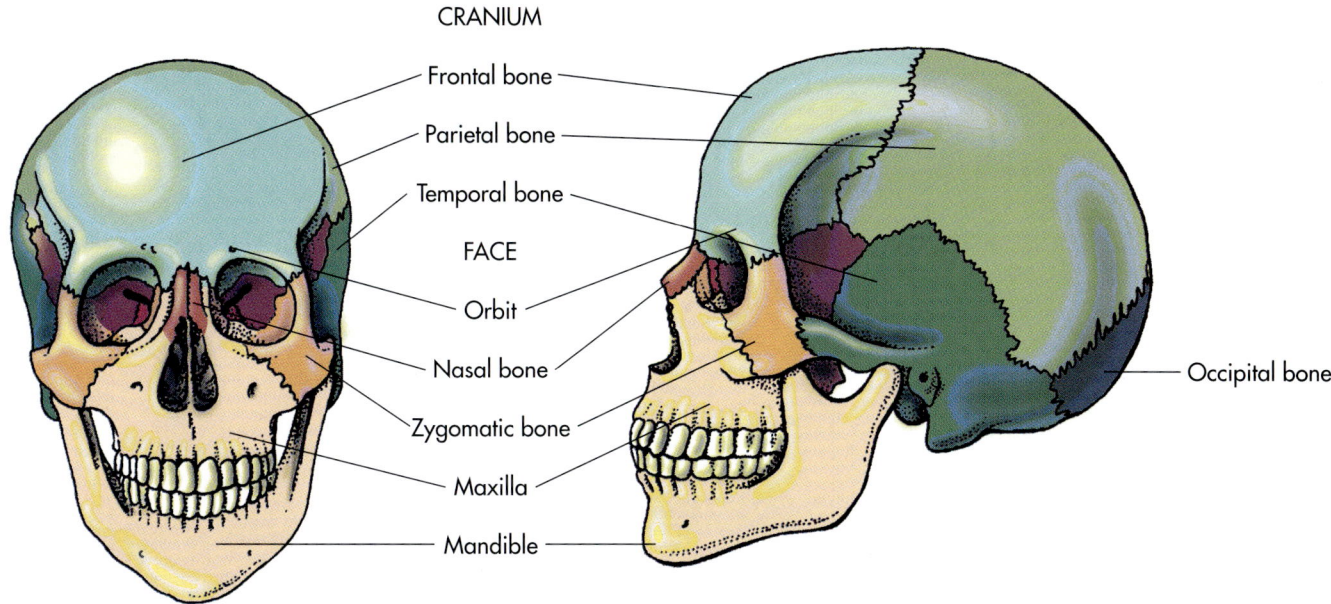

FIGURE 7.5 The skull (cranium and face).

only the upper 10 are attached anteriorly to the sternum; the lower 2 are called floating ribs because they are not attached anteriorly. The **sternum** (breastbone) is divided into three sections: **manubrium** (superior portion), body (middle portion), and **xiphoid process** (inferior portion). The major organs contained within the thorax are the heart, lungs, diaphragm, aorta, and the superior and inferior venae cavae.

Upper Extremities

Each upper extremity consists of the shoulder, arm, elbow, forearm, wrist, and hand (Figure 7.8). The shoulder is formed by three bones. The **scapula** (shoulder blade) lies on either side of the superior back. The **acromion** can be felt at the lateral edge of the shoulder. The **clavicle** (collarbone) runs from the superior sternum to the acromion and attaches the upper extremity to the torso. The bone of the upper arm is called the **humerus**, and the bones of the forearm are called the *radius* and *ulna*. The **radius** is the lateral bone of the forearm, and the **ulna** is the medial bone of the forearm. The joint where the arm and the forearm meet is called the **olecranon** (elbow). **Carpals** are the bones of the wrist, **metacarpals** are the bones of the hand, and **phalanges** are the bones of the fingers.

Pelvis

The pelvis is a cuplike structure resting at the inferior section of the torso. The **iliac crest** makes up the wings of the pelvis. The **ischium** is the lower posterior portion, and the **pubis** is the lower anterior bone that attaches in front to the pubic symphysis (Figure 7.9).

Lower Extremities

The lower extremities are made up of the femur, hip joint, patella, tibia, fibula, ankle, and foot (Figure 7.10). The bone of the thigh is called the **femur**. The **hip joint** is composed of the head of the femur (ball) and the acetabulum (socket of the hip bone). The bones of the lower leg are called the **tibia** (shin bone) and the **fibula** (lateral, smaller bone). The knee joint is where the femur and the tibia come together and are shielded by the **patella**, or kneecap. Distally, the ankle joint is made up of the medial and lateral malleolus. The **tarsals** and **metatarsals** are the bones of the foot, and the bones of the toes are called the *phalanges*.

Muscular System

The muscular system works with the skeletal system to protect the body, give it structure, and provide for movement. **Muscles** are divided into three types: voluntary, involuntary, and cardiac (Figure 7.11).

Voluntary Muscles

Voluntary muscles, also referred to as *skeletal muscles*, are attached to the bones and form the major muscle mass of the body. Voluntary muscles also make up the tongue, eyes, soft palate, pharynx, esophagus, and scalp. They are called *voluntary* because they are contracted and relaxed at the individual's will. Skeletal muscles are attached to bone by tendons. **Tendons** connect bone to muscle, creating a pull between the two bones when the muscle contracts (Figure 7.12).

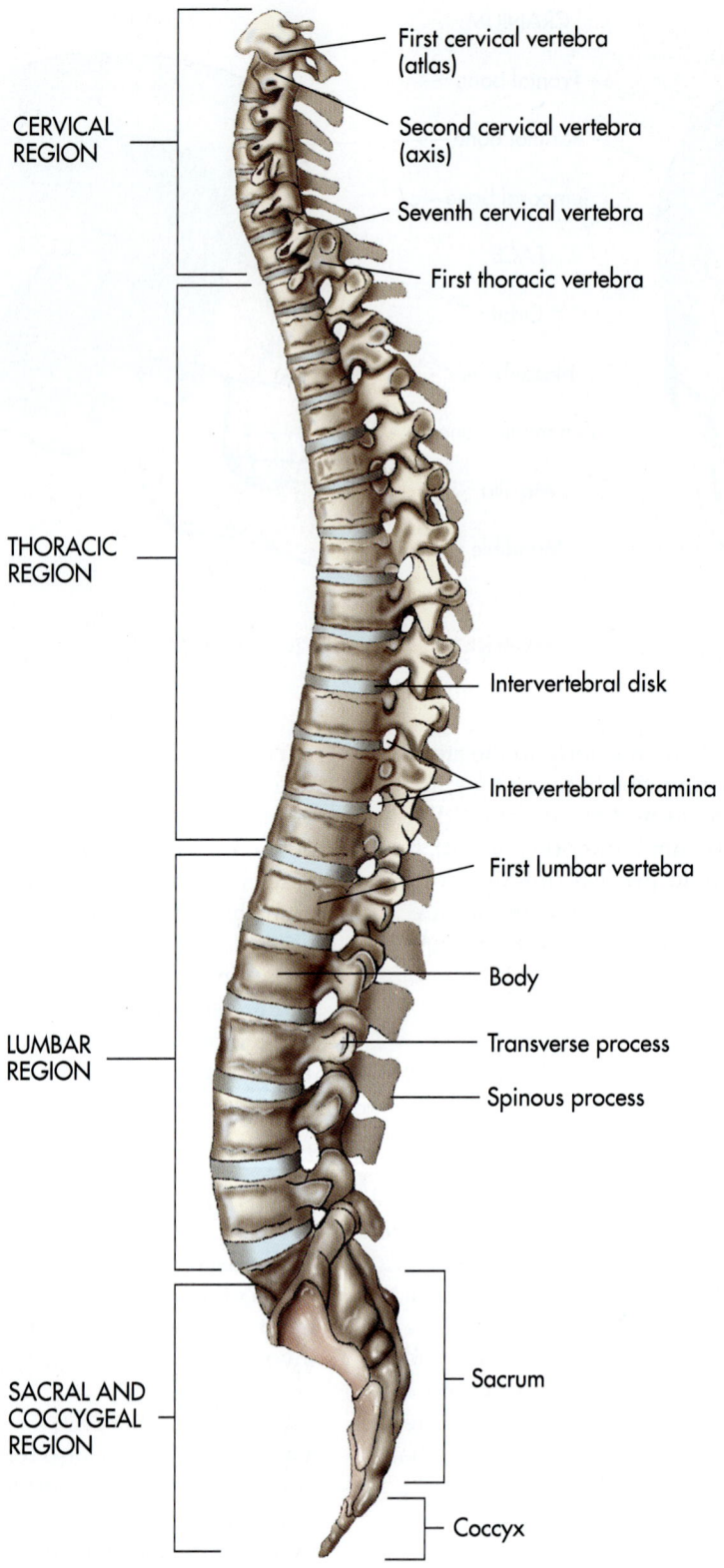

FIGURE 7.6 The vertebral column.

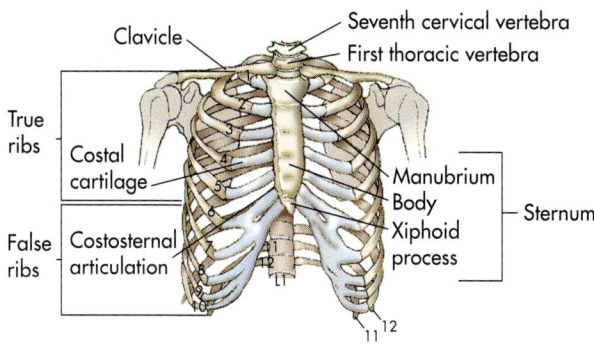

FIGURE 7.7 The thorax.

Involuntary Muscles

Involuntary muscles, also referred to as *smooth muscles*, make up the muscle structure of organs, such as the gastrointestinal (GI) tract, urinary system, blood vessels, and respiratory system. Involuntary muscles control the flow through these structures and carry out the automatic muscular functions of the body. These muscles are not under voluntary control and instead respond to nerve impulses from the nervous system.

Cardiac Muscle

Cardiac muscle is specialized muscle found only in the heart. It functions similarly to involuntary muscle in that it receives automatic stimulation from the nervous system. However, cardiac muscle is unique because it can generate its own contractions, a property known as **automaticity.** Cardiac muscle cannot tolerate interruption of the blood supply for more than a few minutes before death of the muscle occurs.

> ✓ Within the musculoskeletal system, the muscles and bones work together to give the body shape, protect vital internal organs, and provide movement.

Body Systems

Eight major systems in the body work to supply the organs with oxygen, dispose of waste, control the functions of the organs, and regulate temperature.

Respiratory System

The respiratory system carries out the critical function of supplying the body with oxygen and getting rid of carbon dioxide, a waste product generated by metabolism. **Metabolism** is a complex chemical reaction within the body that generates energy. All cells require a constant supply of oxygen to carry out metabolism.

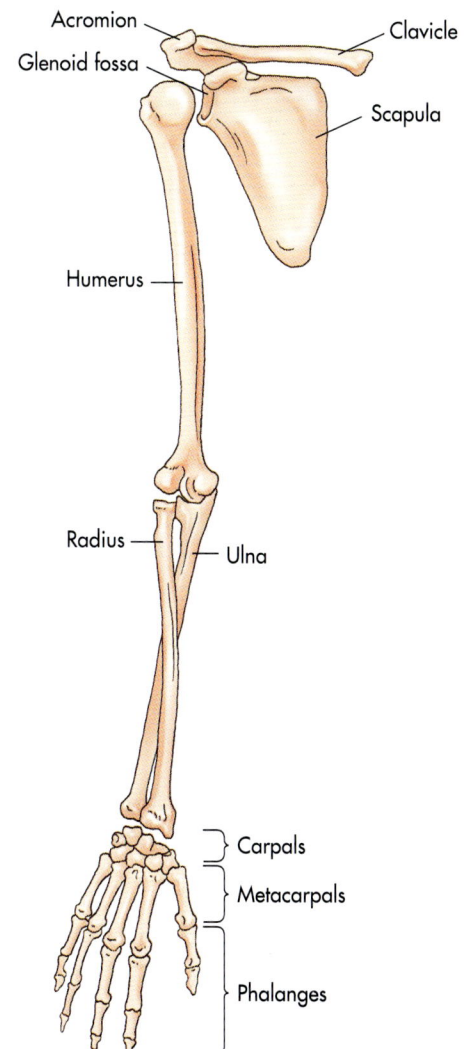

FIGURE 7.8 The upper extremity.

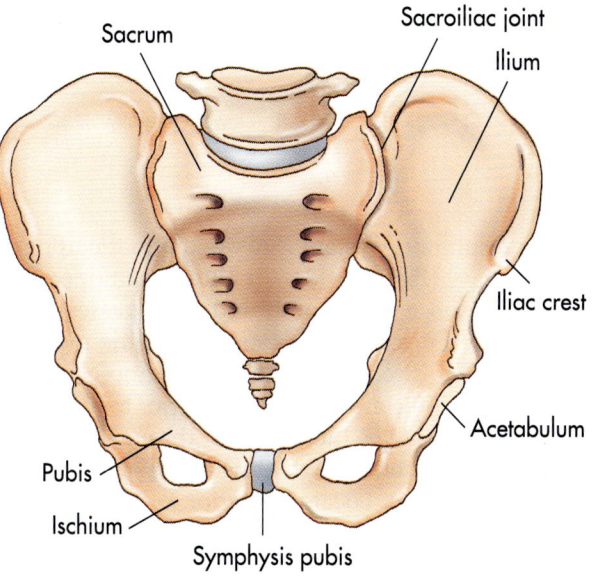

FIGURE 7.9 The bones of the pelvis.

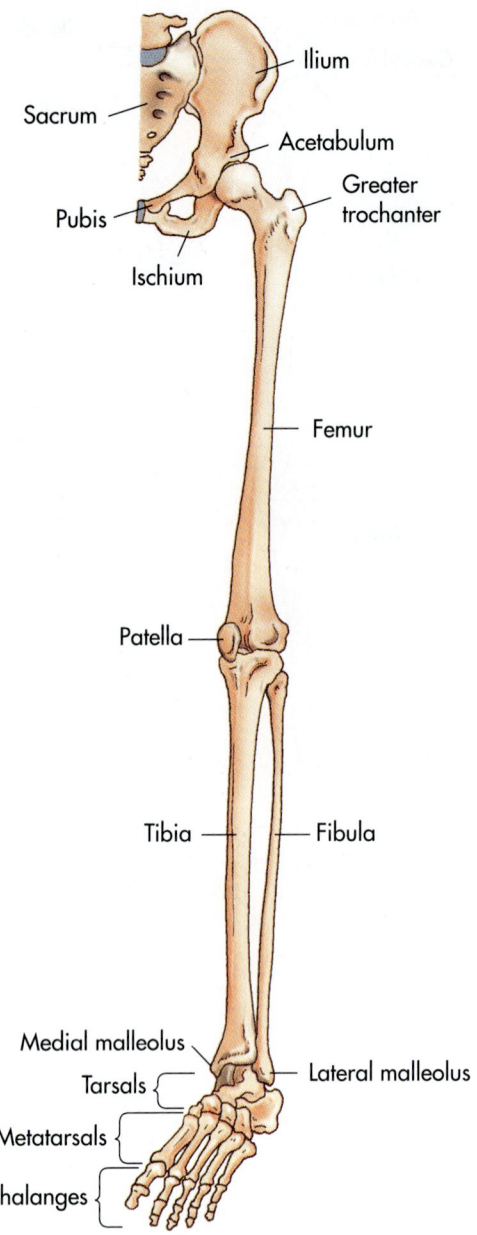

FIGURE 7.10 The lower extremity.

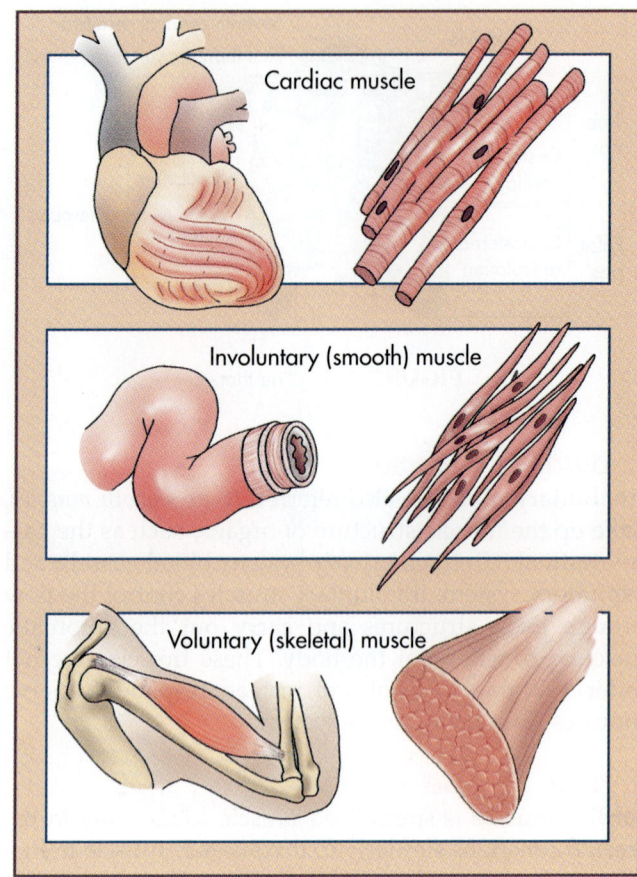

FIGURE 7.11 Types of muscle.

The respiratory system is divided into the upper and lower airways (Figure 7.13). Air enters the upper airway through the nose and mouth and then passes into the **pharynx**, the muscular tube posterior to the mouth and nose. The area directly posterior to the nose is the nasopharynx, and the area directly posterior to the mouth is the oropharynx. Air then passes through the **larynx** (voicebox) before entering the distal airway through the **trachea** (windpipe). Located anterior to the larynx is the **epiglottis**, a leaf-shaped structure that prevents food and liquids from entering the trachea during swallowing. The **vocal cords**, which produce sound, are contained within the larynx. Because air passages must be kept open at all times, the larynx and trachea are composed of cartilage rings connected by ligaments. The thyroid cartilage is the largest and most prominent of the cartilage rings that make up the larynx. The cricoid ring is the cartilage ring that forms the lower portion of the larynx. It is the first ring of the proximal portion of the trachea. The trachea is 4 to 5 inches long and extends from the larynx (distally to the proximal end, the carina) (Figure 7.14).

The trachea divides at the **carina** into two smaller tubes called the **bronchi**, with one bronchus going to each lung. Air moves into the bronchus, which subdivides into smaller tubes within each lung called *bronchioles*, and finally into the alveoli. The **alveoli** are tiny, thin, grapelike clusters contained within the lungs. The alveoli are surrounded by capillaries, which bring oxygen-poor blood to the alveoli. Here carbon dioxide is removed and the blood is resaturated with oxygen. Together, the bronchi, bronchioles, and alveoli make up the lungs. **Lungs** sit on either side of the heart within the rib cage. The lungs are bound superiorly by the clavicles and inferiorly by the **diaphragm**, a dome-shaped muscle used

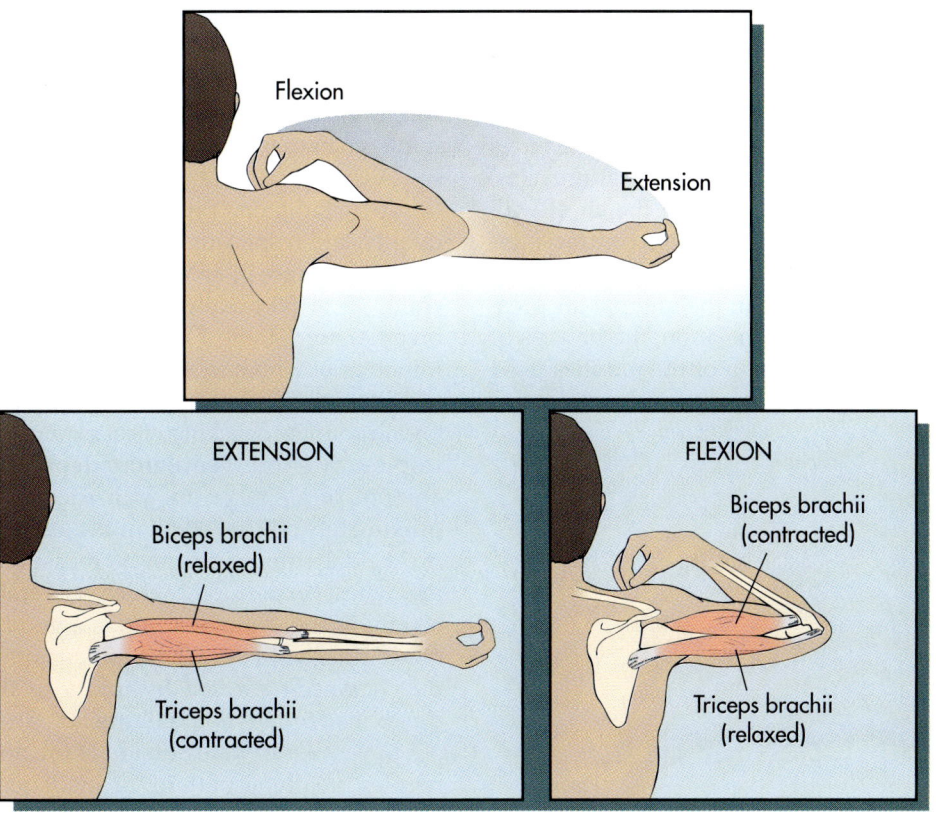

FIGURE 7.12 Voluntary (skeletal) muscle.

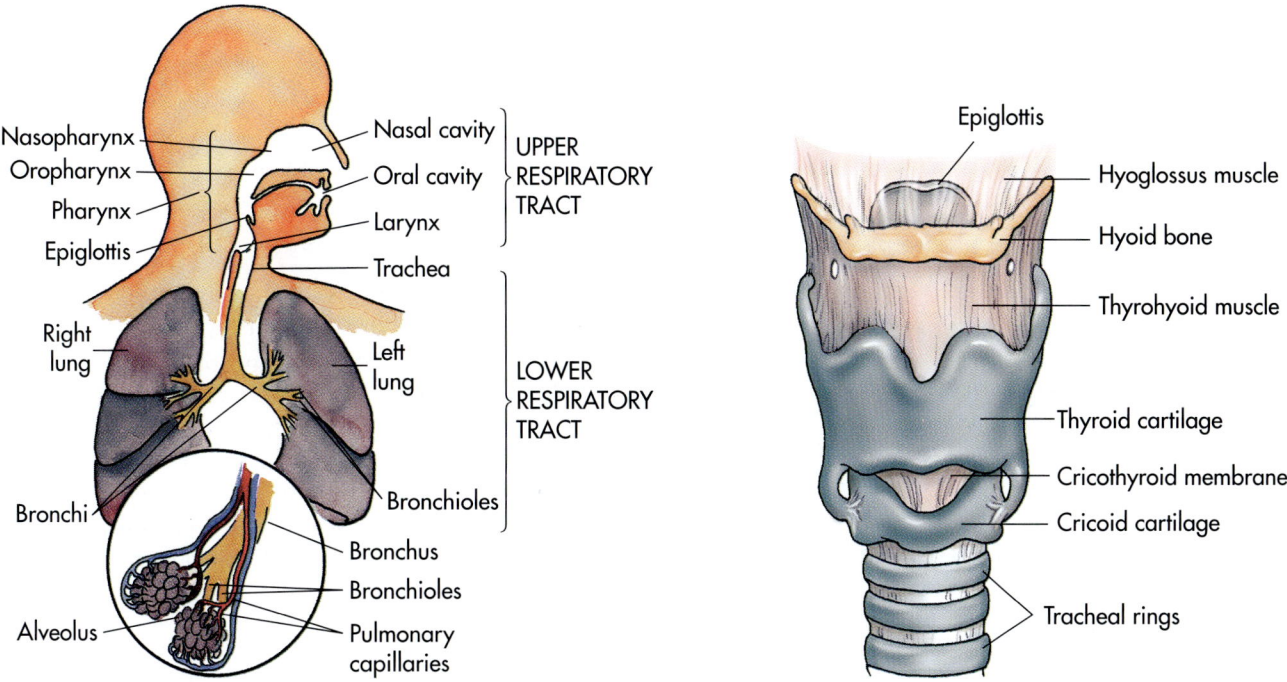

FIGURE 7.13 The upper and lower airways.

FIGURE 7.14 The thyroid and cricoid cartilages.

during respiration. The exterior of the lungs is wrapped with a thin membrane, the **visceral pleura**, which is in contact with the interior lining of the chest wall, the **parietal pleura**. Between the two pleura is a lubricating pleural fluid that prevents friction during respiration (Figure 7.15).

Inhalation is the process of drawing air into the lungs (Figure 7.16). During inhalation the **intercostal muscles**, found between the ribs, contract, pulling the chest wall upward and outward. The diaphragm also contracts, increasing the space in the chest cavity. Because the external air pressure is now greater than the internal air pressure, air rushes into the lungs. Exhalation, the process of air leaving the lungs, is a relaxation of the muscles used for inhalation. As the size of the chest decreases, air is exhaled from the lungs. Respiration is controlled by the central nervous system, which monitors the oxygen and carbon dioxide levels in the blood using sensors located in the aorta, carotid arteries, and brain. In a healthy person, these sensors use the carbon dioxide level to determine when to breathe.

Assessing a patient's breathing requires a determination of ventilatory rate, respiratory rhythm, respiratory quality, and respiratory depth (tidal volume). The normal **ventilatory rate** in an adult is 12 to 20 breaths/min; in a child, 15 to 30 breaths/min; and in an infant, 25 to 50 breaths/min (Table 7.6). **Ventilatory rhythm** is a determination of whether breathing is regular or irregular. The EMT-B measures **ventilatory quality** by listening to breath sounds, checking chest expansion, and monitoring respiratory effort. **Ventilatory depth (tidal volume)** is the amount of air taken in with each breath, which is approximately 500 to 700 ml in the average adult. Although exact tidal volume cannot be measured in the field, normal chest expansion, which generates approximately 600 ml in the average adult, is a good indication of adequate tidal volume. Chest expansion that is shallow or that has been affected by injury to the chest wall produces inadequate tidal volume.

A ventilatory rate outside of the normal ranges, an irregular breathing pattern, or inadequate depth are indications of inadequate breathing. Additionally, inadequate breathing should be suspected if the breath sounds are diminished or absent, chest expansion is unequal or inadequate, or there is an increased effort to breath.

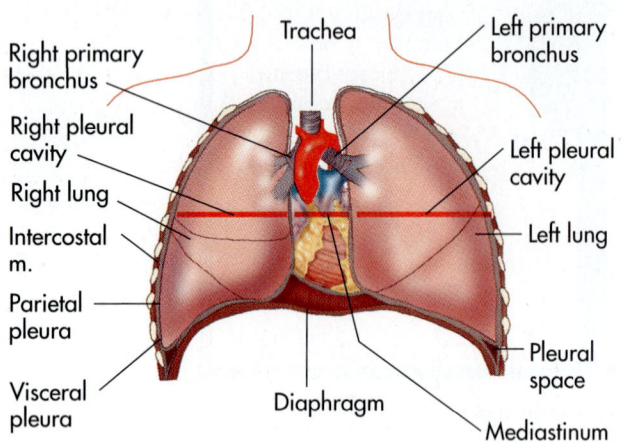

FIGURE 7.15 The lungs and pleura.

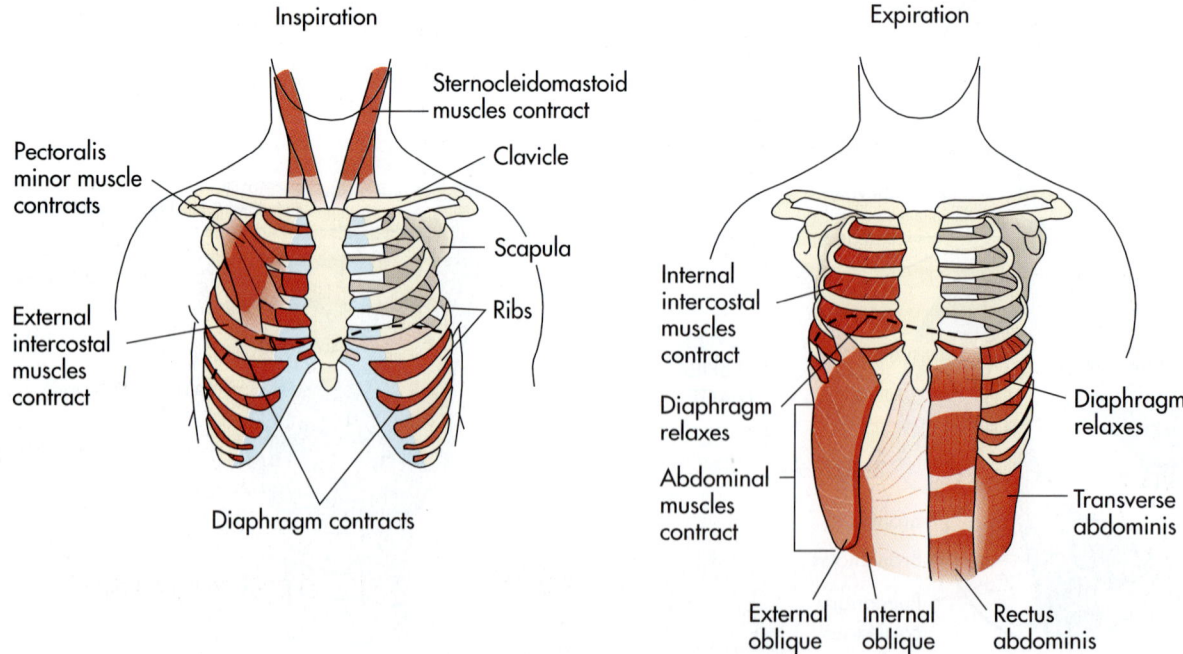

FIGURE 7.16 The mechanics of breathing.

In infants and children, the structures of the mouth and nose are smaller and are therefore easily obstructed. The trachea is narrower, softer, and more flexible than in adults, and infants and children depend more heavily on the diaphragm for breathing because their chest walls are softer.

> ✓ The respiratory system is divided into the upper and lower airways and provides the mechanism for bringing oxygen into the system and expelling carbon dioxide. Adequate ventilation is critical to sustaining life, so early identification of the patient with respiratory difficulty is important.

Cardiovascular System

The cardiovascular system transports oxygen and nutrients to the tissues and removes waste products to be excreted from the body through the lungs. The three major components of the cardiovascular system are the heart, **blood,** and blood vessels. As the centerpiece of the cardiovascular system, the heart functions as a pump that keeps blood moving throughout the body (Figure 7.17).

The **heart** is made up of three layers: the **epicardium** (outer layer), **myocardium** (middle layer), and **endocardium** (inner layer). The myocardium is the actual muscle that contracts. A thin sac, called the **pericardium**, surrounds and protects the heart. The heart is supplied with oxygenated blood by the coronary arteries. In an average adult the heart beats 60 to 80 times per minute, but this rate may be affected by such factors as conditioning, medications, and age.

The heart is located between the sternum and the spine, just lateral to the midline. The heart is divided into four chambers. The two superior chambers are the right and left **atria**, and the two inferior chambers are the right and left **ventricles**. The right atrium receives oxygen-poor blood from the body and pumps it to the right ventricle, where it is pumped out to the lungs through the pulmonary arteries. Oxygen-rich blood returns from the lungs through the pulmonary veins and enters the left atrium. The blood is then pumped into the left ventricle and out to the body through the aorta. Valves guard the entrances and exits of each of the chambers to prevent backflow and to keep the blood moving in the right direction.

The heart is composed of specialized muscle tissue (cardiac muscle) that generates its own electrical impulses. Heart muscle fibers conduct electrical impulses that cause them to contract. Contraction of the heart pumps the blood throughout the body.

Three major types of vessels carry blood: arteries, veins, and capillaries (Figure 7.18). **Arteries** always carry blood away from the heart to the rest of the body. With the exception of the pulmonary artery, arteries always carry oxygen-rich blood. The **coronary arteries** supply the heart muscle with oxygenated blood. The **aorta** is the largest artery, originating from the heart and descending down into the abdominal cavity where it divides into the iliac arteries at the level of the navel (Figure 7.19). The **carotid arteries** originate from the aorta to supply the head with blood. These major arteries of the neck can be palpated on either side of the trachea. The lower extremities receive blood from the **femoral arteries**, the major arteries of the thighs. The femoral artery can be palpated in the groin at the crease between the abdomen and the

TABLE 7.6 Normal Ventilatory Rates

Age Group	Normal Ventilatory Rate
Adult	12-20 breaths/min
Child	15-30 breaths/min
Infant	25-50 breaths/min

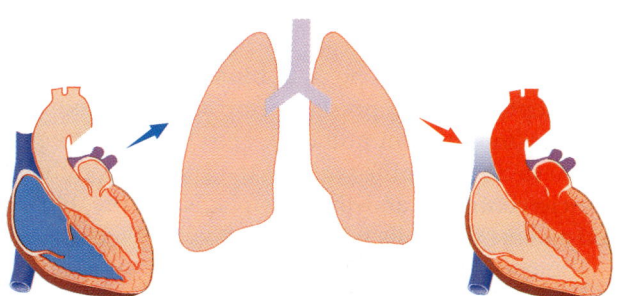

FIGURE 7.17 Internal anatomy of the heart.

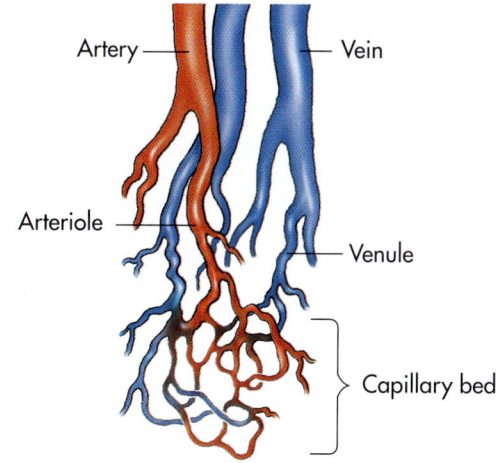

FIGURE 7.18 Arteries, capillaries, and veins.

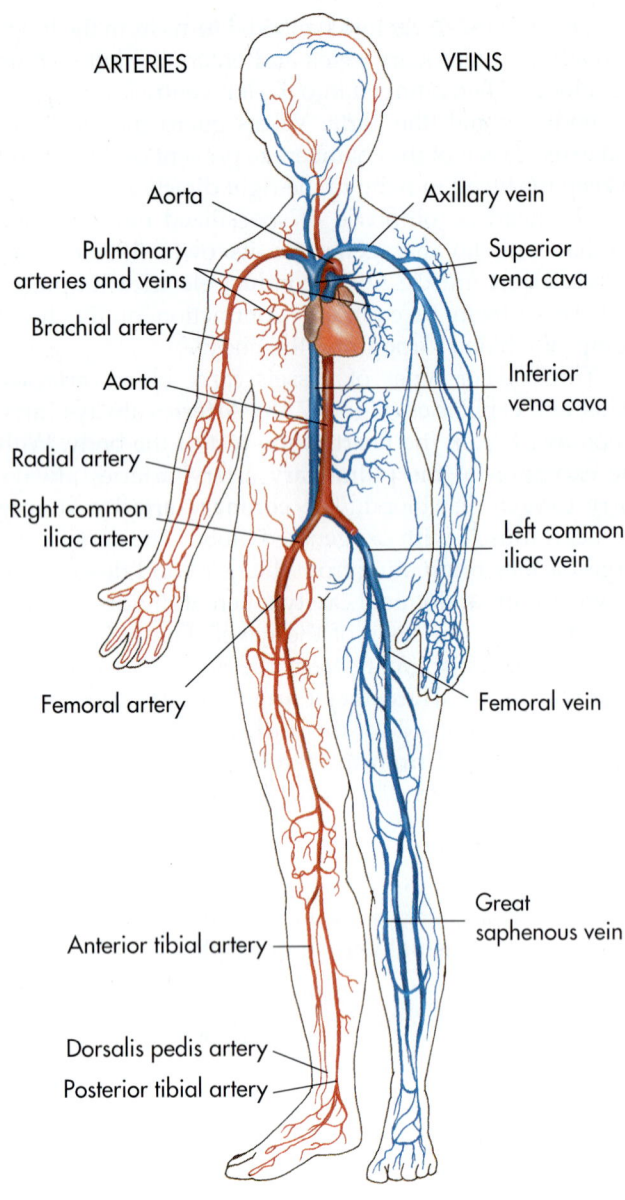

FIGURE 7.19 Major arteries and veins.

thigh. The major artery of the upper arm is the **brachial artery**, which can be felt on the medial aspect of the arm between the elbow and the shoulder. The brachial artery is the primary site at which to measure a patient's blood pressure. The **radial artery** is the major vessel in the lower arm. The radial artery is a common site at which to check a patient's pulse, which can be felt on the thumb side of the anterior aspect of the wrist. In the foot, pulses can be palpated at the posterior tibia, located on the posterior surface of the medial malleolus (ankle), or the dorsalis pedis, located on the anterior surface of the foot.

Arteries subdivide into smaller vessels called *arterioles*, then into capillaries. **Capillaries** are small vessels in which the exchange of nutrients and waste products takes place at the cellular level. Capillaries are located in all parts of the body. Blood flows from the capillaries into the venules, and then into the veins for the journey back to the heart. **Veins** always carry blood back to the heart. With the exception of the pulmonary veins, veins always carry oxygen-poor blood. Blood in veins is not under as much pressure as blood in the arteries because of the distance it has traveled from the heart. Because of this lack of pressure, valves are necessary in the veins to keep the blood from backing up. Two major veins of the body are the **venae cavae**, which deliver oxygen-poor blood from the body into the right atrium. The venae cavae are divided into the superior vena cava, which receives blood from the head and upper extremities, and the inferior vena cava, which receives blood from the torso and lower extremities. **Blood vessels** have the ability to dilate and constrict based on the physiologic needs of the body.

Pulmonary circulation involves the pulmonary arteries, pulmonary veins, and capillaries that surround the alveoli. The **pulmonary arteries** carry carbon dioxide and other waste products to the lungs to be eliminated. The **pulmonary veins** carry oxygen-enriched blood back to the heart to be pumped throughout the body. The exchange of carbon dioxide/waste products and oxygen occurs between the alveoli and the capillaries.

Blood is composed of plasma and three types of cells: red blood cells (**erythrocytes**), white blood cells (**leukocytes**), and platelets (thrombocytes). **Plasma** is a liquid in which the blood cells and nutrients are suspended. Red blood cells make up the largest component of the cell content in blood and are responsible for carrying oxygen and carbon dioxide to and from the tissues. Red blood cells contain a protein called **hemoglobin**, which binds with oxygen to carry it to the tissues. White blood cells exist to fight infection and to establish immunity against certain diseases. **Platelets** are specialized cells that are necessary for the formation of clots, a process that is initiated when the platelets come in contact with a surface other than the normal lining of the blood vessel.

The adult body contains approximately 5 to 6 liters of blood, whereas children have approximately 80 ml of blood for each kilogram of weight. The pulse is generated when the left ventricle contracts, sending a wave of blood through the body, and can be palpated anywhere an artery passes over a bone. The **blood pressure** has two components: **systolic pressure** (top number) and **diastolic pressure** (bottom number). The systolic is the pressure exerted against the walls of the artery when the left ventricle contracts, and the diastolic is the pressure exerted against the walls when the left ventricle is at rest.

The components of the cardiovascular system work together to ensure adequate perfusion of oxygenated blood and other nutrients to the tissues and the elimina-

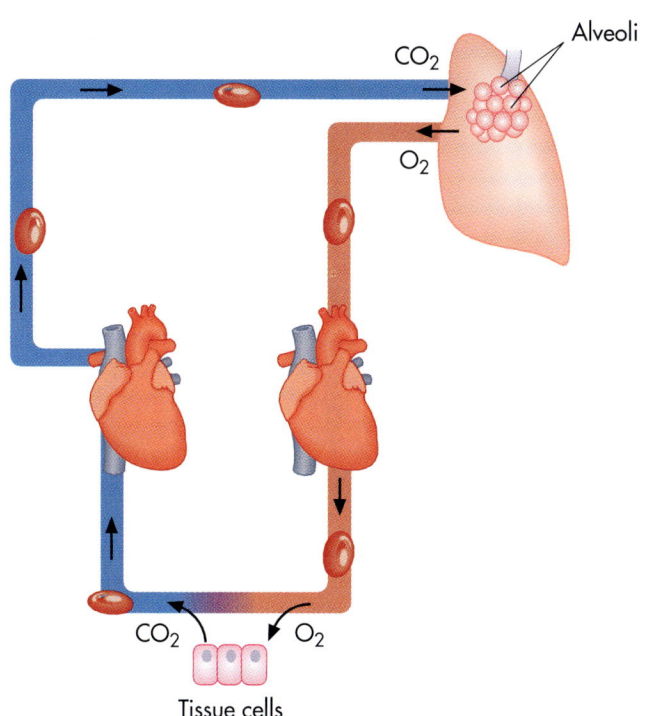

FIGURE 7.20 Main components of the cardiovascular system.

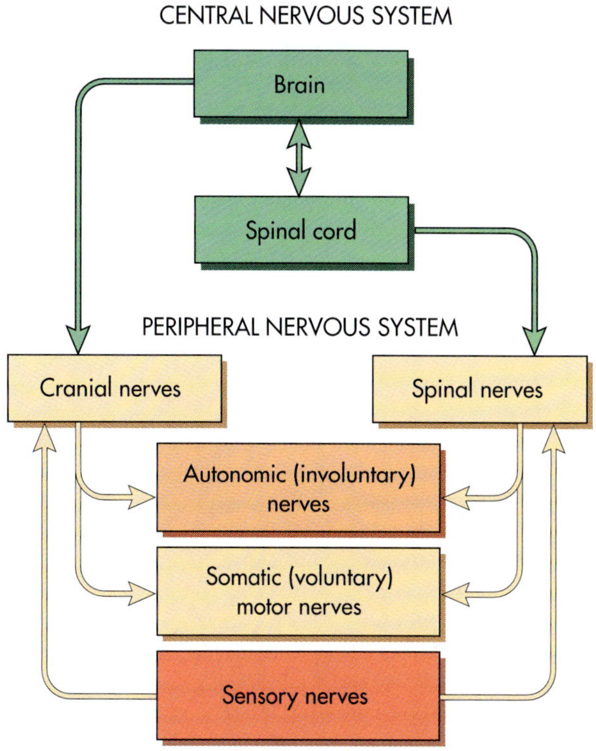

FIGURE 7.21 Divisions of the nervous system.

tion of waste (Figure 7.20). **Perfusion** is the circulation of blood through an organ or structure. When something occurs that prevents circulation, shock (hypoperfusion) can occur. Shock is a serious complication and is addressed in Chapter 9.

> ✓ The cardiovascular system is made up of three major components: the heart, blood, and blood vessels. They work together to adequately perfuse the tissues and to eliminate waste.

Nervous System

The nervous system is the control center of the body, evaluating internal and external stimuli and directing body functions in response to these stimuli. The nervous system has two divisions: the central nervous system and the peripheral nervous system (Figure 7.21). The **central nervous system** is composed of the brain and spinal cord. Together, these structures serve as the command center of the body. The **peripheral nervous system** is composed of the nerves that carry messages to and from the central nervous system. The peripheral nervous system has two types of nerves: sensory and motor. Sensory nerves carry messages from the body to the central nervous system. Motor nerves carry messages from the central nervous system to the body (Figure 7.22, A).

The nervous system performs both voluntary and involuntary functions. Involuntary functions, such as respiration, circulation, and digestion, are carried out by the autonomic nervous system (Figure 7.22, B). The **autonomic nervous system** is divided into two sections, sympathetic and parasympathetic, which have opposite effects on the organs. For instance, the **sympathetic nervous system** speeds up heart rate, and the **parasympathetic nervous system** slows down heart rate, depending on the needs of the body.

> ✓ The nervous system consists of a command center called the *central nervous system*, the brain and spinal cord, and a communications network called the *peripheral nervous system*. Together, they work to keep the body in balance by evaluating internal and external stimuli and controlling the body's responses to these

The brain, or the "hub" of the nervous system, can be separated into three parts, **brain stem**, **cerebellum**, and

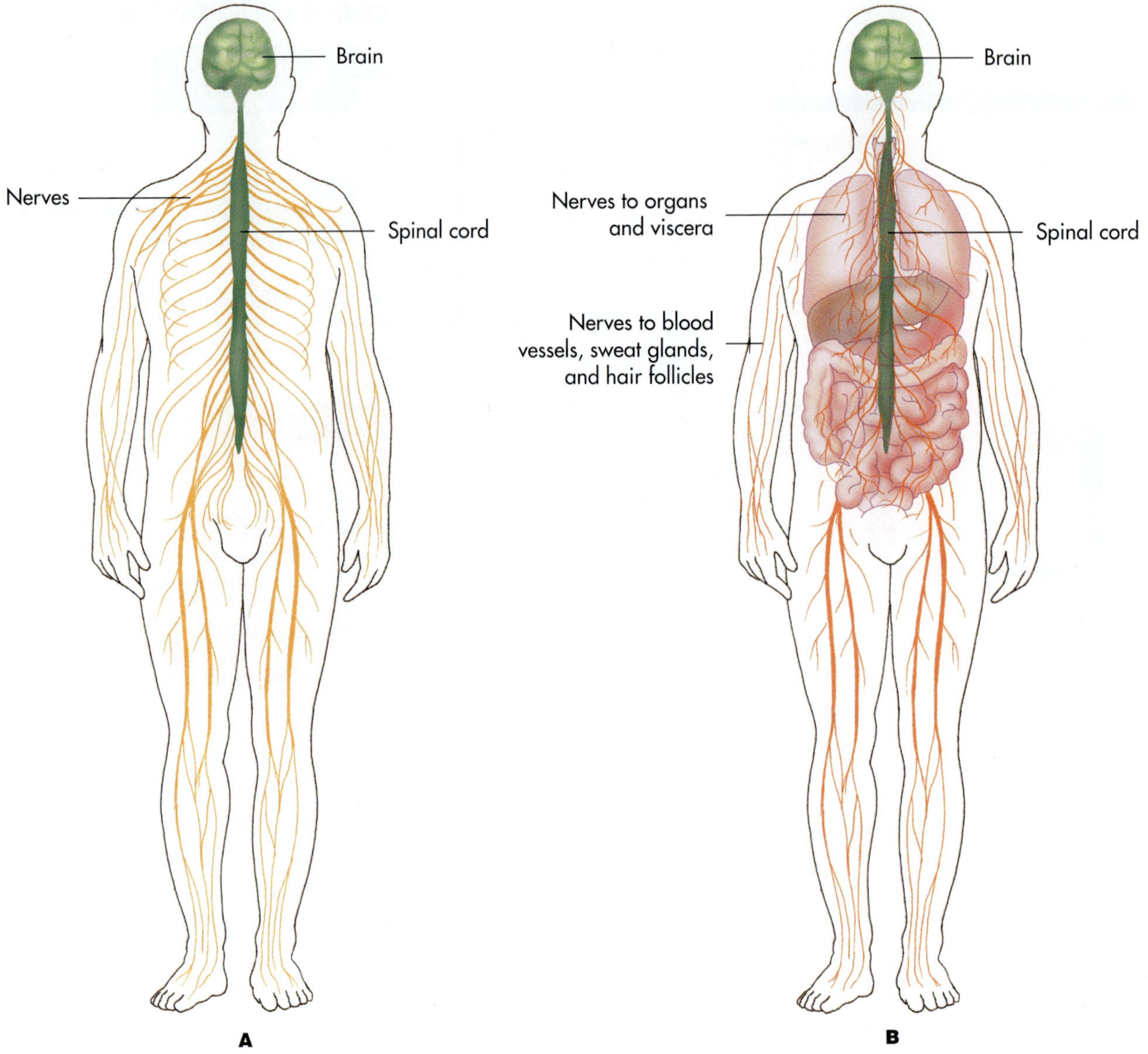

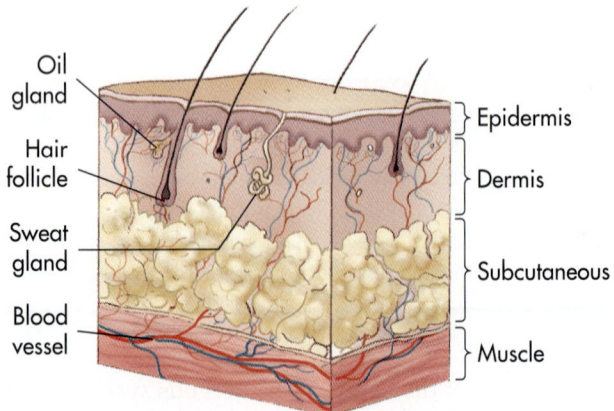

FIGURE 7.22 **A,** The central nervous system consists of the brain (cerebrum, cerebellum, and brain stem) and spinal cord. The nerves make up the peripheral nervous system. **B,** Some of the autonomic nerves, their locations, and their functions.

FIGURE 7.23 The layers of the skin.

cerebrum. Each of these portions of the brain controls different levels of body functions, from basic life functions to complex motor coordination (Box 7.1)

Integumentary System

The skin, also referred to as the **integumentary system,** is the largest organ of the body. The skin protects the body from the external environment (Figure 7.23). It keeps out bacteria and other harmful microorganisms, helps regulate the temperature of the body, prevents water loss, and allows for the transmission of sensations through the motor nerves to the central nervous system. The skin is

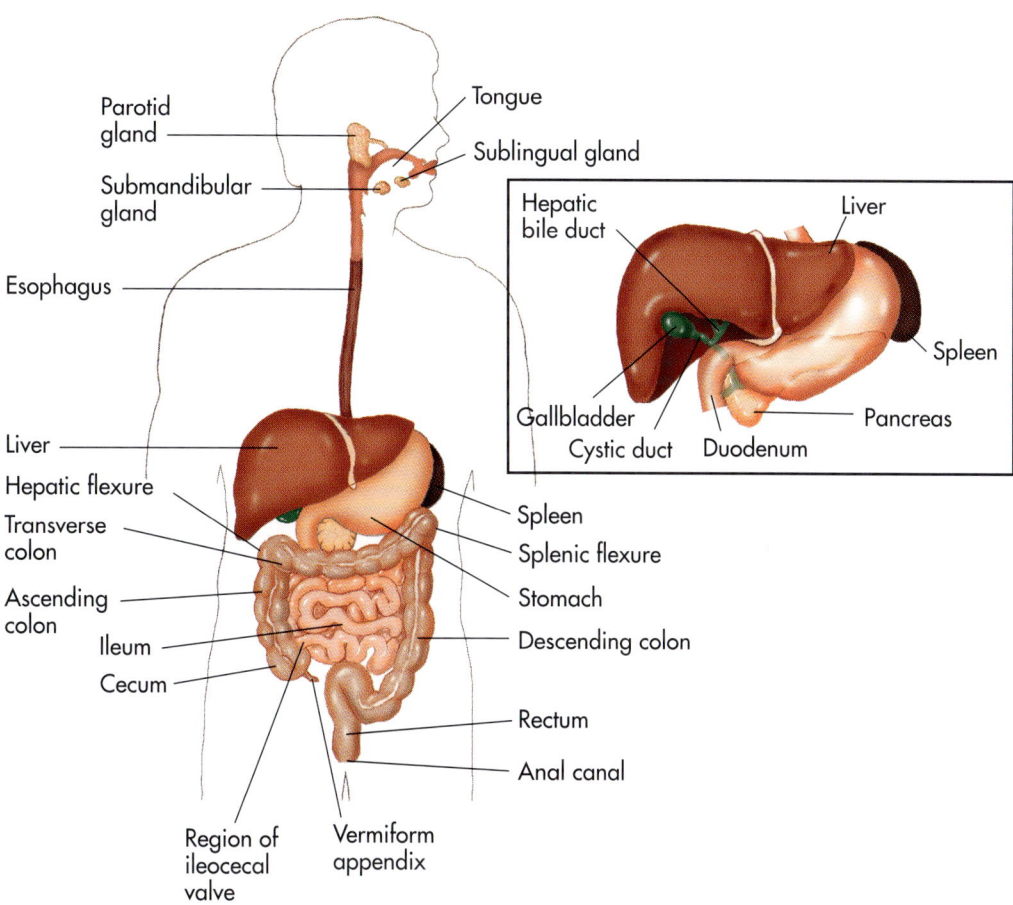

FIGURE 7.24 The digestive system.

made up of three layers: epidermis, dermis, and subcutaneous layer. The **epidermis** is the outermost layer of skin and consists primarily of dead cells, which provide a waterproof barrier. The next layer is the **dermis**, which contains the sweat glands, sebaceous (oil) glands, hair follicles, blood vessels, and nerve endings. The dermis rests on a **subcutaneous tissue** layer, which is made up of adipose (fat) and connective tissue.

✓ The skin covers the body and protects it from the environment, helps regulate the temperature of the body, and transmits sensory information to the central nervous system.

Digestive System

The digestive system processes solids and liquids once they are taken in through the month. It is where food is broken down to provide nourishment at the cell level. This system transcends the oral, thoracic, abdominal, and pelvic cavities. Food is taken into the mouth, passed through the **esophagus** to the stomach, and then passed through the **small intestine** and **large intestine**. Eventually, solid waste is excreted through the **colon** and rectum (Figure 7.24).

> **Box 7.1 Three Main Components of the Brain**
>
> **Brain stem.** Controls basic functions necessary for life, such as breathing and other involuntary bodily functions.
>
> **Cerebrum.** Has numerous functions, including sensory, motor, emotional, and intellectual processes.
>
> **Cerebellum.** Coordinates all activity of the brain. It "fine tunes" all brain functions, making skills that require multiple functions possible (e.g., hand-eye coordination).

Endocrine System

The endocrine system secretes chemicals, called **hormones,** from glands directly into the bloodstream. These

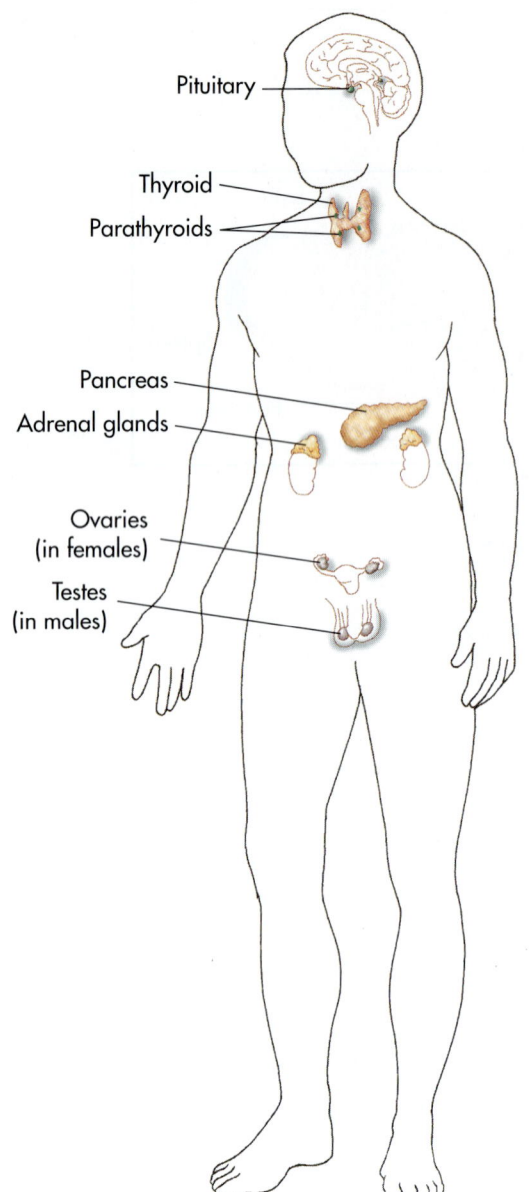

FIGURE 7.25 The location of the endocrine glands in the body.

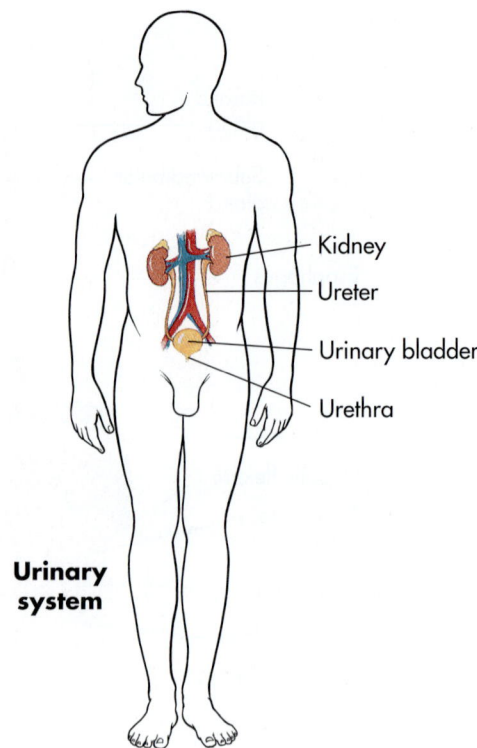

FIGURE 7.26 The kidney with the renal vein, renal artery, and ureter.

✓ The endocrine system secretes hormones necessary to maintain the balance of the body, regulate growth, produce energy, respond to stress, and reproduce.

hormones regulate body activities and functions (Figure 7.25). Hormones are secreted from endocrine glands directly into the bloodstream. The circulatory system delivers the hormones wherever they are needed to regulate growth, produce energy, maintain fluid balance, respond to stress, and manage reproductive functions. Two major hormones are epinephrine (adrenalin) and insulin. Epinephrine enhances the activity of the sympathetic nervous system and is produced in times of stress. Insulin is produced by the pancreas and metabolizes glucose, which is necessary for the production of energy.

Renal System

The renal system collects waste products from the blood stream and excretes them through the renal, or urinary, system. As blood flows into the kidneys through the renal artery, waste products are collected and the "clean" blood is returned from the kidney to the rest of the body through the renal vein. The **kidney** processes the waste product and excretes it through the **ureter** and, eventually, the **urethra** (Figure 7.26)

Reproductive System

The male and female reproductive systems are contained in the pelvic cavity. The female ovaries, fallopian tubes, uterus, and vagina make up the reproductive system. The **ovaries** are where the female's egg is formed (Figure 7.27, *A*).

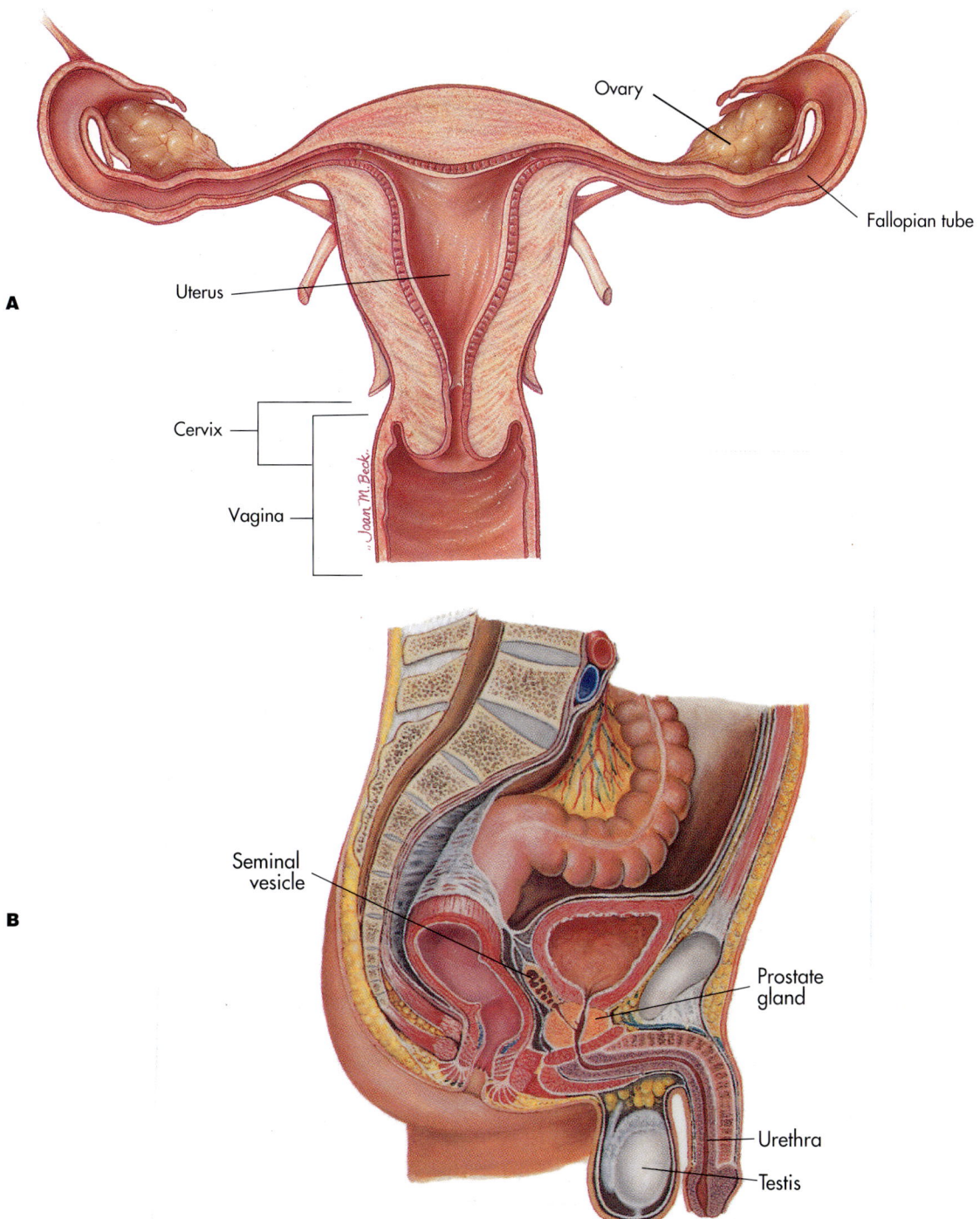

FIGURE 7.27 **A,** Female reproductive system. **B,** Male reproductive system.

The male **testes**, or gonads, are where spermatozoa is created. The rest of the reproductive system is made up of ducts and accessory glands. Externally, the male penis and the scrotum, which contains the testes, are also part of the male reproductive system (Figure 7.27, *B*).

Body Cavities

All of the body systems mentioned previously are contained in various cavities of the body. These systems typically transverse more than one body cavity. A system

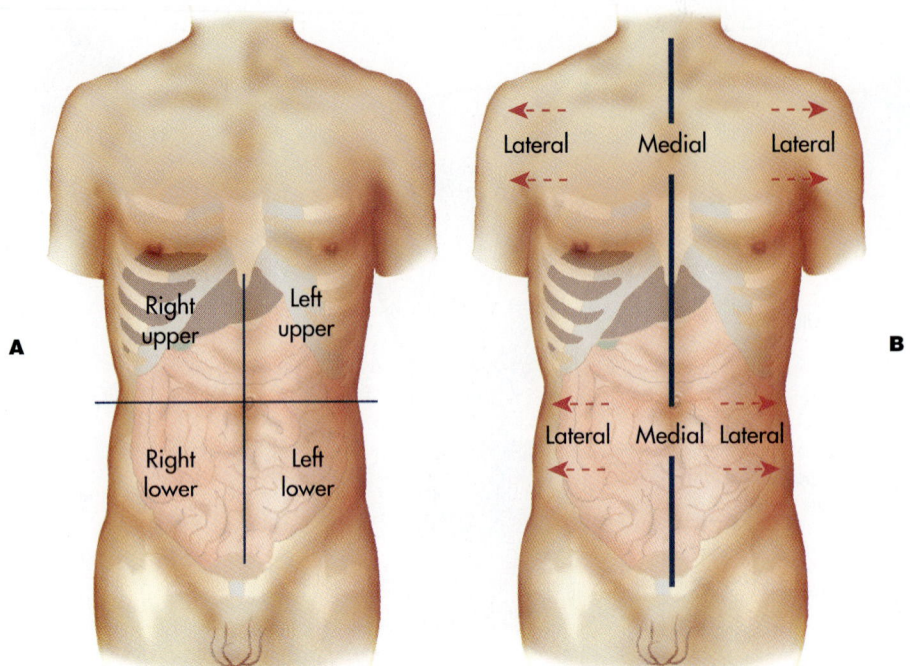

FIGURE 7.28 **A,** The abdomen is divided into four quadrants. **B,** The abdomen can also be divided into lateral and medial portions.

such as the nervous system runs through multiple body cavities.

Skull Cavity

The skull cavity is the area that lies directly beneath the skull bone. The various parts of the brain (cerebrum, cerebellum, and brain stem) fill the skull cavity. Covering the brain is the cerebral cortex. The cerebral cortex is the surface between the brain and the skull. The areas of the cerebrum, or lobes, coincide with the like names of the skull bone areas:

1. Frontal (anterior section)
2. Occipital (posterior section)
3. Temporal (sides)
4. Parietal (top)

Thoracic Cavity

The thoracic cavity lies inferior to the clavical bones and immediately superior to the abdominal cavity and contains the vital organs for circulation and respiration. The thoracic cavity is protected by the ribs anteriorly and medially and by the spinal column and scapulae posteriorly. The diaphragm muscle, which assists with inspiration, is at the base of the thoracic cavity. Imaginary lines can be drawn from the middle of the clavical to the abdomen and are referred to as *midclavicular*. Injures can be noted as medial or lateral to the midclavicular line on the left or right side of the patient.

Abdominal Cavity

The abdominal cavity lies immediately inferior to the thoracic cavity and contains the major organs of digestion and excretion. The abdominal cavity is only partially protected by the ribs, leaving the underlying organs such as the liver, spleen, and intestines vulnerable to injury from direct trauma. The abdominal cavity is divided into four **abdominal quadrants** by imaginary lines that intersect at the umbilicus (Figure 7.28). These quadrants are referred to as the *right upper quadrant* (RUQ), *left upper quadrant* (LUQ), *right lower quadrant* (RLQ), and *left lower quadrant* (LLQ). The major organs contained in the LUQ are the stomach, spleen, and part of the colon (Figure 7.29). The RUQ contains the liver, gall bladder, and part

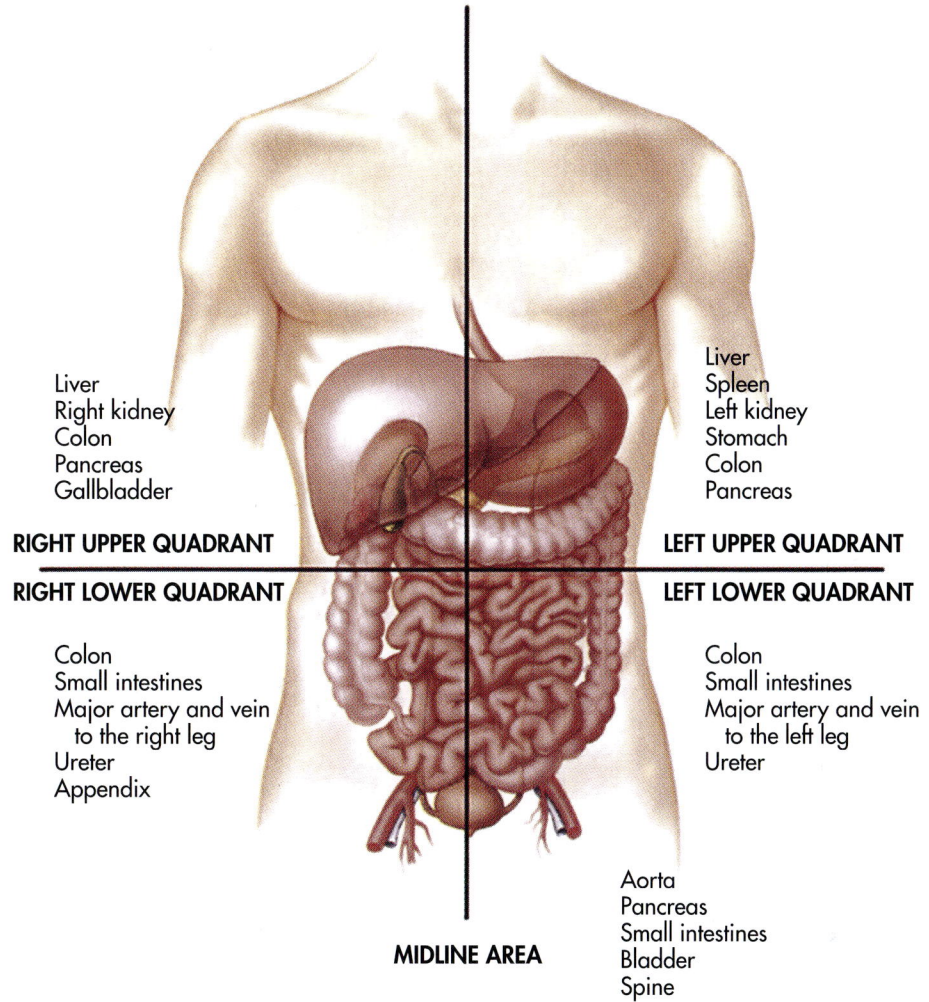

FIGURE 7.29 Major organs contained in each quadrant.

of the colon. Both the LLQ and the RLQ contain part of the colon. The appendix is located in the RLQ. The abdominal cavity is lined by a thin membrane called the **peritoneum**.

The kidneys lie behind the abdominal cavity in what is referred to as the **retroperitoneal space**. This space is located behind the peritoneum superior to the umbilicus from about the third lumbar vertebrae up to the eleventh rib.

> ✓ The abdominal cavity lies inferior to the thoracic cavity and is divided into four quadrants. Many organs are packed into this space with only limited protection from the ribs, increasing the likelihood of internal injury from direct trauma. The kidneys are contained in a space behind the abdominal cavity superior to the umbilicus referred to as the retroperitoneal space.

Summary

- Achieving a good working knowledge of patient anatomy, physiology, and the terminology unique to the medical profession is critical to conducting appropriate patient assessment and communicating vital patient information accurately and concisely.
- The major body systems that the EMT needs to know and understand are the musculoskeletal, respiratory, circulatory, nervous, integumentary, and endocrine systems.
- The musculoskeletal system consists of bones and muscles. Bones support the body and work with the muscles to allow for movement.
- The respiratory system consists of the upper and lower airways. Important structures are the lungs, bronchi, and alveoli. The respiratory system replenishes blood with oxygen and removes carbon dioxide, the waste product of metabolism.
- The circulatory system consists of the heart, blood vessels, and blood. The circulatory system distributes oxygenated blood to all tissues of the body and transports waste products back to the lungs for elimination.
- The nervous system is the control center of the body. The central nervous system, composed of the brain and spinal cord, serves as the command center of the body, and the peripheral nervous system, composed of the nerves, issues these commands to the muscles and organs.
- The integumentary system consists of the skin. The skin protects the internal organs from microorganisms, regulates temperature, prevents water loss, and transmits sensations to the central nervous system.
- The endocrine system secretes hormones from endocrine glands that regulate various processes in the body, such as reproduction and digestion.
- The abdominal, thoracic, and skull cavities are not body systems, but they are important because they contain delicate organs.

Scenario Solution

Several new terms and ideas are brought about in this chapter. As you review this chapter, realize that it is the foundation of your "medical knowledge." It is how you will recognize problems with your patients. It is how you will communicate to other health care professionals. Additionally, it is how you will document your findings on your patient care records or run report, part of the patient's permanent medical record. Using this chapter to build a solid foundation for yourself will allow you to confidently overview the scenario at the beginning of this chapter.

After you package the patient and have begun transportation, you call in to the hospital: "We are en route to your facility with a 35-year-old male patient who was found lying supine in the woods at the base of a tree. The patient was a victim of a hunting accident and was shot out of a tree stand. The patient fell approximately 15 feet to thick brush. The patient is conscious, alert, and oriented, with the following injures: open deformity of the right leg just proximal to the knee, with multiple shotgun pellet wounds to the inferior and lateral portions of the right leg, the inferior and lateral portions of the right buttocks, the right midaxillary portion of his thorax, and the right lateral portion of his neck and jaw. He is immobilized on a long backboard with a cervical collar and a head immobilization device, and the deformed leg has been splinted with a vacuum splint.

Key Terms

Abdominal quadrants Sections of the abdomen; right upper, left upper, right lower, left lower.

Acromion Lateral edge of the shoulder.

Alveoli Small air sacs in the lungs where the exchange of gas takes place.

Aorta Largest artery in the body, extending from the left ventricle through the thorax and abdomen to the navel, where it divides into the iliac arteries; carries blood from the heart to the body.

Key Terms (cont'd)

Arteries Vessels that carry blood away from the heart to the body under pressure.

Atria Upper chambers of the heart; the right atrium receives blood from the superior and inferior venae cavae; the left atrium receives blood from the pulmonary veins.

Automaticity Ability of an organ, such as the heart, to generate an electrical impulse.

Autonomic nervous system Part of the nervous system that regulates involuntary vital functions, including the activity of the cardiac muscle, smooth muscles, and glands; divided into the sympathetic nervous system and the parasympathetic nervous system.

Ball-and-socket joint Joint that moves freely in all directions, such as the shoulder.

Blood Fluid consisting of blood cells and plasma that carries nutrients to the tissues and removes waste.

Blood pressure Pressure that blood exerts on the wall of arteries; measured with a sphygmomanometer.

Blood vessels Vessels that carry blood throughout the body.

Brachial artery Artery located on the inside of the elbow on the same side as the small finger; extends from the elbow to the armpit.

Brain stem Part of the brain responsible for consciousness; contains the medulla oblongata, the pons, and the mesencephalon.

Bronchi Two branches of the trachea. Also known as *bronchial tubes*.

Capillaries Smallest blood vessels in the body; in the tissues, the capillaries surround the cells, allowing gas and nutrient exchange to take place.

Cardiac muscle Made up of three layers—epicardium (external layer), myocardium (middle layer), and endocardium (internal layer).

Carina Division of the lower end of the trachea into the two mainstem bronchi.

Carotid arteries Major arteries of the neck, supplying the face, head, and brain with oxygenated blood.

Carpals Wrist bones.

Cartilage A form of connective tissue that is more elastic than bone and is considered part of the skeleton.

Central nervous system Part of the nervous system comprising the brain and spinal cord.

Cerebellum Portion of the brain located beneath the cerebrum and surrounding the brain stem; coordinates movement.

Cerebrum Portion of the brain divided into left and right hemispheres and further divided into several lobes, each of which has a unique responsibility in the control of specific intellectual, sensory, and/or motor functions.

Clavicle Bone running from the manubruim to the shoulder.

Colon Portion of the large intestine that is divided into three parts—ascending colon, transverse colon, and descending colon.

Coronary arteries First branches off the aorta, which supply the heart with blood; if occluded, a myocardial infarction often occurs.

Dermis Middle layer of the skin that contains the blood vessels, glands, hair follicles, and nerve endings.

Diaphragm Dome-shaped muscle that separates the thoracic cavity from the abdominal cavity; when it contracts, the thoracic cavity enlarges, allowing air to enter the lungs.

Diastolic pressure Pressure in the heart when the heart muscle is relaxing; lower reading of a blood pressure.

Endocardium Inner layer of the heart.

Epicardium Outer layer of the heart.

Epidermis Outermost layer of the skin; consists of cells only.

Epiglottis Leaf-shaped structure just above the larynx that prevents food and liquids from entering the trachea during swallowing.

Erythrocytes Blood cells that contain hemoglobin; primary function is to carry oxygen back to the tissues; also called *red blood cells*.

Esophagus Muscular canal extending from the back of the mouth to the stomach.

Face Bones of the anterior section of the skull.

Femoral arteries Major vessels supplying the legs with oxygenated blood; can be palpated in the groin area.

Femur Bone of the thigh.

Fibula Posterior bone of the lower leg.

Frontal Anterior section of the skull.

Heart Four-chambered organ that pumps blood through the blood vessels to distribute oxygen to the cells of the body.

Hemoglobin Specialized protein that binds to oxygen in red blood cells; gives red blood cells their color.

Hinged joint Joint that moves freely in only one direction.

Hip joint Joint formed by the head of the femur and the acetabulum.

Hormones Chemicals that regulate body activities and functions.

Humerus Bone of the upper arm.

Iliac crest Superior lateral bones of the hip.

Integumentary system Made up of the skin, sebaceous glands, and sweat glands. Its function is to protect

Key Terms (cont'd)

the body and help with temperature and water regulation.

Intercostal muscles Muscles located between the ribs; lift the ribs upward and outward during inhalation, increasing tidal volume.

Involuntary muscles Muscles that carry out the automatic functions of the body.

Ischium Inferior posterior bones of the hip.

Joints Areas where two bones connect.

Kidney Located behind the peritoneum on each side of the vertebral column, the kidneys form urine by the process of filtration, reabsorption, and secretion.

Large intestine Extends from the end of the small intestine to the anus. It is divided into the cecum, colon, sigmoid colon, rectum, and anus.

Larynx Often called the *voice box*, structure consisting of cartilage, muscle, and soft tissues; located between the pharynx and the trachea.

Leukocytes White blood cells; function in the body's immune sytem.

Ligaments Connective tissue that holds bones together at the joint.

Lungs Two large air sacs that are made up of lobes. The right lung has three lobes, and the left lung has two.

Mandible Bone of the lower jaw.

Manubrium Superior section of the sternum.

Maxilla Two bones that form the upper jaw.

Medical terminology Specialized language of the medical profession that allows concise and effective communication.

Metabolism Chemical reactions that take place within an organism to maintain life; the work of cells.

Metacarpals Hand bones.

Metatarsals Foot bones.

Muscles Contractile tissue that works with the skeleton to provide movement and protection for the body.

Musculoskeletal system Includes the muscles and skeletal system and provides a framework for movement and protection for internal organs. The bones are also important in the production of red blood cells.

Myocardium Muscle tissue that makes up the inner layer of the heart.

Nasal bone Bone of the nose.

Occipital Pertaining to the posterior section of the skull.

Olecranon Elbow joint.

Orbit Eye socket.

Ovaries Paired, almond-shaped organs suspended by ligaments in the left and right lower quadrants of the abdomen that release a mature egg once a month in females between approximately 9 and 50 years of age.

Parasympathetic nervous system Part of the autonomic nervous system responsible for returning the body to a normal state after stress.

Parietal Pertaining to the top of the skull.

Parietal pleura Interior lining of the chest wall.

Patella Kneecap.

Perfusion A state of adequate supply of oxygen and nutrients to the tissues; ability of the circulatory system to distribute blood containing nutrients and oxygen to the tissues.

Pericardium Thin sac surrounding the heart.

Peripheral nervous system Part of the nervous system consisting of all nerves that extend from the brain and spinal cord.

Peritoneum Serous membrane covering the organs and lining the abdominal cavity.

Phalanges Bones of the fingers and toes.

Pharynx Hollow space behind the nose and mouth and above the laynx and esophagus; divided into the nasopharynx, oropharynx, and hypopharynx.

Plasma Liquid component of blood that contains proteins such as clotting factors.

Platelets Cellular fragments in the blood that form plugs at the site of bleeding, starting the clotting process.

Prefix Word element placed before the root word that changes the meaning of the word.

Pubis Inferior anterior bone of the hip.

Pulmonary arteries Vessels that cary oxygen-poor blood from the right side of the heart to the lungs; the only arteries in the body that carry oxygen-poor blood.

Pulmonary veins Vessels that carry oxygen-rich blood from the lungs back to the left side of the heart; the only veins in the body that carry oxygen-rich blood.

Radial artery Artery located on the thumb side of the wrist of each arm; extends from the wrist to the elbow.

Radius Bone on the lateral side of the lower arm.

Respiratory depth (tidal volume) Volume of air inhaled with each breath; normally about 500 ml of air in an adult.

Respiratory quality Assessment of breath sounds, chest expansion, and effort.

Respiratory rhythm Measure of the regularity of breathing.

Retroperitoneal space Space posterior to the abdominal cavity that contains the kidneys.

Ribs Twelve pairs of bones that line the wall of the thorax.

Root word Basic stem words used as building blocks for medical terms with the addition of prefixes and suffixes.

Key Terms (cont'd)

Scapula Flat bone located bilaterally in the posterior superior thorax.
Skeleton Major component of the musculoskeletal system; framework for the body.
Skull Bones that house and protect the brain.
Small intestine First portion of the intestine and has three parts—duodenum, jejunum, and iluem. Also known as the *small bowel*.
Sternum Flat bone lying in the anterior center of the thorax.
Subcutaneous tissue Deepest layer of the skin; made up of fatty and connective tissue.
Suffix Word element placed at the end of a root word that serves to form a new word.
Sympathetic nervous system Segment of the autonomic nervous system that works to speed up functions of the body.
Systolic pressure Pressure in the heart when the heart muscle is contracting; upper reading of a blood pressure.
Tarsals Ankle bones.
Temporal Pertaining to the sides of the skull.
Tendons Straps of tissue that attach voluntary muscles to bone.
Testes Two egg-shaped glands that produce spermatozoa (sperm). Also known as the *testicles*.
Thorax Superior two thirds of the trunk.
Tibia Anterior bone of the lower leg.
Trachea Cylinder-shaped tube in the neck composed of cartilage and membrane that extends from the vocal cords to the level of the fifth thoracic vertebra where it divides into two bronchi; also called the *windpipe*.
Ulna Bone on the medial side of the lower arm.
Ureter Narrow tube about 12 cm in length that carries urine from the kidney to the urinary bladder.
Urethra Tube that extends from the bladder to the outside of the body at the urethral meatus. The male urethra is approximately 8 inches long, and the femal urethra is approximately 1.5 inches long.
Veins Vessels that carry blood back to the heart.
Venae cavae Two major veins of the body, the inferior vena cava and the superior vena cava, that return blood to the heart.
Ventilatory rate Breaths per minute.
Ventricles Lower chambers of the heart that pump blood; the right ventricle supplies oxygen-poor blood to the lungs, and the left supplies oxygen-rich blood to the body.
Vertebrae Circular bones that make up the vertebral column.
Visceral pleura Exterior lining of the lungs.
Vocal cords Thin membranes within the larynx that produce sound.
Voluntary muscles Muscles attached to bone that provide for movement.
Xiphoid process Small bony structure located between the costal margins at the lower end of the sternum; used as a landmark for chest compressions and nasogastric tube insertion.
Zygomatic bones Cheek bones.

Review Questions

1. The elbow is located _____ to the wrist.
   a. Distal
   b. Lateral
   c. Proximal
   d. Inferior
2. A patient found lying face up on a couch is in the _____ position.
   a. Prone
   b. Supine
   c. Ventral
   d. Trendelenburg
3. The _____ and _____ are the bones of the lower arm.
   a. Tarsals, metatarsals
   b. Femur, humerus
   c. Radius, ulna
   d. Tibia, fibula
4. _____ muscles are attached to the skeletal system and assist with movement and stability.
   a. Involuntary
   b. Voluntary
   c. Cardiac
   d. Integumentary
5. What is the initial stimulus for the brain to signal breathing in a healthy person?
   a. Oxygen level
   b. Carbon dioxide level
   c. Carbon monoxide level
   d. Intercostal pressure

Review Questions (cont'd)

6. The right ventricle pumps blood to the _____.
   a. Heart
   b. Lungs
   c. Body
   d. Left atrium
7. The nervous system is divided into the _____ nervous system and the _____ nervous system.
   a. Voluntary, involuntary
   b. Vagus, sympathetic
   c. Parasympathetic, voluntary
   d. Central, peripheral
8. The spinal cord is part of the _____ nervous system.
   a. Respiratory
   b. Central
   c. Peripheral
   d. Automatic
9. The reproductive system portion that creates the egg for the female is:
   a. Testes
   b. Ovaries
   c. Ovarian tubes
   d. Pituitary gland
10. The digestive system transverses the following body cavities in order:
    a. Skull cavity, abdominal cavity, reproductive system
    b. Orapharyngeal cavity, thoracic cavity, abdominal cavity, pelvic cavity
    c. Abdominal cavity, pelvic cavity
    d. Thoracic cavity, abdominal cavity, pelvic cavity
11. The key organ of the renal system is:
    a. The renal glands
    b. The gonads
    c. The kidneys
    d. The liver
12. The blood exchanges oxygen for carbon dioxide at the _____.
    a. Venuoles
    b. Heart
    c. Pulmonary artery
    d. Capillaries

Answers to these Review Questions can be found at the end of the book on page 865.

Assessment

Lesson Goal

Assessment is the basis of management. Without proper assessment, correct management plans cannot be developed. The goal of this chapter is to provide the EMT with education pertaining to all phases of assessment and teach the critical skills necessary to identify the subtle findings. These subtle findings separate the EMT who provides outstanding patient assessment and management from the EMT who offers mediocre care.

Scenario

It is 0330 hours on Wednesday morning. You and your partner are dispatched to a private residence on the edge of town in reference to a 72-year-old male who is experiencing shortness of breath. Further information from the communications center reveals that the patient is pale and diaphoretic with a history of congestive heart failure. A first responder has also been dispatched for assistance at the scene. Response time to the scene is 3 minutes. Transportation time to the hospital is 6 minutes. It is a warm summer evening with no weather or traffic issues.

Upon arrival at the residence, the patient's wife meets you and advises you that her husband awakened approximately 15 minutes ago complaining of "not being able to get his breath." He advised his wife, "It's my pulmonary edema again. I can feel it." The patient, who had a double amputation of his legs, is sitting upright in bed with audible wheezes and gurgling on expiration. He looks up as you enter, and you know that he is in trouble. He is pale, diaphoretic, anxious, and breathing at 28 breaths per minute. His wife further advises that he had a double coronary bypass operation 5 years ago, takes digitalis for his irregular heartbeat, is on lasix and potassium, and developed high blood pressure 2 years ago.

 You know your patient is in trouble. What are your first actions? When should you initiate transportation? What useful information did the dispatcher provide to you that will help in treatment and transportation decisions?

Key Terms to Know

Abrasions	Bradycardia	Contusions	Edema
Assessment	Breathing	Crepitus	Exhalation
Auscultation	Capillary refill	Detailed physical examination	Femoral artery
AVPU	Carotid artery	Diastolic pressure	Full pulse
Bounding pulse	Constrict	Dilate	General impression

113

Key Terms to Know (cont'd)

Inhalation
Initial assessment
Interventions
Lacerations
Mechanism of injury
Nature of illness
Ongoing assessment
Oriented
Palpation
Paradoxical motion

Perfusion
Pulse
Pulse character
Pulse pressure
Pulse rate
Pulse rhythm
Radial artery
Rapid trauma- or medical-
   focused history and
   physical examination

Respiration
Retractions
SAMPLE history
Scene size-up
Signs
Sphygmomanometer
Stethoscope
Symptoms
Systolic pressure
Tachycardia

Thready pulse
Triage
Ventilation
Ventilatory character
Ventilatory depth
Ventilatory rate
Ventilatory rhythm

Learning Objectives

As an EMT-Basic, you should be able to do the following:

DOT

- Summarize the reasons for forming a general impression of the patient.
- Discuss methods of assessing altered mental status in adults, children, and infants.
- Discuss methods of assessing and managing the airway in adults, children, and infants (medical and trauma patients).
- Describe methods of assessing and managing difficulty breathing in adults, children, and infants.
- Describe methods used to obtain a pulse in adults, children, and infants.
- Discuss the need for assessing the patient for external bleeding (see Chapter 23).
- Describe normal and abnormal findings when assessing skin (color, temperature condition, and capillary refilling time) in adults, children, and infants.
- Explain the reason for prioritizing a patient for care and transportation (see Chapter 12).
- Describe the areas included in the rapid trauma assessment, and discuss what should be evaluated.
- Describe when the rapid assessment may be altered to provide patient care.
- Discuss the reason for performing a focused history and physical examination.
- Discuss the components of the detailed physical examination and how it is preformed.
- Distinguish between the detailed physical examination that is performed on a trauma patient and that performed on a medical patient.
- Discuss the reasons for repeating the initial assessment as part of the ongoing assessment.
- State the reasons for management of the cervical spine once the patient has been determined to be a trauma patient (see Chapters 10, 11, and 27).
- Describe methods used for assessing whether a patient is breathing.
- State the care that should be provided to the adult, child, and infant patient with adequate breathing.
- State the care that should be provided to the adult, child, and infant patient without adequate breathing.
- Differentiate between a patient with adequate breathing and a patient without adequate breathing.
- Differentiate among methods of assessing breathing in the adult, child, and infant patient.
- Compare the methods of providing airway care to the adult, child, and infant patient.
- Differentiate among methods of obtaining a pulse in the adult, child, and infant patient.
- Demonstrate the techniques for assessing mental status.
- Demonstrate the techniques for assessing the airway.
- Demonstrate the techniques for assessing whether the patient is breathing.
- Demonstrate the techniques for assessing whether the patient has a pulse.
- Demonstrate the techniques for assessing the patient for external bleeding (see Chapter 23).
- Demonstrate the techniques for assessing the patient's skin color, temperature, condition, and capillary refill (infants and children only).
- Demonstrate the ability to prioritize patients.
- Discuss the reasons for reconsideration concerning the mechanism of injury (see Chapter 22).
- State the reasons for performing a rapid trauma assessment.

Learning Objectives (cont'd)

- Recite examples and explain why patients should receive a rapid trauma assessment.
- Demonstrate the rapid trauma assessment that should be used to assess a patient based on mechanism of injury.
- Describe the unique needs for assessing an individual with a specific chief complaint with no known history.
- Differentiate between the history and physical examination that are performed for responsive patients with no known history and those that are performed for responsive patients with a known history.
- Describe the needs for assessing an individual who is unresponsive.
- Differentiate between the assessment that is performed for a patient who is unresponsive or has an altered state of consciousness and the assessment that is performed for other medical patients.
- Demonstrate the patient assessment skills that should be used to assist a patient who is responsive with no known history.
- Demonstrate the patient assessment skills that should be used to assist a patient who is unresponsive or has an altered mental status.
- State the areas of the body that are evaluated during the detailed physical examination.
- Explain what additional care should be provided while performing the detailed physical examination.
- Describe the components of the ongoing assessment.
- Describe trending of assessment components.
- Demonstrate the skills involved in performing the ongoing assessment.

Patient Care Algorithm

Patient Assessment

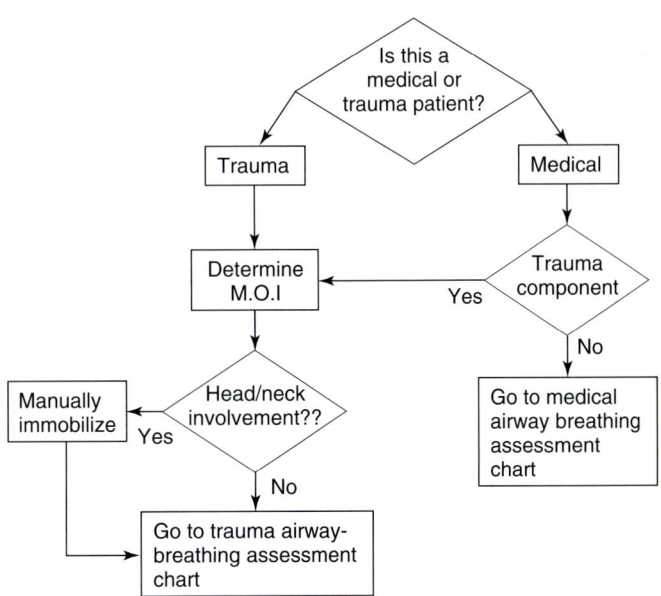

Note: the following patient assessment and management charts are to be used together in an integrated manner. They should not be used as stand alone documents.

Assessment is the basis by which all patients are evaluated, and the initial steps of patient management are based on the results of that evaluation. If the assessment has been done wrong so that the results are incorrect, then the management of the patient may not be correct and the outcome to the patient may be poor. Therefore the assessment chapter is the cornerstone of the emergency medical technician's (EMT's) skills, just as it is the cornerstone of the skills of the nurses and physcians in the emergency department and throughout the hospital. The decisions, whether about safe scene entry, requesting more help, or patient interventions, are guided by evaluation of the scene and assessment of the patient. The EMT must finely hone his or her assessment skills through practice, experience, and ongoing evaluation.

Because assessment and the associated patient management are the essential elements of patient care, this chapter provides only an overview of these skills and management techniques; the rest of the text fills in the details. The EMT must learn and understand the material in this chapter before moving on to the details.

Interventions are actions in response to an assessment of the situation and/or patient. Interventions are intended to achieve specific results. For example, if the assessment of the scene (*scene size-up*) leads to the conclusion that the scene is unsafe, the intervention is either to make the scene safe or to not enter the scene. If the patient assessment findings indicate an airway problem, the intervention is to open and maintain the airway. If continuous assessment indicates that attempts to open the airway are not successful, the next intervention is immediate and safe transportation to a medical facility while continuing to attempt to open the airway.

By design, EMTs do not necessarily diagnose and treat illness and injury; they perform assessment-driven interventions. However, in many instances the EMT will arrive at a conclusion about what is wrong with the patient (*diagnosis*) during the process of assessment. If a patient has no pulse and is not breathing, it is correct to assume that the patient is in cardiac arrest. Although this is making a conclusion (diagnosis) based on the findings, the conclusion is not the important part. It is important to reestablish blood oxygenation and flow. The EMT should carry out the necessary interventions based on the findings identified in the assessment to benefit the patient.

Assessment-driven interventions also occur in the hospital. The physicians and nurses may speculate as to the cause (diagnosis) of the findings, but their first step is to treat the patient. In many instances the diagnosis is not established until after the patient has gone home and other tests are run. A diagnosis assists in the long-term treatment and planning for the patient's care, but that is done later.

Transportation of the patient is in itself an intervention. The point at which the patient is transported, the method by which the patient is transported, and the speed with which the patient is transported are guided by assessment findings. Some patients are so critically ill or injured that the most appropriate care after a rapid initial assessment and management of identified airway problems is early and speedy transportation to an appropriate medical facility.

Assessment and intervention must work hand in hand. Because the purpose of an intervention is to change the status and condition of the patient, its effectiveness must be continuously assessed and reassessed. If an intervention does not have the desired result, different interventions may be required.

Editor's Note

Two formats are used for assessment. One was developed around 1980, is used by physicians and EMS personnel, and was part of the National Standard Curriculum in its first two editions. The other was developed later for EMTs and is now currently taught in the National Standard Curriculum. Because most physicians and nurses are not using the one taught for the EMT-Basic (EMT-B) program, they expect the EMT-B to understand the system that they use. Both are shown in Table 8.1

The two formats are not radically different; the names of the steps are the only difference. Table 8.1 identifies these in a side-by-side manner. The name of the step most often used by hospital personnel is in italics after the EMS name.

This chapter provides information about the various stages of assessment, which are listed sequentially:

1. **General impression and plan of action.** The EMT develops a plan of action while en route to the scene and from the first overview of the situation. This general impression remains fluid throughout the patient management.
2. **Scene size-up.** Immediately on arrival at the scene, a EMT performs a broad overview of the entire situation. The information gathered should include, but not be limited to, the type of emergency, number of patients involved, weather, potential for hazardous

TABLE 8.1 Assessment Step Names

EMS Name	Physician or Nurse Name
Initial assessment	Primary survey
Initial assessment	Resuscitation
Focused assessment	Secondary survey
Detailed history and physical examination	Secondary survey
Management of the problems found	Definitive care
Ongoing assessment	Reassessment

conditions that would affect Emergency Medical Services (EMS), presence or need for law enforcement or fire personnel, length of time required to remove the patients from the scene and transport them to the hospital, and number of EMTs and other rescue personnel that may be required to manage all of the patients and the scene. (Refer to Chapter 12 for detailed information on scene size-up).

3. The EMT can complete the **initial assessment** (*primary survey*) in 60 seconds or less and establish whether the patient has life-threatening conditions that require rapid intervention.
4. The EMT generates a **rapid trauma- or medical-focused history and physical examination** (*part of secondary survey*) based on the patient's chief complaint and physical findings at the scene. The EMT performs the physical examination on those regions of the body that the he or she considers the most likely to have life-threatening conditions. The EMT frequently performs this part of the assessment en route to the hospital.
5. A **detailed physical examination** (*secondary survey*) comprises the region-by-region evaluation of the entire body to look for hidden problems. Because the EMT's goal is to quickly transport the patient to an appropriate medical facility, it is not always necessary to perform a complete evaluation in the field. For critically ill or injured patients, the EMT may never complete this portion of the patient assessment.
6. The EMT performs **ongoing assessment** (*reassessment*) checks for problems that arise after he or she has completed the initial assessment, rapid focused history, and physical examination. Reassessment is an ongoing task in patient care.

■ PATIENT ASSESSMENT
General Impression and Plan of Action

As soon as the EMT receives a call, he or she develops a general impression and plan of action. He or she should discuss them among the team members before arriving on the scene. The **general impression** is the "gut feeling" about the scene and patient based on knowledge and tempered by experience. Developing the plan of action begins with dispatch and continues through scene size-up and patient assessment. The plan of action allows the EMT to make scene management and patient care decisions before his or her arrival at the scene.

A plan of action requires flexibility. The EMT changes the plan as he or she gathers more information. As the EMT receives additional information, he or she evaluates it and fine tunes (or completely changes) the general impression and plan of action. Although subjective, the EMT's general impression is an essential assessment skill that is frequently used to make decisions about scene management or patient care. The following is an example of this type of decision making:

An EMT is called to a motor vehicle accident with an unknown number of victims. While en route, the EMT learns that two vehicles are involved, six victims may be present, and some of the victims may be trapped. Although the injury and damage estimate by the bystanders on the scene may be overstated, the EMT should alert additional personnel. If helicopter backup is available, the EMT should quickly review the dispatch protocols en route. Immediately on arrival, the EMT evaluates the scene and the injured and decides whether additional personnel and what type are needed.

The EMT's ability to form a general impression and develop a plan of action are essential assessment skills that allow early initiation of appropriate interventions, including transportation. **Triage** is the process of sorting patients to determine those who require immediate treatment and transportation. The following is an example of general impression and plan of action in a medical situation:

A patient is experiencing shortness of breath (Figure 8.1). On entering the front door, the EMT observes the middle-age male patient sitting forward in an easy chair, hands on both knees, very pale, sweating heavily, and drawing in each breath by rocking back and forth. Without actually touching or examining the patient, the EMT forms an initial impression of an individual with breathing difficulty

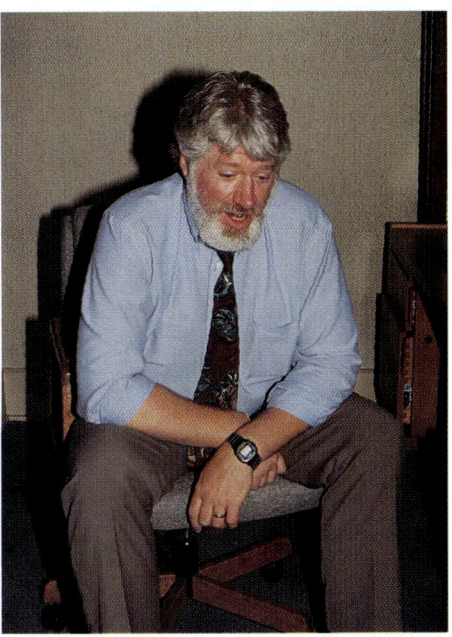

FIGURE 8.1 Scene assessment of breathing difficulty.

and potential cardiac problems and begins to formulate a plan of action. The plan of action should include immediate administration of oxygen, early activation of advanced life support (ALS), limited patient movement, and transfer of the patient to a sitting position. The plan of action also may include preparing for potential complications, including respiratory arrest, cardiac arrest, or airway problems because of decreasing level of consciousness (LOC).

> ✓ A general impression and plan of action are important assessment skills that begin even before examining the patient. They are constantly updated as the EMT receives and evaluates new scene and patient information.

> ✓ The patient assessment consists of initial assessment, rapid focused history and physical examination, detailed physical examination, and ongoing assessment. The EMT may not be able to complete all stages of assessment for every patient.

Scene Survey

Scene survey (assessment of the scene) involves gathering, evaluating, and acting on information from various sources, including dispatch, bystanders, the patient, the family, emergency services workers, and others. Assessment of the scene and the circumstances surrounding the injury or illness are as important as the patient examination. The reliability of the information may vary depending on who acquires or provides the information and his or her level of training and experience. Information obtained from an excited bystander is much less reliable than information provided by an experienced, first responder–trained law enforcement officer or firefighter. Continuous assessment by the experienced EMT provides sufficient information on which to base intervention decisions.

Safety of the Scene

An injured EMT increases the number of patients that must be cared for and decreases the number of personnel available to provide that care. Therefore the EMT's safety is of primary importance. A quick and accurate overview of the scene prevents the EMT, the patient, bystanders, or other emergency services personnel from being injured or exposed to dangerous situations. The safety of all emergency personnel relies on emergency personnel who arrive first on the scene to quickly and accurately determine possible hazards and communicate this information to other responders (Figure 8.2). The EMS personnel who are not the first to arrive should quickly reevaluate the

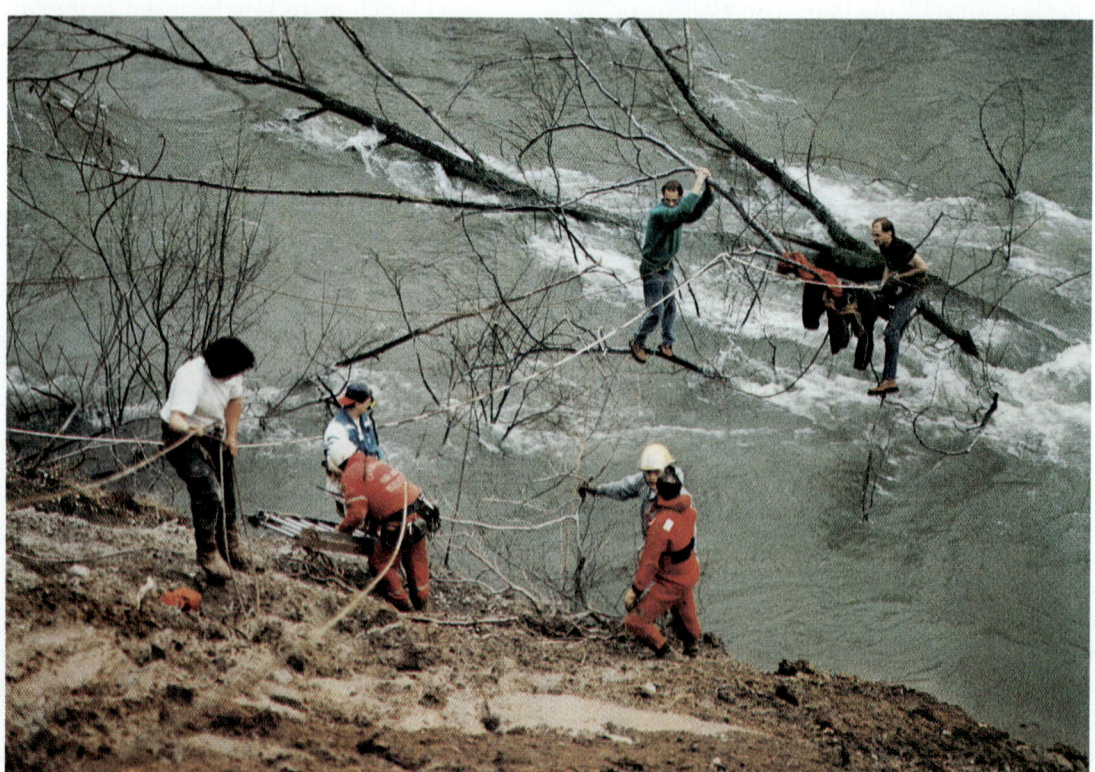

FIGURE 8.2 Hazardous scene.

scene. The adage of "trust no one, check it yourself" holds true at emergency scenes.

Basic scene management requires that the EMT avoid entering an unsafe scene. If the EMT can make the scene safe, he or she should do so. If the EMT cannot make the scene safe, he or she should stop and call for additional assistance. When deciding if the scene can be made safe, the EMT must consider three questions:

1. Does the EMT have the necessary training and/or experience to handle this unsafe scene?
2. Does the EMT have the necessary equipment required to manage this unsafe scene?
3. Does the EMT have the necessary trained personnel to manage this unsafe scene?

> ✓ The EMT should not enter a scene that is unsafe for the EMT or for other EMS personnel. If the EMT cannot make the scene safe, he or she should stop and wait for the scene to be made safe. The EMT should request additional help as required. Do not be a dead hero!

Although an individual EMT may have the training and equipment necessary to manage an unsafe scene, proper management often requires a system of support. Teamwork is critical. Consider a patient found at the bottom of a steep embankment. A single EMT on the initial arriving ambulance may have steep embankment training and may even have ropes and a harness. However, a correct and safe steep embankment rescue requires more

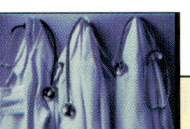

Physician Notes

A situation reported in a newspaper several years ago points out the outcome of bad EMT judgement in scene management:

A person fell into a sewer and was noted to be unconscious when EMS arrived. The senior EMT jumped into the sewer to evaluate the situation and assist the patient. This EMT passed out. The second EMT then jumped in to help them both, but this EMT also passed out. On arrival of the backup unit, the senior EMT jumped into the sewer to provide care. This EMT also passed out. The fourth EMT put on an air pack and brought the three EMTs and the patient out of the sewer. The patient and two of the EMTs died, and one EMT survived. All of these deaths could have been avoided if the senior EMT on the first unit had properly surveyed the scene and not tried to be a hero.

> ✓ Do not attempt to make the scene safe without the appropriate training, equipment, and personnel.

equipment and additional trained personnel. Attempting the rescue with limited resources may jeopardize the safety of the EMTs and the patient. Calling for additional assistance is the correct intervention. The EMT's assessment that the scene is unsafe results in an intervention—make it safe, do not enter the scene, and call for additional help. An injured EMT produces one more patient who must be cared for and one less trained person to provide this care.

Body Substance Isolation Precautions

The EMT's first responsibility is to maintain his or her health. Body substance exposure produces two major problems: (1) the EMT can become infected, and (2) the EMT can transfer infections to other patients, other EMS personnel, or his or her family. The infection transferred to himself or herself or to others may be only a brief inconvenience, such as a cold virus received when the patient coughed during an examination. However, the infection may be life threatening, such as hepatitis or human immunodeficiency virus (HIV).

Total body substance isolation (BSI) is cumbersome, time consuming, and difficult to provide in the field. To determine what level of protection to use in the field, the EMT evaluates the situation, gathers as much information as quickly as possible, and makes a knowledge-based judgment. The more prior knowledge that the EMT has and the better he or she surveys the scene, the more accurate the judgment can be.

The minimum BSI precaution for any emergency response is latex gloves. If exposed body fluids are expected, the EMT should wear eye protection and practical protection of broken skin from these fluids. A gown that is impervious to fluids is a practical solution in the operating room but not in the field. A mask is required, either on the EMT or the patient, if the EMT suspects a respiratory disease such as tuberculosis.

> ✓ Body substance isolation (BSI) precautions protect the EMT and the patient. The EMT should use the appropriate level of BSI precautions. Gloves, masks, eye protection, and open skin protection may be required to protect both the EMT and the patient (see Chapter 6).

Mechanism of Injury (Trauma) or Nature of Illness (Medical)

Mechanism of injury describes how energy of motion is transferred to an individual, resulting in injury. A good understanding of this information allows the EMT to predict up to 90% of injuries before examining the patient. For example, a minor "fender bender" with no damage to the vehicle and no injury to the occupant is one extreme, whereas a front-end collision with significant vehicle damage and potentially serious injury to the occupant's head, chest, neck, and abdomen is the other. Falls generate a different injury pattern. Important information includes height of the fall, the position in which the patient landed, and the number and kind of objects that the patient struck on the way down. Explosions are modified by the distance from the explosion, the amount heat and light, and flying objects (see Chapter 22).

Nature of illness refers to the medical condition causing the emergency that subsequently requires EMS assistance. Examples include the patient who is experiencing chest pain or breathing difficulties. The patient's medical history, as it relates to his or her current chief complaint, is important in the evaluation of medical-related problems.

The EMT can obtain information about mechanism of injury and nature of illness through careful observation of the scene and from the patient, the patient's family, bystanders, and other emergency care providers. The EMT updates the general impression of the patient and the scene and mentally carries out modifications appropriate to the plan of action

Number of Patients

An early determination of the number and severity of the patients assists in the decision to call for more ambulances (air or ground), initiate mutual aid agreements, or activate a major EMS incident or a multiple casualty incident (MCI) plan. Delay in requesting additional help can produce a serious delay in the provision of needed interventions and transportation. The decision to call for additional help may be as important as the actual patient care rendered.

Calling for Additional Help

The EMT generally determines the number of additional ambulances required after identifying the number of patients and seriousness of injuries (the next section on triage explains this in detail). One EMT is usually required for every patient; in rare cases, two patients per EMT can be considered. Although many ambulances can carry up to four patients, this maximum load is usually reserved for MCIs. With four patients in an ambulance, there is limited room to provide patient interventions.

Depending on the local EMS system and the circumstances of the scene, it may be appropriate to request ALS assistance, consider air transport, or request other specialized resources.

If the EMT determines that additional help is required, he or she should request it as soon as possible. Canceling units later is far less problematic than not having them available when needed.

> ✓ The EMT should quickly determine the need for additional resources and call for assistance as soon as possible.

Triage

Triage is the sorting and labeling of patients according to their injuries. If the incident involves multiple patients, a triage area is set up and patients are brought to this location. Patients are placed into one of four categories, and decisions concerning transportation and initiation of care are made from these. Consistent with the local MCI plan, the EMT should coordinate with the incident command system. While triaging patients, the EMT should continue the initial patient assessment to determine life-threatening injuries and their interventions (see Chapter 40 for further discussion).

Initial Patient Assessment

Initial assessment is the rapid evaluation of the patient's major body systems to identify life-threatening problems, initiate interventions, identify priority patients, and determine whether immediate transportation is necessary (Box 8.1).

The EMT's brain gathers information with the eyes (seeing), hands (feeling), ears (hearing), and nose (smelling). This input is analyzed while it is being gathered (simultaneous input and computation). However, because it is impossible for this or any other text to explain the parts of the initial assessment simultaneously, these parts are taught in the following logical steps based on the life-threatening potential of each step:

A—Airway
B—Breathing or ventilation
C—Circulation or perfusion

D—Disability (LOC), at this stage classified according to the AVPU system

E—Exposure of the patient for the rapid focused physical examination and detailed examination, then protection of the patient from the environment (this step is implied in the following sections)

> ✓ During the initial assessment, the EMT should assess for life-threatening problems and provide appropriate interventions, including immediate transportation of priority (critical) patients if needed. The EMT should correct life-threatening problems (intervention) as soon as he or she detects them.

General Impression

This is the same overview as the scene survey, except that in initial patient assessment, a single patient is the object of the EMT's attention rather than the scene.

Initial assessment allows the EMT to form a picture of the patient based on the overall condition (e.g., distress, hemorrhage, pain). A patient who has fallen from a substantial height, was ejected from an automobile, was a passenger in a vehicle in which another person was killed, or is in a vehicle that is severely damaged is probably seriously injured. In addition, if the patient complains of severe pain or is obviously experiencing difficulty breathing, he or she is probably a priority patient.

The patient's reaction further refines the general impression. Does the patient react as expected in this situation? How does the patient generally look? Does the patient look normal or sick? People who are sick usually look sick, and people who look sick usually are sick. Generally, the more sick they are, the worse they look. The sick patient will often have pale, dull skin. The eyes may appear drawn back into their sockets and look hazy or dry. The skin on the face may even appear loose or droopy, and the lips may appear blue.

> ✓ During the initial assessment, the EMT forms a general impression of the patient that helps guide interventions. Patients who look or act sick generally are sick.

Before talking to or touching the patient, the EMT may discover that a patient has breathing difficulty by noting his or her position (sitting up or leaning forward) and listening to the patient's breathing (rapid and labored). Patients with breathing difficulty are high priority, requiring immediate interventions and rapid transportation.

If at any point during the assessment the EMT determines that the patient is a priority or that attempted life-saving interventions are not working, he or she should initiate transportation and ALS activation immediately while continuing assessments and interventions en route.

Calming the Patient

EMTs should identify themselves to all patients and provide reassurance that they are there to help. A patient is often scared and wants to be out of the situation. A calm voice reassures the patient that someone who is knowledgeable and caring is there to help and is usually well received by the patient. For the most part the patient will relax and accept help. A cooperative patient is much easier to care for than one who is fighting the EMT.

Airway Assessment and Intervention (A)

An open airway is the first step in providing oxygen to the lungs and transferring it from there to the tissues of the rest of the body, preventing anaerobic metabolism, and keeping the patient's energy production at an optimum level (see Chapter 9). An airway that is not open or is only partially open is the top priority for management. Jaw thrust, jaw lift, oral or nasal airway, and the steps for airway management are discussed in Chapter 10.

If the patient is talking, screaming, crying, or using expletives, he or she has an open and functional airway. The EMT then can proceed to the next step—assessing

---

Box 8.1   Common Priority Patients

- General impression of a very sick patient
- Unresponsive—no gag or cough
- Responsive but not following commands
- Difficulty breathing
- Shock (hypoperfusion)
- Complicated childbirth
- Chest pain with blood pressure < 100 mm Hg systolic
- Uncontrolled bleeding
- Severe pain anywhere

the patient's breathing. However, if the patient is quiet, the EMT should look for evidence of airway problems. The silent airway may be adequate, but it also may indicate that the airway is not open or the patient is not breathing. A noisy airway generally indicates a problem. Blood or other liquid in the airway will gurgle, and snoring indicates that the tongue is partially occluding the airway. Any airway problem requires immediate intervention (Table 8.2).

If the airway opening intervention does not work, the EMT should prepare for immediate transportation and consider an en route rendezvous with ALS.

> ✓ Airway problems require immediate intervention. If an intervention does not work, the EMT must prepare prompt transportation and consider an ALS rendezvous.

Breathing Assessment and Intervention (B)

The terms **breathing** (**ventilation**) and **respiration** are frequently used interchangeably. However, these terms have different meanings. Breathing is the process of moving air into and out of the lungs. Respiration is the physiologic process of moving oxygen into the cells where it is metabolized and eliminating the waste product of this metabolism (carbon dioxide). Throughout this book ventilation and breathing are used to indicate the mechanical component, and respiration are used to indicate the physiologic component.

Some types of breathing difficulty may be immediately obvious (e.g., wheezing, gasping for air, labored ventilatory movements, or the position of the patient). The general impression of the patient, including skin color, rate and depth of ventilations, effort, and the patient's position, should be the first step in assessing ventilation. With experience the EMT will be able to quickly judge the adequacy of the patient's breathing rate and volume. The EMT should delay counting of the actual rate until the focused part of the examination.

The rates that generally constitute warning signs for breathing difficulty are less than 12 breaths or greater than 24 breaths per minute. The patient's ability to talk is also an indicator of adequate breathing. Talking requires air to be forced across the vocal cords at a smooth and even rate. Breathing difficulty is an indication to institute an intervention. An important intervention is rapid transportation to an appropriate medical facility.

The EMT may rapidly assess the adequacy of the patient's breathing by listening, looking, and feeling the chest (front and back) (Figure 8.3). Breathing problems and interventions are listed in Table 8.3.

A ventilatory rate of greater than 24 breaths per minute should be managed with supplemental oxygen to the lungs (increased oxygenation content to the inspired air). A ventilatory rate of less than 12 or greater than 30 breaths per minute should be managed by assisted ventilation in addition to the increased oxygenation of the inspired air. Assisted ventilations are accomplished by mouth-to-mask; bag-valve-mask; or flow-restricted, oxygen-powered ventilation devices. Unless they are unavailable, all types of assisted ventilation should use supplemental oxygen to increase oxygen concentration (FiO_2) in the ventilated air.

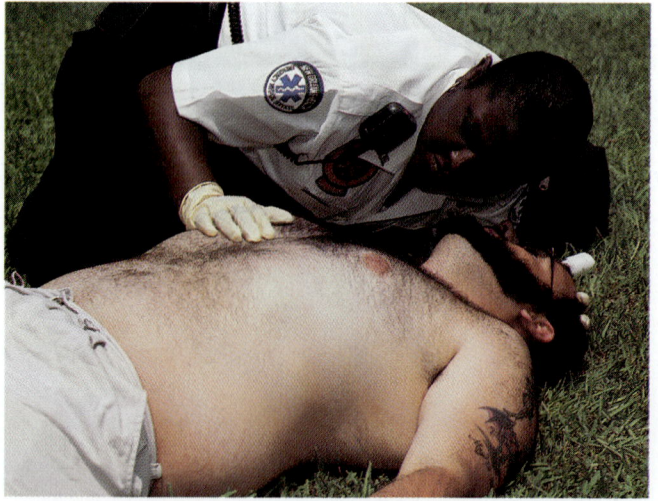

FIGURE 8.3 Look, listen, and feel to evaluate breathing.

TABLE 8.2 Airway Assessment and Potential Interventions

Assessment	Potential Interventions	
No airway	Jaw-thrust Chin-lift Head-tilt/chin-lift	Oropharyngeal airway Nasopharyngeal airway Suction as needed
Snoring	Jaw-thrust Chin-lift Head-tilt/chin-lift Remove pillow from under head	Oropharyngeal airway Nasopharyngeal airway Recovery position Suction as needed
Gurgling	Suction	Recovery position
Vomiting	Suction Finger sweep	Recovery position
Blood in airway	Suction Finger sweep	Recovery position

> ✓ Breathing is assessed by the general impression of the patient, assessment of breathing rates, and feeling the chest. Breathing interventions include transportation to an appropriate medical facility, increased FiO_2 and assisted ventilation.

Circulation Assessment and Intervention (C)

Perfusion

Adequate **perfusion** means that well-oxygenated blood is getting to all of the tissues and organs of the body. Reduction of the ability of the three components of the circulatory system (heart, volume, and vessels) affects perfusion. Many conditions, including major bleeding (external or internal), cold, cardiac failure, and vascular trauma, affect one or all of these components and therefore reduce perfusion. The result of decreased perfusion is anaerobic metabolism and loss of energy production by the body (see Chapter 9). Loss of perfusion and the resultant loss of energy production at the cellular level is one of the most critical conditions that the patient can develop. Loss of perfusion is the condition that the EMT must treat. The diagnosis that leads to loss of perfusion is only important because it may determine the management that is instituted.

Decreased perfusion cannot be observed, the EMT must rely on indirect indications such as pulse, skin color, capillary refilling time, skin temperature, and/or decreased LOC. Because the patient with poor perfusion and hypoxia (lack of oxygen) of the brain may act intoxicated or combative or have a decreased LOC, the EMT must attribute the altered LOC to some cause or condition that prehospital care can influence. The most common of such causes is hypoxia. The correct prehospital care (intervention) for hypoxia is increased FiO_2 in the air that the patient is breathing and assisted ventilation. Other causes of an altered LOC, such as stroke, intoxication, drug overdose, or head injury, are not easily treated in the field. Therefore the emphasis is for the EMT to manage the problem that the patient has and not worry about the etiology (cause). The cause can be determined when the patient arrives in the hospital.

Pulse

The presence or absence of a pulse is determined by feeling for an artery where it is close to the skin and overlies a bone. A pulse should be felt easily at either wrist on the radial side (Figure 8.4, *A*). If a pulse cannot be felt at this location, the carotid artery in the neck should be checked (Figure 8.4, *B*). The femoral artery in the groin is near the midline of the upper thigh. If a patient is 1 year of age or younger, the brachial pulse is felt on the medial surface of the upper arm.

If the EMT cannot find a pulse at any location, he or she should be practical and use judgment based on the information at hand (e.g., Do the rest of the patient's conditions support this assessment?). The patient without a pulse who is not breathing appears to be dead; if not, some important information is missing. The EMT should consider all the possible reasons why the pulse cannot be felt and begin interventions and assessment steps to correct this problem. The absence of a pulse without other signs of death is a clue to check the pulse in another location or have another EMT check the pulse. In the excitement of an emergency scene, it is sometimes easy to miss a pulse. A guaranteed way to assess for a heart beat is to auscultate over the patient's heart. If the heart is beating, it will be heard.

If a pulse and ventilation are absent, the EMT should begin cardiopulmonary resuscitation (CPR) and incorporate the use of an automated external defibrillator (AED). The EMT should initiate immediate transportation and make arrangements for a rendezvous with ALS as appropriate.

The location of the pulse can provide information about the patient's perfusion status. If a pulse is present at the wrist or ankle, the circulatory system is working

TABLE 8.3 Breathing Assessment and Potential Interventions

Assessment	Potential Interventions
No breathing	Mouth-to-mask ventilation Bag-valve-mask ventilation
Wheezing	Oxygen Medication administration
Responsive patient with <12 or >20 respirations per minute	Oxygen (high flow, nonrebreather) Preparation to assist ventilation
Unresponsive patient with inadequate breathing (e.g., <12 or >20 respirations per minute; other signs of respiratory difficulty)	Mouth-to-mask ventilation Bag-valve-mask ventilation
Use of accessory muscles of respiration	Oxygen administration Preparation to assist ventilation
Retractions, uneven chest movement	Oxygen administration Preparation to assist ventilation
Open hole in chest	Oxygen administration Sealing of hole in chest Positioning on injured side
Patient cannot breathe; labored breathing	Oxygen administration Assistance with medication administration
Nasal flaring in children	Oxygen administration

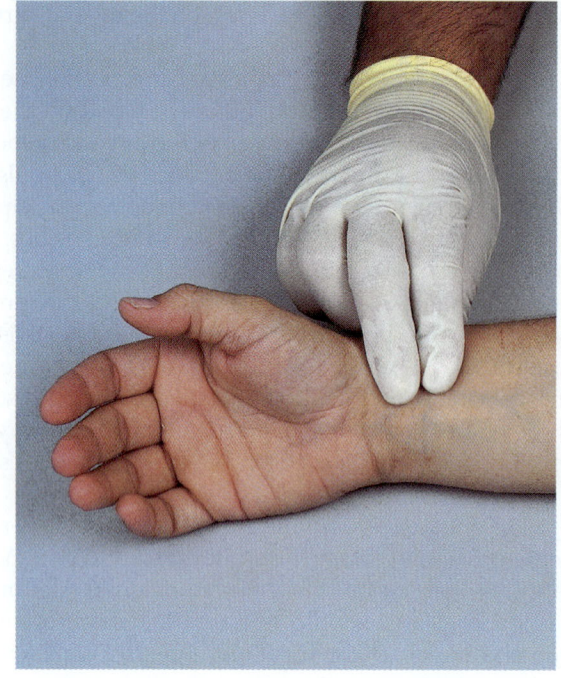
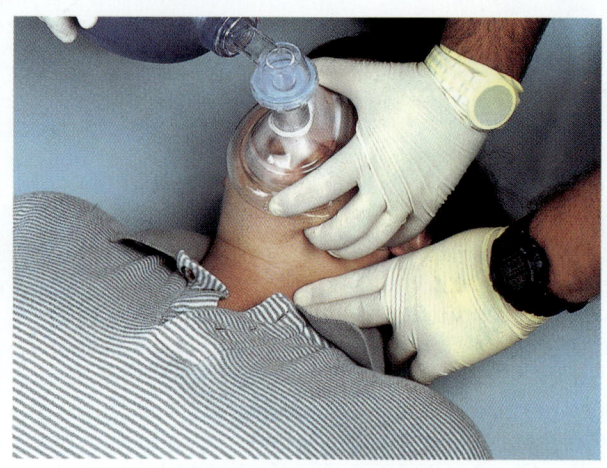

FIGURE 8.4 **A,** Evaluating the radial pulse. **B,** Evaluating the carotid pulse.

sufficiently to supply blood to the most distant parts of the body. However, if the pulse is present only at the carotid or femoral arteries, the body may have begun shunting blood to the more central parts of the body, indicating poor perfusion secondary to a problem with the circulatory system (heart, vascular system, or blood volume).

Capillary Refilling Time

Capillary refilling time is measured by pressing on the skin, compressing all of the blood out of the skin in that area, and estimating the time required to refill the vessels. The normal capillary refilling time is about 2 seconds.

The **capillary refill** test is helpful in evaluating the patient's perfusion. However, like many other signs that the patient may exhibit, several conditions (environmental and physiologic) can alter the results (Figure 8.5). The capillary refill test is a measurement of the time required to reperfuse the skin and therefore an indirect measurement of the acutal perfusion of that part of the body. It is not a diagnostic test of any specific disease process or injury. An absent pulse can result from many of the same conditions as slow capillary refilling time.

Blood Pressure

Blood pressure is not of major importance during the initial assessment and the 60 seconds allotted to that component. The EMT should reserve the blood pressure reading for the focused examination.

Hemorrhage

The EMT should assess for major external bleeding. If major external bleeding is evident, the EMT should control the bleeding with direct pressure, pressure dressing, or pressure point. If the EMT cannot control bleeding with these interventions, he or she should initiate transportation immediately.

Disability (Level of Consciousness) Assessment (D)

During the initial assessment, quick determination of the patient's LOC or responsiveness and use of terms that other members of the health care team can easily understand are important. This is another test, like the capillary refilling time and the pulse, that can be the result of several conditions, the most common of which are hypoxia, brain injury, metabolic conditions such as diabetes, and drug and alcohol overdose. The most critical condition for the patient's survival is hypoxia; therefore LOC in the initial assessment is considered to be an indirect measurement of cerebral oxygenation (brain cell function).

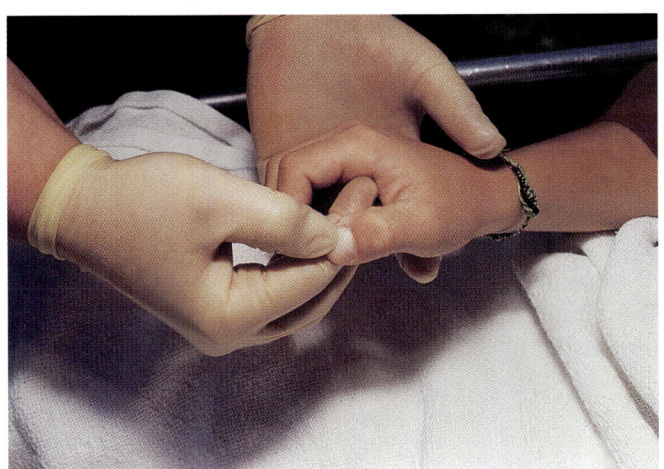 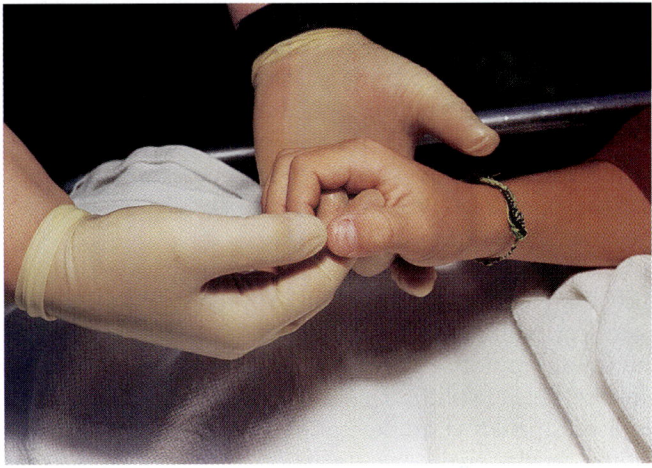

FIGURE 8.5 A, Capillary refill is evaluated by gently pressing on the back of the patient's nail bed or on top of the hand or foot. **B,** The color should return to pink within 2 seconds.

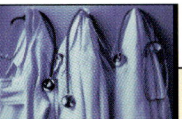 **Physician Notes**

Level of consciousness is abbreviated as *LOC*. *LOC* is frequently misused to represent *loss of consciousness*. A good EMT will use the term correctly but will be aware that others may not and therefore will ask to be sure what is meant when it seems that *LOC* is used incorrectly. The EMT should not assume anything in providing patient care.

The easiest system for defining LOC is the **AVPU** scale:

A—Patient is Alert
V—Patient responds to a Verbal stimulus
P—Patient responds to a Painful stimulus
U—Patient is Unresponsive

A patient is considered to be alert and **oriented** if he or she is aware of the time, place, person, and situation (oriented × 4) and the events surrounding the immediate time. Loss of recall of the event may indicate a period of loss of consciousness. The patient should be verbally responsive and able to answer appropriate questions. Altered LOC may become evident if the patient's responses make no sense.

If the patient is not verbally responsive, the EMT should determine whether the patient responds to painful or uncomfortable stimuli, such as an obvious injury or when the patient's sternum is vigorously rubbed.

> ✓ LOC is assessed using the AVPU system: A = alert, V = responds to verbal stimulation, P = responds to painful stimulus, U = unresponsive.

Priority Patient

Upon completing or during the initial assessment, if the patient's condition is serious, the EMT should postpone the rest of the examination until the patient is en route to an appropriate medical facility. Use of ALS is important but should not delay transportation; if available, early activation of ALS is beneficial. However, the EMT should not delay transportation of the critical patient until the arrival of ALS on the scene. The appropriate intervention for a severely ill or injured patient is rapid transportation to a medical facility; ALS may be able to rendezvous en route.

Rapid Focused History and Physical Examination

Whether en route or on-scene, the rapid focused history and physical examination is the next step in patient assessment. At this point the EMT has completed the initial assessment, and appropriate interventions have been completed or are in progress. The focused history and physical part of the overall assessment means just that—the EMT should focus his or her attention on the region of the patient's body that is most likely responsible for the current condition.

The information gathered during the scene size-up and initial assessment helps the EMT focus on additional historical information and the body systems that he or she should rapidly examine to determine the presence of life-threatening conditions. The EMT directs this part of the assessment toward the trauma or the medical patient. Should the patient have both an illness and an injury, the EMT can gather information on both conditions logically and rapidly. The EMT should perform life-saving interventions as soon as their necessity is determined by the assessment.

Rapid Focused History

The **SAMPLE history** is a tool used to gather pertinent information about the patient and is part of both the trauma and the medical focused assessments. The EMT often takes the history while performing other patient care tasks, such as the physical examination or interventions. The EMT can obtain historical information from the patient, family members, bystanders, and other emergency care providers. The components of the SAMPLE history are as follows:

S—Signs (patient physical findings) and/or symptoms (patient complaints) reported to the EMT
A—Allergies to medications or environment
M—Medications (prescription and over-the-counter [OTC])
P— Pertinent medical history as it relates to the patient's current problem
L—Last oral intake
E—Event (what has happened to the patient)

To further evaluate the patient's chief complaint as defined by signs, symptoms, and events, the EMT can use the mnemonic OPQRST:

O—Onset (When did it start?)
P—Provocation (What makes it worse?)
Q—Quality (How does it feel?)
R—Radiation (Does it move?)
S—Severity (How bad is it?)
T—Time (How long does it last?)

Another mnemonic helpful in remembering to look for signs of trauma in each region or system is DCAP-BTLS:

D—Deformities
C—Contusions
A—Abrasions
P—Punctures/penetrations
B—Burns
T—Tenderness
L—Lacerations
S—Swelling

When taking a history, the EMT should first use an open-ended question, such as, "Can you tell me what happened?" This question gives the patient or other history giver an opportunity to describe what happened or what the problem is without being biased by the way the EMT asks the question. The response can be variable. The patient or other history giver may provide a clear picture of the situation, a minimal response, or a long presentation with little information about the problem at hand. After the EMT asks the open-ended question, he or she should use a more direct line of questioning, including the OPQRST mnemonic to provide more guidance to the patient's response and further define the problem. The objective is to develop a clear idea of the patient's current problem.

> ✓ The rapid focused history is guided by the SAMPLE history system, and the OPQRST evaluation explores the patient's chief complaint.

Rapid Focused Physical Examination

The rapid focused physical examination for the ill or injured patient is a brief look at major body areas to identify life-threatening conditions. If the patient is alert and oriented (can state name, current location, date, etc.), he or she can direct the examination to the appropriate body areas.

If the patient is not alert and oriented, the first intervention should be airway management with increased oxygenation and rapid, safe transportation to a medical facility. While preparing the patient for transportation to the medical facility and while en route, the EMT must rapidly examine all body areas while looking for and correcting other life-threatening conditions. The scene assessment, initial assessment, or general impression may indicate to the EMT that assessment of other regions of the body is needed even if the patient is alert and oriented.

In performing the physical examination, the EMT should use the senses of touch, sight, smell, and hearing to obtain information about the patient. The examination is separated into various body areas: head, neck, chest, abdomen, pelvis, extremities, back, and baseline vital signs.

As the examination progresses, the EMT compares one side of the body against the other, looking for differences. The uninjured or uninvolved side acts as a normal finding for comparison of abnormal findings. For all body areas the EMT should note the presence of skin color changes (pale, yellow, red, or blue) and the presence or absence of sweating. All of these signs are important in determining the accurate condition of the patient.

> ✓ The EMT uses the rapid focused history and physical examination to quickly identify and allow immediate intervention of life-threatening conditions not found in the initial assessment. The focus of the examination (body areas examined) is determined by patient complaint, mechanism of injury or nature of illness, and level of patient responsiveness.

Rapid Focused History and Physical Examination (Trauma)

Physical Examination (Trauma)

In any major trauma patient, the chance of survival is proportional to the length of time between the onset of the incident and the initiation of definitive care. Definitive care for the patient with no airway requires opening the airway and providing oxygenation of the lungs. For the cardiac arrest patient, definitive care involves reestablishment of an effective cardiac output. For the trauma patient, definitive care is hemorrhage control. Control of internal hemorrhage usually cannot be completed outside the operating room. Therefore the EMT must transport the patient to a medical facility with an available operating room. Urban areas usually have trauma centers with available operating rooms. Rural areas may not have a trauma center; therefore the patient is usually transported to the only available hospital in the area. A helicopter response to the scene may be available to transport the patient to an urban trauma center. Each community has its own unique problems. Each EMT must become familiar with the local, regional, and statewide trauma systems.

In the patient with an isolated injury, such as trauma to the arm, the focused examination includes only the arm and is brief. The EMT then proceeds to baseline vital signs, SAMPLE history, and detailed physical examination. The EMT starts transportation immediately when he or she identifies the need.

In the patient with obvious multiple injuries or in the unresponsive patient, the focused examination is still rapid but covers more body systems (Figure 8.6). If the EMT finds life-threatening injuries in the initial assessment, he or she should initiate transportation and perform the focused examination en route to the medical facility. In some instances, the EMT does not perform the focused examination at all if he or she cannot complete the initial assessment and interventions.

Determining whether the patient is alert can help with the assessment. The alert patient can direct the examination with his or her complaints and responses to the examination. Patients with a decreased LOC may still react to an examination with verbal clues, such as moans and groans, or may withdraw from the discomfort caused by examination.

The rapid assessment focuses on those body areas in which the EMT suspects life-threatening injury (Figure 8.7). When examining patients, EMTs should use their senses (smell, hearing, sight, and touch) to assist them. The EMT should first take a moment to identify odors such as gasoline or alcohol (smell). The EMT should then listen for sounds from the patient such as any obvious wheezing, snoring, or other indications of an airway or breathing problem (hearing). The EMT should inspect (sight) and palpate (touch) each body area to identify obvious evidence of injury, such as deformities, **contusions** (deep bruising), **abrasions** (scrapes), punctures or penetrations, burns, tenderness to **palpation**, swelling, or **lacerations** (cuts). Each body area assessment is discussed in the following sections, and additional information is presented.

Head. The EMT should look for obvious evidence of injury. Deformity of the skull, facial bruising, an unstable mandible, teeth that do not oppose or fit together, or movable facial bones are indications of underlying injuries that require an intervention. Some signs indicate old injuries, such as Battle's sign and raccoon eyes (see Chapter 24). Sometimes an altered LOC may be the only indication of a head injury. The size of the pupils and their reactivity to light are important.

Neck. If the mechanism of injury indicates the potential for a head or neck injury, or if the patient is unresponsive, the EMT should immobilize the cervical spine. The EMT should look for obvious evidence of injury. He or she should look for distention of the large neck (jugular) veins indicating a back-up of blood from the heart, which may be due to injury to the chest. If the trachea (windpipe) is not in the middle of the neck as determined by inspection

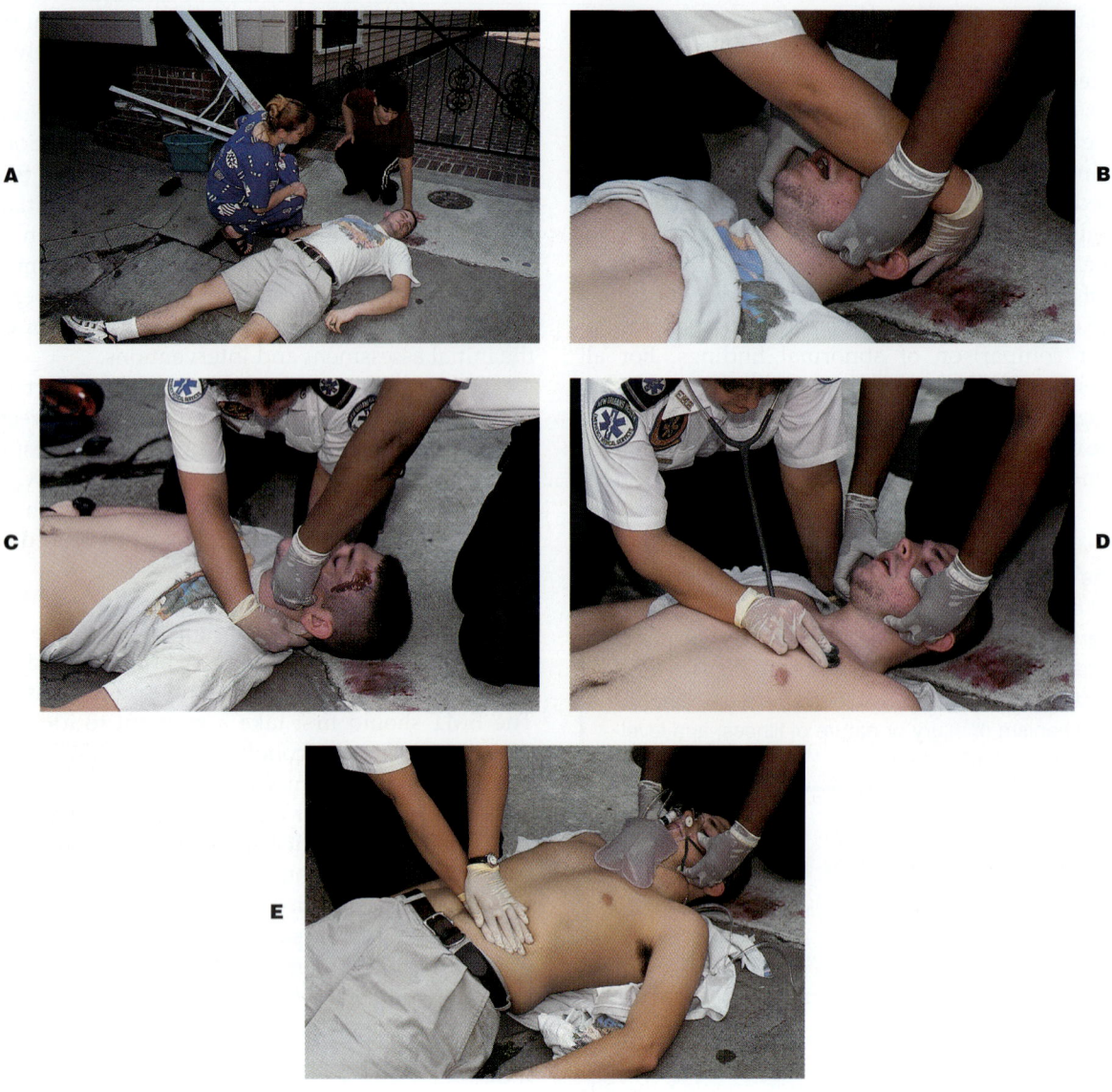

FIGURE 8.6 Focused history and physcial examination—trauma. **A,** Consider the mechanism of injury. **B,** Assess, inspect, and palpate the head. **C,** Assess, inspect, and palpate the neck. **D,** Assess, inspect, and palpate the chest. Check for crepitus. **E,** Assess, inspect, and palpate the abdomen. Is the abdomen soft or rigid?

or palpation, a life-threatening injury to the chest (tension pneumothorax) may be present (Figure 8.8).

Chest. The ribs connect in the back (posterior) to the thoracic spine and in the front (anterior) to the sternum, forming a bony cage. This cage houses the heart, great vessels, and lungs. Under the diaphragm in the abdomen lies the liver on the patient's right, the spleen on the patient's left, and abdominal organs covered by the lower portion of the rib cage (Figure 8.9).

Chest injuries can cause life-threatening damage to many body organs. The EMT should continue to look, listen, and feel for obvious evidence of injury. When the chest is visualized, the EMT should look for any areas that move opposite to the rest of the chest during ventilation. This movement, called **paradoxical motion**, indi-

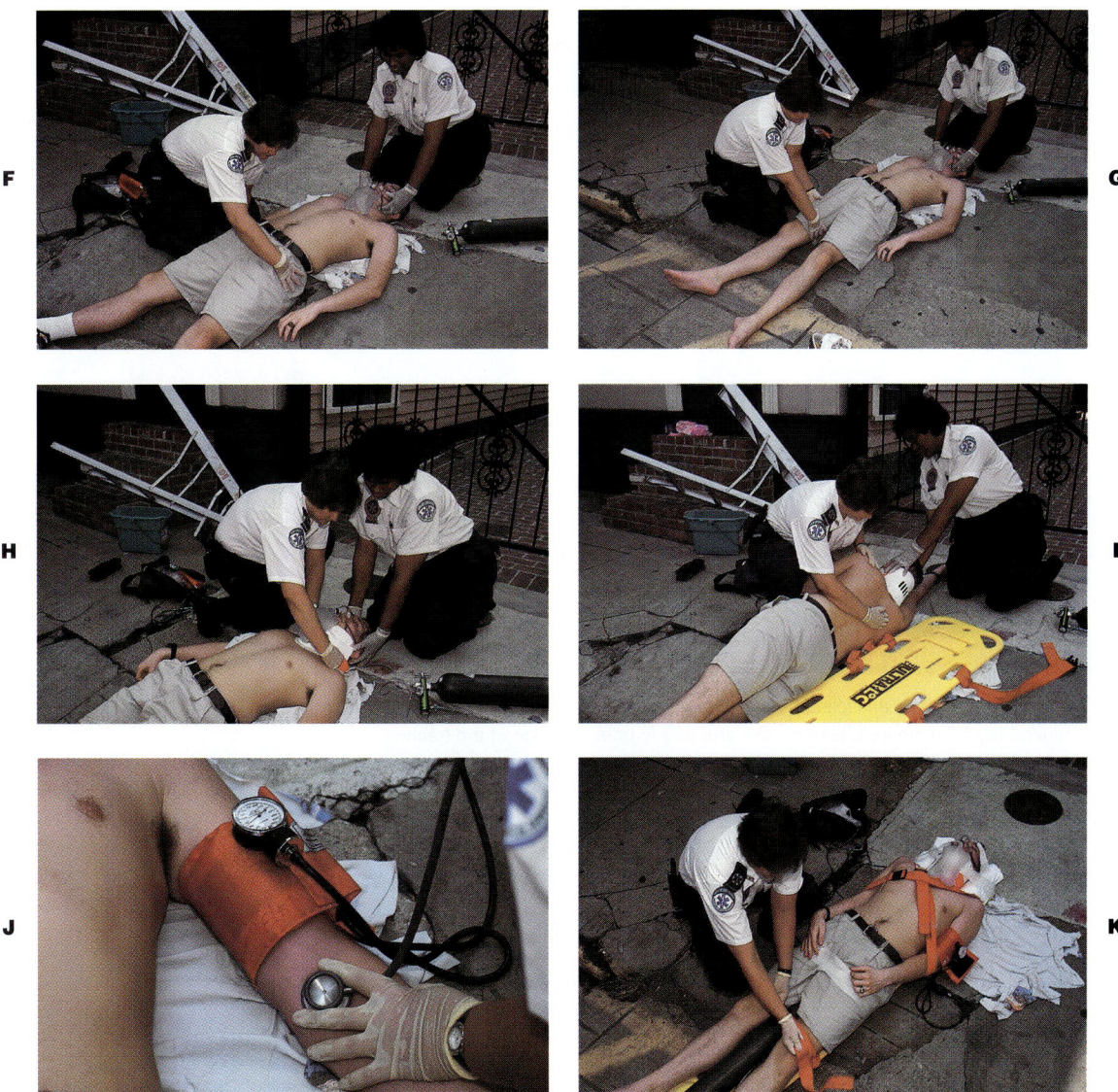

FIGURE 8.6 cont'd **F,** Assess, inspect, and palpate the pelvis. Gently compress the pelvis for tenderness or motion if no pain is noted. **G,** Assess, inspect, and palpate all four extremities. Check for distal pulse, sensation, and motor function. **H,** Apply cervical immobilization device. **I,** Roll the patient with spinal precautions and assess, inspect, and palpate the posterior body. **J,** Assess baseline vital signs. **K,** SAMPLE history.

cates that a section of the bony rib cage has been broken loose by a powerful force and may have damaged the lung underneath (Figure 8.10). The EMT should also check the chest for **crepitus**, which indicates air under the skin and can be felt better than seen (palpating "bubble packs" simulate the feel of crepitus). Crepitus indicates a connection, due to injury, between the air inside the lungs and the skin overlying the chest. During the chest examination, the EMT should use a stethoscope to determine if breath sounds are present and equal on each side of the chest (bilaterally) at the apices, in the midclavicular area, in the midaxillary area, and at the bases (Figure 8.11). In most trauma patients, the patient will be in the supine position when the EMT begins the examination of the chest. The posterior portions of the chest will not be available for the examination. Almost any significant

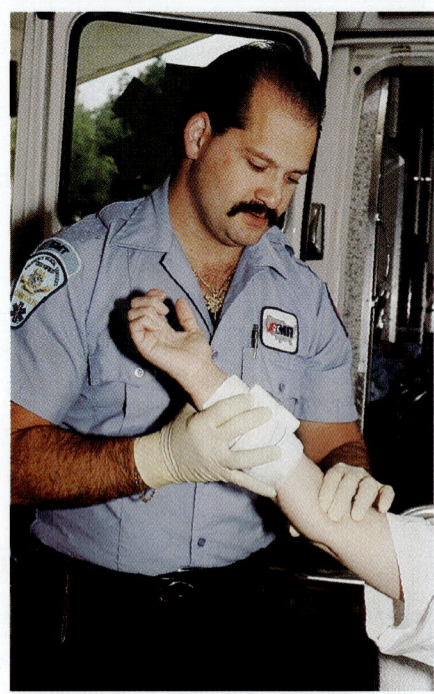

FIGURE 8.7 In the patient with an isolated injury, such as trauma to the arm, the focused examination includes only the arm and is brief. The EMT then proceeds to baseline vital signs, SAMPLE history, and the detailed physical examination, initiating transportation when appropriate.

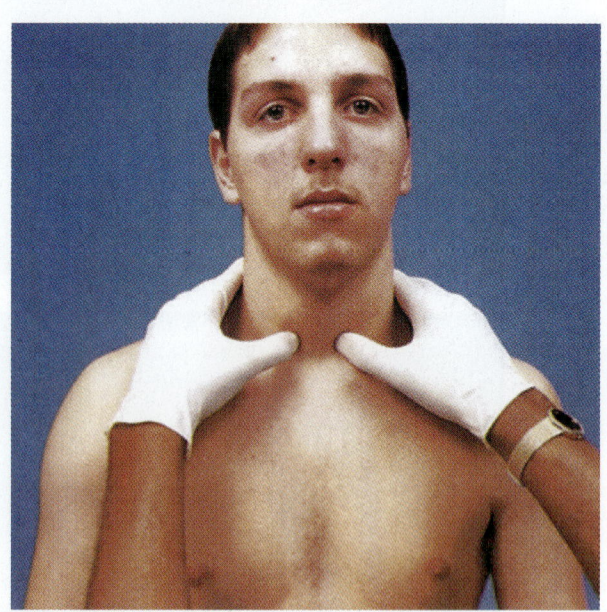

FIGURE 8.8 Position of the thumbs to evaluate the midline position of the trachea.

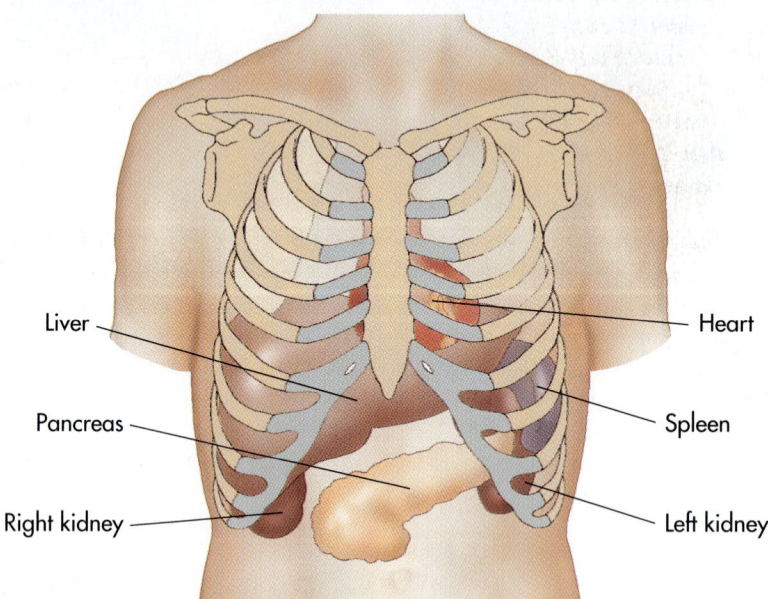

FIGURE 8.9 Organs protected by the rib cage.

injury that can be detected with the stethoscope can be heard from the anterior part of the chest.

Abdomen. In addition to the liver and spleen, which are tucked under the lower rib cage, the abdomen contains other organs that may be injured, including the stomach, pancreas, and portions of the small and large bowel (Figure 8.12). The kidneys, ureters, and large blood vessels (aorta and venae cavae) located behind the organs listed previously also may be injured. In the

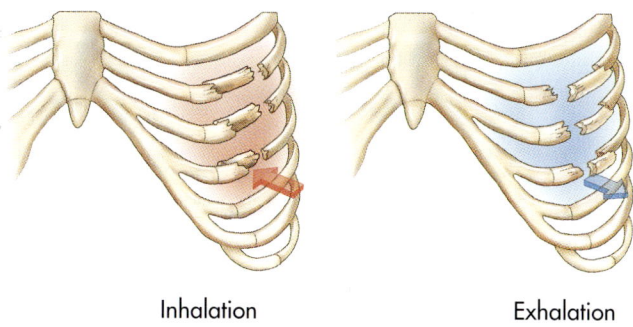

FIGURE 8.10 Paradoxical motion.

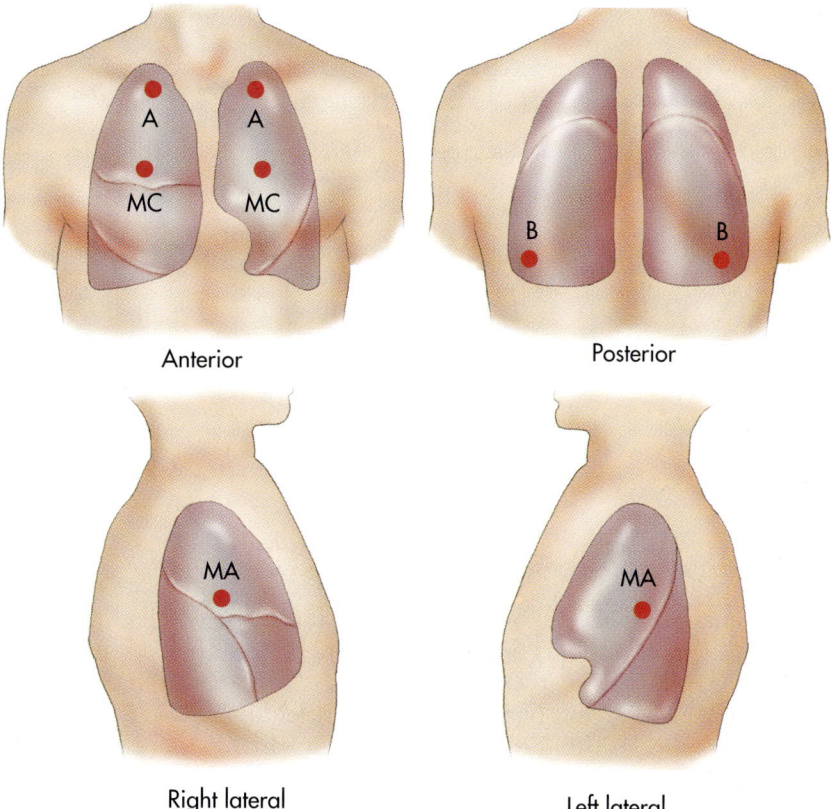

FIGURE 8.11 Listen for breath sounds with the stethoscope at the apex, in the midclavicular line, in the midaxillary line, and at the bases. Compare both sides of the chest at these locations for quality air movement.

later stages of pregnancy, the uterus with the fetus will extend into the abdominal cavity (Figure 8.13).

Distention (swelling) of the abdomen may indicate injury. This sign can be difficult to determine in obese patients. If the patient is alert, the EMT can locate areas that are tender on palpation. A firm abdomen can be an indication that blood, stomach contents, or intestinal contents are present in the abdomen. These substances irritate the abdominal lining and cause the abdominal muscles to tighten (contract).

Bruising and swelling may be a late developing sign of injury. Their absence is unimportant, but their presence is very important. The EMT should look for bruising and swelling and be able to describe them either on the radio or to the emergency department personnel on arrival at the medical facility.

Pelvis. The pelvis is a bony ring into which many blood vessels enter. Some of the blood vessels travel to organs in the pelvis, and some travel through the pelvic ring to

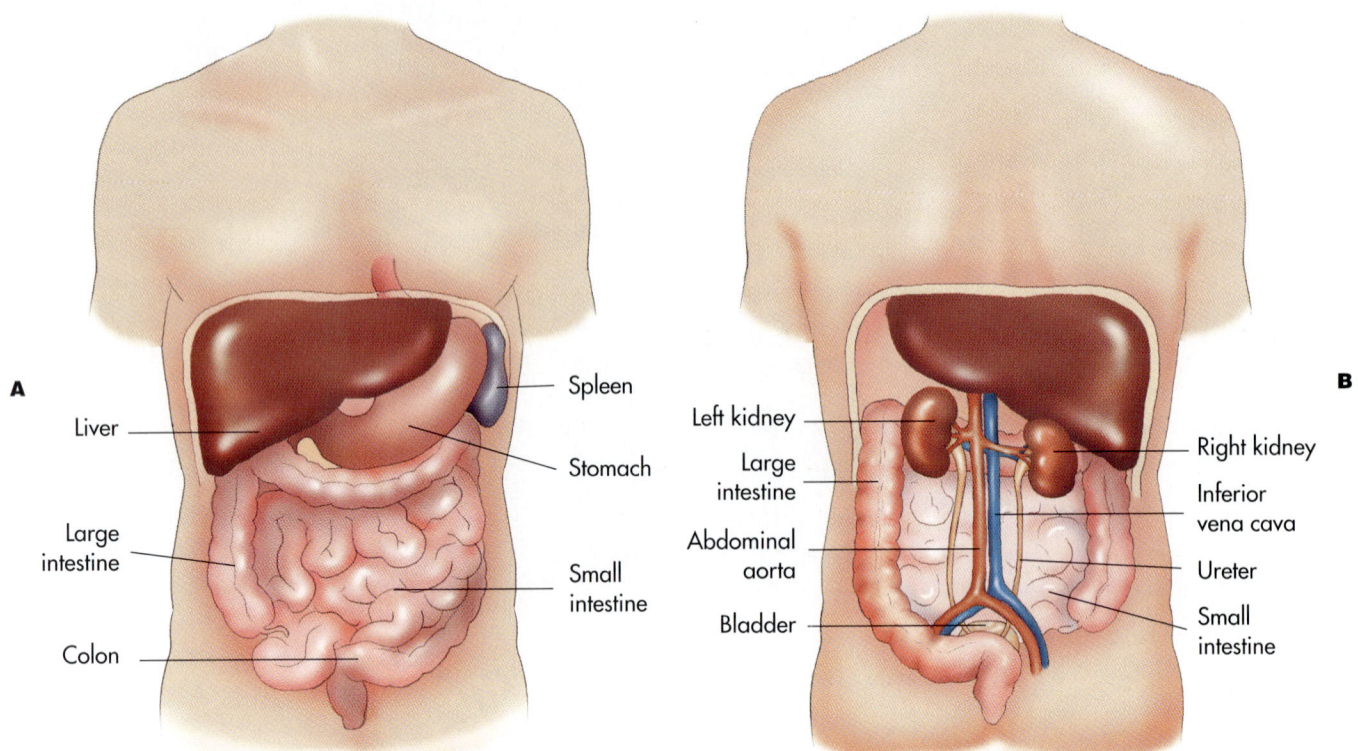

FIGURE 8.12 Organs of the abdomen. **A,** Anterior. **B,** Posterior.

the lower extremities. Located within the pelvic ring is the bladder and, in the female patient, the reproductive organs. In the patient in early pregnancy, a fetus is contained within this ring. The EMT should gently compress the pelvis on the anterior illiac crest and over the symphysis pubis. Tenderness or motion in either area may indicate a damaged ring and injury to structures inside (Figure 8.14).

Extremities. In the alert patient, the EMT should ask for sites of pain or changes in sensation or movement. He or she should look and feel for evidence of injury at these sites. The extremity with obvious or potential injury will need assessment of circulation, sensation, and motor function.

In the unresponsive patient, the EMT should rapidly look at and feel all extremities for evidence of injury. He or she should always check for circulation in the extremities. If the unresponsive patient withdraws an extremity during examination, then sensation and motor function are intact. If no movement occurs, then motor and sensory function cannot be determined.

Tenderness, angulation of the bone, crepitus (palpable), unusual movement, or movement in an unusual area are all signs of extremity injuries, the most severe of which is a fracture. The prehospital provider does not have the equipment or time to determine whether the injury is a sprain, strain, contusion, or fracture. The EMT should manage the injury as if it were severe (e.g., as a fracture).

Back. Examine the back for obvious signs of injury during the most appropriate time, which is often when the patient is log-rolled prior to placement on the cervical spine immobilization device, or if life-threatening injury is suspected.

Baseline vital signs. Lord Kelvin taught that if one can speak in numbers, then one's knowledge is very great. If one cannot speak in numbers, then one's knowledge is weak. At the most appropriate point, the EMT should obtain more exact numbers for the pulse, respirations, and blood pressure than were obtained in the rapid initial assessment. The EMT should determine life-threatening in-

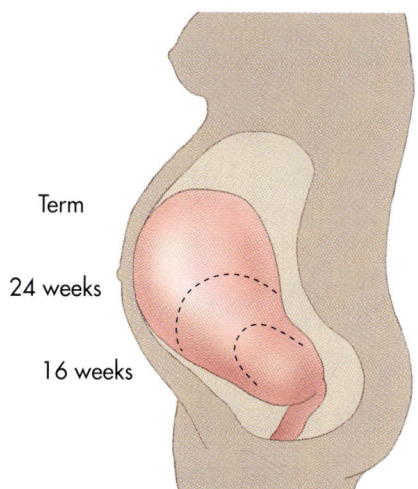

FIGURE 8.13 As pregnancy progresses, the uterus enlarges and becomes an abdominal organ until delivery.

juries before taking baseline vital signs in the injured patient; he or she can obtain baseline vital signs en route to the medical facility.

> ✓ The rapid focused history and physical examination of a trauma patient consists of determining the mechanism of injury and examination of the head, neck, chest, abdomen, pelvis, extremities, and back. The EMT should also obatin accurate vital signs.

Rapid Focused History and Physical Examination (Medical)

Identification of medical problems often requires more diligence on the part of the EMT than identification of problems with the trauma patient. What you see is not often what you get. History plays a much larger part in the assessment of the patient with a medical problem. The EMT must, to an extent, become a detective tracking down a problem without a lot of background information.

EMTs are frequently less comfortable caring for the ill patient than for the injured patient. It is difficult to understand all the medical problems that an EMT may encounter. This difficulty may lead to frustration for the EMT and a sense that he or she is not "doing his or her job." The EMT does not make a specific medical diagnosis but forms a general impression. The assessment approach taught in this chapter allows the EMT to determine problems and provide interventions that help the patient. For example, it does not matter that the patient has congestive heart failure. However, the EMT must assess the breathing problem and provide interventions of

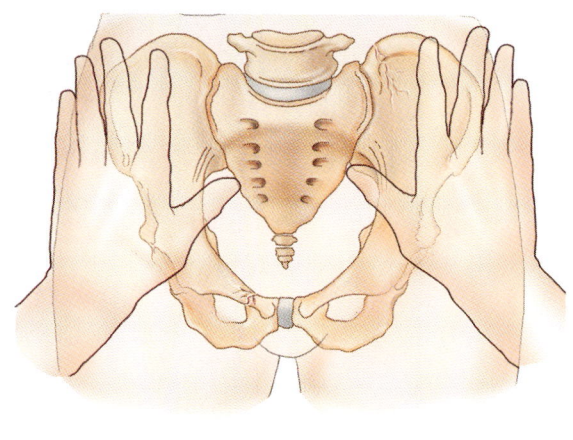

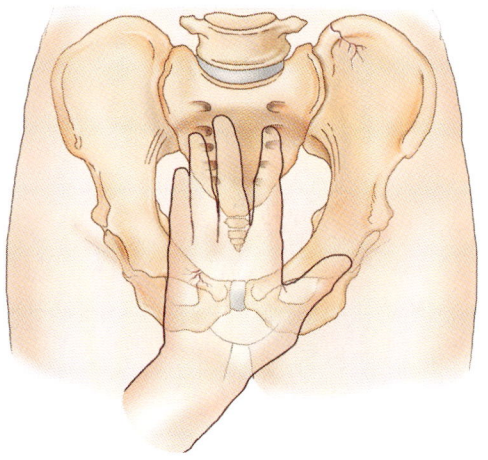

FIGURE 8.14 Gentle compression of the pelvis can reveal damage to the pelvic ring.

oxygen and rapid transportation while closely monitoring the patient until arrival at a medical facility.

Rapid Focused History (Medical)

With the alert and oriented patient, the EMT should use the SAMPLE history and the OPQRST mnemonic to determine the medical problem and direct the rapid focused physical examination. For example, the patient who complains of shortness of breath and reports use of an inhaler requires a rapid assessment of the chest for signs of breathing problems.

In the unresponsive patient, young children, geriatric patients, and patients with an altered LOC, historical information will often come from family members, bystanders, and other providers. Because the patient cannot direct the assessment, the EMT should proceed with a rapid physical examination of all body areas.

Rapid Focused Physical Examination (Medical)

While gathering the information described previously, the EMT should begin the rapid physical examination, providing interventions when they are required (Figure 8.15).

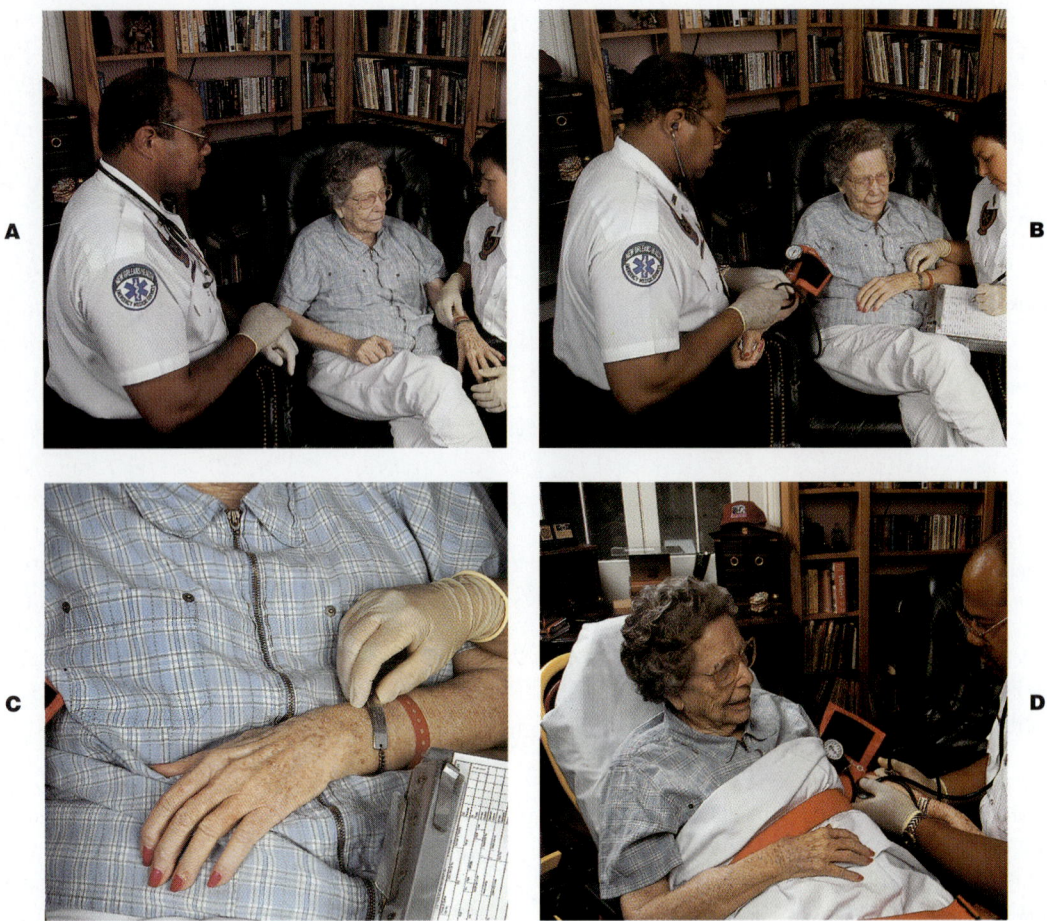

FIGURE 8.15 Rapid focused history and physical examination of a responsive medical patient. **A,** Ask the OPQRST questions and assess SAMPLE history. **B,** The rapid physical examination is directed toward finding life-threatening problems and providing appropriate interventions. **C,** Assess baseline vital signs. **D,** Consult medical direction, and provide emergency medical care based on signs and symptoms.

If the patient appears critical, the EMT should initiate appropriate interventions, including rapid transportation to a medical facility. The EMT directs the examination toward finding life-threatening problems and providing appropriate interventions. The history and examination also allow the EMT to provide an accurate report to medical direction. The accuracy of the report is important; the EMT is in the position of gathering history from the patient, family members, and bystanders and may be the only person able to provide this full range of information to the receiving medical facility. The EMT can complete all or part of this history and physical examination en route to the medical facility.

Head. The EMT should watch the patient's facial expressions and eyes. These areas reflect the level of interest and interaction with the environment and thus are a guide to the severity of the patient's illness. The EMT should check for breath odors such as alcohol. He or she should also note facial weakness or uneven movement.

Neck. The EMT should look for dilated neck veins, which may indicate a poorly functioning heart (see Figure 8.10). He or she should note swelling in the neck and tightening of the neck muscles (accessory muscles of ventilation), which may indicate breathing difficulty.

Chest. The EMT should observe the chest during ventilation, looking for uneven movement or evidence of labored breathing such as **retractions** or abdominal breathing. Retractions occur above the clavicles, between the ribs, or just below the ribs. They appear as indentations, or "sucked in" areas, during inspiration because of the increased work required to breath. Abdominal breathing is the pushing out of the abdomen with inspiration, which helps the diaphragm move downward, causing the lungs to expand. The EMT should also listen for breath sounds.

Abdomen. The EMT should check for distention, tenderness, firmness, and lumps. In the female patient, the EMT should look for obvious pregnancy.

Pelvis. In the pregnant patient in labor, the EMT should check the perineum for evidence of imminent delivery.

Extremities. Cool, clammy extremities may indicate poor perfusion. The EMT should observe extremity movement and extremity **edema** (swelling), which is the result of water leaking from the capillaries.

Back. When edema is present, fluid generally collects in the lower part of the body (the legs in the upright patient and the sacrum in the bed-bound patient).

Baseline vital signs. Medical problems can be less obvious than injuries. Baseline pulse, respirations, and blood pressure can help the EMT determine significant medical illness. The EMT should consider obtaining these values early in the rapid assessment of the medical patient to help focus the physical examination.

Detailed Physical Examination

After the EMT has discovered obvious life-threatening injuries or illnesses and initiated interventions including transportation, he or she performs a **detailed physical examination**. During this phase of assessment, the EMT reevaluates the patient for obvious indications of illness that may have been missed and looks for less obvious evidence of injury or illness to guide additional interventions. The EMT then reevaluates earlier assessment findings and interventions. If the patient is alert and oriented, the EMT performs a detailed examination on the area of concern identified by the patient. In the unresponsive patient, the EMT examines all body areas in detail. Although the findings and/or interpretations may differ, the same examination technique is used for both the trauma and the medical patient. An example is the pediatric patient with a draining ear. In the trauma situation a draining ear indicates a fractured skull, but in the medical setting it is usually the result of a hole in the eardrum from infection. Interventions for these two patients are different. However, interventions are not always different (e.g., a patient with bleeding inside the head that can be caused by either an illness or an injury). Unless other conditions exist, interventions for both patients would be the same except for the addition of cervical spine immobilization for the trauma patient.

Head
The EMT should reassess the patient's LOC, palpate the scalp, and look for new or increased areas of swelling, bleeding, or discoloration.

Face
The EMT should continue to monitor facial expressions and verbal response as a reflection of the patient's LOC. The EMT should check for previously unrecognized facial weakness or uneven movement, color changes, or sweating.

Ears
If drainage is present, the EMT should note the color, odor, and thickness of the drainage. The EMT should also look for discoloration behind the patient's ears.

Eyes
The EMT should check for foreign bodies, equal movement, or color change. The pupils should look the same when compared. Sunlight or a light shined in the eye will cause the pupil to get smaller (**constrict**); if the patient is

> ✓ The rapid focused history of the medical patient plays an important role in patient assessment. The examination includes assessment of facial expression and eyes, neck, chest, abdomen, pelvis, extremities, back, and vital signs.

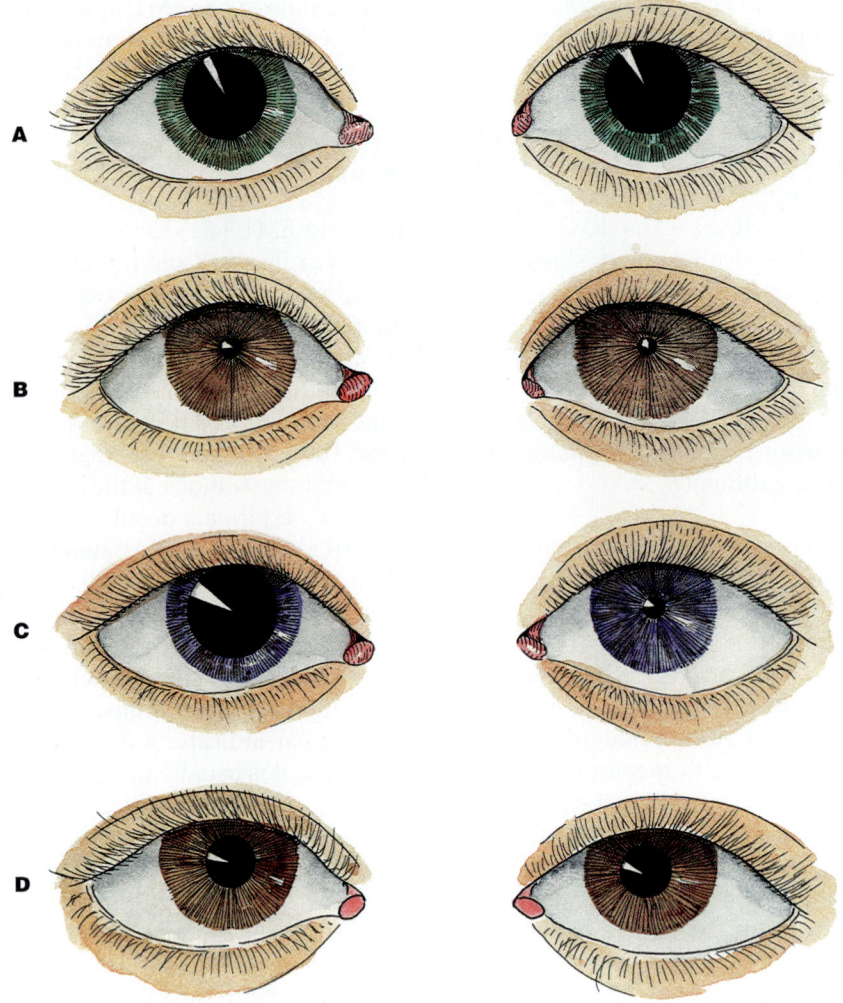

FIGURE 8.16 **A,** Dilated pupils. **B,** Constricted pupils. **C,** Unequal pupils. **D,** Normal pupils.

in dim light, the pupils will be larger (**dilate**). Both are normal reflexes that indicate the eye has the right level of light to function. Abnormal responses are pupils that are dilated in bright light or constricted in dim light. Another abnormal response is one pupil that is larger than the other (Figure 8.16). The EMT should check with the patient because uneven pupils may be a normal variation. Cataract surgery causes an irregular pupil and is seen most often in geriatric patients. As a rough check for vision in each eye, the EMT should have the patient count the EMT's fingers while the EMT's other hand is placed in front of the untested eye but not touching it (Figure 8.17).

Nose
Nasal flaring can be an indication of ventilatory difficulty. The EMT should note drainage from the nose as to color, odor, and thickness.

Mouth
The EMT should look for dentures, loose or broken teeth, or any item that can cause airway obstruction if inhaled. The EMT should note dryness or odors. The lips may demonstrate a color change.

Neck
The EMT should reassess the patient for vein distention, position of the trachea, swelling, and crepitus.

Chest
The EMT should reevaluate earlier findings and interventions. If the patient requires ventilation, the EMT should check effectiveness of air movement with the stethoscope. The EMT should look for labored breathing, such as retractions or abdominal breathing.

Abdomen
The EMT should check for new or changing distention, tenderness, or firmness. He or she should listen to the abdomen with the stethoscope. In the female patient in the later stages of pregnancy, the EMT should feel for the enlarged uterus. It also may be possible for the EMT to feel the fetus move.

Pelvis

If previous palpation of the pelvic ring produced a painful response or movement of the ring, the EMT should not repeat the examination. It provides no further useful information and may cause more pain and possible damage. In the pregnant patient with abdominal pain, the EMT should check the perineum to see if delivery is in progress.

Extremities

The EMT should reevaluate previous findings or interventions. He or she should examine the nail beds for color changes (pink is normal, blue may indicate lack of oxygen, and red may indicate carbon monoxide poisoning). The EMT should look for edema. He or she should check the perfusion and function of an extremity below (distal to) an injury site. Pulse checks, capillary refill, and temperature of the extremity (a warm extremity is adequately perfused) determine perfusion status. Limb movement and feeling demonstrate functional status.

Back

For most patients, the EMT examines the back when the patient is rolled onto a spinal immobilization device or placed on a stretcher. Once the patient is secured to a spinal immobilization device, reexamination of the back is difficult.

Reassessment of Baseline Vital Signs

The EMT should determine what changes, if any, have occurred to the patient's baseline vital signs.

> ✓ The purpose of the detailed physical examination is to discover less obvious evidence of illness and injury so that useful interventions can be initiated and to reassess earlier findings and interventions.

Ongoing Assessment

The purpose of the ongoing assessment is to reassess the patient for changes that may require new interventions, look for omissions, evaluate the effectiveness of earlier interventions, and reassess earlier significant findings. The timing of this ongoing assessment varies with the extent of the patient's injuries. The EMT should reassess critical patients every 5 minutes and stable patients every 15 minutes. The EMT continues the ongoing assessment until the patient is transferred to a higher level of care.

> ✓ During the ongoing assessment, the EMT periodically checks the patient for changes that may require new interventions and reassesses the effectivenes of earlier interventions.

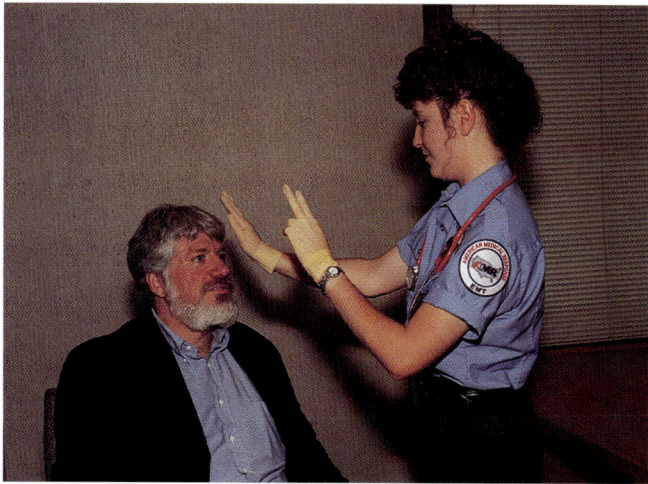

FIGURE 8.17 In suspected visual problems due to illness or injury, a finger count examination provides a quick screen.

■ BASELINE VITAL SIGNS

Vital signs generally include respirations, pulse, blood pressure, and skin color and temperature. In some areas, protocols also call for the patient's level of consciousness (LOC) and pupil reaction to be included in the group of vital signs. Assessing a patient's vital signs generally takes about 2 minutes. An efficient and systematic approach to taking vital signs and history must be developed.

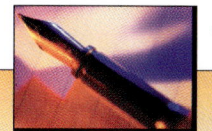 **Tips from the Pros**

In taking vital signs, "practice makes perfect." You will not instantly master these skills; mastery only comes with practice in the field.

Assessing vital signs and obtaining an accurate medical history are the foundation on which the emergency medical technician's (EMT's) treatment of a patient is based in the field. The EMT must take care of many life-threatening problems initially, but the vital signs and history may dictate the course of the treatment for the remainder of the time that the rescuer attends the patient. Therefore the EMT must get accurate and early assessments of vital signs and the patient's medical history.

Vital signs should be assessed and recorded at a minimum of every 15 minutes in a noncritical patient and every 5 minutes in a critical patient and after all medical interventions.

Signs Versus Symptoms

The EMT must be able to distinguish between a sign and a symptom. **Signs** are objective in nature. They can be seen, heard, smelled, measured, or felt concerning a patient's illness or injury. Examples of signs are hemorrhaging, noises from the patient's airway as he or she breathes, an unusual odor on the patient's breath, or deformities of bones. **Symptoms** are purely subjective in nature and have to be related by the patient. Examples of symptoms include nausea, chills, or chest pains.

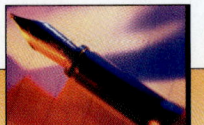

Tips from the Pros

If the patient's condition does not match the vital signs (the patient looks poor, but the vitals are within normal limits) treat the patient, not the vital signs. Always err on the side of caution.

✓ Signs are things that the EMT can observe about a patient's condition; symptoms are things that a patient tells the EMT about his or her condition.

Pulse

Identifying and Locating Pulses

The **pulse** is caused by the wave of blood moving through the vessels of the body as the heart beats. As the heart goes through its cycle of contractions and relaxations, blood is pumped through the circulatory system. Each time the heart contracts, it sends blood through the arteries, and the resulting wave creates the throb of blood that is the pulse. The pulse can be felt wherever an artery that lies close to the skin can be pressed against any underlying firm tissue, such as bone or cartilage (Figure 8.18). Pulses are most often assessed in the **radial artery** in the wrist at the base of the thumb or in the **carotid artery** on either side of the front of the neck. Pulses can also be assessed in the **femoral artery** located in the leg near the groin and in the brachial artery, located on the medial aspect of the upper arm (Figure 8.19).

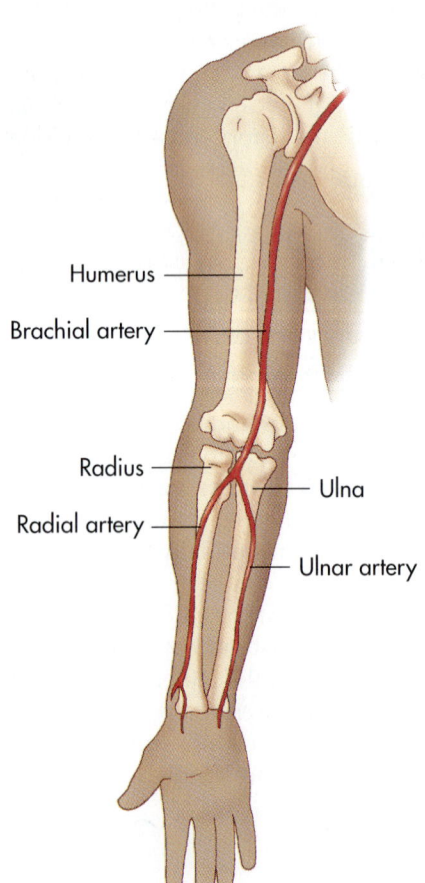

FIGURE 8.18 The radial artery lies just under the skin and over the distal end of the radius.

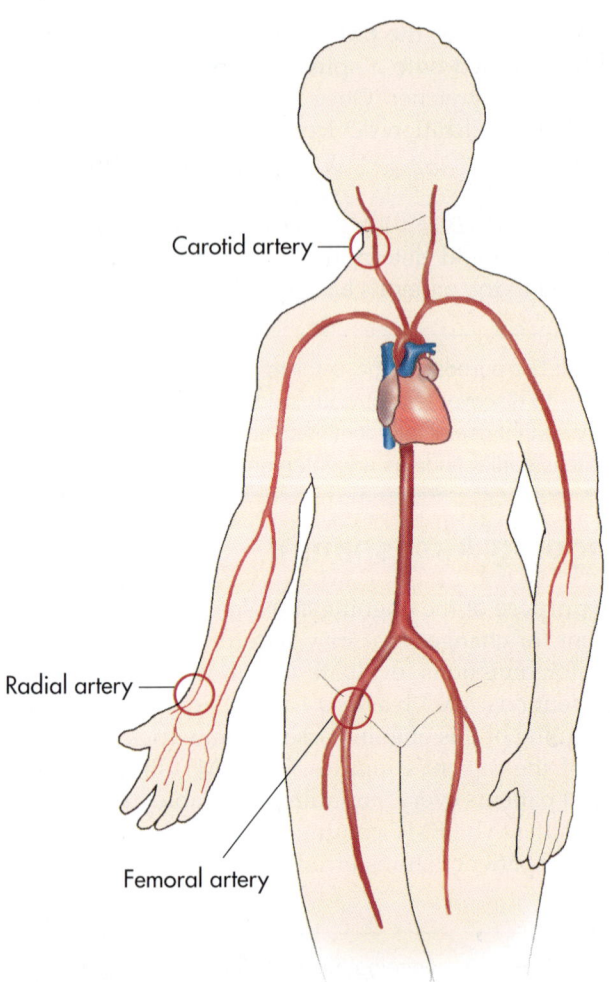

FIGURE 8.19 Pulses may be assessed in the carotid, radial, or femoral arteries.

Rate, Character, and Rhythm

The EMT evaluates the pulse for rate, character, and rhythm. The **pulse rate** is the number of beats per minute and may vary among individuals. Age, sex, physical condition, blood loss, stress, and other factors may have an influence on pulse rate. The normal pulse rate for an adult at rest is 60 to 100 beats per minute. A child's pulse rate may range from 80 to 100 beats per minute, whereas a healthy infant may have a pulse rate of 100 to 120 beats per minute. Rates of 130 to 140 beats per minute are not uncommon in the newborn; however, in adults any rate that exceeds 100 beats per minute is considered rapid. A rapid pulse is called **tachycardia**. An adult's pulse that is below 60 beats per minute, called **bradycardia**, is considered slow.

Pulse character refers to the force of the wave as the blood is pumped through the system. The pulse wave should feel strong. A strong pulse is a **full pulse**, and an extremely strong pulse is a **bounding pulse**. A pulse wave that feels weak and feeble is a **thready pulse**. The pulse rate may affect the character because the faster a pulse beats, the less time there is for the heart chambers to refill with blood. Less blood is pumped from the heart, and the resulting wave of blood may be smaller and weaker.

Pulse rhythm refers to the intervals between the beats of the heart. If the beats are constant, the pulse is regular. If the beats are not constant, the pulse is irregular. Character and rhythm are as important as pulse rate.

Assessing the Pulse

To assess the radial pulse, at least two (but not more than three) fingers are placed in the middle on the anterior side of the patient's arm just above the wrist. (The thumb should never be used to check the pulse because it has its own pulse.) The fingers are slid to the lateral (thumb) side while exerting enough pressure with the fingers to depress the skin of the patient's wrist (Figure 8.20). As the pulse is felt, the number of beats are counted for 30 seconds; that number is then multiplied by 2 to calculate the number of beats per minute, or the rate. If the pulse is irregular or the patient is a child, the EMT should always count for 1 full minute.

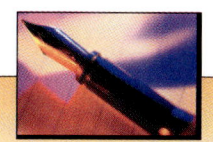

Tips from the Pros

With experience, reduce the count for pulse and respirations to 15 seconds and multiply by 4.

The pulse can be easily assessed at two other anatomic locations: the carotid artery and the femoral artery. The carotid artery is found by placing the fingers on the cricoid (Adam's apple) in the patient's neck. The fingers are slid to the same side of the patient as the assessor is positioned until the groove between the cricoid and muscles are felt. The carotid pulse should be felt in this groove just lateral (to the side) of the cricoid (Figure 8.21). Only one side should be palpated at a time. Sliding the fingers to the opposite side should be avoided. In this position, placing the hand over the throat of the patient may cause airway complications if the neck area is compressed by the force of the hand.

FIGURE 8.20 Assessment of the radial pulse.

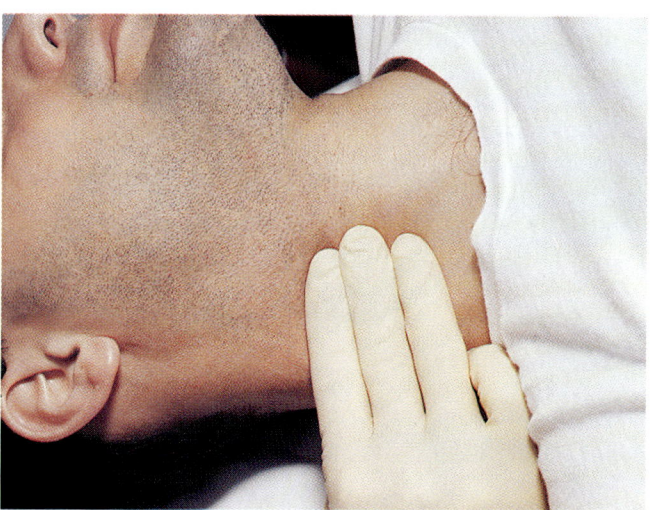

FIGURE 8.21 Assessment of the carotid pulse.

The femoral artery can be located by placing the fingers just lateral to the pubis where the leg and hip are attached. A greater amount of pressure may have to be exerted than at the carotid and radial pulses because the femoral pulse lies deeper below the skin surface than the other pulses. This location is not used often because of the presence of clothing (Figure 8.22). As the beats are counted, the rhythm of the pulse is determined by noticing if the intervals between the beats are approximately the same. If the intervals are about the same, then the pulse is "regular." If the interval changes, then the pulse is "irregular." The quality of the pulse is determined at the same time simply by the feel of the pulse beats. A normal pulse beat feels full and easy to count. A "bounding" pulse feels unusually strong. A weak, or "thready," pulse is hard to detect and count. After the pulse rate and quality have been determined, they should be recorded along with the time that the determination was made.

> ✓ The pulse is the wave of blood as it travels through the blood vessels. It is evaluated for rate, character, and rhythm. Pulse characteristics vary with age.

Ventilations

A single ventilation includes one cycle of breathing in and out. **Inhalation** (inspiration) is the process of taking air into the lungs. **Exhalation** (expiration) is the process of expelling the air that is in the lungs back out into the atmosphere.

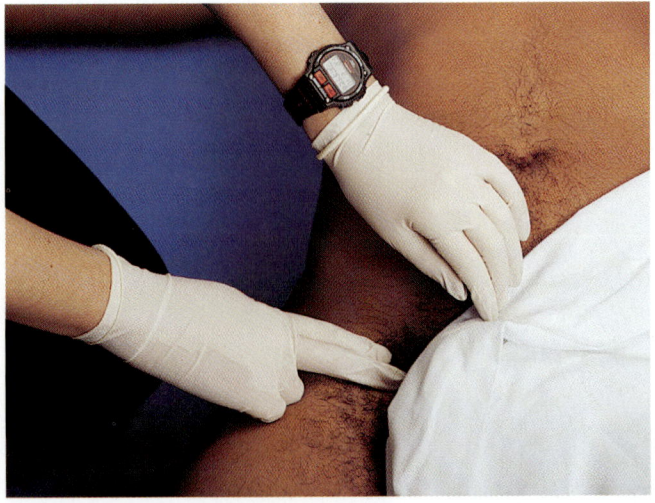

FIGURE 8.22 Assessment of the femoral pulse.

Rate, Character, and Rhythm

The **ventilatory rate** is the number of breaths in 1 minute. The normal ventilatory rate for an adult is between 12 and 20 breaths per minute. Children have a variable ventilatory rate. The smaller the child, the faster the rate of ventilations. An infant may easily breathe 25 to 30 breaths per minute. The EMT should keep in mind that when a person is excited or hurt, the number of ventilations may be increased. In time, the person's rate of ventilations will decrease to a more normal rate.

The EMT should be concerned with ventilatory character and rhythm as the patient's breathing is assessed. The **ventilatory character** includes the depth and the ease with which a patient takes a breath. **Ventilatory depth** refers to the amount of air that is exchanged with each breath. The ease with which a patient breathes determines whether the patient exhibits labored, difficult, or painful breathing. **Ventilatory rhythm** is regular or irregular. Regular ventilations exchange the same amount of air over several cycles in a fairly constant and rhythmic pattern. Any other pattern is irregular.

Assessing Ventilation

The recording of the pulse rate and quality may be delayed until the ventilatory rate and quality have been determined. The reason for delaying is that most patients unconsciously vary their ventilations if they know someone is assessing them. Therefore after the pulse is assessed, the EMT should remain in that position with fingers on the pulse and begin to assess the breathing (Figure 8.23). The ventilatory rate (number per minute) is determined by counting the number of ventilations in 30 seconds, multiplied by 2.

To assess ventilatory character, the EMT should watch the movement of the chest and listen to the patient breathe. If very little air is exchanged, hence little chest wall movement occurs, the ventilations are described as "shallow." If the patient has to exert a lot of effort to take each breath, the ventilations are described as "labored."

As soon as the ventilatory rate and quality have been determined, they should be recorded along with the time that the determination was made. If the recording of the pulse rate and quality have been delayed, then they should also be recorded at this time.

> ✓ Ventilation is the process of taking air into the lungs and expelling it back out. Ventilations are evaluated for rate, depth, rhythm, and character.

Blood Pressure

Systolic and Diastolic Blood Pressures

Blood pressure is a result of the pressure that the blood exerts on the walls of the arteries as blood is forced through the circulatory system by the contraction of the heart. Blood pressure is measured in millimeters (mm) of mercury (Hg). The pressure that is created by the contraction of the left ventricle forcing blood into the body system is called the **systolic pressure**. The systolic pressure is heard first. The **diastolic pressure** is heard second and occurs when the left ventricle is relaxed and refilling with blood. The residual pressure in the system is the diastolic pressure. Blood pressure is usually recorded in even numbers with the systolic pressure stated first and the diastolic pressure second. An example is 130 over 84 (130/84 mm Hg). The difference between the systolic and diastolic pressures is the **pulse pressure**.

An average blood pressure for an adult is 120/80 mm Hg. A widely used rule of thumb is 100 plus the patient's age for systolic pressure up to 150 mm Hg. Women usually range from 8 to 10 mm Hg lower. The diastolic pressure for both men and women is in the 60 to 90 range. Generally, blood pressure is lower in childhood until approximately 14 years of age, when adult ranges will be attained, and higher as age advances.

A popular method to quickly assess the patient's systolic pressure is to assess pulses in specific areas. If a carotid pulse is present, it is assumed the patient has a systolic pressure of at least 60 mm Hg. If a femoral pulse is present, it is assumed the patient's systolic pressure is at least 70 mm Hg. If a radial pulse is present, it is assumed that the patient has a systolic pressure of at least 80 mm Hg.

Equipment

Sphygmomanometers, or blood pressure cuffs, are available in sizes varying from pediatric to large adult. The cuff should completely circle the patient's arm with the bladder covering about half of the arm. The cuff should cover about two thirds of the upper arm, with the bottom about 1 inch above the bend at the elbow. The assessor should ensure that the proper cuff size is used and that he or she can hear the sound of the pulse clearly. Automatic blood pressure monitors are available that measure the pressure and record the reading electronically. However, many automatic monitors may not be suitable for use in a moving vehicle.

Assessing Blood Pressure

Two pieces of equipment are used to assess the blood pressure. The **stethoscope** consists of a bell and a diaphragm on one end of rubber or vinyl tubing and ear pieces on the other end (Figure 8.24, A). Both can be used to pick up sounds within the body. The sounds are transferred to the ear pieces via the tubing (Figure 8.24, B). The sphygmomanometer consists of a vinyl or rubber bladder surrounded by a material sleeve. A gauge and bulb pump are attached to the bladder with hoses (Figure 8.25, A).

Two methods can be used to assess blood pressure. Palpation of a patient's blood pressure is assessed by placing the blood pressure cuff around the patient's upper arm (Figure 8.25, B). The radial pulse is palpated with the assessor's fingers on the patient's same arm on which the cuff is placed. The release valve on the bulb pump is closed and the pump is squeezed repeatedly, filling the bladder with air until a pressure of approximately 200 mm Hg is realized. As the bladder tightens around the arm, the radial pulse will disappear. If the beat of the pulse can be felt when the assessor stops pumping pressure into the bladder, then more pressure should be added until the pulse cannot be felt. The valve on the bulb pump is turned to slowly release the pressure in the bladder. When the radial pulse returns to the arm, the pressure registering on the gauge at that point is the systolic pressure. The rest of the pressure can then be released. This method is not as accurate as auscultation. The systolic reading is generally considered to be 10 mm Hg lower than the same reading that would be obtained by auscultating the blood pressure. The diastolic pressure is not measured. It is recorded as 120/P.

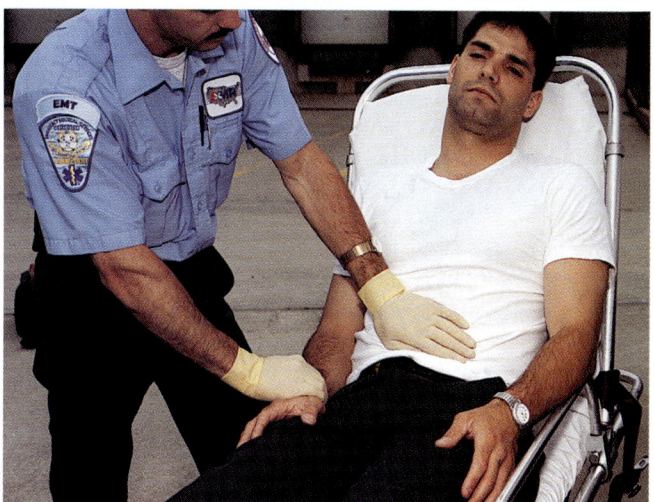

FIGURE 8.23 The assessment of pulse and respiration can be obtained while maintaining the patient in the same position.

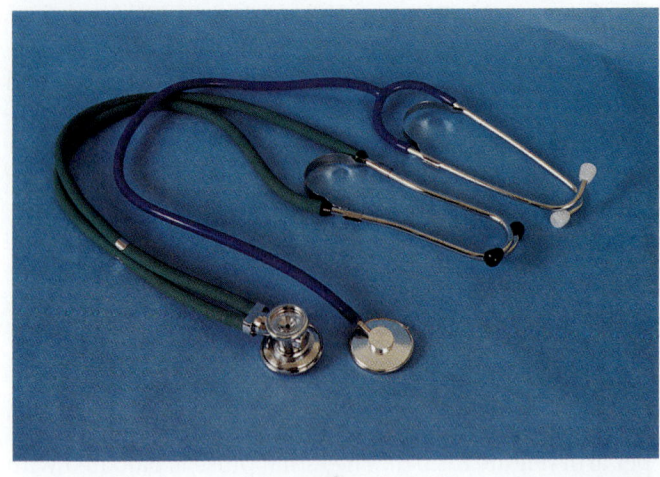
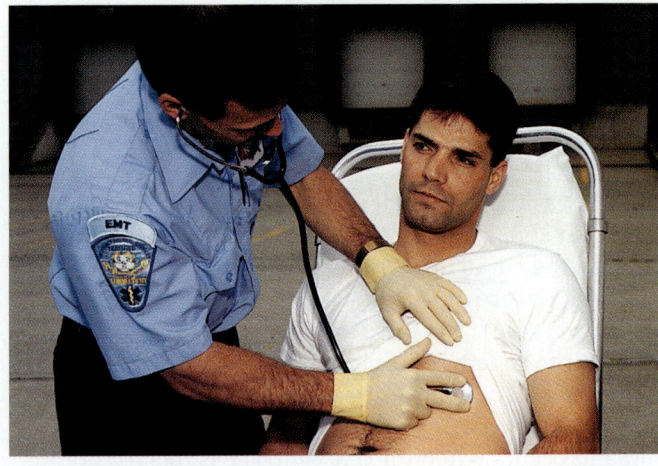

FIGURE 8.24 **A,** Stethoscope. **B,** An EMT using a stethoscope on a patient.

The most accurate method for assessing blood pressure is **auscultation** (Figure 8.25, C). The cuff is applied around the patient's upper arm. The brachial artery is found on the inside of the elbow near where the elbow bends. With the ear pieces in the assessor's ears, the bell of the stethoscope is place where the brachial artery is located. The bulb pump is squeezed with the valve closed so that the bladder fills with air until approximately 200 mm Hg is registered on the gauge. If the beat of the pulse can be heard when the assessor stops pumping the pressure into the bladder, then more pressure should be added until the beat cannot be heard. The valve should be slowly opened to release the pressure. When the heartbeat can be heard again, the pressure that is registered on the gauge is the systolic pressure.

The pressure should be released until a distinct change in sound from loud to soft is noticed. The change in sound may be to silence (no sound). When either of these changes is noticed, the pressure registered on the gauge is the diastolic pressure. A quiet environment is needed to take blood pressure. Obtaining accurate readings takes practice and is not instantly learned.

 Blood pressure measures the force of blood as it travels through the body. It is measured in millimeters of mercury using special equipment. The two methods for taking a blood pressure are palpation and auscultation.

Skin Color and Temperature

Skin color can be a good indicator of heart and lung function. Pale skin may indicate shock, heart attack, or emotional distress. Cyanosis may indicate poor oxygen levels in the blood and first may be noticed in the fingertips or lips and gums. Redness may be caused by high blood pressure, fever, or some types of poisoning. Skin temperature is assessed by touching the patient's skin with the back of the assessor's hand (Figure 8.26). Normal skin is generally warm and dry. A patient with a fever may present with very hot skin. A patient with unusually cool skin may be suffering from shock, heat exhaustion, or exposure to cold. Tympanic thermometers measure the temperature through a sensor placed in the patient's ear. The sensor reads the temperature and displays it digitally.

✓ Skin color and temperature can provide a good indication of the functions of the heart and lungs.

Level of Consciousness

A patient's LOC is assessed by talking to him or her or providing certain stimuli (tapping the feet or shaking the shoulder). The assessment is made to determine if the patient is awake, alert, or confused. The AVPU system is used to determine the patient's state of consciousness:

A—Patient is Alert
V—Patient responds to a Verbal stimulus
P—Patient responds to a Painful stimulus
U—Patient is Unresponsive

The "A" in AVPU represents a patient who is "alert" and "awake." If the patient is aware of the time, the place where he or she is located, and the current date and can recognize persons around him or her, then the patient is said to be alert. If the patient answers all the questions

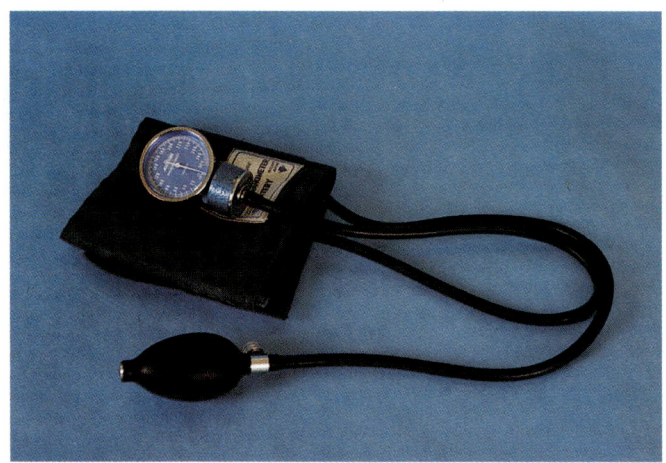
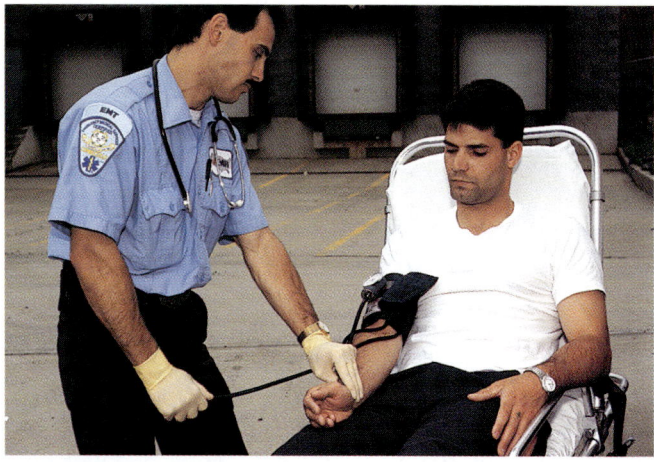
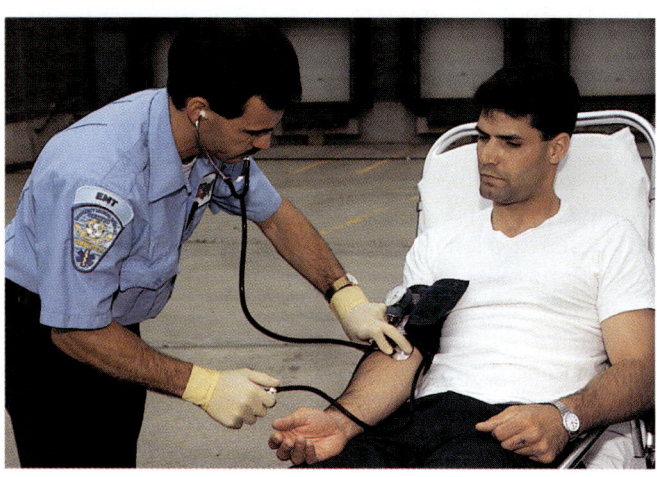

FIGURE 8.25 **A,** Sphygmomanometer. **B,** Measuring the blood pressure by palpation. **C,** Measuring the blood pressure by auscultation.

correctly, he or she is said to be oriented "times four" (written × "4").

The "V" in AVPU represents "verbal stimuli." If the patient responds to the EMT's questions, such as "squeeze my hand," then the patient is considered to respond to verbal stimuli.

The "P" in AVPU represents "painful stimuli." If the patient does not respond to verbal stimuli, often he or she will respond to painful stimuli. There are many humane ways to provide painful stimuli to a patient to assess LOC (e.g., stimulate the bottom of the patient's feet).

✓ The patient's LOC may indicate his or her overall condition. LOC is measured using the AVPU system.

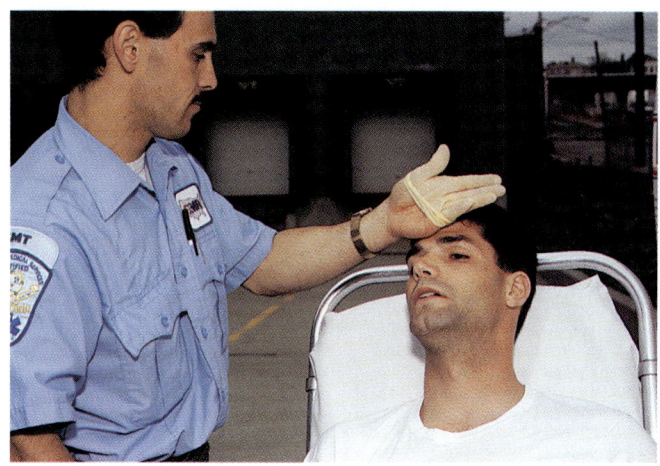

FIGURE 8.26 Skin temperature is evaluated by touching the patient's skin with the back of your hand.

Local protocols should be developed and followed for this assessment. Any response should be documented.

The "U" in AVPU represents "unresponsive." If the patient will not respond to verbal or painful stimuli, then the patient is considered to be unresponsive.

Pupil Reaction

A person's eyes are normally sensitive to the amount of light that enters through the pupils. Pupil size may vary for several reasons (e.g., head injury, drug overdose, or medical complications). Ordinarily when too much light enters the eye, the pupil constricts (shrinks) to limit the amount of light that is allowed to enter. Conversely, when in poor lighting or darkness, the pupil dilates (widens) to allow more light to enter the eye (Figure 8.27). These two functions can be valuable assessment tools. When the pupil constricts, the opening of the eye gets smaller. When the pupil dilates, the opening becomes larger (see Figure 8.16).

Under normal circumstances, the pupils of both eyes will constrict and dilate to the same degree and appear equal in size. The speed at which the constriction or dilation takes place should be the same. Pupils that react differently may indicate injury. They may be slow to react or may not react at all. A person assessing pupil reaction should note if the patient has a prosthetic device (glass eye) or if the patient is blind. Unequal pupil size may be normal in some patients. Cataracts may give the eyes an abnormal appearance.

✓ Pupil size and reaction may indicate potential injuries or illnesses.

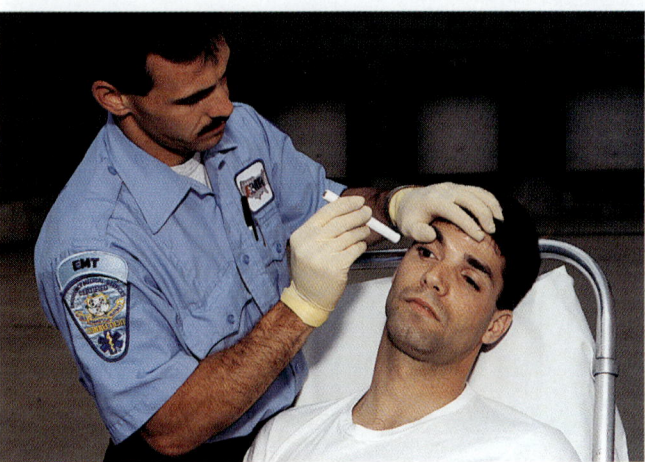

FIGURE 8.27 Examining the pupils.

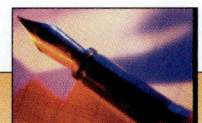

Tips from the Pros

If the patient's vital signs are out of normal range and the patient appears to be in no immediate distress, ask the patient if he or she knows his or her normal blood pressure and pulse.

SAMPLE History

The EMT must obtain a pertinent medical history of the patient. If the patient is conscious, the EMT should try to get the information directly from the patient. If the patient is unconscious or otherwise unable to give the information, the EMT should get the information from relatives or others at the scene. Sometimes when no one at the scene can provide information about the patient, the EMT must seek clues from the residence or from the patient's belongings.

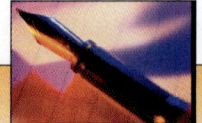

Tips from the Pros

Patients are different ages and come from all types of backgrounds. You must phrase questions in a format that the patient will understand.

To be thorough, the EMT can use the acronym SAMPLE to obtain complete information:

S—*Signs and symptoms.* The signs may include the vital signs that the EMT has taken or is about to take.
A—*Allergies.* Is the patient allergic to any medications or foods, and has the patient ingested any of those things recently? Is the patient allergic to any other substances, bites, stings, or something that could be inhaled or absorbed through the skin?
M—*Medication.* What medications is the patient taking and for what condition are they being taken? Are the medications prescriptions or can they be bought over the counter? Are they illegal drugs?
P—*Pertinent medical history.* Has the patient been experiencing medical problems, diagnosed or not? Has the patient been feeling ill or sought medical assistance from a physician, emergency department, or ambulance? The EMT must get the names of doctors, clinics, or emergency departments visited for similar conditions; they may have information that would be valuable to the physician making a diagnosis at this episode. How long have the problems been occurring, and what were the results from the doctor or emergency department visits? The EMT should at-

tempt to keep the patient focused on the pertinent history; some patients will relate every ache and pain of their entire life.

L—*Last meal.* When did the patient eat his or her last meal? What was eaten? Has anyone else who ate at the same time experienced illness or problems since that meal? This information is important for three reasons: (1) the food itself may be causing the patient's problem; (2) the patient may require surgery on arrival at the emergency department, and this information will be helpful to the surgical staff; and (3) the patient may be diabetic.

E—*Events.* What events led to the decision to summon emergency medial care? Many patients who have medical problems, specific allergies, or other information that may be pertinent in an emergency situation may wear a medical alert necklace or bracelet or may carry a special card in their wallet or purse. If the EMT cannot obtain a history from any other source, he or she should check to see if the patient has any of these items.

> ✓ The history may give the EMT clues to the patient's current condition. The acronym SAMPLE will aid the EMT in gaining a complete history.

Vital Signs Review

1. Signs are things that the EMT can observe about a patient's condition; symptoms are things that a patient tells the EMT about his or her condition.

2. Pulses can be assessed in the radial artery, carotid artery, and less often, the femoral artery. Pulses are assessed for rate (rapid, or tachycardia; or slow, or bradycardia), rhythm (regular or irregular), and character (bounding, full, or thready). The normal pulse rate for an adult is 60 to 80 beats a minute; for a child, 80 to 100 beats per minute; and for an infant, 100 to 120 beats per minute.

3. Ventilation is assessed for rate, character, depth, and rhythm. The normal ventilatory rate for an adult is 12 to 24 breaths per minute; children have higher rates.

4. Blood pressure measurements include the systolic (contraction of the left ventricle) and diastolic pressures (refilling of the left ventricle). The normal adult blood pressure is 120/80 mm Hg. Blood pressure can be approximated by assessing femoral and radial pulses. Blood pressure is more accurately measured by palpation or auscultation.

5. Skin color indicates heart and lung function. Skin temperature can indicate shock, heat exhaustion, or exposure to cold.

6. Level of consciousness (LOC) can be assessed by following the acronym AVPU: *A* (alert and awake), *V* (responds to verbal stimuli), *P* (responds to painful stimuli), and *U* (unresponsive).

7. Pupil reaction may indicate brain function, drug overdose, or medical complications. Pupils that are slow to constrict and dilate or that do not respond at all may indicate different conditions.

8. SAMPLE history includes the following: *S* (signs and symptoms), *A* (allergies), *M* (medication), *P* (pertinent medical history), *L* (last meal), *E* (event).

Summary

- An EMT does not diagnose or treat illness or injury but performs assessment-driven interventions. During assessment and reassessment, the EMT determines the need and appropriate timing for interventions and continually evaluates their effectiveness. Life-threatening assessment findings require immediate intervention. Transportation is an intervention.
- Scene assessment, patient assessment, and the resulting interventions are continuous, not just a one-time event.
- The EMT's ability to form a general impression and develop a plan of action is an essential assessment skill that allows early initiation of appropriate interventions, including transportation.
- A general impression and plan of action are important assessment skills that the EMT can begin even before examining the patient. They constantly are updated as the EMT receives and evaluates new scene and patient information.
- EMTs must consider the source of information and be flexible enough to constantly update their general impression and plan of action based on new information. The EMT should not allow initial information to produce tunnel vision.
- Body substance isolation (BSI) precautions protect the EMT and the patient. The EMT should use the appropriate level of BSI. Gloves, masks, eye protection, and gowns may be required to protect both the EMT and the patient.

Summary (cont'd)

- The EMT should not enter a scene that is unsafe. If the EMT cannot make the scene safe, he or she should stop and wait for the scene to be made safe. The EMT should request additional help as required. The EMT should not be a dead hero!
- The EMT should not attempt to make the scene safe without the appropriate training, equipment, and personnel.
- The EMT should quickly determine the need for additional resources and call for assistance as soon as possible.
- During the initial assessment, the EMT should assess for life-threatening problems and provide appropriate interventions, including immediate transportation for priority (critical) patients if needed. The EMT should manage life-threatening problems (intervention) as soon as they are detected.
- Based on the EMT's knowledge of the mechanism of injury or the nature of illness and overall patient appearance, he or she can form a general impression that will help guide interventions. Sick-looking patients are generally sick.
- If at any point during the assessment the EMT determines that the patient is a priority patient or that attempted life-saving interventions are not working, he or she should initiate transportation and ALS activation immediately while continuing assessments and interventions en route.
- The EMT assesses airway, breathing, circulation, and level of consciousness (LOC) during the initial assessment. If an intervention does not work, the EMT must consider prompt transportation to a medical facility.
- The EMT uses the rapid focused history and physical examination to quickly identify and allow immediate intervention in life-threatening conditions not found in the initial assessment. The EMT determines the focus of the examination (body areas examined) by patient complaint, mechanism of injury or nature of illness, and level of patient responsiveness.
- The mechanism of injury provides valuable information about the injured patient. It guides the assessment and intervention during the focused history and physical examination.
- The purpose of the detailed physical examination is to discover less obvious evidence of illness and injury so that the EMT can initiate useful interventions and reassess earlier findings and interventions.
- The ongoing assessment consists of periodically rechecking the patient at 5-minute intervals to reassess the effectiveness of interventions and uncover emerging problems.

Scenario Solution

The dispatch information is valuable and informative. It has told you that the scene is safe and you should not hesitate to enter. Your general impression of this call is that it may be a bad one. This patient will, if found as described, require immediate intervention to support his airway and rapid transportation with ALS intervention if possible.

Your initial plan of action is to enter the house with oxygen, the automated external defibrillator (AED), a stretcher, and a basic jump kit containing a blood pressure cuff, airways, and a bag-valve-mask. Your partner obtains all relative medical history from the wife while you perform your initial assessment and initiate oxygen at high flow by mask (FiO_2 >0.85).

You initiate rapid transportation. Your First Responder drives so that you can have assistance in the patient compartment from your partner. You place the patient in a sitting position to facilitate fluid accumulation in the bases of his lungs. Your partner assembles a bag-valve-mask unit, out of sight of the patient, and sets out a set of oral airways.

Without going through the process of forming a general impression and developing a plan of action, much on-scene time is lost. The patient's life also can be lost while the you decide what actions to take. Remember that the general impression and plan of action are and should be adjusted as more information becomes available.

Key Terms

Abrasion Damage to the epidermis and dermis from shearing forces; commonly referred to as a *scrape*.

Assessment A process that includes an oral interview and a physical examination. Assessment allows the EMT to gather information or clues that are useful in

Key Terms (cont'd)

deciding which emergency medical interventions will be used. The results of the assessment also are communicated to the medical personnel at the receiving hospital.

Auscultation Listening to sounds of the body with a stethoscope or blood pressure cuff; listening to the blood pressure.

AVPU Acronym for Alert, Verbal, Painful, and Unresponsive; used to describe patient's responsiveness.

Bounding pulse Strong pulse that is easily palpated.

Bradycardia A heart rate less than 60 beats per minute; a patient with bradycardia may or may not have symptoms.

Breathing See *ventilation*.

Capillary refill Time it takes for a patient's skin color to return to normal after the skin or nail bed has been pressed or blanched; normal time is less than 2 seconds; assesses perfusion.

Carotid artery The major artery of the neck, supplying the face, head, and brain with oxygenated blood.

Constrict To make smaller or narrower, as in pupils reacting to light.

Contusion Minor damage in the dermal layer of the skin causing discoloration from blood leaking into surrounding tissue; a bruise.

Crepitus A crackling sensation that can be felt when air escapes from the lungs and gets into surrounding tissue. Similar in feel to pressing on "bubble packs." The sound and the feeling bones can make when they are fractured caused by the rubbing together of loose bone ends.

Detailed physical examination Follows the focused history and physical examination; this portion of patient assessment comprises a region-by-region evaluation of the entire body to check for hidden problems.

Diastolic pressure The pressure in the heart when the heart muscle is relaxing; lower reading of a blood pressure.

Dilate To get larger; as in the pupils reacting to darkness.

Edema Abnormal accumulation of fluid in tissues in response to injury.

Exhalation Breathing air out of the lungs.

Femoral arteries The major vessels supplying the legs with oxygenated blood; can be palpated in the groin area.

Full pulse A strong, normal pulse.

General impression The EMT's overall "gut feeling" about the scene and patient, based on knowledge and tempered by experience.

Inhalation Breathing air into the lungs.

Initial assessment The assessment that is completed by the EMT-Basic after scene size-up. Includes assessment of major body systems (airway, breathing, circulation, and level of consciousness) to identify life-threatening problems and initiation of interventions, including transportation.

Intervention An action or skill performed by the EMT in response to a finding in the initial assessment or focused history and examination.

Laceration A break in the skin of varying depths resulting from a forceful impact with a sharp object; deeper injury than is seen with abrasions, with larger blood vessels involved and more bleeding.

Mechanism of injury The manner in which injuries occur; important in determining whether aeromedical support is needed.

Nature of illness Generally describes the medical condition that prompts an individual to be sick and subsequently request EMS.

Ongoing assessment Follows the detailed physical examination; this portion of the patient assessment checks for problems that arise after the initial assessment and evaluates whether the interventions initiated are working.

Oriented Describes a patient who can state his or her name, current location, date, etc.

Palpation To use the sphygmomanometer and locate the radial pulse with the fingers to obtain a blood pressure.

Paradoxical motion Describes a movement of the chest during respiration when one section of bony rib cage moves in an opposite direction from the rest of the rib cage, indicating that a section of the rib cage has broken loose.

Perfusion A state of adequate supply of oxygen and nutrients to the tissues; ability of the circulatory system to distribute blood containing nutrients and oxygen to the tissues.

Pulse The wave of blood produced by the contraction of the left ventricle; can be felt wherever an artery passes over a bone close to the skin surface.

Pulse character The force of the wave of blood created by the pumping of the heart.

Pulse pressure Difference between the systolic and diastolic pressure.

Pulse rate The number of heart beats per minute.

Pulse rhythm The intervals between the beats of the heart.

Radial artery Artery located on the thumb side of the wrist of each arm; extends from the wrist to the elbow.

Rapid trauma or medical focused history and physical examination Complete evaluation of the patient limited to the area of most concern based on the kinematics of the trauma or the presentation of the medical condition.

Key Terms (cont'd)

Respiration Physiologic process of moving oxygen into the red blood cells and tissue cells and metabolizing the oxygen to make energy (ATP); the process of eliminating the byproducts of metabolism, such as carbon dioxide, in the reverse direction.

Retraction A sign of respiratory distress often seen in infants and children marked by inward pulling of the skin above the clavicles and below the rib cage with inspiration.

SAMPLE history Mnemonic to help EMT-Basics assess history. S—Signs and Symptoms; A—Allergies; M—Medications; P—Pertinent medical history; L—Last oral intake; E—Events leading up to the injury or illness.

Scene size-up Quick, broad overview of the scene that the EMT-Basic performs upon arrival at the scene. During scene size-up, the EMT-Basic checks for scene safety, looks for the mechanism of injury or nature of illness, counts the number of patients, and calls for additional help if needed.

Signs Any observable indication of illness or injury.

Sphygmomanometer A pressure cuff device used on a peripheral extremity to determine the pressure in the heart on relaxation and contraction; also called a *blood pressure cuff.*

Stethoscope A device used to listen to the sounds of the body; consists of a bell and a diaphragm, which pick up the sounds, and rubber or vinyl tubing connected to ear pieces.

Symptoms An indication of illness or injury that is not observable and must be related by the patient.

Systolic pressure The pressure in the heart when the heart muscle is contracting; upper reading of a blood pressure.

Tachycardia Condition in which the heart contracts at a rate greater than 100 beats per minute.

Thready pulse Weak, thin, rapid pulse or heart rate.

Triage A process used to sort patients and determine which will be treated or transported first; often used to describe the sorting process used in a disaster situation but also can apply to any situation in which sorting of patients is necessary.

Ventilation The mechanical process of moving air into and out of the lungs.

Ventilatory character Strength of the ventilations.

Ventilatory depth Depth of each ventilation effort.

Ventilatory rate Number of ventilations per minute.

Ventilatory rhythm Regularity of the ventilations.

Review Questions

1. For the best possible outcome for the patient, the EMT should:
   a. Evaluate the entire body using the look listen feel technique as rapidly as possible.
   b. Look for life-threatening conditions first, and then look for limb threatening conditions.
   c. Evaluate the airway only, and then load the patient into the ambulance for transportation to the hospital.
   d. Load the patient into the ambulance and go to the hospital as quickly as possible without any evaluation or management.
2. Triage in the usual patient care situation is to:
   a. Treat the patient who will most likely survive the incident first.
   b. Treat the patients with the least injuries first.
   c. Treat the most severely injured patients first.
   d. Treat the first patient seen first.
3. On arrival, the view of the scene is the first thing that the EMT notices. The EMT should:
   a. Quell curiosity and look quickly for the patients.
   b. Analyze the scene to identify causative factors of the situation.
   c. First find all of the law enforcement personnel and the bystanders to get the details of what happened before looking at any of the patients.
   d. Ignore everything but the patients.
4. The correct steps for evaluation of the patient condition are:
   i. Check ventilation.
   ii. Check for patent airway.
   iii. Remove the patient's clothes to assess the entire patient.
   iv. Check for perfusion and life-threatening hemorrhage.
   v. Check neurologic status.
   a. v, ii, i, iv, iii
   b. i, ii, iii, iv, v
   c. ii, i, iv, v, iii
   d. iii, ii, i, iv, iii

Review Questions (cont'd)

5. Reassessment of the patient should occur every:
   a. 5 minutes.
   b. 2 minutes.
   c. 3 minutes.
   d. 15 minutes.
6. The prehospital assessment of the patient should be:
   a. Diagnosis driven.
   b. Symptom driven.
   c. EMT best guess driven.
   d. Guided by a call for medical director's opinion each time the unit arrives on the scene.
7. Rapid patient assessment focuses on:
   a. Body areas where the most life-threatening condition probably lies.
   b. Head-to-toe evaluation in that order.
   c. Hemorrhage first, then all other problems.
   d. Load and go so that the physician in the emergency department can evaluate the patient.
8. The EMT-B assessment evaluation and the assessment done by physicians and the nurses in the hospital:
   a. Are not related in any way.
   b. Are the same in every way.
   c. Evaluate the same things but in different order.
   d. Are the same examination but with different titles to the sections.
9. The entire physical examination should be completed in the field because it is the EMT's responsibility to report the entire condition of the patient to the physician in the emergency department.
   The two parts to this statement are:
   a. true, true and related
   b. true, false
   c. true, true and unrelated
   d. false, false

Answers to these Review Questions can be found at the end of the book on page 865.

9

Management of Shock

Lesson Goal

The most critical function of the human body is energy production. The lack of significant energy production, called *shock*, is a result of anaerobic metabolism. The goal of this chapter is to provide understanding of shock as the most important part of physiology and the management of the pathophysiology of the failure to produce enough energy.

Scenario

This scenario is based on an actual patient brought to a level I trauma center by a major city EMS service. You have been called to the scene of a motor vehicle collision. On arrival you see one car upside down off the road. One occupant, the passenger you later learn, is 30 feet behind the car, lying on the ground with a deformed upper leg, alert and talking. The other person, in the driver's seat is pinned by the left leg in the vehicle. On gaining access to the driver, the steering wheel is broken and easily pulled out of the vehicle. Neither occupant was belted at the time of the impact, although both airbags deployed. The driver responds to pain. During the extraction process, which takes about 65 minutes, he is alert with a blood pressure of 128/70 mm Hg, pulse 110 beats/min, and ventilatory rate of 28 breaths/min. Immediately after his leg is free, his pressure drops to 80/60 mm Hg, pulse increases to 130 beats/min, and ventilatory rate increases to 30 breaths/min.

 What is this patient's problem? How should it be managed? Is there anything that should have been done during the prolonged extraction to provide a potentially better outcome?

Key Terms to Know

Aerobic	Brachial artery	Core	Hypoperfusion
Anaerobic	Brachial pulse	Diastolic pressure	Hypotension
Arterioles	Capillaries	Femoral artery	Metabolism
Artery	Capillary refill	Femoral pulse	Penetrating trauma
Atria	Cardiac output	Heart	Perfusion
Auscultation	Cardinal	Heart rate	Periphery
Bicuspid valve	Carotid artery	Hemoglobin	Pneumatic antishock
Blunt trauma	Carotid pulse	Hemorrhage	garment (PASG)

Key Terms to Know (cont'd)

Pulmonary artery
Pulmonary vein
Pulse
Pulse point pressure
Radial artery

Radial pulse
Semilunar valve
Shock
Sphygmomanometer
Systolic pressure

Thready
Trendelenburg position
Tricuspid valve
Vasoconstriction
Vasodilation

Vein
Ventricles
Venules
Volume

Learning Objectives

As an EMT-Basic, you should be able to do the following:

DOT

- Describe the structure and function of the circulatory system and its most important structures: the heart, arteries, veins, and capillaries.
- Identify and demonstrate methods of emergency medical care for internal and external bleeding (see Chapter 23).
- Explain the relationship between body substance isolation and bleeding, and identify the measures that must be taken by the EMT-Basic for self-protection and patient protection (see Chapter 23).
- Identify the relationship between airway management and the trauma patient (see Chapter 23).
- Identify the relationship between mechanism of injury and causes of internal bleeding (see Chapters 22 and 23).
- Identify the signs and symptoms of shock, and describe the appropriate management for internal and external bleeding.
- State the principles of treatment for the patient with signs and symptoms of shock.
- Differentiate among arterial, venous, and capillary bleeding.
- List signs and symptoms of shock (hypoperfusion) (see Chapter 23).
- Demonstrate direct pressure as a method of emergency medical care of external bleeding (see Chapter 23).
- Demonstrate the use of diffuse pressure as a method of emergency medical care of external bleeding (see Chapter 23).
- Demonstrate the use of pressure points and tourniquets as a method of emergency medical care of external bleeding (see Chapter 23).
- Demonstrate the care of the patient exhibiting signs and symptoms of internal bleeding.
- Demonstrate the care of the patient exhibiting signs and symptoms of shock (hypoperfusion).
- Demonstrate completing a prehospital care report for the patient with bleeding and/or shock (hypoperfusion).

Supplemental

- Describe the difference between the systemic and pulmonary circulatory systems.
- Define *cardiac output* and *stroke volume.*
- Describe the difference between anaerobic and aerobic metabolism.
- Describe the Fick principle.
- List indications and contraindications for PASG use.
- Identify the importance of checking pulse of various locations to assess the patient.
- Describe the relationship between cellular energy production and shock.

The most important function of the human body is to produce energy. This energy production occurs at the cellular level and is called **metabolism**. If energy production occurs using oxygen as its driving force, the process is called **aerobic** metabolism. If oxygen is not available, the metabolism occurs without oxygen and is called **anaerobic** metabolism. Aerobic metabolism produces 18 times more energy than does an anaerobic metabolism. Anaerobic metabolism is only a short-term fix that produces energy for a limited period of time before the cells start to die. The cellular biochemistry describing this mechanism is known as the *Krebs cycle*, the details of which are not critical to the EMTs knowledge for the management of a shock patient. However, an overview is pivotal in understanding shock and its management.

Shock is the process by which the body does not produce a sufficient amount of energy because of lack of cellular oxygen and when the energy production has been transferred from the aerobic pathway to the anaerobic pathway. Energy is required for all the body functions that are necessary for life. Failure of energy to be produced in adequate amounts will always result in death. This chapter is more complete than in the previous edition so that

Patient Care Algorithm

Circulatory Assessment

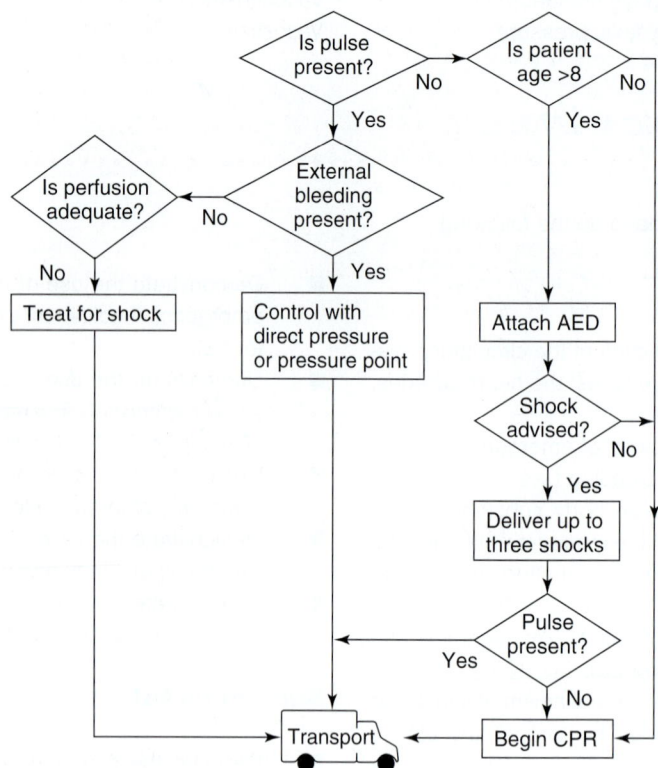

the EMT will have an appreciation for exactly what is happening at the cellular level and will more fully understand the life-threatening condition of shock.

In 1854, an early American surgeon named Samuel Gross described shock as a "rude unhinging of the machinery of life." How that unhinging occurs is explained in this chapter. A more modern definition of shock is "lack of adequate energy production at the cellular level caused by cellular ischemia." A briefer but less descriptive definition is "lack of adequate perfusion of the tissue cells with oxygenated blood." Shock is not low blood pressure, fast **heart rate**, reduced core temperature, low urinary output, or fast ventilatory rate. These are variables by which the physiologic processes may be measured, and therefore they can be defined as some of the

Box 9.1 Stages of Death

- Prolonged anaerobic metabolism reduces energy production.
- Reduced energy production leads to cell death.
- Death of a critical mass of cells within an organ produces organ death.
- Death of critical organs produces patient death.

Physician Notes

The response of each patient is different as to when these signs and symptoms occur. An infant with a very strong heart and very powerful vasoactive vascular system can maintain blood pressure despite the loss of 50% or more of blood **volume**, whereas an older adult with cardiac disease and severe atherosclerosis may show these signs and symptoms with blood volume loss of 10% or less.

symptoms of shock. They do not all have to be present, and in some situations none are present. In some conditions these signs are present but the patient is not in shock. The EMT should not rely on these signs and symptoms, nor their absence, to identify shock.

Failure of the circulatory system in either trauma or medical emergencies is a catastrophic event for all of the body systems because the circulatory system distributes the necessary nutrients (food) and oxygen for adequate energy production. The normal function of all body systems is dependent on proper function of the circulatory system. Failure results in death. The ability to recognize circulatory system failure is a critical skill for the EMT. This chapter provides EMTs with baseline information and an orientation to skills that will assist them in recognizing circulatory system function and failure. This chapter does not address the other critical components of shock: airway and ventilation. These are addressed in Chapters 10 and 11.

Anatomy and Physiology

As identified in the introduction, shock is not the signs and symptoms noted as the EMT examines the patient, but it is the underlying anaerobic metabolism within the cells and the failure of these cells to produce energy for bodily functions. This can involve one cell or many cells, one organ or many organs. Anaerobic metabolism is the first stage of death. If multiple cells die within an organ, that organ dies. If critical organs die, the patient dies (Box 9.1).

The patient may not die immediately when anaerobic metabolism begins. In the first hour that anaerobic metabolism affects the organ, enough cells may not die to immediately kill the organ. Enough cells may have died so that the organ cannot function for a long period of time, but it can continue to function for a short period of time. Even the heart, lungs, kidneys, liver, and immune system may initially survive the anoxic and ischemic event but produce death 2 or 3 weeks later as a result of the initial anaerobic metabolism.

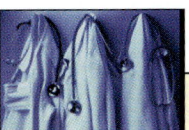 **Physician Notes**

As is discussed later in this chapter, some organs will show signs of cellular death and organ failure earlier and some with show it later. The heart may fail within minutes of onset of ischemia, and death will follow immediately. For other organs it may be 2 to 3 weeks before the patient dies of renal failure or immune system failure. All of these organs were affected by the initial lack of resuscitation in the prehospital portion of patient care that lead to the ischemia of the cells of these organs. Failure of some organs results in death of the patient later than others.

It is therefore the goal of the EMT (and other health care providers) to prevent the progression from anaerobic metabolism to patient death. To accomplish this, anaerobic metabolism must be stopped as quickly as possible. In severe trauma, this process has already begun when the EMT arrives on the scene and continues until the final event. The progression to patient death is interrupted by stopping anaerobic metabolism. Anaerobic metabolism is stopped by making sure that the body delivers enough oxygen to the beleaguered cells so that they once again can produce energy for the body.

Fick Principle

The Fick principle (Box 9.2) defines the necessary steps that the body must go through to prevent anaerobic metabolism.

To understand how oxygenation is achieved at the cellular level and aerobic metabolism is maintained, each step of the Fick principle is discussed. An understanding of the normal anatomy and physiology of the circulatory system and oxygen transportation is a good place to start.

Circulatory System

Survival of humans and other animals depends on the production of energy by and for the cells of the individual organs. If this occurs properly, then the organs can carry out their functions for the body and the body will live. All organs and systems must work together to achieve this goal.

To deliver oxygen and nutrients to the cells to carry out this process, the body has developed an elaborate closed system composed of three parts: a pump (the **heart**), a network of pipes (vessels), and a unique fluid to carry the necessary components (blood).

Oxygen is picked up from the lungs, and glucose and other nutrients are picked up from the gastrointestinal (GI) tract for delivery to the tissue cells. The waste products are picked up from the cells to off-load through the lung and kidneys. Because the normal functioning of the circulatory

---

Box 9.2 Fick Principle

- On-loading of oxygen into the red blood cells (RBCs) in the lungs
- Delivery of those oxygenated RBCs to the tissue cells
- Off-loading of oxygen from the RBCs to the tissue cells

This process is dependent on an adequate RBC mass being present to transport the oxygen.

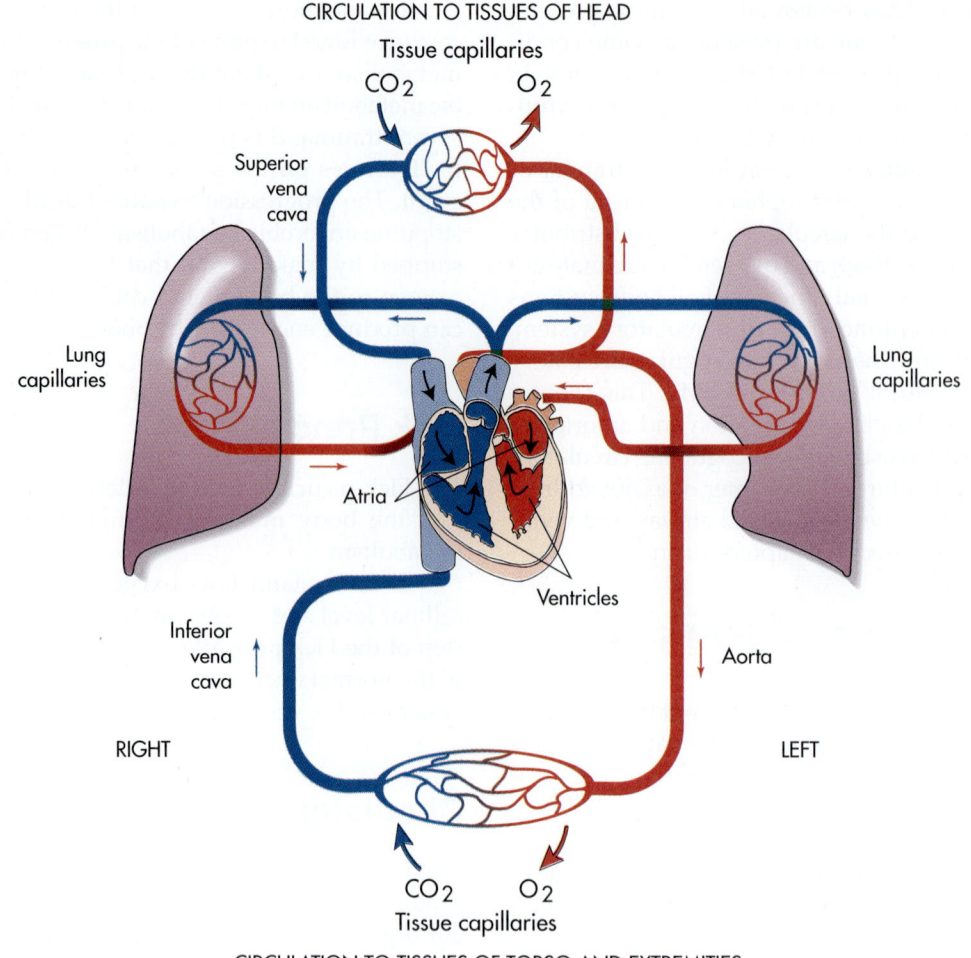

FIGURE 9.1 Blood flow through the circulatory system. Normal functioning depends on the lungs for oxygen.

system depends on the lungs for oxygen, the respiratory and circulatory systems are interrelated. The loss of normal function in one has a profoundly negative effect on the function of the other (Figure 9.1). If this delivery system fails, the cells cannot do their job and death will follow.

To visualize how the three parts of this transport system work, take a 10 ml syringe, connect it to a three-way stopcock, connect the other two parts of the stopcock to a long piece of intravenous administration tubing that has a balloon attached to one of the ports, and fill the whole system with colored water (Figure 9.2). Close the outside wing of the stopcock and draw the plunger. It fills with fluid from the stores in the balloon (diastole). This is similar to the heart relaxing and blood running into it. Then turn the stopcock, and push the plunger in to force the fluid into the loop of tubing. This is like the ventricle emptying and forcing a bolus of blood into the system (systole). The expansion and contracting of the balloon represents the expansion and contraction of the vessels as they absorb the bolus of blood from the heart and distribute it to the rest of the system as blood flows back to the heart. The opening and closing of the stopcock represents the opening and the closing of the valves between the chambers of the heart and between the heart and the outflow arteries. Since there are two halves to the cardiovascular system, add another system of syringes, tubing, and balloon as above and place them side by side. This represents the right and left halves of the heart meeting the needs of the pulmonary and systemic vascular beds and cells. The following sections examine the details of how the individual components work. If it seems too complex, a review of the simple syringe-tube system may help.

Heart

The heart is located in the chest cavity under the breastbone. It is a muscular, hollow organ with many unique and special characteristics. The heart is approximately the the size of the patient's clenched fist. This applies whether the patient is an infant, child, or adult.

The function of the heart is to pump blood through its chambers and push the blood into the vessels so that

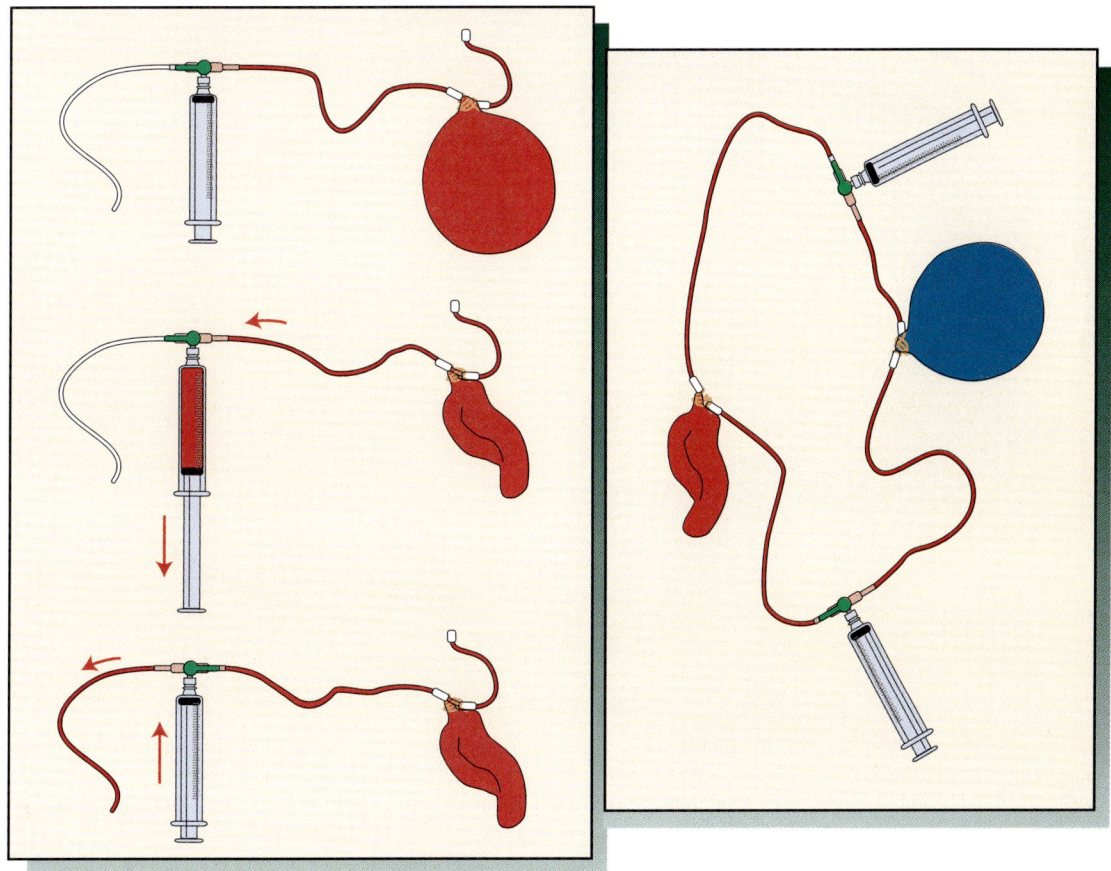

FIGURE 9.2 Syring-tube double-pump system.

it can be moved throughout the body to all areas that need it. The journey that the blood takes starts in the heart and ends in the heart. Although attached as one organ, the heart is actually two separate pumps (think of the syringes) known as the *right heart* and *left heart*. The upper chambers of the heart are called **atria**, divided into the right atrium and the left atrium by a wall of muscle. The lower chambers of the heart are called **ventricles**, divided into right and left sides by a similar wall of muscle.

The right atrium and right ventricle pump blood to the pulmonary beds. The left atrium and left ventricle pump blood throughout the rest of the body, which requires more strength. The muscles of the left heart are larger than those of the right heart, and the pressure is greater in the left heart and systemic vessels than that found in the right heart and pulmonary system. The ventricles of the heart are much larger than the atria, and the muscle walls of the ventricles are much thicker and stronger than the muscle walls of the atria. The right side of the heart receives blood from the body, where much of the oxygen has been extracted into the right atrium. The right ventricle receives this blood from the right atrium and pumps it into the lungs for oxygenation. The left atrium receives the oxygen-rich blood from the lungs, and the left ventricle receives this blood from the left atrium and pumps it out to the body to carry on aerobic metabolism and produce energy. The flow of blood to and from the lungs through the heart is called *pulmonary circulation*. The flow of blood to and from the heart through the body is called *systemic circulation* (Figure 9.3). The right side of the heart receives blood from the systemic system and pumps it, through the lungs (pulmonary), to the left heart.

The openings between the upper and lower chambers of the heart are separated by fibrous tissue called *valves*. The valves open and close during each contraction of the heart muscle, preventing backflow of blood as the muscle squeezes down. The stopcocks that turn in the syringe analogy perform a similar function. As the muscles relax, the chambers are allowed to fill again from downstream. The valves that exist between the atria and the ventricles look like flaps. They attach to the muscles of the heart, and when they open they allow flow of blood

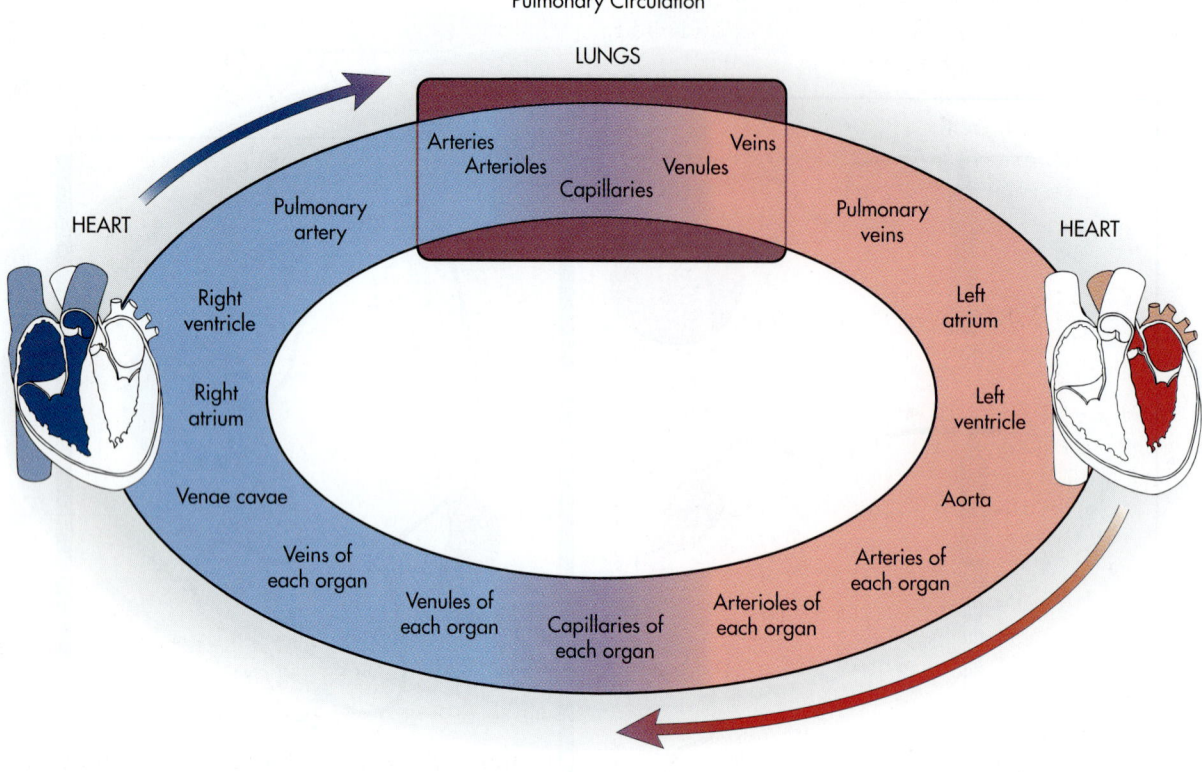

FIGURE 9.3 In the pulmonary system, the blood is pumped from the right side of the heart to the gas-exchange tissues in the lungs. In the systemic circulation, blood is pumped from the left side of the heart to all other tissues of the body. Blood leaves the heart through the arteries, then travels through the arterioles, capillaries, venules, and veins before returning to the opposite side of the heart.

from each atrium into the ventricle below it. As the pressure in the ventricle builds up, the flaps are forced shut, preventing backflow of the blood and forcing it out of the atrium into the ventricles. A similar action occurs in the valve; the blood must pass through as the blood enters into the aorta or pulmonary artery. This valve also closes, preventing backflow into the heart.

Cardiac output. Although the output of the heart is not measured in the field at this time, the process is very important for the EMT to understand in context with the body's ability to profuse the tissues properly. Each contraction of the heart squeezes a bolus of blood into the aorta. As the heart refills and contracts, another bolus of blood in placed into the aorta. This cycle repeats itself with each beat of the heart. The output of the heart is at the crux of circulation and transportation of oxygen to the tissue cells and the removal of waste products.

The arbitrary description of the **cardiac output** is amount of output per minute. The individual output with each beat or contraction of the heart is known as *stroke volume*. To determine the cardiac output, multiply the stroke volume times the number of contractions per minute, or the **pulse** rate. The exact methods of measurement of stroke volume is not easy and is not required of the EMT-B; therefore it will not be explained here. The concept is important, however.

Heart Valves

Between the atrium and ventricles on the right side of the heart is a three-flap valve called the **tricuspid valve**. On the left side of the heart is a two-flap valve called the **bicuspid valve**. The backward flow from the blood vessels back into the ventricles is protected by the aortic and pulmonic **semilunar valves**, which look like half moons (the Latin term for moon is 'luna'). An easy way to remember on which sides of the heart the valves are is to remember that you ride a tricycle before you ride a bicycle.

Blood Vessels

The circulatory system contains three types of vessels:

1. Arteries, which carry blood away from the heart
2. Capillaries, which distrubute the contents of the blood stream through thin walls to the cells
3. Veins, which carry blood back to the heart.

The **artery** is the most muscular vessel. Arteries are composed of several layers of muscle tissue, and their primary function is to carry blood from the heart to the other body systems. Large arteries divide into progressively smaller arteries until they become vessels called **arterioles** (very small arteries). Arterioles become **capillaries** (microscopic vessels). This is much like the branching

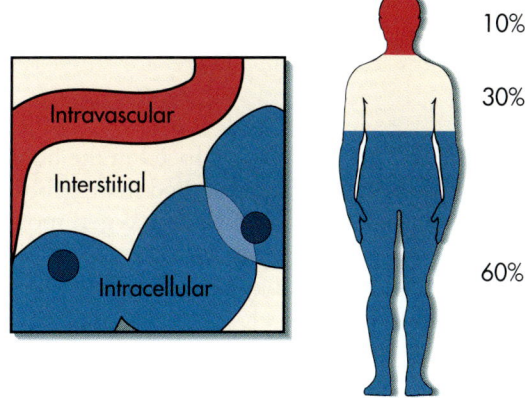

FIGURE 9.4 The three fluid compartments.

> ✓ The structures of the circulatory system include the heart and blood vessels. Blood vessels include arteries, veins, and capillaries. With two exceptions, arteries carry oxygenated blood away from the heart, and veins carry deoxygenated blood to the heart.

of a tree and is called *arborization* Arteries absorb the bolus of blood and modify the force wave by alternately contracting and relaxing with each beat of the heart.

Fluid

The body is approximately 60% fluid. This fluid is housed in three compartments: the intracellular compartment and the extracellular compartment, which is subdivided into the intravascular compartment and the interstitial compartment (Figure 9.4). The fluid moves freely between these compartments, but the contents of the fluid—cellular material (i.e., blood) and protein—do not leave unless there is a hole in the vessel. Some electrolytes can move freely back and forth, whereas others do not. The lack of ability of these non-water materials to move freely creates the force that holds fluid into its own compartment. This force is called *osmotic pressure*. Although this fluid motion is complex, a simplistic explanation is that the cell membrane is freely permeable to water but not to the other components. The body does not like a more concentrated solution on one side of a membrane and a dilute solution on the other. Water tends to cross into the more concentrated side to dilute it, thus equalizing the concentrations on both sides of the membrane.

The membranes between the three compartments are variably permeable. There are some membranes that water and electrolytes can cross but that larger molecules of protein and blood cannot cross. A further complication is that, in severe shock, the capillary membranes can become so damaged that protein can cross. Additional explanation of this concept is discussed later.

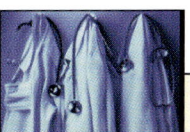

Physician Notes

If the valves become damaged by disease, they may not open or close properly. This produces flow problems into the muscular chambers during the filling part of the cycle or restriction of flow out of the chambers during the contraction part of the cycle.

Capillaries form networks. Under a microscope, a network of capillaries resembles a mesh pot scrubber. Capillaries surround cells and provide oxygen and nutrients (food) to the cells. Only the membrane of the cell and the thin wall of the capillary separate intravascular fluid (containing the supplies) from the fluid in the cell that desperately needs replenishment. The capillaries join, become larger, and are called **venules** (small veins). Venules in turn enlarge and become veins. A **vein,** composed of only one or two layers of muscle cells, is not as thick as an artery. Blood controls the flow through veins with the assistance of surrounding skeletal muscle tissues.

The thicker muscle walls of arteries respond to chemical messages. The message might indicate that the muscles should contract **(vasoconstriction)** or relax **(vasodilation).** A unique difference between arteries and veins is that each vein contains small flap valves similar to those in the heart that close as blood is pushed through, preventing blood from moving backwards. Another major distinction between the two types of large vessels is that, in the systemic complex, arteries carry oxygen-rich blood, whereas veins carry oxygen-poor blood. However, this is the opposite in the pulmonary complex.

Two important vessels in the circulatory system are the pulmonary artery and the pulmonary vein. The **pulmonary artery** is located between the right ventricle of the heart and the lungs and is the only artery that normally carries oxygen-poor blood. Blood depleted of oxygen by the body tissues and carrying carbon dioxide (the waste product of metabolism) is delivered to the right atrium by veins. The pulmonary artery moves oxygen-poor blood from the right ventricle into the lungs to receive oxygen. The exchange of carbon dioxide for oxygen occurs in the capillaries of the lung. The **pulmonary vein** carries oxygen-rich blood back from the lung to the left atrium for circulation back into the system. Thus the pulmonary vein is the only vein that normally carries oxygen-rich blood.

Blood. Blood is in the intravascular compartment and is composed of approximately 55% fluid, which is called *plasma*, and 45% blood cells. There are three types of blood cells:

1. *Red blood cells* (RBCs) are produced in the bone marrow and contain a molecule called **hemoglobin**. Hemoglobin is a protein that binds oxygen molecules. In a sense, hemoglobin acts as a "ferry" for oxygen, carrying it from the lungs to the tissues.
2. There are five types of *white blood cells* (WBCs), which fight infection.
3. The *platelets* produce coagulation, or clotting, at the site of an injury.

Blood may be bright red or dark red in color. The difference in color depends on the amount of oxygen that the blood carries. The blood in arteries should be bright red because it has come from the lungs where it picked up oxygen. Blood in veins (venous blood) is darker because it does not contain as much oxygen. Venous blood is carried to the lungs to rid it of carbon dioxide and pick up more oxygen. The average adult blood volume is approximately 5000 ml, or almost 5 quarts. Blood volume represents only 4.5% of the total body fluid volume. The total blood volume for an child at 1 year of age is 800 ml.

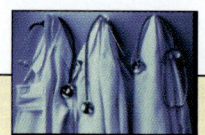

Physician Notes

Blood to be administered to a patients is measured in units. One unit of whole blood equals 500 ml. However, in today's medical practice, whole blood is seldom given to a patient. Blood from donors is separated into its component parts, such as RBCs, platelets, plasma, and clotting factors. This separation makes it possible for more than one person to benefit from the donation of one unit of blood. If an individual has enough red cells but needs platelets, then only platelets are given. After most of the plasma and other cells have been removed, the unit of packed red blood cells (PRBCs) given to the patient has a volume of about 250 ml.

Blood Flow

As described previously, the circulatory (delivery) system is a closed system with all vessels attached to one another. The heart is connected to an artery, which is connected to many arteries, which in turn become arterioles, which eventually become capillaries. The capillaries connect to venules, which are connected to veins, which connect to become one major vein that is connected to the heart. The circulatory system is the human body's internal transportation system. The quality of the heart as a good engine becomes impaired if the blood or vessels are clogged with plaques of cholesterol and other substances. If the heart and vessels become clogged, they will fail to perform effectively as a transportation system for blood.

The circulatory system requires pressure to function, much like a water pump. The chambers of the heart create enough pressure to move the fluid through the entire network of pipes or vessels. The pressure is strongest in the ventricles, which are the chambers of the heart that are the thickest and most muscular.

Heart muscle is unique in that the heart generates electrical impulses on its own. The heart pumps blood in a routine and regular manner. Each pump is called a *beat* of the heart. The volume of blood in the ventricle is forced into the system with each beat of the heart; this is the stroke volume.

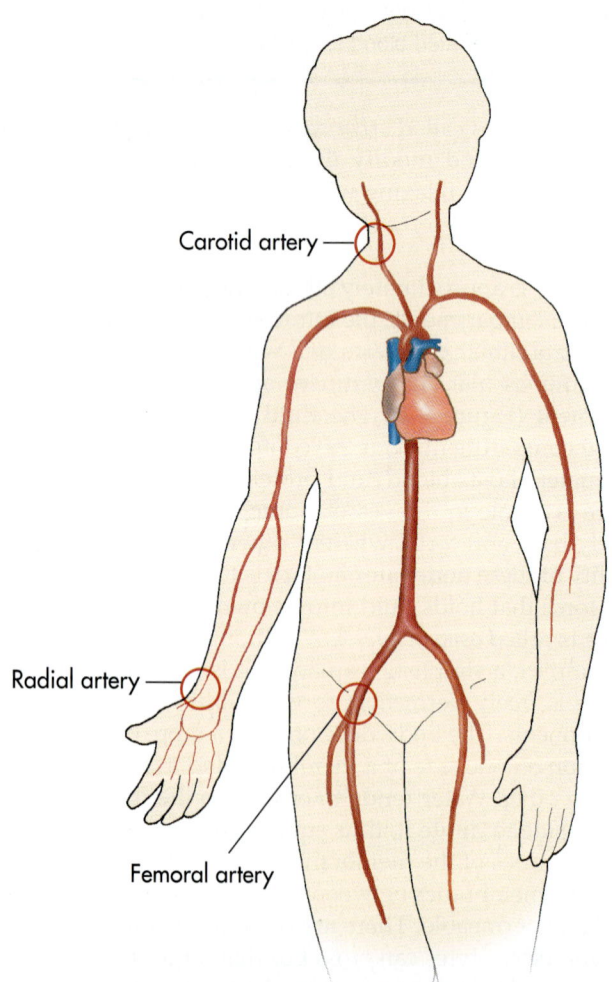

FIGURE 9.5 Easiest locations to find a pulse.

Blood pressure. The pressure inside the arteries can be measured using a **sphygmomanometer** (blood pressure cuff), which measures pressure in millimeters of mercury (mm Hg). Normally two measurements are taken:

1. The pressure in the heart when the muscle is contracting and forcing blood through the arteries is the **systolic pressure**. The systolic pressure is the first, or higher, reading.
2. The pressure in the heart when the muscle is relaxing and pressure in the arteries is at its mininum during the pulse cycle is the **diastolic pressure**. The diastolic pressure is the second, or lower, reading.

This system is analogous to the bagpipe. The piper fills the bag with a large breath of air. This is comparable to the bolus of blood pumped from the heart during systole. While the piper is inhaling to refill the bag, the flow is maintained to the pipes in a constant manner by the pressure within the bag and the compression of the bag by the piper's arm.(diastole) This is like the flow of blood along the vessels by the gradual contraction of the vessel walls and the gradual reduction of the pressure inside the vessels before another bolus of blood replenishes the volume. The muscle cells in arteries contract and assist in the movement of blood through the circulatory system, the distribution of blood flow, and the blood pressure.

Pulse. Some of the larger arteries are under the surface of the skin and directly over the surface of a bone. It is possible to feel the beat (pulse) of the heart at these points. The following are the easiest locations for the EMT to feel the pulse of the heart (Figure 9.5):

1. Thumb (lateral) side of the wrist (**radial artery**)
2. Above the elbow on the inside (medial) of the arm closest to the body (**brachial artery**)
3. Groin area of each leg (**femoral artery**)
4. Either side of the neck, between the Adam's apple (voice box) and the back (**carotid artery**)

Pulse points are named for the artery being palpated. The **radial pulse** is felt at the radial artery, the **brachial pulse** is felt at the brachial artery, the **femoral pulse** is felt at the femoral artery, and the **carotid pulse** is felt at the carotid artery.

Metabolism

As discussed previously, aerobic metabolism uses oxygen to produce energy by a chemical reaction called the *Krebs cycle*. The Krebs cycle is a complicated, multistep chemical reaction that produces molecules of adenosine triphosphate (ATP) within the mitochondria of the cells. When oxygen is not available, lactate and pyruvate are used to produce energy (anaerobic metabolism), but the output is 19 times less than when oxygen is present (Figure 9.6). The complexities of this metabolic process are not important for the prehospital provider, but the use of oxygen to produce energy is very important.

This process can be compared with an automobile using gasoline as its source of energy. As long as there is gasoline in the tank, the car will run fine and can move efficiently. If the gasoline tank is empty, the engine will not run. However, the car can be moved for a short distance and for a limited time using the battery as a source of energy and the starter motor to turn the crankshaft and the wheels. The gasoline as an energy source is comparable with oxygen (aerobic) in the human body, and the battery as an energy source is comparable with the anaerobic cycle.

> ✓ The optimal environment in which human metabolism takes place is aerobic, meaning in the presence of oxygen.

Pathophysiology

The body has several mechanisms for maintaining blood pressure and blood flow to the critical organs for survival (heart, brain, and lungs). These organs are the most sensitive to ischemia and therefore require the greatest attention by the body to preserve blood flow. These organs can survive no longer than 6 to 8 minutes, using anaerobic metabolism, before the cells start to die and proceed toward organ death. The progression to organ death is slower in the GI tract, kidney, and liver, where the tolerance can range from 45 to 90 minutes of ischemia.

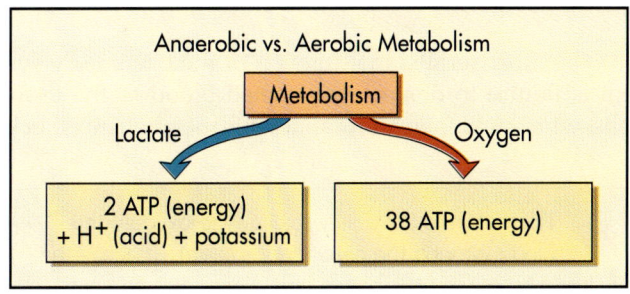

FIGURE 9.6 Anaerobic metabolism produces much less energy and creates potassium and acid wastes.

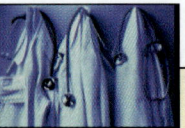

Physician Notes

The diving reflex of some sea mammals, such as the seal, allows them to dive deep and stay for a long time in cold water by diverting the blood supply to the heart and deceasing oxygen consumption. A similar mechanism has been observed occasionally in children who fall into cold water. There have been reports of survival for 45 minutes or longer without long-term brain damage.

One method that the body uses to direct blood flow to the ischemic-sensitive organs is to shut down or reduce the flow of blood to nonvital organs. Checking the blood flow in the hand is an easy way to evaluate if the body has shut down this section. Squeezing the blood from the capillary system in the skin will make that part white (the pink color comes from oxygenated blood). Removing the pressure will allow blood to refill the capillary beds. If the refilling time is slow (approximately 2 seconds is normal), then the body is not allowing blood access to this area of the skin.

This reduced blood flow and poor perfusion is not always a result of shock. Examples of conditions other than shock that will reduce perfusion to the extremities are cold, atherosclerosis, and smoking. Most of the tests that are used to assess patients can be positive in more than one condition. One must use the indication of decreased perfusion in context of the whole patient. Few tests used in patient evaluation can be used alone.

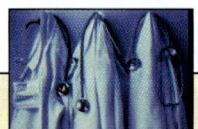

Physician Notes

Refilling time is a function of blood flow to the location being examined and is not always a result of shock. Arteries can constrict as a result of decreased core temperature in a cold environment, obstruction of the vessel secondary to atherosclerosis or trauma, or other causes.

The most serious malfunction of the circulatory system is failure to deliver oxygenated blood to the tissue cells, which will then allow anaerobic metabolism (shock) to develop. The process begins with ischemia of the body cells produced either by hypoperfusion, hypoxia, or both.

Progression of Shock

Shock is often thought to be the collection of signs or symptoms that are the result of a failure to produce enough energy for life processes (anaerobic metabolism) or to perfuse and oxygenate the cells, but this is only partially true. The early stages of shock can exist when all the signs measurable in the field are normal. The terms describing the progression of shock are *compensated*, *uncompensated*, and *irreversible shock*. The first two conditions (compensated and uncompensated) refer to the ability to maintain blood pressure by various means.

1. *Compensated shock* exists when there is hypoperfusion and hypoxia at the cellular level but the body has been able to maintain blood pressure within the normal range by compensating for loss of fluid (traumatic or dehydration) or cardiac failure, reducing the size of the lumen of the vessels (vasoconstriction), increasing heart rate, or providing more forcible cardiac contractions.

2. When these compensatory mechanisms (increased heart rate, arterial constriction, and increased cardiac output [rate and force]) can no longer maintain the blood pressure in the normal range and as pressure drops, it is referred to as *uncompensated shock*. Although the designation is somewhat artificial, it serves as a warning that the situation is quickly becoming worse and that steps must be taken to remedy the condition. This condition of decreased pressure is associated with a diversion of blood from the **periphery** to the **core**. As blood is removed from the general circulation to the core circulation, there is an associated increase in the number of cells undergoing anaerobic metabolism. As the cells of the involved organs are deprived of circulation for an extended period of time, the cells will began to die and the organ cannot function. If only some of the cells die, the organ may survive but will not have the complete function that it had before the insult. Depending on the organ involved, the patient may be negatively affected. For example, if the heart is deprived of circulation and some of the cells die but others remain alive, the heart can still function but not as strongly as before. The patient may be not be able to walk for long distances, or even to the bathroom in severe cases, without developing chest pain or becoming so short of breath that he or she must sit down to rest. The kidneys may function to a limited extent, but if they are taxed by a severe illness, they may lose their function and the patient may need

---

✓ **Perfusion** is the ability to circulate oxygenated blood through the circulatory system. Shock is the failure of the body to perfuse and oxygenate the cells. **Hypoperfusion,** or a decrease in perfusion, is a sign of shock.

dialysis or a kidney transplant to continue to eliminate waste products.
3. Once critical organs can no longer function enough to keep that patient alive, he or she progresses to *irreversible shock*.

Phases of Shock on Cellular Level

Ischemic Phase

Another important pathophysiologic process occurs as blood flow is shunted away from certain cells and these cells become ischemic. As the pressure and flow of blood start to drop, the cells begin to experience reduced blood flow. The muscles in the arterioles and venules close these vessels to shunt blood to the core of the patient, and anaerobic metabolism increases in the affected cells. This causes a buildup of the waste products from anaerobic metabolism (acid and potassium). The capillary lining opens up to allow protein-containing fluid to leak from the intravascular space into the interstitial space.

Stagnation Phase

The arteriole muscles relax next, while the venule muscles remain contracted. This leads to a packing together of the RBCs into clumps. The increased pressure from the open arterioles and the damming force of the closed venules allows more fluid to leak into the interstitial sapce. The fluid in the interstitial space produces an increased space between the cells (edema). This increases the distance between the cells and the capillaries, which results in even less oxygen transportation from the RBCs to the tissue cells.

Washout Phase

The venule muscles relax and the clumps of RBCs are washed out to become emboli in the lungs. The acid and potassium become distributed throughout the body, producing a systemic metabolic acidosis (Figure 9.7).

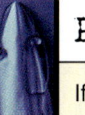

Physician Notes

If this washout situation occurs as a part of reestablishment of oxygenated blood flow, the acidosis and pulmonary emboli are part of the condition known as *reperfusion syndrome*.

Causes of Shock

Shock is caused by an interruption in circulatory function. There are three primary causes of shock in the human body:

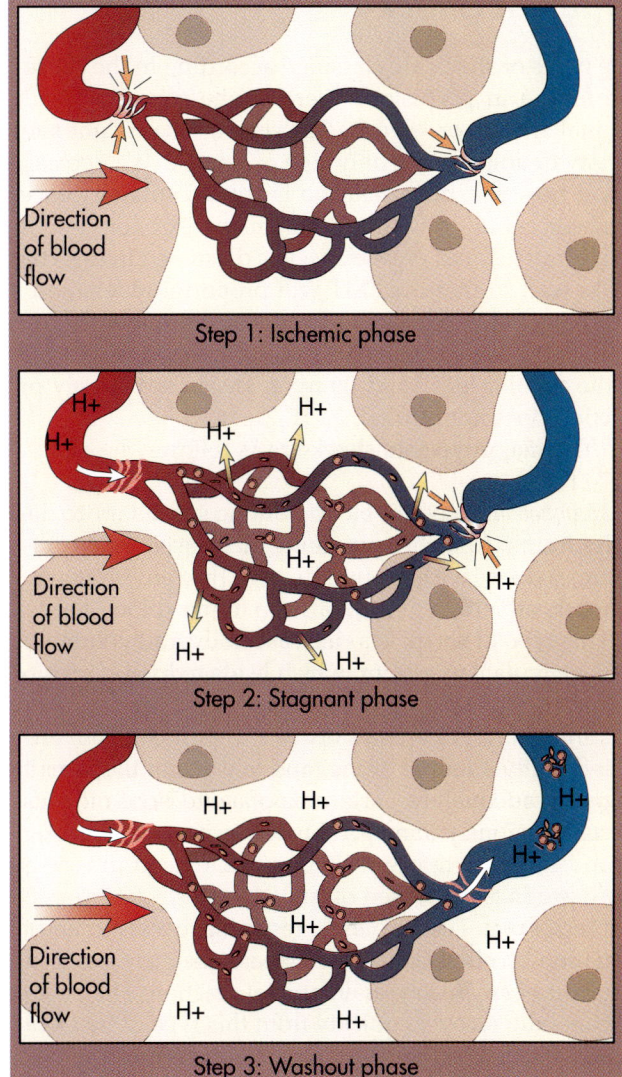

FIGURE 9.7 Phases of cellular shock.

1. *Pump failure* occurs for one of three reasons: decrease in the ability of the muscle to contract, disturbances in heart rate and rhythm (dysrhythmias), or decrease in the ability to receive blood and to pump.
2. *Container failure* occurs when the size of the circulatory system changes without a proportional increase in fluid volume.
3. *Volume failure* occurs when the circulatory system retains its normal size but the fluid volume is decreased.

✓ Shock is caused by a failure of the heart to pump blood efficiently, a change in size of the circulatory system without a proportional increase in fluid volume, or a decrease in fluid volume.

Types of Shock

The types of shock are classified according to the cause of the failure in perfusion. There is one condition, called "spinal shock" or "neurogenic shock," that is not shock by any definition. The only sign of "shock" is a decreased blood pressure, but perfusion is still acceptable. Since it has been confused with shock in many textbooks both for EMTs, nurses, and physicians, it is discussed in this chapter as well so that the EMT will properly understand its pathology. This "shock" is not a result of decreased perfusion and does not cause anaerobic metabolism to occur at the cellular level, and therefore decreased energy production does not result.

The major types of shock are as follows:

- *Hypovolemic*. Loss of blood volume secondary to dehydration (diarrhea, vomiting, decreased intake, increased loss without replacement [hot environment, work, athletic activity]) or from injury (blood loss). This type of shock is a decrease in overall volume in the circulatory system, which leads to hypoperfusion because of lack of blood return to the heart.
- *Cardiogenic*. Failure of the heart to pump effectively. It is usually a failure of the muscle walls of the heart to pump adequately. Large area of acute ischemic muscle, previously damaged heart muscle with scarring, and irregular rate and rhythm of the heart muscle can all produce decreased output.
- *Psychogenic*. The emotional response to a traumatic situation is called *fainting*. The heart rate increases as a result of an anxiety or emotional reaction. The patient generally recovers quickly from this type of incident, and vital signs return to normal. This is a result of vagal stimuli and has been called *vagal-vagal response*.
- *Septic*. Occurs as a result of infection in the body system that causes a vasodilation of the blood vessels. The container increases in size because of toxins in the circulatory system. The normal response to infection is that body systems fight the foreign toxins and the temperature of the body increases in response to this fight. Blood vessels lose their ability to constrict, and therefore hypoperfusion occurs. This type of shock is very seldom seen in the field. Even when seen it is not readily recognized beyond the hypoperfusion state.
- *Anaphylactic*. The result of a foreign protein entering the body to which the immune system establishes a rejection or protection response. In association with the cardiovascular response of hypotension, tachycardia (a generalized or splotchy rash of whelps) develops over the body and the mucus membranes and the muscles of the ventilatory system reduce the airway passages in the hypopharynx, larynx, bronchi, and alveoli. This can be a rapidly fatal condition. Death can occur within minutes as a result of ventilation compromise.

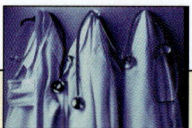

Physician Notes

Neurogenic, or spinal, shock is an interruption in nervous system communication, which results in vasodilatation of the blood vessels. This type of "shock" occurs when the spinal cord is damaged and communication to muscles is interrupted. It becomes a "container" malfunction because the vessels dilate and blood volume becomes entrapped in the extremities. The container enlarges and the blood pressure drops, but hypoperfusion does not occur because the dilated vessels continue to adequately perfuse the tissue cells. Neurogenic shock does not produce a decreased oxygenation of the peripheral tissues.

Neurogenic shock provides a challenge to the EMT and may be confused with true shock because of the vasodilatation that occurs. The heart rate does not increase to compensate for the decrease in blood pressure because the communication of the nervous system to the spinal cord has been interrupted. Therefore the brain does not interpret the crisis in the same manner. The patient in neurogenic shock usually exhibits blood pressure around 80 mm Hg systolic; has a pulse rate of 60 to 80 beats/min; is alert; shows no signs of tachypnea; has warm, dry, pink skin; and has good capillary refilling time.

Neurogenic shock is not shock in true sense. It is usually not a threatening condition to the patient because perfusion is maintained. However, neurogenic shock can be associated with hypovolemic shock.

Each of these causes may occur individually, or they may combine to create a disruption in perfusion. Usually for the prehospital contact, only one will be present when the patient is initially seen. This disruption in perfusion deprives the tissue cells of sufficient oxygen and nutrients to maintain metabolism to produce adequate amounts of energy for cell survival. The EMT most commonly will encounter shock in a traumatic situation that results in blood volume loss, in a cardiac situation from pump failure, in a fainting situation from generalized vasodilatation (container failure), and in acute dehydration secondary to severe diarrhea from fluid failure.

Body's Response to Anaerobic Metabolism

The container (vascular system) can be artificially divided into three physiologic (not anatomic) parts based on the need of the body to survive. The part that serves the heart, brain, and lungs receives the highest priority. The body strives to maintain this perfusion over all the rest since the loss of these organs would deprive the entire body of its supply of oxygenated blood. The blood supply to the abdominal contents and retroperitoneum receives the next highest priority, while the component that serves the extremities is the lowest priority. When the circulation of oxygenated blood is reduced for any reason, the brain prioritizes blood flow among these three physiologic segments of the vascular system. Blood is shunted away from the lowest priority area to those areas that are more sensitive to the loss of oxygenated blood and are essential to maintaining life. Blood is not shunted away from the heart, brain, or lung.

When the blood pressure drops and circulatory flow decreases, the change is detected by the baroreceptors in the carotid artery. This information is transmitted by nerves to the brain, which in turn sends signals to the sympathetic nervous system to release norepinephrine, causing constriction of the smooth muscles in the peripheral arteries and arterioles. This constriction reduces or completely shuts off the flow of blood to the skin and extremities. If this situation continues, blood flow to the GI tract and renal system will be reduced or shut off. This reduction of blood flow is achieved through constriction of diameter of the blood vessels, which increases the resistance to the flow of blood in these vessels.

This selective reduction in blood flow has one helpful effect and one harmful effect on the body. The helpful result is that the vasoconstriction is delayed in the blood vessels that provide circulation to the brain, heart, and lungs. The harmful effect is ischemia in that portion of the body. The vasoconstriction and resultant reduced circulation occur in areas of the body that are not immediately essential to preserving life and that can tolerate ischemia (lack of oxygenated blood) the longest.

Liquids flow along the path of least resistance. Blood is a liquid and follows all the laws of physics for liquids. There is less resistance to the flow of blood to the brain, heart, and lungs than to other parts of the body where the blood vessels have been constricted. The result is improved circulation to the vital organs and decreased circulation to the rest of the body. The increased resistance produced by the peripheral vasoconstriction results in an improved blood pressure. The action of cardiotonic substances such as epinephrine increases cardiac output both in volume and strength, adding to the increase in blood pressure.

There will be decreased or absent blood flow on the distal side of the increased vascular resistance. The decreased circulation through the distal capillary beds and decreased blood flow through distal arteries translates into three of the common signs of shock:

- Loss of normal skin color, moistness, and temperature
- Absent palpable distal pulse
- Delayed capillary refill

The decreased blood flow to the skin, abdomen, and extremities also means that these areas receive less nutrients and oxygen than they need. Rather than "starve," these cells convert from aerobic to anaerobic metabolism to survive. Anaerobic metabolism is not as efficient as aerobic metabolism. Less energy is produced for the body to use, and there is an increase in waste byproducts (principally acids and potassium). The result is a growing state of metabolic acidosis in the peripheral tissues. This acidosis is entirely related to the tissue cells and has no relationship to the regulation of fluids or electrolytes in the kidney.

If, subsequently, adequate circulation is restored and the peripheral cells receive adequate supplies of nutrients and oxygen, they convert back to aerobic metabolism. At the same time, the toxic byproducts of anaerobic metabolism are washed out of the peripheral areas and enter the central systemic circulation. If this accumulation of acids and potassium is large enough, it will now cause systemic metabolic acidosis (reperfusion syndrome).

The result of selective shunting of blood away from noncritical organs and the increased resistance to blood flow is that the heart is forced to junction with three handicaps, all of which decrease its efficiency:

1. The resistance to flow in the vessels of the muscles and capillary beds increases the demand on the heart and increases the amount of work required to force blood through these vessels.
2. The second stressful condition under which the heart must work is decreased oxygenation. The need for oxygen in a harder working (faster beating) heart is greater than for an easier working (slower beating) heart. More work requires more fuel. If the heart must beat faster to overcome the increased afterload, it must have more oxygen. This illustrates the need for the EMT to hyperoxygenate the patient during any period of cardiac stress, thereby helping to prevent further deterioration into shock.

Physician Notes

Although blood pressure is one of the most frequently measured functions of the heart, it is not the most important factor in the management of shock. Delivery of oxygen to the tissues by improving RBC oxygenation in the lungs and perfusion of the cells by these RBCs is the goal of shock management. This chapter is mainly concerned with the perfusion portion of management.

3. The third cardiac difficulty is a lack of available fluid to fill the ventricles during diastole (resting phase). Ejecting blood from the ventricle when the heart is only half full requires more frequent contractions and produces a smaller pulse pressure (and therefore a lower systolic pressure) than when adequate fluid is available. Cardiac work therefore becomes harder but produces less output.

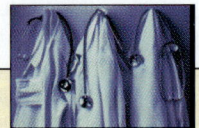

Physician Notes

One sign of shock is a rising diastolic pressure followed by a decline in both systolic and diastolic pressures.

Edema

If a large amount of fluid is present in the interstitial space (a condition known as *edema*), the distance between the capillary wall and the cell membrane becomes much greater. Oxygen must diffuse through the capillary wall, then through the interstitial fluid, and finally through the cell membrane. This increases the amount of fluid separating the capillaries from the tissue cells and increases the amount of distance that nutrients and oxygen must travel to reach the cells. The greater the thickness of interstitial fluid, the more difficult the transfer of the oxygen and other nutrients across this space.

If the left heart has some difficulty and fails to pump out all of the fluid presented to it while the right heart continues to function normally, there will be an overload of fluid into the pulmonary system. This congestion causes a buildup of pressure in the capillary system between the two pumps. This increased pressure forces fluid from the vascular bed into the tissues and the interstitial space. The pulmonary capillary bed is particularly sensitive to these changes because of limited tissue strength in the lungs. Fluid in the interstitial space increases the distance between the alveoli and capillaries, which makes oxygen exchange into the RBCs more difficult. This increased fluid accumulation, if it persists, will

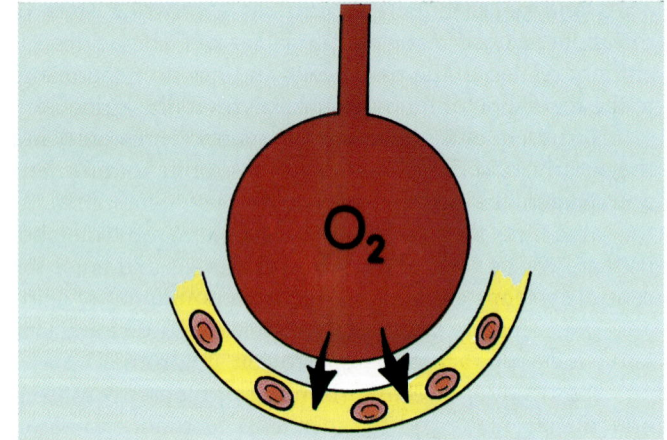
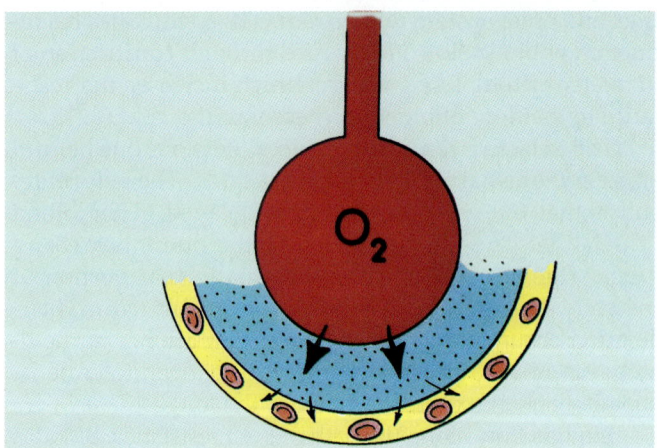
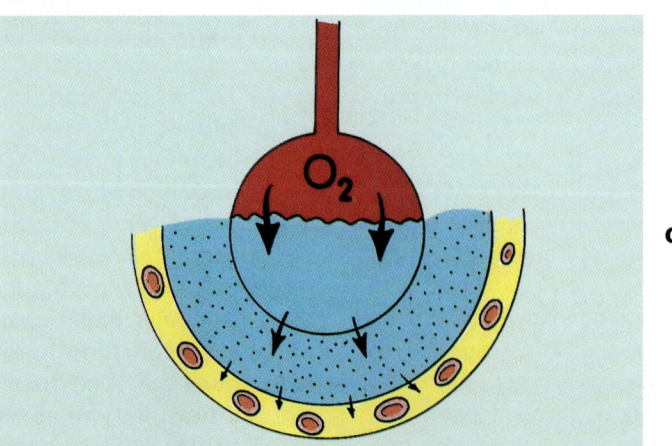

FIGURE 9.8 **A,** Alveolar capillary relationship. **B,** Interstitial area between capillary and alveolus filled with fluid (edema), reducing oxygen diffusion. **C,** Edema fluid fills alveolus, reducing oxygen presence in the alveolus with even more reduction of the body's ability to oxygenate the RBCs.

continue to migrate into the alveoli and produce actual fluid in the space normally occupied by air. This produces even more compromise for the patient because now the inspired air cannot enter the alveoli and be absorbed into the RBCs (Figure 9.8).

Chronic congestion that occurs in the lungs because of failure of the left heart is called *congestive heart failure*. Acute fluid buildup in the interstitial space in the post-trauma patient is known as *acute respiratory distress syndrome (ARDS)*. Congestive heart failure is cardiac in origin, whereas ARDS is a result of leaky capillary syndrome. Although ARDS is not commonly seen in the field because it occurs 24 to 48 hours after admission, the cause is frequently inadequate resuscitation very early in patient care either in the field or in the emergency department. This is one of the causes of death of the patient that can be prevented or reduced by good prehospital care.

The results of such a condition can be rapidly progressive because a vicious cycle quickly develops. The heart does not receive enough oxygen and therefore works harder and pumps more often to remove the deficit. More oxygen is required to provide fuel for the extra work, but the oxygen is not available. This cycle can produce a rapid downward course—even a fatal course—for the patient unless effective treatment is begun quickly to overcome it. Prehospital treatment is best achieved by increasing the oxygen concentration in the inspired air to as close to 100% as possible and by taking the necessary steps to improve perfusion (blood flow).

Severity of Blood Loss

The amount of blood that is lost through injury dictates the severity of the injury or loss. In addition to the amount, the time period over which the blood is lost may also be a factor. One of the compensatory mechanisms that the body uses in shock is to move fluid from the interstitial space into the vascular space when the pressure is low in the vessels. This does not occur instantously but does occur in a matter of an hour or so. The sudden loss of 2 L, or 2000 ml, of blood in the adult produces uncompensated shock and is considered a serious or severe loss, whereas the loss of 1 L, or 1000 ml, over 4 to 5 hours is usually compensated by the movement of interstitial fluid into the vascular system. The results are only moderate since the fluid has been replaced. The loss of blood over an extended period of time does not create hypoperfusion problems for the patient, and the circulatory system continues with minimal compromise. In the child, a sudden loss of 0.5 L, or 500 ml, of blood is considered a severe loss. In the infant, a loss of 150 ml, less than one cup, of blood is considered a severe loss.

The EMT develops a general impression of the patient in shock based on demonstrated signs and symptoms of hypoperfusion. If the signs and symptoms of hypoperfusion exist, the blood loss should be considered severe and the patient will most likely demonstrate signs and symptoms of **hypotension** (low blood pressure). The severity of blood loss is based on the signs and symptoms demonstrated by the patient. Any time the patient demonstrates signs and symptoms of hypoperfusion, the loss is considered severe.

External injury and evidence of blood loss provide visual clues to the EMT that enhance his or her general impression of the patient's condition. The blood losses that occur during internal injury are not always readily identified by the EMT. The general impression of the patient by the EMT will be of signs and symptoms of hypoperfusion other than obvious blood loss.

> ✓ The amount of blood that is lost through injury and the time period over which the blood is lost dictates the severity of the injury or loss.

Assessment

The signs of shock are as follows (Figure 9.9):

- *Rapid ventilatory rate.* The increase that occurs in the rate of breathing during hypoperfusion is a compensatory mechanism of perfusion. A rate of 12 to 20 ventilations per minute is normal. However, a rate

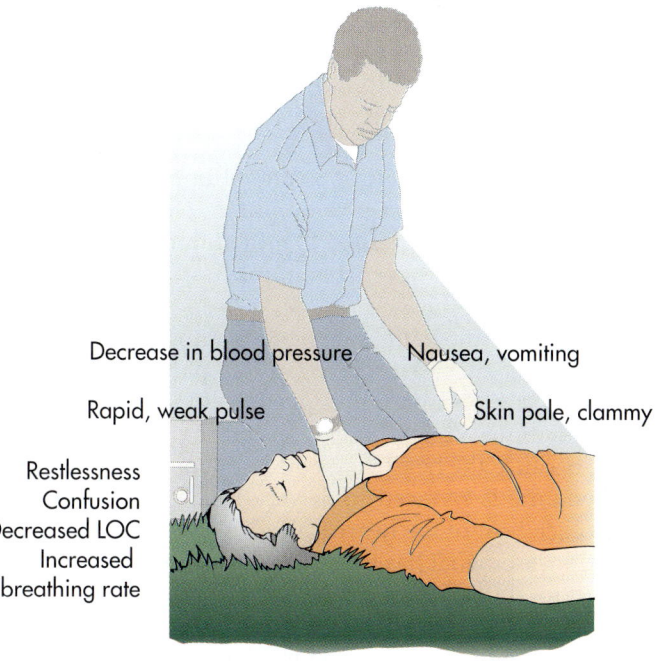

FIGURE 9.9 Common signs of shock.

of 20 to 30 ventilations per minute is concerning. The EMT should keep in mind that anaerobic metabolism increases acid production in the cells. The acid is converted to carbon dioxide (CO_2) by the body's buffer systems. This increased CO_2 is identified by the brain and increases the ventilatory drive to remove it through the lungs. Oxygen is needed to be added to the inspired air. A rate of greater than 30 respirations per minute is very abnormal. Shock is present, and the EMT should provide rapid transportation to a trauma center (if available) while providing assisted ventilation en route. The patient should be placed in the shock position with protection from heat loss.

- *Rapid, weak pulse.* The EMT will often have difficulty palpating a pulse at the end (distal) point of an extremity when the patient is in shock. The further a pulse point is from the heart, the harder it will be to feel when perfusion is poor. Therefore the EMT should attempt to feel pulses close to the core, such as the carotid or femoral pulse. This can actually be of assistance in evaluating a patient. The location at which the pulse is palpated will give a clue as to the blood pressure and therefore the flow. The pulse may be rapid (fast) and weak, often described as a "weak and **thready**" pulse. When volume is lost, the system attempts to compensate for the blood loss as quickly as it can. Each beat of the heart pumps blood into the systemic circulation. The total amount of blood pumped in 1 minute is approximately 5 L, and this amount is called the *cardiac output*. Therefore beats per minute times the volume per beat (stroke volume) equals cardiac output. If the volume decreases with each beat of the heart, the body attempts to maintain cardiac output by increasing the number of heart beats per minute.

$$80 \text{ beats per minute} \times 60 \text{ ml volume} = 4800 \text{ ml cardiac output.}$$
$$120 \text{ beats per minute} \times 40 \text{ ml volume} = 4800 \text{ ml cardiac output.}$$

Therefore the initial safeguard that the system creates is to increase the heart rate in an attempt to maintain perfusion and blood pressure when volume is lost. If the body continues to lose blood, this mechanism eventually fails, because the heart is unable to maintain the rate and the volume is reduced until very little blood is ejected with each beat of the heart.

Consider what has been said about the patient's body trying to shunt blood to the core during shock. If the blood is diverted, then checking the circulation at the periphery could provide a good indication of the body's response to what is happening. If there is shunting in progress, the peripheral pulses should be decreased.

- *Pallor of the skin, which then becomes bluish (cyanotic).* Pallor occurs because the vessels constrict and blood is pushed from the periphery to the core organs. The skin may quickly turn cyanotic because the blood that returns to the periphery is not oxygenated adequately.
- *Pale because all the blood has been shunted away from this area of the skin*
- *Cold and clammy or sweaty (diaphoretic) skin.* Diaphoretic skin is a result of vasoconstriction of vessels in the periphery. The skin becomes cool, and pores open. Again, a decrease in systemic perfusion and a movement of blood to the core organs cause these effects.
- *Decreased level of consciousness.* A decrease in the level of consciousness, or mental confusion, occurs for two reasons: perfusion to the brain is not adequate, and the blood that is perfused is oxygen-poor. Ventilatory effort and the exchange of oxygen in the lungs is critical for the patient in shock. If blood volume is decreased, then the most important treatment is administration of oxygen. The available blood must be well oxygenated if the patient is to improve.
- *Decrease in blood pressure.* A decrease in blood pressure is a late sign of shock. Usually 25% of the total blood volume has been lost when a decrease in blood pressure occurs. In children, a 25% to 50% total volume loss must occur before a drop in blood pressure occurs. Hypotension, or a systolic pressure of less than 100 mm Hg, along with other signs, becomes a significant indicator that the patient is progressively deteriorating and needs immediate treatment and transportation.

Good Rule of Thumb

No pulse at the radial artery = systolic pressure < 80 mm Hg
No pulse at the femoral artery = systolic pressure < 70 mm Hg
No pulse at the carotid artery = systolic pressure < 60 mm Hg

- *Increase in ventilatory rate.* The chemoreceptors located in the circulatory system identify the loss of oxygen and/or the increased amount of acid in the form of CO_2 in the blood and increase the rate of ventilation to obtain more oxygen for the cells and eliminate the CO_2. This increase in the ventilatory rate can be one of the earliest signs of shock.
- **Capillary refill** *time.* Another sign that blood has been shunted to the core is to check the blood flow in

the skin of the periphery. Put pressure on the skin of the great toe or the thumb and squeeze out all of the blood. Estimate the time for blood to flow back into the skin. Greater than 2 seconds is abnormal. This sign of decreased perfusion is present not only in shock, but in many other conditions as well (see discussion in the pathophysiology section on p. 124)

- *Evidence of major blood or nonblood volume loss.* Large amounts of blood lost from a wound or evidence of a rigid, tense abdomen may signal the severity of the trauma that has occurred. If a gunshot wound or stab wound (**penetrating trauma**) is visible, the EMT must suspect that severe damage has occurred internally. The extent of the damage and all organs involved may exceed what can be observed from the exterior.

The signs of shock are the demonstrated effects of hypoperfusion, or the failure to perfuse the body with oxygenated blood. These effects or signs may occur because of blood loss or because the heart fails to pump or the vessels have dilated (vasodilation) and the proportionate expansion is interpreted by the body as a blood loss. Signs of hypovolemic shock may occur after fluid loss of other etiologies such as exposure to heat, severe or prolonged diarrhea and/or vomiting, or reduced fluid intake over an extended period of time. The patient will usually present with the same signs as a trauma patient with significant blood loss.

The symptoms of shock are not always evident because their expression depends on the patient's level of consciousness. The following symptoms may be verbalized by the patient or bystanders:

- Mental confusion
- Feeling of weakness
- Feeling of impending doom
- Nausea and/or vomiting
- Headache

> ✓ Signs of shock include rapid, weak pulse; pallor of the skin, which then becomes cyanotic; cold and clammy or sweaty skin; increase in ventilatory rate; decrease in level of consciousness; and evidence of major blood loss. Symptoms that may be verbalized by the patient or bystanders include mental confusion, feeling of weakness, feeling of impending doom, nausea and/or vomiting, and headache.

The EMT's first impression of a patient will often be determined by the information received from the dispatcher. The potential injuries and mechanism of injury or illness are established by this information. For example, if the dispatcher relates that the patient was shot with a high-velocity weapon in the chest and that the patient is barely breathing and is unresponsive, the EMT immediately knows that the scene may not be safe and that police assistance is necessary. In addition, the signs and symptoms of critical shock and potential for severe injury exist. In a nontrauma situation the dispatcher may describe a patient unconscious in a closed, nonventilated house in the middle of summer, a patient down at work outdoors during the summer, or a patient in bed with several days of GI symptoms. The information provided by the dispatcher is frequently inaccurate, and therefore the EMT must keep an open mind and search for information on arrival.

The obvious loss of blood and the continued loss of blood through open wounds are important in the initial assessment of the patient. The ability to estimate blood loss is an important skill. Increased swelling of muscle tissues is a sign of injury and possible blood loss and must be included in the assessment reported to the physician and nurses receiving the patient. Any blood loss is dramatic and of major concern to the patient. For example, a nosebleed may be interpreted by the patient as a significant blood loss, whereas the EMT may view the blood loss as minor and insignificant. Blood loss is not always evident to the EMT. In **blunt trauma**, for instance, the blood loss may be under the skin and not evident for minutes or hours after the injury has occurred.

In assessing a patient with the signs and symptoms of shock, airway evaluation is the number one priority. Assessment of perfusion is the next priority, which is performed by assessing the presence of a pulse and then the character of the pulse. Ventilatory rate is next on the priority list, and level of consciousness is a **cardinal** indicator of perfusion. Color and temperature of the skin and external bleeding are observable signs that are usefully in the estimation of the level of shock. Next in line to better define shock is blood pressure.

Management

General Principles

General principles of shock management are as follows:

Secure the airway
Heat conservation in the body (energy production is decreased)
Oxygenation of RBCs to replace the tissue deficit
Core perfusion improvement by elevation of the lower extremities
Keep the field time as short as possible and transport the patient to the correct medical facility

- Securing the airway is addressed in Chapters 10, 11, and 14. **Auscultation** of the lungs is important to evaluate the completeness of ventilation.
- **H**eat conservation is very important. As addressed previously, when the metabolism changes from the aerobic to the anaerobic process, the energy production drops 36-fold. One of the results of this situation is the loss of heat production. Since the core temperature is nearly always less than that of the air that surrounds the patient and therefore heat is constantly lost to the environment, steps must be taken to preserve the body heat.
- **O**xygen is the most frequently administrated and the most important drug for prehospital use. When there is decreased blood flow to the tissues, it is critical that every available RBC have the most oxygen that it can carry. After addressing the airway, the second most important step for getting the oxygen to the cells is to provide the largest concentration possible within the alveolus where the exchange of oxygen and carbon dioxide is accomplished.
- Core perfusion preservation is attempted by the body by decreasing the blood flow to the peripherial structures as described previously. The EMT can assist in this process by elevation of the lower extremities. Such elevation will allow the blood that is pooled in the legs to run downhill to the central circulation and will increase the resistance to blood flow into the legs. The blood volume that remains in the trauma or dehydrated patient will be constrained to the core. In the patient whose problem is vasodilitation, such as in fainting, such a maneuver will also restore the core blood flow to the brain.
- Keep the field time as short as possible. The management of shock is to restore the lost volume from whatever the cause and to stop the volume loss as quickly as possible. In most causes of shock this is best accomplished as soon as possible when prolonged field time is not in the best interest of the patient. For example, if the spleen has been fractured and blood loss into the abdominal cavity is 100 ml/min and there is an extra 5 minutes delay in the field to perform an unnecessary test, this will produce a blood loss equal to 10% of the total blood volume in an adult. If the blood loss is faster, this delay will produce even more blood less.

Determining the Cause of Shock

All shock is not a result of blood loss. The first step in patient management is to determine the most likely cause of the shock and then to develop a treatment plan for that etiology. As a general rule these causes can be divided into three categories:

- *Cardiac.* Any type of cardiac failure, either acute or chronic. Most cardiac patients will benefit from oxygen, which should be given quickly. If the patient is currently taking nitroglycerine, the EMT should assist the patient in placing such a pill under his or her tongue. The response to nitroglycerine, especially regarding pain relief, provides significant information as to the etiology of the patient condition. This should be observed, documented, and reported to the emergency department personnel.
- *Medical.* Dehydration secondary to extreme heat or activity without proper intake of fluids; GI dehydration secondary to diarrhea, vomiting, or both; or GI **hemorrhage**. The medical causes of shock are dehydration, fainting, or allergic conditions. These will respond to the general methods of **SHOCK** management outlined previously. The patient with known allergic conditions may have their own "Epi pin" injection device. If such a device is available and the EMT is confident that the shock is a result of an allergic condition and not cardiac, then the patient should be assisted with the administration of the epinephrine.
- *Trauma.* External or internal hemorrhage secondary to a traumatic incident.

Management Steps

Once the EMT has determined that the patient has the signs and symptoms of shock, every effort should be made to transport the patient immediately. Several management steps should be followed in the field and during transport to stabilize the patient's condition. The initiation of this care may also result in the patient's condition improving en route to the hospital, and failure to effectively implement the steps will certainly result in the patient's deterioration. The EMT may only have time to perform a minimal focused assessment of the patient in profound shock. The initial steps for management of shock are as follows:

1. Establishing a patent airway
2. Administering high-concentration oxygen
3. Controlling bleeding
4. Beginning to manage hypotension and continuing during transportation to the hospital
5. Transporting to a medical facility

Establishing a Patent Airway and Administering High-Concentration Oxygen

The patient must have an airway that will support delivery of oxygen. If the patient is not breathing adequately, respiratory effort must be supported by a bag-valve-mask. The rate and depth of ventilations determine the need for assisted ventilation. All patients in a compromised state or potential compromised state should receive high-concentration oxygen. The patient is in a compromised state if his or her ventilatory rate is below 12 breaths per minute or greater than 30 breaths per minute. (Ventilatory rates in excess are a warning that something is amiss. These patients may need assisted ventilation as well.) If the patient is responsive and breathing on his or her own, the preferred method of delivery of oxygen is a nonrebreather oxygen mask at 15 L/min flow. Do not consider the rate of flow alone as the only factor in the amount of oxygen that the patient is getting into his or her lungs. The device used to administer the oxygen is also important. Nasal prongs, for example, can deliver only 24% oxygen no matter how high the flow rate is turned up. A nonrebreather mask will deliver 75% to 90% oxygen to the patient.

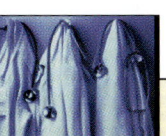

Physician Notes

If the patient is responsive and resists the face mask, this in itself is a sign of hypoxia. Special tender loving care (TLC) on the part of the EMT is required to convince the patient that the mask is important and to allow it to stay in place. Think of how you would feel if you were having difficulty breathing and someone unknown to you put his or her hands or a green plastic mask over your nose and mouth. Your initial action would be to remove it so you could breathe better. This would be even more true if you were frightened and anxious.

The patient who is experiencing shock (decreased energy production) already has a reduced ability to transport oxygen throughout the body. Therefore the EMT must saturate the remaining RBCs with as much oxygen as possible to keep the patient alive. If the patient is unresponsive and breathing at an adequate rate, the nonrebreather oxygen mask at 15 L/min flow should be administered. Any patient who is not breathing adequately on his or her own should receive assisted ventilation with the use of the bag-valve-mask device with accumulator with oxygen at a minimum of 15 L/min flow.

Controlling Bleeding

The control of bleeding is critical for the patient who has experienced blood loss for any reason. The first step in the management of a trauma with blood loss is to determine if it is internal, external, or both. External hemorrhages can be initially addressed in the field, whereas internal hemorrhage cannot. Differentiation between those patients that the EMT can help and those in which the source of blood loss must be treated in the OR is a critical step in management. If the EMT suspects significant blood loss within a body compartment that can only be addressed in the OR, then the management of such patients is rapid transportation to the correct medical facility. This would be a trauma center if one is available in the community. If one is not available, then the patient should be transported to the facility best equipped and staffed for trauma management or the EMT should notify the closest trauma center to provide helicopter intercept if possible. (For further detail, see Chapter 23.)

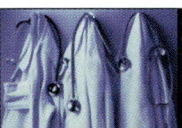

Physician Notes

Completely severed vessels frequently go into spasm and retract into the surrounding muscle tissue. This protective method that the body has developed will, on many occasions, provide complete control over hemorrhage. The injury to the vessels produces only a partial tear in the vessel wall that cannot retract into the surrounding muscle tissue. This injury will more often require extra steps for hemorrhage control.

Managing Hypotension and Transporting to a Medical Facility

Severity of shock is one of the determining factors in the decision for rapid transport of the patient. On determining that the patient is hypoperfused, the EMT should immediately initiate transport to a medical facility. This impression of the patient's condition may occur during the initial assessment, although it may often occur during the focused assessment. If the patient initially is alert and oriented and then becomes less responsive during assessment or if blood pressure drops, the patient has deteriorated and the situation is becoming more critical. This is one indication that whatever is being done for the patient should be completed as soon as possible and transportation should be begun.

Many times the mechanism of injury will indicate the need to rapidly assess, treat, and transport the trauma patient. The patient with cardiac etiology needs drugs that are usually not available to the EMT-B. The patient should get to advanced life support (ALS) care as quickly as possible. ALS care may be quicker in the hospital, or it may be quicker with ALS EMS unit intercept. The EMT must decide which is the quickest and develop a plan toward that goal. This is another of the many situations in which a knowledgeable and thinking EMT can make judgment decisions based on the current conditions. Management can occur during transportation to the hospital, and the EMT should not delay care on the scene when the patient is hypoperfusing. The immediate management of shock is dependent on the overall state of the patient's condition.

The ideal method of controlling hypotension for the patient in hypovolemic shock is to replace the blood volume lost. This replacement can be done at a hospital; however, it is not usually possible for the EMT-B to introduce fluids in the prehospital setting. The delivery of fluids by mouth is not an effective method of replacement, and although responsive patients in severe shock may feel thirsty and request something to drink, the EMT should not allow it. Once the EMT arrives on a scene a patient should never be allowed to eat or drink until the assessment has been completed and permission is given by medical direction for the patient to eat or drink. The following are two methods that will assist the EMT in managing the patient who is in a state of hypoperfusion in the prehospital setting:

1. *Position.* The patient should be placed in the **Trendelenburg position**. Place the patient on the stretcher and raise the foot of the stretcher and/or lower the head of the stretcher. This position allows gravity to assist the movement of blood in the extremities to the core where it is needed (Figure 9.10). The Trendelenburg position increases pressure on the diaphragm and moves the abdominal organs against the diaphragm, making respirations more labored and difficult for the patient in crisis. Therefore the Trendelenburg position should not be used in certain instances.
2. *Use of a* **pneumatic antishock garment (PASG)**. The PASG is a controversial device because its exact role in prehospital care is still not definitively decided. Despite this controversy, it should not be neglected as a prehospital patient treatment tool. Like other medical devices, the PASG should only be used when indicated. Specifically, it is helpful for patients requiring control of blood loss, management of pelvic instabil-

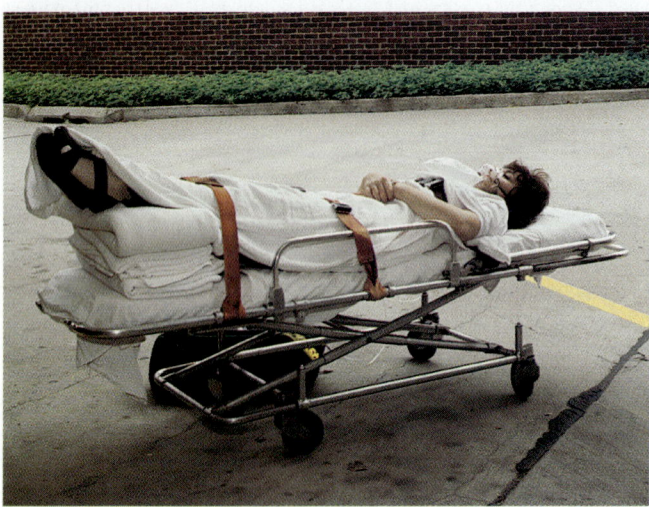

FIGURE 9.10 The patient should be placed in the Trendelenburg position on the stretcher. The foot of the stretcher is raised 8 to 12 inches, or the head of the stretcher is lowered. This position should only be used if there are no apparent injuries to the head, neck, chest, abdomen, pelvis, spine, or lower extremities.

Box 9.3 Recommendations of the National Association of EMS Physicians for the use of the PASG 1996

Usually indicated, useful and effective
Hypotension due to ruptured abdominal aortic aneurism

Acceptable, uncertain efficacy, weight of evidence favors usefullness and efficacy
Hypotension due to suspected pelvic fracture
Anaphylactic shock (unresponsive to conventional therapy)
Otherwise uncontrollable lower-extremity hemorrhage
Severe traumatic hypotension (palpable pulse, unobtainable blood pressure)

Acceptable, uncertain efficacy, may be helpful, probably not harmful
Elderly
History of congestive heart failure
Penetrating abdominal injury
Paroxysmal supraventricular tachycardia (PSVT)
Gynecologic hemorrhage (otherwise uncontrollable)
Hypothermia-induced hypotension

Lower-extremity hemorrhage (otherwise uncontrollable)
Pelvis fracture without hemorrhage
Ruptured ectopic pregnancy
Septic shock
Urologic hemorrhage (otherwise uncontrollable)
Assist intravenous cannulation

Inappropriate option, not indicated, may be harmful
Adjunct to CPR
Diaphragmatic rupture
Penetrating thoracic injury
Splint fractures of lower extremity
Abdominal evisceration
Acute myocardial infarction
Cardiac tamponade
Cardiogenic shock
Gravid uterus

ity, or long transportation times. PASGs may be detrimental to patients with penetrating thoracic trauma or short transportation times. It remains contraindicated in patients with pulmonary edema, traumatic diaphragmatic herniation, or known hemorrhage above the diaphragm (Box 9.3).

The transportation of the patient in shock should be accomplished as soon as possible. It is critical that the patient in any type of shock be constantly reassessed for improvements or deterioration. The EMT should contact medical direction en route to the hospital. The appropriate management of the patient in shock must include notification of the receiving hospital as soon as possible. Although every hospital will treat a patient on arrival, patients will receive the most efficient treatment when hospital staff are able to prepare for their arrival. Physician or hospital communications (medical direction) are necessary for treatment orders,

Editor's Note

The National Association of EMS Physicians (NAEMSP) has published a position paper on the PASG. The following information is compatible with that paper.

Physiology
Pressure applied by the PASG to the legs and abdomen is transmitted directly through the skin, fat, muscle, and other soft tissue to the blood vessels. The vessels are compressed, and their lumen (internal opening) is reduced in size. The physiologic result is twofold. The vascular container in body areas beneath the device is made smaller, increasing the systemic vascular resistance and thereby raising the systolic and diastolic pressures. The remaining fluid can be distributed and better used in the noncompressed upper half of the body.

Hemorrhage
Compression over a bleeding site is the classic method of hemorrhage control. Effective compression can be achieved with the PASG for body areas such as the abdomen, pelvis, and legs. The PASG is just a large pneumatic splint. It should be used to control blood loss and stabilize fractures with the same indications as a pneumatic splint.

Increased bleeding in the noncompressed portions of the body is a potential complication of inflating the PASG. The rate of hemorrhage from an open wound is proportional to the blood pressure inside the injured vessel minus the external pressure on the vessel. Less bleeding occurs with a low blood pressure than with a high blood pressure. Open vessels in the upper half of the body may increase the rate of blood loss when the patient's blood pressure and blood flow are significantly improved, as when the PASG is applied.

Blood Pressure
Reevaluation of several studies indicates that patients with blood pressures below 50 to 60 mm Hg have a better outcome when the PASG is used than when it is not. The increased perfusion of the brain and heart that is provided by the increased vascular resistance in the lower extremities and abdomen is beneficial to such patients.

Immobilization of Fractures
Like any pneumatic splint, the PASG can also be used for fracture immobilization. The two major bones that the PASG immobilizes most effectively are the pelvis and the femur. Because hemorrhage is recognized as a major potential problem with fracture of either of these bones, compression with the PASG provides an extra benefit beyond just immobilizing the fracture. Use of the PASG solely as a splint for isolated lower-extremity fractures where shock is not present or expected, however, is not recommended.

Application
The PASG is applied to the patient as quickly as possible and without delay when indications for its use in hemorrhage control or fracture management are present. The PASG is positioned under the patient in one of several ways. In many cases, it may be simpler to place the patient on the device (as when moving the patient onto a long board) rather than lifting the patient and inserting the garment beneath the patient. The PASG is then securely and snugly fastened and inflated. When the Velcro begins to crackle, between 60 and 80 mm Hg of PASG pressure (not blood pressure) has been achieved (Figure 9.11).

Deflation
Prehospital deflation of the PASG should not be done except in extreme extenuating circumstances, such as evidence of a diaphragmatic herniation, and even then only with on-line medical direction. When deflation is necessary, it should be preceded by assessing the patient and confirming that vital signs are within normal limits. Even with vital signs within normal limits, the patient's blood volume might still be depleted; the inflated PASG has reduced the size of the patient's container, and the available blood volume may just fill the artificially reduced container. As the PASG is deflated, the patient's container size will increase. Unless a sufficient amount of fluid is present in reserve, cardiac preload will decrease, systemic vascular resistance will drop, and the patient's blood pressure and level of perfusion will deteriorate rapidly.

Continued

Editor's Note—cont'd

Contraindications

The current literature does not demonstrate a worse outcome with the use of PASG for the management of intraabdominal, retroperitoneal, and pelvic fracture hemorrhage. In fact it shows improvement in these conditions. However, the published articles demonstrated a worse outcome when the device is placed on a patient with hemorrhage in the chest. This is because pressure and flow are increased in the chest when the device is correctly applied to the lower half of the body. Increased flow and pressure will increase uncontrolled blood loss. Other contraindications include objects impaled in a site that would be covered with the garment, fluid in the lungs, and a patient in the final trimester of pregnancy.

The PASG may create the same difficulty in breathing for the patient that the Trendelenburg position creates, because it may interfere with the movement of the diaphragm. The increase in blood pressure is very quick. It may be sufficient to transport the patient to the hospital, where intravenous fluids will replace the volume that has been lost. If the application of this device results in pulmonary edema or a decrease in blood pressure, the EMT must contact medical direction immediately to obtain orders for deflation of the PASG.

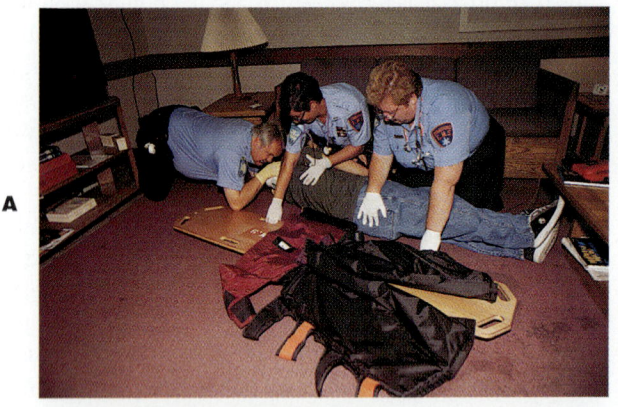
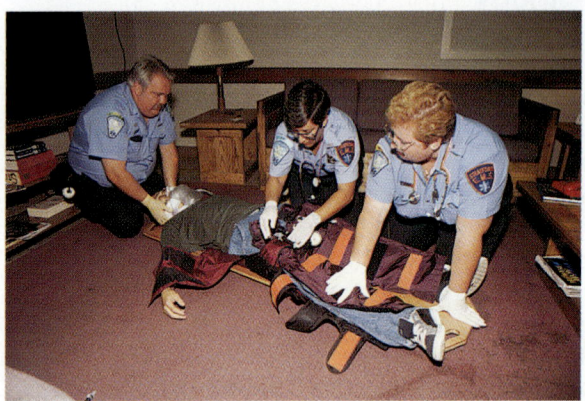
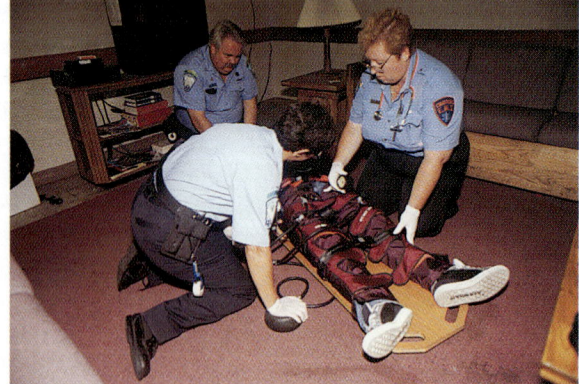
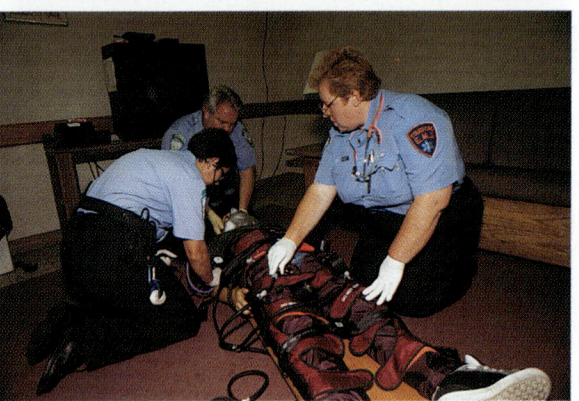

FIGURE 9.11 **A**, Position the pneumatic antishock garment with the top of the abdominal section at or below the last set of ribs. **B**, Enclose both legs and the abdomen. **C**, Inflate with the foot pump. **D**, Close all stopcocks when the patient's systolic blood pressure reaches 100 mm Hg. Do not overinflate.

and medical direction is responsible for selection of the most appropriate treatment facilities for patients.

Hospital facilities should be designated for the patient based on their ability to treat specific types of cases. It is better to transport a patient to a trauma facility that might be farther away than to transport a patient to the closest hospital, which is not prepared to definitively treat the patient. A trauma center has surgeons and ORs that are ready for immediate use, whereas other hospitals may have to call in surgeons and wait for OR staff to arrive from their homes. The key to survival in trauma patients is most often the amount of time that their condition is allowed to deteriorate.

> ✓ Steps for managing shock are establishing a patent airway, administering high-concentration oxygen, controlling bleeding, managing hypotension, and transporting to the hospital.

Summary

- The distribution of oxygen from the respiratory system by the circulatory system is the key factor in shock treatment and care.
- The structures of the circulatory system include the heart and blood vessels. Blood vessels include arteries, veins, and capillaries. In general, arteries carry oxygenated blood away from the heart, and veins carry deoxygenated blood to the heart.
- The optimal environment in which human metabolism takes place is aerobic, or in the presence of oxygen. Perfusion is the ability of the circulatory system to circulate blood and oxygen to the cells.
- Hypoperfusion, or a decrease in perfusion, interrupts body function and the ability to survive. Permanent, irreversible damage occurs when cells function in an anaerobic environment for a prolonged period of time. Hypoperfusion is the cardinal sign of shock, or a failure of the body to perfuse and oxygenate the cells.
- Signs and symptoms of shock include rapid, weak pulse; pallor of the skin, which then becomes cyanotic; cold and clammy or sweaty skin; increase of respiratory rate; decrease in level of consciousness; and evidence of major blood loss. Symptoms that may be verbalized by the patient or bystanders include mental confusion, feeling of weakness, feeling of impending doom, nausea and/or vomiting, and headache.
- In assessing a patient with possible shock, airway evaluation is the number one priority. Assessment of perfusion is the next priority, which is done by assessing the presence and then the character of the pulse. Blood pressure and level of consciousness are cardinal indicators of perfusion. Color and temperature of the skin and external bleeding are also important indicators of shock. It is important for the EMT to estimate blood loss. For the trauma patient, determining the mechanism of injury is essential.
- Steps for managing shock include establishing a patent airway, administering high-concentration oxygen, controlling bleeding, managing hypotension, and transporting to the hospital.
- The EMT must be equipped with the knowledge and skills to readily identify hypoperfusion and treat it quickly. The identification of signs and symptoms of hypoperfusion and the consistent delivery of care using the initial assessment skills are essential to this process. Shock (hypoperfusion) is the most common life-threatening emergency that the EMT will encounter in the prehospital setting. The treatment of the patient who is experiencing this emergency should become an automatic response for the properly educated EMT.

Scenario Solution

Scene safety. The vehicle is in a ditch and has significant damage. There is no water in the ditch, and there is no evidence of a gasoline tank rupture in the car. The scene is reasonably safe, extrication is required, and the EMT should call for assistance of additional tools.

Body substance isolation precautions. The EMT will have gloves on his or her hands and safety goggles on his or her eyes. There is broken glass, and protective clothing is indicated to protect the EMT from injury.

General impression. The EMT will recognize that the patient has sustained significant injury in a single motor vehicle collision and was not wearing a seat belt. The patient is bleeding, appears to be unresponsive, and is pale. This patient is severely injured.

Scenario Solution (cont'd)

Initial assessment. The EMT should provide the following interventions for the patient:

1. Establish level of consciousness (e.g., the patient is unresponsive).
2. Determine airway and ventilation status (e.g., the patient is breathing at 22 breaths per minute, and teeth are broken and bleeding). If this patient stops breathing, the method of choice for securing the airway would be endotracheal intubation.
3. Apply a nonrebreather oxygen mask at 15 L/min flow. If the patient needs support ventilations, the EMT should use a bag-valve-mask device at 15 L/min flow.
4. Obtain a pulse (e.g., the patient has no palpable radial pulse, but there is a rapid and weak carotid pulse; the patient has a low blood pressure).
5. Active bleeding is noted, and the EMT should suspect that the patient may have head trauma, cervical spine trauma, chest trauma, abdominal trauma, and extremity trauma.
6. The patient is severely injured and should be transported as soon as possible.
7. The patient should be rapidly extricated from the vehicle, taking precautions for spinal immobilization using a cervical spine immobilization device and long backboard. Apply the PASG and load on stretcher.

Focused assessment. The patient will be rapidly assessed for signs of injury en route to the hospital in the ambulance. The patient demonstrates profound hypoperfusion and therefore is in shock. A successful outcome for this patient depends on early recognition of the severity of the shock and rapid transport to the hospital for definitive treatment.

Key Terms

Aerobic In the presence of oxygen.

Anaerobic In the absence of oxygen.

Arterioles Smallest branch of an artery; supplies capillaries with oxygenated blood.

Artery Vessel that carries blood away from the heart to the body under pressure.

Atria Upper chambers of the heart; the right atrium receives blood from the superior and inferior venae cavae; the left atrium receives blood from the pulmonary veins.

Auscultation Listening to the sounds of the body with a stethoscope or blood pressure cuff.

Bicuspid valve Two-flap valve that covers the opening between the left atrium and the left ventricle.

Blunt trauma Injury that is not immediately evident to the human eye.

Brachial artery Artery located on the inside of the elbow on the same side as the small finger; extends from the elbow to the armpit.

Brachial pulse Pulse palpated at the brachial artery of the arm, found on the inner aspect of the upper arm.

Capillaries Smallest blood vessels in the body; in the tissues, capillaries surround the cells, allowing gas and nutrient exchange to take place.

Capillary refill Time it takes for a patient's skin color to return to normal after the skin or nailbed has been pressed or blanched; normal time is less than 2 seconds; assesses perfusion.

Cardiac output Total amount of blood pumped in one minute; usually 5 liters.

Cardinal Key, critical, common sign.

Carotid artery Major artery of the neck, supplying the face, head, and brain with oxygenated blood.

Carotid pulse Pulse palpated at the carotid artery of the neck, on either side of the neck beside the larynx.

Core Central part; the heart and lungs of the human body.

Diastolic pressure Pressure in the heart when the heart muscle is relaxing; lower reading of a blood pressure.

Femoral arteries Major vessels supplying the legs with oxygenated blood; can be palpated in the groin area.

Femoral pulse Pulse palpated at the femoral artery of the groin on either side of the pelvis.

Heart Four-chambered organ that pumps blood through the blood vessels to distribute oxygen to the cells of the body.

Heart rate Number of heart beats that occur in one minute.

Hemoglobin A specialized protein that binds to oxygen in red blood cells; it gives red blood cells their color.

Hemorrhage Severe loss of blood.

Hypoperfusion State of inadequate supply of oxygen and nutrients to the tissues, most commonly caused by decreased blood flow. If widespread hypoperfusion exists, the patient is in shock.

Hypotension Abnormally low blood pressure; may be a sign of shock.

Key Terms (cont'd)

Metabolism Chemical reactions that take place within an organism to maintain life; the work of cells.

Penetrating trauma Injury that is evident immediately to the human eye; usually involves a sharp object or high-velocity weapon.

Perfusion State of adequate supply of oxygen and nutrients to the tissues; ability of the circulatory system to distribute blood containing nutrients and oxygen to the tissues.

Periphery Outside part; the legs, arms, abdomen, and brain of the human body.

Pneumatic antishock garment (PASG) Device used to externally vasoconstrict blood vessels for the purpose of moving blood from the periphery to the core of the body.

Pulmonary arteries Vessels that carry oxygen-poor blood from the right side of the heart to the lungs; the only arteries in the body that carry oxygen-poor blood.

Pulmonary veins Vessels that carry oxygen-rich blood from the lungs back to the left side of the heart; the only veins in the body that carry oxygen-rich blood.

Pulse Wave of blood produced by the contraction of the left ventricle; can be felt wherever an artery passes over a bone close to the skin surface.

Pulse point pressure A method of bleeding control in which pressure is applied to the strongest pulse point above an injury.

Radial artery Artery located on the thumb side of the wrist of each arm; extends from the wrist to the elbow.

Radial pulse Pulse palpated at the radial artery of the arm at the wrist, on the outer aspect of the inner arm.

Semilunar valve Two moon-shaped, pocket-like valves; one is located between the right ventricle and the pulmonary artery, and the other is located between the left ventricle and the aorta.

Shock Failure of the circulatory system to perfuse tissues; hypoperfusion of the circulatory system.

Sphygmomanometer Pressure cuff device used on a peripheral extremity to determine the pressure of the heart on relaxation and contraction; blood pressure cuff.

Systolic pressure Pressure in the heart when the heart muscle is contracting; upper reading of a blood pressure.

Thready Weak, thin, rapid pulse or heart rate.

Trendelenburg position Position of stretcher or cot in which the foot of the bed is raised and the head of the bed is lowered; sometimes used to treat shock.

Tricuspid valve Three-flap valve that covers the opening between the right atrium and the right ventricle.

Vasoconstriction Contraction of blood vessels.

Vasodilation Expansion of blood vessels.

Veins Vessels that carry blood back to the heart.

Ventricles Lower chambers of the heart that pump blood; the right ventricle supplies blood to the lungs, and the left supplies the body.

Venules Smallest veins in the body; carry blood from the capillaries to the veins.

Volume Amount of fluid; may be measured in metric or apothecary units.

Review Questions

1. The blood vessel that normally carries oxygenated blood from the lung to the left side of the heart is called the pulmonary _____.
2. The cardinal sign of shock is:
   a. Hypertension
   b. Hypoperfusion
   c. Hypotension
   d. Perfusion
3. Metabolism that occurs in the presence of oxygen is best described by the term:
   a. Acidic
   b. Aerobic
   c. Anaerobic
   d. Apneic
4. Cardiogenic shock is a best described as _____ failure.
   a. Container
   b. Fluid
   c. Pump
   d. Volume
5. _____ is considered severe blood loss in an adult.
   a. 150 ml
   b. 500 ml
   c. 1000 ml
   d. 1500 ml

Review Questions (cont'd)

6. True or False: The mechanism of injury is critical for the EMT to develop a general impression of the patient and his or her condition.
7. The normal rate for capillary refill is:
   a. <1 second
   b. <2 seconds
   c. >2 seconds
   d. >3 seconds

Answers to these Review Questions can be found at the end of the book on page 866.

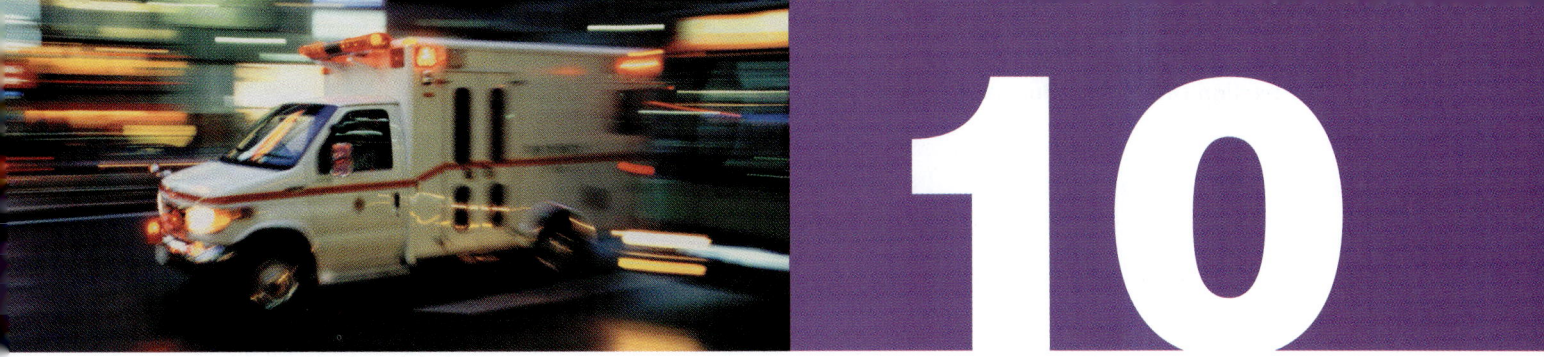

10

Airway Management and Ventilation

Lesson Goal

The first step of the Ficke Principle to prevent anaerobic metabolism is movement of oxygen into the red blood cells (RBCs). Oxygen cannot get to the RBCs if it does not get into the lungs first. There are several ways of opening the airway. Each method has risks and benefits. Each method works well in some situations and not in others. The principle is opening the airway; the preference is how the EMT can do it the best in the particular situation. This chapter presents methods and knowledge so that the EMT can use his or her own judgment to choose the best method for a particular situation.

Scenario

Dispatch sends you to a "man down, not breathing" call. Your response time is 2 minutes. On arrival you note that it is a clear, warm day and there is no evidence of a chemical spill on the scene. A small crowd is gathered. You find a 16-year-old male patient who fell and hit his head on a curb stone. On arrival the patients head is still on the curb and his body is in the street. You note that his head is flexed at about 75 degrees. The patient is blue and seems to be breathing.

Bystanders tell you that he fell while getting out of the way of a speeding vehicle. He was not hit by the car, but he hit his head on the curb. He has not moved since he fell. You determine from his friends that he was in good health before the incident.

 What interventions will you perform when you first arrive? How would you manage this patient's breathing? Do you have other concerns? What do you think the patient's major problem is? Would you call for EMT-Paramedic backup if it was available in your community or is this something that you can handle on your own?

Key Terms to Know

Accessory muscles
Agonal ventilations
Airway adjuncts
Alveolar/capillary exchange
Alveoli
Apnea
Aspiration
Carina
Cellular/capillary exchange
Crackles
Cricoid cartilage
Cyanotic

177

Key Terms to Know (cont'd)

- Dead space
- Diaphoretic
- Diaphragm
- Dyspnea
- Epiglottitis
- Head-tilt chin-lift
- Hemopneumothorax
- Hemothorax
- Hyperventilation
- Hypoventilation
- Intercostal muscles
- Jaw thrust
- Larynx
- Mainstem bronchi
- Minute ventilation
- Nasal prongs
- Nasal flaring
- Nasopharyngeal (nasal) airway
- Nonrebreather mask
- Oropharyngeal (oral) airway
- Pharynx
- Pleura
- Pleural space
- Pneumothorax
- Pulmonary arteries
- Pulmonary veins
- Quality
- Rales
- Rate
- Retractions
- Rhythm
- Sellick maneuver
- Stoma
- Thoracic cavity
- Thyroid cartilage
- Tidal volume
- Trachea
- Tracheostomy
- Wheezing

Learning Objectives

As an EMT-Basic, you should be able to do the following:

DOT

- Identify major respiratory structures, and relate these structures to the function of the respiratory system.
- Identify indications for and demonstrate the proper use of common airway equipment, including the pocket mask, bag-valve-mask device, nasopharyngeal and oropharyngeal airway, and flow-restricted oxygen-powered ventilator.
- Describe and demonstrate techniques for opening and protecting the airway, including the head-tilt chin-lift, jaw thrust, and Sellick maneuvers.
- Describe the importance of suctioning equipment, and demonstrate proper suctioning technique.
- List the signs of adequate breathing.
- List the signs of inadequate breathing.
- Relate mechanisms of injury to opening of the airway.
- Describe the steps in performing the skill of ventilating a patient with a bag-valve-mask while using the jaw thrust.
- List the parts of a bag-valve-mask system.
- Describe the steps in performing the skill of ventilating a patient with a bag-valve-mask for one and two rescuers.
- Describe the signs of adequate assisted ventilation using the bag-valve-mask.
- Describe the signs of inadequate assisted ventilation using the bag-valve-mask.
- Define and describe the steps in providing mouth-to-mouth assisted ventilation with body substance isolation (barrier shields).
- Define and describe the assembly of a bag-valve-mask unit.
- Define and describe the steps in performing the skill of ventilating a patient with a bag-valve-mask for one and two rescuers.
- Define and describe the steps in performing the skill of ventilating a patient with a bag-valve-mask while using the jaw thrust.
- Define and describe assisted ventilation of a patient with a flow-restricted, oxygen-powered ventilation device.
- Define and describe how to ventilate a patient using a stoma.
- Define and describe how to insert an oropharyngeal (oral) airway.
- Define and describe how to insert a nasopharyngeal (nasal) airway.
- Define and describe the correct operation of oxygen tanks and regulators.
- Define and describe the proper use of a nonrebreather face mask and state the oxygen flow requirements for its use.
- Define and describe the proper use of a nasal cannula and state the oxygen flow requirements for its use.
- Demonstrate how to ventilate the infant and child patient.
- Demonstrate oxygen administration for the infant and child patient.

Supplemental

- Explain why assisted ventilation and airway management skills take priority over most other basic life support skills.
- Assess whether a patient is breathing adequately, and appropriately manage a patient who needs ventilatory assistance.
- Explain the rationale for giving a high-inspired oxygen concentration to patients who need it, even if there is a possibility of depression of ventilatory drive.

Airway management and ventilation are the most important components of patient care that an emergency medical technician (EMT) must master. As noted in Chapter 9, for the patient to survive, oxygen must be added to the red blood cells (RBCs) through the lungs and delivered to the tissue cells for aerobic metabolism to produce the energy required to carry on the body functions. Aerobic metabolism cannot occur without oxygen. Airway management is the first step in this process, and ventilation management is the second; without these the patient will die within minutes. The ability to properly and efficiently manage airway and ventilation are the most important skills for any medical care professional who deals with patients. The EMT must learn these skills properly and practice frequently enough so that he or she can carry out the process instantly with out thinking.

> **Editor's Note**
>
> An emergency medical technician (EMT) can be at one of three levels: EMT-Basic (EMT-B), EMT-Intermediate (EMT-I), or EMT-Paramedic (EMT-P). The term EMT is used in this text to mean any person working as an emergency medical technician at any of the three levels.

Patient Care Algorithm

Airway and Breathing Assessment

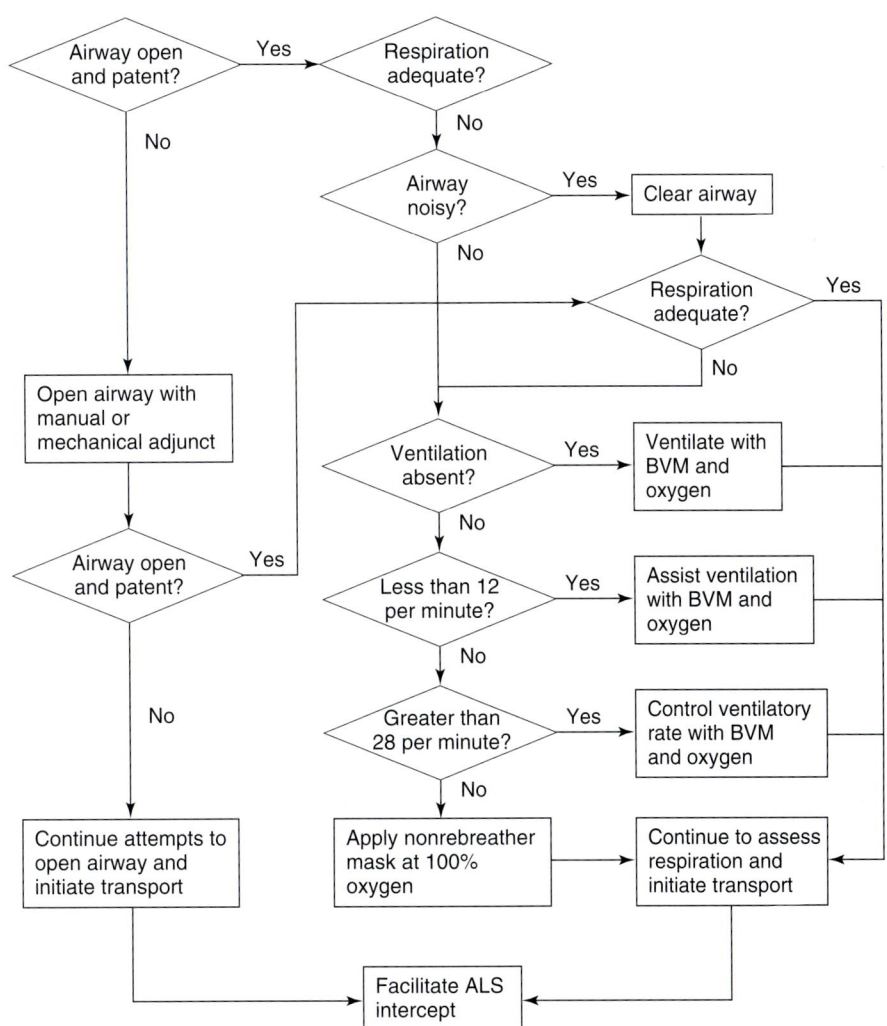

Proper assessment of airway compromise and rapid interventions have a dramatic influence on patient outcome. An EMT must be able to recognize a patient who needs help with airway control and/or ventilation. Airway and ventilation assessment take place on every call. Many times the experienced EMT evaluates the airway subconsciously. Often, the EMT must provide supplemental oxygen or perform airway interventions. Examples include an unconscious trauma patient who needs an artificial airway, an asthma patient who needs oxygen, or a patient in cardiac arrest who needs assisted ventilation.

Airway management techniques change rapidly. The EMT who is constantly thinking about his or her patients will keep up on these changes. For example, the esophageal obturator airway is used infrequently because newer alternatives have become available. However, there are certain situations in which nothing else will work and the EMT must be confident that he or she can use it effectively. Endotracheal intubation is the procedure of choice in patients who need airway protection and/or assisted control of ventilation. Performance of this skill requires special training, more initial practice, frequent use, and retraining to maintain efficiency. Endotracheal intubation is now an optional skill used by many EMT-Bs and is discussed in Chapter 11.

This chapter begins with an overview of the anatomy, physiology, and pathophysiology of the respiratory system. Airway and ventilatory assessment is discussed, with an emphasis on common problems that the EMT must manage in the field. The equipment and skills needed for airway management and assisted ventilation are described.

Anatomy and Physiology

Because this complicated process of respiration is more that just the moving of air into and out of the lungs, the movement of air in and out will be called *ventilatory rate* and not *respiratory rate*. Although the term *respiratory rate* is commonly used, this text uses *ventilatory rate* so that the EMT will understand the correct physiology.

The respiratory system serves three main functions:

1. *Supplies oxygen to the blood, which then carries the oxygen to the body tissues and off-loads the oxygen into the cells.* During normal metabolism,

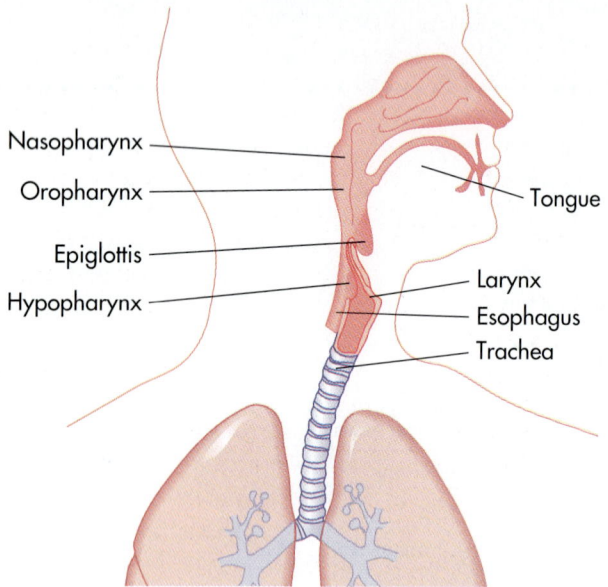

FIGURE 10.1 Lateral view of the pharynx.

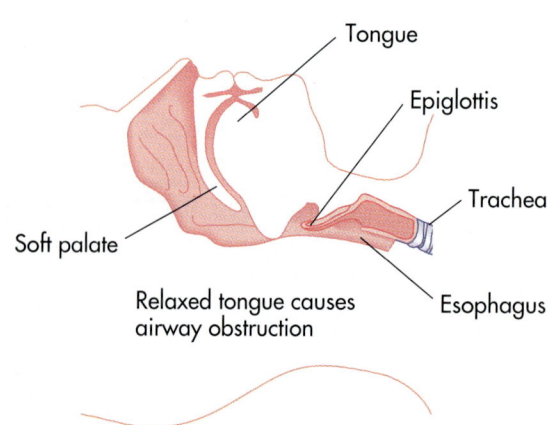

FIGURE 10.2 Airway obstruction by the tongue in an unresponsive, supine patient.

the body cells use oxygen to generate energy (aerobic and anaerobic metabolism; see Chapter 9). This process produces waste products, one of which is acid (H^+) that is converted by the body's buffer system to carbon dioxide and water (see Chapter 9).
2. *Serves to exhale the carbon dioxide brought back to the lungs by the blood.* The supply of oxygen and removal of carbon dioxide are critical processes that normally take place automatically. Any disruption of the respiratory system can lead rapidly to a decrease in oxygen and increase in carbon dioxide in the tissues, which may lead to death if the disruption is not corrected.
3. *Metabolizes oxygen in the Krebs cycle for energy production* (see Chapter 9). Energy is a force that drives all the cells in the body. Unless the respiratory system produces this energy, the body dies.

Anatomy

The ventilatory system consists of the upper airway, lower airway, and lungs. The respiratory system includes the ventilatory system and the metabolism that occurs within each cell of the body. Each of these structures of the ventilatory system plays an important role in supplying oxygen to and removing carbon dioxide from body tissues. Ventilation is a mechanical process; respiration is a physiologic process.

Upper Airway

The EMT must be familiar with the structures of the upper airway because he or she directly controls and maintains the patient's upper airway. During normal breathing, air enters the nose, where it is warmed and humidified by the nasal passages. Air then enters the **pharynx**, which is a hollow cavity that separates the mouth and nose from the larynx and esophagus. The part of the pharynx behind (posterior to) the nose is the nasopharynx, and the part posterior to the mouth is the oropharynx. The lowest (most inferior) part of the pharynx is the hypopharynx (Figure 10.1). In conscious patients the pharynx is a hollow space. In an unconscious, supine patient the tongue often collapses into the hypopharynx, causing obstruction (Figure 10.2). The most common cause of an obstructed airway in an unconscious patient is the tongue.

The **epiglottis** is a leaf-shaped structure located just above the larynx that prevents food and liquids from entering the **trachea** (windpipe) during swallowing. The **larynx** is a structure made of cartilage, muscle, and soft tissue. It contains the vocal cords and is commonly referred to as the *voice box*. The **thyroid cartilage** ("Adam's apple") and **cricoid cartilage** are important structural components of the larynx (Figure 10.3). The vocal cords are suspended between cartilage and are controlled by several small muscles. The fine movements of the vocal cords are important for speaking and protecting the airway from liquids or solids. **Aspiration** describes the accidental inhalation of liquids or solids into the lower airway.

> ✓ The upper airway extends from the mouth and nose to the larynx. In unconscious supine patients, the tongue commonly causes partial or complete upper airway obstruction.

Lower Airway

The firm ring of the cricoid cartilage is the inferior (lower) boundary of the upper airway and the beginning of the lower airway. The trachea, or windpipe, is a tube that is supported by C-shaped rings of cartilage in the front and on the sides. The cricoid cartilage is the only complete ring of cartilage around the airway. The esophagus lies posterior to the trachea. At the level of the sternal angle, the trachea divides into left and right **mainstem bronchi**. This division is called the **carina** (Figure 10.4). Note the angle formed at the carina by the two mainstem bronchi. The right mainstem bronchus is more directly in line with the trachea. Because of this relationship, foreign bodies aspirated into the trachea are more likely to enter the right mainstem bronchus than the left. For the same reason, an endotracheal tube inserted too far is more likely to enter the right than the left mainstem bronchus.

The bronchi divide into smaller airways until they connect with the **alveoli**, which are small air sacs with

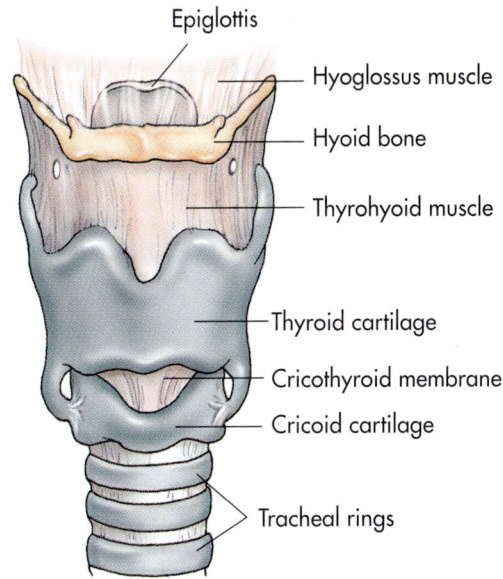

FIGURE 10.3 Anterior view of the larynx.

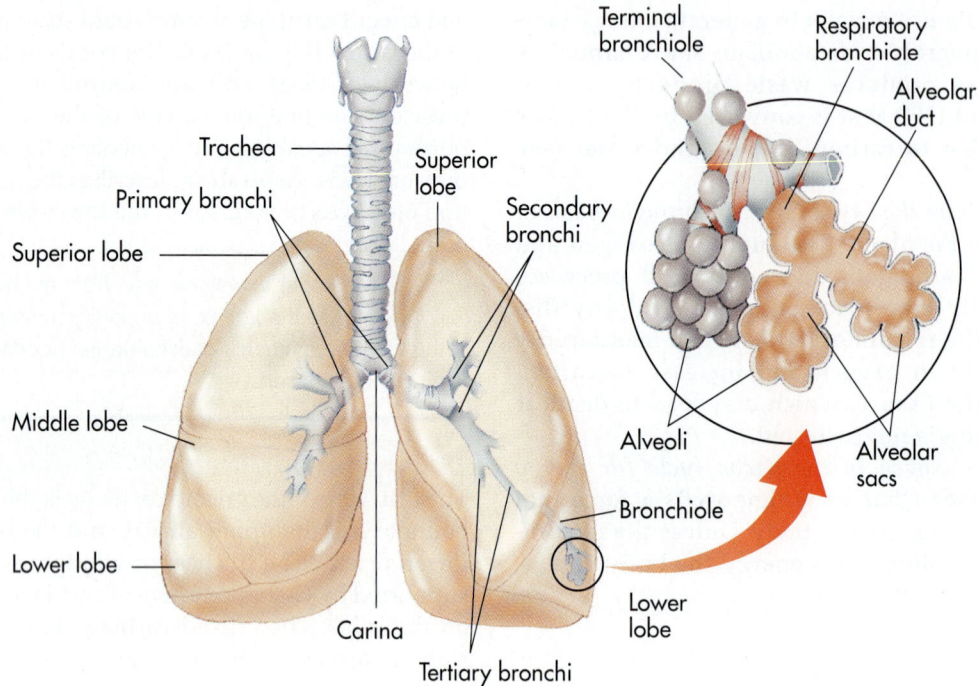

FIGURE 10.4 Anterior view of the trachea, mainstem bronchi, and alveolar sacs.

very thin walls surrounded by capillaries. When air reaches the alveoli, oxygen is transferred into the capillaries where it binds to a protein called *hemoglobin* in the RBCs. Carbon dioxide collected by RBCs is transferred from the plasma (the liquid part of blood apart from the RBCs and white blood cells [WBCs]) to the alveoli. This exchange of oxygen for carbon dioxide takes place in millions of alveoli throughout the lungs with each breath and is called the **alveolar/capillary exchange**. After this exchange, carbon dioxide is exhaled and oxygen is transported to the tissues by the RBCs.

> ✓ The lower airway begins at the cricoid cartilage and extends to the lungs, where the alveolar/capillary exchange occurs.

Lungs

The lungs lie in the **thoracic cavity**, a protective bony structure formed by the ribs, sternum, and spinal column. Each lung is divided into lobes. The right lung has three lobes, and the left lung has two lobes. Note the position of the lungs in relationship to the heart and airway structures (Figure 10.5). The thoracic cavity is a sealed space lined by a thin membrane called the **pleura**. Each lung is also covered by a pleural membrane. These pleural membranes slide smoothly against each other during respiration. The space between them, called the **pleural space**, is normally filled with a small amount of fluid.

Sometimes air or blood enters the pleural space, causing it to enlarge. Because the lungs are soft structures, an enlargement of the pleural space may collapse all or part of a lung. Lung collapse can cause respiratory distress and even death if not recognized. Air in the pleural space is called a **pneumothorax**, and blood in this space is called a **hemothorax**. If both blood and air are present, it is called a **hemopneumothorax** (Figure 10.6). Most patients with a pneumothorax or hemothorax have sustained a traumatic injury to the thoracic cavity.

Infant and Child Anatomy

Infants and children are more susceptible to airway obstruction because they have smaller airway structures and a proportionally larger tongue. The smaller size of the mouth, nose, and trachea makes it easier for a foreign body to cause obstruction and for swelling to obstruct the airway. Infants and children with an upper respiratory infection such as croup or epiglottitis (discussed later) develop airway compromise much more quickly than adults. Also, because infants and children use energy at a relatively higher rate, they have less reserve and are less able to compensate when they experience difficulty

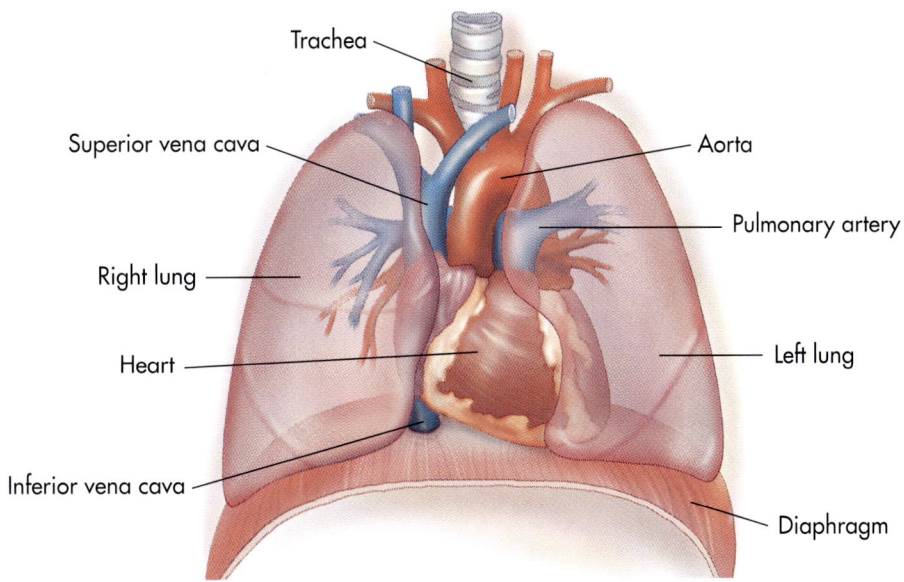

FIGURE 10.5 Thoracic cavity.

breathing. In addition to being smaller, the trachea and cricoid cartilage are softer structures than in adults, again making them more susceptible to obstruction. Because of the smaller size of the chest wall, infants and children depend more heavily on the diaphragm for breathing.

> ✓ Smaller airways and a proportionally larger tongue make infants and children more susceptible to airway obstruction by foreign bodies and swelling.

Physiology

The **diaphragm** is a thin, dome-shaped muscle that separates the thoracic cavity from the abdominal cavity. When the diaphragm contracts, it moves downward, the thoracic cavity enlarges, and air enters the lungs. The **intercostal muscles** also enlarge the thoracic cavity during inspiration by moving the ribs upward and outward (Figure 10.7). In contrast to inhalation, which is an active process using muscles, exhalation is passive. The diaphragm and intercostal muscles relax, causing the thoracic cavity to become smaller and forcing air out of the lungs.

The venous system returns oxygen-poor blood back to the right side of the heart. The heart pumps this blood to the lungs through the **pulmonary arteries** (see

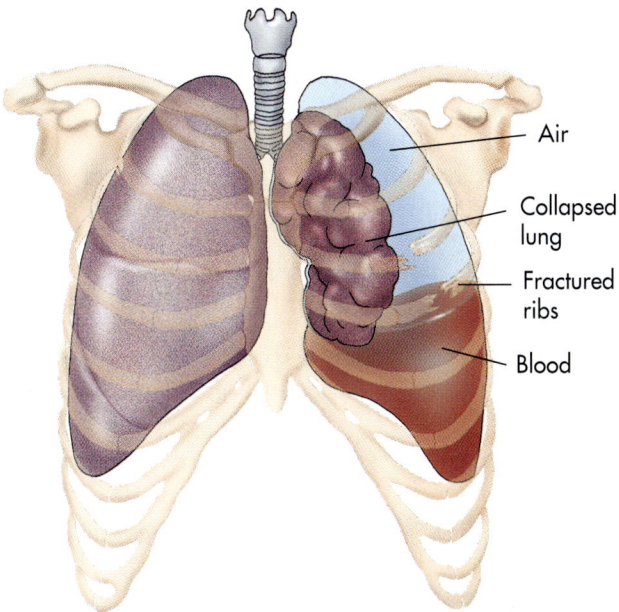

FIGURE 10.6 Hemopneumothorax.

Figure 10.5), which are the only arteries in the body that carry oxygen-poor blood. The pulmonary arteries divide, forming pulmonary capillaries. During the alveolar/capillary exchange, oxygen enters the capillaries and carbon dioxide enters the alveoli. The pulmonary capillaries join together, eventually forming four large **pulmonary veins**, which enter the left atrium of the heart. The heart

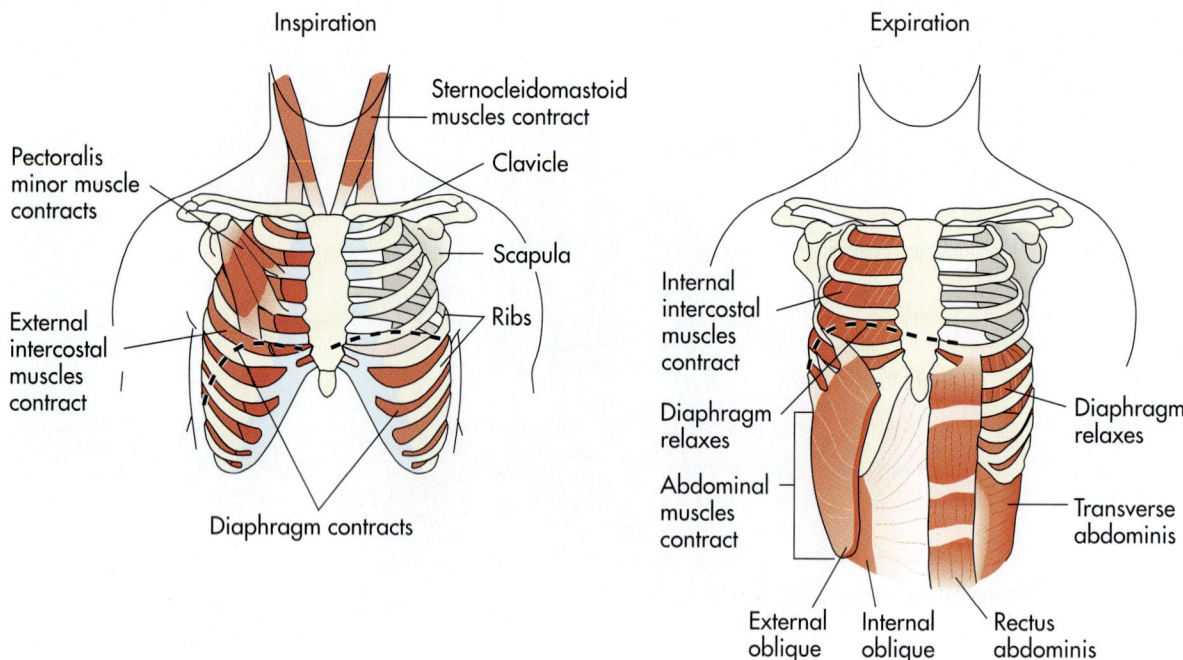

FIGURE 10.7 Muscles of inspiration. During inspiration, the diaphragm moves downward, intercostal muscles lift the ribs upward and outward, and accessory muscles lift the sternum and upper ribs.

then pumps the blood to the body tissues through the arteries. Note that the pulmonary veins are the only veins in the body that carry oxygen-rich blood.

A similar exchange of oxygen and carbon dioxide takes place in the tissues. The **cellular/capillary exchange** provides oxygen to cells and removes carbon dioxide. Every living cell depends on this exchange.

> ✓ The alveolar/capillary and cellular/capillary exchanges provide a constant supply of oxygen to the tissues.

Assessment

Assessment of Breathing

During the initial assessment of the patient, the EMT assesses the adequacy of breathing and determines the need for intervention. The **rate**, **rhythm**, **quality**, and depth of ventilation are the primary factors on which to focus when assessing breathing. The normal ventilatory rate depends on the patient's age. A ventilatory rate of 34 breaths per minute is normal for an infant and above normal for an adult. The normal ventilatory rate is 12 to 20 breaths per minute for adults, 15 to 30 for children (1 to 8 years of age), and 25 to 50 for infants.

The rhythm of ventilations may be regular or irregular. An irregular breathing rhythm may be a sign of damage to respiratory control centers in the brain, as is seen in some head injuries.

The quality of breathing depends on factors such as breath sounds, chest expansion, and ventilatory effort. The EMT student should listen to breath sounds of classmates to become familiar with normal breath sounds. Abnormal breath sounds include wheezing, crackles, and rales. **Wheezing** is a high-pitched noise that is caused by air traveling through constricted bronchi. Wheezing most commonly occurs in asthma patients. **Crackles** are lower-pitched noises that are caused by a collection of fluid in the smaller airways. They are often heard in patients who have an infection of the lungs, or pneumonia. Crackles are further described as being either fine (a softer sound caused by a small amount of fluid) or coarse (a harsh gurgling sound heard with larger amounts of fluid). Coarse crackles are a more serious sign of respiratory compromise. **Rales** (pronounced 'rauls,' not 'rails') are heard when areas of collapsed alveoli expand with inhalation or when fluid collects in the smaller airways. Rales can be simulated by rubbing hair between the thumb and fingers next to your ears. The terms *rales* and *fine crackles* are sometimes used interchangeably.

Sometimes breath sounds cannot be heard in a part of the lung. Lack of breath sounds means air is not moving through that part of the lung. Absent breath sounds often are a sign of lung collapse, as is seen with a pneumothorax or hemothorax. Other causes of absent breath sounds are pneumonia and severe asthma. The absence of breath sounds on one side of the chest in a patient who is acutely short of breath is a very serious sign because it can indicate impending respiratory failure.

Other signs that the EMT should look for when assessing the quality of breathing include chest expansion and ventilatory effort. In normal breathing, the chest cavity expands smoothly and evenly as air enters the lungs. Chest expansion should be the same on both sides. If one side of the chest does not expand on inspiration, a collapsed lung or painful rib fractures may be present, preventing the patient from expanding that side of the chest. The amount of effort required for breathing is another important sign of pulmonary difficulty. Normal breathing requires little effort. A patient in respiratory distress often uses extra muscles to assist in breathing, known as **accessory muscles**. These muscles are located in the neck and in the back. During inspiration they contract to help lift the ribs upward and outward in an attempt to increase the volume of each breath. Noisy breathing is another abnormal sign of respiratory distress.

The color cyanotic (blue) and the temperature of the skin (cool) are frequent indicators of decreased perfusion of the skin in the area being evaluated. This if frequently due to decreased oxygenation.

The depth of breathing depends on the **tidal volume**, which is the volume of air inhaled with each breath. Tidal volume is normally about 500 ml per breath in an adult. Some of the air inhaled with each breath anatomically must stay in the upper and lower airways. It does not get to the alveoli for gas exchange. The space in which this air is contained is called **dead space** and normally contains approximately 150 ml of air (Figure 10.8).

The tidal volume multiplied by the ventilatory rate for 1 minute is called the **minute ventilation**. For example, if the tidal volume of each breath is 500 ml and the ventilatory rate is 12 breaths per minute, then the minute ventilation (500 × 12) is 6000 ml/min, which converts to 6 L/min.

Minute ventilation is important because it includes both the tidal volume and the ventilatory rate. For example, a patient with a ventilatory rate of 40 breaths per minute may have a low minute ventilation if the depth of ventilation is very shallow (i.e., the tidal volume is low). The EMT must assess the depth of breathing in addition to the rate. Patients with shallow breathing may not have adequate tidal volumes to maintain minute ventilation. In shallow volume ventilation, much of the air movement just moves the dead space up and down and does not bring in much new well-oxygenated air into the lungs. A decline in either the ventilatory rate or the tidal volume can decrease minute ventilation. A decrease in minute ventilation is called **hypoventilation**. Hypoventilation

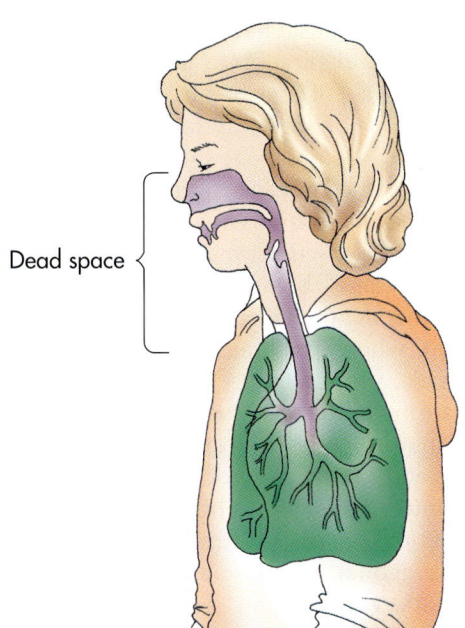

FIGURE 10.8 Diagram demonstrating dead air space. Dead air space never reaches the alveoli for gas exchange.

can impair carbon dioxide elimination and oxygenation, leading quickly to lack of oxygenated RBCs and thus decreased oxygen delivery to the tissue cells, resulting in decreased energy production (shock).

> ✓ The rate, rhythm, quality, and depth of ventilations are signs used to assess the adequacy of breathing. Minute ventilation is calculated by multiplying the tidal volume by the ventilatory rate.

Signs and Symptoms of Inadequate Breathing

The most obvious symptom of inadequate breathing is shortness of breath. The symptom of shortness of breath is called **dyspnea**. Patients with dyspnea usually sit upright and breathe through the mouth instead of the nose. They may support their elbows on the arms of the chair to allow more lift during assessory muscle contraction. They will often speak in short sentences with one or two words between breaths. The ventilatory rate of patients who are not breathing adequately is usually faster than normal; however, patients with a depressed level of consciousness (LOC) may breathe slowly and irregularly. Slow, irregular breathing can often be observed in patients with severe head injury or drug overdose.

In addition to ventilatory rate, the EMT must assess the quality and depth of the ventilations. **Nasal flaring** may be seen in patients with dyspnea, especially in infants and children. Nasal flaring is simply a widening of the nostrils with inspiration, a process intended to increase the volume of the breath. Another sign of increased respiratory effort is retractions. **Retractions** are indentations of the skin above the clavicles, between the ribs, and below the rib cage during inspiration. Retractions are especially common signs in infants and children. In infants, retractions may become severe enough to produce "seesaw" breathing, in which the abdomen and chest move in opposite directions with each breath.

A patient who is not breathing adequately will often have cool, pale, and sometimes **diaphoretic** (sweaty) skin. If inadequate breathing continues, the patient may become **cyanotic** (blue). The first areas to become cyanotic are usually the lips and fingers. Any patient with cyanosis needs aggressive intervention with a high percentage of inspired oxygen (FiO_2). The most extreme form of inadequate breathing is **agonal ventilations**, which are occasional gasping breaths occurring just before death, usually with little or no air movement. A complete lack of ventilatory effort is called **apnea**. Patients with agonal breathing or apnea require airway management and assisted ventilation.

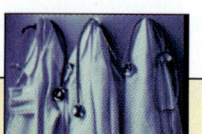

Physician Notes

Although somewhat expensive and not available on many ambulances, the pulse oximeter is an excellent device to determine the oxygenation of the tissue of the fingers and toes. It is an indicator of the amount of oxygen saturation in the blood, not an indication of the oxygenation content, and should not be confused with the measurement of the Pao_2 as determined by the blood gas measurement. The use of the pulse oximeter will assist the EMT in evaluating the patient's oxygenation status.

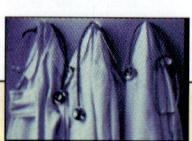

Physician Notes

One of the most important questions that the EMT can ask is "Why?"
1. Why is the patient cyanotic (blue)? Because unoxygenated blood looks blue through the skin. This requires approximately 5 grams of unoxygenated hemoglobin in the arterial system. Unoxygenated hemoglobin means lack of adequate oxygen delivery to the tissue cells, therefore decreased energy production (shock)
2. Why is the patient cool? Lack of energy production leads to reduced body heat, and reduced circulation to the periphiphery leads to decreased oxygen delivery, which leads to decreased oxygen to the cells and more decreased production and more severe shock.

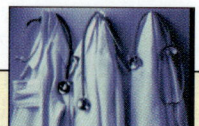

Physician Notes

The amount of oxygen delivered to the patient for inspiration is important. The delivery of oxygen depends on two factors: (1) the delivery device and (2) the rate of flow of the oxygen to the delivery device.

The inspired gas or air that the patient takes in with each breath is known as the percentage of inspired air or the fraction of the air that is oxygen. The medical abbreviation for this percentage is FiO_2. Each type of delivery device provides a different FiO_2.

The EMT must not connect an oxygenation delivery device to a patient without knowing how much oxygen that the specific type of device should deliver. The following table provides the maximum percentage of oxygen that each device should deliver assuming optimum oxygen flow rate:

Device	FiO_2	Percentage
Nasal prongs	0.24	24
Nasal cannula	0.30	30
Ventura mask	0.35-0.45	35-45
Nonrebreathing mask	0.85	85
Bag-mask		
Without supplemental oxygen	0.21	21
With supplemental oxygen	0.40	40
With accumulator	0.95	95
Anesthesia gas machine	1	100

✓ Patients with inadequate breathing will usually complain of shortness of breath. Ventilatory effort may be increased, and the skin may be cool, diaphoretic, and/or cyanotic.

Management

Airway Management

Opening the Airway

Assessing the patient's airway is the first step in the initial assessment. The EMT must intervene immediately if a patient does not have an open airway. In an unconscious patient the most common cause of airway obstruction is the tongue. The **head-tilt chin-lift** maneuver is the easiest technique for opening an airway in patients without a suspected spinal injury (Figure 10.9, A). An unconscious patient should be placed in a supine position if possible. The EMT should place one hand on the patient's forehead and the other under the chin. The EMT should position the hand under the chin carefully so that it does not compress the larynx and cause partial

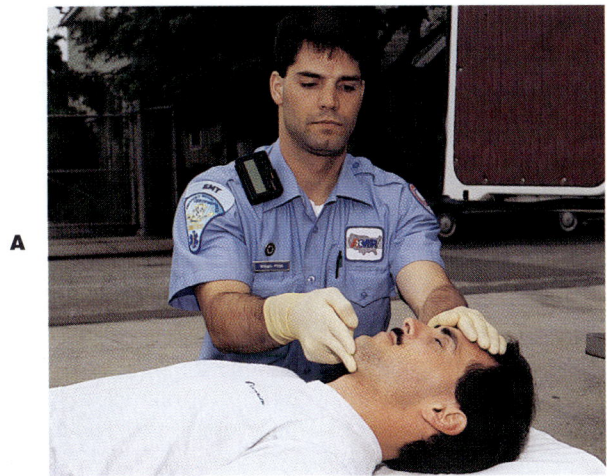
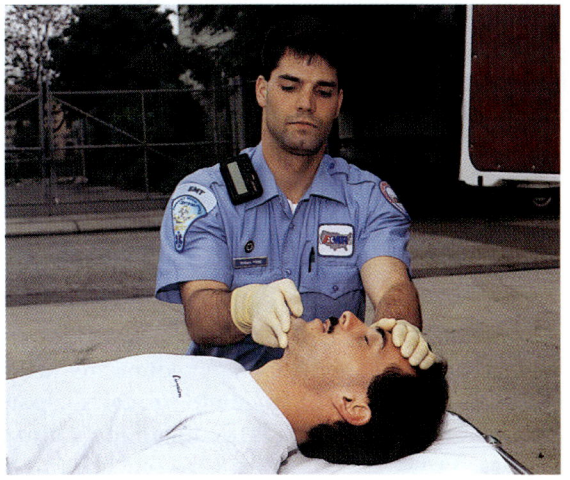

FIGURE 10.9 Head-tilt chin-lift maneuver. **A,** Place the patient in a supine position and kneel at the patient's side with one hand on the patient's forehead and one hand below the patient's chin. **B,** Gently lift the chin and tilt the head back. This maneuver pulls the tongue forward and opens the airway.

airway obstruction. Gentle extension of the neck, combined with upward pulling of the chin, lifts the tongue out of the pharynx (Figure 10.9, B). When the EMT suspects a cervical spine injury, he or she must hold the patient's neck in a neutral in-line position and use the **jaw thrust** maneuver to open the airway (see Jaw Thrust Skill Sheet at the end of this chapter). While maintaining cervical stabilization, the EMT thrusts the jaw forward using upward pressure on the angles of the jaw (mandible). The tongue is firmly attached to the mandible; therefore forward movement of the jaw lifts the tongue out of the pharynx.

The EMT must be comfortable with both the jaw thrust and the head-tilt chin-lift maneuvers. If these maneuvers do not open the airway, the EMT should proceed with standard basic life support (BLS) procedures for managing an obstructed airway. The EMT should reposition the head and attempt to open the airway. If ventilation is still unsuccessful, the EMT should perform up to five abdominal thrusts, along with attempts to ventilate and finger sweeps of the mouth (in adults). In addition to aggressively attempting to open the airway, the EMT must prepare the patient for immediate transportation to a medical facility. He or she should perform three cycles of abdominal thrusts and finger sweeps, then transport the patient, continuing attempts to clear the airway during transportation. In the presence of a cervical spine injury, the EMT should carry out these procedures with spine protection considerations.

Unresponsive patients with dentures or partial dental plates are at risk for airway obstruction. Usually dental appliances can be left in place without obstructing the airway. They may actually assist in mask seal maintenance during assisted ventilation. The EMT should remove them only if they are causing airway compromise.

> ✓ The head-tilt chin-lift and jaw thrust maneuvers are important techniques for opening the airway.

Suctioning

Suctioning is used to clear an airway obstructed by oral secretions, blood, other liquids, or food particles. A patient requires suctioning whenever other attempts to clear the airway fail, when a gurgling sound is heard during breathing, or when fluid is seen in the airway of an unresponsive patient. The EMT should always use body substance isolation (BSI) techniques while suctioning because contact with respiratory secretions is likely (see Suctioning Skill Sheet at the end of this chapter).

Several types of suction devices are available to the EMT. All ambulances have a mounted suction device that uses an electric pump. In addition, portable suction must be available with either battery-powered or hand-operated units. Suction devices are used with two main types of suction catheters. Rigid catheters are used to suction the mouth and oropharynx of infants, children, and unresponsive adults. Soft catheters are used to suction the nose, nasopharynx, and other areas that cannot be suctioned with a rigid catheter. Soft catheters should be measured so that they are not inserted beyond the base of the tongue. A useful guide is to measure from the tip of the nose to the tip of the ear. In intubated patients, soft catheters are used to suction the endotracheal tube.

The EMT should insert the appropriate catheter to the base of the tongue. Suction is applied while withdrawing the catheter in a side-to-side motion for a maximum of 15 seconds. Because of their small respiratory reserve, infants and children should be suctioned for shorter periods of time. If emesis or secretions cannot be cleared in 15 seconds, the EMT should log roll the patient and clear the oropharynx manually. Although it is important not to delay assisted ventilation for more than 15 seconds, it is also important not to force secretions or emesis into the lungs during assisted ventilation. Therefore the EMT must use the 15-second maximum suctioning time as a guide, only exceeding it in situations in which assisted ventilation would be ineffective without further suctioning. Patients with large amounts of frothy secretions (as in pulmonary edema) may require frequent suctioning. If this occurs, the EMT should suction the patient for a maximum of 15 seconds, ventilate for 2 minutes, suction for up to 15 seconds, and so on. The EMT should continue this pattern and contact medical direction during rapid transportation to a medical facility.

The EMT should inspect suctioning devices on a regular basis. A wall-mounted device should generate 300 mm Hg vacuum when working properly. The EMT should recharge battery-powered units regularly. During suctioning the EMT must observe the catheter and tubing for patency and flush them with water or replace them if they are obstructed.

> ✓ Portable suction units are devices used to clear the airway. Soft or rigid catheters are used for up to 15 seconds to remove secretions and/or blood.

Assisted Ventilation

Assisted ventilation is one of the most important skills that an EMT performs. Proper technique takes diligent practice. Inexperienced EMTs should rely on their more experienced colleagues to monitor and evaluate their assisted ventilation skills. The ability to effectively ventilate patients saves more lives than almost anything else an EMT does. This section begins by discussing airway adjuncts used in assisted ventilation, followed by a discussion of the devices and techniques used for assisted ventilation.

> **Editor's Note**
>
> The terms *artificial ventilation* and *assisted ventilation* have similar meanings. *Artificial ventilation* is an older term that has has been replaced in this text by *assisted ventilation*. *Assisted ventilation* identifies the skill required to "assist" the patient when his or her own ventilation is inadequate in either volume or rate. If the patient has no ventilation effort, *assisted* can mean to completely replace the absent ventilations.

The EMT should exercise BSI whenever ventilating a patient. Because of concerns about tuberculosis and other infectious organisms, the EMT should use mouth-to-mouth ventilation with caution. Although barrier devices have been produced that protect the rescuer during mouth-to-mouth ventilation, an EMT responding in an ambulance has more effective methods of assisted ventilation, which are discussed in the following sections.

Airway Adjuncts

Airway adjuncts are devices used for assisting upper airway control in patients who cannot control their own airways. Most unconscious patients and many patients with a decreased LOC require an airway adjunct. The primary function of adjuncts is to prevent obstruction of the upper

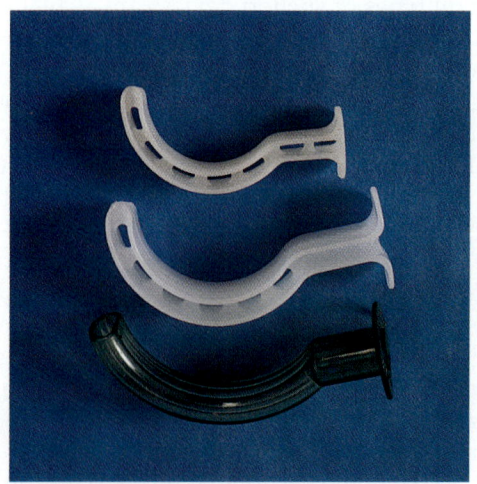

FIGURE 10.10 Oropharyngeal airways.

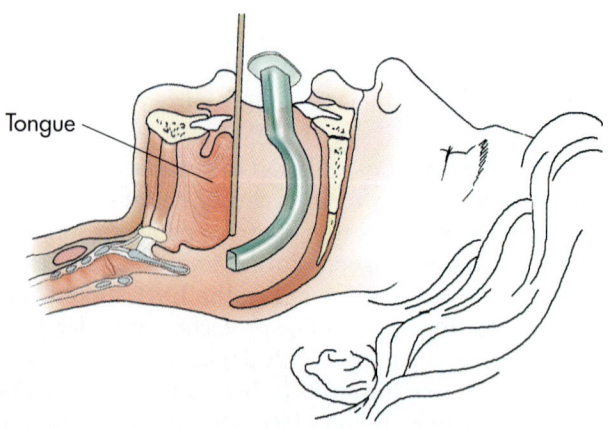

FIGURE 10.11 Insertion of the oropharyngeal airway using a tongue depressor.

airway by the tongue. The effectiveness of assisted ventilation is greatly improved by the use of airway adjuncts.

Oropharyngeal airway. The **oropharyngeal (oral) airway** (Figure 10.10) is used to assist in maintaining an open airway in unresponsive patients who do not have an intact gag reflex. If a patient is responsive or if an unresponsive patient begins to gag during insertion, the oropharyngeal airway should not be used (see Oropharyngeal Airway Insertion Skill Sheet at the end of this chapter). The proper size is selected by measuring from the corner of the mouth to the angle of the jaw. In adults, the airway is inserted upside down, then rotated 180 degrees so that the flange rests on the patient's teeth. This technique prevents the tongue from being pushed posteriorly during insertion, causing obstruction. Another method for inserting the oropharyngeal airway is to use a tongue depressor to push the tongue down and forward during insertion (Figure 10.11). This technique prevents airway obstruction and is the preferred technique for oropharyngeal airway insertion in infants and children.

Nasopharyngeal airway. The **nasopharyngeal (nasal) airway** (Figure 10.12) is a semirigid device that can be inserted into the nose of patients who cannot tolerate an oropharyngeal airway. Typically, patients who need a nasopharyngeal airway are responsive but not alert enough to adequately control their own airway. The nasopharyngeal airway is measured from the tip of the nose to the tip of the ear. Before insertion, the airway should be lubricated with a water-soluble lubricant. The airway is inserted into the nostril and advanced posteriorly, with the bevel toward either the base of the nose or the nasal septum (Figure 10.13). Often, one nasal passage is considerably larger than the other; therefore if the airway cannot be advanced in one nostril, an attempt should be made in the other nostril. If the airway cannot be advanced easily, it should not be forced, because this may cause bleeding, pain, and/or further airway obstruction (see Nasopharyngeal Airway Insertion Skill Sheet at the end of this chapter).

> ✓ Commonly used airway adjuncts include oropharyngeal and nasopharyngeal airways. The oropharyngeal airway should only be used in patients who do not have a gag reflex.

Assisted Ventilation Techniques

Techniques used by EMTs for assisted ventilation include the following:

1. Mouth-to-mask
2. Bag-valve-mask (one-person or two-person)
3. Flow-restricted oxygen-powered ventilator
4. Sellick maneuver

Mouth-to-mask ventilation. Mouth-to-mask ventilation is the most effective method of assisted ventilation for a single EMT. The EMT is positioned behind the supine patient's head. To maintain an effective seal, the EMT first applies the apex of the mask over the bridge of the nose and then lowers it over the face and mouth. The EMT applies pressure behind the mandible with the fingers and seals the mask against the face with the thumbs. When performed properly, the technique results in an effective mask seal and opens the airway with a jaw thrust maneuver. If the EMT suspects a cervical spine injury, he or she should maintain the neck and head in a neutral position and use an oropharyngeal or nasopharyngeal airway

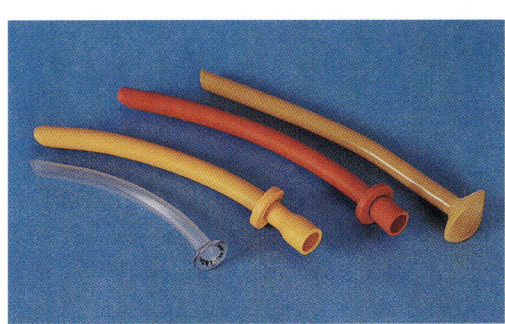

FIGURE 10.12 Nasopharyngeal airways.

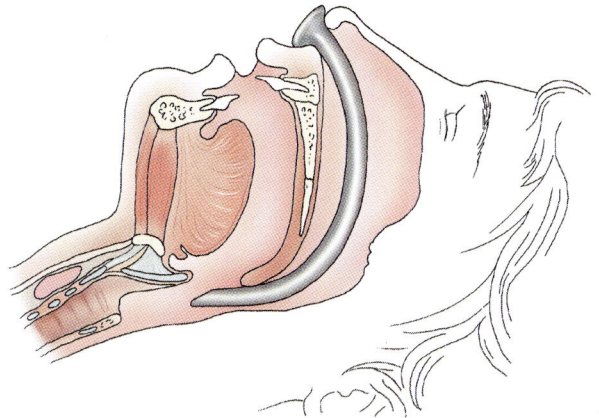

FIGURE 10.13 The nasopharyngeal airway in proper position.

(see Mouth-to-Mask Ventilation Skill Sheet at the end of this chapter).

The EMT performs ventilation by blowing through a one-way valve (Figure 10.14) using an even breath with moderate pressure. If the EMT uses excessive force, air will enter the esophagus and stomach, increasing the risk of regurgitation and aspiration. Without supplemental oxygen, the patient receives a 16% concentration of oxygen from the EMT's breath. This low concentration of inspired oxygen is the main disadvantage of mouth-to-mask ventilation. To increase the inspired oxygen concentration, the EMT can connect the mask to high-flow oxygen at 15 L/min.

Assessing ventilation. The EMT should monitor the effectiveness of assisted ventilation by watching for chest rise and listening for breath sounds. If the chest does not rise and fall with ventilation, the EMT should reposition the head. He or she should first return the head to a neutral position and then reopen the airway using the head-tilt chin-lift maneuver. If air leaks around the mask, the EMT must reposition his or her fingers and the mask to obtain an airtight seal. If breath sounds and chest rise are still not present after repositioning the head and adjusting the mask seal, the EMT must rule out an airway obstruction. The pharynx and mouth often need suctioning before effective assisted ventilation can occur. If the airway is patent (open) but the EMT still cannot confirm adequate ventilation, he or she should use a different assisted ventilation device, such as a bag-valve-mask or flow-restricted oxygen-powered ventilator. The EMT must continually assess the effectiveness of assisted ventilation, regardless of what technique is being used. If assisted ventilation appears ineffective, the EMT must perform the above interventions to improve effectiveness.

During assisted ventilation, the EMT gives breaths every 5 seconds for adults and every 3 seconds for infants and children. Patients requiring assisted ventilation are likely to have very low levels of oxygen in their blood, especially patients in cardiac arrest. Therefore the EMT may need to increase the rate of assisted ventilation, especially during the first several minutes. Increasing

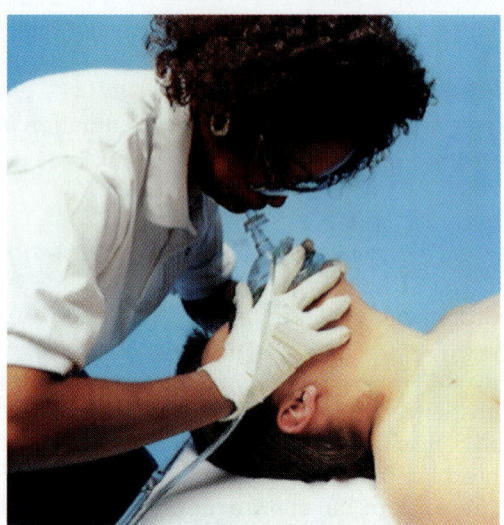

FIGURE 10.14 Mouth-to-mask ventilation. Kneel behind the supine patient's head. Open the airway using the jaw-thrust maneuver. Apply the apex of the mask over the patient's nose, then lower the mask over the face and mouth to obtain a tight seal. Deliver slow, steady breaths at an age-appropriate rate through a one-way valve. Supplemental oxygen can be connected to the mask to increase the inspired oxygen concentration.

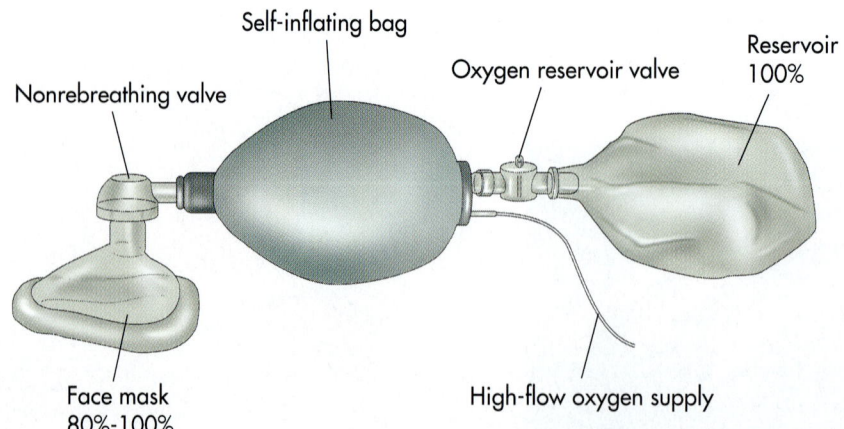

FIGURE 10.15 The bag-valve-mask consists of a face mask, one-way (nonrebreathing) valve, self-inflating bag, and oxygen reservoir.

minute ventilation above normal is called **hyperventilation**. Hyperventilation is especially important in the management of patients with head injuries.

> ✓ Mouth-to-mask ventilation is an effective method for one EMT to ventilate an apneic patient. The effectiveness of assisted ventilation is assessed by listening to breath sounds and watching for chest rise.

Bag-valve-mask ventilation. The bag-valve-mask (BVM) consists of a face mask, one-way valve, self-inflating bag, and oxygen reservoir (Figure 10.15). It is available in infant, child, and adult sizes. The BVM should not have a pop-off valve, or else the pop-off valve should be disabled. Failure to do so could result in inadequate assisted ventilation. The oxygen inlet and reservoir allow for high concentrations of inspired oxygen (80% to 100%). The BVM device should be used with high-flow oxygen. The device should also have a nonrebreather valve to maintain high concentrations of inspired oxygen.

The volume of most adult BVMs is approximately 1600 ml. Despite what appears to be a large volume for ventilation, the BVM provides less volume than mouth-to-mask ventilation if an airtight seal is not obtained between the mask and face. An airtight seal is difficult to maintain unless a second EMT squeezes the bag to deliver ventilations. Because of the difficulty of maintaining an airtight seal while squeezing the bag, a single EMT should perform mouth-to-mask ventilation or use a flow-restricted oxygen-powered breathing device before using the BVM alone (see Bag-Valve-Mask [One Person] Skill Sheet at the end of this chapter).

When two EMTs are available, the BVM can be a very effective device. One EMT kneels behind the patient's head and inserts an oropharyngeal or nasopharyngeal airway. This EMT obtains an airtight mask seal with the same technique used for mouth-to-mask ventilation (Figure 10.16). The second EMT squeezes the bag with both hands for ventilations (see Figure 10.16). Both EMTs should watch for chest rise and listen for breath sounds to ensure adequate ventilation. With an airtight seal it is possible to give a tidal volume that is too large, forcing air into the stomach. If the abdomen becomes distended during ventilation, the EMT should extend the patient's neck slightly and give breaths less forcefully, provided that there is adequate chest rise.

If alone, the EMT should form a "C" around the ventilation port with the thumb and index finger and then use the middle, ring, and little fingers to lift the jaw and form a seal with the mask. The second hand is then used to squeeze the bag. The most commonly encountered problem with this device is maintaining an airtight seal between the mask and face. For this reason, the use of the BVM system is best when two people are available.

If a trauma patient requires assisted ventilation, the ETM should assume a cervical spine injury until proven otherwise. The EMT must maintain the head and neck in a neutral position. The EMT opens the airway with a jaw thrust maneuver, inserts an airway adjunct, and applies the mask from behind the patient's head. Ideally, an assistant maintains cervical spine stabilization while the EMT seals the mask. Alternatively, the EMT can stabilize the patient's head between his or her legs. An assistant then squeezes the bag for ventilation. Trauma patients often require suctioning and should be assessed frequently for airway compromise. See the Bag-Valve-Mask Skill Sheet at the end of this chapter.

> ✓ Bag-valve-mask ventilation is most effective when one EMT obtains a mask seal and another delivers ventilations. The cervical spine of trauma patients must be kept neutral during assisted ventilations.

Flow-restricted oxygen-powered ventilators. Flow-restricted oxygen-powered ventilators provide 100% oxygen at a maximum flow rate of 40 L/min. Flow rates greater than 40 L/min inevitably cause gastric distention, increasing the risk of regurgitation and aspiration. Flow-restricted ventilators are designed to prevent this problem, which frequently occurred with older "demand valve" devices. They also have an inspiratory pressure relief valve that opens at pressures of 50 to 60 cm H_2O. This

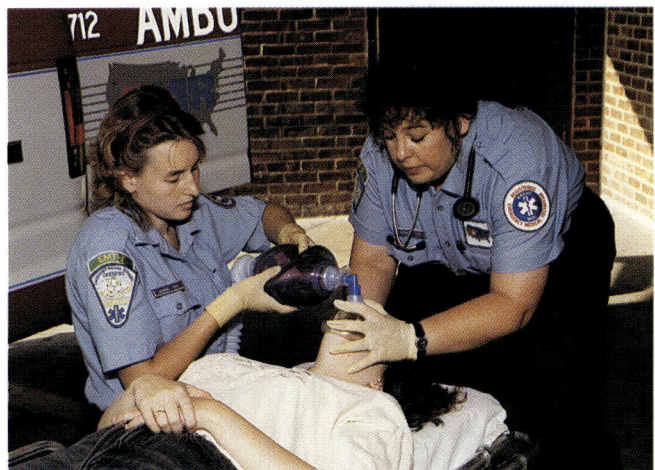

FIGURE 10.16 Bag-valve-mask ventilation. One EMT kneels behind the supine patient's head, opens the airway with the jaw thrust maneuver, and inserts an oropharyngeal airway. After an airtight seal is obtained, the second EMT squeezes the bag to deliver ventilations.

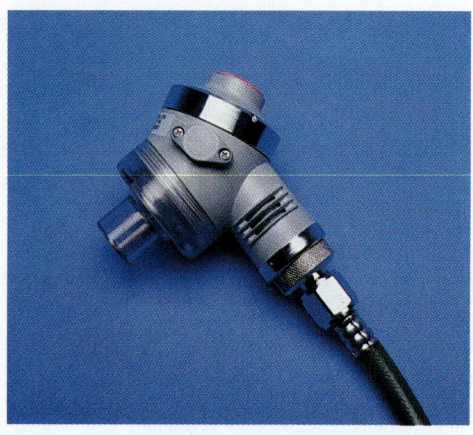

FIGURE 10.17 Manually cycled flow-restricted oxygen-powered ventilator. This device is used with a face mask and airway adjunct. Open the airway with the jaw thrust maneuver. Insert an airway adjunct and seal the mask in place. When the mask is in place, trigger the device to deliver ventilations.

valve either vents the remaining oxygen to the atmosphere or ceases gas flow. Most devices have an audible alarm that sounds when air is vented to the atmosphere. The EMT must know how his or her device operates. If an EMT is not familiar with the relief valve mechanism, ventilations can be lost to the atmosphere.

If a patient's airway is obstructed, the maximum airway pressure should be reached during inspiration, triggering the relief valve to either stop gas flow or vent the remaining volume to the atmosphere. However, if an airtight seal is not obtained with the face mask, air can leak into the atmosphere. If air leaks around the mask, the maximum inspiratory pressure is never reached, the relief valve does not open, and the alarm does not sound despite the airway obstruction. Therefore an airway obstruction can go unnoticed if the EMT relies solely on the pressure relief valve to recognize problems with ventilation. Maintaining an airtight seal, watching for chest rise, and listening for breath sounds will confirm adequate ventilation. The EMT should be aware that with these ventilators, the chest often does not rise as high as with BVMs or older "demand valve" devices. This difference is an important point to remember when assessing the adequacy of ventilation with flow-restricted ventilators.

Flow-restricted oxygen-powered ventilators should only be used with adults. The EMT first opens the airway and inserts an appropriate adjunct. The EMT then seals the mask in place with two hands. Most of these units have a trigger positioned so that the EMT can use both hands to maintain the mask seal. The device is triggered, allowing oxygen to flow until the chest rises (approximately 1 to 2 seconds) (Figure 10.17). As with other methods of assisted ventilation, if the chest does not rise and breath sounds cannot be heard, the EMT must reassess the patient. If the abdomen is distended, the EMT should reposition the head. If air leaks around the mask, the EMT should reposition the mask and fingers. If trauma is involved, the EMT should protect the cervical spine using the same technique used with other methods of assisted ventilation.

 Flow-restricted oxygen-powered ventilators deliver 100% oxygen at a maximum flow rate of 40 L/min.

Sellick maneuver. During assisted ventilation the EMT may use the **Sellick maneuver** to decrease the likelihood of regurgitation and aspiration. Aspiration of stomach contents can cause severe inflammation in the lungs and even death. The Sellick maneuver is a technique used in operating rooms to prevent passive regurgitation during intubation. The maneuver is performed by applying firm pressure on the cricoid cartilage (see Figure 10.3). The complete ring of the cricoid cartilage occludes the esophagus, which is located just posterior to it. The cricoid cartilage can be found just below (inferior to) the thyroid cartilage in the neck. The small depression below the thyroid cartilage is the cricothyroid membrane. The EMT applies pressure on the cricoid cartilage with the thumb and index finger just lateral to the midline. The EMT should maintain this pressure until the patient has spontaneous respirations, is intubated, or becomes responsive by moving, coughing, or gagging. This technique relies on the proper identification of anatomic structures, which can be difficult, especially in children. The technique also requires extra personnel and should not take the place of acquiring and maintaining an airtight seal for effective assisted ventilation.

Special assisted ventilation situations. A **tracheostomy** is a surgical opening in the neck that opens the trachea to the atmosphere. Tracheostomies are placed in patients who require long periods of assisted ventilation or in patients with cancer of the neck. A tracheostomy tube is often inserted in the opening (Figure 10.18). The EMT can attach the tracheostomy tube directly to the bag-valve device after the mask is removed. The EMT can then ventilate patients provided that there is not an obstruction at or below the tracheostomy. If secretions are present, the EMT can use a soft suction catheter to suction the tracheostomy.

If no tracheostomy tube is present, the opening in the neck is referred to as a **stoma**. Several options exist for ventilating a patient with a stoma. If the airway is not obstructed, the EMT can seal the stoma and ventilate the patient through the mouth and nose with one of the previously mentioned techniques. Other techniques include

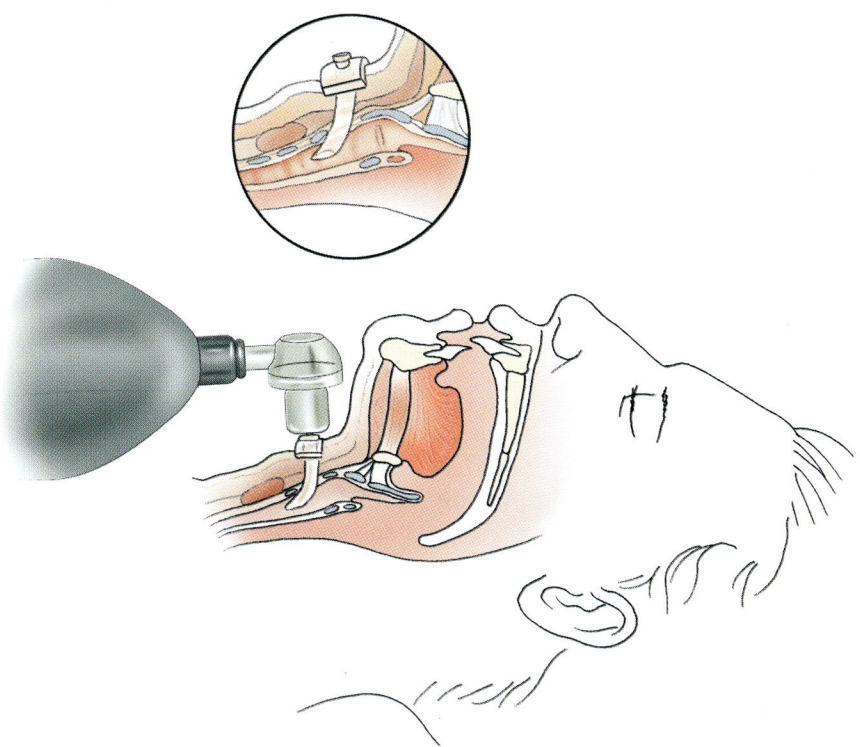

FIGURE 10.18 A tracheostomy is a surgical opening in the neck. The tracheostomy tube can be used for ventilation with a bag-valve-mask or flow-restricted oxygen-powered ventilator.

mouth-to-stoma, BVM-to-stoma, or oxygen-powered ventilation device-to-stoma ventilation. Because of infection precautions, mouth-to-stoma ventilation is not routinely performed. If it is performed, the EMT should use a plastic barrier device. With a BVM, the EMT can use an infant or child mask to form a seal over the stoma. Because the stoma provides a direct opening into the lower airway, the EMT does not need to position the head and neck. If air leaks out the mouth and nose while ventilating, the EMT must place a seal over the mouth and nose with a second face mask.

Assisted Ventilation in Infants and Children

The EMT must manage infants and children differently than adults. When opening an infant's airway, the EMT should keep the patient's neck in a neutral position. Hyperextension of the neck of an infant can cause airway obstruction because of the size and flexibility of the airways. In a child, the neck can be extended slightly past neutral. During assisted ventilation in infants and children, the EMT should avoid excessive bag pressure and tidal volumes. Gastric distention occurs more easily; therefore smaller, more frequent breaths (every 3 seconds) are more effective using a smaller BVM. BVM ventilation is much easier with pediatric patients and is usually preferable, even with a single EMT.

Assisting a Patient's Ventilation

Some patients may be breathing but not with a sufficient minute ventilation to maintain adequate gas exchange. With these patients, the EMT should assist the patient's breathing by giving assisted breaths with 100% oxygen at the same time that the patient inhales. Depending on the patient's LOC and airway control, an airway adjunct may be required. Generally, patients with a depressed LOC and a ventilatory rate less than 12 or greater than 20 breaths per minute are likely to require assisted ventilations. The EMT must use clinical judgment to decide which patients require assisted ventilation. As discussed in the section on the assessment of breathing, the EMT should monitor the rate, rhythm, quality, and depth of spontaneous respirations to decide whether assisted ventilations are required.

To assist ventilation, the EMT may use any of the assisted ventilation techniques discussed. After obtaining a mask seal, the EMT gives assisted breaths with the patient's spontaneous ventilatory effort. It is important to assist the patient's breaths once the mask seal is obtained because the patient will feel suffocated if not assisted when the mask is in place.

> ✓ Patients with a depressed LOC and a ventilatory rate less than 12 and greater than 20 breaths per minute may require assisted ventilation to improve oxygenation.

Supplemental Oxygen

EMTs frequently administer supplemental oxygen to patients in the field. The indications for giving supplemental oxygen are discussed in Chapter 14. This section discusses the equipment and techniques for providing supplemental oxygen.

Oxygen cylinders are produced in several sizes, each of which is designated with a letter (Figure 10.19). Any cylinder that contains oxygen is green in color. EMTs must handle oxygen cylinders carefully and secure them properly during transportation because their contents are under very high pressure. Each tank is connected to a pressure regulator and flowmeter for oxygen administration. The pressure of a full cylinder is approximately 2000 psi (pounds per square inch). This pressure can vary with the temperature of the environment. Warmer temperatures cause oxygen to expand, increasing the pressure in the cylinder.

The EMT must change the pressure regulator and flowmeter quickly between oxygen cylinders (Figure 10.20). Oxygen cylinders have a protective seal when fully pressurized, which the EMT must remove before attaching the regulator. After removal of the seal, the EMT should open and shut the valve quickly to remove any particles that may have been present under the seal. The EMT then attaches the regulator to the cylinder. The regulator is designed so that it can only be attached to the oxygen cylinder in one direction and cannot be applied to pressurized tanks containing other gases. After the regulator is applied, the EMT attaches an oxygen device to the flowmeter and adjusts the oxygen flow rate to the desired setting. After administering oxygen to a patient, the EMT should remove the device from the patient and close the valve on the oxygen cylinder. After closing the valve, the EMT should leave the flowmeter on until oxygen flow stops. This relieves all pressure from the regulator before the oxygen cylinder is stored.

Many ambulances are now carrying liquid oxygen tanks. These tanks can hold more oxygen than pressurized gas cylinders. Another advantage is that refilling can be done without removing the tank from the ambulance. For these reasons, liquid oxygen tanks will likely become more common in the future (see Application of Oxygen Regulator to Tank Step-by-Step Procedure and Turning on Oxygen Tank Step-by-Step Procedure at the end of this chapter). Tanks should be positioned to prevent falling and blows to the valve and gauge assembly and secured during transportation.

Use of a humidifier is recommended for long-term use.

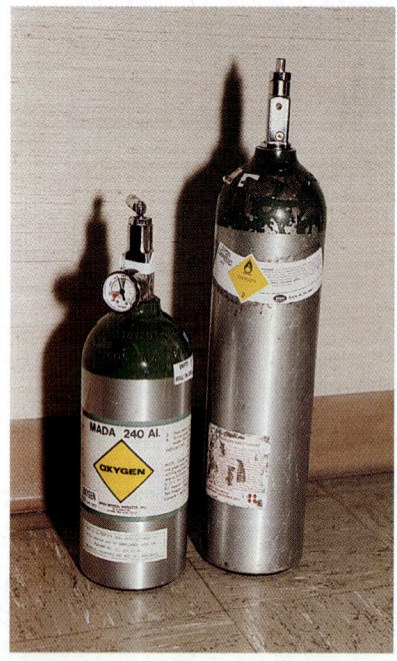

FIGURE 10.19 Aluminum oxygen cylinders.

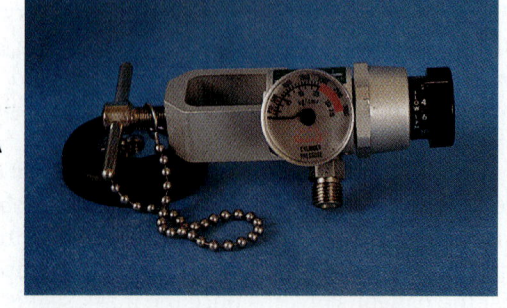 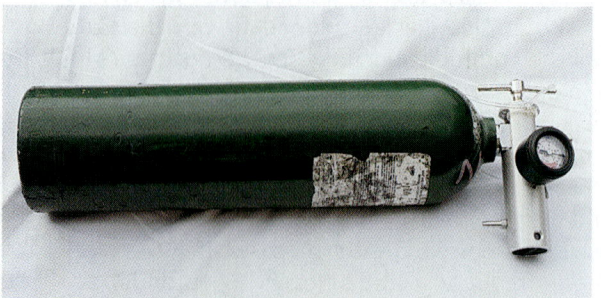

FIGURE 10.20 Oxygen regulator and flowmeter.

Nasal Prongs

Nasal prongs (Figure 10.21) are connected to the oxygen tank and have two "prongs" that insert into the nares of the patient. Even at very high flow rates, the amount of oxygen that the patient breathes in with each ventilation cycle is minimal. This is for two reasons:

1. The volume of the space at the nasal opening is so small that there is no accumulation of oxygen during exhalation. As the patient breathes in, there is rapid mixing of the oxygen from the prongs with the ambient air so that the FiO_2 is not much different from that of the external air. The maximum amount of increased oxygen is just 24% ($FiO_2 = 0.24$).
2. If the patient is breathing mostly from the mouth and not through the nose (as happens with many frightened patients), there is even less oxygen taken into the lungs with each breath.

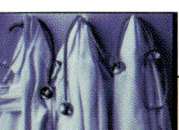

Physician Notes

Much confusion comes from the fact that most manufacturers of nasal prongs label the device as a nasal cannula. The true nasal cannula delivers a higher percent of oxygen up to 30% ($FiO_2 = 0.30$). The difference is that the nasal prongs insert only into the nares and deliver only 24% oxygen ($FiO_2 = 0.24$). A nasal cannula is a long tube that inserts through the nose into the back of the nasopharynx or even down into the oropharynx. Currently most ambulances do not have a nasal cannula as part of their supplies. Rather, they have nasal prongs that are labeled as a nasal cannula.

Nasal Cannula

Nasal prongs may be called "nasal cannula" by some manufacturers. The true nasal cannula should only be used in stable patients who are not in acute respiratory distress. The maximum flow rate with the nasal cannula is 5 to 6 L/min. Flow rates greater than this dry out the nasal passages, causing discomfort for the patient. The nasal cannula delivers about 35% inspired oxygen concentration. If a patient with chronic obstructive pulmonary disease (COPD) is not in severe distress, a nasal cannula can be used at a flow rate of 1 to 4 L/min. However, patients with acute respiratory distress should be given high concentrations of oxygen with a nonrebreather mask, even if they have a history of COPD (see Application of Oxygen Nasal Prongs Step-by-Step Procedure at the end of this chapter).

Nonrebreather Mask

The **nonrebreather mask** (see Figure 10.21) is the best method of providing high concentrations of supplemental oxygen to the spontaneously breathing prehospital patient. With high-flow rates (15 L/min), the mask can deliver up to 90% oxygen. Because the nonrebreather mask can feel restrictive to the patient, it should not be used with flow rates less than 10 L/min. The mask has a reservoir bag and a one-way valve that minimizes rebreathing of expired air. Before placing the mask on the patient, the reservoir bag should be full. The flow rate is then adjusted so that the bag does not completely collapse during respirations. The mask is available in adult, child, and infant sizes. The EMT should use the appropriate size and make sure that the mask fits snugly on the nose to maximize effectiveness (see Application of Nonrebreather Mask Skill Sheet at the end of this chapter).

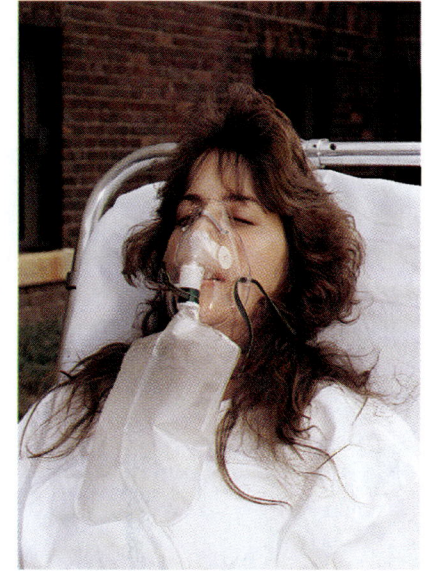
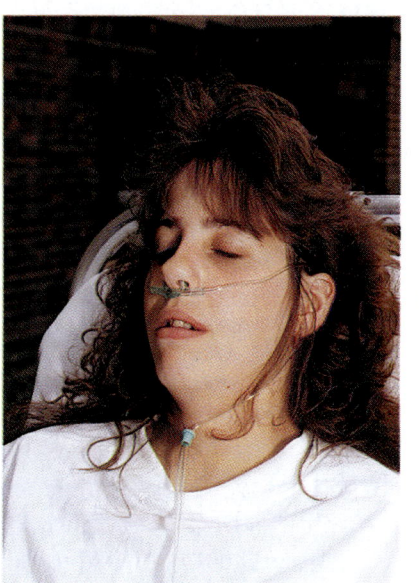

FIGURE 10.21 **A,** Nonrebreather mask. **B,** Nasal prongs.

Patients who are cyanotic, cool, clammy, or extremely short of breath need oxygen. Many concerns have been raised about giving patients with a history of COPD too much oxygen, which can decrease their respiratory drive. These legitimate concerns have not been shown to be valid in the prehospital setting. A patient with signs and symptoms of serious respiratory compromise should be given high concentrations of oxygen even if he or she has COPD. Similar concerns have been raised about giving infants and children high concentrations of oxygen. Again, in the prehospital setting, infants and children who require oxygen should receive high concentrations of oxygen.

✓ The nonrebreather mask and nasal cannula are used to provide supplemental oxygen. Patients with signs or symptoms of acute respiratory distress need high concentrations of oxygen with a nonrebreather mask.

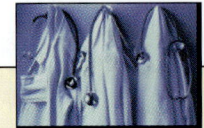

Physician Notes

The bag-valve-mask device is most effective when used by two people. It can be very difficult to obtain and maintain an effective mask seal with one hand while ventilating with the other. Therefore the use of these devices by two EMTs is strongly encouraged.

The advantages of newer flow-restricted oxygen-powered ventilators need emphasis. Contrary to older "demand valve" ventilators, which used flow rates in excess of 100 L/min, the newer flow-restricted ventilators are much less likely to cause abdominal distention. The use of flow-restricted ventilators is encouraged to decrease the likelihood of complications from abdominal distention, such as emesis, aspiration, and difficulty with assisted ventilation.

Step-by-Step Procedure

Jaw Thrust

1. Ensure scene safety.

2. Initiate body substance precautions.

3. Lightly place thumbs on the zygomatic arch.

4. Place middle fingers on either side of the angle of the mandible with ring and little fingers for support (see Step 4).

5. Thrust the jaw forward by pushing middle fingers up on the angle of the jaw and using thumbs on the zygomatic arch for leverage if needed (see Step 5).

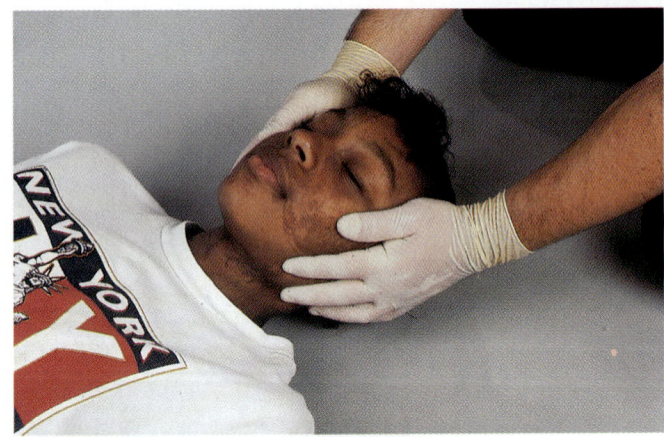
Step 4

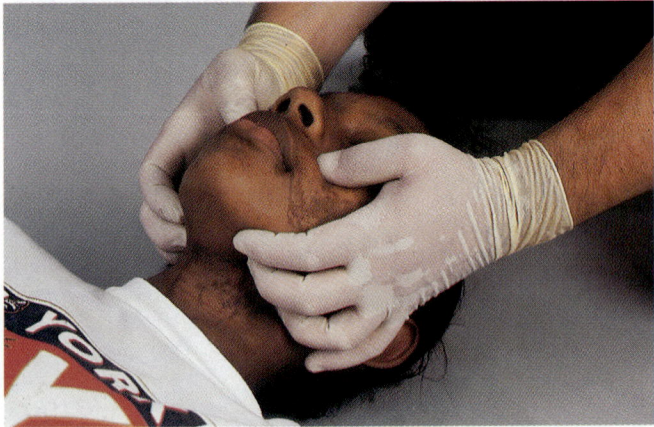
Step 5

Step-by-Step Procedure

Suctioning

1. Ensure scene safety.

2. Initiate body substance precautions.

3. Gather equipment (Figure 10.22):
   Suction device
   Rigid-tip catheter
   Soft-tip catheter
   Suction tubing

4. Connect suction tubing to the suction device.

5. Turn suction device on to check efficacy.

6. Turn suction device off once efficacy has been established.

7. Select rigid- or soft-tip catheter and connect to suction tubing.

8. Place catheter inside mouth or nose.

9. Place index or middle finger of hand holding suction catheter over the opening on the suction catheter. This procedure initiates suctioning.

10. Hold finger over opening and retract catheter from orifice.

11. While withdrawing from orifice, sweep catheter from side to side to clear airway.

12. Document treatment and findings. Caution: Suction for 15 seconds, ventilate for 2 minutes, and suction for 15 seconds. Repeat cycle as necessary. The pharynx should be cleared of all debris so as to not push it into the lungs during ventilation.

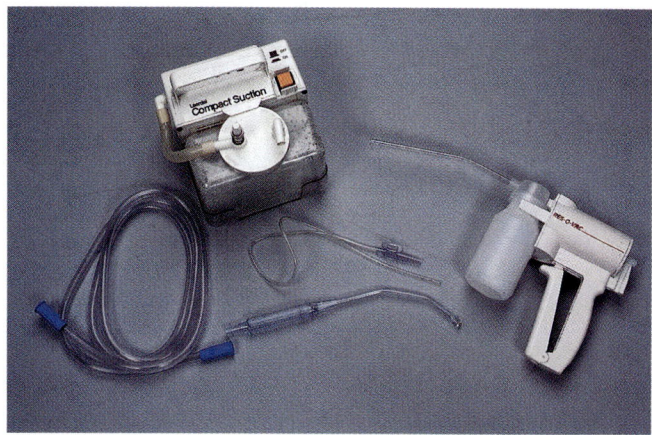

FIGURE 10.22 Suctioning device, rigid-tip catheter, soft-tip catheter, and suction tubing.

Step-by-Step Procedure

Oropharyngeal Airway Insertion

1. Ensure scene safety.

2. Initiate body substance precautions.

3. Gather equipment:
   Oropharyngeal airways
   Suction
   Oxygen mask
   Oxygen tank with regulator
   Tongue depressor

4. Select proper size of oropharyngeal airway by measuring from the corner of the mouth to the angle of the jaw.
   a. Airway too short (see Step 4a)
   b. Airway correct size (see Step 4b)
   c. Airway too long (see Step 4c)

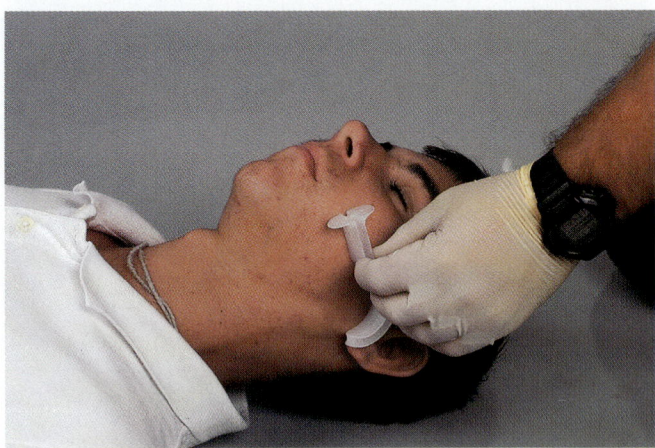

Step 4a

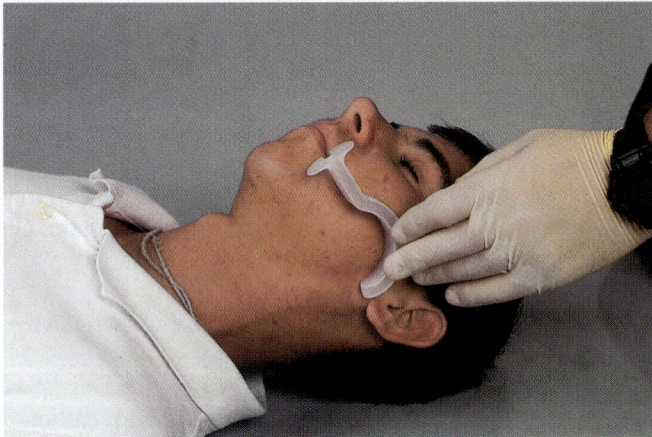

Step 4b

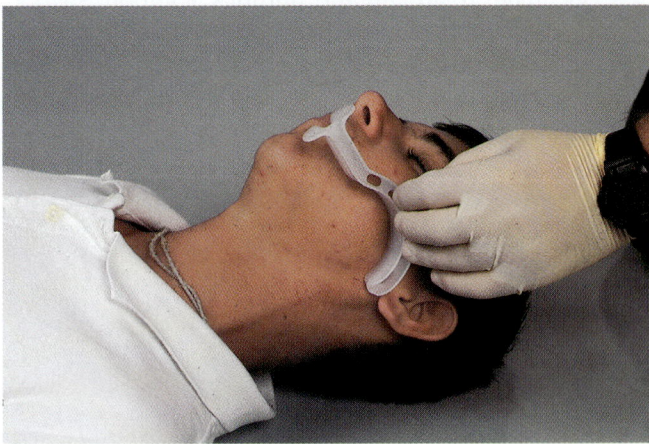

Step 4c

Oropharyngeal Airway Insertion (cont'd)

5. Two techniques are used to insert the oropharyngeal airway. The first technique is to begin to insert the airway opposite of the anatomic position in which it will rest (see Step 5a). This is accomplished by guiding the curved end of the airway along the hard palate. Once the tip reaches the back of the patient's mouth, the airway is rotated 180 degrees and dropped into the oropharyngeal region of the throat so the phalange of the airway is resting on the patient's teeth (see Step 5b).

6. A modification is the use of a tongue depressor. In this technique the tongue is physically pressed downward to allow the passage of the oropharyngeal airway into its anatomic position (see Figure 10.11).

The second technique is to pass the oropharyngeal airway in the anatomical position. The EMT must take care to not push the tongue into the back of the oropharynx and block the airway (see Step 6).

7. The airway is in its final position when the flange rests comfortably on the patient's teeth (see Step 7).

8. Initiate suction if necessary to clear airway.

9. Initiate oxygen therapy with nonrebreather mask or BVM assistance.

10. Document findings and treatment.

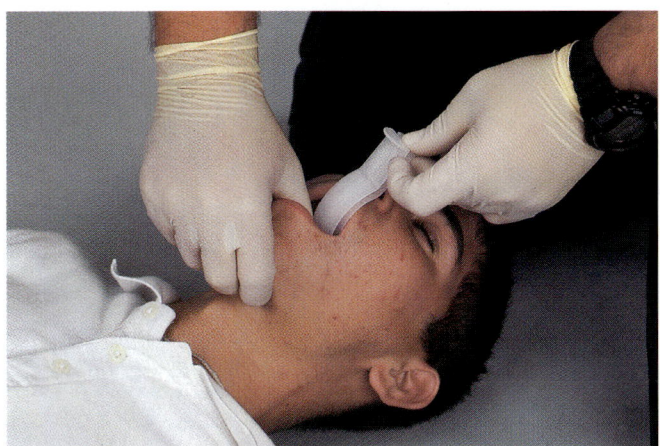

Step 5a

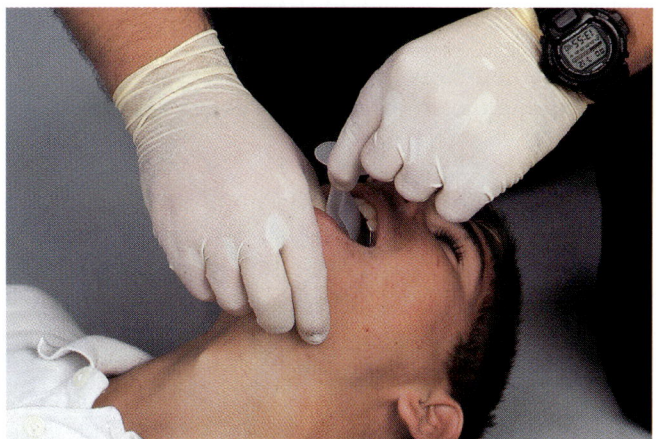

Step 5b

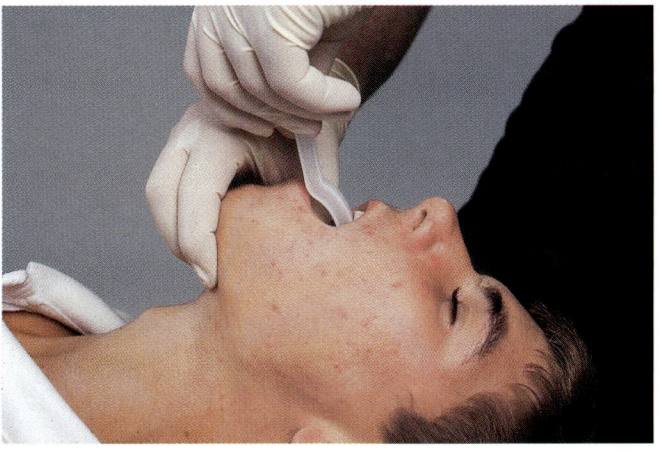

Step 6

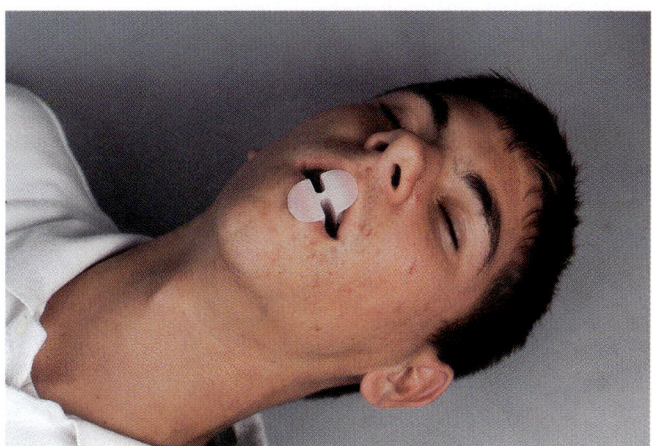

Step 7

Step-by-Step Procedure

Nasopharyngeal Airway Insertion

1. Ensure scene safety.

2. Initiate body substance precautions.

3. Gather equipment:
   Nasopharyngeal airways
   Suction
   Oxygen masks
   Oxygen tank with regulator
   Water-soluble lubricant

4. Select proper size of the nasopharyngeal airway by measuring from the tip of the nose to the tip of the ear (see Step 4).

5. Lubricate the appropriate size nasopharyngeal airway with a water-soluble lubricant.

6. Insert the airway into one nare with bevel of airway toward either the base of the tongue or the nasal septum (see Step 6).

7. Advance airway posteriorly until phalange of airway is resting on the nose. If resistance is met, remove the airway and attempt to insert in other nare (see Step 7).

8. Initiate suction if necessary to clear airway.

9. Initiate oxygen therapy using nonrebreather mask or BVM assistance.

10. Document findings and treatment.

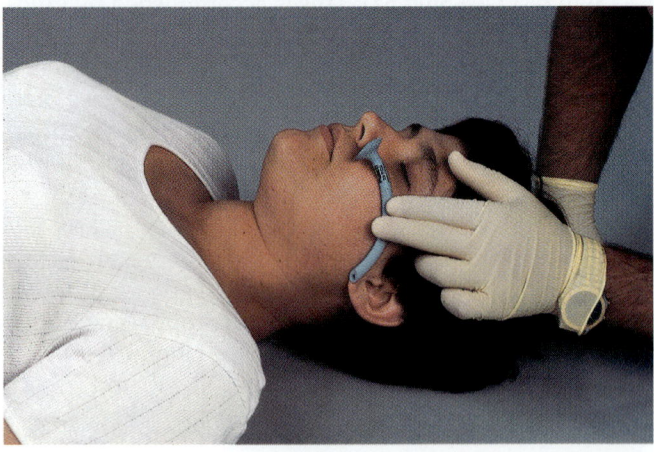
Step 4

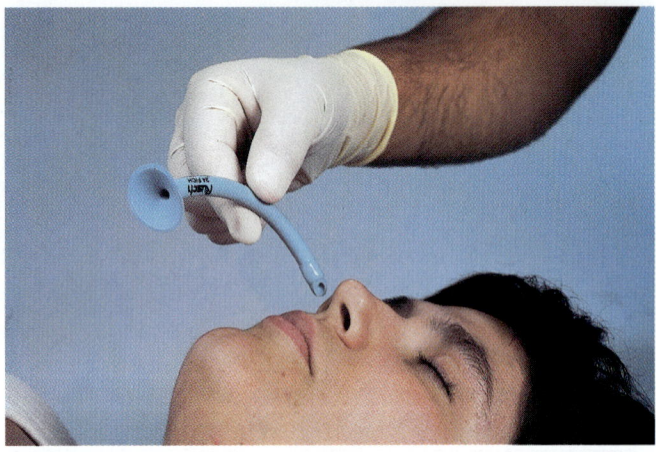
Step 6

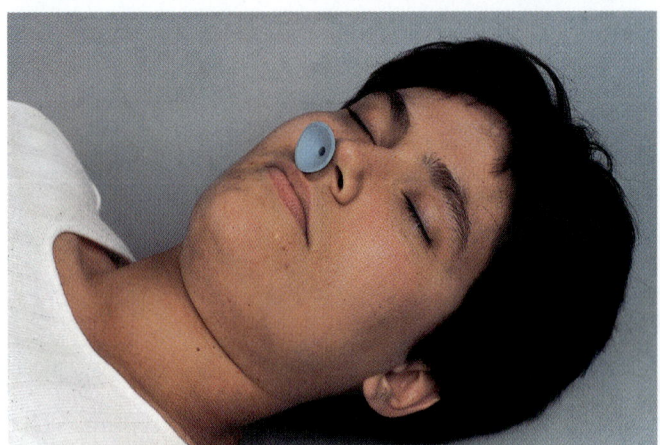
Step 7

Step-by-Step Procedure

Application of Oxygen Regulator to Tank

1. Gather equipment:
   Oxygen regulator
   Oxygen tank
   Oxygen key

2. Remove plastic tab from around the stem of oxygen tank (see Step 2).

3. Be careful not to lose the O-ring inside plastic tab (see Step 3).

4. Fit oxygen regulator into oxygen tank. The regulator fits like a lock and key into the tank. It will not have a snug fit if not placed exactly right.

5. Make sure the O-ring is placed between the regulator and tank properly. The O-ring acts as a gasket between the two pieces of equipment (see Step 5).

6. Tighten screw into tank. Hand tighten the regulator to the oxygen tank. Do not use a great deal of force to tighten regulator (see Step 6).

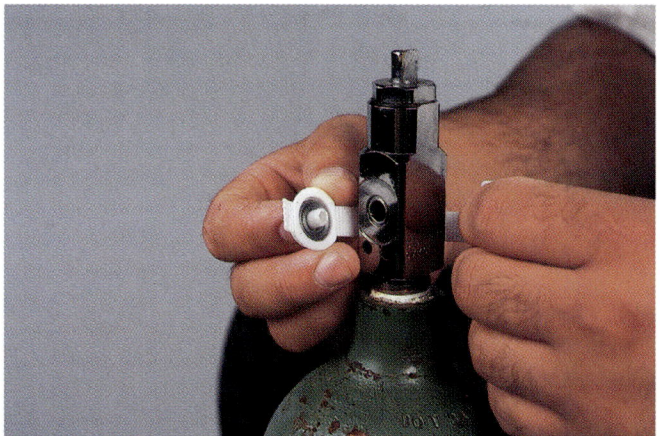
Step 2

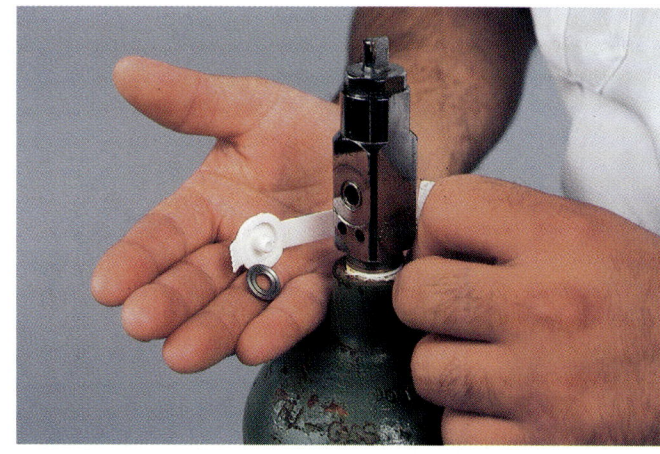
Step 3

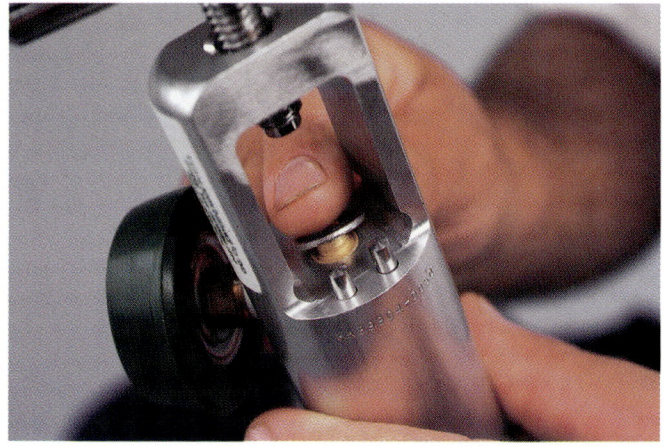
Step 5

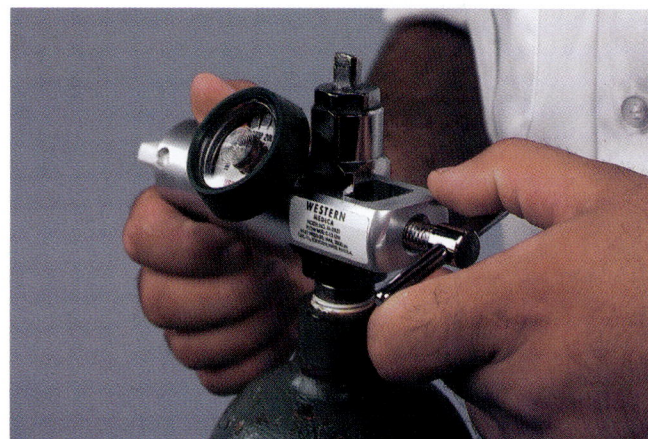
Step 6

Step-by-Step Procedure

Turning on Oxygen Tank

1. Gather equipment:
   Oxygen tank with regulator
   Oxygen key
   Oxygen mask or cannula

2. Attach oxygen tubing to "Christmas tree" (the green cone-shaped attachment to the regulator). Place oxygen key on the rectangular shaped stem of the oxygen tank.

3. "Crack" the oxygen tank open by using the oxygen key and rotating the stem. Do not turn the valve all the way open (only a quarter turn will do).

4. Check for leaks by listening by the regulator for a "hiss" of air escaping (see Step 4).

5. Check volume of oxygen tank by reading the gauge on regulator (see Step 5).

6. Using the flow valve, turn the regulator on to the desired flow rate (this will depend on the patient and the type of oxygen device used) (see Step 6).

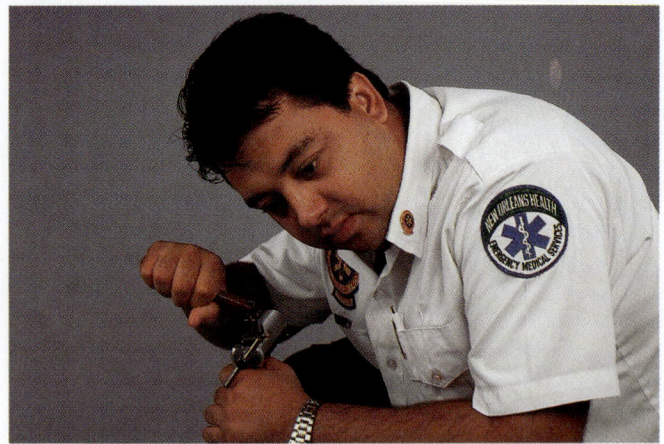
Step 4

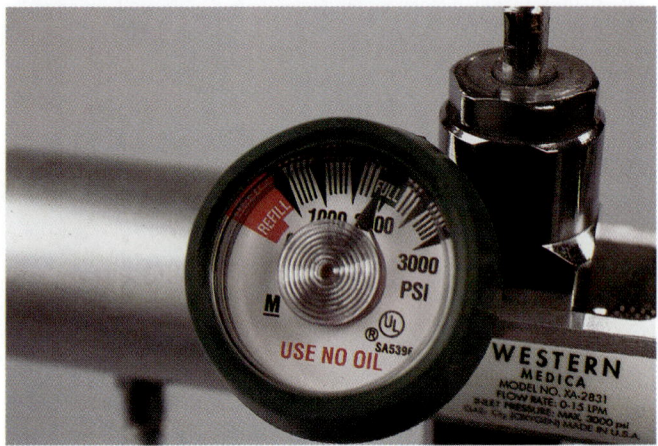
Step 5

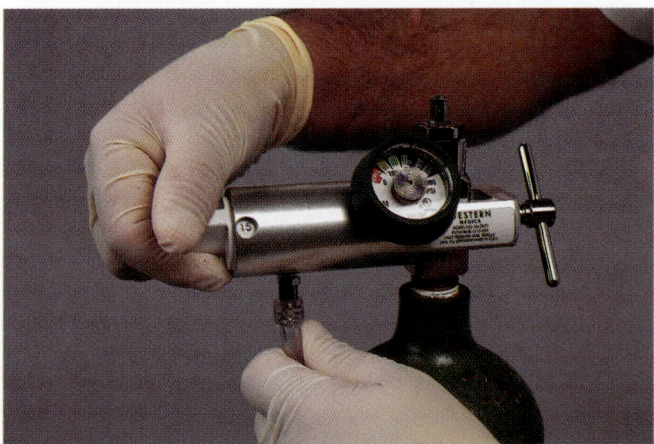
Step 6

Step-by-Step Procedure

Mouth-to-Mask Ventilation

1. Ensure scene safety.

2. Initiate body substance precautions.

3. Gather equipment:
   Face mask
   One-way breathing valve
   Oxygen tank with regulator
   Oxygen tubing

4. Kneel behind the patient's head, with patient in supine position.

5. Apply one-way valve to mask (see Step 5a) and attach oxygen with tubing to the mask if possible (see Step 5b).

6. Open the airway using the appropriate airway opening maneuver as dictated by the patient's injuries and mechanism of injury.

7. Apply the pointed or apex portion of the mask over the patient's nose and the base of the mask over the patient's mouth (see Step 7). Obtain a tight seal by placing thumbs toward the nose of the patient and index fingers toward the chin of the patient. Use the middle, ring, and little fingers to open the airway as indicated.

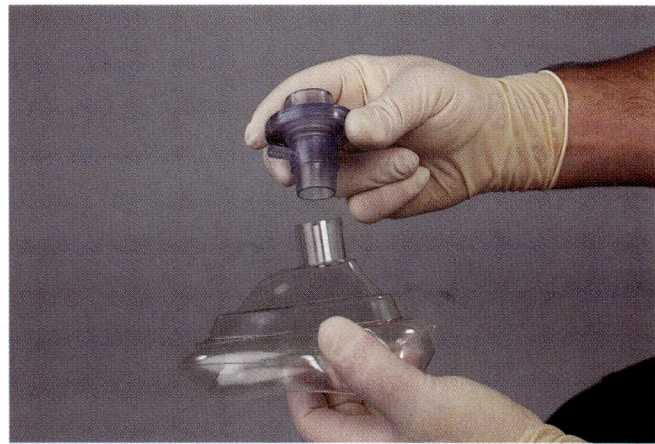
Step 5a

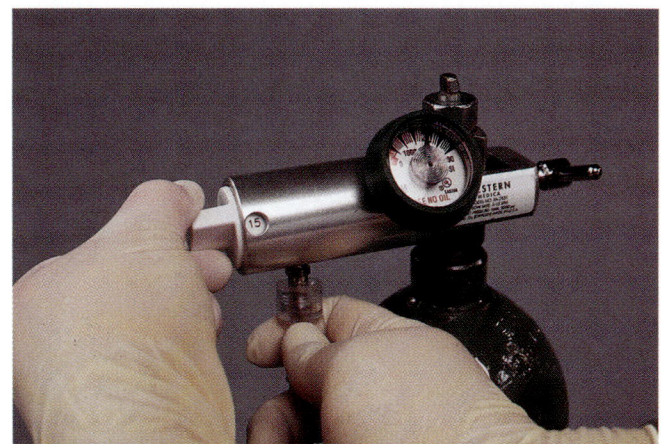
Step 5b

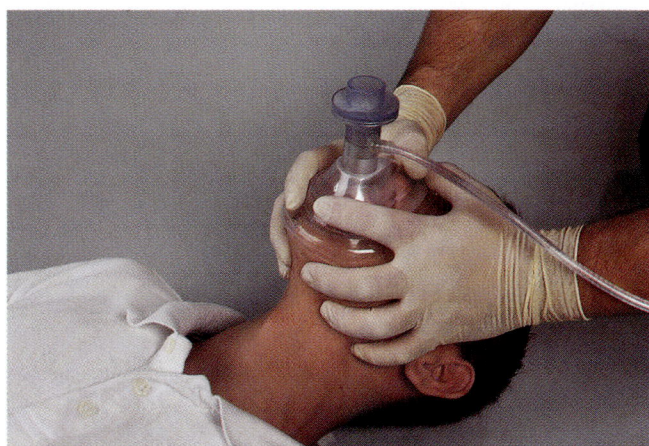
Step 7

continued

Mouth-to-Mask Ventilation (cont'd)

8. Deliver slow and steady breaths at an age-appropriate rate with supplemental oxygen (see Step 8).

9. Document findings and treatment.

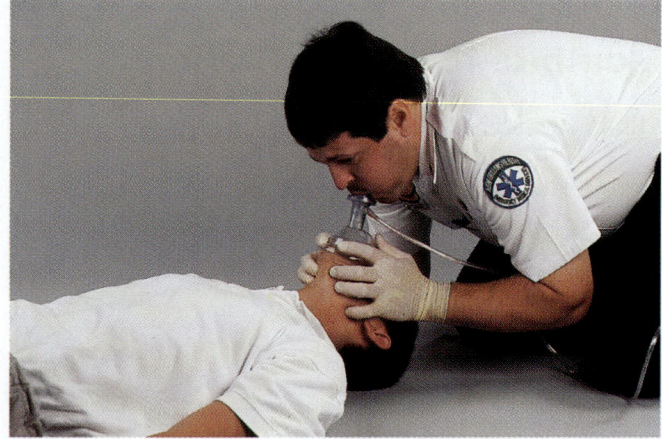

Step 8

Airway Management and Ventilation | Chapter 10

Step-by-Step Procedure

Bag-Valve-Mask (One Person)

1. Ensure scene safety.

2. Initiate body substance isolation.

3. Gather equipment:
   Oxygen tank with attached regulator
   BVM
   Nasal/oral airway

4. Establish unresponsiveness by shake and shout.

5. Establish breathlessness by opening airway, looking, listening, and feeling (see Step 5).

6. Select appropriate size mask for the patient.

7. Insert nasal/oral airway (see Step 7).

8. Attach BVM to oxygen and turn oxygen on with high concentration (10 to 15 liters per minute) (see Step 8).

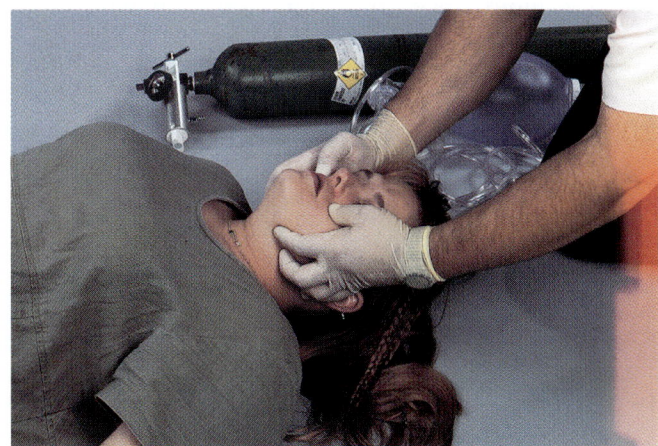
Step 5

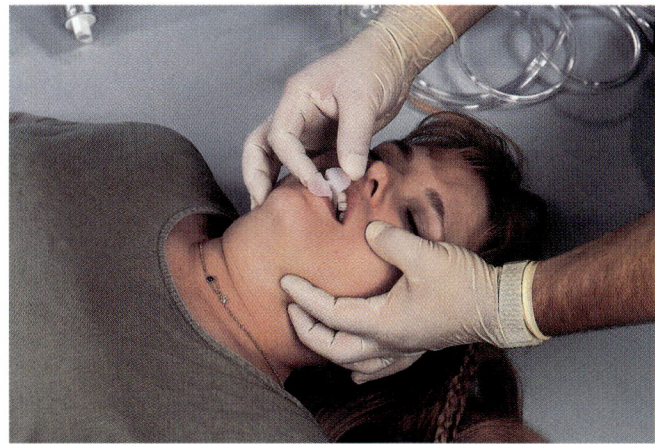
Step 7

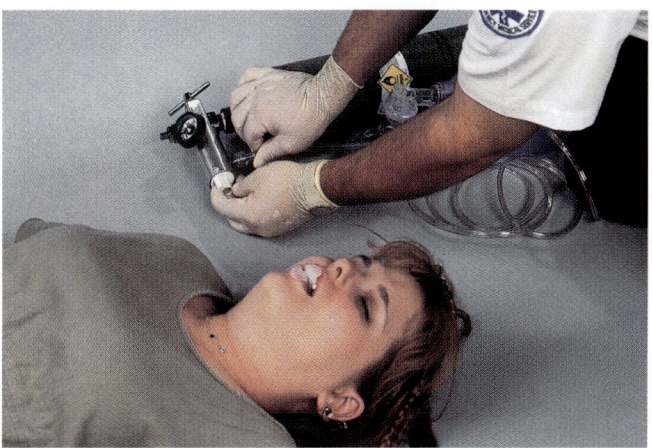
Step 8

continued

Bag-Valve-Mask (One Person) (cont'd)

9. With non-dominant hand, use small, ring, and middle fingers to lift mandible up to open airway.

10. Use index finger and thumb (also known as "C" clamp) to secure seal of BVM by placing thumb toward nose and index finger over chin (see Step 10).

11. With dominant hand, squeeze bag of BVM to empty oxygen from bag as much as possible.

12. Use thigh or body to adequately empty bag of oxygen. Ensure that the BVM completely refills.

13. Document findings and treatment.

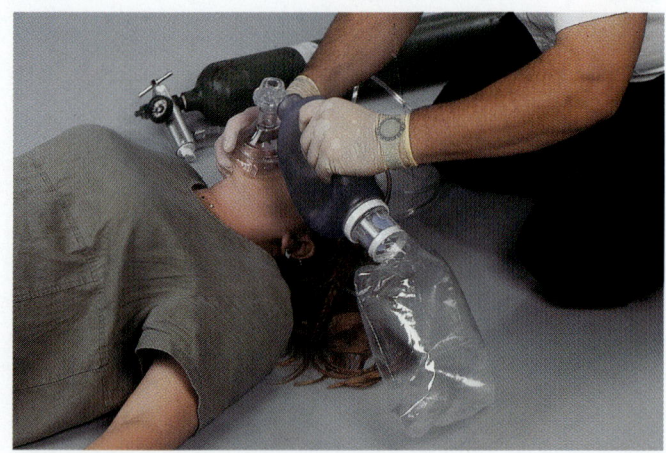

Step 10

Step-by-Step Procedure

Application of Oxygen Nasal Prongs

1. Gather equipment:
   Oxygen regulator with tank
   Oxygen nasal prongs

2. Remove oxygen nasal prongs from plastic wrapping.

3. Extend tubing away from nasal prongs.

4. Attach tubing to "Christmas tree" (nipple) on the oxygen regulator.

5. Adjust oxygen regulator to the desired flow rate (2 to 6 liters per minute).

6. Place nasal prongs just inside each nare with the plastic tab laid on top to the upper lip.

7. Bring nasal prongs around each of the ears and down the anterior region of the neck.

8. Pull plastic sliding cylinder to cinch the nasal prongs to maintain position (see Step 8).

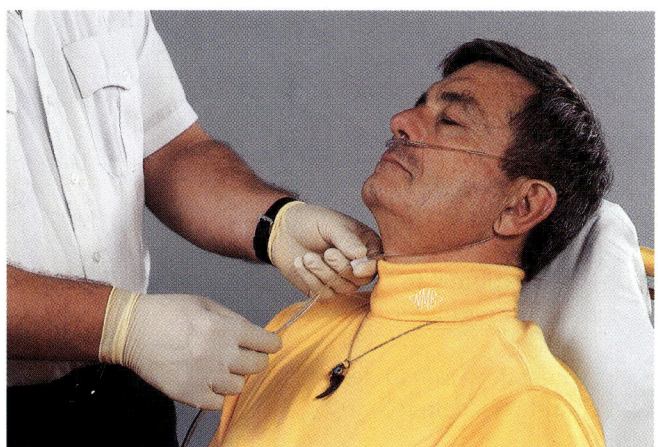

Step 8

Step-by-Step Procedure

Application of Nonrebreather Mask

1. Gather equipment:
   Oxygen tank with regulator
   Oxygen nonrebreather mask

2. Remove nonrebreather mask from plastic wrapping.

3. Extend tubing away from mask.

4. Attach tubing to "Christmas tree" (nipple) attachment on regulator.

5. Adjust flow rate to desired setting (10 to 15 liters per minute) (see Step 5).

6. Firmly place two fingers inside the mask and hold pressure on the plastic flap to allow the plastic bag part of the mask to inflate. This will take about 5 to 10 seconds. This step is the most important to ensure correct flow rate to the patient (see Step 6).

7. Extend green elastic band and place mask over the patient's head (see Step 7).

8. Cinch the metal band above the patient's nose to ensure an adequate seal around nose.

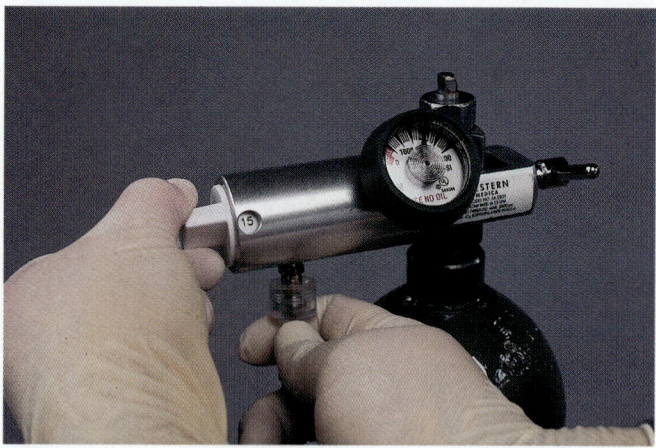
Step 5

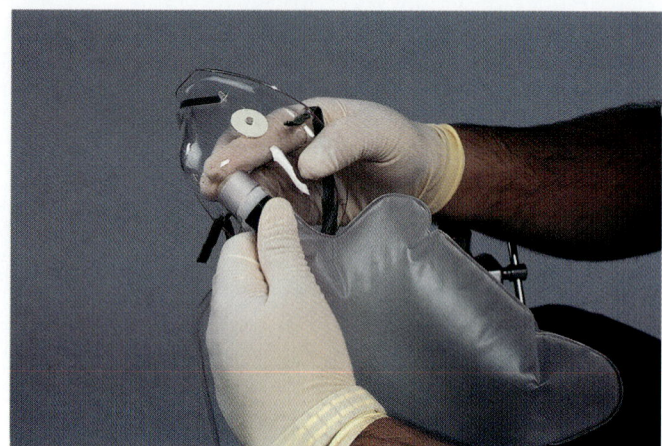
Step 6

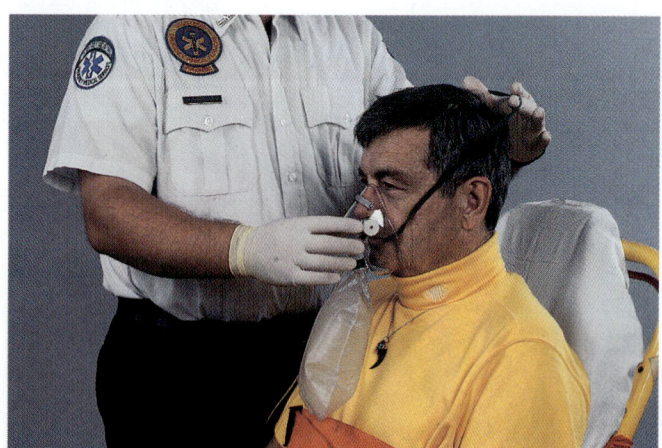
Step 7

Summary

- Airway management and assisted ventilation take priority over all other basic life-support skills. A patient without an airway is a dead patient.
- The most common cause of an airway obstruction in an unresponsive patient is the tongue.
- The respiratory system is designed to supply oxygen to and remove carbon dioxide from the body. The alveolar/capillary and capillary/cellular exchanges enable this interchange between oxygen and carbon dioxide to take place.
- Proper assessment of breathing includes determination of the rate, rhythm, quality, and depth of ventilations.
- Techniques for opening the airway of an unresponsive patient include the head-tilt chin-lift and jaw thrust maneuvers. Trauma patients with a suspected spinal injury should be managed with in-line immobilization of the cervical spine.
- Airway adjuncts such as oropharyngeal and nasopharyngeal airways should be used to maintain the airway of patients during assisted ventilation.
- Assisted ventilation techniques include mouth-to-mask, bag-valve-mask (one-person and two-person) ventilation, and the flow-restricted oxygen-powered ventilator. The most difficult part of assisted ventilation is maintaining an airtight seal between the mask and face.
- Patients who are in acute respiratory distress should be given high concentrations of oxygen, even if they have a history of COPD.
- Frequent reassessment of ABCs (airway, breathing, and circulation) during transportation prepares the EMT to manage airway problems and/or patient deterioration en route.

Scenario Solution

Scene safety is the first concern at any scene. With this particular scenario, the scene seems to be safe. The second initial concern upon arrival at the scene is with universal precautions. You should wear gloves, at the very least, until the scene and patient mandates more precautionary equipment.

Because the patient fell and hit his head, you must take C-spine precautions. After you have immobilized the patient's C-spine, you must assess the airway and patency. If the patient is not breathing, then you must initiate rescue breathing, preferably with a bag-valve-mask (BVM) and oxygen supplementation. Once you have opened the airway with assisted breathing, you must check for circulation. The easiest access for checking pulse is from the carotid artery. If you do not detect a pulse, you must initiate cardiopulmonary resuscitation (CPR).

This patient is breathing but needs assistance because his ventilatory rate is 8 breaths per minute. You should give assistance with a BVM and supplemental oxygen at a rate of 15 L/minute. The patient has a pulse rate 60 beats per minute, and when you assess "D" (disability, or LOC) the patient is unresponsive. You disrobe the patient ("E"; exposure) and note no obvious trauma.

The patients vital signs are the next priority. His blood pressure is 160/50 mm Hg, his pulse rate is 60 beats per minute, his ventilatory rate is 8 breaths per minute, and his skin is cool and dry. You notes no obvious trauma on the quick secondary survey, so you direct you treatment toward head injury. While the patient's C-spine is maintained, you place the patient on a long spine board (LSB) and a stretcher. You transport the patient to the emergency department while continuing to ventilate him and monitoring his vital signs and responsiveness.

Key Terms

Accessory muscles Muscles located primarily in the neck that contract to increase tidal volume during respiratory distress.

Agonal ventilations Occasional gasping breaths that occur just before death.

Airway adjuncts Devices such as oropharyngeal and nasopharyngeal airways that are designed to prevent airway obstruction by the tongue.

Alveolar/capillary exchange Gas exchange that occurs in the lungs; oxygen enters the capillaries and is transported by the blood, and carbon dioxide enters the alveoli and is exhaled.

Alveoli Small air sacs in the lungs where the exchange of gas takes place.

Apnea Complete lack of respirations.

Key Terms

Aspiration Accidental inhalation of fluid or other particles into the lower airway.

Carina Division of the lower end of the trachea into the two mainstem bronchi.

Cellular/capillary exchange Exchange of oxygen that occurs in the body tissues; oxygen enters the cells to be metabolized, and carbon dioxide enters the capillaries to be carried to the lungs.

Crackles Lower-pitched bubbling sounds produced by fluid in the lower airways; often described as either fine or coarse.

Cricoid cartilage Complete ring of cartilage at the lower end of the larynx that marks the beginning of the lower airway; compressed during the Sellick maneuver.

Cyanotic Blush color of the skin associated with unoxygenated hemoglobin.

Dead space Space in the lungs that contains air that is inhaled but does not reach the alveoli for exchange; includes the upper and lower airways and is usually about 150 ml in volume.

Diaphoretic State of sweating (e.g., patients with cardiac chest pain are often diaphoretic).

Diaphragm Dome-shaped muscle that separates the thoracic cavity from the abdominal cavity. When it contracts, the thoracic cavity enlarges, allowing air to enter the lungs.

Dyspnea Symptom of having difficulty breathing or shortness of breath.

Epiglottitis Inflammation of the epiglottis; a bacterial infection seen most often in children. The epiglottis becomes swollen and may cause airway obstruction; patients often have excessive drooling.

Head-tilt chin-lift Maneuver that opens the airway of unconscious patients; the neck is extended with one hand on the forehead and one hand under the chin.

Hemopneumothorax Collection of both blood and air in the pleural space; always abnormal and may cause collapse of the underlying lung.

Hemothorax Accumulation of blood and fluid in the pleural cavity usually caused by trauma.

Hyperventilation Process in which minute ventilation is increased above normal; purposely done for patients with head injuries or with prolonged apnea.

Hypoventilation Process of lowering minute ventilation below normal. Patients who are hypoventilating have higher carbon dioxide and lower oxygen levels than normal.

Intercostal muscles Muscles located between the ribs that lift the ribs upward and outward during inhalation, increasing tidal volume.

Jaw thrust Maneuver for opening the airway in unconscious patients; enables cervical spine stabilization and is often used with trauma patients.

Larynx Often called the *voice box,* structure consisting of cartilage, muscle, and soft tissues; located between the pharynx and the trachea.

Mainstem bronchi Two primary divisions of the trachea that supply the lungs with oxygen.

Minute ventilation Amount of air inhaled in 1 minute; calculated by multiplying the tidal volume by the respiratory rate

Nasal prongs Device used to deliver low concentrations of oxygen to patients who need supplemental oxygen but who are not in acute respiratory distress.

Nasal flaring Widening of the nostrils that occurs during inhalation in patients with respiratory distress.

Nasopharyngeal (nasal) airway Airway adjunct inserted into a nostril and designed to prevent airway obstruction by the tongue.

Nonrebreather mask Device used to deliver high concentrations of oxygen to patients in acute respiratory distress; has a reservoir bag and one-way valve to prevent rebreathing.

Oropharyngeal (oral) airway Airway adjunct designed to prevent airway obstruction by the tongue in unconscious patients; inserted upside down and rotated 180 degrees.

Pharynx Hollow space behind the nose and mouth and above the larynx and esophagus; divided into the nasopharynx, oropharynx, and hypopharynx.

Pleura Thin membrane that covers the lungs and lines the thoracic cavity

Pleural space Potential space between the two layers of pleura surrounding the lungs.

Pneumothorax Collection of air in the pleural space; always abnormal and may cause collapse of the underlying lung.

Pulmonary arteries Vessels that carry oxygen-poor blood from the right side of the heart to the lungs; the only arteries in the body that carry oxygen-poor blood.

Pulmonary veins Vessels that carry oxygen-rich blood from the lungs back to the left side of the heart; the only veins in the body that carry oxygen-rich blood.

Quality In patient assessment, strength, depth, and completeness of assessment. In patient care, accuracy, completeness, and correctness of care.

Rales Fine breath sounds that represent opening of collapsed alveoli or fluid in the small airways near the alveoli; simulated by rubbing hair between the fingers.

Key Terms (cont'd)

Rate Number of occurrences in a period of time, such as ventilations per minute.

Retractions Sign of respiratory distress often seen in infants and children marked by inward pulling of the skin above the clavicles and below the rib cage with inspiration.

Rhythm Cadence or equality in repetition.

Sellick maneuver Maneuver designed to prevent passive aspiration during assisted ventilation; performed by applying posterior pressure to the cricoid cartilage.

Stoma Artificially created opening between two passages or body cavities or between a cavity or passage and the body's surface.

Thoracic cavity Bony structure made of ribs, muscle, and cartilage that protects the lungs and vital organs.

Thyroid cartilage Often referred to as the *Adam's apple*; most prominent part of the larynx.

Tidal volume Volume of air inhaled with each breath; normally about 500 ml in an adult.

Trachea Cylinder-shaped tube in the neck composed of cartilage and membrane that extends from the vocal cords to about the level of the fifth thoracic vertebra where it divides into two bronchi; also called the *windpipe*.

Tracheostomy Surgical opening through the neck into the trachea through which an indwelling tube may be inserted.

Wheezing High-pitched sounds heard when air moves through constricted airways; commonly occurs in patients with asthma.

Review Questions

1. The most common cause of an obstructed airway in an unresponsive patient is:
    a. Respiratory secretions
    b. Tongue
    c. Foreign body
    d. Heart attack
2. Infants and children are more susceptible than adults to airway compromise for all of the following reasons except:
    a. Smaller airway size
    b. Proportionally larger tongue
    c. Airway cartilage is more firm than in adults
    d. Upper respiratory infections are more common
3. True or False: The pulmonary arteries carry oxygenated blood from the lungs to the left atrium of the heart.
4. Which of the following is *not* used to assess the adequacy of breathing?
    a. Ventilatory rate
    b. Depth of ventilations
    c. Skin color
    d. Blood pressure
5. Which of the following is an appropriate use of assisted ventilation?
    a. Using a flow-restricted oxygen-powered ventilator with an infant
    b. Assisting ventilations in an unresponsive patient with a ventilatory rate of 34 breaths per minute
    c. Using bag-valve-mask ventilation with a single EMT
    d. Ventilating a semiresponsive patient with a gag reflex using an oropharyngeal airway and bag-valve-mask
6. A patient with COPD who is in acute respiratory distress with cyanosis should be given:
    a. High concentration of supplemental oxygen
    b. Low concentration of supplemental oxygen
    c. No oxygen
    d. BVM ventilation
7. One of the earlist indicators of anaerobic metabolism is:
    a. Hypotension
    b. Tachypnea
    c. Decreased capillary refill time
    d. Decreased ventilation rate
8. The most common reason for BVM ventilation failure is:
    a. No oral airway
    b. Poor mask-face seal
    c. Small hands on the bag
    d. Wrong bag

Answers to these Review Questions can be found at the end of the book on page 866.

11

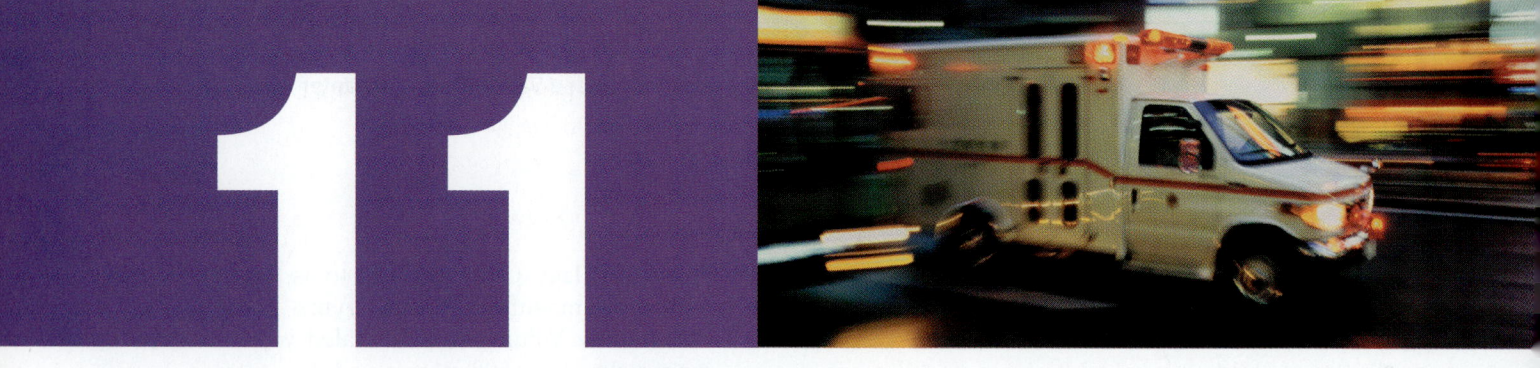

Advanced Airway Management Skills

Lesson Goal

The most important skill that an EMT needs to improve survival is airway management. If oxygenation of the patient fails, the patient will not survive. Other techniques are available to make airway management easier and more convenient and allow the EMT to do more than one job. This chapter addresses those advanced techniques. Just because they are included in this text does not mean that they will be included in each service at the EMT-B level. The techniques used on each EMS service depends on local protocols, city or county (parish) ordinances, and state laws. Reading and learning the skills does not mean that the EMT will be allowed to perform the technique. However, the EMT may be better able so assist the EMT-P when both services are available on each call. This chapter presents those advanced techniques.

Scenario

You and your partner respond to the scene of a 65-year-old male who was "found down" by family members. They reported to the dispatch that they saw the patient collapse on the floor. He has not spoken since he fell. He is unresponsive but is breathing at a rate of 6 breaths/min and gurgling with mucus around his closed lips, he has a carotid pulse rate of 40 beats/min, and his pupils are 6 mm not fixed. You are in charge.

 What is your first priority? What will be your first steps to assess and manage the patient? What are the potential associated problems that require management?

Key Terms to Know

Advance directive	Endotracheal tubes	Esophageal intubation detection device	Laryngoscope
Arytenoid cartilage	Endotracheal tube cuff	Extubation	Living will
Automated transport ventilators	End-tidal carbon dioxide	Glottic opening	Nasogastric (NG) tube
Compliance	Epigastrium	Hypoxia	Nasotracheal intubation
			Occiput

Key Terms to Know (cont'd)

Orogastric tube
Pilot balloon
Preoxygenation

Sellick maneuver
Sniffing position

Stylet
Uvula

Vallecula
Xiphoid process

Learning Objectives

As an EMT-Basic, you should be able to do the following:

DOT

- Describe and identify the anatomic structures involved in performing endotracheal intubation in the infant, child, and adult.
- Describe and demonstrate the techniques used for endotracheal intubation in the infant, child, and adult, which include choosing an appropriate-size endotracheal tube, inserting a stylet, using both curved and straight blades for intubation, securing the endotracheal tube, and demonstrating endotracheal suctioning.
- Recognize the complications of advanced airway management, including the consequences of unrecognized esophageal intubation.
- Differentiate between the airway anatomy in the infant, child, and adult.
- Explain the pathophysiology of airway compromise.
- Describe the proper use of airway adjuncts (see Chapter 10).
- Review the use of oxygen therapy in airway management (see Chapters 9 and 10).
- Describe the indications, contraindications, and technique for insertion of nasal gastric tubes.
- Describe how to perform the Sellick maneuver (cricoid pressure).
- Describe the indications for advanced airway management.
- List the equipment required for orotracheal intubation.
- List complications associated with advanced airway management.
- Describe the skill of orotracheal intubation in the adult patient.
- Describe the skill of orotracheal intubation in the infant and child patient.
- Describe the skill of confirming endotracheal tube placement in the infant, child, and adult patient.
- Describe the skill of securing the endotracheal tube in the infant, child, and adult patient.
- Demonstrate how to perform the Sellick maneuver (cricoid pressure).
- Demonstrate the skill of orotracheal intubation in the adult patient.
- Demonstrate the skill of orotracheal intubation in the infant and child patient.
- Demonstrate the skill of confirming endotracheal tube placement in the adult patient.
- Demonstrate the skill of confirming endotracheal tube placement in the infant and child patient.
- Demonstrate the skill of securing the endotracheal tube in the adult patient.
- Demonstrate the skill of securing the endotracheal tube in the infant and child patient.

Supplemental

- Recognize and respect the feelings of the patient and family regarding advance directives as they apply to endotracheal intubation.
- Describe and demonstrate the skill of confirming endotracheal tube placement, including the use of end-tidal carbon dioxide detection or other detection techniques.
- Explain and recognize the pathophysiology of airway compromise, including the indications and rationale for advanced airway management by EMT-Bs.

Successful management of a critical illness or injury depends on accurate airway assessment and appropriate management. Airway management is the first priority of patient care for any patient. There are basic life support (BLS) and advanced life support (ALS) steps in the management of this critical skill. In the past, only ALS personnel have been allowed to perform advanced airway procedures such as endotracheal intubation. However, since the emergency medical technician-basic (EMT-B) is often the first to arrive at the scene, many emergency medical services (EMS) systems are teaching the EMT-Bs to perform advanced airway management techniques.

With proper training and skills maintenance, the use of advanced airway management skills by EMT-Bs should improve patient care and outcomes. EMT-Bs who

Patient Care Algorithm

Medical Patient Airway-Breathing Assessment

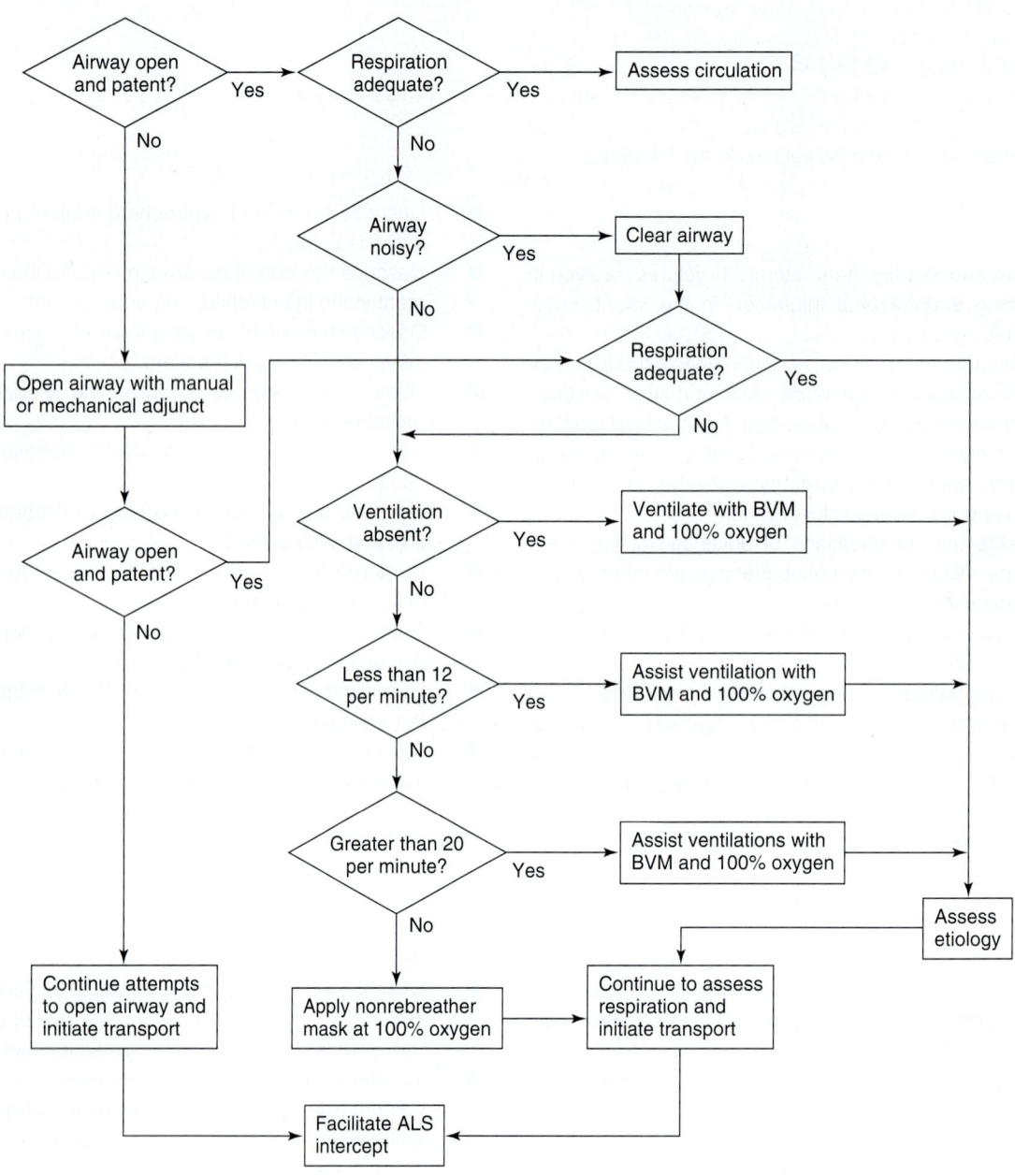

perform endotracheal intubation need thorough initial training, frequent practice, and close supervision by medical control in the classroom and in the field. The skills themselves are not difficult for the EMT to learn; however, since the EMT-Bs who need these techniques are usually in areas of small population, the skills are used infrequency. Any skill that goes unused for a long period of time will deteriorate. The EMT-Bs who use the skills the least but need them the most are the most likely to forget how to do them quickly and efficiently. The most dangerous EMT is the one who has been taught a skill but who neglects to maintain efficiency and cannot perform to the needs of the patient at the critical time. Therefore the EMT must refresh the skill frequently in the classroom, emergency department, and operating room. The EMT-B who learns this skill must promise himself or herself and the patient that he or she will always be able to do it correctly and quickly.

This chapter begins with a review of anatomic structures important for endotracheal intubation. The signs and symptoms of airway compromise and the indications for advanced airway management are discussed. Endotracheal intubation skills for the infant, child, and adult are described in detail. Emphasis is placed on recognizing the complications of intubation, especially the consequences of unrecognized esophageal intubation. The EMT must recognize when an attempt at intubation is unsuccessful.

Advanced airway management remains an optional skill for good reason. The absolute priorities for patients with airway and respiratory compromise are airway management and ventilation. Although endotracheal intubation is the preferred airway for many critically ill or injured patients, *ventilation takes priority over intubation*. Almost all patients can be ventilated without an endotracheal tube by using BLS skills. Therefore intubation is still considered an optional skill for EMT-Bs.

The ability to use advanced airway management skills is an exciting step for EMT-Bs that should have a positive influence on patient care and outcomes. To maximize this positive influence, EMT-Bs must recognize the degree of initial training and persistent practice required to successfully and consistently perform endotracheal intubation in the field. Many data in the EMS and other literature documents that without continous practice both in the field and in the laboratory, skill deterioration will occur and the patient will suffer. If the EMT-B is not sure that he or she can preform advanced airway management well, he or she should not attempt it. Recent studies have identified that bag-valve-mask (BVM) ventilation is equal to endotracheal tube ventilation in most circumstances.

Anatomy and Physiology

The anatomy of the respiratory system is discussed in detail in Chapter 10. The EMT student should review that chapter before studying advanced airway management. This section focuses on the anatomic structures of the upper airway that are directly involved in endotracheal intubation.

Upper Airway

The mouth and nose are the beginning of the upper airway. The **uvula** is a small structure made of soft tissue that is suspended from the roof of the mouth just in front

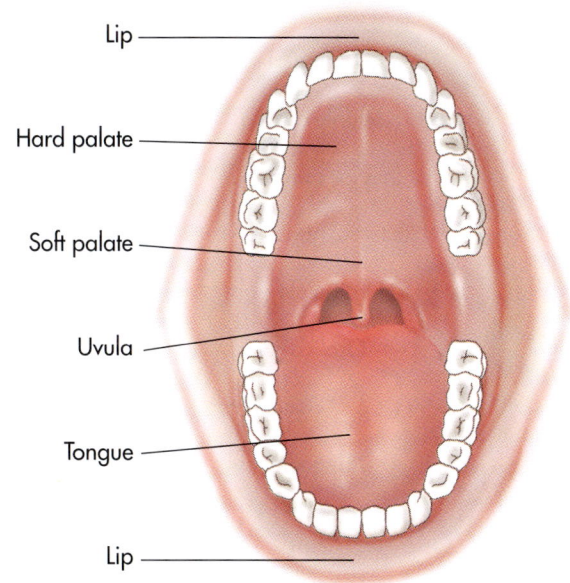

FIGURE 11.1 The uvula is suspended from the roof of the mouth posteriorly. The teeth, tongue, and soft tissues of the oral cavity present potential barriers to endotracheal intubation.

of the oropharynx (Figure 11.1). It is easily visualized when the mouth is opened widely and can be used to determine how far to insert the instrument used for intubation. The tongue is a much larger structure than most people realize. Figure 11.2 shows that the base of the tongue extends down to the epiglottis. Patients who need endotracheal intubation usually do not have control of the tongue, and it often collapses into the back of the pharynx, causing airway obstruction. During intubation the tongue is moved to the side of the mouth with a laryngoscope blade. The size of the tongue in some patients makes this task difficult. At the base of the tongue, a valley is formed between the tongue and the epiglottis called the **vallecula** (see Figure 11.2), which is used as a landmark during endotracheal intubation.

The vocal cords are located within the larynx at the beginning of the trachea. They protect the opening of the trachea from aspiration of liquids and foreign material. During endotracheal intubation the vocal cords are visualized with a laryngoscope and a tube is passed between them into the trachea. The vocal cords are shaped in an upside down "V," with the apex facing anteriorly. Figure 11.3 demonstrates the vocal cords as seen with a laryngoscope during intubation. The opening between the vocal cords is called the **glottic opening**. Each vocal cord is attached posteriorly to an **arytenoid cartilage**, which functions as a "pivot point" for vocal cord movement. The arytenoid cartilages are located at the two bases of the "V" formed by the vocal cords. The esophagus is located just posterior to the glottic opening. The close proximity of the esophagus makes inadvertent esophageal intubation easy if the vocal

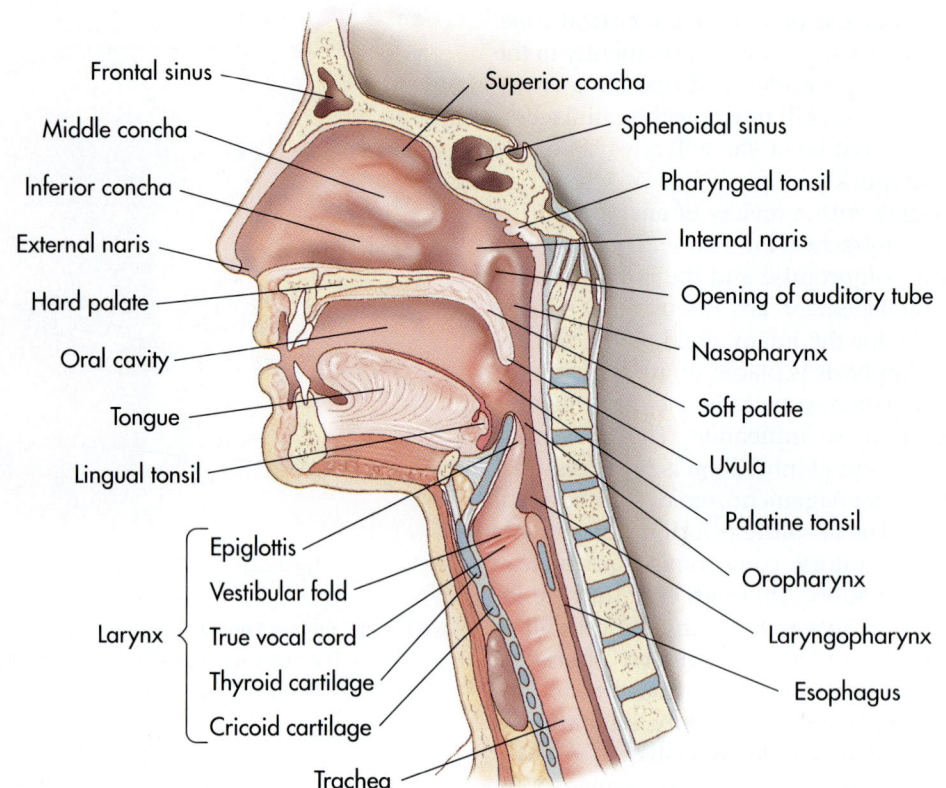

FIGURE 11.2 The base of the tongue extends to the epiglottis, forming the vallecula. The large size of the tongue can interfere with visualization during intubation.

cords are not adequately visualized before tube insertion. *Unrecognized* esophageal intubation is fatal. Familiarity with the anatomy of the upper airway decreases the likelihood of successful esophageal intubation.

Infant and Child Anatomy

The upper airway structures of infants and children are softer and more fragile than those of adults. Therefore the EMT must take care not to damage structures during intubation. The combination of a proportionally larger tongue and a smaller larynx makes the vocal cords appear more anterior in infants and children than in adults. The anterior location of the vocal cords can make intubation difficult, especially when the EMT is inexperienced. The EMT should practice with appropriate models to become familiar with infant and child upper airway anatomy before gaining experience on live patients in the operating room. For further information, see Chapter 10.

> ✓ Familiarity with the anatomy of the upper airway is essential for successful endotracheal intubation. To visualize the vocal cords for tube placement, the EMT must recognize the anatomic landmarks of the larynx.

Pathophysiology of Airway Compromise

Airway compromise quickly leads to shock and death if not corrected. The most common cause of an obstructed airway in an unconscious patient is the tongue (Figure 11.4). Other causes of airway obstruction include respiratory secretions, gastric contents, and foreign bodies. In trauma patients, blood and teeth can obstruct the airway. Any of these materials can be aspirated into the lower airway, inhibiting air movement and gas exchange. When a patient has an obstructed airway, ventilation of the alveolae cannot be done and O_2/CO_2 exchange is not accomplished. Until the airway obstruction is corrected the patient will continue to deteriorate; therefore other interventions by the EMT are meaningless unless the airway is controlled.

Assessment: Indications for Endotracheal Intubation

Signs and symptoms of airway compromise are discussed in Chapter 10. Most unconscious patients will require some form of airway control. An airway adjunct such as

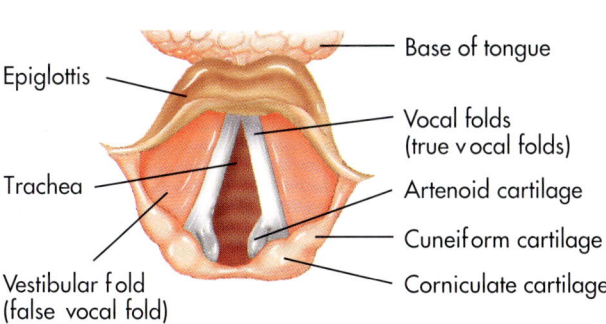
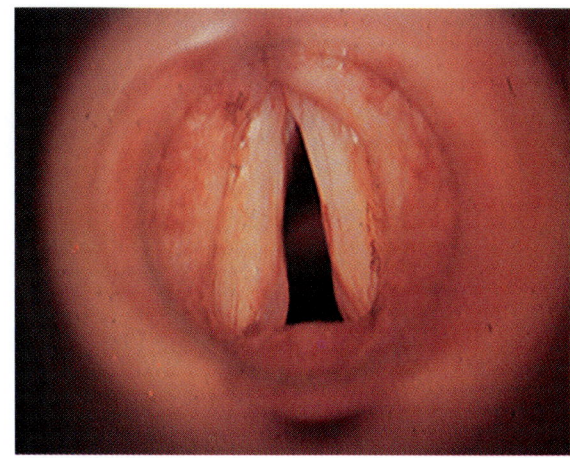

FIGURE 11.3 Illustration of the larynx as seen during endotracheal intubation.

an oropharyngeal or nasopharyngeal airway is the initial step to keep the airway open. Suctioning is another important BLS skill frequently needed in unconscious patients. A patient with noisy breathing, especially gurgling sounds during respiration, probably needs suctioning.

Endotracheal intubation is indicated when the following criteria exist:

1. EMT is unable to adequately ventilate the apneic patient with a BVM
2. Patient is unresponsive to painful stimuli
3. Patient has no gag reflex or coughing
4. Patient is unable to protect the airway (e.g., cardiac arrest)

Patients who have an intact gag reflex and are partially responding may not tolerate endotracheal intubation without the administration of medications that are not available to the EMT-B. Therefore intubation by EMTs is more easily preformed (without the use of Rapid Sequence Intubation drugs [RSI]) in patients who are unresponsive and do not have an intact gag reflex. The patient with a head injury needs oxygen to reduce the effect of **hypoxia** on the brain. Survival without significant residual neurologic defects depends on this respiration process in the brain. Patients with a Glasgow Coma Scale score of <8 do considerably better when intubated in the field before arrival in the emergency department.

Most patients intubated by EMT-Bs in the field will be apneic. Some patients will be breathing and still meet the above indications for endotracheal intubation. In a patient who is spontaneously breathing, the EMT should assess the patient by monitoring the rate, rhythm, quality, and depth of respirations. If the patient has signs of poor airway control such as noisy breathing, vomiting, or evidence of hypoxia (e.g., poor skin color or cyanosis), the EMT should first intervene with BLS airway techniques.

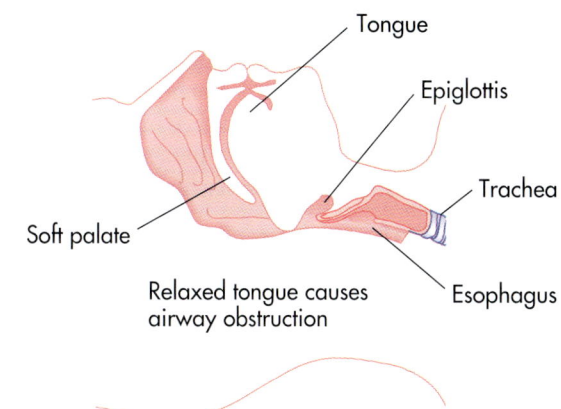

FIGURE 11.4 In unconscious patients, the tongue often collapses into the back of the pharynx, obstructing the airway.

If the patient's condition remains unchanged, the EMT should perform endotracheal intubation for definitive airway control.

> ✓ Endotracheal intubation is indicated in unresponsive patients without a gag reflex who need assistance with airway control. The EMT uses BLS airway techniques before intubation.

Management

Control of the airway is the most critical intervention of prehospital care because a patient without an airway is a dead patient. The BLS skills covered in Chapter 10 are the most important airway skills used by the EMT, and they must be mastered before the EMT attempts advanced airway management techniques. This section describes the techniques of advanced airway management, beginning

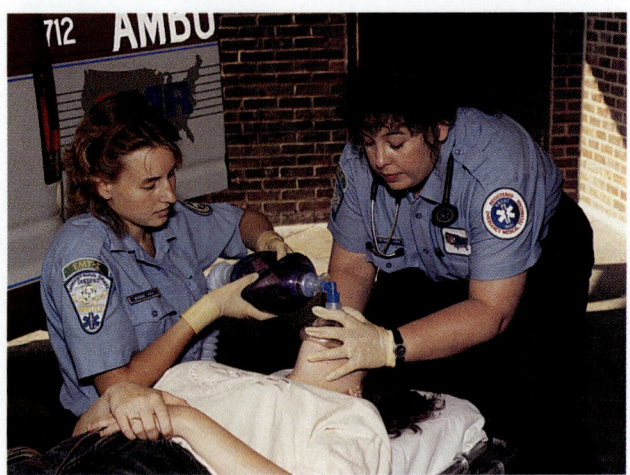

FIGURE 11.5 Two-person bag-valve-mask ventilation is an effective preoxygenation technique.

with the role of BLS skills in endotracheal intubation. Nasogastric tube placement; endotracheal intubation in adults, infants, and children; alternative airways when endotracheal intubation is not achievable; endotracheal suctioning; and automated transport ventilators are discussed.

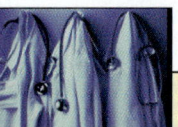 **Physician Notes**

The EMT cannot expect to learn and maintain airway management skills without consistent practice. The EMT who takes on this advanced skill must commit to his or her patients that he or she will be dedicated to keeping these skill sharp and well honed. EMTs performing advanced airway skills in the field should practice regularly with airway models and perform the procedure on patients in the controlled environment of an operating room with direct supervision by an anesthesiologist. Failure to maintain these skills can result in the death of patients.

Basic Airway Techniques

The EMT should open the airway of an unconscious patient using the head-tilt/chin-lift or jaw thrust maneuver. Before intubation, the EMT should ventilate the patient with BLS techniques. The EMT should insert an oropharyngeal or nasopharyngeal airway and ventilate the patient with mouth-to-mask, BVM, or flow-restricted oxygen-powered ventilation. The immediate concern in a patient with poor or absent respirations is hypoxia. The quickest way to correct hypoxia is to ventilate the patient with BLS techniques using 100% oxygen. Since assisted ventilation must be withheld during endotracheal intubation, initial BLS ventilation is critical for **preoxygenation**, the process of increasing the oxygen content in the lungs before intubation (Figure 11.5).

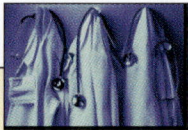 **Physician Notes**

Endotracheal intubation is an aggressive intervention that should not be performed by every EMT-B. This skill is optional, and local medical direction should consider several factors before proceeding with the training. Endotracheal intubation is a difficult skill. Even EMT-Ps who intubate relatively frequently are unsuccessful at times. EMT-Bs who intubate should have the opportunity to perform the skill regularly. If the call volume does not provide an adequate opportunity to maintain skills, the EMT must have other opportunities to intubate. The EMT cannot maintain adequate skills for performing endotracheal intubation in the prehospital environment without having opportunities to intubate in more controlled settings. The emphasis during training should be on recognizing when to suspend intubation attempts if unsuccessful and how to confirm endotracheal tube position. Endotracheal intubation by EMT-Bs has the potential to improve patient care and outcomes; however, the EMT should only attempt it with an awareness of the potential for complications and need for ongoing training.

Endotracheal Intubation

The EMT can perform endotracheal intubation using either an orotracheal or a nasotracheal technique. **Nasotracheal intubation** involves insertion of a tube through the nose into the trachea and is only performed on patients who are breathing. This form of intubation is more difficult than endotracheal intubation. Only EMTs who are experienced in the orotracheal technique should use the nasotracheal technique.

Endotracheal intubation is performed for complete airway control. The tube that is inserted into the trachea has a cuff that is inflated to prevent aspiration around the tube. This method minimizes aspiration and gastric distention, improves oxygenation, and allows for suctioning of the lower airway. Endotracheal intubation is the definitive advanced airway technique in the apneic patient.

Complications of Endotracheal Intubation

Although endotracheal intubation provides many advantages, it is a technically challenging procedure that carries several significant risks, some of which are life-threatening (Box 11.1). The most critical complication of the procedure is esophageal intubation which is fatal if unrecognized.

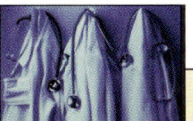

Physician Notes

Esophageal intubation is not a complication. Unrecognized and unresolved esophageal intubation is a fatal complication.

Box 11.1 Complications of Endotracheal Intubation

- Unrecognized esophageal intubation
- Hypoxia from prolonged unsuccessful attempts
- Trauma to lips, teeth, tongue, and larynx
- Emesis
- Right mainstem bronchus intubation
- Inadvertent extubation

A second life-threatening complication of endotracheal intubation is that prolonged unsuccessful attempts at the procedure lead to inadequate oxygenation. To avoid this complication, any single attempt should be limited to 30 to 45 seconds. A single EMT should not attempt to intubate a patient more than twice. Before each attempt, the EMT *must* ventilate the patient with 100% oxygen to provide adequate preoxygenation for the next intubation attempt. Although local protocols may vary, the EMT should perform a maximum of three attempts at a scene with assisted ventilation before each attempt. If still unsuccessful, the EMT should transport the patient with BLS-assisted ventilation en route. The priority for an apneic patient is *ventilation,* not intubation. Although an endotracheal tube is the definitive airway, prolonged unsuccessful attempts at intubation do the patient more harm than good.

The third life threatening complication of the use of endotracheal intubation is unrecognized **extubation**. Despite the fact that the tube may still be taped in the mouth, movement of the head can pull the endotracheal tube out of the trachea and into the esophagus. The motion of extension, flexion, and lateral rotation move the tube significantly in relationship to the trachea.

Each time the patient is moved, there is a risk of displacement After moving the patient, the EMT should confirm endotracheal tube placement by listening to breath sounds, watching for chest rise, and documenting end-tidal carbon dioxide (CO_2) or using another method of confirming correct tube position (see "Confirming Endotracheal Tube Placement" on page 225).

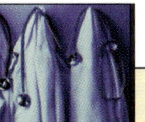

Physician Notes

The EMT must understand that extubation can occur without complete removal of the endotracheal tube. The end of the tube can slip out of the trachea and enter the esophagus while the patient is being moved. If the EMT does not reconfirm tube position in this situation, hypoxia and death can occur quickly. A recent article by Matera on the problem of unrecognized extubation recommends that all field intubated patients be transported taped to a backboard to reduce the incidence of this complication.

If a patient becomes responsive after being intubated, he or she often will try to remove the tube. If this occurs, the EMT should restrain the patient's hands to prevent extubation.

If the EMT does not handle the laryngoscopy carefully during endotracheal intubation, trauma to the lips, teeth, gums, tongue, and airway structures may result. The difficulty of intubation in the prehospital environment makes these complications more likely unless the EMT takes care to avoid them.

Endotracheal intubation can also affect the cardiovascular system. During intubation the heart rate may slow down as a result of stimulation of the nerves that regulate heart rate. If the patient becomes more responsive during the procedure, the heart rate may increase because of anxiety, pain, and hypoxia. Therefore the EMT should monitor and document vital signs before and after the procedure. The patient also may vomit during the procedure, so suction must be available.

An endotracheal intubation placed too far down may go into the main stem bronchus and ventilate only one lung. Because of the angle formed by the main stem bronchi at the carina, an endotracheal tube that is inserted too far will likely enter the right main stem bronchus. The EMT can recognize this complication by hearing breath sounds on the right but not on the left. To correct the problem, the EMT deflates the cuff on the tube and pulls the tube back until he or she hears breath sounds bilaterally. The EMT should be aware that

✓ Endotracheal intubation is the definitive airway in an apneic patient; however, it is a technically challenging procedure that has several potential complications. Two life-threatening complications of endotracheal intubation are unrecognized esophageal intubation and hypoxia from prolonged unsuccessful intubation attempts.

the tube can occasionally enter the left main stem bronchus instead of the right and breath sounds are heard on the left side, not the right. Again, the EMT should pull the tube back until he or she hears breath sounds on both sides. The EMT must reinflate the cuff after pulling the tube back.

Equipment for Endotracheal Intubation

To perform endotracheal intubation the EMT needs the equipment shown in Figure 11.6 and Box 11.2. The EMT must exercise body substance isolation (BSI) precautions, including masks and protective eye wear, when attempting endotracheal intubation. The **laryngoscope** is the instrument used to visualize the vocal cords for endotracheal tube placement (Figure 11.7, *A*). It has two components: a handle and a blade. Two primary blades are used for intubation: the curved blade and the straight blade. Both blades have a notch that attaches to a locking bar on the laryngoscope handle (Figure 11.7, *B*). Locking the blade in place illuminates a light for vocal cord visualization. Both curved and straight blades are available in assorted sizes. The curved blade is designed to be inserted into the vallecula, which pulls the epiglottis anteriorly to allow vocal cord visualization. The straight blade is designed to directly lift the epiglottis during endotracheal intubation. To ensure proper performance in an emergency, the EMT should regularly inspect the laryngoscope handle and blades. The EMT should carry spare batteries and light bulbs with the advanced airway kit.

Endotracheal tubes are available in several sizes based on the internal diameter of the tube in millimeters. The tube sizes are in 0.5 mm increments. Adult females generally require a 7 to 8 mm tube, and adult males require an 8 to 8.5 mm tube. (An emergency rule is that a 7.5 mm tube fits most adults.) An advanced airway kit should have multiple tube sizes available. Other components of an endotracheal tube are seen in Figure 11.8, *A*. The 15 mm adapter on the tube is designed to fit standard airway attachments, such as a BVM. The **endotracheal tube cuff** holds approximately 5 to 10 ml of air. It should be inflated until there are no air leaks around the tube during assisted ventilation. If air leaks persist despite 10 ml of air in the tube, either the cuff on the tube has ruptured or the patient needs a larger endotracheal tube. The EMT should check the cuff for leaks before attempting intubation. A **pilot balloon** is attached near the ventilation adapter to verify cuff inflation.

Endotracheal tubes have centimeter markings along the length of the tube, which the EMT can use to determine how far the tube has been inserted. Endotracheal tubes may be up to 33 cm in length for an adult. With orotracheal intubation, the tube is rarely inserted beyond 25 cm from the front teeth. On average, the following distances exist in an adult:

Teeth to cords	15 cm
Teeth to sternal notch	20 cm
Teeth to carina	25 cm

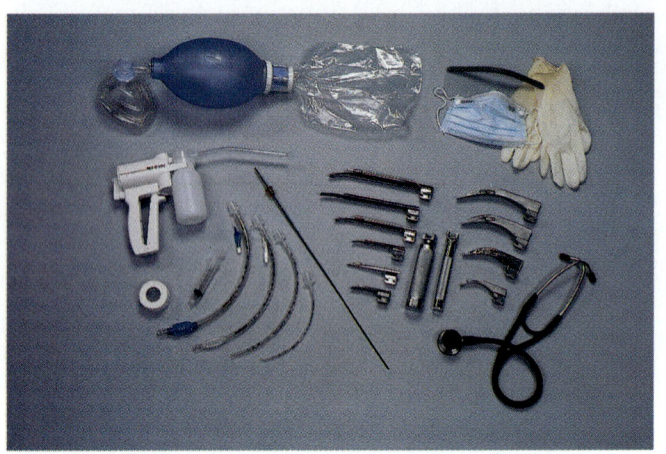

FIGURE 11.6 Equipment for endotracheal intubation.

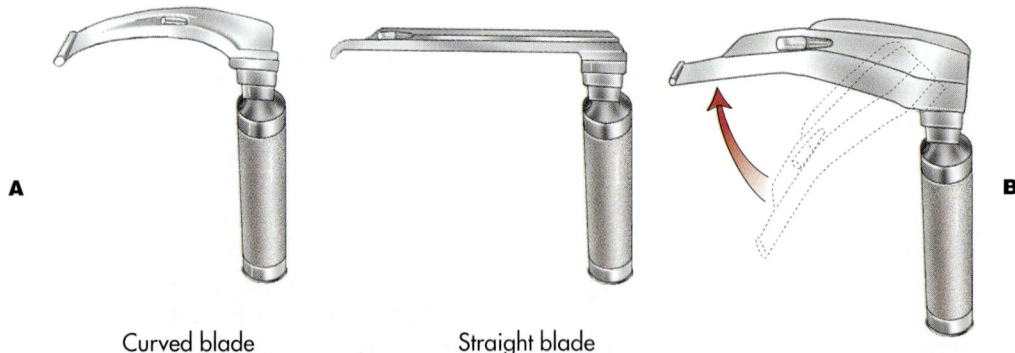

Curved blade   Straight blade

FIGURE 11.7 **A,** Laryngoscope handle and blades. Attach the laryngoscope blade to the handle. **B,** Lock the laryngoscope blade in place by aligning the notch of the blade with the locking bar of the handle. Elevating the blade to a right angle locks the blade in place and turns on the light.

Since the length of tube insertion is measured using centimeter markings at the front teeth, a helpful hint is to think "teeth and tube at 22." In most adults, proper endotracheal tube position is confirmed between 20 and 25 cm. Beyond 25 cm, main stem bronchus intubation, usually right, is likely.

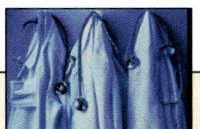

Physician Notes

In the phrase "average distances," the important term is "average." Some patients will have the tube in the right main stem bronchus at 19 cm. The EMT should perform careful auscultation to ensure correct placement.

A **stylet** is used to provide stiffness to the endotracheal tube during insertion (Figure 11.8, B). This allows the tube to be directed toward the vocal cords more easily. Stylets are malleable metal rods that are inserted into the endotracheal tube and molded to the desired shape for insertion, usually a gentle curve. They should not be inserted beyond the end of the endotracheal tube. A stylet that protrudes from the end of the endotracheal tube can injure airway structures during insertion. Other equipment needed for endotracheal intubation includes a suction unit, a 10 ml syringe for cuff inflation, water-soluble lubricant for the endotracheal tube and stylet, towels to raise the patient's **occiput** (back of the skull) for airway alignment (nontrauma patients only), and a securing device for the endotracheal tube (e.g., tape or a commercial securing device).

Adult Endotracheal Intubation

Anyone who performs endotracheal intubation must be familiar with the anatomy of the upper airway. Before intubating, the EMT should evaluate the general appearance of the patient. Possible barriers to intubation include loose dentures, large or displaced teeth, and stiffness in the neck and/or jaw caused by arthritis. All patients need to be ventilated with BLS skills before intubation. The EMT should assess the anatomy of the patient's upper airway during BLS ventilation to identify potential problems. If the EMT has difficulty inserting an airway adjunct

Box 11.2 Equipment Needed for Endotracheal Intubation

- Gloves
- Mask
- Goggles
- Laryngoscope blades and handle
- Assorted endotracheal tubes
- Stylet
- Water-soluble lubricant
- 10 ml syringe
- Tape and/or commercial securing device
- Towel
- Suction unit

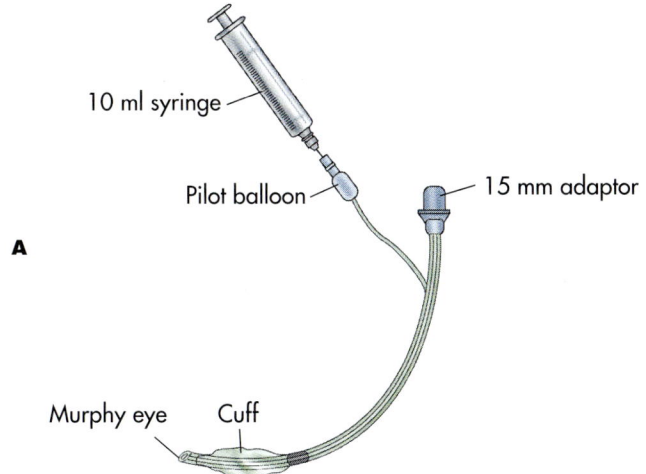
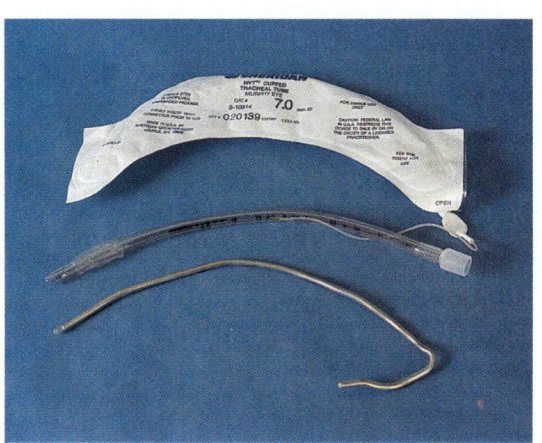

FIGURE 11.8 **A,** The endotracheal tube. **B,** A stylet is used to provide stiffness to the endotracheal tube during insertion.

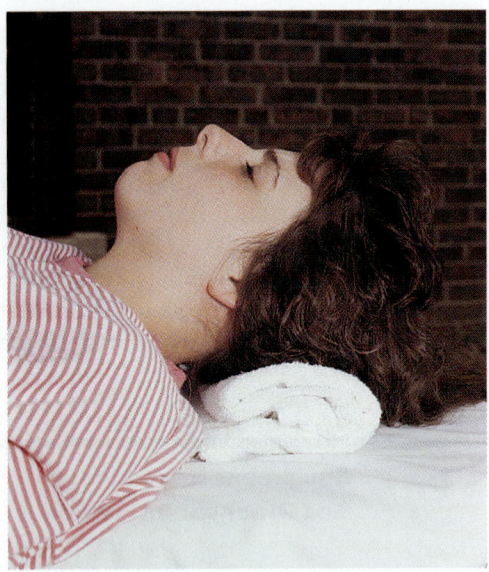

FIGURE 11.9 Sniffing position.

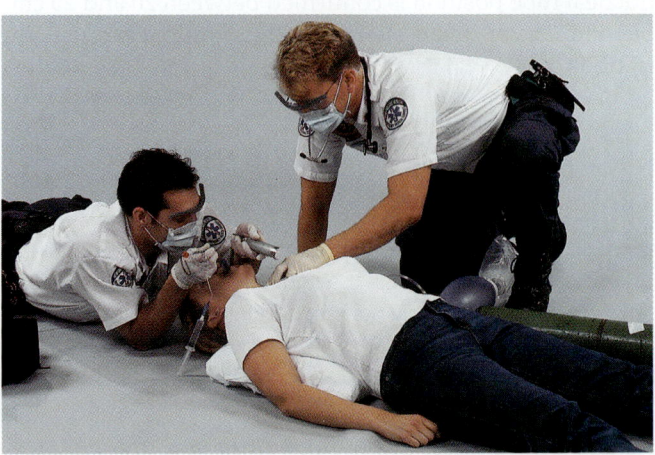

FIGURE 11.11 Prone intubation position. The EMT lies prone and supports the laryngoscope arm on the elbow.

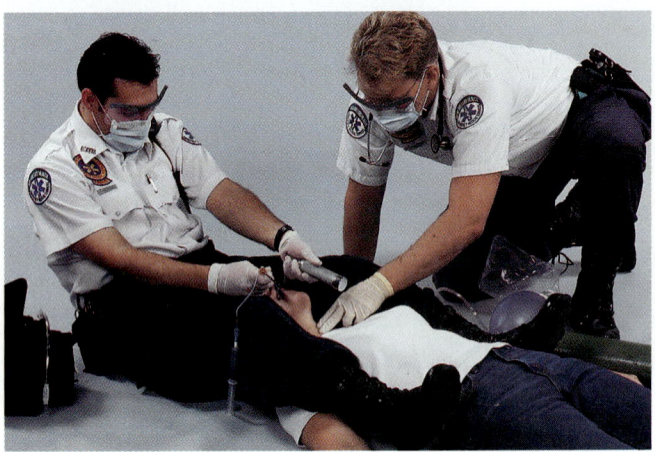

FIGURE 11.10 Sitting intubation position. The EMT holds the head tightly between the legs, leans back at a 45-degree angle to properly visualize the cords, and inserts the endotracheal tube into the trachea.

because of the anatomy of the mouth or because of arthritis in the jaw, endotracheal intubation will likely be difficult. Patients that grow beards frequently do so to disguise a "small chin." During the elevation of the mandible to visualize the cords, the mandible moves back rather than up. Extra lift or laryngeal compression may be required to properly see the opening in the trachea.

> ✓ The success of intubation depends on adequate preparation. Preparation includes having the proper equipment available and assessing the patient for anatomic barriers to intubation.

Before attempting endotracheal intubation, the EMT must take BSI precautions. The EMT should preoxygenate the patient using 100% oxygen and assisted ventilation and hyperventilate the patient during preoxygenation. The EMT should confirm the adequacy of assisted ventilation by listening to breath sounds and watching for chest rise. The EMT should assemble and test the equipment needed. Adequate preparation is paramount to successful endotracheal intubation. Specifically, the EMT should assemble the laryngoscope and check the light, check the cuff on the endotracheal tube for leaks, have a suction device readily available, and insert a stylet into the tube. One of the easiest steps to forget is inserting the stylet. It is extremely frustrating to have an adequate view of the vocal cords and not be able to insert the endotracheal tube because of its flexibility. Although it is not always needed, a stylet is usually helpful for endotracheal tube guidance.

Patient position. Patient position is an important component of successful endotracheal intubation. In non-trauma patients, the head is placed in the **sniffing position.** The neck is flexed and the head is extended at the base of the skull (Figure 11.9). This position provides the best alignment for vocal cord visualization. The sniffing position is obtained in a supine patient by placing a towel underneath the occiput. An alternative to this position is to place a towel or other support beneath the shoulders and hyperextend the neck.

Intubation in the field is more difficult that intubation in the hospital. In the field, the patient is frequently on the ground or floor. The patient is not usually at the correct height for the EMT to intubate as would be con-

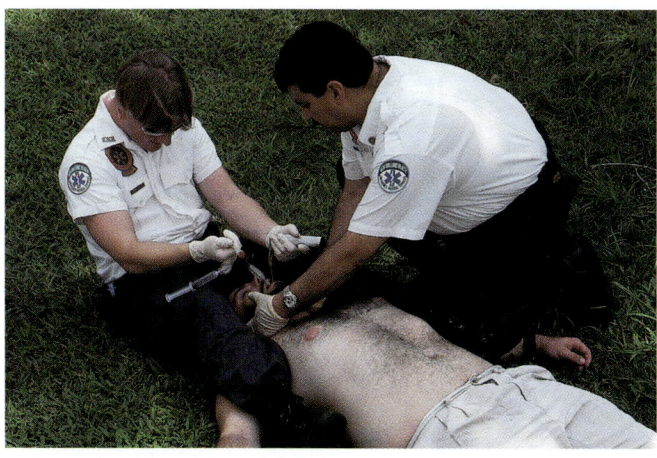
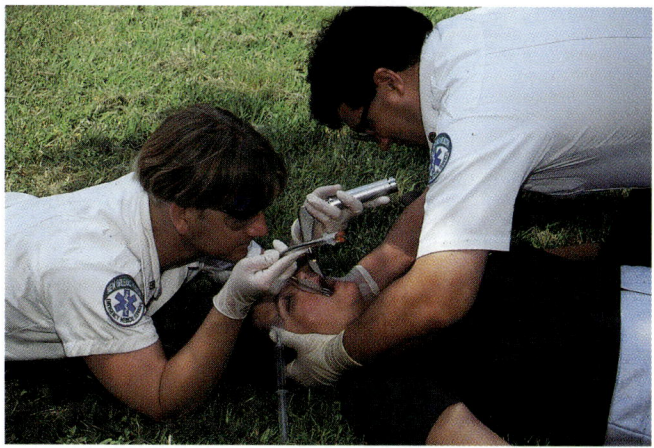

FIGURE 11.12 **A,** Sitting intubation position for trauma patient; note spinal immobilization. **B,** Prone intubation position for trauma patient; note spinal immobilization.

vient in the hospital or emergency department. Therefore the EMT must position himself or herself on the ground or floor so that the EMT's head is near the head of the patient yet allowing for the correct movment of the hands and arms of the EMT. The two postions most often used are as follows:

1. The EMT sits on the ground with one leg over each of the patient's arms and gently moves forward until the patient's head can be secured high between his or her thighs. The EMT applies firm pressure with the thighs to the sides of the patient's head. The grip of two EMTs will keep the head from moving about or rotating to hyperextension during intubation. In Figure 11.10, EMT #1 supports the patient's head with his thighs and begins to position the laryngoscope. If the EMT leans back at about a 45-degree angle, the cords are more easily visualized. EMT #2 provides pressure on the trachea **(Sellick maneuver).**
2. Figure 11.11 shows EMT #1 in the prone position at the patient's head. EMT #1 intubates the patient while EMT #2 provides tracheal pressure (Sellick maneuver).

In trauma patients, the EMT must maintain in-line neutral cervical spine immobilization. This added challenge makes endotracheal intubation even more difficult (Figure 11.12).

Laryngscope. The laryngoscope is designed to be held in the left hand. The blade is inserted into the right corner of the mouth, taking care not to damage the teeth or soft tissues. The tongue is swept to the left with the laryngoscope blade. This step is critical. If the tongue is not displaced, the vocal cords will not be visualized. After displacing the tongue, the blade is inserted to the proper anatomic landmark. For the curved blade, this is the vallecula (Figure 11.13, A). The straight blade directly lifts the epiglottis for vocal cord visualization (Figure 11.13, B). A helpful hint when using the straight blade is to initially insert the blade to the uvula, then attempt to lift the epiglottis after the tongue has been displaced. A common mistake with the straight blade is to insert the blade too far, which makes landmarks difficult to find.

Intubation procedure. Figure 11.14 illustrates the steps of endotracheal intubation. After insertion, the tongue and mandible are lifted up and away from the patient using the laryngoscope. This should lift the epiglottis and reveal the vocal cords. The EMT must not to use the patient's teeth as a fulcrum, since this can damage them and eliminate the space needed to pass the endotracheal tube through the mouth. Once the glottic opening is visualized, the EMT should not take his or her eyes off of the vocal cords if possible. An assistant should hand the endotracheal tube to the EMT, who should gently pass it through the glottic opening. The EMT should insert the tube so that the cuff just passes the vocal cords. The EMT should visualize the endotracheal tube passing between the vocal cords—this is the most effective way of confirming tube placement. The EMT should record the length markings on the tube at the upper front teeth.

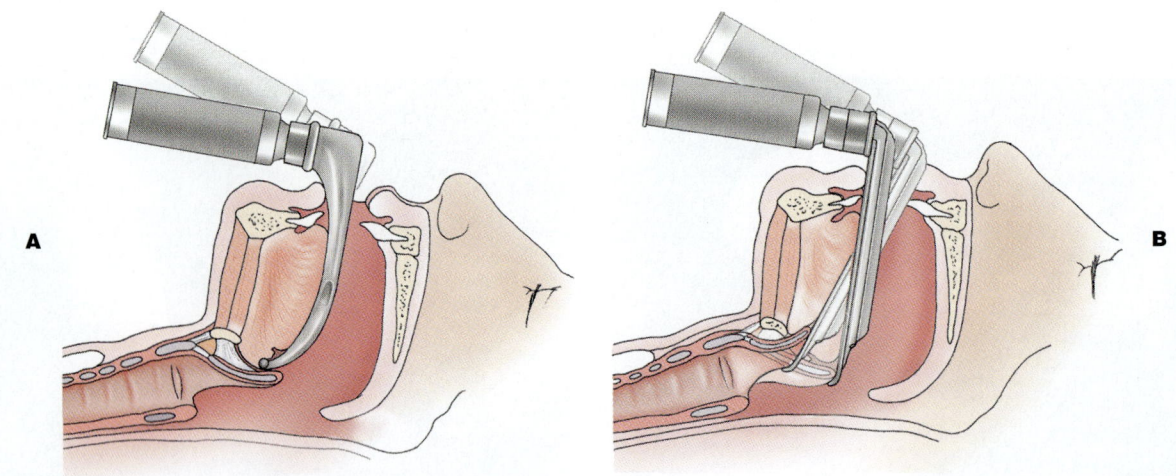

FIGURE 11.13 **A,** The curved blade is inserted into the vallecula. **B,** The straight blade directly lifts the epiglottis.

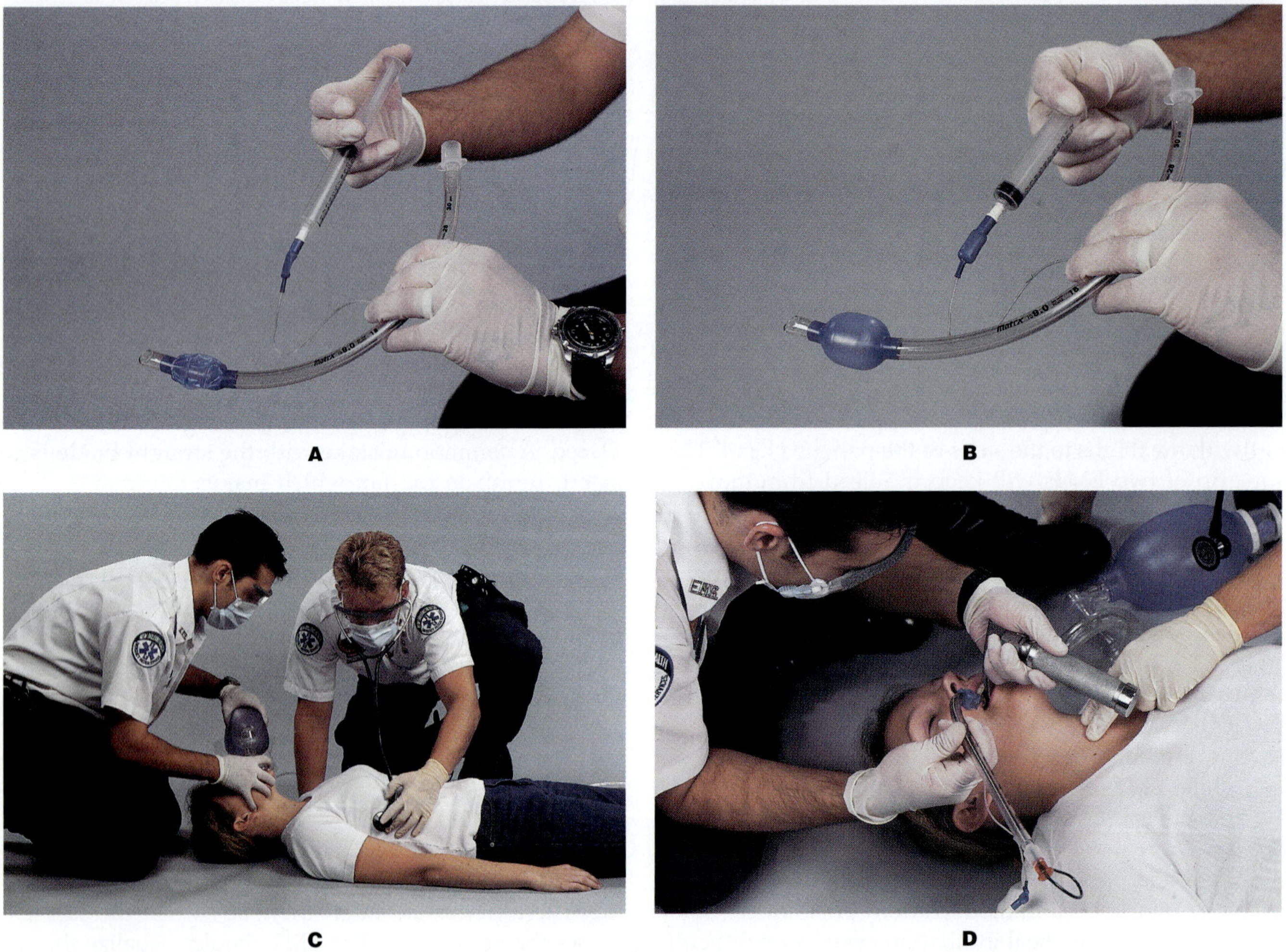

FIGURE 11.14 **A** and **B,** Assemble and check all equipment. **C,** Hyperventilate the patient with 100% oxygen. Position the patient's head and neck. **D,** With the laryngoscope held in the left hand, insert the blade into the right side of the mouth, displacing the tongue to the left.

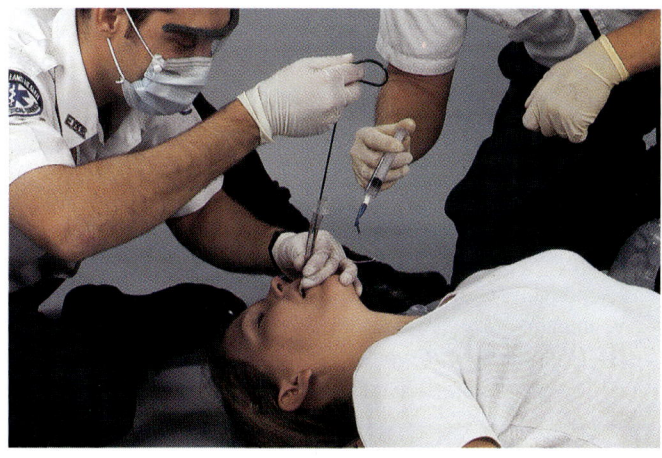

E

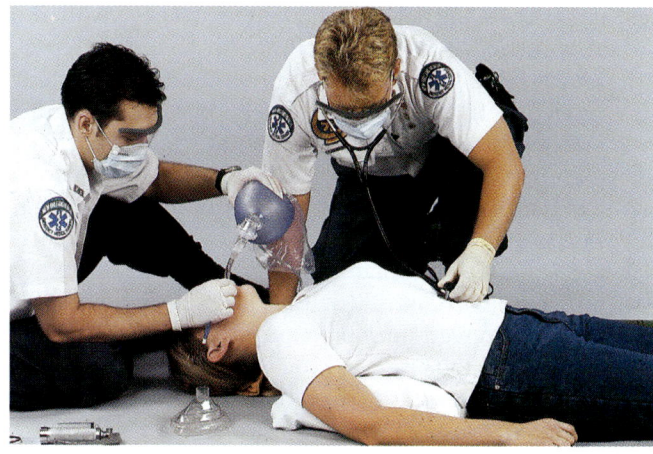

F

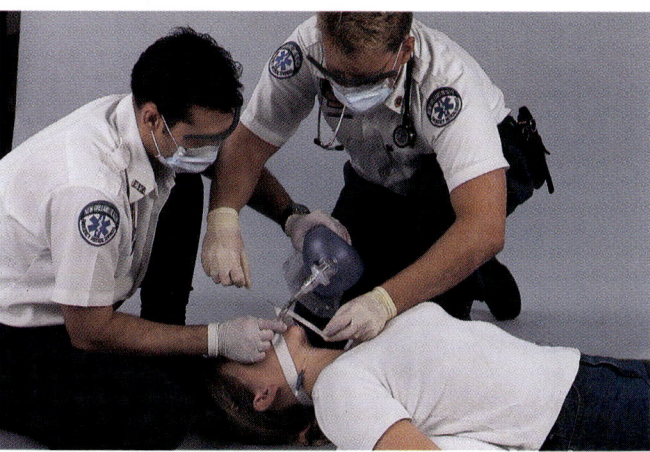

G

FIGURE 11.14, cont'd **E,** Advance the endotracheal tube through the right corner of the mouth and through the vocal cords. **F,** Inflate the endotracheal tube cuff, remove the stylet, and ventilate the patient. **G,** Confirm placement of the tube by auscultating the epigastrium and lungs. Secure the tube in place if proper placement is confirmed.

After passing the endotracheal tube between the cords, the EMT should remove the laryngoscope carefully. Again, the teeth and soft structures of the mouth can be damaged if the laryngoscope is removed too quickly. The EMT should remove the stylet from the endotracheal tube and inflate the cuff with 5 to 10 ml of air. The tube must be held in place until its position has been confirmed and it has been secured. The EMT's partner should attach a BVM and begin assisted ventilation.

The Sellick maneuver can be used to help prevent passive regurgitation and aspiration during endotracheal intubation. This maneuver, discussed in Chapter 10, involves applying pressure to the cricoid cartilage. The Sellick maneuver may also assist in vocal cord visualization, although thyroid cartilage pressure may be more helpful in this respect (see Figures 11.10 and 11.11).

Confirming endotracheal tube placement. Perhaps the most important component of endotracheal intubation is confirming tube position. Anyone who regularly performs this skill has occasionally intubated the esophagus. Though undesirable, esophageal intubation by itself is not a life-threatening complication. On the other hand, *unrecognized* esophageal intubation is fatal. Therefore it is important that the EMT be skillful in the process of confirming endotracheal tube position. If an EMT cannot confirm that a tube is in the trachea, he or she should remove it and ventilate the patient with BLS skills. The following steps help the EMT confirm correct endotracheal tube placement:

1. Confirm that the tube enters the trachea by visualizing it as it passes between the vocal cords.
2. Observe for chest rise and fall with each assisted ventilation.

> ✓ Successful endotracheal intubation in the adult is dependent on adequate preparation, proper patient position, and detailed knowledge of upper airway anatomy. To be successful in the field, consistent practice is required.

3. Auscultate the lateral and anterior chest wall for breath sounds bilaterally. If breath sounds are present on one side but not on the other, a main stem bronchus intubation has likely occurred (Figure 11.15). This usually occurs on the right side, and therefore breath sounds are absent on the left until the tube is withdrawn from the bronchus. In this case, note the length marking on the tube at the upper front teeth, deflate the cuff, and slowly pull the tube back 1 to 2 cm. Auscultate breath sounds as the tube is removed until they are equal bilaterally.
4. Listen over the **epigastrium**, where only faint transmitted breath sounds should be heard during ventilation. If loud gurgling breath sounds are heard over the epigastrium, an esophageal intubation has probably occurred and the tube should be removed immediately.
5. Look for condensation inside the endotracheal tube.
6. Assess presence of CO_2 in expired air.

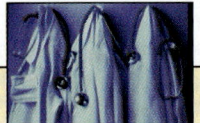
Physician Notes

As in many medical situations, there are principles and preferences. The *principle* here is that both lungs and the epigastrium should be auscultated. The order in which this is done is ones personal *preference*.

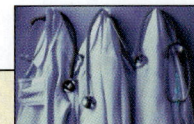
Physician Notes

The first steps that should always be done after endotracheal intubation are as follows:

R—Recognition that the tube has passed through the cords
I—Inflation (rise) and deflation (fall) of the chest during ventilation
S—Sounds of air movement in both lung fields
E—Epigastrium auscultation (no air sounds)

The following are other signs that indicate proper placement of the chest tube:

- Expired CO_2 detection device
- Esophageal intubation detection device
- Pulse oximeter

When the tube is in the trachea, CO_2 is exhaled with each breath. The CO_2 exhaled at the end of each expiration is called **end-tidal carbon dioxide** (ETCO$_2$) and can be measured as a method of verifying endotracheal tube placement. Commercial ETCO$_2$ detectors are placed directly on the endotracheal tube during assisted ventilation (Figure 11.16). If ETCO$_2$ is present, a color change occurs in the detector. Quantitative ETCO$_2$ detectors

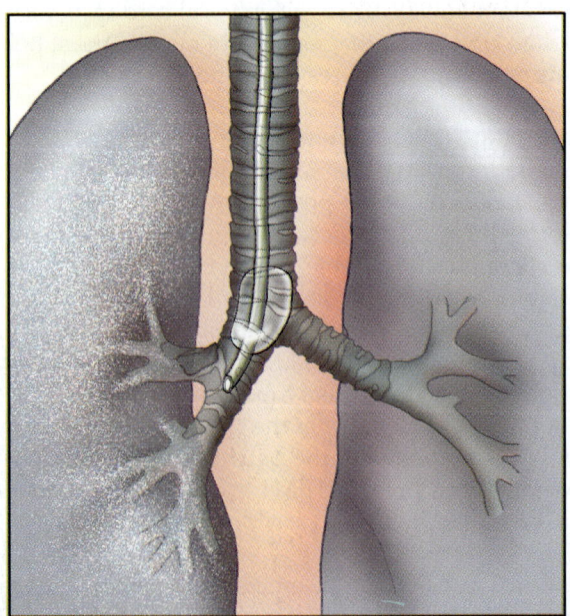
FIGURE 11.15 After intubation, if breath sounds are present on one side but not the other, a mainstem bronchus intubation has likely occurred. This usually occurs on the right side.

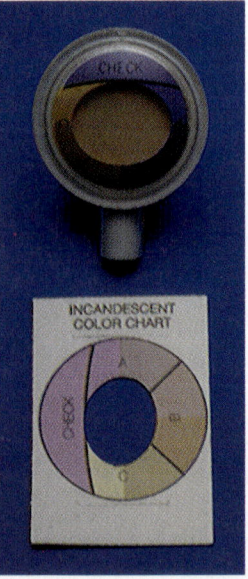
FIGURE 11.16 A qualitative end-tidal CO_2 detector.

measure and report a specific pressure of $ETCO_2$. $ETCO_2$ monitoring is a routine technique in the operating room. It is now being used to verify endotracheal tube position in other settings as well, including prehospital care.

Another method used to help verify proper endotracheal tube position is placement of an **esophageal intubation detection device** on the end of the tube. This can be a self-inflating bulb or a commercially available syringe. The principle that underlies this device is that if the tube is in the trachea, air can be aspirated freely. If the tube is in the esophagus, the wall of the collapsible esophagus is drawn against the tip of the endotracheal tube by the negative pressure of the self-inflating bulb or syringe. Therefore air cannot be withdrawn with the syringe or the self-inflating bulb does not reexpand.

Another method of confirming endotracheal tube position is to reinsert the laryngoscope blade and visualize the tube in the glottic opening. This technique is helpful when the environment is too loud to hear breath sounds. When using this technique, the EMT must not dislodge the tube with the laryngoscope blade. After confirming proper endotracheal tube position, the EMT should secure the tube in place and ventilate the patient at an age-appropriate rate. The EMT can insert an oropharyngeal airway to serve as a bite block (i.e., to prevent the patient from biting on the tube and causing airway obstruction).

> ✓ Confirmation of endotracheal tube placement is best done by visualizing the endotracheal tube as it passes between the vocal cords. Other techniques for verifying placement include auscultating over the lungs and epigastrium, watching for chest rise, and using devices such as $ETCO_2$ detectors or esophageal intubation detection devices.

No one sign or test is 100% reliable. At least three should be used, but more is better. Each time the position of the endotracheal tube is changed or the patient is repositioned, the EMT should use at least three of these methods to recheck the position and document (Box 11.3).

If the EMT cannot successfully intubate the trachea, there are various methods to continue to manage the airway. There is not a true standard currently in use. Some options are a multilumen airway (MLA), continued assisted airway management with a BVM, oral airway, and a combination of these. Many medical directors choose to have EMT-Bs trained to insert MLAs to control the airway and protect against initial or recurrent regurgitation of gastric contents. The esophageal-tracheal tube (Combitube) is an example of such a device. These devices are not included in the curriculum, but many systems will include them and therefore require training in their use, especially in situations in which attempts at endotracheal intubation fail. Therefore Combitube is discussed briefly in this section.

Combitube is an alternative airway device that can be used as a primary airway or in cases of failed endotracheal intubation. The Combitube is a double-lumen ventilation tube that can be inserted without direct visualization of the airway. The device has two inflatable cuffs (Figure 11.17). The larger (pharyngeal) cuff, when inflated, provides an airway seal, whereas the other, at the tip of the tube, occludes the esophagus. Should the tube enter the trachea, this cuff acts as an endotracheal tube cuff. Thus this device minimizes the risk of aspiration of gastric contents and permits ventilation without the need for a mask seal. There are two ventilation ports on the Combitube; therefore the device can be used for assisted ventilation when inserted into either the trachea or the esophagus. Further training with this airway is required before attempting its use in the field. The pharyngeal-tracheal lumen (PTL) airway is a

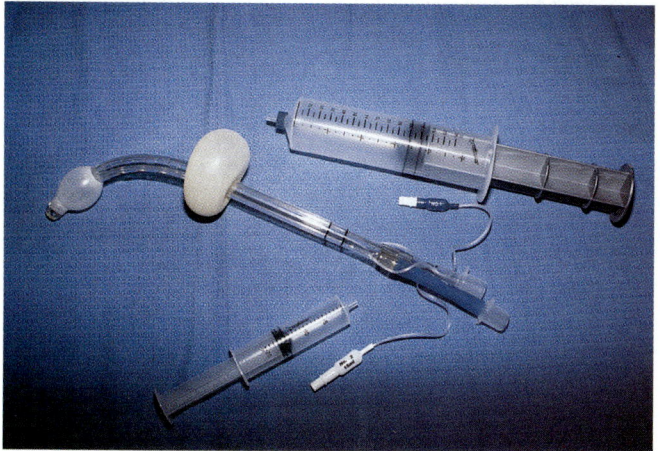

FIGURE 11.17 The esophageal-tracheal Combitube, shown with both the pharyngeal and distal cuffs inflated. There are two ventilation ports, one for esophageal placement and one for tracheal placement.

> **Box 11.3 Confirming Endotracheal Tube Placement**
>
> - Visualize the tube as it passes through the vocal cords
> - Auscultate breath sounds
> - Auscultate over the epigastrium
> - Watch for chest rise and fall
> - End-tidal carbon dioxide
> - Moisture condensation inside tube
> - Esophageal detection device
> - Pulse oximeter

device similar in design and function, although somewhat more complicated to use.

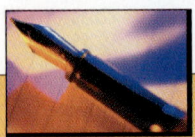

Tips from the Pros

- When inserting a straight blade during intubation, initially insert the blade to the uvula, then sweep the tongue to the left. The easiest mistake to make with a straight blade is inserting the blade too far.
- If the tongue is not adequately swept to the left with the laryngoscope blade, reposition the patient and attempt to move the tongue again. It is pointless to even attempt to look for the vocal cords if the tongue has not been moved out of the way.
- The key to intubating is to have everything prepared *before* the attempt is made. The easiest steps to forget are placing a stylet in the endotracheal tube and properly positioning the patient. It is easy to become rushed and settle for an inadequate patient position. Taking a little extra time to place the patient in the sniffing position with the occiput elevated will probably decrease the overall time needed to place the endotracheal tube.
- Another trick for confirming endotracheal tube placement is to watch for vapor condensation in the tube when the patient exhales. If the tube is in the trachea, saturated air from the lungs may condense during exhalation. This condensation is helpful when present; however, it is not always present, even when the tube is in the trachea. This method is not as reliable as the other methods of confirming endotracheal tube placement.
- When checking the laryngoscope light, think "bright, white, and tight." The bulb must be working properly before attempting to intubate.
- It may be useful to hold your breath as you attempt to intubate. If you have to take a breath during insertion, then the patient has to take a breath too. If the patient has not been intubated at this point, stop and hyperventilate the patient before continuing intubation attempts.

Infant and Child Endotracheal Intubation

Infants and children are not simply "little adults," and special consideration must be taken for endotracheal intubation in this age group. Anatomically, the cricoid cartilage is the narrowest part of the airway in infants and children; therefore endotracheal tube size should be based on the cricoid ring rather than the glottic opening. Also, it is difficult to obtain a single visual plane from the mouth through the pharynx to the glottic opening for endotracheal intubation because of the relatively larger tongue and the small, anterior larynx.

When selecting equipment, a straight blade is often preferred for intubating infants because of better tongue displacement and vocal cord visualization. In older children the curved blade is used because its broad base and flange provide better control and displacement of the tongue. Appropriate endotracheal tube size is much more variable in children; therefore it is best to have a chart available for assistance. A tube with a 3 to 3.5 mm internal diameter (ID) is used for newborns and small infants. A tube with a 4 mm ID is used in infants up to 1 year of age. The following formula is useful for selecting endotracheal tube size in children:

$$\text{Endotracheal tube size} = \frac{16 + \text{Age in years}}{4}$$

Another method for estimating endotracheal tube size is to use the size of the infant's little finger as an estimate. The EMT must have a range of sizes available in case he or she encounters difficulties with placement.

In children younger than 8 years of age, uncuffed endotracheal tubes are used. The narrow ring of the cricoid cartilage provides a functional cuff around the tube in this age group. Most endotracheal tubes used in infants and children have a vocal cord marker that is used to ensure placement of the tip of the tube in the midtrachea. The tubes also have centimeter markings to document length of insertion. The following guidelines can be used for insertion length from midtrachea to teeth:

6 mo to 1 yr	12 cm
2 yr	14 cm
4 to 6 yr	16 cm
6 to 10 yr	18 cm
10 to 12 yr	20 cm

To perform endotracheal intubation in infants and children, the EMT should align the patient's head to allow visualization of the vocal cords. The EMT can visualize the vocal cords with a laryngoscope if the child is in a head-tilt/chin-lift position. If the vocal cords cannot be visualized, the EMT can place a towel under the child's shoulders and make a second and final attempt at intubation. If the EMT suspects trauma, he or she must maintain the cervical spine in a neutral position. Little force is needed to intubate infants and children. The EMT must take care not to damage upper airway structures with the laryngoscope.

The best method for confirming endotracheal tube position is visualizing the tube as it passes between the vocal cords. In infants and children, the symmetric rise and fall of the chest during assisted ventilation is an important verification of tube placement because breath sounds can be misleading. The EMT should auscultate over the epigastrium and both lung fields. The heart rate and skin color of the patient should also improve after endotracheal intubation provided the patient has a perfusing cardiac output. If the tube is in the proper place but adequate lung expansion does not occur, the tube may be too small and an air leak may be present at the glottic opening. If auscultation at the neck reveals a loud air leak, the tube should be replaced with a larger tube, perhaps one with a cuff if the child is older than 8 years of age. Other reasons for inadequate lung expansion include BVM dysfunction and inadequate assisted breaths by the ventilator.

> **Physician Notes**
>
> Overinflation of the lungs in a pediatric patient is easy to do since much less volume is required than in an adult. The EMT should pay careful attention to this difference.

✓ Endotracheal intubation in infants and children requires careful selection of proper endotracheal tube size, knowledge of anatomic structures, and careful technique to avoid damaging airway structures.

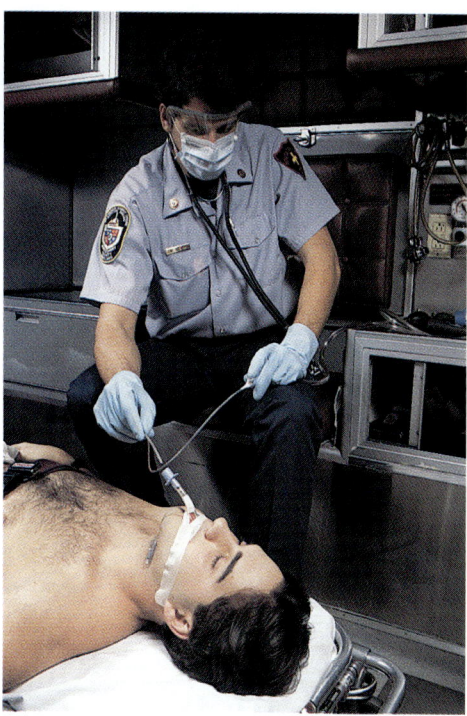

FIGURE 11.18 To perform endotracheal suctioning, a sterile flexible suction catheter is inserted without suction to about the level of the carina. The catheter is then withdrawn with suction using a twisting motion.

Endotracheal Suctioning

Once an endotracheal tube is in place, the EMT can suction the patient's lower airway. Although this gives the advantage of clearing deep secretions from the lower airway, there are complications from suctioning through an endotracheal tube. Patients may have arrhythmias, hypoxia, or bronchospasm from airway stimulation. Also, the catheter may stimulate the cough reflex and cause damage to the mucosa of the respiratory tree.

At the time that endotracheal intubation is complicated, there may be debris, vomitus, blood, or other secretions that block the visualization of the cords and the laryngeal opening. The EMT can remove these obstructions with a yanker suction tip and the unit suction. These obstructions can be voluminous, especially if the patient vomits when the laryngoscope is inserted. The available suction should be strong enough to remove this material quickly.

Indications for endotracheal suctioning include the presence of obvious secretions or the development of poor **compliance** while ventilating with a BVM device. When the lungs become less compliant, they are more stiff, and more pressure is required for inspiration. To perform endotracheal suctioning, the EMT should hyperventilate the patient for preoxygenation using sterile technique. The EMT inserts a sterile flexible suction catheter without suction to about the level of the carina. The EMT then withdraws the catheter with suction using a twisting motion (Figure 11.18).

Automated Transport Ventilators

After endotracheal intubation, the EMT must maintain assisted ventilation. The standard BLS devices used for performing assisted ventilation are the BVM and the flow-restricted oxygen-powered ventilator. Both of these devices can provide adequate assisted ventilation. **Automated transport ventilators** (ATVs) are alternative devices for ventilating intubated patients (Figure 11.19). These devices are oxygen-powered ventilators with settings for tidal volume and respiratory frequency. They provide a set tidal volume of 100% oxygen during a predetermined inspiratory cycle time. The use of an ATV frees the EMT from manually ventilating the patient. Although the EMT does not have to directly ventilate the patient, he or she must monitor the ATV closely to ensure proper function. The EMT should auscultate breath sounds frequently and observe the patient for symmetric chest rise. ATVs are useful devices for delivering consistent minute ventilation in intubated patients. They can

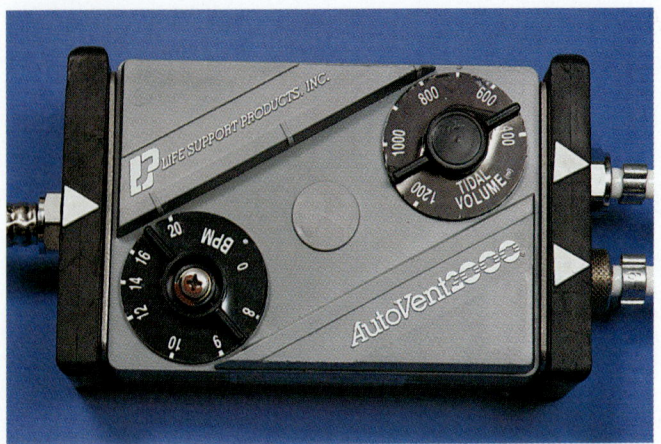

FIGURE 11.19 Automatic transport ventilators have settings for tidal volume and respiratory frequency.

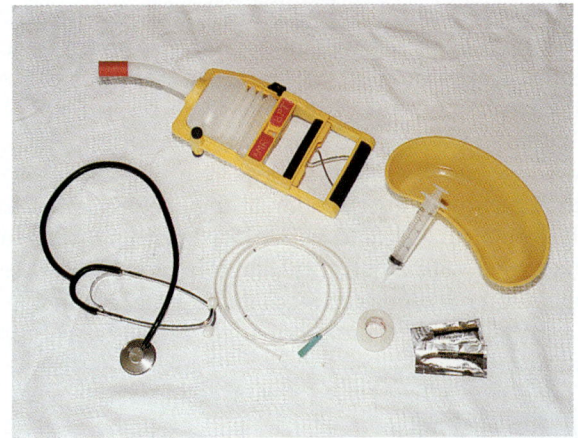

FIGURE 11.20 Equipment for nasogastric tube placement.

also be used during chest compressions, which makes cardiopulmonary resuscitation (CPR) easier to perform.

Nasogastric Tube Placement

A **nasogastric (NG) tube** is used for stomach and proximal small bowel decompression, medication administration, nutrition, and gastric lavage. Gastric lavage is a process in which the stomach is flushed with fluid and then emptied, and it is used to prevent absorption of ingested substances or to control bleeding. The NG tube is placed through the nose and esophagus into the stomach. Once in place, it can be connected to a suction device for stomach decompression.

An NG tube is indicated when gastric distention makes assisted ventilation difficult. Decompression of the stomach in this setting improves ventilation by decreasing pressure below the diaphragm and decreases the risk of vomiting and aspiration of gastric contents. An NG tube should be placed after the patient has been successfully intubated. Although stomach decompression is helpful during assisted ventilation, airway control takes priority over NG tube placement.

A contraindication for NG tube placement in the field is the presence of major facial trauma and/or the possibility of a basilar skull fracture (see Chapter 24). An NG tube placed in a patient with facial and skull fractures may penetrate a fracture of the cribriform plate and enter the cranial cavity, producing brain damage. In patients with suspected skull or facial fractures, the NG tube should be placed through the mouth (i.e., an **orogastric tube**) to decompress the stomach. Other complications of NG tube placement include tracheal intubation, nasal trauma, and vomiting.

The equipment needed for NG tube placement includes an NG tube, 20 ml syringe, water-soluble lubricant, stethoscope, suction unit with tubing, tape, and emesis basin (Figure 11.20). Nasogastric tubes are available in several sizes, designated by the French catheter size system. In the French system, the diameter increases as the number increases. The following sizes are appropriate:

Age	French size
Newborn/infant	8
Toddler/preschooler	10
School-age child	12
Adolescent/adult	14 to 16

To insert an NG tube, the tube should be measured from the tip of the nose, around the ear, to below the xiphoid process (Figure 11.21, *A*). The end of the tube is lubricated, and the patient is placed in a supine position with the head turned to the left side in anticipation of emesis. If trauma is suspected, the cervical spine must be maintained in a neutral position. The tube is inserted along the floor of the nose and passed until the measured length has been inserted. If the tube cannot be passed in one nostril, the other nostril should be used. If no trauma is involved, slight flexion of the neck often helps guide the NG tube into the esophagus. When the tube enters the stomach, a return of gastric contents is usually seen. To confirm NG tube placement, 10 to 20 ml of air should be injected into the NG tube while auscultating (listening with a stethoscope) over the epigastrium (Figure 11.21, *B*). The EMT should easily hear the air as it enters the stomach. Water should not be used to confirm placement because the NG tube may have inadvertently entered the lungs. If position cannot be confirmed, the NG tube should be removed. After confirming placement, the tube

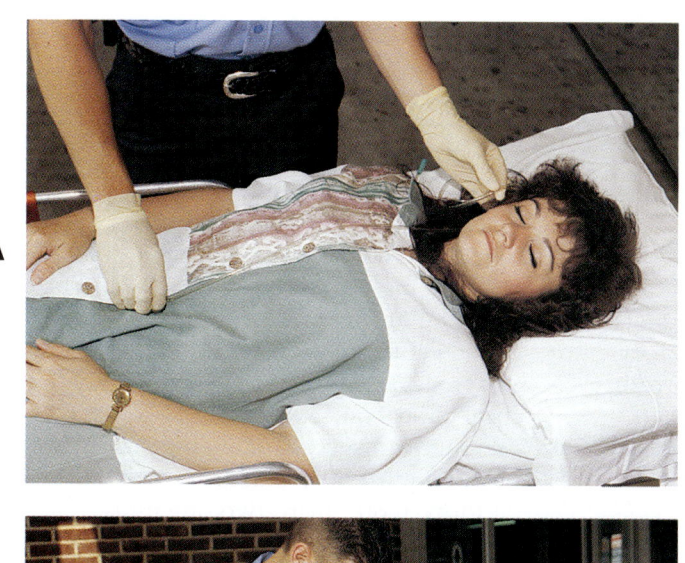
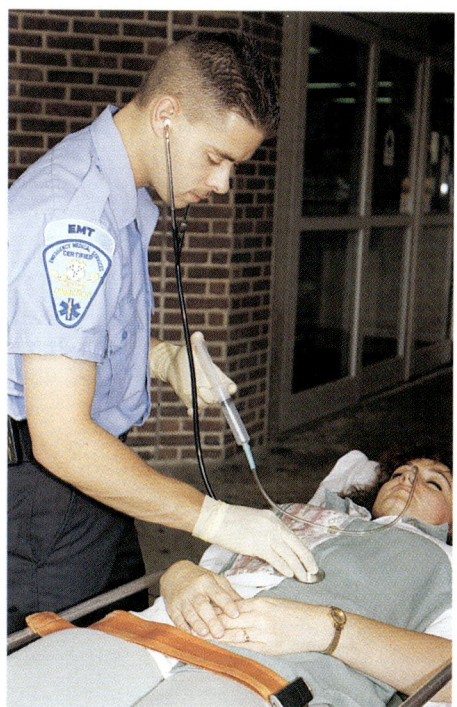
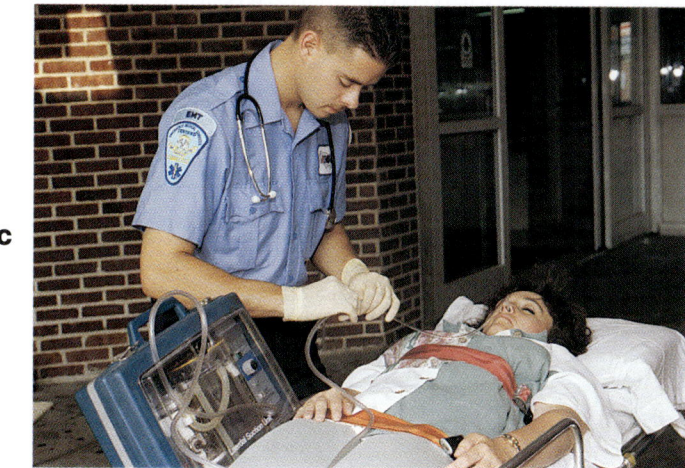

FIGURE 11.21 **A,** Nasogastric (NG) tube placement. The NG tube is measured from the nose and the ear to below the xiphoid process. **B,** To confirm NG placement, the EMT injects air with a syringe while listening over the epigastrium. **C,** The NG tube is secured in place and connected to suction.

is secured in place with tape and low intermittent suction is applied for gastric decompression (Figure 11.21, C).

Advance Directives

An **advance directive** is a document that a patient prepares regarding his or her wishes for medical care and other issues should he or she become unable to make decisions. A **living will** is an example of an advance directive. Many patients have living wills that specify the interventions they wish to receive in the event of an emergency such as cardiac arrest. Often, these living wills state that the patient does not want to be intubated and/or resuscitated in the event of a cardiac arrest. The EMT is often placed in a difficult situation because the document may not be immediately available when the emergency occurs. If there is any question about the patient's wishes, the EMT should attempt to perform all the interventions that are indicated for proper patient care. If the patient's wishes are clearly against endotracheal intubation or other resuscitative measures, the EMT should respect the patient's wishes and not perform the interventions. To be sure of the patient's wishes, it is helpful to see the actual document that outlines what the patient wants. This material is covered in detail in Chapter 3.

Summary

- Endotracheal intubation by EMT-Bs is a challenging procedure that requires thorough initial training, frequent practice, and dedicated supervision by the EMS medical director and the local supervising authority for EMS.
- Many critically ill and injured patients require advanced airway management. Since the EMT-B is often the first to arrive, endotracheal intubation by EMTs has the potential for improving patient care and outcomes.
- Endotracheal intubation is the definitive airway in the apneic patient; however, ventilation takes priority over intubation.
- The EMT who is unable to intubate a patient must recognize this problem and promptly return to BLS assisted ventilation for transportation.
- Endotracheal intubation can be a lifesaving procedure; however, it also has significant potential complications. The two most serious complications of endotracheal intubation are unrecognized esophageal intubation and hypoxia from prolonged unsuccessful intubation attempts.
- Anyone who performs this skill regularly has intubated the esophagus. The critical skill needed by the EMT is the ability to recognize an esophageal intubation when it occurs. The best way to avoid this complication is to visualize the endotracheal tube as it passes between the vocal cords. Listening to breath sounds, watching for chest rise, documenting end-tidal carbon dioxide ($ETCO_2$), or using esophageal intubation detection devices are other methods for confirming a tracheal intubation.
- Prolonged unsuccessful attempts at endotracheal intubation must be avoided. A single EMT should not perform more than two attempts. Each attempt should be no longer than 30 seconds and should be preceded with preoxygenation by hyperventilation.
- An NG tube can be used to decompress the stomach after a patient has been successfully intubated.
- Some patients have advance directives, such as living wills, that indicate a desire not to be intubated. The EMT should act according to local protocols for managing patients with living wills.

Scenario Solution

You should insert an oropharyngeal airway. The patient requires ventilation with 100% oxygen using a technique such as BVM ventilation. These interventions are BLS procedures. If you do nothing more for this patient, you already may have saved the patient's life.

The indications for advanced airway management in this patient include slow spontaneous ventilations, unresponsiveness, and the risk of vomiting with aspiration of gastric contents. This patient clearly cannot control his own airway. The definitive airway in this patient is an endotracheal tube.

No apparent contraindications for endotracheal intubation exist in this patient. The only possible contraindication at this point is an advance directive by the patient that clearly documents a desire not to be intubated. However, the patient's age makes this unlikely. You should assume that the patient desires a full resuscitation unless told otherwise by family members.

While preoxygenating the patient with BLS assisted ventilation, you should set up for endotracheal intubation, including inspection of the needed equipment. You should place the patient's head in the sniffing position and proceed with endotracheal intubation, visualizing the tube as it is passed between the vocal cords. You should confirm tube position by listening to breath sounds, watching for chest rise, and documenting end-tidal carbon dioxide or using an esophageal intubation detection device. You should ventilate the patient en route to the medical facility using a BVM or an automated transport ventilator.

Key Terms

Advance directive A legally binding document prepared and signed by an individual that clearly states his or her personal wishes regarding implementation of lifesaving techniques in the event that the individual is severely injured or terminally ill and cannot make decisions at that time.

Arytenoid cartilage Small structures that serve as the posterior attachments for the vocal cords; located behind the glottic opening on each side of the larynx

Automated transport ventilators Oxygen-powered devices with settings for tidal volume and respiratory frequency designed to provide assisted ventilation for intubated patients.

Compliance When used to describe the lungs, this term refers to the relative stiffness of the lungs. As compliance decreases, the lungs become more stiff and difficult to ventilate.

Endotracheal tube A specialized tube designed to definitively control the airway. The tube has a cuff that is inflated in the trachea to prevent aspiration and improve oxygenation.

Endotracheal tube cuff A small balloon that is inflated with 5 to 10 ml of air to prevent aspiration around the endotracheal tube; it should be checked for leaks before insertion.

End-tidal carbon dioxide The carbon dioxide that is exhaled with each breath. After endotracheal intubation, documenting the presence of end-tidal carbon dioxide helps confirm tube position.

Epigastrium The area between the umbilicus and the xiphoid process. The EMT auscultates in this area after endotracheal intubation to ensure that an esophageal intubation has not occurred.

Esophageal intubation detection device A specially designed syringe or a self-inflating bulb used to determine whether air can be aspirated freely; used to help confirm correct endotracheal tube placement.

Extubation The process of removing an endotracheal tube. If a patient becomes more responsive after endotracheal intubation, he or she may attempt self-extubation because of discomfort.

Glottic opening The opening between the vocal cords through which an endotracheal tube is passed.

Hypoxia A condition in which the patient has a shortage of oxygen at the cellular level. Signs and symptoms of hypoxia include dyspnea, restlessness, confusion, lethargy, and poor skin color.

Laryngoscope The instrument used to visualize the vocal cords for endotracheal tube insertion; it has two parts: a handle and a blade.

Living will A legal document, signed and witnessed, outlining the types of medical interventions that may or may not be implemented on the signer who may or may not have been diagnosed with a terminal or permanently disabling injury or medical condition.

Nasogastric (NG) tube A tube that is placed through the nose and esophagus into the stomach; can be used for gastric decompression, medication administration, nutrition, or gastric lavage.

Nasotracheal intubation A type of endotracheal intubation in which the tube is passed through the nose and into the trachea; performed only by advanced life support personnel in patients who are breathing.

Occiput Posterior part of the skull that rests on the ground when a patient is supine; a towel is placed under the occiput to put the patient in the sniffing position.

Orogastric tube The same tube as used for nasogastric insertion, only placed through the mouth instead of the nose; orogastric route is required in patients with suspected facial or skull fractures.

Pilot balloon The small balloon near the adapter end of the endotracheal tube that verifies inflation of the endotracheal tube cuff.

Preoxygenation The process of hyperventilating a patient with 100% oxygen before attempting endotracheal intubation; should occur before each attempt.

Sellick maneuver Maneuver designed to prevent passive aspiration during artificial ventilation; performed by applying posterior pressure to the cricoid cartilage.

Sniffing position The desired patient position for endotracheal intubation; the patient's neck is flexed slightly and the head is extended at the base of the skull.

Stylet A malleable metal rod that is inserted into the endotracheal tube to provide stiffness for intubation; it should not extend beyond the tracheal end of the tube during insertion.

Uvula The small grapelike structure made of soft tissue that hangs from the roof of the mouth just in front of the oropharynx.

Vallecula The valley formed between the base of the tongue and the pharyngeal surface of the epiglottis; the curved laryngoscope blade is inserted into the vallecula during endotracheal intubation.

Xiphoid process The small bony structure located between the costal margins at the lower end of the sternum; used as a landmark for chest compressions and nasogastric tube insertion.

Review Questions

1. Which of the following is incorrect regarding the vallecula?
   a. It is a valley between the base of the tongue and the pharyngeal surface of the epiglottis.
   b. It cannot be visualized without a laryngoscope.
   c. The straight blade is inserted here during endotracheal intubation.
   d. The curved blade is inserted here during endotracheal intubation.
2. Which of the following indicates that the patient is not a candidate for endotracheal intubation by an EMT-B?
   a. Gag reflex
   b. Vomiting
   c. Gurgling sounds
   d. Spontaneous reduced rate of ventilation
3. The most serious complication of endotracheal intubation is:
   a. Hemorrhage
   b. Unrecognized esophageal tube placement
   c. Right main stem bronchus placement of the tube
   d. Lack of suctioning after placement of the tube
4. Which of the following is not a good method for confirming endotracheal tube placement?
   a. End-tidal carbon dioxide
   b. Lung sound auscultation
   c. Chest expansion with assisted ventilation
   d. Waiting for a chest x-ray examination at the hospital
5. Which of the following is incorrect regarding automated transport ventilators?
   a. The batteries must be frequently recharged for proper function.
   b. They have settings for tidal volume and respiratory frequency.
   c. They deliver 100% oxygen over a fixed inspiratory cycle time.
   d. They can be used for assisted ventilation during CPR in intubated patients.

Answers to these Review Questions can be found at the end of the book on page 866.

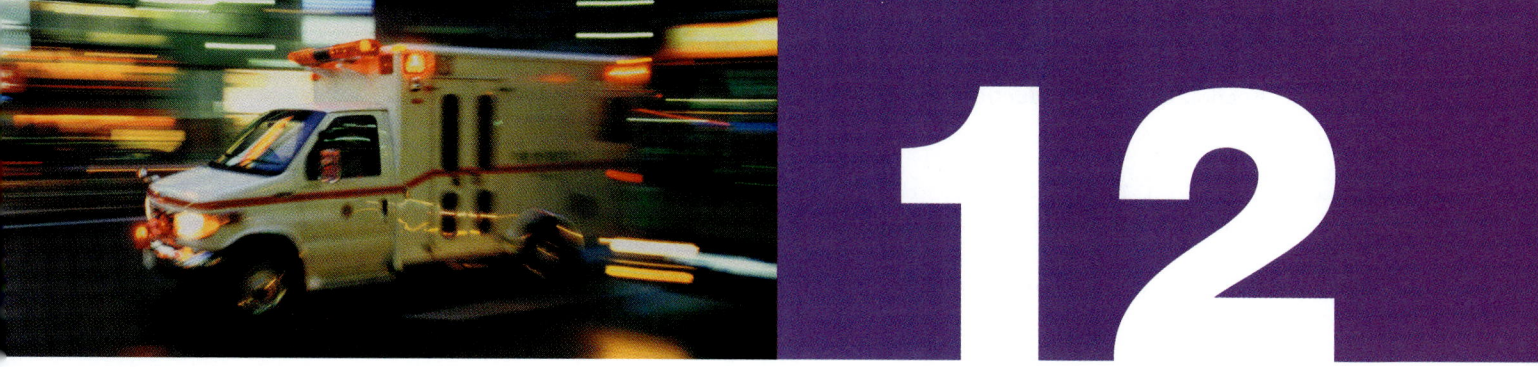

Scene Size-up and the EMS Call

Lesson Goal

A lot is always happening on the scene of any call. Some occurrences are very important to the EMT and others are not. This chapter sets the stage for the EMS run and points out high priorities. Understanding and not just memorizing this material will play an important role in the EMT's time in the field or in a supervisory position within the EMS.

Scenario

It is a warm early fall evening and you have been dispatched to a residence approximately 30 miles outside of town in reference to a 62-year-old woman who is experiencing "severe chest pain and shortness of breath." The weather is good and you have paved highway to both the scene and the hospital. Transportation time from the hospital to the scene is approximately 45 minutes.

En route to the call the dispatcher advises that the daughter, who initiated the 911 call, has advised that there is an EMS DNR order present at the scene.

On arrival you are met at the door by the daughter who is in possession of the EMS DNR order that was signed 5 days ago when her mother was brought home from the hospital. The mother is suffering from terminal cardiovascular disease and was ruled out as candidate for a heart bypass procedure due to the advanced stages of her disease process. The doctors, at the request of the family, sent the patient home to die with her family.

The patient is lying in bed with home oxygen at 4 liters by nasal cannula. She is observed to be diaphoretic and pale and in obvious pain. Her airway is intact; respirations are 24 and shallow; pulse is 128, weak, and irregular at the radius; and blood pressure is 96/62. Pulse oximetry shows a reading of 84%. She is oriented times 4 and clearly states to you that she does not want to be resuscitated if she arrests. She further states that she had her daughter call because of the increasing pain, unrelieved by morphine, and she did not want her daughter to be alone if she dies. She is requesting transportation to the hospital and asks for more morphine to control the pain, if possible.

 What are the correct and medically appropriate steps to be taken for this patient?

Key Terms to Know

Advance directive
Cerebrovascular accident
Computer-aided dispatch
Criteria-based dispatch
Do-not-resuscitate (DNR) order
Durable power of attorney
Emergency medical dispatch

235

Key Terms to Know (cont'd)

EMS do-not-resuscitate legislation
Enhanced 911
Living will
Mass casualty incident
Medical direction
Prehospital care
Resuscitation not indicated (RNI)
Special needs patient
Trauma center

Learning Objectives

As an EMT-Basic, you should be able to do the following:

DOT

- Recognize hazards and potential hazards.
- Describe common hazards found at the scene of a trauma and a medical patient.
- Determine if the scene is safe for the EMT to enter.
- Discuss common mechanisms of injury and natures of illnesses.
- Discuss the reason for identifying the total number of patients at the scene.
- Explain the reason for identifying the need for additional help or assistance.
- Observe various scenarios and identify potential hazards.

Supplemental

- Identify the various phases of an EMS call and the different scenarios that can occur with each.
- Describe the interaction among the public, the dispatcher, EMTs, and other responding agencies.
- Describe the importance of effective communication in the processing of the EMS call.
- Describe the importance of scene evaluation, both while en route to and on arrival at the scene, and the impact on the outcome of the patient.
- Describe emergency medical dispatch and its role in helping the emergency medical technician (EMT) develop strategies for delivery of the best possible patient care.
- Describe the key elements of the scene survey, gained from both the dispatcher and the survey of the scene on arrival, that can affect the outcome of patient care.
- Describe the potential threat hazardous materials present to both the EMT and the patient at the scene of a medical emergency.
- Describe the necessary safety measures to be taken for protection of both the patient and EMTs at a scene.
- Describe the importance of personal protective equipment to the EMT's safety and reduction of contamination by bloodborne pathogens or other potentially infectious materials in caring for a patient.
- Describe how bioethical considerations affect the resuscitation of patients in the prehospital setting.
- Assess the appropriateness of a do-not-resuscitate (DNR) order, a living will, advance directives, or a durable power of attorney and describe how it is used to implement or withhold resuscitation.

There is perhaps no more unsafe time for the emergency medical technician (EMT) than arrival at the scene. The EMT must rapidly assess any risks that may be present, quickly make appropriate decisions, and take actions to ensure that neither the patient nor the EMTs become unnecessarily exposed to increased hazard.

Because of the advancements in dispatch information and techniques, today's EMTs have more information available to help them make these determinations before they arrive at the scene. Even with these advances and new technology, EMTs still must ensure their own safety on arrival at the scene.

The growth of medical knowledge about the management of patients, in both the prehospital and hospital settings, is increasing at a rapid rate as well. EMTs must keep pace with this explosion of knowledge in order to be able to provide the best possible patient care. This includes the latest patient treatments, as well as both medical and nonmedical problems that can arise.

Evaluation of the trauma scene and determination of the forces involved are essential parts of patient care. Knowledge of concepts that may affect management of a scene and delivery of patient care is an important part of this base, such as scene management, threats to the safety of the patient and EMTs, hazardous materials, weather, environment, and the location of the scene. The issue of either not starting resuscitation or discontinuing it once it has been initiated has been debated for as long

Patient Care Algorithm

Scene Size-up

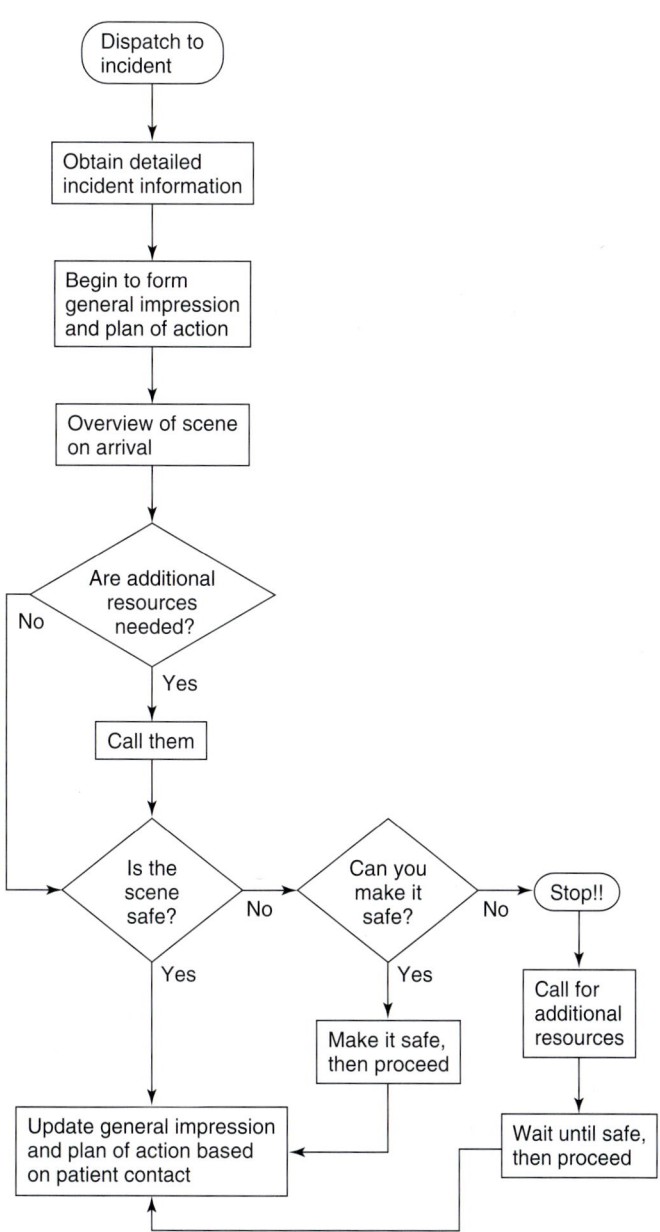

as emergency medical services (EMS) has existed. In recent years, several states have initiated legislation that allows EMS providers and **medical direction** physicians to address this issue. Because this is a limited issue it is not addressed in this chapter, but the EMT must be aware of the rules and regulations that apply locally.

Because of the many threats to personal safety that exist today, the EMT must be prepared to identify scene hazards quickly and determine if and how the scene can be made safe. EMTs who deliver complete, competent care are aware of resources in their community that can be called on for assistance and help. Some scenes are beyond the EMT's ability to make safe. This determination must be made quickly to avoid unnecessary risk or injury. EMTs should not enter these unsafe scenes.

Types of EMS Calls

Patients come in all varieties with varying degrees of severity of their presentations (appropriate hospital, appropriate method of transportation, etc.). The EMT's ultimate goal is to provide efficient, high-quality patient care.

Different EMS systems have a higher percentage of specific types of incidents. Examples include higher numbers of violence-related trauma in an urban setting, more cardiac emergencies in retirement communities, more injuries related to machinery in a farming or ranching area, and more recreational-related emergencies in a remote or wilderness area. Examples of the types of patient presentations that the EMT is likely to encounter are presented in the following sections.

Cardiovascular

The American Heart Association has determined that approximately 1 million Americans die annually from cardiovascular disease (Figure 12.1). One half of these deaths are attributed to coronary artery disease, with approximately 300,000 being sudden death. Approximately 160,000 of these deaths occur in patients under age 65 years. Nationally, multiple studies have shown that the types of patients can be divided into thirds: approximately one third cardiovascular disease, one third trauma, and one third medical.

Medical

Medical calls consist of diabetics, seizures, drug overdoses, respiratory calls, gastrointestinal disorders, and brain attacks, to name but a few. Many of these patients

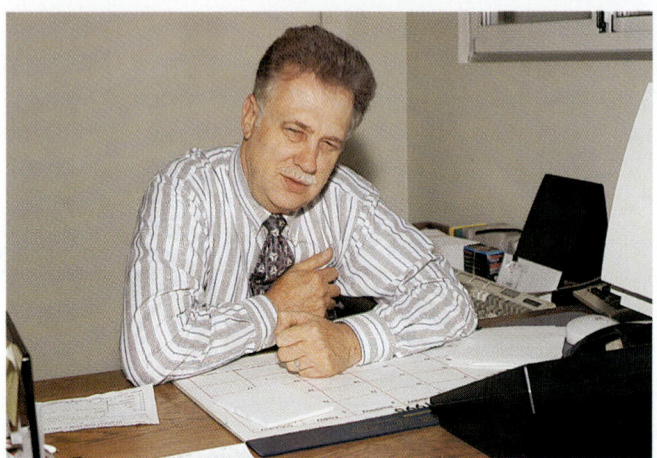

FIGURE 12.1 Approximately one third of EMS calls are for patients with symptoms related to cardiovascular disease.

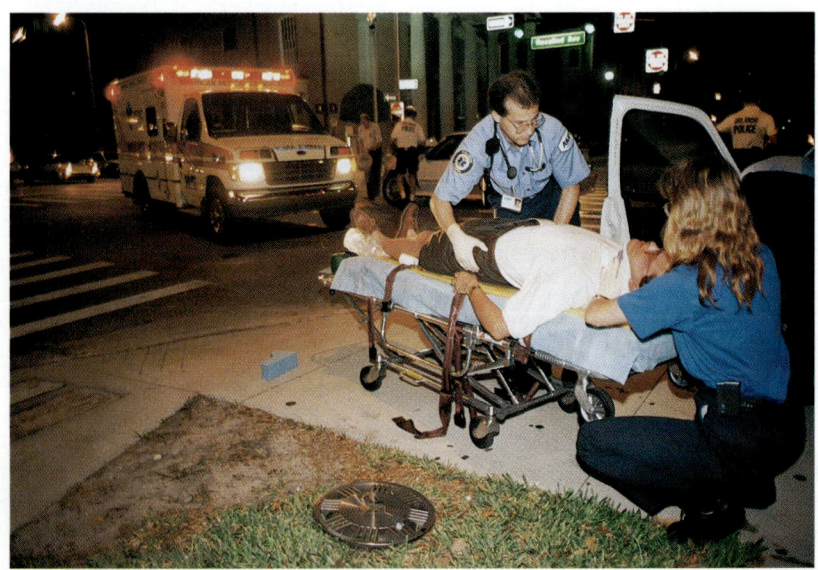

FIGURE 12.2 Trauma is the leading cause of death for children and adults under age 45. EMTs respond to a variety of trauma calls. Traumas represent approximately one third of EMS runs.

have more than one pathology. It is common to arrive at the scene of this type of call and find that the patient has an extensive medical history and is experiencing multiple medical problems at this time. As the population ages, patients with multiple problems will become even more common. These patients often put off calling for assistance until the complications have become severe.

Trauma

In a landmark report published in 1966 by the National Academy of Sciences, "Accidental Death and Disability: The Neglected Disease of Modern Society," trauma was listed as the leading cause of death in the first half of the life span. At the beginning of the new millennium, trauma continues to be the leading cause of death for children and adults under age 45 years, and it is the third-leading cause of death for all age groups. EMTs respond to a variety of trauma calls (Figure 12.2). Because trauma patients are usually younger than patients experiencing cardiac-related illness, they represent a greater loss of productive years, require longer rehabilitation, and negatively affect the production of a strong tax base.

Pediatric

Although pediatric patients make up approximately 30% of the population, they account for only approximately 10% of the call volume of the EMS system (Figure 12.3). Unintentional injuries are the leading cause of death in children over age 1 year. Other causes of death for children include injuries from burns, drowning, child abuse, and poisoning. Calls for respiratory difficulty and seizures are the most common medical problems that the EMT encounters. Motor vehicle collisions (MVCs) and falls account for the bulk of the injuries. These calls relate to the time of day and the season of the year. During the daytime hours of 6 AM until midafternoon to late afternoon, the calls for injuries rise dramatically; this time frame coincides with the school day. Pediatric calls for illnesses show a greater incidence during the afternoon and evening hours.

Geriatric

The EMT can expect the unique challenge of treating the elderly to grow (Figure 12.4). Currently, 11% of the U.S. population is made up of individuals over age 65 years; by 2030 the number will be approximately 18%. The major causes of illness and death in the geriatric population

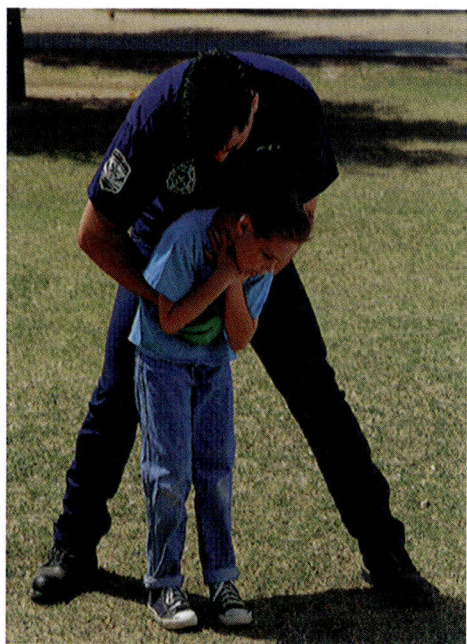

FIGURE 12.3 Pediatric illnesses and injuries require prompt attention by the EMT and transport to an appropriate facility.

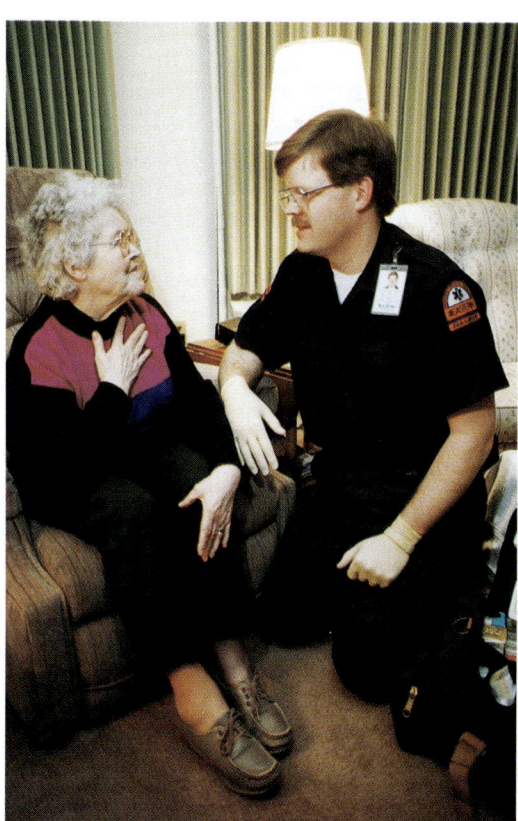

FIGURE 12.4 EMTs will most likely encounter elderly patients.

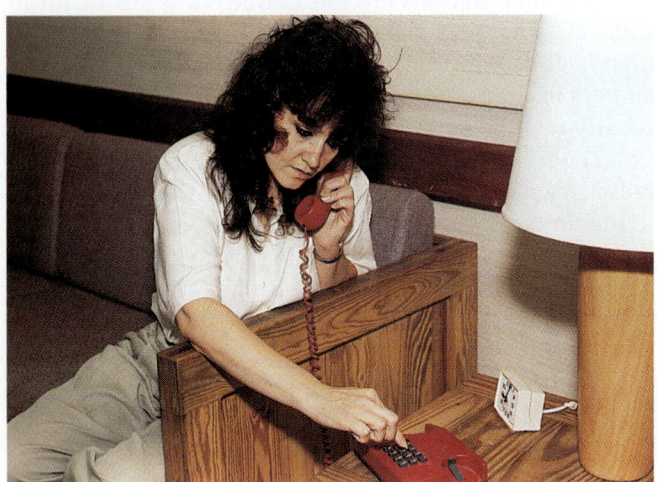

FIGURE 12.5 Any call for emergency care begins with citizen access.

are related to cardiovascular disease, **cerebrovascular accident** (brain attack), altered mental status, and pneumonia. Trauma is the fifth-leading cause of death in the elderly. Falls are the leading cause of trauma deaths and disability in the geriatric age group.

Because of changes in metabolism that occur with aging, drug doses prescribed for the elderly may need to be reduced by one third to one half of the usual adult dose. Geriatric patients may experience polypharmacy, in which medications are overprescribed, multiple medications are prescribed by different physicians, medications are given to them by well-meaning friends, or medications are taken in very high doses. These situations increase the risk of drug interactions. Chapter 30 discusses the unique challenges of this growing and specialized group of patients.

Special Needs Patient

An additional category of patients that the EMT is likely to encounter is the **special needs patient**, previously referred to as handicapped or disabled persons. During assessment and treatment, such patients may appear defensive or uncooperative. The EMT should take extra time to assure these patients and to make them comfortable. Do not to allow previous misunderstanding, personal bias, or misperceptions to detract from the patient's needs.

Citizen Access and Communication

Any call for emergency care begins with citizen access. The public plays a vital role as a member of the emergency health care team (Figure 12.5). Accessing EMS through the standard or **enhanced 911** system (a 911 system that is fully computerized) or a seven-digit telephone number is the standard method for obtaining assistance (see Chapter 34). Because valuable time may be lost before 911 is called, it is imperative that EMS access begin as soon as possible.

Many communities throughout the United States have some coverage by the standard or enhanced 911 system. Only six states currently have 100% coverage of 911. Cellular technology has allowed citizens to access 911 from mobile and cellular phones. Many EMS services have introduced cellular technology as an alternative to traditional two-way radio use for their communications.

Combined with significant improvements in the field of emergency medicine, this translates to changed prehospital care. Improved care cannot be accomplished without rapid access to prehospital care. Definitive treatments that previously had been the domain of the emergency department are now beginning in the prehospital setting. Two examples are the use of thrombolytic agents for the myocardial infarction patient and the use of whole blood and packed cells for trauma patients. It is becoming common to see these definitive interventions begun by prehospital providers during long or delayed transportation. Quick transportation of patients allows definitive treatments to be initiated as early as possible. The key to minimizing delay rests with the initial access and ongoing communications that occur between the EMT in the field and the physician at the hospital.

> ✔ Regardless of which category of patient is encountered or what symptoms are presented, the EMT's standard approach and goal should remain the same. The EMT must prepare for the call but must be able to adjust to a variety of patients and environments once he or she arrives on the scene. Chapter 32 focuses on the special needs patient.

> ✔ Citizen access and communication is the latest growth area regarding EMS response. Continued implementation of 911 systems coupled with the phenomenal growth of cellular telephones has dramatically compressed the time frame between incident occurrence and agency dispatch. Shortening time between occurrence and treatment has proven critical for both heart attack and trauma patients.

Dispatching the Ambulance

The goal for EMS systems is to have an EMT crew on the scene within 4 to 6 minutes from the time the call is received at the emergency communications center. Financial, geographic, and other constraints increase this target to 6 to 9 minutes in urban areas. Sparsely populated and wilderness areas are unable to meet this goal in even a small percentage of cases because of long access and transportation times. Some communities use a tiered response system that can send both a basic life-support team and an advanced life-support team to each emergency. Fire service personnel and police officers may also be dispatched, either as first responders or as the primary EMS provider.

Emergency medical dispatch (EMD) and citizen use of 911 (or enhanced 911) have evolved as key components of an effective EMS system. These components have improved early access for emergency care. EMD training programs have emerged that provide dispatchers with training in quality assurance, total quality management, and medical direction (Figure 12.6) (see Chapters 4 and 36). Today, more and more states are passing legislation that require dispatchers be able to give prearrival instructions to the callers. These include instructions on how to perform cardiopulmonary resuscitation or position the unconscious medical patient to protect the airway.

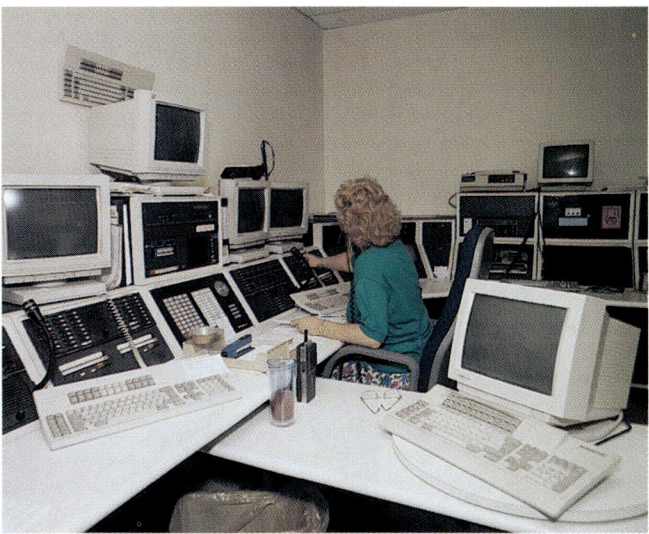

FIGURE 12.6 Emergency medical dispatch and citizen use of 911 (or enhanced 911) have evolved as key components of an effective EMS system.

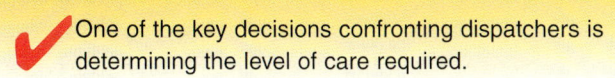
One of the key decisions confronting dispatchers is determining the level of care required.

To assist dispatchers in deciding the level of care needed, medical criteria have been developed to guide the dispatcher in his or her questioning of the caller and, based on the answers provided, in making dispatch decisions as to the level of care needed and required resources. One of several commercially available EMD programs is called **criteria-based dispatch** (CBD). Additionally, **computer-aided dispatch** (CAD) systems combine both prearrival instructions and priority dispatch and are being integrated into EMS communication systems. It is the responsibility of the EMT to work with the emergency communication center and to recognize the importance of functioning as a team.

En Route to the Scene

Development and continued improvements in EMD have done much to improve EMS response (Figure 12.7). EMD is designed to ensure that the EMT receives appropriate information so that he or she is prepared to manage the scene on arrival.

Good EMD includes the following:

- Complete and accurate call information (described further in the following section)
- All pertinent weather information that could delay response or transportation
- Traffic delays en route to the scene due to roadways blocked by construction or heavy commuter traffic
- Delays that can be anticipated because of blocked railroad crossings or raised bridges
- The fastest, safest route to follow
- Identified alternative routes for the responding unit(s) so that delays are kept to a minimum
- Prearrival instructions to the caller regarding care for the patient while the EMS unit is en route

Dispatch Information

Essential information includes as full and complete a description of the scene as the dispatcher has been able to gather from the caller. Depending on the completeness of the caller's description, dispatch information enables the EMT to determine whether the call

- Is a trauma or medical call. The EMT then can make informed decisions as to what type of equipment must be taken from the unit. The EMT can review the possible conditions that the patient may have and formulate an evaluation and treatment plan.

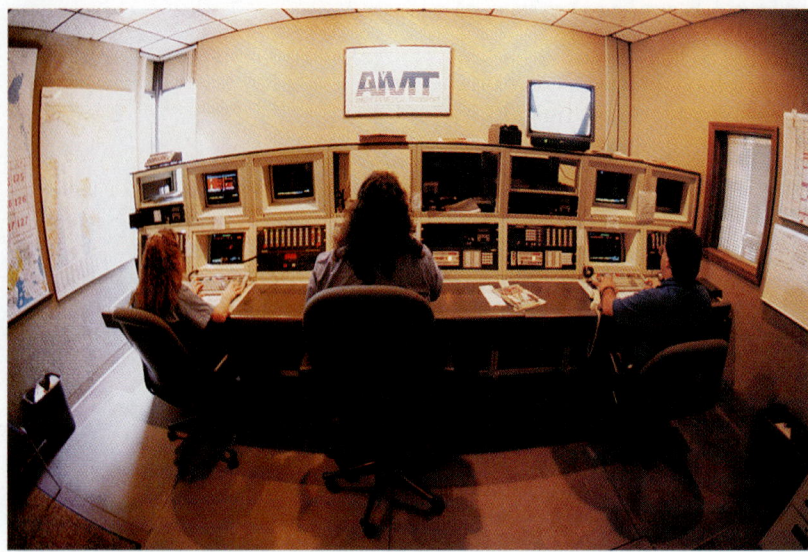

FIGURE 12.7 Emergency medical dispatch ensures that the EMS unit receives the appropriate information so EMTs can arrive at the scene quickly and be prepared to manage the scene when they arrive.

- Includes any life-threatening conditions (e.g., patient having chest pain, difficulty breathing, severe bleeding).
- Involves fire or building hazards.
- Involves other hazards such as downed power lines, broken gas transmission lines, volatile or toxic substances that have been spilled on the ground or released into the air, and even vicious or threatening animals.
- Requires special rescue equipment, such as heavy extrication, high-angle rescue, or water rescue equipment.
- Involves multiple vehicles or otherwise indicates that more medical personnel may or will be needed on the scene.
- Involves the possibility of helicopter evacuation.
- Requires special personnel and equipment. Waiting until arrival on the scene and then requesting these needed resources could result in unnecessary delay in patient care. These resources easily can be canceled when the EMT arrives on the scene.
- Will be affected by weather conditions. If the roads are wet, icy, or snow covered, additional time will be needed for response and transportation. In rural areas, roads may become impassable to regular EMS vehicles, requiring specialized vehicles to get access to and transport the patient.
- Involves environmental conditions such as very hot or very cold climates. The medical condition of the patient may be aggravated by the environment, and treatment plans may have to be altered to avoid unnecessary exposure to the elements.
- Involves any type of reported violence. EMTs should never enter such situations until the dispatcher confirms that law enforcement officers are on the scene and that it is secure.
- Includes prearrival instructions that have been given to the caller to provide care to the patient until EMS arrives.

A review of the initial dispatch and any subsequent information given to the unit while en route to the scene can be very helpful to the EMT. The first two elements, location and type of call, help determine whether an immediate need for additional or specialized resources exists. If the EMT believes that aeromedical transportation may be indicated, he or she should ask for the status of the helicopter as soon as possible. Early notification is important, because helicopters have a mandatory warm-up period before they can lift off for the scene. Calls involving any type of reported violence should never be entered until the dispatcher confirms that law enforcement personnel are on the scene and that it is secure. Calls that involve respiratory, cardiac, or motor vehicle collisions

> ✓ EMD can provide valuable information to EMTs before they arrive on the scene. Such information may be invaluable in preparing the EMTs for the equipment, extra resources, and extra personnel that a scene may require. EMD also provides prearrival instructions to the caller as to how to care for the patient until EMS arrives.

often require additional personnel, who should be dispatched immediately.

Hazardous Materials

Twenty years ago, hazardous materials were not included in training programs for EMTs. Today, hazardous materials are being transported daily on commercial carriers and are becoming a regular part of EMS scene response and management. All hazardous materials should be considered a threat to the EMT until proven otherwise (Figure 12.8). As the types and numbers of hazardous material shipments grow each year, more accidents occur and more EMS personnel are dispatched to these accidents. EMTs must recognize their own limitations in both training and equipment to properly manage these calls. Ludwig Benner, a hazardous materials specialist with the National Transportation Safety Board, has perhaps the simplest yet most graphic definition of hazardous materials. According to Benner, a hazardous material is "any substance that jumps out of its container at you when something goes wrong and hurts and harms the things it touches."

Most larger urban fire departments have specialized hazardous materials units and specially trained personnel to handle these types of calls. Many large industrial plants that use hazardous materials have their own in-house teams. In many cases, these experts will leave the plant site and assist with the call if agreements have been made beforehand. Most states, by law, have a designated agency that often is responsible for managing hazardous material calls. The EMT should remember that even when a state agency has been designated as the lead agency for these types of incidents, often the personnel are not the best trained, best equipped, or most qualified to handle the scene. A good example is a situation in which state police have been designated as the lead agency for management of a hazardous materials incident, but their training is limited to a total of 16 hours. The EMT should make a point to establish who the lead agency is and what protocols are in place for this type of incident. A good EMD center must have all the necessary resources available for immediate contact once the determination is made that a hazardous materials incident has occurred. For more information about hazardous materials incidents, see Chapter 40.

> ✓ Hazardous materials may make a scene dangerous. Sometimes expert personnel are available to manage these scenes, but sometimes they are not. EMTs must learn how to handle hazardous materials scenes before expert help arrives.

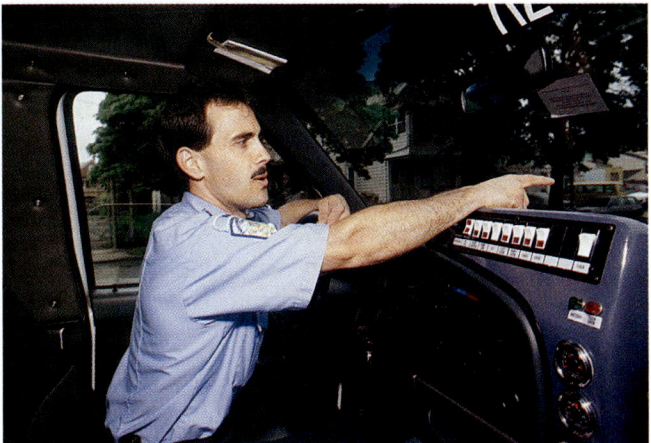

FIGURE 12.8 On approaching the scene, the EMT should first determine that the scene is secure and safe to enter.

At the Scene

As the EMT approaches the scene, he or she first should determine that the scene is secure and safe to enter. If the scene is a medical call in a residential neighborhood, it may only be necessary to determine the presence of traffic on the street before exiting the vehicle. At a trauma call, the EMT should determine if scene hazards still exist, such as explosions, an unstable building, downed power lines, or spilled gasoline. In the case of an assault, it is important to know if the perpetrator has left the scene or is in custody. In the case of an assault involving either a gun or knife, the EMT needs to know where the weapon is.

Appropriate scene control is the responsibility of police, fire, and EMS personnel. Interagency communication and coordination are vital to a smooth operation. Managing any scene involves clearly defined leadership roles and responsibilities for all personnel. Resolution of any conflicts regarding scene control and management should be accomplished before the response in the quiet of a conference room. If conflicts still exist, they must be dropped while on the scene. The reason that you are on the scene is the patient. Do not forget that important fact.

Once on the scene, the EMT begins to assimilate information that is observed, reported, and gathered firsthand. The original dispatch information should not bias conclusions or create tunnel vision but should complement the findings that are presented to the EMT. After exhausting these avenues of collecting pertinent information, speak directly with the patient. If the situation and the patient's condition permit, talk with first responders, friends, relatives, and co-workers who are present on the scene.

Trauma Scene Evaluation

Trauma scenes present somewhat of a different challenge from that of a medical call to the EMT in assessing the scene. The total scene must be quickly evaluated to determine the probable mechanism of injury. At the scene of a motor vehicle collision, for instance, this evaluation involves determining how the vehicle or vehicles collided, the speed involved at the time of impact, and whether seat belts or air bags restrained the victims. At an industrial accident, evaluation includes determining the height from which the victim fell, the amount of debris that fell on the victim, or the type of machinery involved in the accident. If the call is one that involves penetrating trauma, the evaluation must include the type of weapon involved and ballistics if a firearm was used. Evaluation is important because it serves to guide the EMT during the physical examination of the patient in looking for and identifying possible injuries. Chapter 22 discusses kinematics of injury in detail.

> ✓ On entering a trauma scene, the EMT should evaluate the mechanism of injury to determine what injuries exist.

Establishing Control of the Scene

Immediately on entering the scene, the EMT should establish control, if this has not already been done. Patients, family members, and bystanders may be frightened or anxious. Chaos is common at an emergency scene, and the EMT must firmly take charge of medical care at the scene. If the call is to a crime scene, law enforcement personnel are concerned with preservation of the crime scene. Being sensitive to crime scenes allows the EMT to evaluate and treat victims, if indicated, while preserving as much of the crime scene as possible. Any scene that involves fire, or the threat of fire, should be controlled by the fire department to allow safe entry by the EMT. In some cases a family physician or another physician who has stopped to render assistance may be present. The EMT must be responsive to the physician-patient relationship. At the same time the EMT should explain that he or she is under medical direction, either on- or off-line, and should attempt to put the physician at the scene in touch with the medical direction physician. If direct contact is not possible, the EMT must explain to the physician at the scene that if the physician asumes control and responsibility, he or she must accompany the EMT to the hospital to directly hand off care to the physician in the emergency department (especially if the physician has initiated treatment beyond that of current licensure/certification of the EMT).

Perhaps the key element to gaining control of a scene is the confidence with which the EMT interacts with the patient and also with support personnel, family mem-

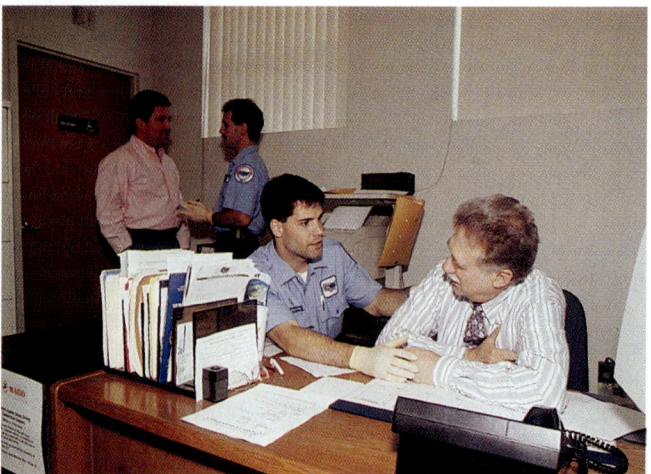

FIGURE 12.9 Communication will take the form of face-to-face conversations with patients, family, bystanders, and staff.

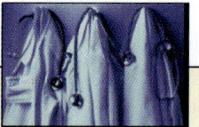 Physician Notes

The presence of a physician on the scene can be a blessing or a major hazard with which the EMT must deal. This pressure can create more frustration than the bystanders. The physician may believe that he or she has a responsibility to become involved, despite having no knowledge of prehospital care, being unused to dealing with the emergency patient, or having knowledge that is limited to one part of the anatomy.

This situation requires much tact on the part of the EMT. The best solution is to have a policy that addresses the presence of a physician on the scene.

A suggested approach for these protocols is as follows. The physician must identify his or her presence to the EMT and show proper identification. The physician then should be informed that the scene is under the control of the medical direction physician and that all care is being directed by that physician and the protocols that have been approved by the appropriate authority in that community. If the physician on the scene wishes to provide medical care for the patient, the physician must also accept the medical and legal responsibility for the outcome of the care given to the patient. In addition, the physician must accompany the patient to the hospital.

bers, and other medical personnel on the scene. If a physician is present at the scene and is providing care for the patient, EMTs should always identify themselves and their level of training. Ask what can be done to assist in the care of the patient. If something should be done, ask rather than direct. Care of the patient must be the guiding factor.

Better results in patient care can be obtained by demonstrating respect. Identify yourself and state your qualifications. Most people do not understand what "EMT" means. Many people do not like strangers calling them by their first names, so be polite and ask first. One example of an introduction is, "Hello, my name is Larry, and I'm an emergency medical technician. I'm trained to assist you and am here to help you. Can you tell me what your problem is today?"

Taking Command of the Scene

A critical component of being an EMT and responding to an EMS call involves the ability to take command of the situation. Leadership is the ability to influence others to carry out assigned tasks and to perform as required according to job assignments. In an emergency situation, the need to delegate authority is critical. For directives to be carried out, each EMT and other members of the team must understand their assignment and believe that they can carry out their tasks.

An EMT learns to lead by following the examples set by other leaders and being sensitive to the cues sent forth by these leaders. Before the EMT can begin to exercise authority over others at the scene of an emergency, he or she should give some thought to how those on the scene (both above and below in the chain of command) will react. Before the response, EMTs must also explore how they feel about taking command of the scene. Because prehospital care often requires working with limited support under perhaps very adverse conditions, the EMT must accept command positions as a necessary fact of prehospital organization. An EMT who does not come to grips with his or her own emotional reactions to being a leader will find it difficult to employ authority prudently and productively with others. EMS must be a paramilitary organization to function properly. There are always situations in which to take orders and to give them.

> ✓ Leadership is not a result of one's position but is the ability to influence others. An EMT may have the authority to direct others; however, unless he or she is able to influence people to make things happen, no action will occur.

Communicating Effectively

Another important component of scene management is the ability of the EMT to communicate effectively. Communication is a form of influence. It involves a relationship in which all parties play distinct but complementary roles. Effective communication is not unilateral bludgeoning, in which one person is active while the other is passive.

The purpose of effective communication is the transmission of information. For the EMT, communication takes the form of face-to-face conversations with patients, family members, bystanders, and staff (Figure 12.9). It also involves written reports in which patient care information, radio transmissions for medical direction, memos, or additional directives are documented.

Patient Interaction

The EMT is the physician surrogate in the prehospital setting and becomes the physician's eyes, ears, voice, and hands. A good EMT assists the remote physician in developing a mental picture of what is occurring. The ability to be able to transmit this information accurately and quickly depends in large part on the EMT's assessment skills (Figure 12.10).

Accurately assessing a patient in the field while minimizing delay in transportation separates the good EMT from the excellent one. All of the information (data) gathered by the EMT during the various phases of assessment must be documented and communicated to the emergency department staff.

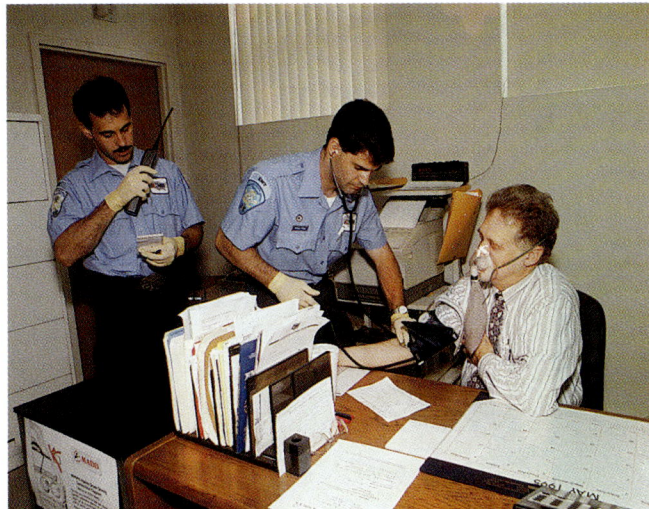

FIGURE 12.10 The ability to transmit patient information to medical direction accurately and quickly depends, in large part, on the EMT's assessment skills.

As with any skill, patient assessment requires practice to attain a level of expertise and proficiency. Although previous experience may prepare the EMT for many of the patients he or she will encounter, there will always be EMT calls that contain the unexpected. In these situations, acquired field knowledge, continuing medical education, assessment skills, and leadership qualities will be put to the ultimate challenge.

The Role of Compassion

EMTs who feel and exhibit confidence must also demonstrate competence and compassion for their co-workers and other medical personnel, as well as for the patient and family. Competence is best demonstrated by directing and initiating care in a smooth and direct manner that tells both your co-workers and the patient that you know what you are doing and how to do it. Compassion for the patient and his or her family is demonstrated by actions and words. Patiently explaining to the patient and family what is happening and what is needed can go far in gaining acceptance and cooperation. Removing sunglasses, looking at the patient or family when speaking, holding the patient's hand, and letting a sick or injured child sit on a parent's lap are all indicators of the compassionate EMT. These small gestures, while they may appear insignificant, can do much to promote good interactions and patient care. Of course, the safety of the scene and the welfare of the patient and the caregivers take precedence over everything else. There are times when compassion must come after lifesaving techniques. Also, never let compassion interfere with personal safety!

> ✓ The EMT should establish control over the scene early but should also show compassion toward patients, family members, other EMS personnel, and police and fire personnel on the scene.

Other Scene Considerations

Personal protective equipment (PPE) is designed to protect emergency personnel from the risk of contamination by blood, airborne contaminants, or other potentially infectious materials and should always be worn (Figure 12.11). Minimally, PPE includes gloves when dealing with any situation in which EMTs could be at risk from blood or other potentially infectious materials. When appropriate, full face protection and gowns should be worn. Any EMT involved with rescue or extrication should always be in full protective clothing (turn-out gear of pants, boots, helmet with eye and face protection, coat, and heavy gloves) as indicated by the conditions at the scene.

> ✓ The EMT should consider any bodily fluid from a patient as potentially infectious.

A **mass casualty incident** (MCI) is discussed in detail in Chapter 40, but it is extremely important to note that the EMT must recognize (even before leaving the unit) that if additional personnel and equipment are needed they must be summoned early. One good definition of an MCI is any scene that the initial responding unit cannot handle alone (Figure 12.12). Two seriously injured patients may generate an MCI call if one unit cannot provide adequate care. The same can be said for a call in which the EMTs are not equipped to handle the hazards. With multiple patients, the EMT first must survey the scene so that all patients can be identified and any previously unreported hazards found. At this point, additional resources, fire and police personnel, hazardous materials units, or additional units that may be required can be requested. Triage is the sorting and allocation of treatment to patients to maximize the number of survivors. Stop-

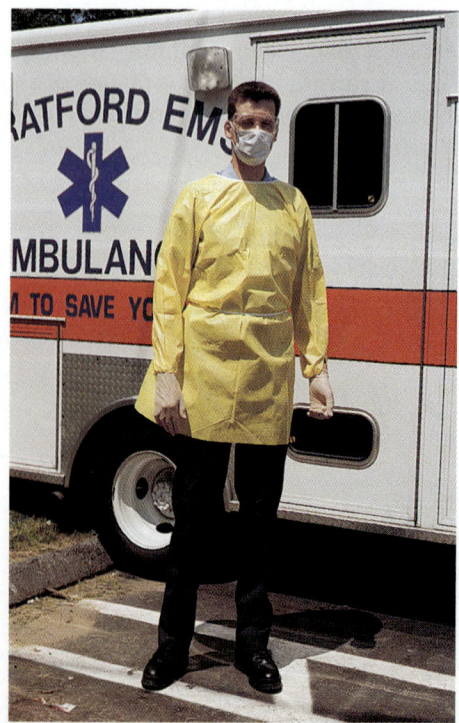

FIGURE 12.11 Personal protective equipment is designed to protect emergency personnel and should always be worn when a risk of contamination from either bloodborne or airborne contaminants exists.

ping at the first patient and beginning treatment prevents the assessment of other patients and delays the calling of additional resources and the performance of lifesaving interventions. By surveying the entire scene, the EMT has a better idea of how to use the available resources, particularly if the scene is an MCI.

The EMT must know what agencies to contact (and how to contact them) for appropriate backup units in that community. There is no consistency across the United States as to what service is provided by whom. Each community is different. Know your own resources.

> ✓ Once the EMTs put on protective equipment, scene hazards have been neutralized, and appropriate background information has been obtained, patient evaluation can begin.

Bioethical Considerations

Primum no nocere, Latin for "first do no harm," has been the first tenet of patient care since the Romans and Greeks began writing about medicine. It has long guided the profession of medicine, including prehospital care, and training programs for the EMT have used this tenet as a major theme. **Bioethical considerations**, long discussed and debated in medicine, have recently become a major consideration in prehospital care and are involved in the first interactions that the EMT will have with the patient.

One problem that the EMT has always had to face is the question of whether resuscitation is appropriate to begin or to continue once started. Certain trauma patients cannot be saved no matter what level of care is immediately available to them.

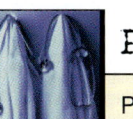

Physician Notes

Patients injured by blunt trauma to the chest or abdomen or penetrating trauma to the abdomen and without vital signs on the scene are considered by most trauma surgeons, and with adequate support in the literature, to be nonsurvivors. Local protocols should prevail.

Patients with certain preexisting medical conditions that have been identified by their physician as terminal may not wish to have life-sustaining care initiated. Beginning resuscitation or terminating it once begun has long been a gray area in prehospital medicine. No legislative guidelines are in place in some states, whereas others have adequately addressed the question. Some physicians are not comfortable making these kinds of decisions without being present at the scene or without specific legislation to back them up. Although resuscitation issues have always been discussed and debated, decisions are usually reached in an informal manner by physicians and families and, as stated previously, in many cases without supporting legislation. At the time of writing of this book, legislation is in place in 17 states (and pending in 14 others) that provides guidelines for resuscitation.

The **do-not-resuscitate (DNR) order**, durable power of attorney, **advance directive**, and **living will** are traditionally associated with hospital and long-term care facilities and may not have relevance to EMS. New legislation

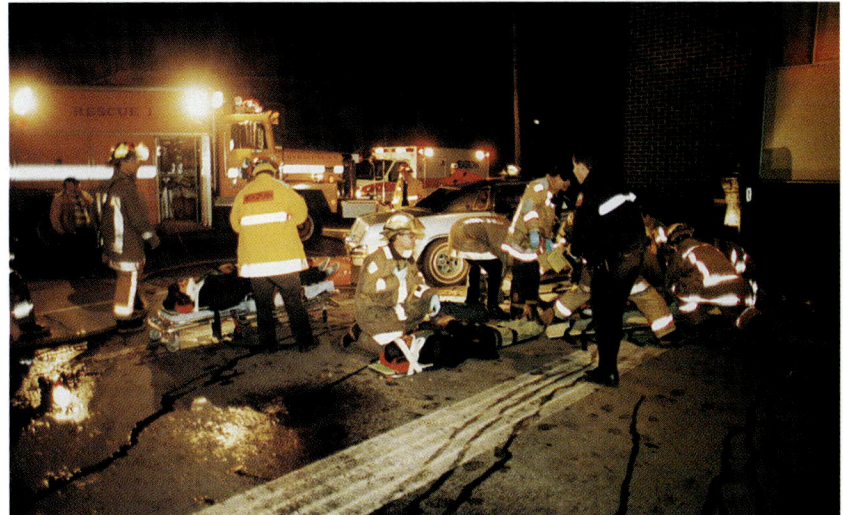

FIGURE 12.12 A *mass casualty incident* is defined as any scene that requires additional resources or units other than the initial responding unit.

dealing with prehospital care and its initiation and termination are known as **EMS do-not-resuscitate legislation** or **resuscitation not indicated (RNI)**.

RNI legislation is designed to give patients the opportunity to express their wishes, in writing, concerning resuscitation efforts and to give prehospital care providers the legal support to follow these resuscitation decisions. Generally, the laws provide specific instances in which the EMT may, in direct contact with a physician, determine that initiating or continuing resuscitative efforts is futile and unnecessary. Because these decisions must be made in concert with medical direction, the EMT must complete a rapid evaluation and be prepared to give an accurate yet brief description of the scene and the patient(s). In these situations, the EMT becomes the eyes and ears of the physician. The EMT must give enough information that the physician gains an accurate picture of the scene.

EMS DNR orders have been designed to prevent unnecessary or futile interventions in the case of the terminally ill patient or the patient who has injuries of such proportion that he or she will never regain a quality of life. Although designed to prevent unwarranted interventions by EMS personnel (e.g., cardiopulmonary resuscitation, intubation, defibrillation, and medication administration), they do not preclude the administration of procedures intended for the comfort of the patient (e.g., oxygen, suctioning, administration of analgesics, controlling bleeding, and generally making the patient comfortable).

The proper procedure for the EMT to follow if he or she encounters an EMS DNR order is to

1. Perform initial assessment.
2. Verify identification of patient by driver's license or other signed photo identification or family member or other party who can positively identify the patient.
3. Administer oxygen by mask or cannula.
4. Suction the airway.
5. Manage airway with basic procedures (no intubation or other advanced procedures).
6. Control bleeding.
7. Administer analgesics (EMT-Paramedic skill level only).
8. Make the patient comfortable.
9. Support family members and make them comfortable.

If there are any questions about the validity of an EMS DNR order or there is evidence of an attempted homicide, initiate resuscitation until such time that the questions have been answered. If possible, contact medical direction for consultation.

Most of the states that have this type of prehospital advance directive legislation in place have provisions for the patient to wear a special identification bracelet. Some states have a central registry so that immediate verification can be obtained.

The relationship between EMS DNR orders and durable powers of attorney is important. Durable powers of attorney are legally binding documents that give the person named the power to make decisions on behalf of the person who authorizes it. This power can include decisions related to health care. If an EMT encounters a situation involving both a durable power of attorney and an EMS DNR order, the EMS DNR order shall prevail for EMS treatment.

The proper procedure for the EMT to follow if he or she encounters either an EMS DNR order or a durable power of attorney is as follows:

1. Perform initial assessment.
2. Verify, using a driver's license or other signed photo identification, family member's positive identification, or identification by a person who knows the person, that the person is the one who executed the durable power of attorney.
3. Verify the identification of the person identified in the durable power of attorney as the authorized health care decision maker, by photo identification or other positive means.
4. Determine that the identification bracelet or document is original and not defaced in any way. (If defacement is found, resuscitation must be initiated.)

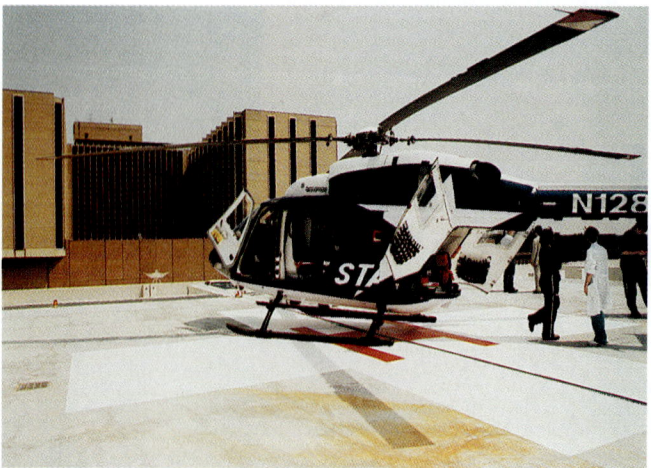

FIGURE 12.13 When considering aeromedical transportation, the risk-benefit ratio must be weighed.

> ✔ Emergency medical services do-not-resuscitate (EMS DNR) legislation, also called resuscitation not indicated (RNI) legislation, prevents unnecessary, futile interventions in the cases of terminally ill or fatally injured individuals. Only care that contributes to patient comfort should be given.

5. Ask family members to make a reasonable search if no bracelet or document is immediately available. (If a document cannot be found immediately, initiate resuscitation and contact medical direction.)
6. Initiate comfort measures as appropriate if patient has not yet expired.

This new legislation has two benefits for EMS. First, the laws allow the EMS unit and personnel to return to service more quickly. In smaller services, this rapid return can be important to the system if personnel and other resources are limited. Second, the laws reduce the risk involved in driving to the hospital using the siren and warning lights (i.e., reducing the probability of an automobile collision, injury, or death).

The EMT is trained in and expected to provide lifegiving care. Police officers are trained to investigate and solve crimes. Often these two areas collide at a scene. The police sometimes call an EMS unit to a scene solely for the purpose of determining the absence of life. They are most interested in preserving the crime scene, and the EMT should respect this goal. However, if the patient in question shows signs of life, the EMT has a duty to act and must initiate care and transportation of the patient. Cooperation and preplanning between all agencies that may interact at the scene of a medical emergency is the best way to avoid conflicts occurring at the scene. A plan agreed on ahead of time as to how they will deal with this type of incident will make the situation more comfortable for all involved.

Transportation Considerations

The method of transportation should be considered as soon as enough information is gathered and life-threatening conditions are managed. Transportation is an intervention that, like all interventions, must be prioritized and accomplished in a safe manner. The most appropriate mode of transportation and the destination hospital are often determined long before the patient has been assessed, treated, and packaged. Choosing one hospital over another depends on patient request, proximity, specialized care, emergency department patient diversion status, and any local protocols. Local (city, county, state) laws and rules may vary regarding hospital bypass. Some legislation forbids it, some permits it, and some requires bypass of one hospital and transportation to a **trauma center**.

When considering aeromedical transportation, the risk-benefit ratio must be weighed (Figure 12.13). Usually a helicopter is warranted if rapid access to a higher level of care is required (hospital to hospital) or for scene response when hospital access time to the correct hospital can be shortened. Another consideration is access to an appropriate landing zone (see Chapter 39). For most patients the best and most commonly used method of transportation is the ground ambulance.

For the new EMT (and the old), mastering and maintaining safe driving techniques are as important as understanding clinical care. All of the prehospital care and transportation decisions are worthless if the patient never arrives at the hospital or the crew is injured in the process.

> ✓ An EMS response usually involves dispatch, prearrival instructions, scene, and transportation considerations. Emergency medical dispatchers are specially trained telecommunicators who receive the call for assistance, dispatch the correct EMS response, and provide prearrival instructions to the caller. Additionally, EMD provides the EMT with valuable prearrival information that will aid the initial scene size-up. The decision to transport the patient will then be made in relationship to the patient's best interest, which may or may not be the closest medical facility to the incident. Last, patient transportation is an important function of the EMT; in actuality, it is a treatment intervention.

Emergency Department

Arrival at the emergency department (ED) does not mark the end of the EMT's responsibility. The EMT must report to and discuss the findings and treatment rendered with the nurse and emergency physician (Figure 12.14). To ensure continuity of care, it is important that the EMT remain with the patient throughout the transfer process in the ED.

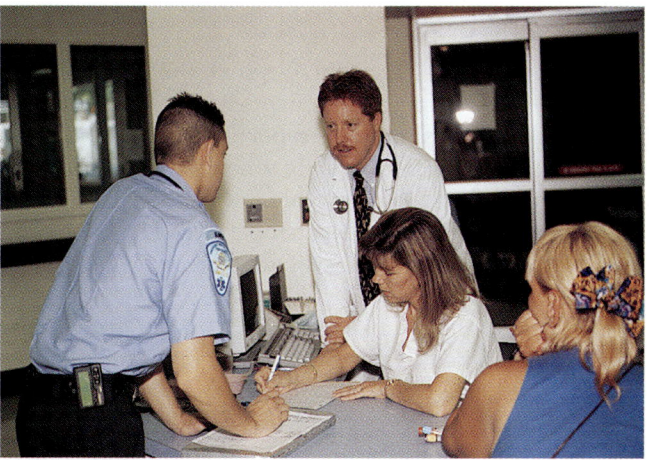

FIGURE 12.14 The EMT must report and discuss his or her findings and the treatment rendered with the triage nurse and emergency physician.

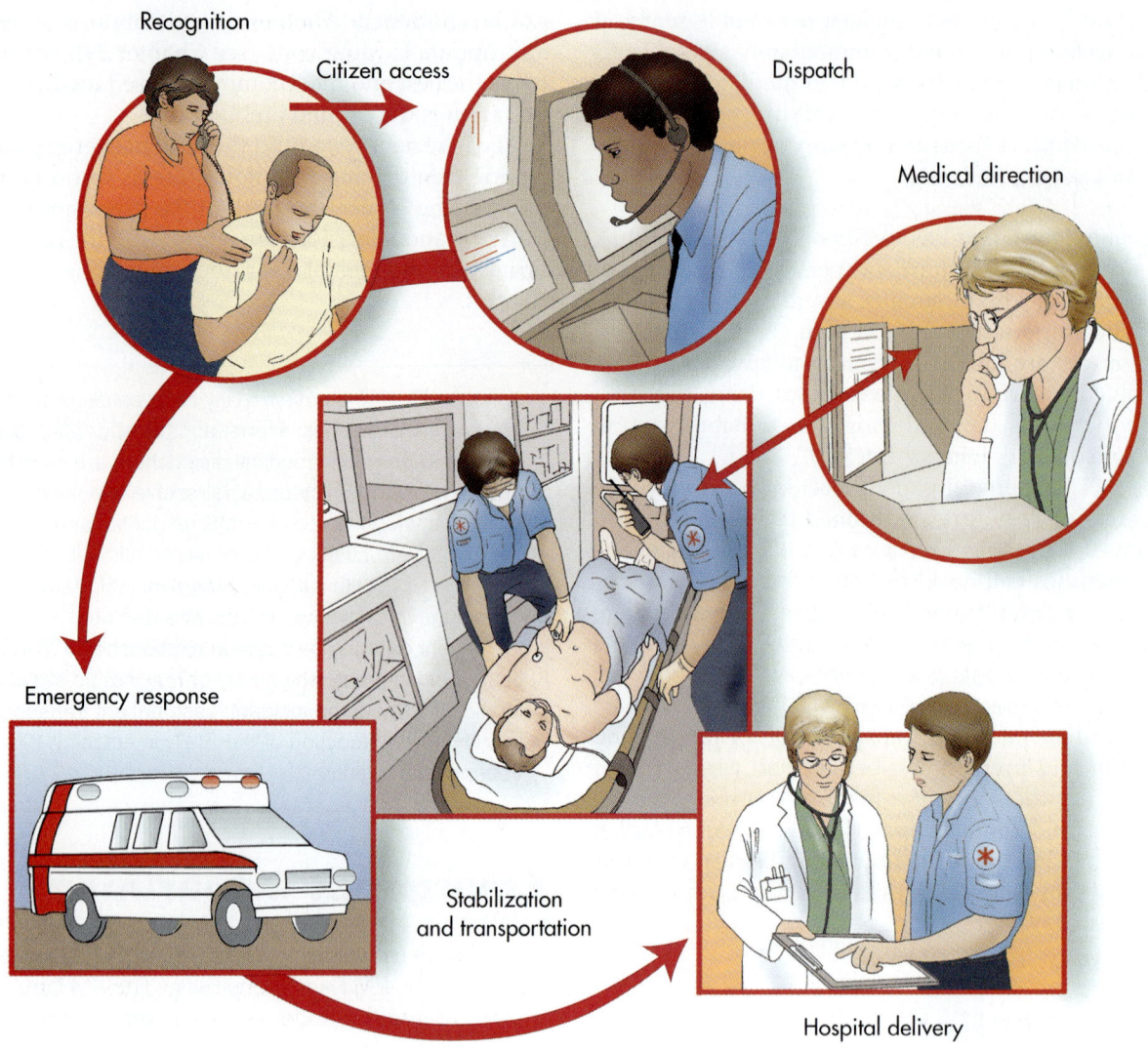

FIGURE 12.15 Anatomy of an EMS call.

After the EMT leaves the hospital, the only way the ED staff can determine what happened before arrival is through the **prehospital care** report (PCR). It is therefore imperative that all findings, treatments, and procedures be documented and that any valuables or personal effects be left with the ED staff. Remember, what has not been documented on the PCR is assumed not to have been done (see Chapter 35).

Before leaving the ED, the EMT must be sure that the vehicle is prepared in the event that another incident occurs. Properly dispose of contaminated sharps, biohazardous waste, and linen in a designated (red) biohazard bag. Nondisposable equipment such as traction splints, pneumatic antishock garments, and trauma boards should be disinfected. Once the EMT has reported "clear and available" to the dispatcher, the EMT must be prepared to respond to the next EMS call.

✓ Although formal EMT intervention stops on arrival at the hospital, the patient's care continues. It is imperative that the EMT give a full report to the emergency department representative, usually a nurse or physician. This report is usually verbal at first and then documented on the prehospital care report. The patient's return to normal function in a timely and productive fashion will depend on the prehospital intervention you render, as well as the care delivered by the members of the health care team in the hospital.

Continuum of In-hospital Care

For the patient, the ED may represent only one more vital step in the continuum of care. An EMT should be aware of what services are offered in the local hospitals. Many hospitals offer specialized critical care units for trauma/surgical, cardiac, neonatal, pediatric, burn, and medical patients. Remember, a total EMS system includes not only first responders, basic life-support units, advanced life-support units, and EDs, but also critical care units and rehabilitation services.

Ultimately, the patient's return to normal function in a timely and productive fashion will depend on the prehospital intervention that you render, as well as the care delivered by the other members of the health care team in the hospital (Figure 12.15).

Summary

- The EMT should review the dispatch information to ensure the safest and quickest route to the scene.
- The EMT should evaluate the scene to the determine the need for additional resources and/or the presence of hazardous materials.
- The EMT should know who and what resources are available in the area that can be called for assistance.
- The EMT should take control of the scene, exhibiting confidence to the patient, family, and other members of the EMS team.
- The EMT should always protect himself or herself from threats at the scene, whether it is a domestic, traffic, hazardous materials, or bloodborne pathogens scene.
- The EMT should know and understand the law as it relates to stopping or not starting resuscitation.
- If the EMT cannot make a scene safe, he or she should get out before he or she becomes part of the problem.

Scenario Solution

Your first priority is to the patient. A thorough and complete primary assessment has revealed that your patient is not perfusing well. You should consider increasing her oxygen concentration, including switching her to a mask to increase her FiO_2. An intravenous line should be started, but large amounts of fluid should not be given, even though the physical findings indicate a low perfusion state, due to her history and lung sounds indicating fluid buildup.

Consideration of requesting an EMT-Paramedic intercept should be made and, if possible, initiated at this time to administer analgesics to give pain relief and comfort.

You must verify the patient's identity and that the EMS DNR order is correctly filled out. Verification of the patient's wishes, per the DNR order, should be verbally verified with the patient and while the daughter is present in the room.

Transportation should be initiated as soon as possible, allowing the daughter to ride in the vehicle to the hospital. Notification to the receiving hospital of necessary information should be made before arriving at the facility.

Patient comfort should be your overriding concern.

Key Terms

Advance directive A legally binding document prepared and signed by an individual that clearly states his or her personal wishes regarding implementation of lifesaving techniques in the event the individual is severely injured or terminally ill and cannot make decisions at that time.

Cerebrovascular accident (CVA) Medical term for stroke.

Computer-aided dispatch (CAD) A computerized dispatch communications program.

Criteria-based dispatch (CBD) Type of dispatch based on the recognition that the level of care at either the EMT-Basic or EMT-Paramedic level required for patients and the urgency of prehospital care can be identified by established medical criteria.

Key Terms (cont'd)

Do-not-resuscitate (DNR) order Instructions to withhold resuscitation efforts issued by a physician after consultation with the patient or surrogate decision maker.

Durable power of attorney Legally binding document signed by a party that designates an individual to make health care decisions for the person executing the document.

Emergency medical dispatch (EMD) An approach to the dispatch functions of an EMS system that involves the dispatcher in making decisions about the type and priority of EMS response that is necessary, providing critical information to responding units while they are en route, and providing prearrival instructions to callers until the EMS units are on the scene.

EMS do-not-resuscitate legislation Legislation providing for a legally binding order signed by a physician and by the person that precludes any lifesaving techniques being started on a patient who has terminal illness and who arrests.

Enhanced 911 (E-911) A fully integrated, computerized 911-access telephone system.

Living will Legal document (signed and witnessed) outlining the types of medical interventions that may or may not be implemented on the signer, who may or may not have been diagnosed with a terminal or permanently disabling medical condition.

Mass casualty incident (MCI) Any incident involving one or more patients that cannot be handled by the first responding unit(s) to the scene.

Medical direction Various duties that a physician provides in support of an EMS system, including protocols, case reviews, and educational programming.

Prehospital care Health-related services provided to the patient outside of the hospital, generally at home, at work, or in the field.

Resuscitation not indicated (RNI) Term applied in the prehospital setting to those patients who, because of their medical condition or injuries, have no chance of survival and in whom resuscitative efforts would be futile; sometimes termed *futile intervention*.

Special needs patient Patient who has any condition with the potential to interfere with usual growth and development; may involve physical disabilities, mental disabilities, or chronic illness, as well as forms of technological support.

Trauma center A hospital equipped and staffed to handle trauma patients. Trauma centers are divided into three levels based on response capability. Level I: a hospital staffed and equipped to place the patient in the operating room within minutes of arrival. All staff members are available in the hospital 24 hours per day. Level II: a hospital staffed and equipped to place the patient immediately in the operating room if necessary. Some staff members may not sleep in the hospital but are available in the emergency department when patients arrive. Level III: a hospital with emergency department staff members who are available to the hospital 24 hours per day, but the operating room, surgical, and anesthesia staff members may be at home and on call for rapid response when the need exists.

Review Questions

1. From the following list, identify those elements that are considered part of the scene survey: (1) number of patients, (2) hazards or potential hazards that exist, (3) need for additional resources, (4) cancellation of additional resources that have been dispatched and are not needed.
   a. 1, 3
   b. 2, 3
   c. 1, 2, 3, 4
   d. 3, 4
2. On arriving at a scene, different hazards can be present that pose a threat to the safety of an EMT. Which type of call can present the greatest number of risks to the EMT?
   a. Medical patients
   b. Trauma patients
   c. Respiratory patients
   d. Geriatric patients
3. What is the benefit of evaluating the mechanism of injury at a scene?
   a. It helps the EMT determine the number of patients that are involved.
   b. It helps the EMT evaluate the patient(s) for possible injuries.

Review Questions (cont'd)

   c. It determines whether or not the EMT should initiate resuscitation.
   d. It determines the type and amount of fluids the patient should receive in the prehospital setting.
4. There are two main reasons for the EMT to review the dispatch information while en route to a call and perform a quick yet thorough scene survey on arrival. The first is to ensure that the best and most complete care can be given in the shortest time frame. The second is:
   a. To cancel any unneeded resources that have been dispatched.
   b. To ensure the EMT's own safety.
   c. To provide a complete and comprehensive radio report to the emergency medical dispatch center on arrival.
   d. To identify reasons not to transport the patient(s).
5. Considering the traditional EMS response, number the following call segments in the correct sequence.
   a. Emergency department
   b. Continuing in-hospital care
   c. Citizen access to EMS
   d. Prearrival considerations
   e. Dispatching the ambulance
   f. Scene assessment and control
   g. Transportation considerations
   h. Interaction with the patient
6. True or False: Knowledge that a scene is unsecured is critical for the EMT.
7. True or False: Scene control is the sole responsibility of the EMS agency.
8. In which way does an EMT communicate?
   a. Face to face
   b. Written reports
   c. Radio transmissions
   d. Memos and directives
   e. All of the above
9. True or False: Transportation of the patient is considered *after* the patient has been assessed, treated, and packaged.
10. Which of the following statements best describes the position the EMT should take regarding bodily fluids?
    a. Only blood should be considered as a threat to the EMT.
    b. Vomit or other fluids from the gastrointestinal tract should be considered as a threat to the EMT.
    c. All bodily fluids from the patient should be considered a risk to the welfare of the EMT.
    d. Only airborne fluids from the patient's coughing and that can be inhaled by the EMT should be considered as dangerous.
11. The role of emergency medical dispatch (EMD) is to provide early access to prehospital care. Which of the following statements best describes the overall role EMD plays in patient care?
    a. The EMD center is responsible for assuming complete control over all EMS scene responses and direction of medical care.
    b. The EMD center is responsible for providing prearrival instructions to callers and providing as much information as possible on the nature of the call and any special situations that may exist to the responding unit(s).
    c. The EMD center is responsible for determining the mode of transportation for the patient and which hospital the patient is to be transported to.
    d. The EMD center is responsible for maintaining current files of prehospital EMS DNR orders and, further, for determining their current validity.
12. Which of the following statements most accurately reflects the purpose and intent of EMS DNR and RNI orders?
    a. EMS DNR and RNI orders allow the EMT to make on-scene determination of whether to initiate resuscitation procedures.
    b. EMS DNR and RNI legislation is designed to give patients the opportunity to express their wishes in writing concerning resuscitation efforts on their person.
    c. EMS DNR and RNI orders allow family members to make all medical care decisions for the patient regardless of the patient's mental condition.
    d. The EMT has the right to disregard any EMS DNR or RNI order that is correctly filled out and presented by the patient or family member if the EMT feels that resuscitation should be undertaken.

Answers to these Review Questions can be found at the end of the book on page 866.

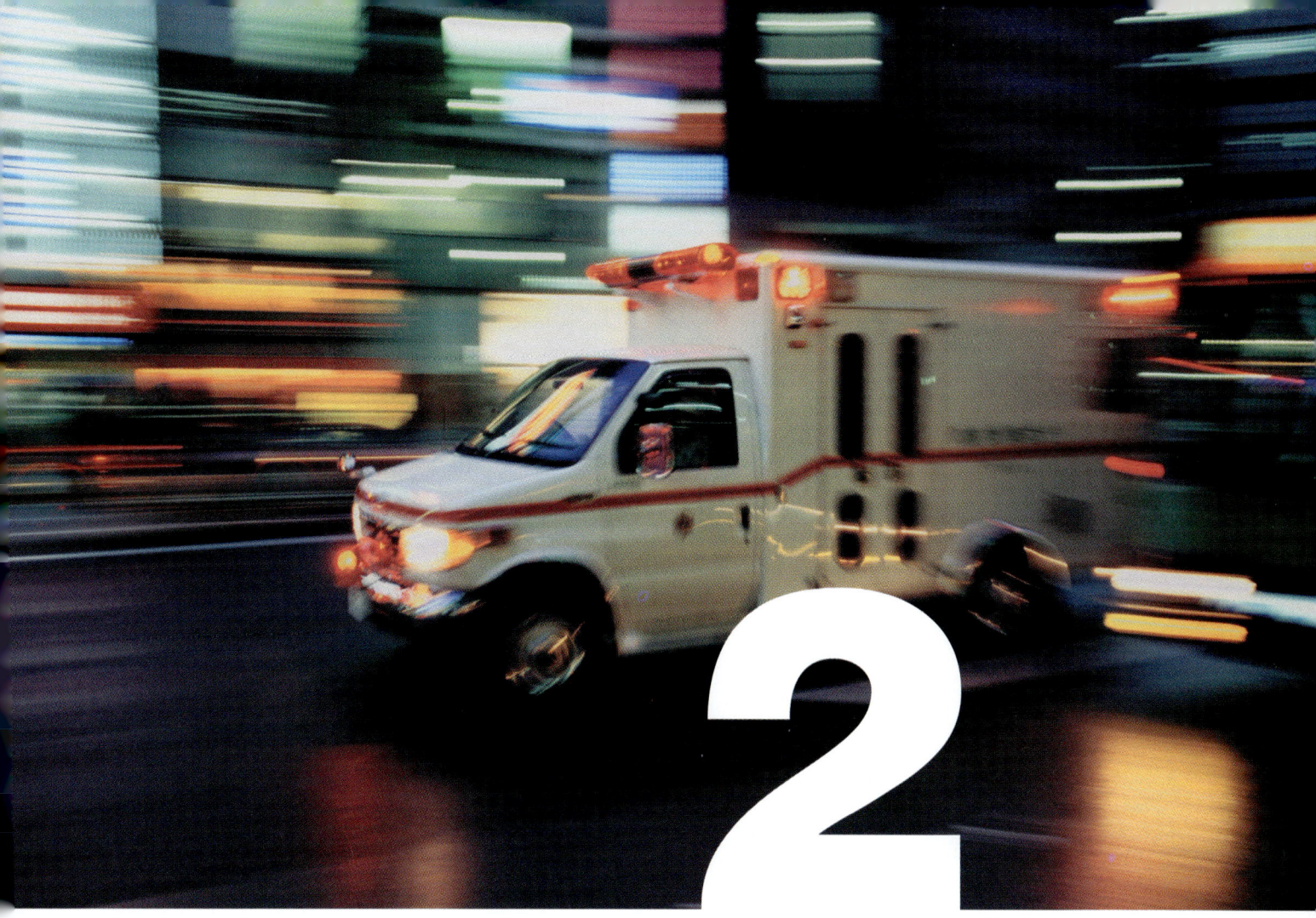

Section Two

Nontraumatic Emergencies

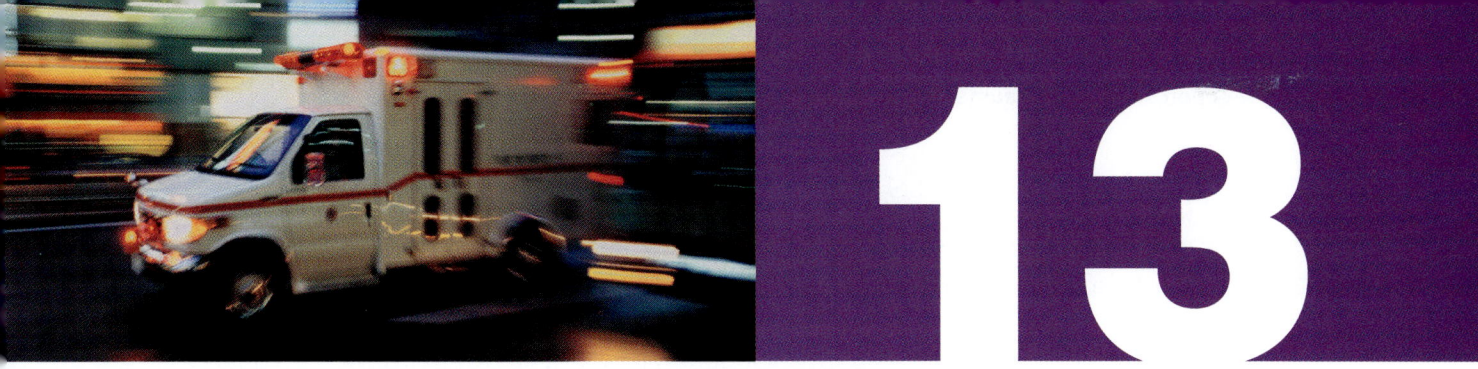

General Pharmacology

Lesson Goal

The goal of this chapter is to familiarize the EMT-Basic with the principles of patient-assisted administration of medications. This chapter also reviews the basic fundamentals of pharmacology.

Scenario

You have just been dispatched to a call for assistance in the mountains on the east edge of town in reference to a 23-year-old female who has been stung by an unknown insect and is experiencing shortness of breath. Further information indicates that the patient has a known allergic reaction to insect bites and reportedly has suffered acute allergic reactions in the past. Currently, the patient is awake and is experiencing moderate shortness of breath, complaining of severe itching in her throat, and developing hives, according to the caller.

You have good access roads to the patient with a response time of 18 minutes and a transport time of 30 minutes to the hospital.

On arrival you find the patient on the ground, supine, pale in color, and experiencing shortness of breath and hives on both arms, the upper chest, and the neck area. She has a pulse of 122 at the carotid, has respirations of 28 with expiratory wheezing, and is responsive, appropriately, to voice. A Medic Alert tag stating "allergic to bee stings" is noted on her right wrist. She is holding some type of pen in her hand, which, on further examination, is revealed to be an "epi-pen" with her name on it. She is asking you to administer the drug to her.

 Can you do this? What is the correct procedure? What steps will you take if you do administer the medication, both during and after injection? What medications can the EMT administer?

Key Terms to Know

Absorption	Generic name	Pharmacology	Systemically acting
Actions	Indications	Protocols	medication
Availability	Locally acting medication	Route of administration	Trade name
Contraindications	Medical direction	Side effects	
Duration of action	Medications	Standing orders	

Learning Objectives

As an EMT-Basic, you should be able to do the following:

DOT

- Identify which medications will be carried on the unit.
- State the medications carried on the unit by their generic names.
- Identify the medications that the EMT-Basic may assist the patient in administering.
- State the medications that the EMT-Basic may assist the patient in administering by their generic names.
- Discuss the forms in which the medications may be found.
- Demonstrate general steps for assisting patients with self-administration of medications.
- Read the labels and inspect each type of medication.

Medications are used extensively in emergency situations to treat the cause of the disease or to relieve symptoms of an underlying problem. Although drugs are intended to be beneficial, the EMT must also understand and remember that they can be dangerous if used incorrectly. Even if used correctly, there are known complications to every type of drug that the EMT must know and understand. An EMT should not give a patient a medication or drug if the EMT does not know that drug's expected outcome, the potential complications, and how to manage adverse effects if they occur.

The emergency medical technician (EMT) has select drugs available on the unit and can also assist with the patient's own prescription medications, depending on state and local treatment guidelines. Drugs are referred to by **trade name, generic name,** and chemical name. Drugs are available in many different forms (tablet, capsule, liquid, etc.). The way the drug is given, the **route of administration,** depends on the type of drug and its form. Speed of **absorption** and **availability** of any given drug are related to the route of administration and the type of drug.

Actions, side effects, indications, contraindications, and dose are critical characteristics of each medication. Federal regulations require the name, strength, dose, and directions to be listed on the label of each drug container.

Before giving a medication, the EMT must take an initial history and assess the patient to determine the correct course of action. This is true for giving a medication to any patient under the EMT's care. After giving the medication, the EMT must continue to reassess the patient for effects of the drug.

Overview of the Use of Medications by the EMT

Health care providers use a variety of medications to treat their patients. Medications are chemicals that change the way the body functions, and the study of these medications is termed **pharmacology.** Many illnesses are due to changes in the normal chemical functions of the body. These broken chemical "machines" can be fixed or improved with the correct medications.

Drugs are used to treat either the cause of the illness or the symptoms. For example, diabetes is a disease caused by insufficient insulin in the blood. Providing insulin in drug form corrects the chemical abnormalities of diabetes. A heart attack is usually caused by narrowing of the blood vessels in the heart. Nitroglycerin reduces the pressure in the system that decreases the workload of the heart and therefore relieves the pain caused by insufficient blood flow through the diseased vessels, but it does not fix the narrowed vessels that cause the disease.

Medications have a variety of useful effects, such as relieving pain, decreasing the work of the heart, or absorbing poisonous materials from the stomach. However, drugs can be dangerous if used incorrectly. A patient's condition can be made worse by giving the wrong drug, giving the wrong amount, or using the wrong technique.

Two groups of medications are available to the EMT-Basic. The first group consists of medications carried in the ambulance by the EMT; these medications can be given to the patient. The availability of these drugs on the emergency medical services (EMS) unit is permitted by

TABLE 13.1 Medications Available to the EMT

Medications Carried in the Ambulance	Medications in the Patient's Possession
Activated charcoal	Epinephrine
Oral glucose	Nitroglycerin
Oxygen	Prescribed inhaler

state law or local treatment guidelines. EMTs must have the legal authority to administer any drug to a patient.

The second group consists of medications prescribed for the patient. These drugs have been prescribed by a physician for the patient to treat a specific condition or disease. The EMT may only assist the patient in taking these medications with approval by **medical direction**. A list of these medications is provided in Table 13.1.

> ✓ Medications can be beneficial but may also cause injury or death if used incorrectly. Medications in the ambulance may be given by the EMT, but the EMT may only assist patients in taking certain medications in their possession.

Medication Names

All medication has several names (at least three). The chemical name is the long, complex description of the structure of the drug. This name is not used in clinical medicine. The two most recognized kinds of names are the generic name and the trade name.

The generic name is a simple form of the complex chemical name. The generic name is assigned by the government and is officially listed in the *United States Pharmacopeia*. Each drug has only one generic name.

The trade name, or brand name, is given to a drug by the companies that sell the drug. Each drug can have more than one trade name because it can be made or sold by different companies. The trade name is often a word that is easy to say, spell, and remember. Trade names belong to the company that registers them and can be recognized by the trademark symbol (®) at the end of the name.

Tips from the Pros

Do not be embarrassed or think that you lose respect in the eyes of the patient because you do not know all of the names of a drug. Simply say to the patient, "I'm not sure about that drug. What does it do?" If still uncertain, call medical control before giving the patient any medication, even if the patient insists that the medication is correct. Patients commonly confuse the symptoms of a condition and believe that one drug is good for all conditions.

Several pocket guidelines are available commercially that provide the names of drugs (all three names) and their actions.

> ✓ A single medication has many names. Each drug has one generic name but can have more than one trade name. The trade name, recognized by the trademark (®) symbol, is used by drug companies in marketing the drug.

Thus any given drug will have a chemical name, a generic name, and possibly several trade, or brand, names. For example, a common medicine found in drugstores is ibuprofen. Ibuprofen is the generic name. The trade names are Advil®, Motrin®, Nuprin®, and others. All of these names refer to the same drug. Another example is a type of inhaled medicine often used to treat asthma. The generic name is albuterol, and it has two trade names, Proventil® and Ventolin®. Again, these trade names refer to the same medicine (Figure 13.1).

Forms of Medications

Each medication is prepared in a form that allows safe storage, handling, and use. The form of the medicine depends on the chemical nature of the drug and the planned route of administration. The route of administration and form of the specific drug are designed to allow proper concentrations of the drug to enter the bloodstream.

A drug may be available in a variety of forms, and each form has a specified route of administration. Each form of the drug should be used only through the appropriate route of administration. For example, the liquid form of nitroglycerin is designed for use sublingually (under the tongue) as a spray. It should never be given by

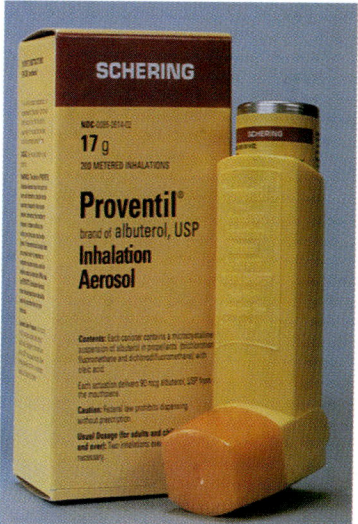

FIGURE 13.1 Albuterol (generic name) is an inhaled medicine used to treat asthma.

injection. Some examples of the different forms of medications follow.

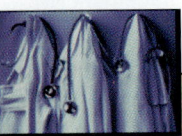

Physician Notes

The chemical composition of a drug determines whether it is inactivated by the digestive enzymes in the stomach or intestine and therefore cannot be taken orally; whether it is rapidly absorbed by the mucosa lining of the mouth; whether it is absorbed rapidly into the bloodstream when given by intramuscular injection but is not absorbed into the mucosa of the gastrointestinal tract; or whether the lining of the lungs rapidly absorbs it if it is inhaled.

Tablets

Tablets are made from a compressed powder, may be coated, and come in a variety of shapes. Tablets are given orally and may be swallowed or placed sublingually. Aspirin is an example of a tablet that is swallowed, and nitroglycerin is an example of a sublingual tablet (Figure 13.2, *A*).

Gels

A gel is a semiliquid that contains a dissolved medication (Figure 13.2, *B*). Gels may be placed between the gum and cheek or under the tongue. They can also be swallowed or rubbed on the skin for transdermal absorption.

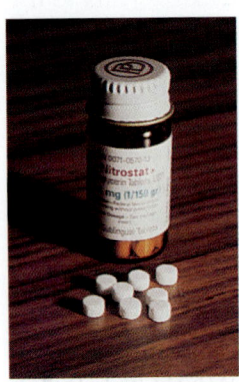

A

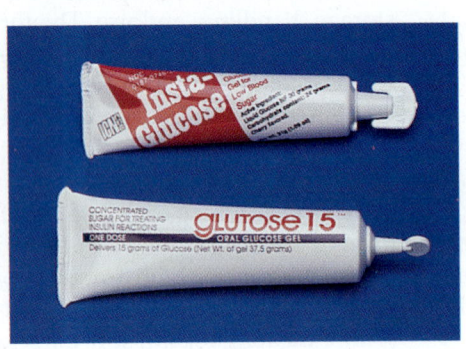

B

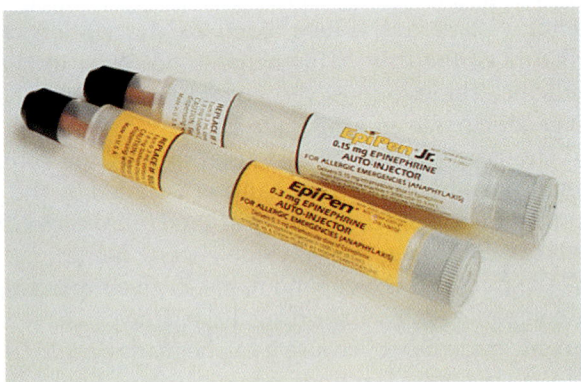

C

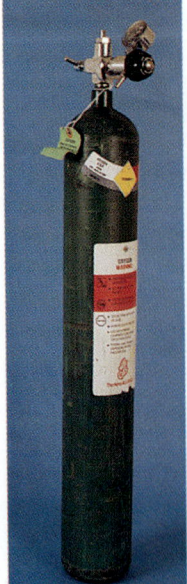

D

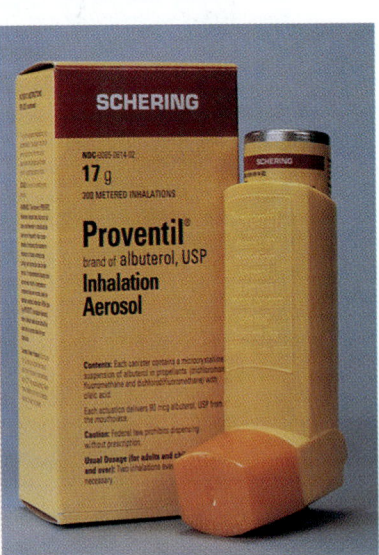

E

FIGURE 13.2 Medication forms. **A,** Nitroglycerin (dry tablets). **B,** Glucose paste (gel). **C,** Epinephrine autoinjector (liquid). **D,** Oxygen (gas). **E,** Albuterol inhaler (liquid powder).

Glucose gel is one example and is administered to patients who are hypoglycemic.

Liquid for Sublingual Spray

Many drugs are in a liquid form, and each liquid is designed for a specific route of administration. Nitroglycerin is available in a liquid and designed to be sprayed under the tongue. The liquid is converted to a spray by chemical reaction in the container. This type of liquid is not suitable for injection and is not effective if swallowed.

Suspensions

A suspension is a mixture of particles of the drug in a liquid. The particles do not dissolve. A suspension is often given by mouth and must be shaken before administration. An example of a suspension is activated charcoal.

Liquid for Injection

Medications that are injected usually are in liquid form. These liquids are sterile and designed to be injected safely into the body through different routes of administration; subcutaneous, intramuscular, intravenous (IV) push, and IV infusion are the most common. An example of an injectable liquid is epinephrine (Figure 13.2, C). Only liquids specifically designed for injection should be used for that purpose.

Gases

Oxygen is a useful "medication" that is in the form of a gas (Figure 13.2, D). It requires special storage tanks and regulator equipment to provide the correct flow to the patient.

Fine Powder for Inhalation

A mechanical inhaler produces a puff of very fine powder that is inhaled by the patient. The powder is carried into the lungs by the inhaled breath. Various medications used for asthma, such as albuterol, are prepared in this form (Figure 13.2, E).

Liquid for Nebulizers

A nebulizer is a machine that transforms a liquid medication into a mist. The mist is given to the patient to breathe through a mask or mouthpiece. Nebulizers are another method of getting a drug into the lungs in high concentrations.

> ✔ Drugs are produced in many forms (tablets, liquids, fine powders, etc.). A drug may be available in more than one form. Each form is designed to be used in a specific manner.

Drug Dynamics

Many medications must enter the bloodstream to be effective. Once in the blood, the drug is carried to all the organs of the body and acts on many different systems. Such drugs are said to act systemically. Some of the effects are beneficial, and some are undesirable (adverse effects). An example of a **systemically acting medication** is glucose. Glucose given by mouth is absorbed and enters the blood. Once in the blood the glucose is carried to the brain and other organs, where it is used by the cells to create energy.

Other medications are designed to act locally. They are applied directly to the diseased area. Some examples are inhaled medicine for asthma, which acts directly in the lungs, and steroid cream for the skin, which acts at the site of a rash. Every **locally acting medication** has some absorption into the blood, which may cause systemic side effects.

Each drug has defined indications (conditions when the drug should be used), contraindications (conditions when the drug should not be used), side effects (problems produced by the drug), actions (what the drug does and why), and synergistic effects (how the drug acts in the presence of other drugs).

> ✔ Systemically acting drugs are absorbed into the bloodstream and carried to all parts of the body. Locally acting drugs are placed directly on the involved area, and only small amounts enter the blood.

Administration

Drugs are administered by many different routes. The route is determined by the dose to be administered; the type of drug to be given; the effects desired; and the effects on the body of the breakdown, distribution, and elimination of the drug. The route of administration influences the speed of absorption, the availability, and the **duration of action.**

Most drugs used by EMS providers are given either as an aerosol mist or by injection, either subcutaneous, intramuscular, or intravenous. This is because drugs used in the prehospital setting are generally lifesaving in nature and must be quickly absorbed into and distributed by the blood. The advantages and disadvantages of the major routes are discussed in the following sections (Table 13.2).

Intravenous Injection

Drugs can be placed directly into the blood through an intravenous (IV) line and catheter. The advantages of this route are rapid effect and good availability with high levels of drug in the blood. The disadvantages are the need to have an IV line in place and the possibility of serious side effects caused by a high concentration of some drugs.

Intramuscular Injection

A drug can be injected directly into the muscle tissue by placing a needle into the patient's muscle. The drug is then absorbed from the muscle into the blood. The advantages of this route are easy access (no IV line is needed) and fairly rapid absorption. The main disadvantage is pain with some drugs. Intramuscular injection cannot be used with patients taking blood thinners, and it may disrupt blood tests used to diagnose a heart attack.

In addition, in patients who are in shock, the poor blood circulation causes slow absorption and therefore delayed drug action.

Subcutaneous Injection

A drug can be injected just under the skin into the fat and connective tissue above the muscle. The rate of absorption varies depending on the form of the drug. Many drugs can be used with this kind of injection, including liquid solutions, which are absorbed quickly, and solid pellets, which are absorbed very slowly. The disadvantages are that large volumes cannot be given and the drug must be nonirritating. An automatic epinephrine injection pen is an example of a subcutaneous medication.

Oral

Medications are often given by mouth (orally) because it is easy and does not require an injection, IV access, or patient discomfort. Once the drug is swallowed, it is absorbed from the stomach and intestines. Absorption is slower than with an injection. The disadvantages are that some medications are not absorbed well from the stomach and unresponsive patients cannot be given oral medications. Glucose is an example of an oral medication.

Rectal

Some medications can be given rectally, and these drugs generally take the form of suppositories or liquid. The medicine is placed through the anus into the space just inside (the rectum). Rectally administered drugs are absorbed at a speed similar to oral medications. An advantage is that even an unresponsive patient can safely receive rectal medications.

Sublingual

Sublingual medications are placed in the mouth but are not swallowed. They are held in the mouth under the tongue and allowed to dissolve. Sublingual medications are absorbed much faster than swallowed medications. Unresponsive patients should not be given sublingual medications. Nitroglycerin is an example of a medication that can be given sublingually.

TABLE 13.2 Routes of Administration

Route	Advantages	Disadvantages
Intravenous injection	100% availability Very rapid effect	Need intravenous access High concentration of drug can cause serious side effects
Intramuscular injection	Rapid absorption Easy access	Disrupts laboratory tests for heart attacks Contraindicated in patients on blood thinners
Subcutaneous injection	Can use a variety of drugs Easy access	Variable absorption Only for small volumes
Oral	Easy Noninvasive	Slower absorption Responsive patients only Low availability of some medications
Sublingual	More rapid absorption Better availability of some drugs	Responsive patients only
Inhalation	Very rapid absorption Local or systemically acting drugs	Certain drugs only Patient must be alert and able to use inhaler

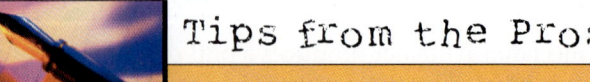

Tips from the Pros

When assisting patients with sublingual medications, it is important that they do *not* swallow the medicine. Sublingual medications such as nitroglycerin do not work when swallowed.

Inhalation

Inhaled medications reach the lungs immediately and can have rapid systemic effects. They often are used to treat asthma or other breathing disorders. The patient must be alert and able to use the mechanical inhaler. Only specifically designed drugs can be administered by this route.

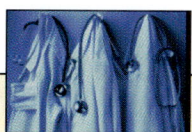

Tips from the Pros

Most inhalers are difficult for patients to use correctly. It is helpful if the EMT becomes familiar with the proper technique to assist the patient in using the inhaler correctly.

Topical

A topical medication is applied as a cream or patch to the skin. Topical medications have delayed effects and slow systemic absorption. They are rarely used in emergency situations. Examples of topical medications are nitroglycerin patches or paste used to treat patients with angina and steroid creams such as hydrocortisone used to treat skin rashes.

✓ The route of administration is the way the drug is put into the body. Each route has advantages and disadvantages.

Absorption

A critical characteristic of a systemic drug is its absorption. The speed of absorption is how fast the drug leaves the site of administration and enters the blood. Rapidly absorbed drugs enter the blood in a short time. Aerosol mists and intramuscular injections are examples of rapid absorption. Appendices A through F at the end of this chapter list all routes of administration for drugs.

In addition to the speed of absorption, it is also important to know how much of the drug is absorbed. This characteristic is called the availability. If a drug has high availability, most of the drug will eventually enter the blood. If the drug has low availability, only a small amount of the drug will enter the blood. For example, if a pill is taken orally and half of it is absorbed from the stomach and the other half is excreted in the feces, the drug has 50% availability.

The speed of absorption and availability depend on three factors: the kind of drug, the route of administration, and the form of the drug. In many cases, the route of administration is the most important factor in speed and availability.

Elimination

The body begins to remove a medication as soon as it enters the blood. The liver, kidneys, and lungs filter the blood in different ways to help remove all types of drugs. Some drugs are removed more by the liver, others more by the lungs or kidneys. The duration of action of a drug is how long its main action lasts after one dose. The duration of action depends on the specific way the drug works, the dose, the route, and how fast the drug is eliminated.

Physician Notes

Almost all drugs and medications have a toxic level at which the drug has a higher negative effect than a positive one. When a drug or medication is given to a patient before the last dose has been eliminated, such problems can occur. Even if the drug is given in a correct manner and dosage, if the body's elimination system is impaired, the drug's concentration can build up to toxic levels.

Reading Labels and Prescriptions

Each prescription medication has a label on the container with a description of the drug and directions for its use. This information is critical for the safe use of any drug. Careful reading of the label of a patient's prescription container over the radio to medical direction may provide valuable information for patient care.

The components of a drug label include the patient's name, name of the drug, medication strength, number of pills, route, and directions.

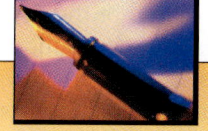

Tips from the Pros

Always ask the patient for all of his or her medications and bottles. These containers should be taken with the patient on any transport because they provide valuable information on specific medication types and dosages.

Patient's Name

The patient must be identified and the name matched with that on the drug label.

✓ The speed of absorption is how fast the drug leaves the site of administration and enters the blood. This rate depends on the route of administration.

Name of Drug

This name may be the trade or generic name.

Strength of Medication

The amount of medication in each tablet, capsule, injection, or puff is measured in milligrams (mg), grams (g), or micrograms (μg).

Number of Pills

The total number of pills in the bottle is often written on the label. This information can be helpful in overdose situations to help determine how many pills may have been taken.

Route

The route of administration is often abbreviated. Oral—PO, sublingual—SL, subcutaneous—SQ or SC, rectal—supp., inhaled—puffs.

Directions

This part of the label typically includes when to take the medication and how much to take at each time. Abbreviations are often used in this section of the label. Every day—qd, twice a day—bid, three times a day—tid, four times a day—qid, at bedtime—hs, every 4 to 6 hours—q4-6h, and as needed—prn.

Specific Medications

The medications carried in the EMS vehicle and those medications that the EMT may assist the patient with taking are shown in Table 13.3. The main action of the drug and its side effects are listed. All drugs have indications, which are the conditions and situations in which the drug should be given. For example, chest pain is an indication to give nitroglycerin. Contraindications are conditions and situations in which a drug should not be given. Low blood pressure, which is often defined as a systolic pressure lower than 100 mm Hg, is a contraindication to using nitroglycerin. The common contraindications and the usual dose and route of administration are shown in Table 13.3.

The indications for using the drugs are discussed in detail in the relevant chapters:

Oxygen: see Chapter 10.
Glucose: see Chapter 17.
Activated charcoal: see Chapter 19.
Nitroglycerin: see Chapter 15.
Epinephrine: see Chapter 18.
Inhaler: see Chapter 14.

Assessment and Management

A patient must be thoroughly assessed both before and after a medication is given. Knowledge of the indications, contraindications, actions, and side effects of the drugs is critical for this evaluation.

Initial Assessment

The purpose of an initial assessment is to identify which medications might be helpful and to identify conditions that change the way the drugs are used. The initial assessment should include the following:

- Current problem: what are the symptoms and main problems at this time?
- Background history of current event.
- Medications: current and recent medications. It is especially important to note whether the patient has already taken the prescribed drug and, if so, how many times and over what time period.
- Allergies to any medications.
- Past medical history, including alcohol use, asthma, chronic obstructive pulmonary disease (COPD), diabetes, heart disease, hypertension, kidney disease, liver disease, and stroke.
- Physical examination: vital signs, mental status, and general examination.

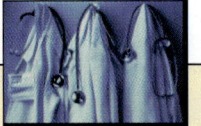

Physician Notes

Medications can be helpful and even lifesaving in the right situation, but they can also be dangerous. It is important to follow the algorithm and look for indications, allergies, and *any* contraindications before giving a medicine or assisting with administration of a medicine. Have a routine series of questions to ask for each medicine to cover these areas. A systematic approach is the only way to avoid medication error.

TABLE 13.3 Specific Medications

Medication	Action	Side Effects	Contraindications	Administration Route	Common Dose
Oxygen	Increased oxygen pressure and oxygen content in the blood	High concentrations may decrease respiratory drive in COPD patients	None	Inhaled, via mask or nasal cannula	2-15 L/min
Glucose	Raises blood glucose levels	Possible hyperglycemia	Unresponsive patients should not be given oral medication	Oral paste is rubbed inside the cheeks and mouth and swallowed	25 g; repeat as needed
Activated charcoal	Absorbs many poisons from the stomach and intestine and binds them to surface of charcoal	If it enters the lungs, it can cause severe pneumonitis; deactivates ipecac syrup	Never give oral charcoal to an unresponsive, semiresponsive, or convulsing patient	Oral	25-100g in a water slurry
Nitroglycerin	Dilates large veins and decreases the workload on the heart; dilates large coronary arteries; helps relieve the pain of angina	Hypotension Increased heart rate Headache	Allergy to nitrates Hypotension Increased intracranial pressure	Sublingual tablets or oral spray	Tablets: 0.3, 0.4, or 0.6 mg; given one at a time every five minutes or as directed Spray: 0.4 mg per spray
Epinephrine	Increases blood pressure by constricting arteries and opens the airways of the lungs	Increased heart rate Hypertension Arrhythmias Tremor	Increased risk of injury in patients with hypertension, heart disease, or stroke; use of monoamine oxidase inhibitor–type drugs; *never* contraindicated in severe anaphylaxis	Subcutaneous injection	0.2-0.5 ml of a 1:1000 dilution (0.2-0.5 mg)
Albuterol Terbutaline Metaproterenol	Inhaled, causes opening of airways in the lungs allowing for easier breathing	Tremor, arrhythmias, palpitations, and hypertension are prominent; increased heart rate and blood pressure are rare	Allergy to the drug; use of monoamine oxidase inhibitor–type drugs	Inhaled into the lungs from a variety of mechanical inhalers	Two to three deep inhalations every 4 hours

Many of these items are covered in the initial evaluation of the patient. The most important areas are current symptoms, vital signs, major medical problems, and allergies. Patients should not be given medications to which they are allergic or for which they have a major contraindication.

Management

Once the EMT determines that an intervention with a medication may be indicated, the next step should be to obtain authorization for administration, or assistance with administration, by contacting medical direction. Medical direction refers to the directives for patient care provided by physicians. These can be given by radio or telephone. In some cases, written **standing orders,** contained within patient care **protocols,** may authorize interventions with medications without contacting medical direction. The specific medications that can be used and the exact standing orders vary with different medical directors and EMT services. Medical direction should be contacted whenever the EMT has questions about assessment or management of a patient.

For many medications, the EMT-Basic may only assist the patient in taking the medication from the patient's own supply. Assisting means finding the bottle, getting some water for pills, and helping the patient to hold a glass or read a label. The EMT-Basic cannot give these medications directly to the patient.

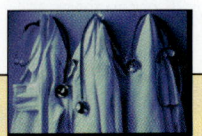

Physician Notes

It is important to realize that the EMT and the medical direction physician are working together to provide the best care possible to the patient. Medical direction is always available when there are questions or problems. EMTs are encouraged to contact medical direction whenever the appropriate action is unclear based on prior instruction or training. This two-way contact is how the EMT and medical direction physician can best work together.

Continuing Assessment

After a medication has been given, the assessment process continues. This evaluation should not delay appropriate transport to a medical facility. Continuing assessment should include the following:

- Repeating vital signs and mental status
- Observing for specific desired actions of the medication (i.e., relief of symptoms)
- Observing for unwanted side effects
- Documenting the patient's response to the intervention as it occurs
- Intervening again if the patient fails to respond, has side effects, or has changing symptoms

Summary

- Drugs are beneficial for many patients but are dangerous if used incorrectly.
- The EMT is able to give patients the drugs carried in the ambulance and may assist the patient in taking some personal medications.
- Each drug has only one generic name, which is a simple form of the chemical name. Each drug may have several different trade names.
- The route of administration is how the drug is put into the body. There are important advantages and disadvantages to each route.
- Oral medications should never be given to an unresponsive patient or a patient with a decreased level of consciousness.
- Medications come in many forms, including tablets, liquids, gels, powders, and gases. Each form is designed to be used by a specific route and should not be used by a different route.
- Before giving medications, the patient is assessed for allergies, contraindications, and major medical problems by medical history and physical examination. Medical direction must be contacted before giving certain medications and at any time when the appropriate action is unclear.
- The assessment process includes continuous monitoring of vital signs and patient response to medications.
- The continuing assessment of response to medications leads to appropriate changes in intervention.

Scenario Solution

This patient has signs and symptoms consistent with an acute allergic reaction, also called anaphylaxis. Your primary survey reveals the patient to be in distress, and immediate action is needed. She indicates that her shortness of breath has gotten worse, her throat now feels like it is swelling, and the hives are increasing. She further tells you that this feels like the last time she was stung by a bee, when her throat "swelled shut." The physical examination reveals a small puncture-like wound on the side of her neck with a stinger still visible.

As your partner prepares oxygen for the patient, you read the epi-pen. It has her name on it, it is current with the expiration date, and the patient advises you that she has carried one for 3 years, since the last episode like this. She asks you to open it for her and put it in her hand so she can inject it into her thigh.

Scenario Solution (cont'd)

She tells you this is the same drug that she used last time. Your current treatment guidelines allow you to assist patients in the use of an epi-pen in this type of situation.

Your patient is able to self-administer the epinephrine. As you place her on the ambulance gurney and administer oxygen, you begin to see the results of the drug. Her breathing is slowing and becoming more regular. She says that her throat feels a little better and the tightness in her chest is not as bad. You are able to remove the stinger from the injection site, and your patient shows great improvement by the time you reach the hospital.

Key Terms

Absorption The uptake of medications into tissues.

Actions The desirable effects of a drug (e.g., the action of oral glucose is to raise the blood sugar level).

Availability Amount of drug that is absorbed from the site of administration.

Contraindications Conditions or situations in which a drug should not be given (e.g., lack of consciousness is a contraindication to the administration of oral medications).

Duration of action The length of time a drug is effective after one dose.

Generic name A simple form of the chemical name of a drug; each drug has only one generic name.

Indications Conditions under which a drug is given (e.g., chest pain is an indication for giving nitroglycerin).

Locally acting medication Drug that is applied directly to an affected area; it usually has a very low absorption into the bloodstream.

Medical direction Various duties that a physician provides in support of an EMS system (protocols, case reviews, educational programming, etc.).

Medications Chemicals that change the way the body functions; used to treat a variety of diseases and symptoms.

Pharmacology Study of how chemicals work in the human body.

Protocols Written or printed instructions or plans for carrying out an activity. In EMS, a protocol is a document that describes, usually in a step-by-step manner, the method that is used to deal with a particular set of symptoms or conditions.

Route of administration The way a drug is put into the body.

Side effects Unwanted or harmful effects of a drug. Almost all medications have some side effects, the severity of which often depends on the dose of the drug.

Standing orders Patient care directions in writing that authorize specific steps in patient assessment and intervention without the requirement of direct medical direction contact by radio or telephone; usually highly specific in what can be done and contained within the patient care protocols.

Systemically acting medication A drug that enters the bloodstream and is transported throughout the entire body.

Trade name Drug name created by the company that sells the drug; one drug may have many trade names.

Review Questions

1. Medications are designed:
   a. To have as few side effects as possible.
   b. So that they can be used safely in all situations.
   c. Without testing and are taken at the patient's risk, just like over-the-counter health supplements.
   d. Without regard for safety of the patient.
2. Drugs have:
   a. Only one trade name but several generic names.
   b. Only one generic name but several trade names.
   c. One generic name and one trade name.
   d. Several generic names and several trade names.
3. Liquid epinephrine designed for a nebulizer:
   a. Can safely be given by subcutaneous injection.
   b. Can only be used in a nebulizer.
   c. Has no restrictions on its use.
   d. Should never be used by an EMT.
4. The major side effect of albuterol/terbutaline is:
   a. Hypoglycemia.
   b. Sleepiness.
   c. Tachycardia and cardiac complications.
   d. Analgesia.

Review Questions (cont'd)

5. The usual route of administration of albuterol/terbutaline is:
   a. By mouth.
   b. By inhaler.
   c. Subcutaneously.
   d. Intravenously.
6. The major contraindication to the use of activated charcoal is:
   a. Tachycardia.
   b. Unresponsive patient.
   c. Hypotension.
   d. Vomiting.
7. The reason for continuing assessment after medications are given to a patient is to:
   a. Ensure that the patient has taken the medication.
   b. Identify complications tha result from the medication.
   c. Decide whether to transport the patient to the hospital.
   d. Call the patient's private physician and get further instructions for patient care.

Answers to these Review Questions can be found at the end of the book on page 866.

Appendix A: Oral Glucose Agents

I. Generic Name: Oral glucose
II. Trade Name: Glutose, Insta-Glucose, Insulin Reaction
III. Type of Drug: Nutrient
IV. Mechanism of Action: Oral glucose is absorbed from the intestine after administration and then used by tissues. Direct absorption occurs, resulting in a rapid increase in blood glucose levels, making it very effective in small doses.
V. Prehospital Indications:
    A. To treat coma caused by hypoglycemia
    B. To treat coma of unknown origin
    C. To treat seizures of unknown etiology
    D. To treat new onset of seizures
    E. To treat known diabetics actively seizing
VI. Contraindications:
    A. Stroke
    B. Delirium tremens with dehydration
VII. Precautions/Incompatibilities:
    A. Blood sugar documented before administration
    B. Pregnancy
    C. Wernicke-Korsakoff syndrome
    D. Alcoholism
VIII. Administration: 10 to 20 g orally (1 tube), repeat in 10 minutes if necessary. Response should occur in 10 minutes.
IX. Side Effects/Adverse Reactions: Nausea
X. Overdose Therapy: Not an issue with oral glucose agents

Appendix B: Activated Charcoal

I. Generic Name: Activated charcoal
II. Trade Name: Charcola, Arm-a-Char, Charcoaide, Instachar
III. Type of Drug: Adsorbent
IV. Mechanism of Action: Activated charcoal binds to and absorbs ingested poisons, which inhibits their absorption in the gastrointestinal tract. It forms a barrier between the substance and the gastric mucosa.
V. Prehospital Indications: Activated charcoal is used in the treatment of certain cases of poisoning and overdoses in the alert patient. It is most commonly given in the hospital after gastric lavage but is appropriate to give in the prehospital setting before lavage if long transportation is anticipated.
VI. Contraindications:
    A. Oral administration to the comatose patient
    B. Patients who have ingested cyanide, mineral acids, strong bases, methanol, ethanol, lithium, or iron because it does not bind to these agents
VII. Precautions/Incompatibilities:
    A. Will bind with ipecac and other oral drugs given simultaneously; must be given after emesis has occurred if being used with ipecac
    B. Works best if given without the use of ipecac
    C. May cause vomiting
VIII. Administration:
    A. Comes unmixed or "blended" in a sorbitol syrup
    B. Adults: 60 to 100 grams
    C. Children: 30 to 60 grams
    D. If unmixed product is used, should be mixed in a glass of water
IX. Side Effects/Adverse Reactions: Constipation, diarrhea; large doses may cause vomiting
X. Toxic Effects: Extremely rare; bowel obstruction and aspiration are major concerns
XI. Overdose Therapy: Airway should be managed if aspiration occurs

Appendix C: Epinephrine

I. Generic Name: Epinephrine
II. Trade Name: Adrenalin
III. Type of Drug: Sympathomimetic
IV. Pharmacology: Epinephrine is a catecholamine that stimulates both alpha-adrenergic and beta-adrenergic receptors in the sympathetic nervous system. Stimulation of beta receptors is significantly more profound than its effect on alpha receptors. Stimulation of cardiac beta$_1$-receptors increases the rate and force of contractions and increased atrioventricular conduction, resulting in an increase in cardiac output. Epinephrine can cause spontaneous firing of Purkinje fibers and has been shown to initiate spontaneous

Appendix C: Epinephrine (cont'd)

myocardial contraction in asystole. Stimulation of beta$_2$-receptors relaxes the bronchial smooth muscles, thereby increasing vital lung capacity. Stimulation of alpha receptors causes vasoconstriction.
  A. *Alpha:* Bronchial, cutaneous, renal, and visceral arterial constriction
  B. *Beta 1:* Positive inotropic and chronotropic actions; increases automaticity
  C. *Beta 2:* Bronchial smooth muscle relaxation and dilation of skeletal vasculature; blocks histamine release
V. Pharmacokinetics: Subcutaneous or intramuscular injection gives a rapid onset with longer duration; half-life is short (minutes); epinephrine is degraded in the liver with renal excretion
VI. Prehospital Indications:
  A. Severe bronchospasm; bronchiolitis and asthma
  B. Anaphylaxis
VII. Contraindications:
  A. Hypertension
  B. Narrow-angle glaucoma
  C. Pulmonary edema
VIII. Precautions/Incompatibilities:
  A. Autooxidation of catecholamine is pH dependent
  B. Potentiates other sympathomimetic
  C. Incompatible with sodium bicarbonate, nitrates, lidocaine, and aminophylline
IX. Interactions: Patients on monoamine oxidase (MAO) inhibitors, antihistamines, or tricyclic antidepressants may have heightened effects
X. Administration: Single-dose prefilled syringe delivers 0.3 mg in 1 ml (1-1000)
XI. Side Effects/Adverse Reactions:
  A. CNS: Psychomotor agitation, anxiety, headache
  B. Cardiovascular: Tachycardia, hypertension, ventricular dysrhythmia, palpitations
XII. Toxic Effects:
  A. Uncontrolled effects on myocardium and arterial system, including myocardial ischemia and lethal dysrrhythmias
  B. Increased stimulation of the CNS
XIII. Overdose Therapy: Supportive care of signs and symptoms

Appendix D: Nitroglycerin

I. Generic Name: Nitroglycerin (NTG)
II. Trade Name: Nitro-bid, Nitrostat, Nitrogard, Nitro, Dur, Nitrolingual, Nitrol, Tridil
III. Type of Drug: Antianginal
IV. Pharmacodynamics: Nitroglycerin works to relax smooth muscle of the vasculature. While venous effects predominate, nitroglycerine produces a dose-dependent dilation of both arterial and venous beds. Dilation of the postcapillary sphincter produces a venous pooling effect, decreasing venous return to the heart, thereby reducing left ventricular end diastolic pressure (preload). Arteriole relaxation reduces systemic vascular resistance, thereby reducing afterload. Although nitroglycerin will relax the large epicardial arteries, the exact contribution to relieving exertion angina is unknown. Effective coronary perfusion pressure is normally maintained but can be compromised if blood pressure falls excessively or increased heart rate decreases diastolic filling time.
V. Pharmacokinetics: Nitroglycerin is readily absorbed through the sublingual mucosa and the skin. Nitroglycerine has a short half-life estimated at 1 to 4 minutes and is metabolized in the liver.
VI. Prehospital Indications: Chest pain, anginal pain
VII. Contraindications:
  A. Known hypersensitivity to drug
  B. Increased intracranial pressure
  C. Hypovolemia
  D. Hypotension
VIII. Precautions/Incompatibilities:
  A. Excessive use may lead to tolerance
  B. May cause a rapid decrease in blood pressure
  C. Patient should be prone or supported while medication is given
  D. Patients with postural hypotension
IX. Administration:
  A. Adults (sublingual): 0.3 to 0.4 mg tablets; repeat at 3 to 5 minutes as needed to a total of three tablets (or more by MCEP order)
  B. Adults (lingual spray): 0.4 mg/spray, sprayed directly under the tongue; additional one or two sprays every 3 to 5 minutes for a total of three sprays
X. Side Effects/Adverse Reactions:
  A. CNS: Headache, dizziness, weakness
  B. Cardiovascular: Hypotension, reflex tachycardia, fainting
  C. Gastrointestinal: Nausea, vomiting, dry mouth

Appendix D: Nitroglycerin (cont'd)

XI. Toxic Effects:
   A. Cardiovascular: Hypotension, tachycardia, heart block
   B. Respiratory: Hyperpnea, dyspnea
   C. Gastrointestinal: Nausea, vomiting, anorexia
   D. CNS: Flushing, diaphoresis, dizziness, syncope, confusion, fever

XII. Overdose Therapy:
   A. Decrease or discontinue drip rate
   B. Treat hypotension with fluids and elevation of legs

Appendix E: Oxygen

I. Generic Name: Oxygen
II. Trade Name: Oxygen
III. Type of Drug: Atmospheric gas
IV. Mechanism of Action: Supports cellular life and function as it is transported through the body on hemogolbin found in red blood cells
V. Prehospital Indications:
   A. Hypoxemia
   B. Ischemic chest pain
   C. Respiratory distress
   D. Carbon monoxide poisoning
VI. Contraindications: None
VII. Precautions/Incompatibilities: None in prehospital setting
VIII. Administration:
   A. High concentration: 10 to 15 L/min via mask
   B. Low concentration: 1 to 4 L/min via nasal cannula
IX. Side Effects/Adverse Reactions:
   A. High-flow oxygen may cause respiratory depression in patients with CO_2 poisoning
   B. Oxygen supports combustion
X. Toxic Effects: None

Appendix F: Bronchodilators

I. Generic Name: Albuterol
II. Trade Name: Proventil, Ventolin
III. Type of Drug: Adrenergic, beta$_2$ agonist
IV. Pharmacology: Bronchodilators work to produce bronchodilation by relaxing smooth muscle tissue of the bronchioles associated with asthma, bronchitis, emphysema, or bronchiectasis. Additionally, bronchodilators may facilitate expectoration. Pharmacologic actions include alpha-adrenergic, B$_1$, and B$_2$ stimulation.
V. Prehospital Indications: Albuterol is used to treat reversible airway obstruction caused by:
   A. Wheezing associated with asthma
   B. Chronic obstructive pulmonary disease (emphysema)
   C. Chronic bronchitis
VI. Contraindications:
   A. Patient with known sensitivity to drug (adrenergic amine)
   B. Not to be used with other beta-agonist aerosols
VII. Precautions/Incompatibilities:
   A. To be used with caution in patients with heart disease, hypertension, and diabetes
   B. To be used with caution in patients who have taken other sympathomimetic agents
   C. Incompatible with tricyclic antidepressants and monamine oxidase inhibitors
VIII. Administration: Comes as metered dose inhaler (MDI) and can be given 1 to 2 inhalations (90 mg/spray) (two puffs from an MDI is a very small dose; 10 to 15 puffs is probable safe); *patient should be sitting up and encouraged to breath deep and occasionally hold his or her breath*
IX. Side Effects/Adverse Reactions:
   A. CNS: Nervousness, tremor, headache
   B. Cardiovascular: Hypertension, dysrhythmias, chest pain
   C. Gastrointestinal: Nausea, vomiting
X. Toxic Effects:
   A. Paradoxical bronchospasm
   B. Worsened ischemia in the acute myocardial infarction setting
XI. Overdose Therapy:
   A. Discontinue drug
   B. Treat signs and symptoms per protocol

14

Respiratory Emergencies

Lesson Goal

Next to airway problems, breathing difficulty is on of the more common life-threatening conditions that the EMT will encounter and probably the most common in nontrauma patients. This chapter addresses those nontrauma conditions. Sometimes the signs may be subtle and difficult to identify. These are the situations in which the EMT needs to have a strong fund of knowledge to provide the best chance for the patient to survive.

Scenario

You are dispatched to a 25-year-old woman who has suddenly become short of breath. She is outside in a very dusty field that is the site of a local music festival. On arrival you find a patient who appears anxious and short of breath. Her friends tell you that she has a history of asthma, but the patient is unable to give you any additional information because of her respiratory distress. The friends are very anxious and want you to take the girl to the hospital as fast as you can.

The patient is responsive and alert, with respiratory rate of 40 breaths per minute and pulse rate of 50 beats per minute.

The patient's skin color is pale, and her lips are starting to turn slightly blue. As you continue your assessment you find that she is using the muscles in her neck during inspiration and that the skin below her rib cage moves in and out with her breathing. On auscultation you hear high-pitched noises during both inspiration and expiration; normal breath sounds are difficult to identify. As you place the oxygen mask on the patient, she grabs it and pulls it off. During your assessment the patient's friends become more anxious, loudly asking you to just leave for the hospital.

 What signs and symptoms of respiratory distress are present in this patient? What questions would you ask at this point? Are there any barriers to proper patient management at this scene? If so, what can you do about them? Outline the steps you would take to manage this patient effectively during transport.

Key Terms to Know

Accessory muscles
Agonal ventilations
Alveolar/capillary exchange
Apnea

Bronchodilators
Bronchospasm
Cellular/capillary exchange
Chronic bronchitis

Crackles
Croup
Cyanosis
Dyspnea

Emphysema
Epiglottitis
FiO_2
Hyperventilation

Key Terms to Know (cont'd)

Hypoxia
Metabolism
Metered dose inhaler
Mottling

Nasal flaring
Paresthesia
Pneumonia
Pulmonary edema

Pulmonary embolism
Rales
Respiratory alkalosis
Retractions

Stridor
Tachypnea
Ventilatory arrest
Wheezes

Learning Objectives

As an EMT-Basic, you should be able to do the following:

DOT

- List the indications and contraindications for inhaler medications and demonstrate the steps required to assist with inhaler administration.
- List the structure and function of the respiratory system.
- Establish the relationship between airway management and the patient with breathing difficulty.
- List signs of adequate air exchange.
- State the generic name, medication forms, dose, administration, action, indications, and contraindications for the prescribed inhaler.
- Differentiate among the emergency medical care of the infant, child, and adult patient with breathing difficulty.
- List the signs and symptoms of respiratory distress and demonstrate the ability to intervene appropriately with supplemental oxygen or airway management and artificial ventilation.

Supplemental

- Define FiO_2 and discuss why it is a more descriptive term than *high-flow oxygen* when addressing the needs of the patient with respiratory distress or potential respiratory distress.
- Describe the assessment and prehospital care of the patient with breathing difficulty.
- Describe the special considerations needed to care for infants and children with respiratory emergencies.
- Relate the physiology of the respiratory system to the signs and symptoms of inadequate breathing.

One of the most common chief complaints encountered by the emergency medical technician (EMT) is shortness of breath. Every year more than 200,000 people die from respiratory emergencies. The EMT plays an important role in the care and transport of patients with respiratory distress. Careful assessment and prompt intervention in the prehospital setting can have a dramatic impact on patient outcome. The goal of the EMT is to maintain and, if possible, improve the patient's condition during transport. With respiratory emergencies, this goal often can be achieved by administering oxygen, maintaining patient comfort, and assisting with the administration of the patient's inhaler medications.

Although the EMT frequently will hear that the EMT should not make diagnoses, that statement is not true. The EMT makes diagnoses every time he or she comes into contact with a patient. They may not be the detailed diagnoses that appear on the patient's discharge summary from the hosptial, but neither are many of the diagnoses made by the physician in the emergency department. The are "working diagnoses," not final diagsoses. The EMT makes a diagnosis of the patient's condition and how critical that condition is. This statement applies to respiratory problems perhaps more than any other situation the EMT may encounter. When the EMT sees such a patient as described in the opening scenario, the initial diagnosis is *respiratory distress*. The next responsibility that the EMT has is to identify the probable reasons for this distress, formulate a treatment plan, and begin treatment. The assessment that the EMT performs is to identify which anatomic structures (larynx, trachea, bronchi, bronchioles, alveolus) are producing the patient's symptoms. Once this has been determined, the EMT must formulate a plan to relieve the patient's symptoms while transporting the patient to the hospital. To carry out this responsibility the EMT must understand the anatomy, physiology, pathology, and pathophysiology that produce these conditions in order to make rational judgements for patient care.

In Chapter 10 it was noted that there is a significant difference between ventilation (breathing) and respiration. *Respiration* is the entire process of oxygenation of the tissue cells for metabolism and removal of the waste products of metabolism. It begins with the fractional inspired oxygen

Patient Care Algorithm

Respiratory Distress Patient Assessment

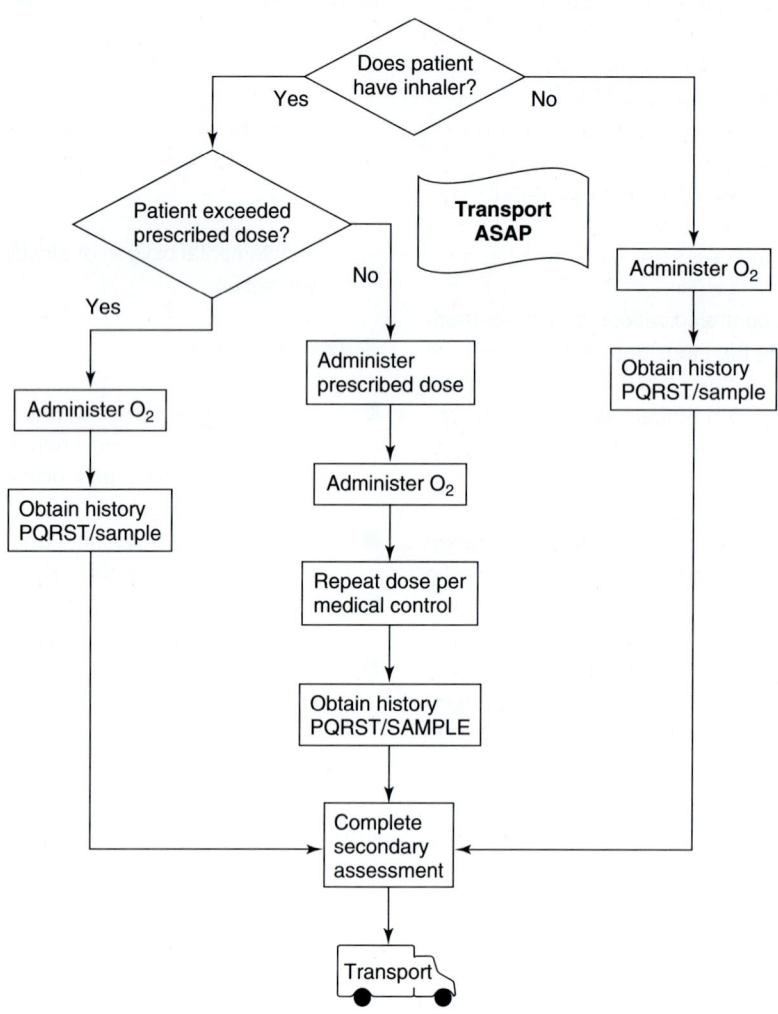

concentration **(FiO$_2$)** of the air coming in through the mouth and nose, continues through the utilization of oxygen in cells, and ends as the by-product of metabolism is exhausted through the mouth and nose into the ambient air. *Ventilation* is the mechanical movements of the chest and lungs that facilitate this portion of respiration. This text will adhere to that distinction for educational purposes.

Respiratory emergencies are particularly common in infants and children. Because of their relatively small respiratory reserve, infants and children with severe respiratory distress deteriorate quickly. If not stopped, this deterioration leads to respiratory and cardiovascular collapse. The use of oxygen can slow or stop this rapid progression. This chapter reviews some of the more common respiratory emergencies of childhood and discusses appropriate management.

The anatomy and physiology of the respiratory system are discussed in Chapters 7 and 10. The EMT student should review that material before reading this chapter. After a brief review of respiratory physiology, the assessment of a patient with respiratory complaints is discussed in detail. The common respiratory disorders encountered by the EMT are discussed, focusing on important signs and symptoms that require intervention by the EMT. The management of prehospital respiratory emergencies is covered, including oxygen therapy and the techniques for assisting with inhaler administration.

Respiratory System

This chapter briefly reviews the physiology of the respiratory system and then focuses on the pathophysiology of respiratory emergencies. Airway and ventilation are covered in other chapters and are not repeated here. The emphasis of the pathophysiology section is on disorders the EMT frequently encounters. The role of the EMT is to recognize signs and symptoms of respiratory compromise and intervene appropriately. The pathophysiology of common respiratory emergencies is discussed so that the EMT will have a better understanding of respiratory signs and symptoms and why these signs and symptoms occur. With that understanding the EMT can make decisions for patient care more accurately and quickly.

The respiratory system serves two basic functions: it supplies oxygen to and removes carbon dioxide from the tissue cells. Oxygen is used by the body's cells to make energy, and carbon dioxide is produced as a by-product. Body tissues rely on a continuous supply of oxygen to maintain this energy-producing process, which is termed **metabolism**. Any interruption of the supply of oxygen or removal of carbon dioxide can quickly lead to shock and death.

To maintain metabolism the body relies on two exchanges of oxygen and carbon dioxide (Figure 14.1). The first exchange occurs in the lungs and is termed the **alveolar/capillary exchange**. In this exchange oxygen moves from the alveoli into the blood, where it is taken up by the red blood cells. Carbon dioxide moves from the plasma of the blood into the alveoli to be exhaled. The second exchange is the **cellular/capillary exchange**. This exchange occurs throughout the body tissues. It involves the transfer of oxygen to the body cells and the removal of carbon dioxide.

Pathophysiology

The common medical emergency conditions that the EMT encounters affect the oropharynx, the larynx (vocal cords), the bronchioles, and the alveoli. The etiology is most often related to swelling, spasm, fluid, interruption of blood supply, or reduction of the surface area for the exchange of oxygen and carbon dioxide.

Among the most common disorders the EMT encounters in the field are chronic obstructive pulmonary disease and asthma. Other respiratory emergencies include hyperventilation, pulmonary edema (usually secondary to congestive heart failure), pulmonary embolism, pneumothorax, and hemothorax. Respiratory infections can also cause acute shortness of breath (**dyspnea**), including croup and epiglottitis in children and pneumonia in patients of any age.

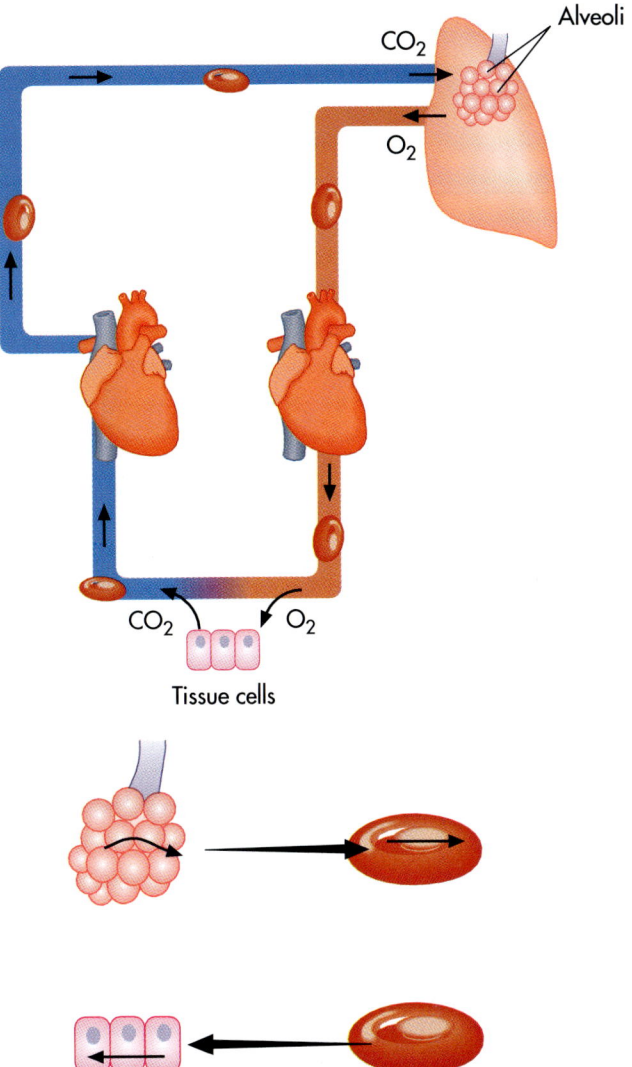

FIGURE 14.1 Alveolar/capillary exchange occurs in the lungs, where carbon dioxide is exhaled and oxygen is picked up by the blood. Cellular/capillary exchange occurs in the body tissues, where oxygen is released to the tissues and carbon dioxide is picked up by the blood.

Chronic Obstructive Pulmonary Disease

Chronic obstructive pulmonary disease (COPD) is a common disease most often seen in older patients who smoke. There are three components to this condition:

1. In **emphysema**, the alveoli in the lungs are destroyed. This reduces the alveolar/capillary surface area for gas exchange. Although the remaining alveoli stretch and enlarge to fill the space in the thoracic cavity, the exchange surface has been significantly reduced (Figure 14.2). There is also collapse of the airways in the lungs.

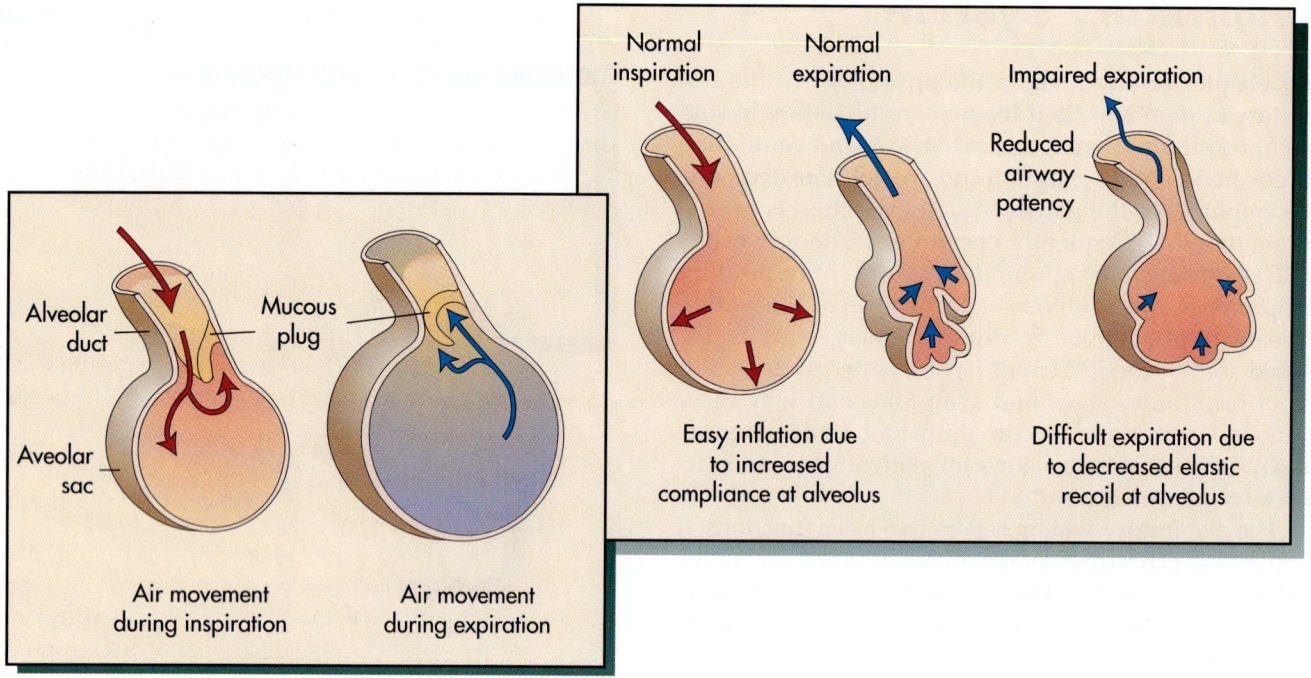

FIGURE 14.2 Mechanism of air trapping in COPD: Mucous plugs and narrowed airways cause air trapping and hyperinflation on expiration. During inspiration, the airways enlarge, allowing gas to flow past the obstruction. This mechanism of air trapping occurs in asthma and chronic bronchitis. Mechanism of air trapping in emphysema: Damaged or destroyed alveolar walls no longer support and hold open the airways, and alveoli lose their property of elastic recoil. Both of these factors contribute to collapse during expiration.

2. **Chronic bronchitis** is a form of obstructive disease characterized by excess mucus production in the airways, causing cough and airway obstruction.
3. In the alveoli that cannot completely empty secondary to obstruction by mucus, bacteria grow and produce infections.

Patients with COPD tend to function with mild dyspnea as a baseline condition and then have an increase in symptoms over hours to days. The increase in symptoms is often due to a respiratory infection.

Patients often have several signs and symptoms of respiratory distress, such as dyspnea, productive cough, agitation, and possibly cyanosis. Patients with COPD often develop a unique shape in the thoracic cavity termed *barrel chest deformity*. The upper part of the chest becomes expanded from constant overinflation of the lungs, caused by the trapping of air in obstructed airways (Figure 14.2).

Asthma

Asthma is most common in children and young adults but can occur at any age. Asthma is caused by airways that are oversensitive to stimuli in the environment and to emotional states. The airways suddenly narrow, a reaction termed **bronchospasm**. The airways then become swollen and filled with mucus, producing additional obstruction to the bronchioles. This make the movement of air very difficult. The movement of air through these areas of obstruction produces a high-pitched sound termed *wheezing*.

These small airways open more as the thoracic cavity expands to develop the negative pressure, but as the pressure becomes positive, the lung paryenchyma starts to collapse and the additional pressure forces the small airway closed. Therefore air moves in at a faster rate than it can move out. Asthmatics especially have difficulty exhaling.

Persons with asthma may have long periods of time without symptoms and then suddenly have a severe attack. Asthma patients frequently have prescribed inhalers that dilate the bronchi to help relieve an acute attack. Signs and symptoms of asthma include dyspnea, wheezing, dry cough, and an overexpanded chest. If the asthma attack is severe, the patient may not move enough air to cause wheezing. Therefore on examination of the patient, the EMT may not detect the classic sound associated with the disease. The loss of wheezing in an asthma patient is a sign for which to watch, because it may indicate a severe attack and not a resolution of symptoms.

Other signs of a severe asthma attack are changes in level of consciousness, such as confusion, irritability, or lethargy. These signs indicate **hypoxia**, a condition in which the patient has a shortage of oxygen. Asthma patients with signs of hypoxia are having a severe attack and may deteriorate rapidly to ventilatory arrest, followed by cardiac arrest if hypoxia is not corrected. Severe attacks of asthma, accompanied by uncorrected hypoxia, can lead to cardiac arrest. In these situations, hypoxia causes severe slowing of the heart rate, followed by asystole. Therefore patients having an asthma attack should be treated as rapidly as possible to prevent lethal hypoxia.

Asthma is a commonly encountered condition that can cause death. Asthma is believed to be increasing among adults, and there is some evidence that deaths from asthma are increasing. The EMT should be familiar with the assessment and management of an asthma patient.

Asthma is not a simple process and has been broken down into four stages. The interested EMT is referred to an EMT-Paramedic textbook or a medicine textbook for further education on this process.

Hyperventilation

> **Tips from the Pros**
>
> If an anxious patient is complaining of tingling hands and feet, think of hyperventilation first. Because an injury to the spinal cord can produce similar symptoms, it is important to look for evidence of a neck or back injury; however, hyperventilation is a much more common cause of these symptoms and is often missed in the field.

The EMT encounters hyperventilation syndrome frequently in the field; however, it is often unrecognized. The patient breathes faster than normal for a variety of reasons (see following discussion). The increased ventilatory rate drives off carbon dioxide faster than the body's metabolic rate produces it. Because CO_2 comes from the buffer system as a method of eliminating acid (one of the by-products of metabolism), the total body acid becomes lower than normal, the pH rises, and the system becomes alkalotic. Because this is produced by the respiratory system, it is termed **respiratory alkalosis**. The result of this change is twofold: nerve endings registering the stimuli incorrectly produce the symptom of tingling, and spasm of the forearm muscles draws the hands into a claw. The most common location for the tingling (**paresthesia**) is in the fingertips and around the mouth.

There are two major causes of hyperventilation: (1) anaerobic metabolism secondary to hypoxia and decreased oxygen delivery to the tissue cells and (2) the hyperventilation syndrome that results from pain and anxiety. Anaerobic metabolism is not usually associated with the tingling around the mouth and at the fingertips or the carpopedal spasm of respiratory acidosis (see Chapter 9).

Pain and anxiety may worsen respiratory acidosis. The following examples illustrate this process:

1. A patient recieves a blow to the chest causing a fracture. Pain causes the patient's breathing to become shallow and rapid.
2. A patient is worried and anxious because of stress, family emergency, or the death of a loved one. The patient unknowingly begins to ventilate faster.
3. A patient notices a sharp stabbing pain in his chest. The pain is caused by intercostal muscle spasm. To the patient, all chest pain is cardiac. Concern and worry are immediately present. Both pain from the muscle spasm and worry about the possibility of a heart attack increase the ventilatory rate, driving off carbon dioxide.

Hyperventilation is an abnormal increase in ventilatory rate and tidal volume (the volume of air inhaled with each breath). The anxiety of an emergency often leads to hyperventilation. Patients who are hyperventilating may or may not complain of dyspnea, and they often are in pain from other injuries. Signs and symptoms of hyperventilation include increased respiratory rate, tingling in the hands and feet (paresthesia), hunger for air, and agitation. The management of hyperventilation includes calm reassurance and "talking down" the patient. Patients can be instructed to breathe into a small bag, forcing the patient to breathe a higher concentration of carbon dioxide ($FiCO_2$). The EMT should be persistent with patients, instructing them to relax and slow down their breathing. This approach does work, although it can be difficult and very slow with some patients.

> **Physician Notes**
>
> Unless the EMT is very sure that this is an isolated hyperventilation syndrome that is not associated with another condition, management with a paper bag can be dangerous. The "paper bag trick" is an effective method of controlling the CO_2 level, but it must be used with caution.

It is important to realize that an abnormally high ventilatory rate (**tachypnea** or hyperventilation) is not always caused by anxiety. For example, patients in diabetic coma (ketoacidosis) will hyperventilate as a natural response to their disease state. It is important not to withhold oxygen from patients when the cause of tachypnea is unknown.

Pulmonary Edema

Pulmonary edema is a condition in which fluid accumulates in the airways. Many conditions cause pulmonary edema, but the most common is congestive heart failure (see Chapter 15). Other causes include severe infection, smoke or toxin inhalation, high altitudes, narcotic overdose, and fluid overload. The fluid causes decreased air movement in the lungs and an impaired alveolar/capillary exchange. The patient usually has severe dyspnea and possibly hypoxia. The symptoms of pulmonary edema may begin suddenly or develop over days. The patient's breath sounds will have coarse crackles, especially in the lower part of the lungs. Other signs of pulmonary edema are pink frothy sputum (material produced with coughing) and distended veins in the neck. Neck veins become distended because of congestion in the heart and lungs, causing blood to back up into the neck. Patients in pulmonary edema should be given high-flow oxygen and transported immediately.

Pulmonary Embolism

Pulmonary embolism most commonly occurs when a blood clot in a deep leg vein breaks off and travels to the lungs. The clot lodges in a branch of the pulmonary arteries, causing decreased blood flow to part of the lung. The decreased blood flow disrupts the alveolar/capillary exchange, leading to hypoxia. If the clot is large enough, pulmonary embolism can cause sudden death. Patients with pulmonary embolism usually become suddenly dyspneic and often have tachycardia.

Pneumothorax and Hemothorax

Pneumothorax and hemothorax are discussed in Chapter 25. They are caused by an accumulation of air (pneumothorax) or blood (hemothorax) in the pleural space. The pleural space is the space between the lungs and the thoracic cavity. Normally, it is filled with only a small amount of fluid, allowing the lungs to slide freely against the thoracic cavity during breathing. When air or blood enters this space, the lung collapses on the affected side, leading to hypoxia. The most common cause of a pneumothorax or hemothorax is trauma; however, some patients develop a spontaneous pneumothorax without any history of trauma. Patients are usually highly dyspneic and often have chest pain. Their ventilatory rate is often abnormally high (tachypnea or hyperventilation), breath sounds are diminished on the affected side, and they may appear to be deprived of oxygen (agitated, hungry for air, disoriented, and poor skin color or cyanosis).

Respiratory Infections

Respiratory emergencies due to infections are most commonly seen in infants and children. The two most common respiratory infections encountered by the EMT in children are croup and epiglottitis. **Croup** is an infection caused by a virus that affects the upper airway. Children with acute croup are often agitated and have a characteristic "barking" cough, as well as low-grade fever and cold symptoms. Croup usually affects children ages 6 months to 3 years. **Epiglottitis** is an infection of the epiglottis caused by bacteria. The epiglottis becomes swollen and may obstruct the upper airway. Children are especially susceptible to airway obstruction by epiglottitis because of the smaller size of the upper airway. A child with epiglottitis often sits still, has an excessive amount of saliva drooling from the mouth, and may have a high fever. The EMT must be careful not to place anything in the mouth of a child who may have epiglottitis, because this can cause spasm and obstruction of the upper airway. Adults can also develop epiglottitis, but this is less common.

An infection of the lung tissue is termed **pneumonia**. (Occasionally the EMT will hear the term *pneumonitis*, which essentially means the same thing.) Pneumonia usually develops over a period of days and most often affects young children and older adults, although patients of any age may be affected. It can be caused by bacteria, viruses, or fungi. The infection may be limited to part of the lung or may involve the entire lung. The alveoli and small airways become filled with the infecting organisms and large numbers of white blood cells, causing decreased oxygenation of the blood and dyspnea. Signs and symptoms include fever, chills, cough with sputum production, and dyspnea. In severe cases, which are most often seen in the elderly, pneumonia may progress rapidly and cause severe hypoxia.

> ✓ The respiratory system supplies oxygen to the blood, metabolizes the oxygen, and removes carbon dioxide through the alveolar/capillary exchange. Any condition that impairs this exchange can cause signs and symptoms of inadequate breathing.

Assessment

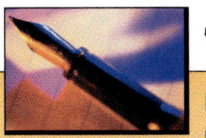

Tips from the Pros

Listen to breath sounds before transporting the patient. It is often difficult to hear breath sounds once the ambulance is moving.

When assessing an infant or child for respiratory distress, have a parent hold the child while you listen to breath sounds. This decreases anxiety for the child and gives the EMT a much more accurate assessment of respiratory status.

A thorough assessment of the patient with a respiratory emergency leads to appropriate management. Few situations are more frightening than not being able to breathe. A calm and reassuring attitude during the assessment and initial care will help decrease the patient's anxiety. The assessment of breathing, including the signs and symptoms of inadequate ventilation, is discussed in Chapter 10. This material is reviewed here because of its importance and also to relate specific signs and symptoms of inadequate breathing to the respiratory emergencies encountered by the EMT in the field.

After the initial assessment, the EMT should take a brief history from the patient using the SAMPLE format discussed in Chapter 8. Important information includes the onset and duration of symptoms, the presence of associated symptoms, the patient's past medical history, and a list of medications and drug allergies. The onset of symptoms may be abrupt (pneumothorax, pulmonary embolism) or gradual (pneumonia). This information is important, because the receiving physician will use it to make a diagnosis. Important associated symptoms include fever and cough, which might suggest pneumonia. If the patient has a cough, it is important to know if the cough produces sputum. The appearance of the sputum (clear or colored) can also be important information. A list of the patient's medications is helpful to the physician in making a diagnosis. Drug allergies are always important to know, because the patient may be given medications in the emergency department.

After arriving on the scene to began the scene survey, trying to get a grasp on exactly what is going on, the EMT does not have time to try to think of all the components of the physical examination that may be important. In fact all are important and must be considered, although many may be normal. Therefore if the EMT has a system that is always used each time he or she arrives on the scene and must deal with a respiratory problem or evaluate for the possibility of such a problem, having the format memorized will be of great benefit. Trying to memorize multiple formats can be difficult; therefore the format outlined in Box 14.1 was developed. It is easy to learn and difficult to forget because it follows the alphabet and the logical look-listen-feel approach to patient care.

To assess the adequacy of breathing, the EMT monitors the rate, rhythm, quality, and depth of ventilations. The normal ventilatory rate varies with age: for adults it is 12 to 20 breaths per minute, for children 15 to 30 per minute, and for infants (less than 1 year of age) 25 to 50 per minute. Patients with dyspnea are often tachypneic, which means their ventilatory rate is abnormally high.

The ventilatory rate is driven by two main forces: the level of oxygenation and the level of carbon dioxide. In the normal patient with normal metabolism it is the level of carbon dioxide that is the most powerful. As an example, the swimmer who purposefully hyperventilates under the mistaken belief that this is loading extra oxygen into the system to allow the swimmer to stay under water without breathing for a longer period can achieve this goal, but it is not safe. Hyperventilation reduces the CO_2 in the system; therefore it will require longer for the levels to reach the threshold to stimulate the drive to ventilate. This comes at a price because the oxygen level was not increased by the hyperventilation, and the swimmer may become hypoxic and lose cerebral function without ever feeling the need to breathe and therefore will not surface until he or she becomes unconscious.

As in any part of assessment there are no exact cutoff lines in patient function. It is a continuum of variables. However, to make judgements one must have some type of gauge. Table 14.1 shows an acceptable gauge of the rate of adult ventilation.

The rhythm of ventilation may be regular or irregular. A patient with a head injury or drug overdose may have an irregular pattern of ventilations. The quality of ventilation is determined by listening to breath sounds, watching for even chest expansion, and assessing the effort required for breathing.

The depth of ventilation is important to assess, because insufficient tidal volumes can lead to hypoxia if not corrected. Abnormally shallow breathing is a common response to pain. For example, a patient with rib fractures or severe abdominal pain is more likely to take rapid, shallow breaths. In the severely ill or injured patient, shallow breathing can contribute to shock if not corrected.

Patients with a ventilatory emergency often have abnormalities of rate, rhythm, quality, and depth of breathing. The ventilatory rate is usually elevated, although patients with head injuries or those who are close to ventilatory arrest may have an abnormally slow or irregular rate. In **ventilatory arrest**, the patient stops breathing. Just before ventilatory arrest the patient may have **agonal ventilations**, which are occasional gasping breaths that occur before death. A patient with agonal ventilations or

Box 14.1 McSwain-Paturas Respiratory Assessment System (MPRAS)

Look
A—Alert EMT finds the important signs that may not be obvious to the casual EMT.*
B—Breathing rate and patterns.†
C—Color of the skin of the patient.
D—Deviated posture. Is the patient erect and straight, or must he or she support the arms on the legs for support of the shoulders to improve the effectiveness of the accessory muscles?
E—Effort of ventilation.
F—Framework of the chest, barrel chested? Narrow, pigeon chested? Asymmetric chest wall?
G—Great additional muscles of the neck, back, and shoulders needed for pulmonary expansion muscles?
H—Huffing through pursed lips?
I—Intercostal space retraction. Also note subcostal and supraclavicular spaces for retraction.

Listen
Sounds heard *without* assistance of stethoscope
  Airway sounds
  Sonorous sounds
  Wheezes
  Difficulty in speaking because talking requires too much effort or reduces the rate of ventilation.
Sounds heard *with* the assistance of the stethoscope
  Crackles or rales
  Rhonchi
  Wheezes
  Present, absent, or decreased
  Bronchial sounds

Feel
Subcutaneous air
Abnormal chest wall motion
Grating ribs to palpation
Pain associated with chest wall or rib palpation

---
*The astute and caring EMT wants to identify everything that is going to affect patient care. By looking for subtle signs and symptoms the astute EMT can many times find bits of information that lead to diagnoses and treatment patterns sooner than would otherwise be expected and therefore lead to improved outcome. Any EMT can manage a patient based on the gross signs. An outstanding EMT is alert and finds the subtle signs that can truly make a difference in the outcome. Therefore the outline for patient care starts with *alert* as reminder to look for the small things.

†There are several components to breathing: rate, rhythm, quality, and depth. The analysis of ventilation plays an important role in determining the status of the respiratory system in patients.

---

ventilatory arrest requires immediate assisted or controlled ventilation with an FiO_2 as high as possible.

Color

Other signs of inadequate breathing include poor skin color and signs of hypoxia. The skin of dyspneic patients is often cool, clammy, and pale. A more serious sign is **cyanosis** (blue skin), a late finding in severe respiratory distress (Figure 14.3). Hypoxia is a condition in which the patient has a shortage of oxygen. Patients who are deprived of oxygen are often confused, restless, lethargic, or irritable. They have pale or cyanotic skin color and appear to be in shock. Their heart rate is often elevated (tachycardia). In addition to cyanosis, patients with severe hypoxia may have patches of white and pink skin, a process termed **mottling**. Mottling is seen most often in patients with COPD or patients in shock. A patient with cyanosis or mottling is severely deprived of oxygen and requires immediate administration of high-concentration oxygen, regardless of COPD history.

TABLE 14.1 Ventilatory Rate

Rate	Situation	Management
0-8	Slow, needs assistance	FiO_2 0.85 or greater
8-20	Normal	No assistance required
20-30	Borderline (Is something going on? What is about to happen next?)	FiO_2 0.35-0.45; consider assisted ventilation
30-40	Condition is serious	FiO_2 0.85 or greater
>40	Condition is very serious	FiO_2 1.0; if possible, consider immediate intubation

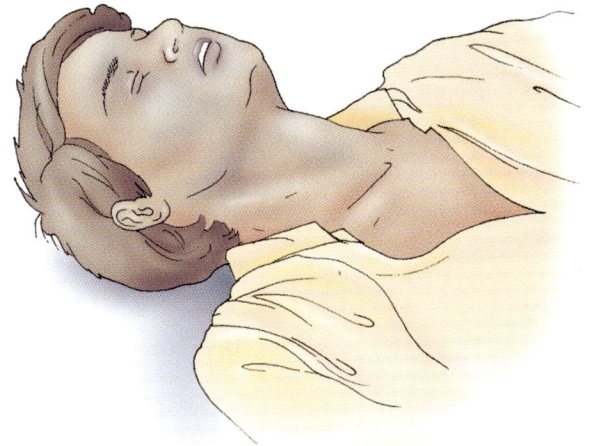

FIGURE 14.3 Cyanosis is a late sign of respiratory distress.

Deviated Posture

Patients who are using **accessory muscles** to breathe prefer to sit upright and lean forward—a position that makes the accessory muscles most effective for increasing tidal volume. To assist in the effect of these muscles, the patient rests elbows on knees or on the arm of the chair. This position allows the muscles that are attached to the shoulder girdle, such as the pectoralis major and minor and the latissimus, to provide assistance in the expansion of the lungs.

Effort of Breathing

The effort required to breathe can be estimated by the patient's ability to talk. Patients who are in acute respiratory distress are often unable to talk. If they can talk, they often speak in short one- or two-word sentences. **Nasal flaring** is another sign of increased ventilatory effort, especially in children. In infants, the abdomen and chest may move in opposite directions during respiratory distress, resulting in "seesaw" breathing.

Framework

As the alveoli break down with emphysema and the patient chronically uses accessory muscles for breathing, keeping the chest expanded more and more to take in enough air with each inhalation, the chest wall becomes rounded in appearance (barrel chest). This is highly indicative of COPD.

Great Acessory Muscles

Ventilatory effort can be assessed by watching for the use of accessory muscles during inspiration, a finding that is especially common in infants and children.

In addition to listening to breath sounds, the quality of breathing is assessed by looking for even chest expansion during inspiration and by assessing ventilatory effort. Accessory muscles are used during acute respiratory distress to increase the tidal volume of each breath. They are located primarily in the neck and are especially prominent in patients with COPD and in infants and children.

Huffing

A patient who has COPD or other severe pulmonary problems will assist the breathing effort by exhaling through pursed lips.

Intercostal Muscles

Retractions are indentations of skin that occur above the clavicles, between the ribs, and below the rib cage. They occur as the patient works harder to breathe, a process that pulls in the soft tissues of the chest wall (Figure 14.4).

Listen

If the ventilatory condition is severe, the abnormal sounds of breathing frequently can be heard while standing next to or even some distance from the patient. This should be a warning sign that the patient is in significant difficulty and may require immediate intervention. Most often, however, abnormal sounds can be detected only with the stethoscope (auscultation).

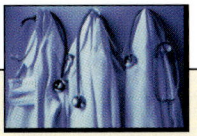 **Physician Notes**

Identifying the sounds of normal and abnormal breathing is among the most critical skills that the EMT must master. This will require several hours of practice. One way to improve one's skill and knowledge is to ask the emergency department nurse every time you bring in a patient, "Are there any patients with abnormal breath sounds here today that I can listen to?"

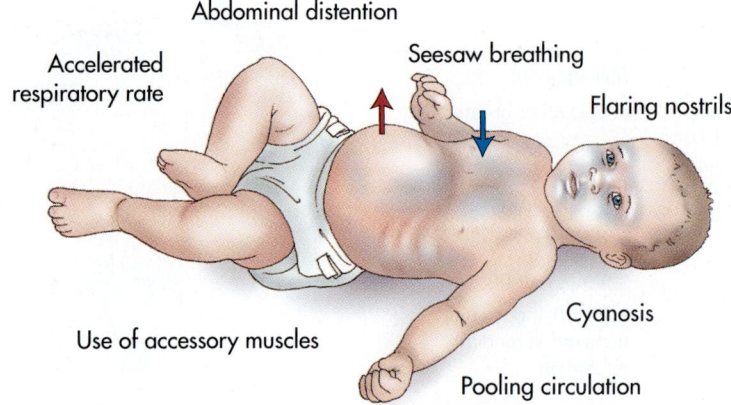

FIGURE 14.4 An infant in respiratory distress with flaring of the nostrils and retraction of soft tissues on inspiration. The abdomen may distend, causing "seesaw" breathing. Cyanosis or ashen color and accelerated ventilatory rate with expiratory grunt or whimper are additional signs of respiratory distress.

During inadequate breathing, breath sounds may be abnormal or absent. Audible **wheezes** are a common sign of ventilatory distress during an acute asthma attack. These high-pitched breath sounds occur as air moves through constricted airways. They are especially common during exhalation but also occur during inhalation in an acute attack. **Crackles** are breath sounds caused by fluid in the airways, as in pneumonia or pulmonary edema. They can be fine or coarse, depending on the amount of fluid present. **Rales** are fine sounds that can be simulated by rubbing hair between the thumb and fingers. They are heard when areas of collapsed alveoli expand with inhalation or when fluid is present in the smaller airways. The term *fine crackles* is now being used more frequently than *rales*; however, they refer to the same abnormal breath sound. Absence of breath sounds is a worrisome sign, especially in a patient who is acutely short of breath. A pneumothorax, a hemothorax, or pneumonia may result in absent breath sounds. A patient with absent breath sounds over part of the chest and acute shortness of breath requires immediate transport with administration of high-flow oxygen.

Noisy breathing is a sign of respiratory distress. Sometimes wheezing can be heard without using a stethoscope. **Stridor** is a high-pitched, harsh sound heard during inspiration that results from a narrowing in the upper airway. It is often heard in children and may be due to a foreign body that is partially obstructing the airway or an infection such as croup or epiglottitis. Snoring or gurgling sounds during breathing suggest inadequate upper airway control. A patient with snoring or gurgling first needs to have the airway opened. An artificial airway adjunct or suctioning may also be needed, depending on the patient's level of consciousness.

> ✓ A careful assessment by the EMT is needed to properly intervene during a respiratory emergency. To evaluate breathing the EMT monitors the rate, rhythm, quality, and depth of ventilations. The EMT should also observe the patient's general appearance, looking for signs and symptoms of hypoxia such as confusion, restlessness, dyspnea, and pale or cyanotic skin color.

Management

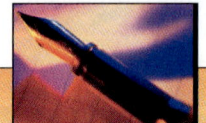 **Tips from the Pros**

Encourage the use of a spacer device when administering bronchodilators. Spacers make handheld inhalers much more effective because of improved absorption.

General Respiratory Care

The most important interventions for a patient with inadequate breathing are to establish and maintain an adequate airway, administer supplemental oxygen, and provide assisted ventilation when needed. Other interventions include monitoring vital signs, maintaining patient comfort, and assisting with inhaler medications as indicated. The EMT must be familiar with the techniques of airway control, suctioning, artificial ventilation, and oxygen administration, which are discussed in Chapter 10. A patient in respiratory distress may require intervention with airway management and assisted ventilation at any time.

After arriving at the scene of a respiratory emergency the EMT should begin assessment and management with the initial assessment. After assessing the patient's airway, the adequacy of breathing should be assessed. Any problems discovered during the initial assessment require prompt intervention; therefore if the patient has signs and symptoms of respiratory distress, oxygen should be administered immediately. Most patients with a respiratory emergency should be given high-concentration oxygen in the prehospital setting. In patients with COPD, some concern exists about giving too much oxygen. These patients are chronically deprived of oxygen, and they rely on this hypoxia to stimulate breathing. Therefore the administration of high-concentration oxygen can take away their stimulus to breathe, causing **apnea** (no respirations). This concern has led to recommendations not to give high-concentration oxygen to patients with COPD. However, experience has not shown this concern to be a problem during the relatively short transport times seen in prehospital care. Furthermore, patients with COPD can become severely hypoxic during acute episodes of increased shortness of breath. These acute episodes are sometimes termed *exacerbations of COPD*. Any patient with signs of hypoxia needs high-flow oxygen, regardless of a history of COPD. If a patient with COPD has only mild symptoms of respiratory distress, low concentrations of oxygen may be given by cannula. Keep in mind that most patients with COPD who require emergency care because of respiratory symptoms are in moderate to severe respiratory distress, requiring high-concentration oxygen for adequate treatment. It is important to ask the patient or family members how much worse the patient is compared with his or her condition before the onset of symptoms, because this will help the EMT decide how aggressive to be with oxygen therapy.

In addition to providing oxygen, the EMT should monitor vital signs frequently, keep the patient comfortable, and reassure the patient. Patients with hypoxia are often tachycardic. By monitoring vital signs, the EMT can assess the patient's response to therapy. If a patient's hypoxia is improved by administering high-flow oxygen, the heart rate may return to normal. Patients in respiratory distress will usually not be comfortable in a supine position. They often prefer to sit up, which is the best position for accessory muscles to assist with breathing. The EMT should let the nontrauma patient stay in whatever position is most comfortable, because this will decrease the patient's anxiety. Calm reassurance by the EMT will also help relieve anxiety. As the patient calms down, the feeling of dyspnea often improves.

TABLE 14.2 Common Bronchodilator Medications

Generic Name	Trade Name
Albuterol	Ventolin®
	Proventil®
Isoetharine	Bronkosol®
	Bronkometer®
Metaproterenol	Alupent®
	Metaprel®

Inhaler Medications

Many patients with asthma or COPD use inhaler medications called **bronchodilators** to relieve acute symptoms. Part of the EMT's role is to assist patients with inhaler administration. The medications have several different names (Table 14.2); however, all of them work by dilating constricted airways, making breathing easier. The medications come in **metered dose inhalers**, which are small devices designed to give a fixed dose of medication with each puff (Figure 14.5, *A*). The patient must have a prescription for the medication, which gives the recommended number of puffs for each administration.

The following indications must be met before the EMT can assist with an inhaler:

1. The patient exhibits signs and symptoms of ventilatory distress.
2. The patient has a currently prescribed handheld inhaler.
3. The EMT has specific authorization from medical direction to assist with inhalers.

Physician Notes

Major changes in the prehospital care of patients with respiratory emergencies include the change in management of COPD patients and new options for EMTs in airway management (see Chapter 11). EMTs in the past were strongly discouraged from giving high-concentration oxygen to patients with COPD in the past because of a concern about causing apnea from decreased ventilatory drive. This concern has not been shown to be a major problem in the prehospital setting; however, hypoxia among patients with COPD continues to be a problem. Based on this experience, patients with hypoxia should be given high-concentration oxygen, even if they have COPD. Despite this change in recommendations, EMTs should continue to be informed about the potential for decreased ventilatory drive after oxygen administration in patients with COPD. The EMT should promptly intervene with assisted ventilation if a patient's ventilatory drive is suppressed.

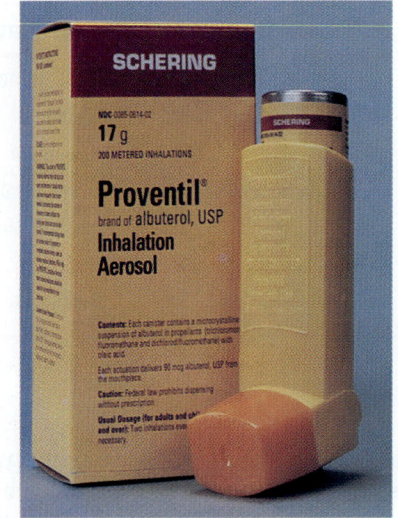
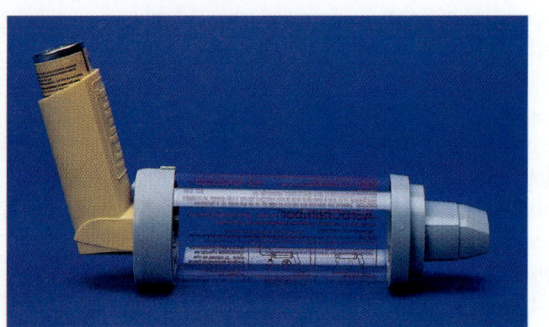

FIGURE 14.5 **A,** A metered dose inhaler delivers a fixed dose of medication with each puff. **B,** A spacer device increases the amount of medication reaching the lungs.

The following are contraindications for assisting with handheld inhalers:

1. The patient is unable to use the device (e.g., due to severe symptoms).
2. The inhaler is not prescribed for the patient (e.g., a family member has an inhaler).
3. The patient has already taken the maximum prescribed inhaler dose.
4. The EMT does not have authorization from medical direction to assist with inhalers.

To assist with an inhaler the EMT should first ensure that the prescription is for the patient, that the medication has not expired, and that the patient is alert enough to use the inhaler. The EMT should ask the patient how many doses he or she has already taken and verify the prescription to ensure that the maximum dose has not been reached. To use an inhaler most effectively, it should be at room temperature or warmer. The EMT should shake the device vigorously several times, remove any oxygen adjunct from the patient, and have the patient exhale deeply. Most patients use a spacer device between the inhaler and the mouth. A spacer is simply a tube that is attached to the inhaler (Figure 14.5, *B*). It is used to help increase the amount of medication that becomes airborne and reaches the lungs. Without a spacer, most of the medication strikes the walls of the mouth before it can be completely aerosolized (airborne) for inhalation. The patient places his or her lips around the opening of the spacer device (or inhaler if no spacer is available) after exhaling. Shortly after the patient begins to inhale, the device should be triggered by the patient. The patient should hold his or her breath as long as possible after the medication has been delivered to improve absorption. After using the inhaler, oxygen again should be given to the patient. After several seconds the dose may be repeated as allowed by medical direction and the patient's prescription.

Bronchodilators act to dilate constricted airways by stimulating specific receptors in the airways. Receptors are areas on the bronchi where drugs attach and produce their effects. These medications are similar to epinephrine, a substance that is released in the body during times of stress. Therefore it is not surprising that the side effects of bronchodilators include increased pulse rate, tremors, nervousness, and agitation. The EMT should carefully monitor and record the patient's vital signs before and after administering a bronchodilator. The patient's ventilatory status must also be reassessed after an inhaler is used. The EMT should be prepared to intervene with assisted ventilation at any time should the patient deteriorate.

> ✓ The care of a patient in respiratory distress includes administering oxygen, maintaining comfort, and providing reassurance. The EMT can assist with the administration of inhaler medications in patients who have a prescription.

Managing Childhood Respiratory Emergencies

The management of infants and children with respiratory emergencies requires careful assessment and calm reassurance by the EMT. The anxiety of the patient and family members may aggravate the patient's condition;

therefore the EMT should carefully explain everything that he or she intends to do for the patient. The most common emergencies encountered in children are asthma, croup, and epiglottitis. Asthma now is becoming more common and accounts for more deaths than either croup or epiglottitis. A child with a severe asthma attack will have wheezing, agitation, and possibly retractions. The child with croup will have a characteristic "barking" cough and is often agitated and restless. A child with epiglottitis often remains still and may have inspiratory stridor, but usually not a cough. In epiglottitis, the patient has difficulty swallowing saliva and therefore has excessive drooling. The EMT's role is not to diagnose croup, epiglottitis, or any other disorder in the field; however, if epiglottitis is suspected, the child should be handled very carefully, because aggravation of the upper airway may cause spasm of the larynx and complete airway obstruction. The EMT should not examine the airway or lay the child down. Often, the best position for transporting children with respiratory distress is in a parent's lap. The management of these disorders includes an assessment of the degree of respiratory distress and the administration of oxygen. No contraindication exists to giving high-concentration oxygen to children in the prehospital setting. Children who will not tolerate a mask will often tolerate blow-by oxygen. The ability to reassure the patient and family when appropriate makes the management of childhood respiratory emergencies much more successful.

Handheld inhalers are commonly used by children, and the indications are the same for these patients. Rather than wheezing, children may have frequent coughing as a sign of constricted airways. The EMT should ask family members what symptoms the inhaler is prescribed for. Keep in mind that children have less respiratory reserve than adults, and they may deteriorate rapidly. Cyanosis is a late finding in children and indicates impending respiratory collapse. The EMT should look for earlier signs of respiratory distress, such as nasal flaring, retractions, and noisy breathing. Proper intervention with oxygen or inhaler administration can prevent respiratory decompensation.

Summary

- The body relies on two exchanges of oxygen and carbon dioxide to maintain metabolism. The respiratory system is directly involved in both of these exchanges.
- The most common respiratory emergencies encountered by the EMT are acute exacerbations of COPD and asthma attacks.
- Croup and epiglottitis are common respiratory infections in children that may cause acute respiratory distress. Asthma is another cause of respiratory distress in children. It is becoming more common and results in more deaths than croup or epiglottitis. Infants and children have less respiratory reserve than adults and may deteriorate quickly.
- When assessing breathing, the EMT monitors the rate, rhythm, quality, and depth of ventilations. Each of these areas has specific signs and symptoms that may indicate inadequate breathing. In addition, the EMT should assess the general appearance of the patient, including skin color and mental status.
- The management of patients with respiratory emergencies involves oxygen administration, maintaining patient comfort, and assisting with bronchodilator administration. The EMT must be ready to intervene with assisted ventilation at any time when caring for a patient in acute distress.
- When caring for infants and children in respiratory distress, it is especially important to provide reassurance when appropriate.

Scenario Solution

The patient in this scenario has several signs and symptoms of ventilatory distress. Her ventilatory rate is elevated (i.e., she is tachypneic), she is becoming severely hypoxic (pulse rate low), she has audible wheezes and poor air entry with breath sounds, she is using accessory muscles for inspiration, and retractions are present. Furthermore, she is anxious and unable to talk and her skin is becoming cyanotic. The overall initial assessment indicates that this patient is rapidly deteriorating and requires prompt intervention and transport.

Based on the initial assessment, this patient needs an inspired oxygen content as close to FiO_2 as possible started immediately (nonrebreather mask with O_2 flow at 15 L/min). After starting oxygen therapy, a brief history should be taken. Because this patient has evidence of constricted airways (i.e., wheezing),

Scenario Solution (cont'd)

it is important to know if she has a prescription for an inhaler. Other important questions include when and how her symptoms started, whether she has had a similar episode in the past, what her past medical history is, and what her current medications and drug allergies are.

The patient's friends are appropriately anxious during this obvious respiratory emergency. If the EMT remains calm and intervenes promptly, the friends' anxiety may be partially relieved. Although it is important to reassure both the patient and the patient's friends, statements such as "Everything is going to be fine" are not always appropriate, especially in a situation such as this when the patient appears to be in severe distress. The best way to relieve the patient's and the friends' anxiety is to remain calm and intervene promptly and efficiently and transport as quickly as the patient's management permits.

This patient should receive immediate high-flow oxygen by nonrebreather mask. The patient should be kept in a position of comfort and transported promptly, with frequent vital sign checks en route. If the patient has an inhaler, the EMT should assist with administration en route. The EMT should be prepared to perform artificial ventilation if needed.

Key Terms

Accessory muscles Muscles located primarily in the neck that contract to increase tidal volume during respiratory distress.

Agonal ventilations Occasional, gasping breaths that occur just before death.

Alveolar/capillary exchange Gas exchange that occurs in the lungs; oxygen enters the capillaries and is transported by the blood, and carbon dioxide enters the alveoli and is exhaled.

Apnea Complete lack of respirations.

Bronchodilators Medications that relax constricted airways, making airflow easier; commonly used in patients with chronic obstructive pulmonary disease and asthma.

Bronchospasm A condition seen in patients with asthma in which airways constrict tightly in response to irritants, cold air, exercise, or unknown factors.

Cellular/capillary exchange Exchange of oxygen that occurs in the body tissues; oxygen enters the cells to be metabolized, and carbon dioxide enters the capillaries to be carried to the lungs.

Chronic bronchitis A form of chronic obstructive pulmonary disease commonly seen in smokers, characterized by a chronic productive cough and obstructive airway symptoms.

Crackles Low-pitched bubbling sounds produced by fluid in the lower airways; often described as either fine or coarse.

Croup A viral infection seen in children, characterized by a "barking" cough and moderate to severe ventilatory distress.

Cyanosis Slightly bluish, grayish, slatelike, or dark purple discoloration of the skin due to a deficiency of oxygen and excess of carbon dioxide in the blood.

Dyspnea The symptom of having difficulty breathing or shortness of breath.

Emphysema A form of chronic obstructive pulmonary disease characterized by destruction of alveoli and obstructive airway symptoms; commonly seen in smokers.

Epiglottitis Inflammation of the epiglottis; a bacterial infection seen most often in children. The epiglottis becomes swollen and may cause airway obstruction; patients often have excessive drooling.

FiO_2 Percentage of inspired oxygen.

Hyperventilation A process in which minute ventilation is increased above normal; it is purposely done for patients with head injuries or with prolonged apnea.

Hypoxia A condition in which the patient has a shortage of oxygen at the cellular level. Signs and symptoms of hypoxia include dyspnea, restlessness, confusion, lethargy, and poor skin color.

Metabolism Chemical reactions that take place within an organism to maintain life; the work of the cells.

Metered dose inhaler Device designed to give a fixed dose of inhaled medications with each puff; most inhalers are used by patients with chronic obstructive pulmonary disease or asthma.

Mottling A condition seen in patients with severe hypoxia; skin has diffuse patches of red and white discoloration.

Nasal flaring Widening of the nostrils that occurs during inhalation in patients with respiratory distress.

Paresthesia Any subjective sensation experienced as numbness, tingling, or a "pins and needles" feeling; may be a symptom of hyperventilation or a spinal cord injury.

Key Terms (cont'd)

Pneumonia An infection of the lungs that may be caused by bacteria, viruses, or fungi; patients often have fever, dyspnea, and a cough.

Pulmonary edema A condition in which fluid builds up in the alveoli and small airways, causing hypoxia and dyspnea; most commonly caused by congestive heart failure.

Pulmonary embolism A blood clot in the lungs, reducing blood flow in the affected lung.

Rales Fine breath sounds that represent opening of collapsed alveoli or fluid in the small airways near the alveoli; simulated by rubbing hair between the fingers.

Respiratory alkalosis Caused by excessive elimination of carbon dioxide when the patient's ventilatory rate increases.

Retractions A sign of respiratory distress often seen in infants and children marked by inward pulling of the skin above the clavicles and below the rib cage with inspiration.

Stridor An abnormal, high-pitched, musical sound caused by an obstruction in the trachea or larynx; usually heard during inspiration.

Tachypnea A rapid ventilatory rate.

Ventilatory arrest Lack of breathing. A patient in ventilatory arrest may have agonal respirations; however, these are not effective breaths.

Wheezes High-pitched sounds heard when air moves through constricted airways; commonly occurs in patients with asthma.

Review Questions

1. Which of the following is true regarding the alveolar/capillary exchange?
   a. Oxygen enters the blood and carbon dioxide enters the alveoli.
   b. This exchange occurs primarily in the body tissues.
   c. Hypoventilation will not impair this exchange.
   d. Children can tolerate an interruption of this exchange longer than adults.

2. The disappearance of wheezing during an acute asthma attack:
   a. Is always a sign of improvement.
   b. Is never a sign of improvement.
   c. May be a sign of improvement.
   d. Has no relevance to this situation.

3. Signs and symptoms of hypoxia include all of the following *except*:
   a. Restlessness
   b. Dyspnea
   c. Warm and pink skin
   d. Confusion
   e. Lethargy

4. Which statement is the most accurate?
   a. A child with epiglottitis is more likely to cough than a child with croup.
   b. A child with croup is more likely to cough than a child with epiglottitis.
   c. Neither condition is likely to cause the child to cough.
   d. Both conditions are equally likely to cause the child to cough.

5. Which of the following **IS NOT** a contraindication to inhaler administration?
   a. The patient is not alert enough to use the device.
   b. The EMT does not have authorization from medical direction to assist with inhalers.
   c. The patient does not have a current prescription.
   d. The patient has audible wheezing with respirations.

6. All of the following are true regarding respiratory emergencies in children *except*:
   a. Children have less respiratory reserve than adults.
   b. Children are often frightened and need careful reassurance during care.
   c. Parents usually increase the patient's anxiety and should be removed if possible.
   d. Children are more likely to have retractions, nasal flaring, and the use of accessory muscles during breathing.

Answers to these Review Questions can be found at the end of the book on page 866.

15

Cardiovascular Emergencies

Lesson Goal

Cardiovascular emergencies represent almost one third of the patients seen in the field. This chapter describes those problems and their management.

Scenario

You are called to the scene of a 48-year-old woman who is complaining of a crushing chest sensation. "It feels like someone dropped a rock on my chest," she tells you. She also tells you that because of her family history of cardiac problems, she runs 5 miles each day. She has just come in from her daily exercise. You find her sitting in a chair wet with sweat "from the run," but she has cool skin. It is almost blue in color. She appears short of breath. "Also from the run," she tells you. Her respiratory rate is 32, and her blood pressure is 90/54. Her radial pulse is 110 ("from the run"). Although her pulse is irregular and weak, she tells you that it is often this way when she finishes her run.

After your initial assessment, the patient tells you that she is thirsty and wants a drink of water. You send your partner for water and the patient suddenly becomes unresponsive. After placing her supine on the floor, you find the patient to be pulseless and apneic. Although an advanced life support ambulance is on its way to the scene, it will be 10 minutes before it arrives.

? **Is this a cardiac problem, or one of dehydration? When you first arrived, should you have suspected that this problem was of cardiac origin? When you arrived on the scene, could you have prevented this outcome? Should you immediately transport or wait for the arrival of the advanced life support unit? If you elect to wait, what should you do while the unit is en route? If you elect to transport, what are the immediate steps that you take?**

Key Terms to Know

Angina pectoris	Automated external defibrillator	Cardiac arrest	Coronary arteries
Aorta		Cardiogenic shock	Defibrillation
Arterioles	Blood pressure	Carotid arteries	Diaphoretic
Atherosclerosis	Brachial artery	Case reviews	Diastolic pressure
Artery	Bradycardia	Chain of survival	Dorsalis pedis artery
Atrium	Capillaries	Congestive heart failure	Dysrhythmia

Key Terms to Know (cont'd)

Electrocardiogram	Nitroglycerin	Pulse pressure	Veins
Femoral arteries	Perfusion	Radial artery	Ventricle
Hemoglobin	Plasma	Red blood cells	Ventricular fibrillation
Hypertension	Platelets	Shock	Ventricular tachycardia
Hypotension	Posterior tibial artery	Standard cardiac care	Venules
Inferior vena cava	Pulmonary arteries	Sublingually	White blood cells
Ischemia	Pulmonary edema	Superior vena cava	
Myocardial infarction	Pulmonary veins	Systolic pressure	
Myocardium	Pulse	Tachycardia	

Learning Objectives

As an EMT-Basic, you should be able to do the following:

DOT

- Describe the anatomy and function of the cardiovascular system.
- Identify signs and symptoms of patients experiencing a cardiovascular problem and perform the necessary interventions for standard cardiac care.
- Describe the emergency cardiac care system, including the rationale, indications, and contraindications for early defibrillation; the importance of early advanced cardiac life support (ACLS); the relationship between basic life support and ACLS providers; and the role of the emergency medical technician within this system (see Chapters 12 and 16).
- Explain the rationale for facilitating the use of nitroglycerin for patients with chest pain, including the indications, contraindications, and side effects of the drug.
- Discuss the position of comfort for patients with various cardiac emergencies.
- Establish the relationship between airway management and the patient with cardiovascular compromise.
- Predict the relationship between the patient experiencing cardiovascular compromise and basic life support.
- Explain that not all chest pain patients progress to cardiac arrest and do not need to be attached to an automated external defibrillator.
- Explain the importance of urgent transportation to a facility with advanced cardiac life support if it is not available in the prehospital setting.
- Discuss the components that should be included in a case review.
- Recognize the need for medical direction of protocols to assist in emergency medical care of the patient with chest pain.

Each year nearly 500,000 people die in the United States as a result of coronary heart disease. Half of these deaths occur outside the hospital. Sudden death is the first sign of cardiac disease in 50% of prehospital deaths. Early defibrillation with an **automated external defibrillator** (AED) has changed the role of the emergency medical technician (EMT) in emergency cardiac care. The outcome of prehospital cardiac arrest depends on four components of the emergency medical services (EMS) system known as the **chain of survival**: early access, early cardiopulmonary resuscitation (CPR), early defibrillation, and early advanced cardiac life support (ACLS). In the past, EMTs were limited to performing CPR for the management of prehospital cardiac arrest. Although CPR continues to be a critical life-sustaining component of emergency cardiac care, it is only a holding pattern. The best cardiac output (CO) (pulse times stroke volume) that can be achieved by CPR is 30% of normal or less. Most CPR, according to the American Heart Association, is in the range of 15% to 20%. In most patients this will not provide enough CO to oxygenate the brain and heart for more than a few minutes. The normal muscular contractions of the heart must be reestablished. Rapid defibrillation is recognized as the major determinant of survival for patients in cardiac arrest caused by ventricular fibrillation. Defibrillation with AEDs has added an exciting challenge to the role of the EMT in managing prehospital cardiac arrest.

Although the management of cardiac arrest is emphasized in this chapter, the majority of patients with cardiovascular problems are not in cardiac arrest. The role of the EMT in managing patients with cardiovascular complaints such as chest pain or discomfort is one of supportive care. This chapter briefly discusses some of the

Patient Care Algorithm

Chest Pain Patient Assessment

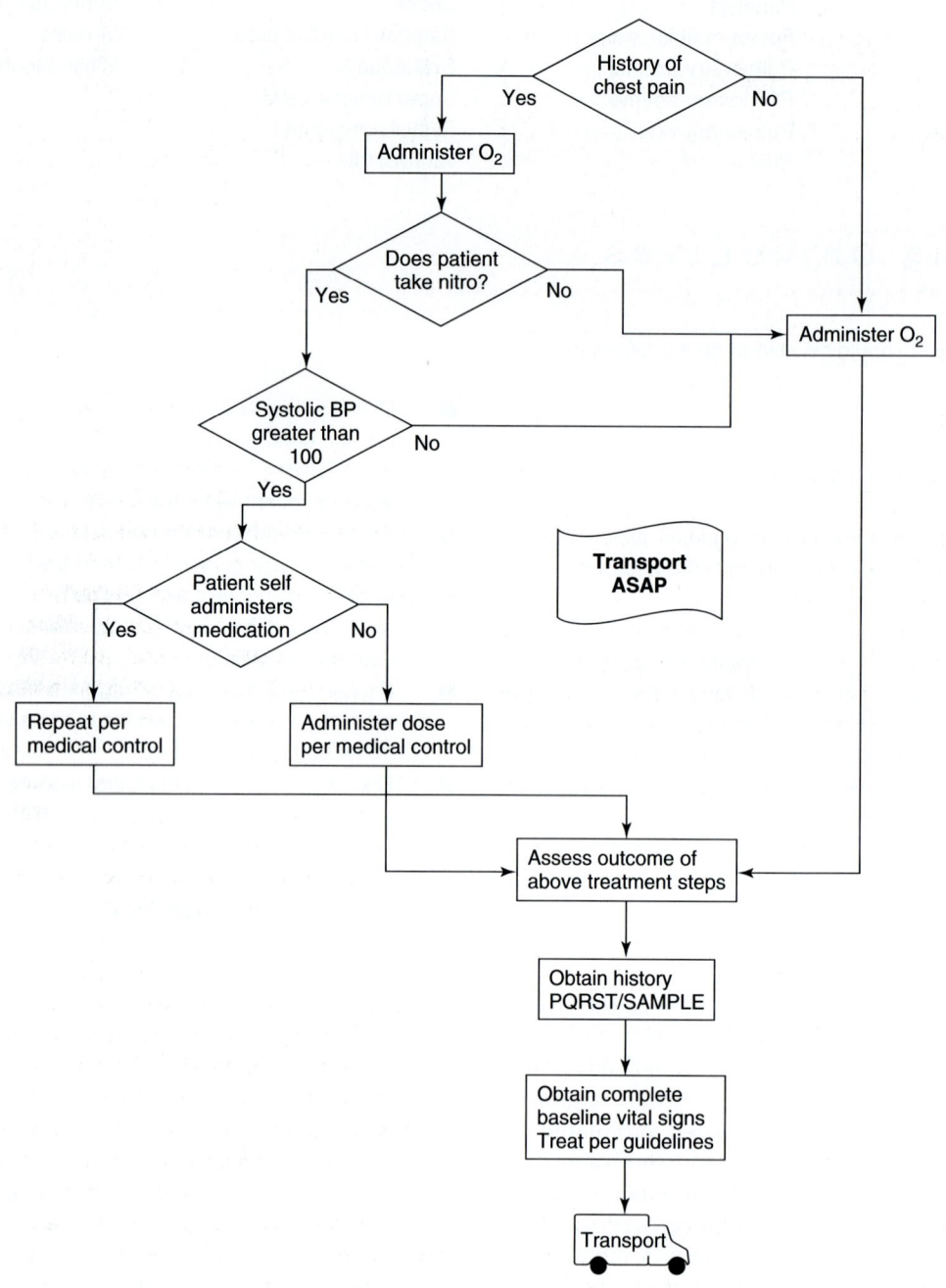

causes of cardiac symptoms, such as acute myocardial infarction and congestive heart failure. The emphasis for the EMT is on assessing the patient and making appropriate interventions based on that assessment, not on diagnosing a specific problem. A careful cardiovascular assessment leads to appropriate supportive and therapeutic interventions.

This chapter begins with a discussion of the anatomy and physiology of the cardiovascular system. A brief discussion of cardiovascular pathophysiology follows, including acute myocardial infarction and congestive heart failure. The assessment of the cardiac patient is then discussed. The rationale and components of standard cardiac care are described, including the appropriate use of nitroglycerin. Cardiac arrest management is then discussed in detail, emphasizing the use of AEDs. Basic life-support skills are reviewed, focusing on the coordination of CPR with the use of AEDs.

Anatomy

Heart

The heart is a specialized muscle with four chambers designed to maintain blood flow to the lungs and body. Functionally, the heart can be divided into right and left halves, each of which has an upper chamber called an **atrium** and a lower chamber called a **ventricle**. The right half of the heart receives blood from the veins of the body, which empty into the right atrium through the **superior vena cava** and **inferior vena cava**. The right ventricle then pumps this oxygen-poor blood to the lungs through the **pulmonary arteries**. After receiving oxygen and eliminating carbon dioxide in the lungs, the blood enters the left atrium via the **pulmonary veins**. The left ventricle then pumps this oxygen-rich blood to the body. In simplified terms, the right half of the heart pumps blood to the lungs, and the left half of the heart pumps blood to the body (Figure 15.1).

Four valves in the heart prevent backflow of blood. Two of these valves are located between the atria and ventricles, one in each half of the heart (tricuspid on the right and the mitral on the left). The other two valves prevent backflow of blood into the ventricles. One valve is located between the right ventricle and the pulmonary artery (pulmonic valve), and the other is located between the left ventricle and the aorta (aortic valve) (Figure 15.2).

Arteries

An **artery** is a blood vessel that carries blood away from the heart. All arteries carry oxygen-rich blood except for

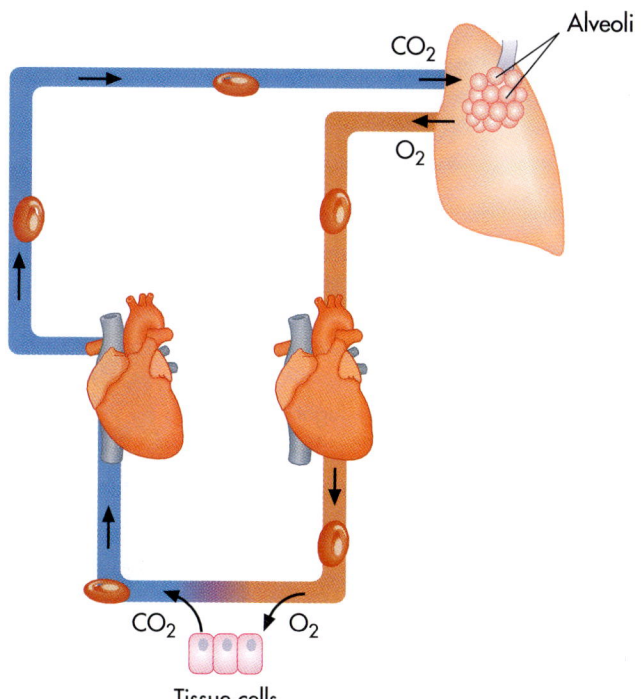

FIGURE 15.1 The heart is a double pump. One half pumps blood through the systemic circulation, and the other half pumps blood through the pulmonary circulation.

the pulmonary arteries, which carry deoxygenated blood from the right ventricle to the lungs. Figure 15.3 demonstrates the major vessels of the cardiovascular system. A working knowledge of the location of major arteries can be used by the EMT to monitor the rate and quality of a patient's pulse, assess blood supply to an injured extremity, and control bleeding through the use of pressure points. The **aorta** is the largest artery in the body, extending from the left ventricle to the navel, where it divides into the iliac arteries. Throughout the thoracic and abdominal cavities the aorta lies just in front of the vertebral column. The aorta supplies blood to all other arteries. The **coronary arteries**, the first branches of the aorta, supply the myocardium with blood. When these arteries become occluded, the myocardium is deprived of blood supply, which may lead to a **myocardial infarction** (heart attack).

The **carotid arteries** carry most of the blood supply to the head (face, scalp, pharynx mouth, bone, eyes, and brain). They are the major arteries of the neck and can be palpated under the large muscle (sternocleidomastoid). The **brachial artery** supplies the upper arm and can be palpated on the inside of the arm approximately one third of the distance between the elbow and shoulder. Brachial artery pulsations are heard when auscultating a blood pressure with a sphygmomanometer (blood pressure cuff) and stethoscope. The **radial artery** is one of two major arteries of the lower forearm and hand. Pulsations

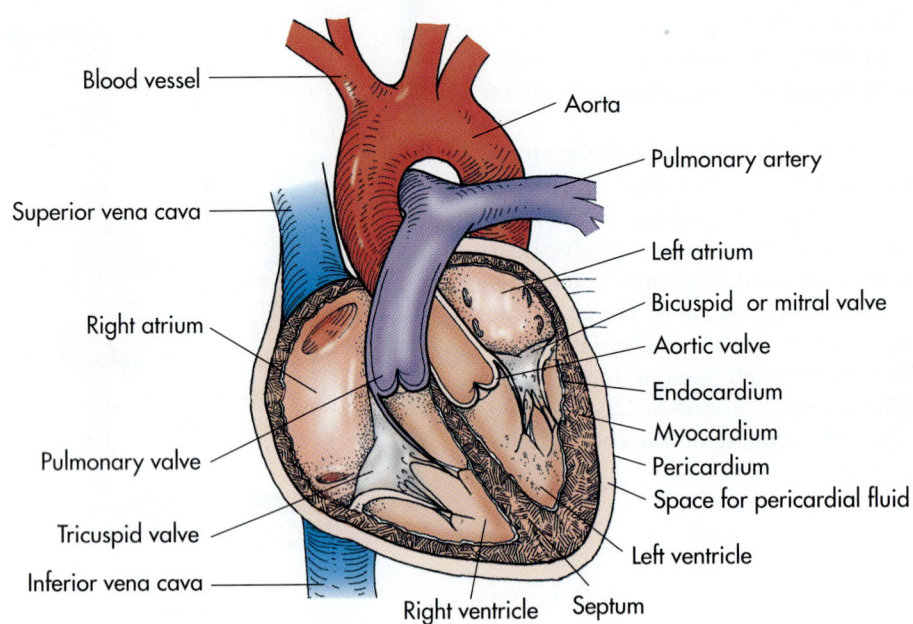

FIGURE 15.2 The heart valves prevent backflow of blood while the heart chambers refill.

can be felt on the anterior surface of the wrist on the thumb side. The **femoral arteries** are the major vessels supplying the lower extremities and groin area. They can be palpated in the groin area on both sides. The **posterior tibial artery** is located just behind the medial malleolus at the ankle. The **dorsalis pedis artery** is located on the upper surface of the foot. In some patients with vascular disease, the posterior tibial and dorsalis pedis pulses are difficult to palpate. The EMT is most interested in palpating these pulses when there is an injury to the lower extremity, requiring assessment of the blood supply distal to the site of injury. If pulses cannot be palpated distal to an injury, the color, temperature, and capillary refill of the extremity should be assessed (see Chapter 8).

Arterioles are the smallest branches of arteries and eventually become capillaries. **Capillaries** are very small blood vessels located between arterioles and venules (Figure 15.4). Capillaries surround the body cells and supply them with oxygen and nutrients. They are the site of the capillary/cellular exchange (see Chapters 9 and 10).

The walls of the arteries have a muscular layer that contracts and dilates based on the presence of epinephrine, norepinephrine, and nitric oxide. Contraction of these vessels has two results: reduced volume in the vascular system and increased blood pressure produced by the increased force required to push blood through the smaller vessel. Dilation of the vessels creates the opposite effect. This change has a major effect on the heart by increasing or decreasing the amount of work and therefore its oxygen consumption.

Veins

Veins are vessels that carry blood toward the heart. Except for the pulmonary veins, which carry oxygenated blood from the lungs to the left atrium, all veins carry deoxygenated blood. The smallest veins in the body are the **venules**. Venules receive blood from the capillaries and begin the transfer of blood back to the heart. The largest veins in the body are the superior vena cava and inferior vena cava, which carry blood to the right atrium (Figure 15.5). The forward flow of the blood in the veins is maintained by three factors: force of the blood coming through the capillary beds; valves in the veins that prevent backflow (in the same fashion as the valves in the heart); and squeezing action on the veins as the muscles of the extremity contract, such as during walking.

> ✔ The heart maintains a constant blood supply to the body tissues. Arteries carry oxygenated blood away from the heart, and veins carry deoxygenated blood to the heart.

Physiology

The heart relies on a conduction system to coordinate the contraction of the atria and ventricles. Specialized conduction pathways carry electrical impulses from the atria to the ventricles. These electrical impulses occur in

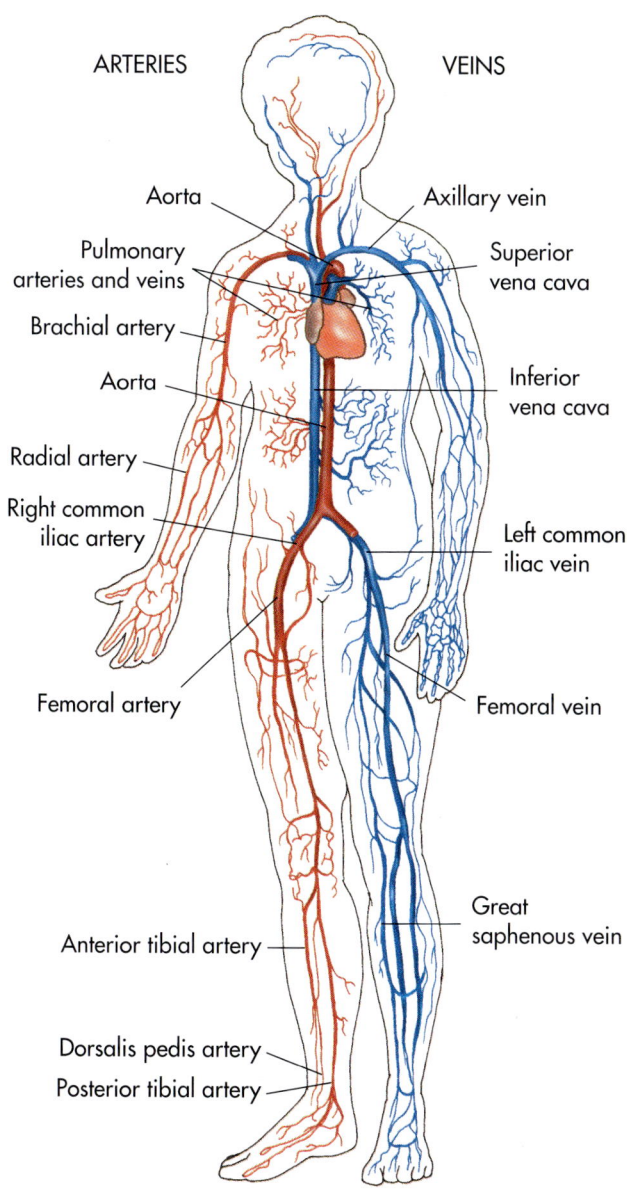

FIGURE 15.3 Major arteries of the cardiovascular system.

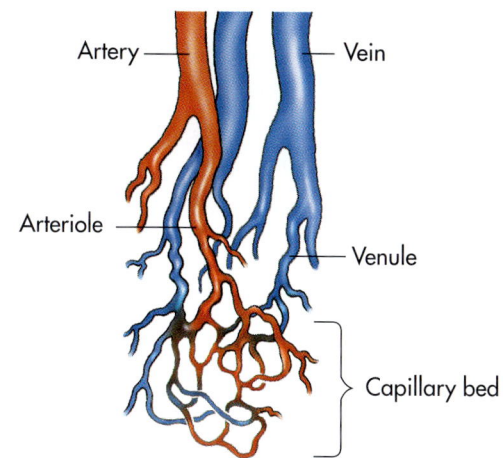

FIGURE 15.4 The vessels branch into smaller and smaller tubes until they are capillaries that are so small that perhaps only one red blood cell can pass at a time.

predictable patterns and are observed on the **electrocardiogram** (ECG). The electrical rhythm of the heart is measured by electrodes that are placed on the chest wall and extremities. A normal ECG rhythm strip is shown in Figure 15.6.

Heart Rate and Rhythm

Normally, an electrical impulse begins in the right atrium at the sinoatrial (SA) node. The impulse quickly travels from the SA node throughout both atria. After a short pause in a node of tissue between the atria and ventricles, the impulse spreads through the ventricles. This node of tissue between the atria and ventricles is called the atrioventricular (AV) node. Contraction of the heart muscle **(myocardium)** occurs shortly after the electrical impulse travels through the heart. Because of the delay in the electrical impulse at the AV node, the atria contract before the ventricles. This is important, because the contraction of the atria helps fill the ventricles with blood.

Sometimes the conduction system of the heart malfunctions, causing symptoms. An abnormal rhythm of the heart is termed a **dysrhythmia**. A block in the electrical conduction system may slow the heart rate. A heart rate less than 60 beats per minute is called **bradycardia**. Sometimes part of the heart will begin to produce electrical impulses too quickly, causing the heart to beat rapidly. A heart rate greater than 100 beats per minute is called **tachycardia**. Patients may be bradycardic or tachycardic without having symptoms. For example, tachycardia is considered a normal response to exercise. Also, some people, particularly athletes, may be bradycardic while at rest without having symptoms. Thus it is important to interpret bradycardia and tachycardia in the context of the patient's activity level and symptoms.

Ventricular fibrillation (VF) is a dysrhythmia in which the electrical conduction system is overwhelmed by impulses throughout the heart (Figure 15.7). Because the entire heart is receiving random, disorganized electrical impulses, coordinated contraction cannot take place. The heart simply fibrillates (quivers in a disorganized fashion) and does not generate blood flow. Patients in VF do not have a pulse and require prompt

294 Section Two | Nontraumatic Emergencies

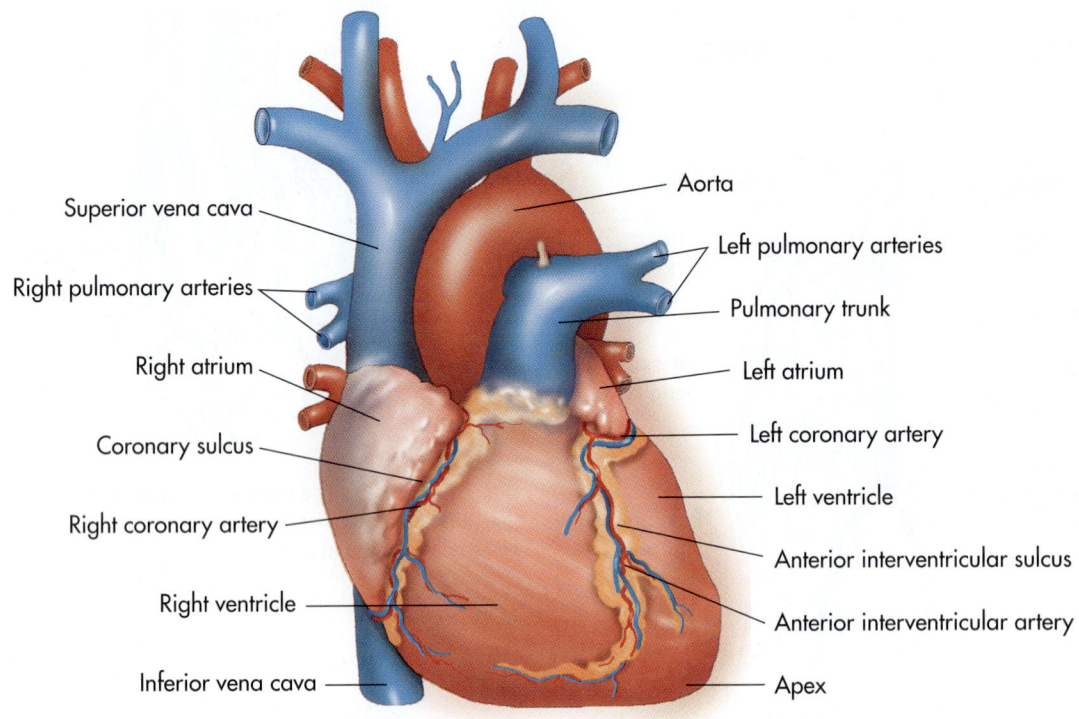

FIGURE 15.5 The superior and inferior venae cavae return deoxygenated blood to the right atrium.

Normal Sinus Rhythm (NSR)

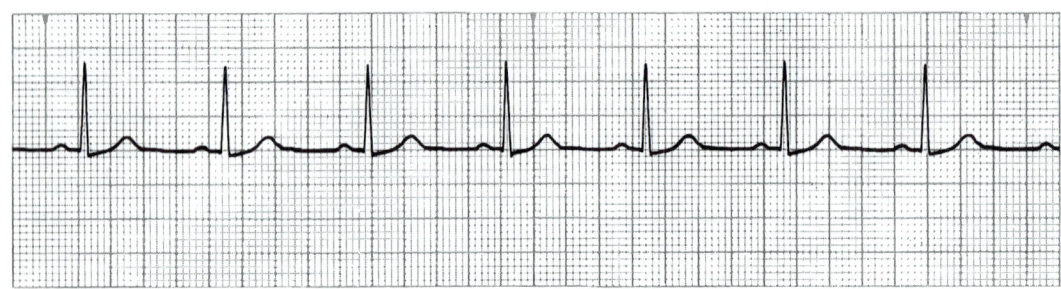

FIGURE 15.6 Normal sinus rhythm.

defibrillation as a lifesaving intervention. **Defibrillation**, the delivery of an electrical shock to the myocardium, temporarily stops electrical activity in the heart. This temporary halt is designed to allow the normal conduction system to regain control in the heart, enabling effective contraction.

Another dysrhythmia that may require defibrillation is **ventricular tachycardia** (VT). In VT, the ventricles are driven by an electrical impulse that is independent of the normal conduction system (Figure 15.8). Patients may be in VT and still maintain a normal blood pressure. However, if the VT is too fast or if the myocardium is damaged, the dysrhythmia may not allow for effective contraction of the ventricles, resulting in decreased or absent blood flow. Pulseless VT is another dysrhythmia that requires prompt defibrillation. It is treated with the same protocol as VF.

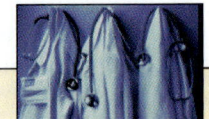 **Physician Notes**

Disruptions of the conduction system in the heart are termed *dysrhythmias*. The two life-threatening dysrhythmias treated with defibrillation are ventricular fibrillation and pulseless ventricular tachycardia.

Arrhythmia means "without rhythm." Asystole is an example of this condition.

Ventricular Fibrillation (VF)

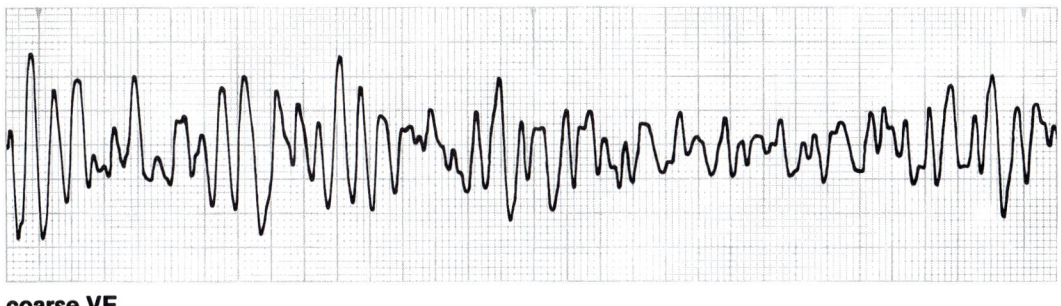

coarse VF

FIGURE 15.7 Ventricular fibrillation.

Ventricular Tachycardia (VT)

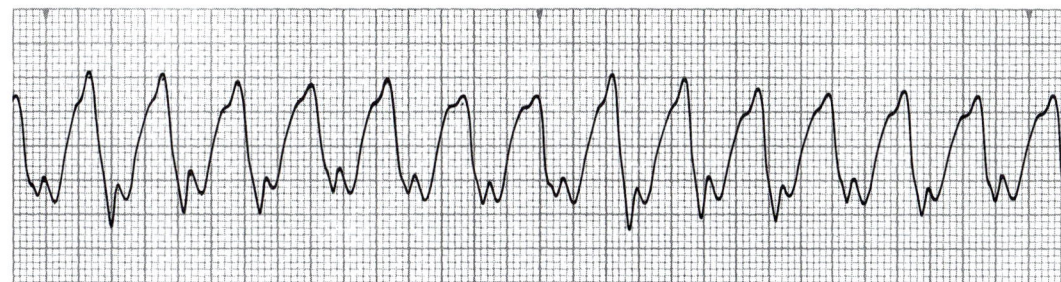

FIGURE 15.8 Ventricular tachycardia.

Blood

Blood is a specialized fluid that carries oxygen and nutrients to the body tissues and removes carbon dioxide and other waste products. Oxygen is absorbed into the hemoglobin molecule that is carried within the red blood cell from the lungs. Carbon dioxide is removed from blood and exhaled through the lungs. Waste products are removed through the kidneys and liver. Blood is composed of two major parts: the fluid component, or **plasma**, and the cellular component, which contains several types of cells. Red blood cells give blood its color and carry oxygen. **Red blood cells** (erythrocytes) contain **hemoglobin**, a specialized molecule designed to bind oxygen for transport. **White blood cells** (leukocytes) are an important part of the body's immune system, which defends the body against infections. **Platelets** are small cellular fragments that function in clotting. After a vessel is injured and bleeding begins, platelets are attracted to the area and form a plug on which a blood clot forms.

Pulse and Blood Pressure

A **pulse** is formed when the left ventricle contracts, sending a wave of blood throughout the arterial system. Pulses can be palpated in areas where arteries travel and over a bone. The closer to the skin surface that the artery lies, the smaller the vessel and the weaker the pulse that can be felt. The carotid and femoral pulses are central pulses. Peripheral pulses are felt on the extremities. Radial and brachial pulses are felt in the upper extremities and posterior tibial, and dorsalis pedis pulses are felt in the ankles and feet.

Blood pressure is a measurement of the force applied to the arterial walls by the blood. **Systolic pressure** is exerted against the walls of the arteries when the left ventricle contracts and forces blood out of the heart. It is the pressure that circulates the blood throughout the body. **Diastolic pressure** is the pressure that remains in the blood vessels when the left ventricle is refilling from the left atrium. **Pulse pressure** is the difference between the systolic and diastolic pressures. Normally, systolic blood pressure is approximately 120 mm Hg, and diastolic pressure is approximately 80 mm Hg. A patient with a blood pressure of 120/80 would have a pulse pressure of 40 mm Hg (120 − 80 = 40). Mean arterial pressure (MAP) is the diastolic pressure plus one third of the pulse pressure. In a patient with a blood pressure of 120/80, the MAP is 80 + (40/3) = 93.3.

Blood pressure increases gradually with age. Abnormally high blood pressure is termed **hypertension**, and abnormally low blood pressure is termed **hypotension**. Under normal conditions, all of the peripheral pulses can be palpated. When a patient is hypotensive, it may become difficult to palpate peripheral pulses. In general, a systolic pressure of 80 mm Hg is needed to palpate a radial pulse, 60 mm Hg to palpate a carotid pulse, and 70 mm Hg to palpate a femoral pulse. These values can be used as a helpful estimate of blood pressure, especially in trauma patients; however, it is best to measure blood pressure directly with a sphygmomanometer whenever possible.

Physician Notes

Although the terms *mean arterial pressure* and *pulse pressure* are not part of the EMT-Basic National Standard Curriculum, they are words that the EMT will hear in the emergency department and in the hospital as nurses and physicians talk about patients. Understanding what they mean will help the EMT understand what is happening to the patient and become a more educated EMT and provide better patient care.

> ✓ Blood pressure is a measurement of the force applied to the arterial walls by the blood. Pulse pressure is the difference between systolic and diastolic blood pressures.

Pathophysiology

Although the EMT is not expected to diagnose the different cardiovascular disorders, they are described to aid in understanding the cause of cardiovascular signs and symptoms. The prehospital management of many of these disorders is termed **standard cardiac care**. The EMT should focus on assessing signs and symptoms and then intervening as necessary to improve the signs and relieve the symptons when possible.

Angina Pectoris

The most common cause of signs and symptoms in a patient with cardiovascular compromise is inadequate blood flow to the myocardium. Inadequate blood flow to a tissue is termed **ischemia**. When an area of the heart becomes ischemic, the patient may develop chest pain. Chest pain brought on by exercise and relieved by rest is termed **angina pectoris**. In anginal pain, the blood supply to the heart is sufficient for resting conditions but becomes inadequate during exercise or stressful events, usually because of narrowed coronary arteries secondary to atherosclerosis. **Atherosclerosis** is a condition in which cholesterol and cellular debris form a plaque on the insides of arteries, narrowing the area through which blood flows and making ischemia more likely. Many patients with a history of anginal pain take nitroglycerin tablets to help relieve the pain. Nitroglycerin is discussed in detail later in this chapter.

Myocardial Infarction

Sometimes the blood supply to part of the myocardium is completely stopped, usually because of a blockage in one of the coronary arteries. Unless blood flow is restored quickly, part of the myocardium dies, resulting in a myocardial infarction (MI). Unlike angina pectoris, in which the myocardium survives intermittent periods of ischemia, an MI results in irreversible death of part of the heart muscle. An MI, or heart attack, is not the same as cardiac arrest. In **cardiac arrest**, the heart stops pumping blood and the patient becomes unresponsive, pulseless, and apneic. Although an MI is not the same thing as car-

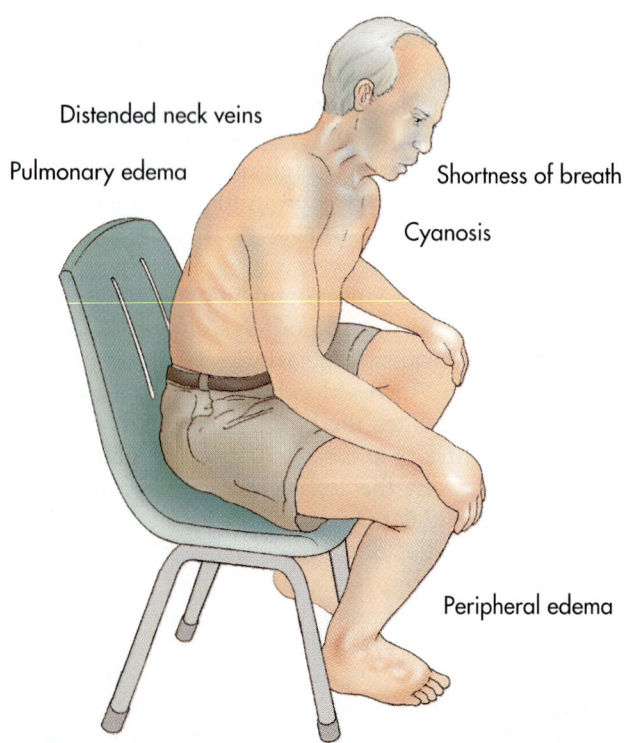

FIGURE 15.9 Congestive heart failure. Inadequate pumping by the heart causes fluid to back up in the lungs, neck veins, and extremities.

diac arrest, it may lead to cardiac arrest, either through an arrhythmia such as VF, or secondary to the death of a large part of the myocardium.

Congestive Heart Failure

Congestive heart failure (CHF) is a condition in which the left side of the heart cannnot pump out all of the blood that the right side of the heart pumps into the lungs. This flooding of the lungs and accumulation of fluid, termed *congestion*, results in shortness of breath because of the accumulation of fluid in the alveoli preventing adequate oxygen and carbon dioxide exchange. Fluid in the lungs is termed **pulmonary edema** and may be heard as coarse rales when listening to breath sounds. If the right side of the heart pumps inadequately, blood backs up into the venous system, causing congestion and the loss of fluids into the tissues. The most common signs of right-sided heart failure are distended neck veins and swelling (edema) in the lower extremities (Figure 15.9).

Cardiogenic Shock

The supply of oxygen and nutrients to the tissues by blood is termed **perfusion**. During failure of the cardiovascular system, a state of widespread decreased perfusion may develop, which leads to anaerobic metabolism and lack of adequate energy production; this condition is termed **shock** (see Chapter 9). **Cardiogenic shock** is a state of hypoperfusion caused by inadequate pumping action by the heart. It is an extreme form of CHF. The most common cause of acute cardiogenic shock is an MI. A patient in cardiogenic shock is often pale, cyanotic, diaphoretic, and restless. The pulse is often weak and rapid, respirations are shallow and rapid, and blood pressure is decreased. Unless corrected quickly, cardiogenic shock leads to cardiac arrest and death.

> ✓ Important cardiovascular disorders that will be encountered by the EMT include angina pectoris, myocardial infarction, congestive heart failure, and cardiogenic shock.

Assessment

The assessment of a patient with cardiac symptoms begins with the initial assessment, focusing on airway, breathing, and circulation. Appropriate interventions should be made if problems are found. For example, if a patient complains of severe substernal chest pain and

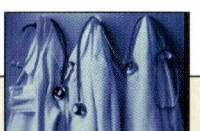

Physician Notes

The prehospital care of patients with cardiovascular complaints depends on a thorough history and patient assessment. A complete description of the patient's pain, including location, quality, severity, aggravating and relieving factors, presence of radiation, and associated symptoms, will give the receiving physician a great deal of information about the patient. The medical history obtained during the assessment and the interventions of standard cardiac care give the receiving physician a head start on patient management.

shortness of breath, the EMT should administer high-concentration oxygen as part of the "breathing" step in the initial assessment.

Although a wide variety of complaints are associated with the cardiovascular system, the most common complaint is chest pain that may or may not be accompanied by shortness of breath (dyspnea). When interviewing a patient with chest pain, it is important to characterize the pain as much as possible. The pain should be assessed and documented by determining its location, quality, and severity; presence of radiation; aggravating and relieving factors; and associated symptoms (Box 15.1). Classically, cardiac pain is located in the center of the chest (i.e., substernal, or below the sternum), is a dull or squeezing pressure, is severe, and often radiates down one or both arms (the left more often than the right) or to the jaw. The pain may be brought on by exercise (anginal pain) or may occur at rest. This is frequently attributed to indigestion by the patient as a method of denial. To rate the severity of pain, it is often helpful to use a scale from 1 to 10, with 10 being the worst pain the patient has ever had or could imagine. (Some patients have never experienced severe pain and have little or no reference point.) The EMT should obtain a baseline pain rating at the beginning of the assessment and then use subsequent ratings to monitor the patient's condition and response to care.

Box 15.1 Characteristics of Pain

- Location
- Quality
- Severity
- Presence of radiation
- Aggravating factors
- Relieving factors
- Associated symptoms

Box 15.2 Signs and Symptoms of Cardiac Compromise

- Substernal chest pain (crushing or squeezing)
- Radiation of pain to jaw or arm
- Shortness of breath
- Anxiety
- Nausea and vomiting
- Cool, clammy skin
- Abnormal pulse rate or rhythm
- Indigestion

The most common symptoms associated with cardiac chest pain are shortness of breath and nausea. Patients experiencing cardiac symptoms may be anxious and have a feeling of impending doom. Their skin is often cool and may be **diaphoretic** (sweaty). The pulse rate may be abnormal or irregular. The patient may also have an abnormal blood pressure (either high or low) (Box 15.2).

The signs and symptoms just described are the classic features of cardiac chest pain, but many times patients complain of chest pain that is atypical. For example, the pain may be sharp or burning in nature, may become worse with deep inspiration, or may be located in the back. Although these symptoms are less suggestive of a cardiac problem, the EMT in the field should not try to diagnose the cause of the patient's symptoms but should assess the patient and make appropriate interventions based on that assessment. Therefore any patient who complains of chest pain must be taken seriously. The pain should be assumed to be cardiac in origin and treated as such.

Management

Standard Cardiac Care

After performing the initial assessment and determining that the patient has signs or symptoms consistent with a cardiovascular problem, the EMT should begin standard cardiac care (Box 15.3). Standard cardiac care for the EMT-Basic (EMT-B) involves placing the patient in a position of comfort and providing supplemental oxygen (FiO_2 should be greater than 0.35). This can easily be achieved with a nonrebreathing mask at 10 L/min flow. The patient should be rapidly transported to the closest appropriate medical facility. Vital signs should be monitored frequently on the scene and en route. The new recommendations of the American Heart Association (2000) include the use of aspirin in the immediate management of chest pain in the field. The benefit is to decrease plate stickiness and therefore to decrease the clot propagation in the coronary arteries. The dosage is 160 to 325 mg (one half or one whole adult aspirin). The EMT should listen to breath sounds to check for signs of pulmonary edema. The EMT should also look for distended neck veins and swollen extremities, which are signs of CHF.

Supplemental oxygen increases the content of oxygen in the blood, which helps deliver oxygen to areas of decreased blood flow. For example, increasing the content of oxygen in a narrowed coronary artery with poor blood flow helps maintain the myocardium supplied by that coronary artery. Supplemental oxygen may increase arterial oxygen content enough to adequately supply the myocardium, relieving the patient's chest pain. Placing the patient in a comfortable position is also important. Most patients with chest pain and shortness of breath prefer a sitting position. Accommodating the patient as much as possible may alleviate anxiety and help reduce pain.

> ✓ Common signs and symptoms of cardiovascular compromise include chest pain, shortness of breath, cool and sweaty skin, irregular pulse, abnormal blood pressure, anxiety, and a feeling of impending doom.

> ✓ Standard cardiac care includes maintaining patient comfort, providing supplemental oxygen, assisting with nitroglycerin administration, delivering the patient quickly to the hospital, and monitoring vital signs.

Tips from the Pros

When the potential of a cardiac condition exists, use this easy-to-remember mnemonic of the steps of the history and management:

O—Onset of the pain.
P—Provoke. What causes the pain to worsen or be alleviated?
Q—Quality of the pain.
R—Radiation. Does the pain radiate to another part of the body?
S—Severity of the pain.
T—Time/Treatment. When did the pain start? What treatment has been used? Did it make the pain better or worse?

Nitroglycerin Administration

The EMT-B cannot administer medications that have not previously been prescribed for the patient. However, a patient can be assisted with medication administration; therefore EMTs should have a basic understanding of a few common medications. These are discussed in detail in Chapter 13.

The most common medication with which EMTs assist patients is **nitroglycerin** (NTG). Trade names for NTG include Nitro-Bid® and Nitrostat®. NTG relaxes and dilates blood vessels, decreasing the workload of the heart. With a decreased workload, the heart's demand for oxygen decreases, often leading to a relief of symptoms. NTG also dilates the coronary arteries, improving blood supply to the myocardium. The side effects of NTG include decreased blood pressure, headache, and changes in pulse rate. It is important to monitor and record the patient's vital signs and symptoms while administering the drug.

To administer NTG, all of the following criteria must be met:

- The patient has signs and symptoms of chest pain.
- The patient has a current prescription for NTG.
- The EMT has authorization by medical direction to administer the drug.

Contraindications to NTG include the following:

- Systolic blood pressure less than 100 mm Hg
- Head injury
- Infant or child patient
- Patient has taken three NTG tablets before EMT arrival

The dosage of NTG is one tablet (or one to two puffs of NTG spray), administered **sublingually** (under the tongue) every 3 to 5 minutes until pain is relieved, up to a maximum of three doses. The EMT must reassess vital signs and chest pain after each dose. The systolic blood pressure must be greater than 100 mm Hg before each dose. The EMT should assess the patient carefully before giving each dose, making sure the patient remains alert. The expiration date on the nitroglycerin bottle should be checked before administration. If the medication is working properly, the patient may feel a burning sensation under the tongue or develop a headache or flushed face. These side effects are usually not severe.

To administer NTG, the EMT first documents a blood pressure greater than 100 mm Hg. The EMT then checks the patient's prescription to ensure that it is accurate. The EMT places the tablet under the tongue and has the patient close his or her mouth. The patient should not chew the tablet—it should dissolve and be absorbed under the tongue. If the patient has NTG spray instead of tablets, the patient should hold his or her breath and administer one to two puffs under the tongue. The blood pressure should be taken 2 minutes after giving the dose. The EMT should record the vital signs, symptoms, and time of administration for each dose. It may be helpful to use a pain rating scale (from 1 to 10) to monitor the patient's pain relief with the drug.

Box 15.3 Standard Cardiac Care

- Make the patient comfortable
- Administer oxygen
- Monitor vital signs
- Aspirin
- Assist in administration of nitroglycerin when indicated

The patient must have a current prescription in his or her name. Often, family members of patients have their own prescriptions for NTG, but the EMT cannot assist with NTG administration unless the prescription is for the patient.

✓ With authorization from medical direction, the EMT may assist a patient in taking his or her nitroglycerin when the patient has a current prescription and has chest pain consistent with angina. The EMT must be familiar with the contraindications and side effects of nitroglycerin.

Cardiac Arrest Management

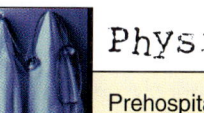

Physician Notes

Prehospital cardiac arrest is best managed by implementing the four links in the chain of survival. Early defibrillation and ACLS care in the field provide the best chance for patient survival. When pulselessness and apnea are confirmed, defibrillation with an automatic external defibrillator has priority over all other patient interventions. Efficient management of prehospital cardiac arrest relies on the coordination of basic and advanced life-support providers through the establishment of local protocols. Frequent training using cardiac arrest scenarios provides the EMT with the skills necessary to perform in the field. Thorough review of cases is needed to reinforce proper procedures and correct performance deficiencies. Dedicated involvement by local medical direction is the best way of ensuring appropriate EMT management of cardiovascular emergencies in the field.

Basic life-support skills are a critical component of cardiac arrest management. EMTs must review and practice CPR, especially artificial ventilation skills using airway adjuncts. Mouth-to-mask, bag-valve-mask, and flow-restricted oxygen-powered ventilation are discussed in Chapter 10.

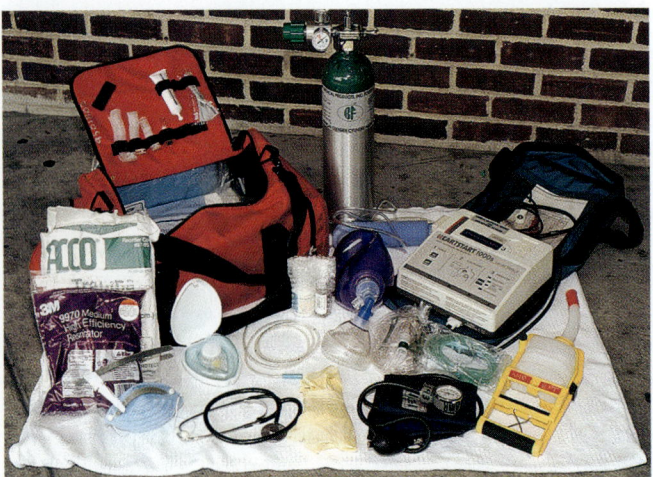

FIGURE 15.10 Equipment for cardiac arrest management. An automated external defibrillator (AED) and jump kit should be available for the initial management of cardiac arrest. A jump kit should include body substance isolation equipment, face mask, airway adjuncts, stethoscope, and blood pressure cuff.

While en route to the scene of a possible cardiac arrest, body substance isolation precautions should be used, including the use of gloves and other protective clothing. All of the equipment needed for the initial management of the patient should be easily accessible in a "jump kit" along with an AED (Figure 15.10). The EMTs should define the roles each crew member will perform at the arrest scene by establishing practice protocols for managing cardiac arrest. In general, one EMT should be assigned to the airway and one assigned to operate the AED. If other EMTs are available, they should assist the EMT at the airway and perform chest compressions. The EMT operating the AED generally has control of the arrest scene, because this person stops CPR for pulse checks and ensures that the patient is clear when delivering shocks. If possible, this EMT should not perform CPR, because this activity may interfere with operation of the AED and make overall scene management difficult.

After confirming pulselessness and apnea, CPR should be performed until an AED is available. If the patient is less than 8 years of age or less than 55 pounds, CPR should be performed en route to the nearest hospital. If the patient is more than 8 years of age, the AED electrodes should be attached. One-rescuer CPR is performed only while one partner is preparing equipment or during transport. In general, EMTs perform two-rescuer CPR in the field. The optimal use of personnel is having two EMTs at the airway (one to maintain a mask seal and one to ventilate the patient) and one EMT doing chest compressions.

Automated External Defibrillation

The most common initial rhythm in cardiac arrest is VF, and the definitive treatment for VF is defibrillation. These two facts have led to an emphasis on early defibrillation for the management of cardiac arrest caused by VF. Although VF is the most common initial rhythm, the likelihood of successful defibrillation diminishes rapidly after onset of VF. Thus a critical window of time exists in which defibrillation has the greatest potential for improving patient outcome. All emergency personnel who respond to patients in cardiac arrest should be trained to operate a defibrillator. AEDs have been shown to be effective when used by personnel with a wide variety of medical training, including fire and police department first responders and EMTs. Early defibrillation by non-ACLS personnel has been shown to decrease the time needed for other ACLS interventions, such as endotracheal intubation, intravenous (IV) line placement, and drug administration. AEDs enable widespread implementation of early defibrillation and are now a standard part of the EMT-B curriculum.

Survival of prehospital cardiac arrest depends on a combination of key interventions known as the chain of survival (see Figure 16.1). The four links in the chain of survival are early access, early CPR, early defibrillation, and early ACLS. Access to EMS has dramatically improved since the implementation of the 911 communication system. Further public education is needed to continue improvements in early access. The importance of early access is emphasized by the recent change in adult CPR guidelines, which instruct a single rescuer to access the system immediately on confirming pulselessness and apnea, rather than doing CPR for 1 minute and then calling.

Early CPR is the second link in the chain of survival. CPR is recognized as an important life-sustaining, but usually not lifesaving, intervention. Prompt and effective CPR allows time for interventions such as defibrillation and ACLS to be effective. Although early defibrillation is a lifesaving intervention, the first two links are also critical in the chain of survival. Without early access and early CPR, defibrillation and ACLS are often ineffective. Also, once defibrillation has removed VF, patients often require further CPR before the pulse returns because the shock delivery can be followed by asystole (electrical "flat line") or a very slow pulseless rhythm. With CPR this pulseless electrical state can become reorganized, with restoration of pulses.

> ✓ Basic life-support skills are a critical component of cardiac arrest management. An AED and the equipment needed for CPR should be in a jump kit that is used for every potential cardiac arrest call.

Before the onset of automated external defibrillation by EMTs, the responsibility of the EMT-B ended with performing CPR with supplemental oxygen. AEDs have enabled EMTs to provide early defibrillation, the third critical link in the chain of survival. Many EMS systems have shown increased survival rates from prehospital cardiac arrest in patients who are found in VF. These increased survival rates have occurred since the development of early defibrillation programs using AEDs.

Early ACLS care with IV placement, endotracheal intubation, and drug administration is the final link in the chain of survival. The new curriculum now includes endotracheal intubation as an option for EMT-Bs, further expanding their role in cardiac arrest management. Because EMT-Bs are beginning to perform roles that were previously reserved for ACLS providers, the interaction between ACLS personnel and EMT-Bs during the management of cardiac arrest must be redefined. The importance of definitive ACLS care still exists despite the expanded role of the EMT-B and should continue to be emphasized as a critical link in the chain of survival.

> ✓ The four links in the chain of survival are early access, early CPR, early defibrillation, and early ACLS.

Tips from the Pros

> It is helpful to have one's own jump kit available. This kit, which may be a vest or pack that goes around the waist, should have a pair of gloves, oral airway, and mask with a one-way valve. This jump kit allows the EMT to initially manage any patient in cardiac arrest until an AED arrives. Jump kits are especially helpful when a "patient down" call turns out to be a cardiac arrest. The EMT should never go to a patient scene without an appropriately equipped jump kit.

In EMS systems using both EMTs and advanced life-support (ALS) personnel, protocols should be established for the coordination of patient care. EMT operation of an AED does not require ALS personnel on scene. After arrival, ALS personnel should continue to use the AED for defibrillation as indicated until the initial set of stacked shocks is delivered. At that point ALS personnel may wish to change to a conventional defibrillator for further monitoring. EMS systems that routinely use a two-tiered BLS/ALS system may consider equipping the EMTs with AEDs that have monitor screens to facilitate the coordination between EMTs and ALS personnel. Many nonmedical buildings have AEDs available for use in case of emergency. These are available to nonmedical personnel.

Postresuscitation Care

Once VF or pulseless VT has been removed by defibrillation and pulses have returned, management of the patient depends on the use of effective basic life-support (BLS) skills. If a pulse is present at any time, breathing should be assessed. If the patient is breathing adequately and the airway is patent, high-concentration oxygen is given during transport. If the patient is apneic, airway control and artificial ventilation with 100% oxygen is performed during transport. Some patients may be breathing, but not with an adequate rate or tidal volume. In general, if a patient's ventilatory rate is less than 12 or greater than 20 breaths per minute, assisted ventilation with $FiO_2 > 0.85$ (85% to 100% oxygen in inspired air) is given with the patient's spontaneous breaths. After assessing breathing and intervening appropriately, the patient's vital signs are obtained. During transport the AED should remain attached to the patient. Vital signs should be reassessed frequently during transport.

> ✓ After a return of pulses, patient management relies on the effective use of BLS skills, including airway management, artificial ventilation, and frequent vital sign checks.

Cardiac Arrest in Children

The most common cause of cardiac arrest in children is respiratory compromise. It has been assumed that children rarely die from VF; therefore AEDs are not presently used in children younger than 8 years of age or weighing less than 90 pounds. The primary interventions for children in cardiac arrest have been airway management and assisted ventilation with 100% oxygen and chest compressions. Although these interventions continue to be important, recent evidence suggests that VF is not rare in child and adolescent cardiac arrest. Therefore it is possible that AEDs that deliver lower-energy shocks may be used in the future for children in VF or pulseless VT.

Continuing Education

Successful use of AEDs depends on thorough initial training and continuing education. The American Heart Association publishes a variety of guidelines and additional information on AEDs. Many EMS systems require practice drills to assess competency in AED operation every 90 days. Quality improvement with AEDs requires dedication on the part of the EMTs in the field, managers of the EMS system, and medical directors in charge of AED protocols. AED operation by EMTs can take place

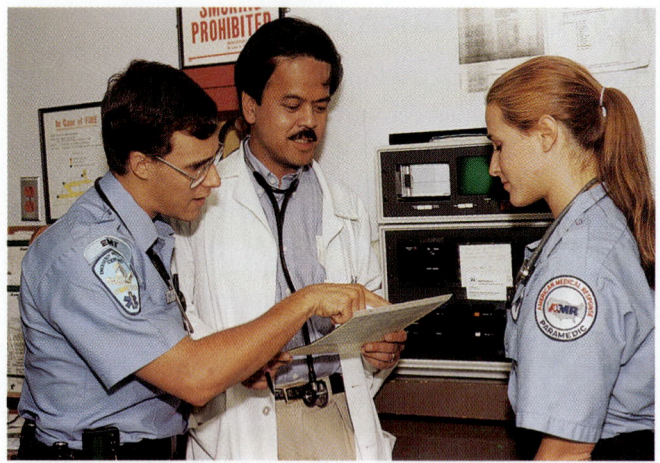

FIGURE 15.11 Case reviews reinforce proper interventions and help correct performance deficiencies. Case reviews depend on thorough documentation using written reports, voice electrocardiogram recordings, and AED data stored in memory modules or event cards.

only under the authority of local medical direction. Every case in which an AED is used must be reviewed by the local medical director. Documentation of events should be performed through written reports, voice and ECG tape recordings, solid-state memory modules, or memory cards containing digitized ECG recordings and, with some devices, digitized voice recordings (Figure 15.11). These **case reviews** allow for continuous improvement in AED operation and cardiac arrest management. The ultimate goal of AED education and case reviews is to improve patient survival from prehospital cardiac arrest.

> ✓ AEDs enable EMTs to perform a lifesaving intervention for patients in VF or pulseless VT. Proper use of AEDs depends on thorough training, established protocols, frequent practice, and proper defibrillator maintenance.

Summary

- The heart is a specialized muscle that provides blood flow to the lungs and body. The right half of the heart supplies the lungs and the left half supplies the body.
- Arrhythmias occur when the conduction system of the heart is disrupted. The two arrhythmias that are treated by AEDs are ventricular fibrillation and pulseless ventricular tachycardia.
- When assessing a patient with chest pain, the location, quality, severity, presence of radiation, aggravating and relieving factors, and associated symptoms are used to characterize the pain.
- Patients experiencing cardiac ischemia often have substernal chest pain with radiation to the jaw or left arm, cool and sweaty skin, a rapid or irregular pulse, nausea or vomiting, and a feeling of impending doom.
- Congestive heart failure and cardiogenic shock occur when the pumping action of the heart is inadequate, causing fluid to back up in the lungs and extremities. Patients will be short of breath and may have abnormal breath sounds such as crackles. Cardiogenic shock is an extreme form of congestive heart failure that is life threatening.
- Standard cardiac care involves placing the patient in a position of comfort, administering oxygen, and assisting with the administration of nitroglycerin when indicated.
- Survival from prehospital cardiac arrest depends on the four links in the chain of survival: early access, early CPR, early defibrillation, and early ACLS care.
- Proper AED operation depends on a thorough knowledge of established protocols, frequent practice with the device, and routine defibrillator and battery maintenance.
- When an AED is available, defibrillation takes priority over all other interventions in a patient who is in VF or pulseless VT.

Scenario Solution

1. This is a cardiac problem.
2. You should suspect this as a cardiac problem because of the cyanotic color of the patient and the low blood pressure. Although it could be dehydration and both should be included in your thought process, the most life-threatening condition is that of cardiac origin, so you should address this first.
3. You can potentially prevent the outcome by treating it as a cardiac condition, starting oxygen at a high concentration ($FiO_2 = \geq 0.85$) and using nitroglycerin if the patient had been using it in the past and had some of her own. You should also give aspirin.

Scenario Solution (cont'd)

4. You should start transportation immediately with advanced cardiac life support (ALCS) intercept, if available.
5. While waiting for the arrival of ALCS, you should continue cardiopulmonary resuscitation (CPR) with a high concentation of oxygen in the bag-valve-mask system ($FiO_2 = 0.95$) and use of an automated external defibrillator (AED) as appropriate.
6. You should give the same type of care to the patient en route to the hospital.

Key Terms

Angina pectoris Chest pain or pressure frequently brought on by exercise and relieved by rest; caused by ischemia in the heart and often treated with nitroglycerin.

Aorta The largest artery in the body, extending from the left ventricle through the thorax and abdomen to the navel, where it divides into the iliac arteries; carries blood from the heart to the body.

Arterioles The smallest branch of an artery; supplies capillaries with oxygenated blood.

Artery Vessel that carries blood away from the heart to the body under pressure.

Atherosclerosis A disease in which arteries are narrowed by collections of cholesterol and cellular debris; it increases the risk for angina pectoris and myocardial infarction.

Atrium One of the upper chambers of the heart; the right atrium receives blood from the superior and inferior venae cavae; the left atrium receives blood from the pulmonary veins.

Automated external defibrillator (AED) A device used in cardiac arrest to perform a computer analysis of the patient's cardiac rhythm and deliver defibrillatory shocks when indicated.

Blood pressure The pressure that blood exerts on the walls of arteries; measured with a sphygmomanometer.

Brachial artery Artery located on the inside of the elbow on the same side as the small finger; extends from the elbow to the armpit.

Bradycardia A heart rate less than 60 beats per minute; a patient with bradycardia may or may not have symptoms.

Capillaries The smallest blood vessels in the body; in the tissues, capillaries surround the cells, allowing gas and nutrient exchange to take place.

Cardiac arrest A condition in which the heart no longer generates blood flow, causing pulselessness and apnea; two of the many causes are arrhythmias and myocardial infarction.

Cardiogenic shock A condition in which the heart's output is not strong enough to meet the body's needs, causing widespread hypoperfusion.

Carotid arteries The major arteries of the neck, supplying the face, head, and brain with oxygenated blood.

Case reviews A method of quality assurance that involves reviewing actual cases with EMTs in order to review the quality of care delivered by the EMS system.

Chain of survival The critical interventions needed to improve survival from prehospital cardiac arrest, including early access, early cardiopulmonary resuscitation, early defibrillation, and early advanced cardiac life support.

Congestive heart failure A condition in which the heart is an inadequate pump, causing fluid to build up in the lungs (pulmonary edema) and venous system (distended neck veins).

Coronary arteries The first branches off the aorta, which supply the heart with blood. If occluded, a myocardial infarction often occurs.

Defibrillation The delivery of an electrical shock to the myocardium in an attempt to convert ventricular fibrillation or ventricular tachycardia to a normal rhythm.

Diaphoretic State of sweating (e.g., patients with cardiac chest pain are often diaphoretic).

Diastolic pressure The pressure in the heart when the heart muscle is relaxing; lower reading of a blood pressure.

Dorsalis pedis artery An artery located on the upper surface of the foot; usually palpable and can be used to assess blood supply distal to the leg injury.

Dysrhythmia Abnormal rhythm.

Electrocardiogram (ECG) The tracing of the electrical conduction system in the heart; normally occurs in predictable patterns.

Femoral arteries The major vessels supplying the legs with oxygenated blood; can be palpated in the groin area.

Hemoglobin A specialized protein that binds to oxygen in red blood cells; it gives red blood cells their color.

Hypertension Abnormally high blood pressure; it is a risk factor for atherosclerosis, stroke, and other vascular events.

Hypotension Abnormally low blood pressure; may be a sign of shock.

Key Terms (cont'd)

Inferior vena cava The major vein of the abdominal cavity; returns blood from the lower extremities, pelvis, and abdomen to the right atrium.

Ischemia Inadequate blood flow to a tissue; can cause anginal pain or a myocardial infarction.

Myocardial infarction (MI) A condition in which part of the heart muscle (myocardium) dies because of inadequate supply of oxygen and nutrients; also called *heart attack.*

Myocardium Muscle tissue that makes up the inner layer of the heart.

Nitroglycerin A medication that dilates blood vessels and decreases the workload on the heart; often used to treat angina pectoris.

Perfusion A state of adequate supply of oxygen and nutrients to the tissues; ability of the circulatory system to distribute blood containing nutrients and oxygen to the tissues.

Plasma The liquid component of blood that contains proteins such as blood clotting factors.

Platelets Cellular fragments in the blood that form plugs at the site of bleeding, starting the clotting process.

Posterior tibial artery An artery located on the inside of the ankle.

Pulmonary arteries Vessels that carry oxygen-poor blood from the right side of the heart to the lugs; the only arteries in the body that carry oxygen-poor blood.

Pulmonary edema A condition in which fluid builds up in the alveoli and small airways, causing hypoxia and dyspnea; most commonly caused by congestive heart failure.

Pulmonary veins Vessels that carry oxygen-rich blood from the lungs back to the left side of the heart; the only veins in the body that carry oxygen-rich blood.

Pulse The wave of blood produced by the contraction of the left ventricle; can be felt wherever an artery passes over a bone close to the skin surface.

Pulse pressure The difference between the systolic and diastolic pressures.

Radial artery Artery located on the thumb side of the wrist of each arm; extends from the wrist to the elbow.

Red blood cells Blood cells that contain hemoglobin; primary function is to carry oxygen to the tissues.

Shock Failure of the circulatory system to perfuse tissues; hypoperfusion of the circulatory system.

Standard cardiac care Management of a patient with cardiac complaints; includes maintaining patient comfort and administering oxygen.

Sublingually Under the tongue (e.g., nitroglycerin is often administered sublingually).

Superior vena cava Large vein that returns blood to the right atrium from the thorax, arms, head, and neck.

Systolic pressure The pressure in the heart when the heart muscle is contracting; upper reading of a blood pressure.

Tachycardia Condition in which the heart contracts at a rate greater than 100 beats per minute.

Veins Vessels that carry blood back to the heart.

Ventricle One of the lower chambers of the heart that pump blood; the right ventricle supplies blood to the lungs and the left supplies the body.

Ventricular fibrillation (VF) An arrhythmia in which the heart is in a state of disorganized electrical and mechanical activity, resulting in a lack of blood flow; treated with defibrillation.

Ventricular tachycardia (VT) An arrhythmia in which the ventricles are driven by an electrical impulse separate from the normal conduction system; pulses may or may not be present; if there are no pulses, defibrillation is necessary.

Venules The smallest veins in the body; carry blood from the capillaries to the veins.

White blood cells Blood cells that function in the body's immune system.

Review Questions

1. Which of the following is not in the correct order?
   a. Pulmonary artery, lungs, left atrium
   b. Aorta, femoral artery, dorsalis pedis artery
   c. Pulmonary vein, right atrium, right ventricle
   d. Arteriole, capillary, venule

2. Hemoglobin is a specialized molecule designed to carry oxygen, which is found in which of the blood cells?
   a. White cells
   b. Red cells
   c. Leukocytes
   d. Platelets

Review Questions

3. A patient's blood pressure is 120/80 mm Hg. Which of the following is incorrect?
   a. The systolic blood pressure is 120 mm Hg.
   b. The pulse pressure is 40 mm Hg.
   c. The diastolic blood pressure is 80 mm Hg.
   d. The pulse pressure cannot be determined from the given data.
4. Which of the following is not a common sign or symptom of an acute MI?
   a. Sudden onset of severe headache
   b. Crushing substernal chest pain
   c. An aching pain in the shoulder
   d. Cool and sweaty skin
   e. Shortness of breath
5. A patient is found unresponsive. Pulselessness and apnea are confirmed. Which of the following is the most appropriate immediate action?
   a. Call for ALS backup
   b. Perform aggressive CPR
   c. Consult medical direction for advice
   d. Attach an AED as soon as possible and press "analyze"
6. Which of the following is a contraindication to assisting with nitroglycerin administration?
   a. Diastolic blood pressure of 70 mm Hg
   b. The patient has taken one nitroglycerin tablet before arrival
   c. Local medical direction does not allow EMTs to assist patients with medications
   d. The patient is having severe substernal chest pain

Answers to these Review Questions can be found at the end of the book on page 866.

16

Early Defibrillation

Lesson Goal

The goal of this chapter is to help the student understand the indications for and operation of the automated external defibrillator in accordance with accepted safe standards of use and care.

Scenario

On a warm, sunny, spring morning you and your partner are dispatched to a local church in response to a reported "72-year-old male who has collapsed and is not breathing. CPR is in progress." Response time is 4 minutes, and two police officers have arrived 2 minutes before your unit. They have assessed the patient, assumed CPR, and used their automated external defibrillator (AED) one time. They advise you that the patient is still in cardiac arrest as you walk into the room. Further information reveals that the patient was not feeling well early in the morning but insisted on going to church anyway. His wife states that he suddenly turned very pale, began sweating, and grabbed at his chest as he attempted to get up from his seat. He collapsed almost immediately but did not hit his head as he fell. He was caught by bystanders who lowered him to the floor. Citizen CPR was begun immediately.

 Your unit carries an AED, and you have been certified in its use. You have your usual complement of patient care equipment. What would you do next?

Key Terms to Know

Advanced life support
Atherosclerosis
Automated external defibrillator (AED)
Cardioversion
Defibrillation
EMT-Defibrillation
Medical command authority
Myocardial infarction
Pacing
Permanent vegetative state
Ventricular fibrillation

Learning Objectives

As an EMT-Basic, you should be able to do the following:

DOT

- List the indications for use of the automated external defibrillator (AED).
- List the contraindications for use of the AED.
- Explain the roles of age and weight in use of the AED.
- Discuss the fundamentals of and explain the rationale for early defibrillation.
- Explain the importance of early ALS interventions to the cardiac arrest patient, if available.
- Discuss the types of AEDs.
- Differentiate between a fully automatic and a semiautomatic AED.
- Discuss procedures that must be taken into account for use of the AED.
- Discuss circumstances in which inappropriate shocks could occur while using the AED.
- Discuss advantages and summarize speed of operation in use of the AED.
- List the steps in use of the AED.
- Discuss procedures for management of a patient who remains in cardiac arrest after use of the AED.
- Discuss the importance of postresuscitation patient care.
- List the importance of regular skills practice in using the AED and the methods of accomplishing this.
- Explain the role that medical direction plays in the use of the AED.
- Discuss the components of and why case reviews are important in the use of the AED.
- Define the function of all controls found on an AED.
- Demonstrate the application and use of the AED.
- Demonstrate the maintenance procedures for the AED.
- Demonstrate patient assessment during and after use of the AED.
- Demonstrate skills to complete the operator's skills checklist for the AED.

Cardiac emergencies are the leading emergency in the United States. Each year 1.5 million individuals suffer a **myocardial infarction** (heart attack), with some 500,000 deaths resulting. Most of these sudden death episodes occur outside of a medical facility. Rapid defibrillation with an **automated external defibrillator** (AED) is the only treatment that can save an individuals life. AEDs have become smaller, lighter, and smarter than any previous device and can be used by anyone with minimal training. Using an electrical shock (**defibrillation**), the AED can stop chaotic and unorganized heart rhythms that lead to death. For an adult who is in cardiac arrest, defibrillation is the priority in their care. It should be administered as soon as practical and without delay. Early defibrillation is a vital link in the chain of survival (Figure 16.1).

Sudden Cardiac Death

In the United States approximately 1000 adults die each day from *sudden cardiac death* (cardiac arrest). Many of these patients die outside of a medical setting (e.g., at work, at play, while traveling, or while sitting in their homes). If an individual remains in cardiac arrest without definitive treatment (defined as a combination of basic life support [BLS] and **advanced life support** [ALS]), his or her chance for survival diminshes (Table 16.1).

> ✓ For every minute that a patient remains in cardiac arrest, his or her chance for survival diminishes.

Myocardial infarction occurs for a variety of reasons (Box 16.1). One of the most common causes is **atherosclerosis**, the buildup of plaque within the lumen of the coronary arteries, leading to decreased blood flow and oxygen

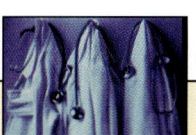

Physician Notes

The Fick principle demonstrates that the three elements that must be met to prevent anaerobic metabolism and to continue the body's ability to produce energy are (1) oxygenation of the red blood cells (RBCs) in the lungs, (2) delivery of the RBCs to the tissue cells, and (3) offloading of the oxygen from the RBCs to the tissues cells. Three parts of the cardiovascular system are necessary to accomplish the delivery: the heart (pump), blood (fluid), and vessels (pipes). Without oxygen the cells convert from aerobic metabolism to anaerobic metabolism to produce energy. Anaerobic metabolism, which uses 38 energy molecules of adenosine triphosphate (ATP), is much less efficient than aerobic metabolism, which uses only 2 (see Chapter 9).

Patient Care Algorithm

Circulatory Assessment

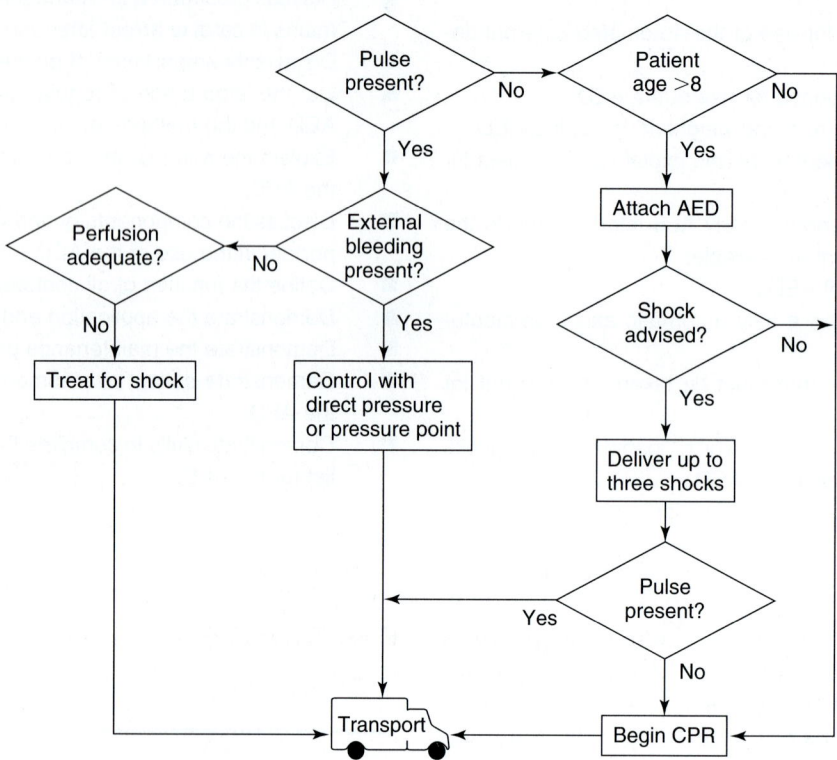

TABLE 16.1	Survival Rates between Cardiac Arrest and Delivery of CPR and Defibrillation	
Time to CPR (min)	Time to ALS (min)	Survival Rate (%)
0-4	0-8	43
0-4	16+	10
8-12	8-16	6
8-12	16+	0
12+	12+	0

Data from Eisenberg MS, Bergner L, Halstrom A: Cardiac resuscitation in the community: importance of rapid provision and implication for program planning, *JAMA* 241:1905, 1979.

supply to the heart muscle. When heart muscle is deprived of oxygen and other nutrients it becomes irritable and will cause the electrical rhythm of the heart to become irregular and unstable. This irregularity deprives the myocardial muscles of oxygen, producing anaerobic metabolism. The resultant lack of energy production in the heart muscles causes the heart to stop its pumping action (cardiac arrest).

The second major cause of cardiac arrest is electrical disturbances within the heart, which accounts for approximately 80% of cardiac arrests. The normal electrical rhythm becomes chaotic and unorganized, producing no cardiac output and resulting in **ventricular fibrillation** or asystole. The only effective treatment to reestablish the normal prodcutive rhythm and cardiac output is *defibrillation*. The heart is no longer able to pump blood, and death will result if the normal heart rhythm cannot be restored. Without adequate blood flow, the patient's cells are deprived of oxygen, which is the most important nutrient to produce energy (see Chapter 9).

> ✓ The only definitive treatment for a patient who is in ventricular fibrillation is *defibrillation*. Without defibrillation, the heart is no longer able to pump blood and death will result if the normal heart rhythm cannot be restored.

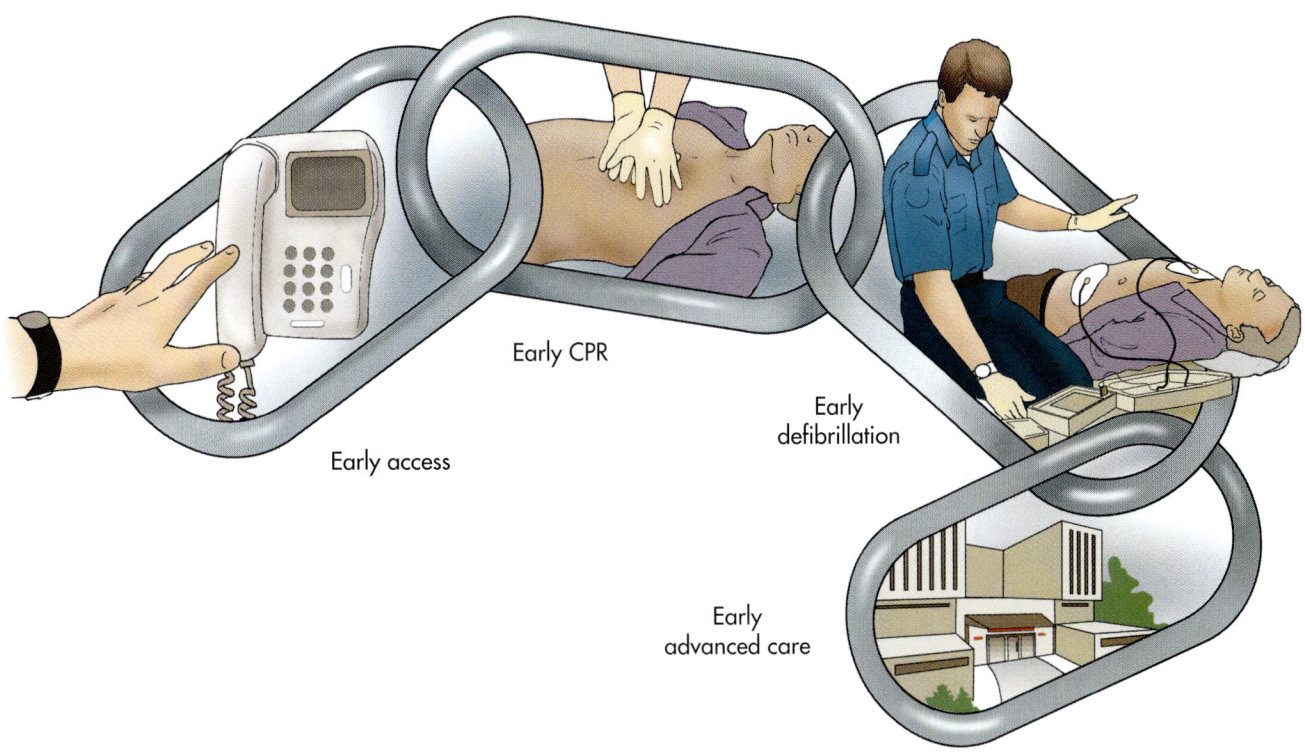

FIGURE 16.1 The chain of survival.

The brain is more sensitive to oxygen deprivation than any other tissue in the body and will suffer permanent injury when it is left without oxygen for 4 to 6 minutes. A person whose brain is deprived of oxygen for 10 minutes generally will not recover; the oxygen deprivation can lead to a **permanent vegetative state**. Given that the average response time in the United States for an EMS unit to arrive at a scene is over 5 minutes, early defibrillation is imperative.

Physician Notes

Permanent vegetative state describes a patient with no brain function except for the portion that controls autonomic system functions, such as breathing and cardiovascular action. This is the lowest brain level short of brain death.

Approximately 500,000 individuals who suffer from a myocardial infarction or fatal dysrhythmia heart attack succumb to cardiac arrest each year. These patients need to have immediate access to a defibrillator if they are to have a good chance of survival. Although there are no absolute ages in which a cardiac arrest occurs, most appear in patients who are in their fifties and sixties. Historically, cardiac arrest occurs more often in males than in females, but the incidence in women increases after menopause. A nonarrest situation is manifested by chest pain that may or

Box 16.1 Risk Factors for Sudden Cardiac Death

Heredity
Gender
Age
Cigarette smoking
High blood pressure
Inactivity
High cholesterol level
Diabetes
Obesity
Excessive stress

may not be accompanied by nausea, sweating, shortness or breath, and vomiting (see Chapter 15 for further review).

As knowledge of medical science grows, the equipment that prehospital providers have available to use in the field improves. This knowledge (provided by this text and the emergency medical technician–basic [EMT-B] course) and the equipment required to allow medical and nonmedical responders reverse ventricular fibrillation helps the EMT restore cardiac output and provide blood flow throughout the body. AEDs use computer technology to help the EMT diagnose and determine treatment for the patient who is in cardiac arrest. This treatment is called *defibrillation* and uses electricity to eradicate the nonfunctional heart rhythm.

Automated External Defibrillator

History of Defibrillation

The practice of BLS, cardiopulmonary resuscitation (CPR), and defibrillation is only 40 years old. The first experiments with the use of electricity to correct abnormal electrical patterns were performed in Russia. These early machines were large and nonmoveable, required alternating current (AC) electricity, and were difficult to use. Perhaps the largest drawback was that the patient had to be brought to the device, which added to the delay in treatment time.

The first battery-powered defibrillator were released in 1963. Although this was the first portable device, it was large, weighed more than 50 pounds, and could only be used for defibrillation of a patient, not **cardioversion** or **pacing** like current devices. In 1980 a new company was formed in Oregon to develop a more sophisticated defibrillator that was portable and made most of the treatment decisions for the rescuer. Working under the premise that most cardiac arrests occur outside of a medical facility, the physician running this program wanted defibrillation to be as available as portable fire extinguishers. In other words, the goal was to provide lay rescuers with a computerized defibrillator that would recognize and interpret ventricular fibrillation and determine whether to defibrillate.

Chicago's O'Hare International Airport was one of the first sites in which security personnel were trained in the use of the AED. Success was quickly demonstrated as lay rescuers with only 4 hours of training in the use of the AED could safely and efficiently use the device on a cardiac arrest patient. Most of the early successes and use of the AED in the 1980s were in the private sector. Large corporations were quick to recognize the value of the having an AED in the workplace and provided training to employees who volunteered to be part of an emergency response team. However, the EMS community continued to rely on paramedics providing defibrillation.

The idea of training EMT-Bs to use a defibrillator was beginning to emerge in the 1980s. Between 1985 and 1988 the number of **EMT-Defibrillation** programs in the United States grew from 225 to 690, and the first EMT-Defibrillation programs for first responders were being initiated. Developed primarily for law enforcement in rural or wilderness areas that had long response times for volunteer services, EMT-Defibrillation programs grew rapidly, with over 1000 reported programs in place by 1995.

Defibrillation was not new to the EMS community during the 1980s and 1990s. A physician who understood that the treatment needed to be taken to the patient introduced the concept of mobile coronary care in Belfast, Ireland in 1966. The idea of ALS care being provided by paramedics in the United States was beginning to grow. Early programs in Miami, Kansas City, Kansas, and Seattle were being put into place and providing evidence of good success. Early defibrillation in the prehospital setting was provided only by ALS personnel, which meant that delay of treatment was often because first responders could only perform CPR while awaiting the arrival of a paramedic unit.

In 1988 the American Heart Association released its interim report on the use of defibrillators by EMT-Bs. Studies conducted at several sites showed that individuals with minimal training and background could be trained to safely use a defibrillator. This was the beginning of the revolution in both the design and use of AEDs by medical and nonmedical personnel. The fourth generation of AEDs are smaller, lighter, and smarter than previous versions, and they require little maintenance. Advances in battery technology have provided energy sources that are good for 3 years without routine charging. As designs have improved and technology has advanced, AEDs has become simpler to use. Today, individuals with little or no medical background can safely use an AED with only 3 to 4 hours of training (Figure 16.2).

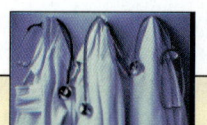
Physician Notes

CPR is a holding pattern that can maintain marginal cardiac output and oxygen delivery. It is not definitive care. The definitive care of cardiac arrest is reestablishment of cardiac output and the delivery segment of the Fick principle. CPR cannot be used as a tool to continue oxygenation of the heart and brain for more than a few minutes. This is the benefit of the use of the AED by EMT-Bs and appropriately trained lay personnel.

Functions of the AED

Defibrillation is accomplished by the delivery of high-voltage current through the patient's skin. The current traverses the myocardium and terminates ventricular fibrillation by stopping the chaotic electrical pattern that has developed as a result of either an anoxic myocardium or electrical system instability. Delivery of the defibrillation current temporarily paralyzes the heart muscle and the electrical system. This action allows the heart's natural pacemaker system to begin working

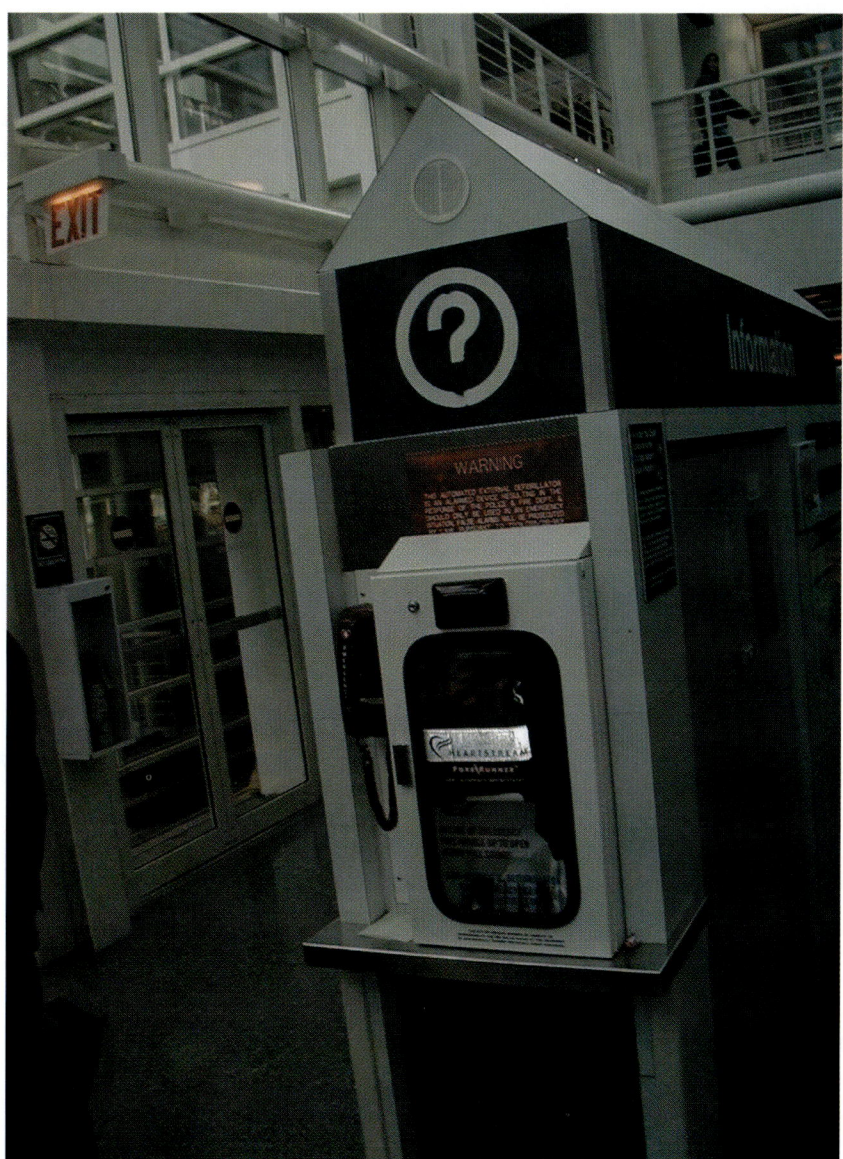

FIGURE 16.2 Public access to an AED at O'Hare International Airport in Chicago. The AED is becoming a part of many public areas. The EMT-B may arrive at the scene when the AED sequence has already been started by someone on the scene. The EMT-B should be prepared to take over the patient management unless the person on the scene is more knowledgeable than the EMT-B. In this situation, the EMT-B should assist.

again, resulting in an orderly firing of the heart muscle cells and restoration of normal blood flow.

BLS and CPR are integral to the successful use of an AED. CPR does not reverse a cardiac arrest and therefore cannot be used alone to resuscitate a patient in cardiac arrest. However, CPR slows the process of dying by artificially keeping the heart marginally oxygenated and in a state of ventricular fibrillation, thus allowing a greater window of opportunity for resuscitation. The most important part of CPR occurs before the arrival of the AED by increasing the probability that a patient's heart will still be in ventricular fibrillation when the AED arrives.

The current generation of the AED is a combination of a standard defibrillator and a computer. The computer analyzes the patient's rhythm and determines whether it fits within preset guidelines and thus can be treated with defibrillation energy. The AED diagnoses either ventricular fibrillation (Figure 16.3) or nonventricular fibrillation (Figure 16.4) and provides a defibrillation current when ventricular fibrillation is present. The energy level delivered (measured in Joules) is identical to that delivered using a manual defibrillator.

The AED looks for a certain waveform pattern and duration that meets the criteria for ventricular fibrillation. Using two pregelled pads applied to the patient's chest and to the device by a cable (Figure 16.5), the AED both analyzes and, if appropriate, treats the patient.

The rhythm strip shown in Figure 16.3 represents a regular sinus rhythm, or one that is occurring naturally within the heart's pacemaker system. An indication of regular sinus rhythm is the tall QRS complex, which is the part of the electrical impulse that indicates the movement of electrical energy through the heart muscle. Figure 16.4, A shows an electrocardiograph (ECG) tracing of a patient who is in ventricular fibrillation. The organized rhythm found in the regular ECG tracing is absent, and that the QRS complex cannot be easily identified. The QRS does not exist because there is no orderly firing of the heart's electrical system. Detecting the presence or absence of the QRS complex is the primary method used by the AED's electronic protocol to identify the presence or absence of ventricular fibrillation.

Another technique that AED uses to determine whether the patient is in ventricular fibrillation is determination of the height of the QRS complex, called *amplitude*. A vertical height of less than 1 mm (Figure 16.6) (one small box on the ECG paper) is cosidered a nonventricular fibrillation rhythm, and thus the AED will not defibrillate the patient (Box 16.2).

Although each type of AED has its own internal circuitry for the detection of sinus rhythm, most use the same principles of patient application and use. An AED is

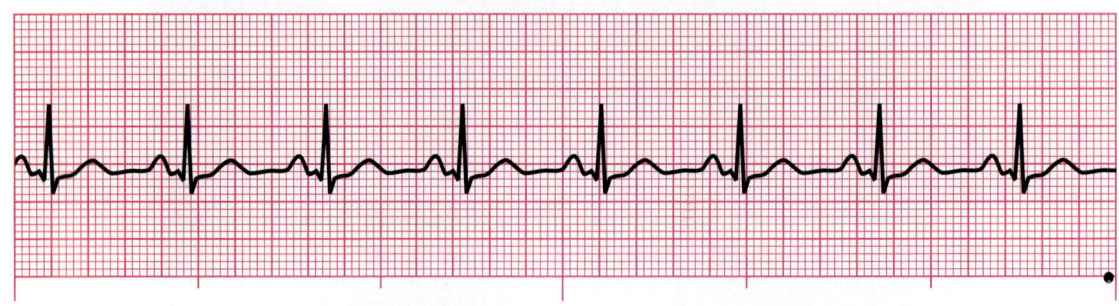

FIGURE 16.3 Normal sinus rhythm.

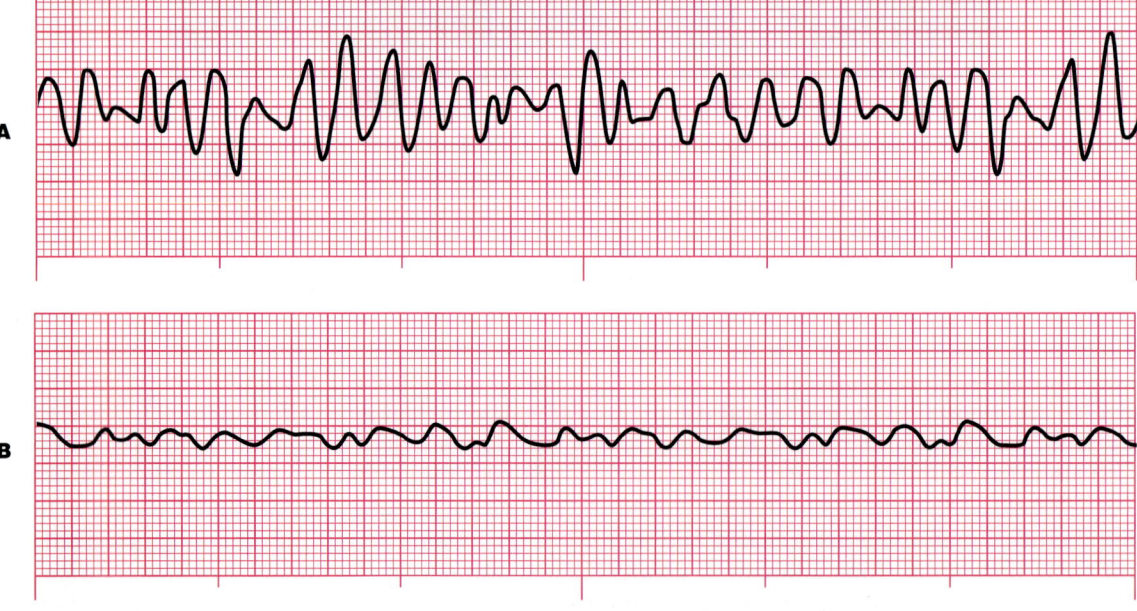

FIGURE 16.4 **A,** Coarse ventricular fibrillation. **B,** Fine ventricular fibrillation.

either fully automatic or semiautomatic in its operation, depending on whether the operator has to manually push the shock delivery button (semiautomatic) or the device will perform the delivery automatically (fully automatic). All other operations of the device are the same.

Use of the AED

The EMT should perform body substance isolation procedures when using an automated external defibrillator (AED). Upon arrival at the scene, the first member of the EMS team must preform a primary patient assessment to determine the status of the patient. The EMT must recheck this primary survey frequently throughout care of the patient ("Trust no one, do it yourself"). CPR should be continued until the AED is attached to the patient and ready for use.

 The AED should only be applied to a patient who is unconscious, unresponsive, and pulseless.

To use the AED, the EMT should first bare the patient's chest. The EMT should be aware of modesty issues for female patients, especially in a public location. Often the monitoring/treatment electrode pads can be placed on the patient under his or her blouse or sweater. However, the EMT should not allow modesty concerns to interfere with proper patient care. It is important that the pads are applied directly to the patient's skin. If the patient's chest is wet, either from sweating or other sources of water, the EMT should dry the chest before attaching the monitoring/treatment electrode pads. It may even be necessary to clip the hair of a patient with excessive chest hair.

Next the EMT should turn on the AED and follow the voice prompts and commands. The AED is designed to work with the rescuer by giving voice commands. These voice commands vary among machines but consist of five basic prompts:

1. *"Attach electrode pads."* This statement is given if the device is turned on before application of the monitoring/treatment pads and serves as a reminder to do so. Additionally, this command plays if the pads become loose or disconnected after they are applied to the patient, such as when moving the patient.

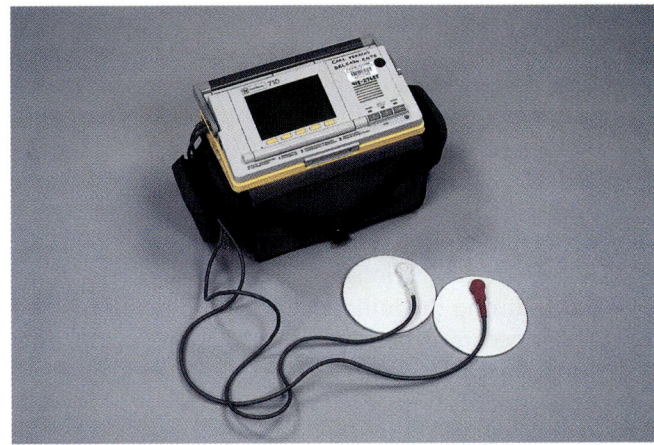

FIGURE 16.5 Pregelled pads are applied to the patient's chest and attached to the AED by cables.

> **Box 16.2 ECG Rhythm Strip Interpretation by the AED**
>
> - Size and form of the patient's QRS complex
> - Organization of ECG rhythm
> - Measurement of height of QRS on ECG (amplitude)
> - Patient's heart rate as measured on the QRS

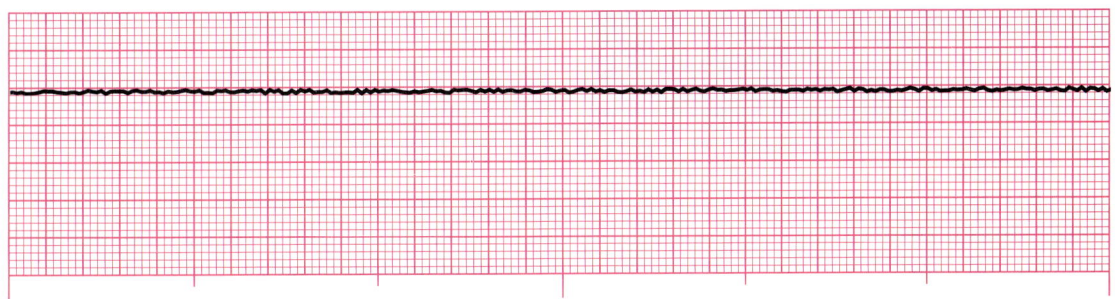

FIGURE 16.6 Asystole is not considered ventricular fibrillation. Note the lack of a QRS complex.

2. *"Assessing—do not touch patient."* This prompt is given after the device has been turned on, has completed its self-test, and is beginning analysis of the patient's ECG. During this time the EMT cannot perform CPR on the patient; move the patient in any way, including a moving ambulance or patient gurney; or perform any other patient care procedures. Any movement of the patient can cause the AED to determine a false positive and fail to treat a patient who is in ventricular fibrillation.
3. *"Charging—stand back."* This command is given each time the AED determines that ventricular fibrillation is present and the device is charging its capacitors to deliver a pre-determined energy level. This serves as a warning to all members of the resuscitation team, but the AED operator must ensure that no one is touching the patient at this point. Because the electrical energy moves through the patient's entire body, anyone who is in contact with the patient will receive a jolt of energy as well. *If the resuscitation team is using a fully automated AED, this voice prompt will be the only warning that a shock is going to be delivered.*
4. *"Push to shock."* This command is announced once the AED is fully charged and ready for treatment of the patient. The AED operator should survey the patient from the head to the toes and then back to the head before pushing the shock button to ensure that no one is in contact with the patient. On a fully automated AED, this command is not announced and their is no flashing button for the operator to push.
5. *"Check breathing and pulse."* This prompt occurs in one of two situations. It occurs after every third shock during the initial defibrillation of the patient, and it occurs if the initial analysis of the patient's heart rhythm reveals a nonventricular fibrillation pattern or if the patient's ECG rhythm is changed from a ventricular fibrillation to a nonventricular fibrillation pattern by any single defibrillation shock.

All AEDs are programmed to deliver defibrillatory shocks in stacked sets of three. This means that the patient receives three successive defibrillation shocks if the heart rhythm remains unchanged. This means that a patient receives three defibrillation shocks initially, after the device is attached and turned on, unless the heart rhythm is changed by any one electrical shock.

Treatment protocols for use of the AED have been designed using the guidelines of the American Heart Association. These research-based guidelines indicate that a patient in cardiac arrest with ventricular fibrillation should receive a series of three stacked defibrillation shocks upon initiation of treatment. If the rhythm has not changed during these initial shocks, the patient should receive 1 minute of CPR and an additional three stacked shocks. The rationale for the use of 1 minute of CPR between the third and fourth shocks is because a myocardium that is not oxygenated will not respond to defibrillation. Therefore if the patient remains in ventricular fibrillation after the third shock, the myocardium needs to be oxygenated with CPR before any further attempts at defibrillation are made. More detailed information can be found in the AED Skill Sheet at the end of this chapter.

The rescuer on scene with an AED should follow the guidelines listed in the previous paragraph and in the AED Skill Sheet, except for performing CPR. The EMT should attach the AED to the patient as soon as practical and initiate treatment of the patient. The EMT should not take time to call for additional help or to contact **medical command authority** until after the first three shocks have been given, the voice prompt to "check breathing and pulse" is heard, or additional help has arrived on scene.

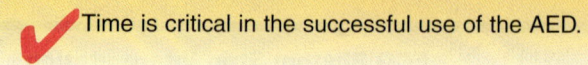

> Time is critical in the successful use of the AED.

EMTs must always follow established local patient treatment guidelines for use of the AED. The local medical director will have the final say in how and when the AED can be used. Use of an AED does not require the presence of ALS personnel on scene, but they should be notified, if they are available in the area, as soon as possible upon arrival at the scene or even by the dispatcher at the receipt of the initial call if the determination is made that a cardiac arrest is in progress. The EMT Paramedics (EMT-Ps) have advanced skills and knowledge, and administration of drugs is often necessary in a postresuscitation situation.

> The EMT-P's advanced skills, knowledge, and ability to administer drugs are often necessary in a postresuscitation situation

Voice Commands and Prompts Given by the AED

- Attach electrode pads.
- Analyzing—Stop CPR
- Charging—Stand clear
- Push flashing button to shock
- Check breathing and pulse

Safety Issues

The currently available AED should not be used on a patient who is under 8 years of age or who weighs less than 41 kg (90 lb). The amount of electrical energy delivered to the body can produce significant damage to the heart and nervous system in these patients.

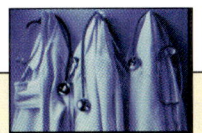

Physician Notes

An AED will probably not be effective on patients who are in cardiac arrest secondary to major trauma because the usual cause is either blood loss or airway compromise. Defibrillation is not the method of management for these conditions

> **Box 16.3** Safety in the Use of the AED
>
> - Do not use on patients who weigh less than 25 kg (55 lb).
> - Do not use in a wet environment because it can result in energy being transferred to the rescuers.
> - Ensure that no one is touching the patient at the time of energy delivery.

Safety issues indicate that the AED should not be used on a patient in a wet medium; he or she should be moved to a dry environment. Because the AED is an electrical device, if the EMT using the device is standing in water, the shock will go to the rescuer as well. This also applies if the patient is on a metal surface and someone is in contact with the metal during defibrillation (Box 16.3).

Postresuscitation Care

The EMT will be prompted at different points in the resuscitation effort to evaluate the patient for return of breathing and pulse. This occurs after the third defibrillation and sixth defibrillation and at any point where the AED detects a change in the patient's rhythm and determines that it will not shock the patient.

If the patient regains a spontaneous pulse, the rescuers continue with BLS and CPR and contact medical control or refer to their treatment guidelines for consideration of termination of resuscitation efforts. This decision must always be made with the best interests of the patient and family in mind and generally is not done without direct communication with the medical director or *medical control emergency physician (MCEP)*.

If there is return of a spontaneous pulse, the first step is to ensure that the patient has a patent airway and that ventilations are adequate. If the ventilations are inadequate, the patient should immediately receive ventilatory assistance with supplemental oxygen. Even if the ventilations are adequate, supplemental oxygen must be applied as soon as possible. Continuous monitoring of the patient's airway, ventilations, and pulse are mandatory during the immediate postresuscitation phase. The AED should remain applied to the patient so that immediate defibrillation can be delivered again if necessary. However, the patient cannot be moved with the AED in the on position. Any movement of the patient requires that the AED be turned off to avoid error in interpretation of the patient's cardiac rhythm by the device.

All treatments given to the patient with the AED must be documented on the patient run report. This includes times; number of shocks given; any treatment given before, during, or after resuscitation; and any ECG tracings from the AED if the machine is so equipped. Additionally, the EMT should document any interactions with family, bystanders, or other rescuers on the patient run report. If the AED has a tape recorder built in, the EMT should remove the tape immediately and place it with the patient run report for review by the medical director.

Maintenance of the AED

Each AED manufacturer has recommended inspection and maintenance procedures to ensure the constant state of readiness for their device. EMTs who are trained and allowed to use the device should familiarize themselves with their machine's recommended procedures and ensure that they are completed and documented. Figure 16.7 provides an example of a recommended operator skills checklist for use of the AED. One of the most important maintenance items for the AED is to ensure that the batteries are up-to-date and fully charged to ensure optimal device function.

Maintaining AED Skills

Although the advent of the AED and its use by lay rescuers and EMTs has proven to be a major step forward in the care of the cardiac patient, it is not used on a regular basis by most rescuers. Because the proper and safe use of the device requires both cognitive and psychomotor skills, it is imperative that all EMTs who are authorized to use the AED participate in regular skill maintenance

Automated Defibrillators: Operator's Shift Checklist

Date _____ Shift _____ Location _____

Mfr/Model No. _____ Serial No. or Facility ID No. _____

At the beginning of each shift, inspect the unit. Indicate whether all requirements have been met. Note any corrective actions taken. Sign the form.

	OK as Found	Corrective Action/ Remarks
1. Defibrillator Unit Clean, no spills, clear of objects on top, casing intact		
2. Cables/Connectors a. Inspect for cracks, broken wire, or damage b. Connectors engage securely and are not damaged*		
3. Supplies a. Two sets of pads in sealed packages, within expiration date* b. Hand towel c. Scissors d. Razor e. Alcohol wipes* f. Monitoring electrodes* g. Spare charged battery* h. Adequate ECG paper* i. Manual override module, key, or card* j. Cassette tape, memory module, and/or event card plus spares*		

4. Power Supply
a. Battery-powered units
  (1) Verify fully charged battery in place
  (2) Spare charged battery available
  (3) Follow appropriate battery rotation schedule per manufacturer's recommendations
b. AC/battery backup units
  (1) Plugged into live outlet to maintain battery charge
  (2) Test on battery power and reconnect to line power		

5. Indicators*/ECG Display a. Remove cassette tape, memory module, and/or event card* b. Power-on display c. Self-test OK d. Monitor display functional* e. "Service" message display off* f. Battery charging; low battery light off* g. Correct time displayed; set with dispatch center		
6. ECG Recorder* a. Adequate ECG paper b. Recorder prints		
7. Charge/Display Cycle a. Disconnect AC plug – battery backup units* b. Attach to simulator c. Detects, charges, and delivers shock for VF d. Responds correctly to nonshockable rhythms e. Manual override functional* f. Detach from simulator g. Replace cassette tape, module, and/or memory card *		
8. Pacemaker* a. Pacer output cable intact b. Pacer pads present (set of two) c. Inspect per manufacturer's operational guidelines		
Major Problem(s) Identified (Out of Service)		

*Applicable only if the unit has this supply or capability

Signature _____

FIGURE 16.7 Typical AED operator skills checklist.

practice. This ensures that when the EMT needs to use the AED, he will be able to do so without hesitation and in the proper sequence. Current guidelines recommend that skill review and practice be conducted every 90 days.

 Every event in which the AED is used should have medical director review.

The EMT can accomplish these reviews by examining the run report, listening to audio tape recordings made by the device, and having the crew reenact the scene. This type of quality assurance involves all players of the team and promotes optimal use of the device in patient care.

Step-by-Step Procedure

Automated External Defibrillator

1. Ensure scene safety.
2. Initiate body substance isolation.
3. Establish unresponsiveness with shake and shout.
4. Open airway and determine breathlessness.
5. Using BVM or one-way valve face mask, give two quick breaths with high concentration of oxygen.
6. Feel for carotid pulse and determine pulselessness (see Step 6).
7. Initiate CPR.
8. Turn defibrillator on (see Step 8).
9. Attach automated defibrillator pads to patient with pads in correct position (see Step 9).
10. Rescuer directs to stop CPR and ensures that no one is touching patient (see Step 10).

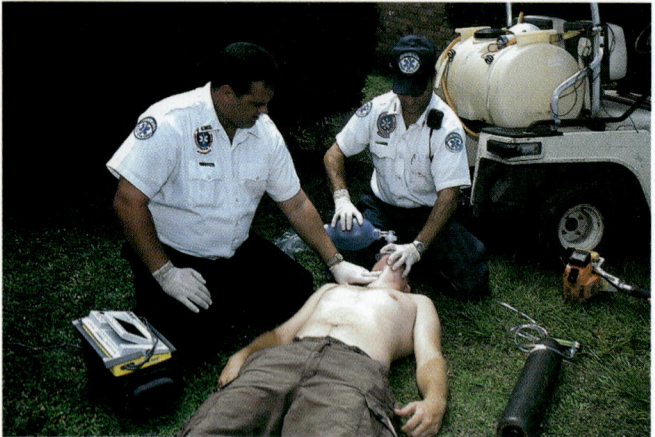
Step 6

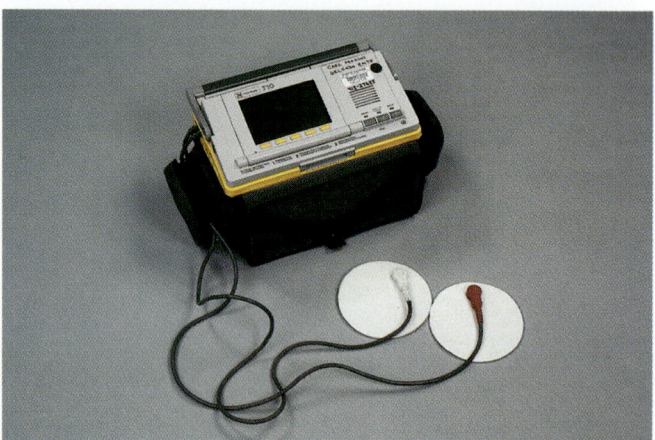
Step 8

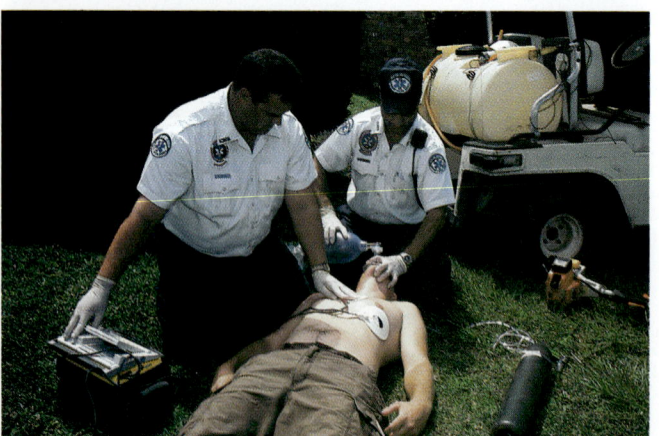
Step 9

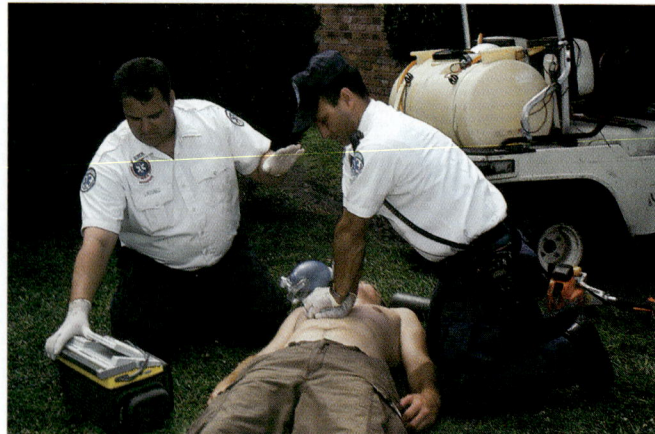
Step 10

continued

Automated External Defibrillator (cont'd)

11. Depress ANALYSIS button on the AED so the machine can analyze rhythm.
12. If shock is advised the rescuer yells, "CLEAR", and the partners response should be "CLEAR" and ensures no one is touching patient (see Step 12).
13. Depress the SHOCK button if so indicated by machine (see Step 13).
14. Deliver three successive shocks if so indicated by the AED while ensuring that no patient contact exists.
15. Check for pulselessness and breathlessness.
16. If no pulse or breathing exists, insert nasal or oral airway and resume CPR.
17. Ensure that CPR is done effectively by checking carotid pulsation and effective breaths by ensuring rise and fall of the chest (see Step 17).
18. Gather information of events from family or bystanders.
19. Repeat defibrillator sequence as necessary (see Step 19).

NOTE: In a moving vehicle the AED motion sensor may prohibit the AED from recognizing a rhythm.

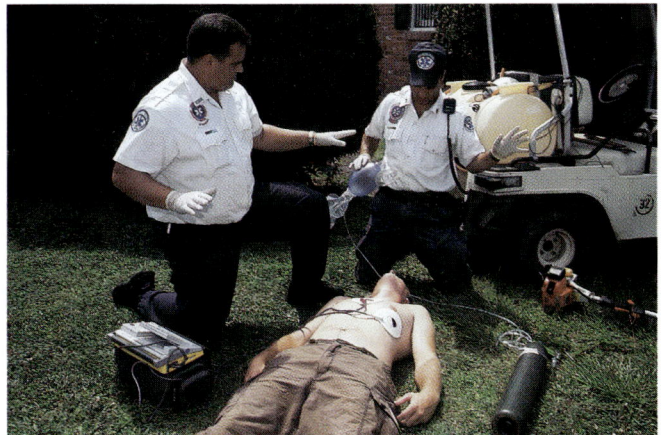

Step 12

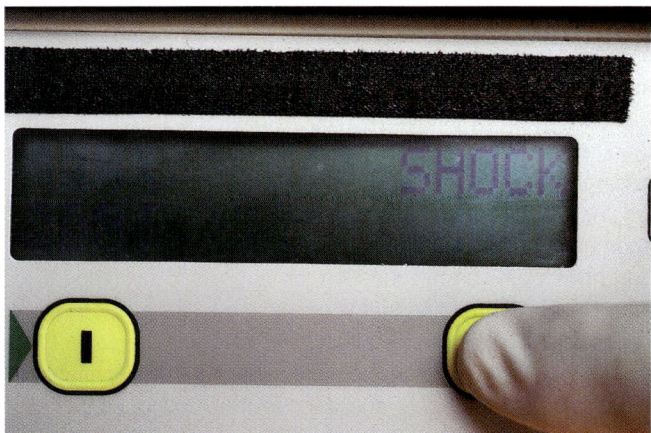

Step 13

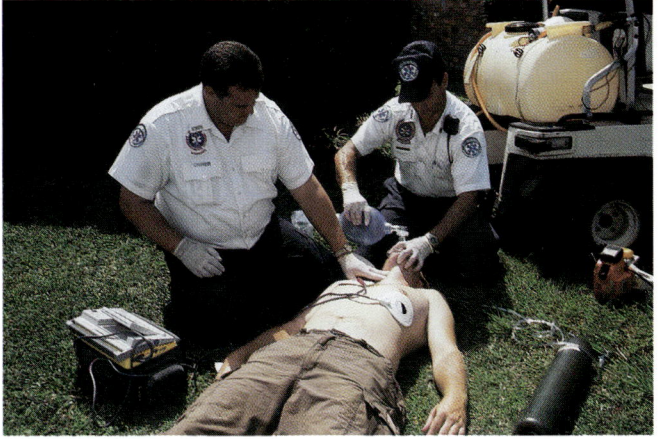

Step 17

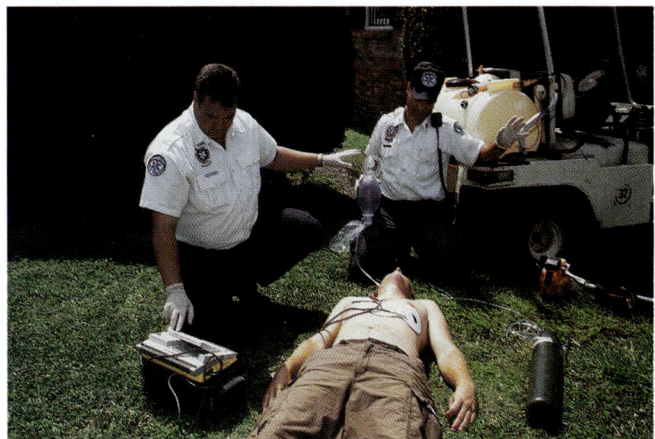

Step 19

Summary

- Restoration of cardiac output is the only method of definitive care of the cardiac patient in the field.
- Automated defibrillation is a simple and effective method of restoration of cardiac output and rhythm.
- CPR is only a holding pattern until normal cardiac output can be reestablished.
- AED can be used by personnel with minimal cardiac training without the assistance of drugs.
- Many lives can be saved with the use of AED and assisted ventilation with a high concentration of oxygen (FiO_2) during the prehospital period.

Scenario Solution

As you and your partner enter the scene, you observe two first responders who have assumed CPR and are using a bag-valve-mask (BVM) with supplemental oxygen. You should ensure that adequate room is available to work on the patient. If inadequate space is found, you must immediately stop the resuscitation effort long enough to get the patient moved and then resume CPR. Additionally, if there are any safety issues present, these must be dealt with before using the AED.

As you confirm that the patient is pulseless and without spontaneous ventilations, prepare the AED for its second use and have your partner question the family and bystanders for any relevant information that you may need. This includes pertinent medical history, medications, and how long the patient has been down. You should connect the pads to the AED patient cable or connect the cable and pads to the AED, depending on your particular device. Turn the AED on and listen for voice prompts. Ensure that CPR has been stopped when you activate the device and that no one is touching the patient.

Follow the voice prompts given by the AED. While the device is assessing the patient and delivering treatment, you, as the team leader, should be thinking ahead to your next sequence of events. This includes 1 minute of CPR after the third shock, evaluation of pulses and ventilations if prompted by the device, and whether you want to load the patient for transportation to an appropriate facility or ALS intercept or remain at the scene.

After analyzing the patient's rhythm and determining that it is ventricular fibrillation, the AED delivers two successive shocks. After the second shock has been delivered, the machine advises to "check breathing and pulse." Assessment reveals a weak, regular pulse at the carotid artery. The rate is approximately 110 beats/min. The patient is attempting to breathe on his own, but the depth and rate are inadequate. The partner begins assisted ventilations with a BVM and supplemental oxygen.

As you prepare the patient for transportation, his pulse becomes stronger and is now present at the radius with a rate of 92 beats/min. His ventilations are now 18 per minute and regular as you switch to a nonrebreather mask, which delivers oxygen of at least 0.85. His oxygen saturation is at 96%, his color is good, and he is warm to the touch. He is beginning to move his lips and hands as his wife kisses him while being loaded into your vehicle for transportation.

Because bystander CPR was initiated immediately on the patient, first responders were on the scene in less than 2 minutes to continue BLS with supplemental oxygen, your response time was under 5 minutes, and you had an AED available for immediate use, your patient was given all the opportunities for survival.

Key Terms

Advanced life support Care provided to patients using drugs or for advanced invasive airway procedures using cardiac monitor defibrillators designed to stabilize or restore normal functioning within the body. These skills are generally reserved for prehospital care providers trained above the EMT-Basic level.

Atherosclerosis Form of arteriosclerosis in which deposits of yellowish plaques containing cholesterol and lipid materials become deposited within the intima and media layers of arteries, generally resulting in decreased blood supply

Automated external defibrillator Device that uses computer technology to automatically interpret a patient's electrical heart rhythm and can also deliver a defibrillatory shock when indicated.

Cardioversion Restoration of normal cardiac function and rhythm to the heart using electrical energy.

Defibrillation Use of electroshock to terminate ventricular fibrillation.

EMT-Defibrillation Use of a defibrillator by EMT's trained at the basic level to treat patient's who are in cardiac arrest with ventricular fibrillation.

Key Terms (cont'd)

Medical command authority Base station physician to which the EMT can communicate by telephone or radio for directions in delivery of patient care.

Myocardial infarction Death to a portion of the heart muscle caused by interruption of normal blood supply and oxygen. May be caused by a thrombosis, coronary artery spasm, or emboli.

Pacing Regulation of the rate of contraction of the heart muscle by use of an artificial cardiac pacemaker. These devices can be external or internal.

Permanent vegetative state Condition in which the human body no longer exists in a conscious state. This condition is caused by massive trauma to the brain or by extended periods of anoxia to brain tissue, resulting in no conscious activity within the nervous system.

Ventricular fibrillation Dysryhthmia caused by fibrillatory contractions of ventricular muscle due to rapid repetitive excitation of myocardial fibers without coordinated contraction of the ventricle.

Review Questions

1. The automated external defibrillator is designed to be used by the EMT-Basic in the treatment of certain cardiac patients. Which of the following patients fits into this category of use:
   a. Unconcious patient with a pulse and needs monitoring
   b. Unconscious patient without a pulse and is not breathing
   c. Concious patient who is experiencing severe head pain
   d. Concious patient with chest pain and needs monitoring

2. The design of the automated external defibrillator (AED) is such that individuals can learn to operate it safely in a relatively short period of time. There are two types of AEDs that have been specifically built for this purpose. Which statement best describes the operation of the AED?
   a. "The AED operator must set all parameters for the machine to operate before initiating its use."
   b. "The AED operator must be able to interpret the patient's ECG to determine if the device should be activated."
   c. "The AED operator must reset the correct energy setting between each shock delivered by the device."
   d. "The AED operator need only be able to turn the device on and off and manually discharge the energy if the device is semiautomatic."

3. Early defibrillation has been identified as a key component of the chain of survival. Which statement best describes the rationale for early defibrillation training?
   a. Defibrillation is the first step to a successful resuscitation of all patients who are in cardiac arrest.
   b. Defibrillation is the only intervention to a successful resuscitation of a patient who is in cardiac arrest.
   c. Early defibrillation significantly increases the chances of survival for a patient in cardiac arrest.
   d. The training of personnel in early defibrillation has proven to be so effective that all patients who are unconscious and unresponsive should receive this life-saving procedure.

4. Evaluation of training programs for the use of AEDs has demonstrated that it is primarily a psychomotor (hands-on) type skill and as such regular review sessions should be held. Current standards suggest that all providers who use the AED should be involved with review training a minimum of every _____ days.
   a. 60
   b. 90
   c. 120
   d. 80

5. Criteria and treatment guidelines for the use of the AED have been developed to ensure safe and quick use of the device. Which statement best describes the rationale for having voice commands incorporated into the device?
   a. Because the AED is used so rarely by the EMT-Basic, the voice commands are necessary to ensure correct use.
   b. Voice commands are incorporated into the AED so that all individuals present at a resuscitation will know what is occurring.
   c. Voice commands of the AED are recorded on the internal computer to ensure correct use and functioning of the device.
   d. Voice commands serve as a backup for the device operator to assist in the application and use of the device.

Review Questions (cont'd)

6. The first step in the use of the AED is to confirm that the patient is unconscious and unresponsive. Once the EMT has confirmed that the patient is in cardiac arrest, what is the next step for the operator of the device?
   a. Turn on the AED and wait for a voice prompt to continue.
   b. Bare the patient's chest for electrode application.
   c. Call for ALS intercept, if available, to assist in care of the patient.
   d. Perform 1 minute of CPR before attaching electrode pads to patient.

Answers to these Review Questions can be found at the end of the book on page 866.

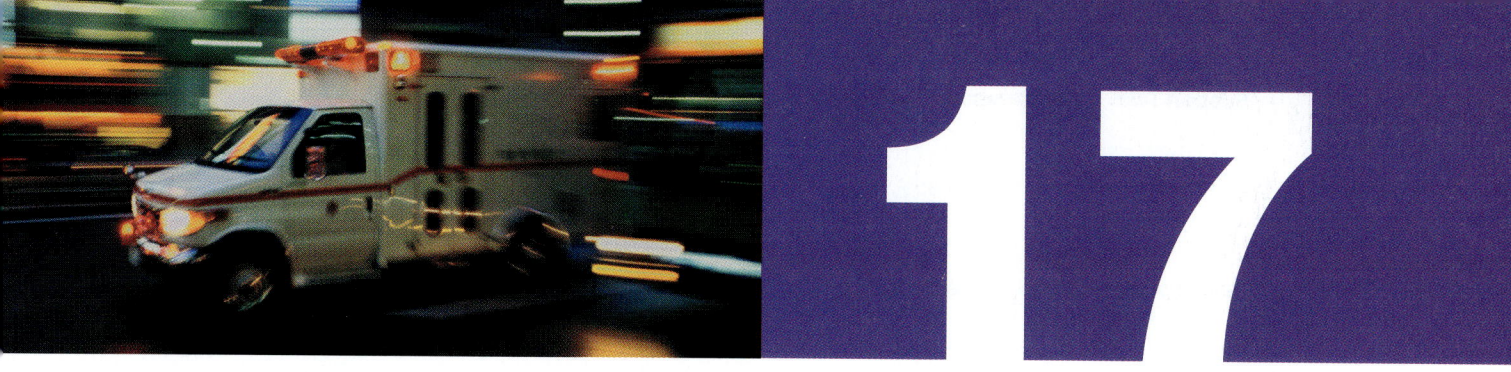

17

Altered Mental Status

Lesson Goal

The goal of this chapter is to help the EMT-Basic understand the causes of altered mental states so that he or she can assess and treat these patients quickly and appropriately.

Scenario

You are called to the scene of a "man down." You arrive to find a well-dressed man on a park bench, and bystanders tell you that he is unresponsive. He appears to be breathing, and there are no clues at the scene as to whether he has been injured.

As you approach the patient, another man runs up and tells you that he was the one that called the ambulance. He tells you that the man was talking to him when his speech suddenly became slurred. He also states that the patient complained of being tired but did not seem to be having any other difficulties.

The patient responds when you grasp his shoulder, his airway is open, and he is breathing without difficulty. His radial pulse is strong and regular, although maybe a little fast. His skin is cool, moist, and pale. He is trying to talk to you, but his speech is slurred and difficult to understand.

 How would you approach this man? How would you begin your assessment? What types of injuries or conditions can cause this presentation? What else would you look for? Can you do anything for him now?

Key Terms to Know

Cushing's triad
Diabetes
Epilepsy
Glasgow Coma Scale
Glucagon
Glucose
Glycogen
Grand mal
Hemiparesis
Hemiplegia
Hyperglycemia
Hypoglycemia
Insulin
Insulin-dependent diabetes mellitus
Ischemia
Islets of Langerhans
Kussmaul's respirations (air hunger)
Non–insulin-dependent diabetes mellitus
Oral hypoglycemics
Pancreas
Paralysis
Parasthesia
Petit mal
Polyuria
Postictal state
Status epilepticus
Tonic-clonic
Transient ischemic attack (TIA)

323

Learning Objectives

As an EMT-Basic, you should be able to do the following:

DOT

- Identify the patient taking diabetic medications with altered mental status and the implications of a diabetes history.
- State the steps in the emergency medical care of the patient taking diabetic medicine with an altered mental status and a history of diabetes.
- Establish the relationship between airway management and the history of diabetes.
- State the generic and trade names, medication forms, dose, administration, action, and contraindications of oral glucose.
- Evaluate the need for medical direction in the emergency medical care of a diabetic patient.

Supplemental

- Describe the different levels of altered mental status.

- Describe and differentiate among the following possible causes for altered mental status:
    - Neurologic (stroke, seizure, organic brain syndrome, Alzheimer's disease)
    - Toxicologic (drug or alcohol induced)
    - Traumatic (injury)
    - Hypoxia (impaired respirations or circulation)
    - Metabolic or organic (diabetes)
- Demonstrate the assessment and documentation process of patients with altered mental status.
- Identify the appropriate prehospital management of patients with altered mental status.
- Identify specific prehospital management appropriate for patients with diabetes.
- Identify medications that reveal important history regarding patients with altered mental status.
- Identify special safety concerns for the patient and rescuer when working with patients with altered mental status.

The hardest patient for which to care is the patient who does not tell the emergency medical technician (EMT) what he or she needs. If the patient is unconscious or responding inappropriately, it is difficult for the EMT to determine what is happening and what the patient needs.

However, the situation usually provides clues. If the EMT is thorough in his or her assessments and understands the causes of altered mental status, he or she can assess and treat these patients quickly and appropriately.

Causes of Altered Mental Status

Altered mental status can be a result of many or even multiple causes. The most obvious cause is head injury, but metabolic causes are another common cause of altered mental status.

Diabetes

The most common metabolic cause of altered mental status is **diabetes**. More than 10 million Americans are affected by diabetes, many of whom may be unaware of their disease. In the diabetic patient, metabolic problems prevent the body from using sugar properly. This is important because sugar is the body's primary fuel. The sugar that the body uses is called **glucose**. The digestive system breaks down the complex sugars in food into glucose so that it can be absorbed into the body's cells. Glucose cannot get across the cell membrane and into the cell unless it is accompanied by the hormone insulin. **Insulin** is secreted by the pancreas in amounts appropriate to the needs of the body and the amount of glucose to be transported into the cells.

In diabetic patients, the level of glucose in the body's cells is low because of either low circulating glucose levels or ineffective action of existing insulin. Either of these conditions will lead to abnormally high levels of circulating glucose in the blood. Insufficient circulating glucose will produce low cellular glucose, which stimulates more glucose production by the liver. Insufficient insulin to transport glucose produces low cellular glucose levels, which also stimulates more glucose production by the liver.

Diabetic patients can present with emergencies related to either high or low blood glucose levels. High blood glucose levels can damage cells and upset normal body functions as the body attempts to compensate for the impaired membrane transfer of glucose. When diabetes is treated, medications are given to improve movement of circulating glucose into cells. If too much medication is given or not enough food is eaten, the blood glucose level may drop to abnormally low levels. To function appropriately, all cells in the body must have a supply of oxygen and fuel to create energy. Most cells in the body can use other fuels such as fats or proteins, but brain cells are unique because they can only use glucose. For this reason a patient with a low blood glucose level has dysfunctioning brain cells. Clini-

Patient Care Algorithm

Altered Mental Status Patient Assessment

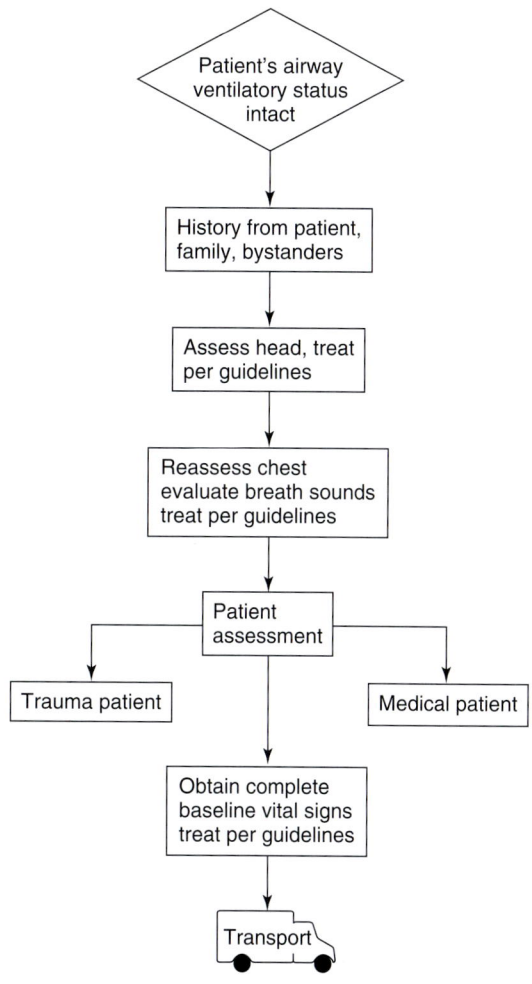

cally this dysfunction may result in lethargy, confusion, combativeness, or coma.

The normal blood glucose level is 80 to 120 mg/dl. High blood glucose is known as **hyperglycemia**, and low blood glucose is known as **hypoglycemia**.

The EMT can start treatment of low blood glucose in the field. High blood glucose must be treated in the hospital, and the primary intervention by the EMT involves appropriate assessment and transportation.

Anatomy and Physiology

Glucose metabolism. All cells of the body use sugar (glucose) and oxygen as fuel for energy. Glucose is primarily acquired from the digestion of carbohydrates, which include starches and complex sugars. Starches and complex sugars must be converted to the simple sugar glucose before being absorbed into cells. When no immediate source of glucose is available from recent ingestion of carbohydrates (as in fasting), the body has two alternate sources of glucose. The first is the breakdown of **glycogen**, a storage form of carbohydrate contained in the liver. The

> ✓ Diabetes is a disease resulting from problems with the metabolism of glucose. Problems can result from glucose levels that are abnormally high (hyperglycemia) or low (hypoglycemia).

second is the breakdown of protein by **glucagon** in the liver to glucose and a series of acids known as *ketone bodies*.

Insulin. For the glucose to pass from the blood stream into the cell, a hormone called *insulin* is needed. Insulin is made in special cells in the **pancreas** called *beta cells*. The beta cells are contained in clusters, called the **islets of Langerhans**, in the pancreatic tissue. These islets were first described by a German pathologist Paul Langerhans in the late 1800s. The pancreas also makes digestive enzymes that are secreted through the pancreatic duct into the intestine. Insulin is secreted directly into the blood stream.

Classifications of Diabetes

Diabetic patients may not make enough insulin or may have cells that do not respond to the insulin that is available. These two circumstances are called, respectively, Type I or **insulin-dependent diabetes mellitus** (IDDM), and Type II or **non–insulin-dependent diabetes mellitus** (NIDDM). Patients with IDDM usually require insulin treatment. The onset of IDDM usually occurs in adolescence or early adulthood, although some patients may be very young. The cause of IDDM in many patients is the result of a virus that damages the pancreas, leading to a lack of adequate insulin production. NIDDM is more common in older patients and is frequently associated with obesity. Obesity causes increased resistance to the action of insulin on the cell membrane.

> 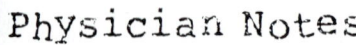 **Physician Notes**
>
> A history of increased frequency of urination often is difficult to assess. Asking if the patient is waking up several times during the night to urinate when he or she previously did not have to may be a better indicator of polyuria.

Because of the limited ability of cells to use glucose in diabetes, blood glucose levels are frequently elevated. When blood glucose exceeds 200 mg/dl, the excess is excreted by the kidney, producing more urine. This loss of glucose and water leads to the classic triad of diabetic symptoms: increased urination (**polyuria**), increased thirst to replace the water lost in urine, and increased hunger and calorie intake to replace the glucose calories lost in urine.

Pathophysiology

Metabolic effects of diabetes. Most of the effects of diabetes can be attributed to the effects of low insulin levels. These effects include the following:

1. *Increased blood glucose levels.* Hyperglycemia is toxic to cells, particularly nerve cells and vascular (blood vessel) cells.
2. *Increased fat use.* In the short term, increased fat use causes acid buildup in the bloodstream because fat breakdown products are acidic. In the long term, this acid buildup may accelerate atherosclerosis, or hardening of the arteries.
3. *Increased protein use.* Increased protein use may lead to tissue and muscle wasting and poor healing of injuries.

Major Types of Diabetic Emergencies

Three major types of emergencies are specific to patients with diabetes: (1) diabetic ketoacidosis, (2) nonketotic hyperosmolar syndrome, and (3) hypoglycemia.

Diabetic ketoacidosis. In diabetic ketoacidosis (DKA), cells fail to metabolize glucose. DKA may be caused by lack of adequate insulin, as in known diabetic patients who stop taking medication. DKA also may be the presenting problem of a previously undiagnosed diabetic patient. However, DKA most commonly is seen in known diabetic patients who develop an increased need for insulin to respond to an infection or significant stress.

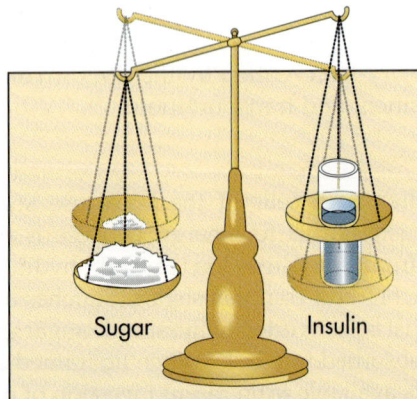

HYPERGLYCEMIA/HYPOGLYCEMIA	
Nausea and vomiting or hunger	Frequent urination
Abdominal pain	Weakness, incoordination
Cold, clammy skin	Headache, drowsiness, seizures
Weak, rapid pulse	Normal, elevated or low blood pressure
Normal or rapid breathing	Confusion, coma, appearance of intoxication
Intense thirst, acetone breath	Altered consciousness

FIGURE 17.1 Signs and symptoms of hyperglycemia and hypoglycemia.

Because the cells are not able to metabolize glucose, the body begins to metabolize fats and protein to provide an energy source for the cells. Using fats and proteins for energy results in the production of ketone bodies, some of which are acidic and lead to acidosis. Another ketone body is acetone, which may cause the patient to have a fruity odor on the breath. The blood glucose level is usually moderately elevated, causing diuresis (loss of body water) and dehydration. Severe dehydration can lead to decreased tissue perfusion, decreased oxygen delivery to the tissue, and shock.

Nonketotic hyperosmolar syndrome. In nonketotic hyperosmolar syndrome (NKHS), insulin is low but not completely absent. The fat and protein breakdown that characterizes DKA does not occur or occurs to a much lesser extent. Nevertheless, these patients may become very dehydrated and may be hyperglycemic, with extremely high blood glucose levels of 1000 mg/dl or higher. NKHS is more common in older adults and NIDDM patients. These patients will present with altered mental status as s result of the extreme hyperglycemia (Figure 17.1).

Hypoglycemia. Paradoxically, hypoglycemia, or low blood glucose, may occur in diabetic patients, usually as a result of treatment with insulin or **oral hypoglycemics**. Frequently, a missed meal or increased caloric need, as in illness or extraordinary exercise, leads to hypoglycemia. Low blood glucose results in altered mental status because neurons (brain cells) need glucose as fuel. Prolonged lack of fuel to neurons can result in seizures or brain damage (see Figure 17.1).

> ✓ Diabetic emergencies can be related to hypoglycemia or hyperglycemia. Hyperglycemia can result in dehydration and a buildup of acid in the blood. Hypoglycemia, which is most often a complication of the treatment of diabetes, deprives the brain of fuel, leading to changes in the patient's mental state.

Management of Patients with Diabetes

Prehospital management of diabetic problems is generally directed at the management of altered mental status and, if possible, replacement of fluid to correct dehydration. The management of altered mental status must include meticulous attention to airway. If the patient is cool, pale, or tachycardic, the EMT should provide supplemental oxygen. If the airway is patent and breathing is adequate, the EMT should assess the patient's ability to swallow safely. Patients who are not effectively swallowing their saliva (drooling) generally should not be given anything by mouth. Patients who are responsive and only mildly lethargic or confused may be given some glucose-containing food; juice with added sugar is a standard choice. Small quantities of granulated sugar or commercially available high-glucose gels (Insta-glucose, Glutose) in the mouth may be sufficient to restore the patient to a normal level of consciousness (LOC). Once the patient's LOC has improved, the patient will be able to safely ingest larger amounts of sugar-containing liquids or solids (Figure 17.2).

In the unresponsive patient or the patient who is assessed to be at risk for aspiration, the EMT should give nothing by mouth. In those systems in which EMT-Bs are permitted to initiate intravenous (IV) lines, a standard IV with a 5% glucose-containing solution may provide enough glucose to the brain cells to rouse the patient. However, this will likely require an order from medical direction. In systems that have a tiered response and a paramedic-level provider available, a patient with altered mental status and a history of diabetes should prompt an advanced life support (ALS) response because IV glucose can immediately resolve hypoglycemia and limit potential damage to brain cells.

Because many other reasons for altered mental status exist besides hypoglycemia, including hyperglycemia, concerns arise about giving glucose without a blood glucose test. In circumstances in which no blood glucose test is available, a small additional rise in hyperglycemia is much less dangerous than continued hypoglycemia. Therefore treating any diabetic patient who has altered mental status by administering sugar is appropriate.

Neurologic Causes of Altered Mental Status

Strokes

Strokes, or cerebral vascular accidents (CVAs), can affect any part of the brain and are caused by a disruption of the blood supply to the affected area of the brain. They are also called *brain attacks* because of the similarity to the causes of heart attacks. Much like heart attacks, atherosclorotic disease contributes to the potential for strokes. The interruption of blood supply to brain tissue causes **ischemia**, which will cause infarction or death of brain cells if unrelieved. Strokes present with signs and symptoms relative to the specific part and amount of the brain involved. The patient may present with an altered LOC and or **paralysis, parasthesia, hemiparesis, or hemiplegia**. The EMT should keep in mind that the left side of the brain controls the right side of the body and the right side of the brain controls the left side of the body. This means that paralysis of the left side implies damage to the right side of the brain and vice versa. The patients condition can progressively worsen but typically will stabilize within 72 hours.

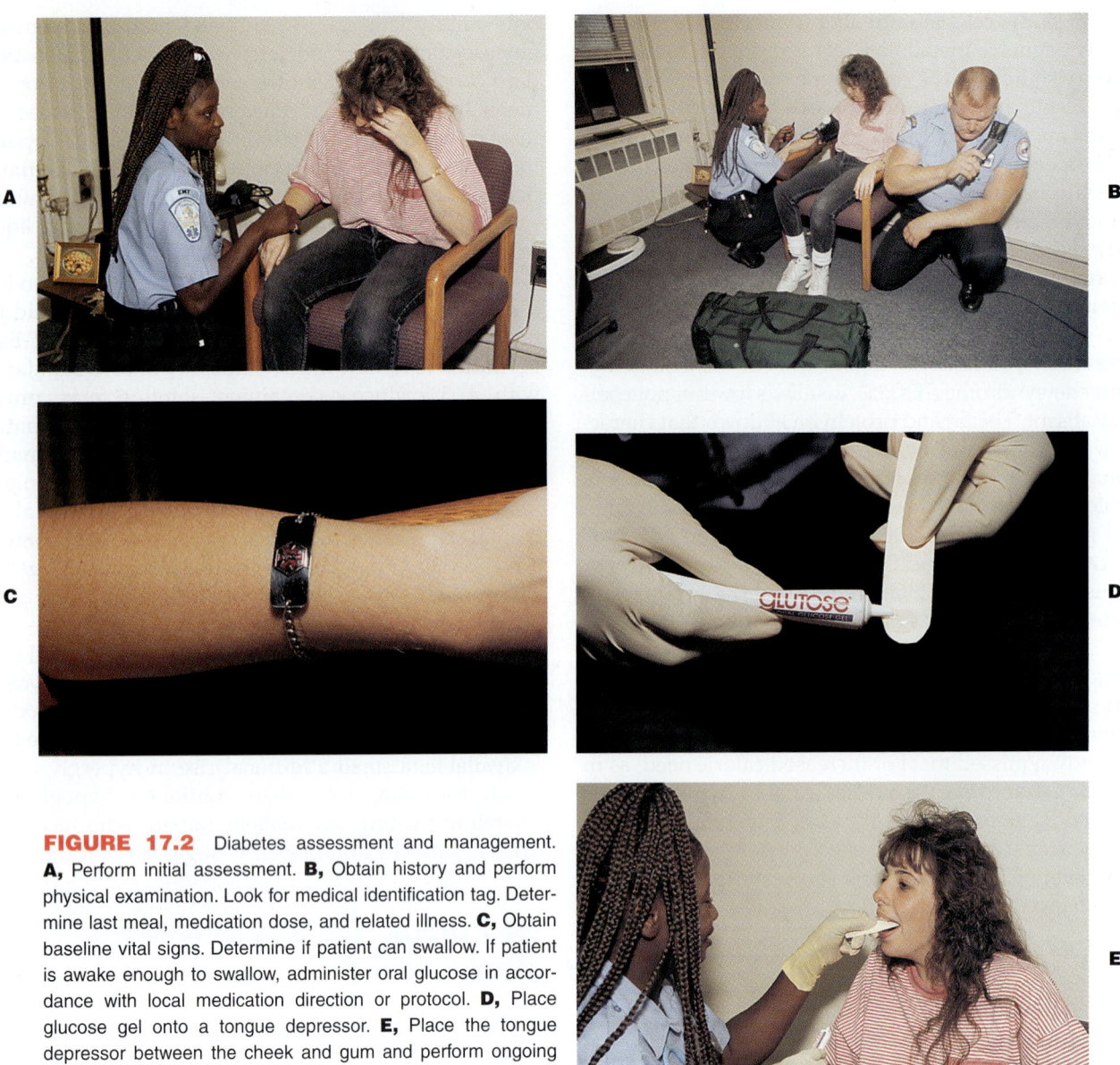

FIGURE 17.2 Diabetes assessment and management. **A,** Perform initial assessment. **B,** Obtain history and perform physical examination. Look for medical identification tag. Determine last meal, medication dose, and related illness. **C,** Obtain baseline vital signs. Determine if patient can swallow. If patient is awake enough to swallow, administer oral glucose in accordance with local medication direction or protocol. **D,** Place glucose gel onto a tongue depressor. **E,** Place the tongue depressor between the cheek and gum and perform ongoing assessment.

The most common cause of stroke is the occlusion of a blood vessel leading to the brain by either a clot that forms within the cerebral blood vessel (thrombus) or a clot that forms elsewhere in the body and travels to the brain (embolus). In either case, the blood flow is cut off and the cells become ischemic and infarct (die). Often patients or their families describe a gradual progression of signs and symptoms as the clot slowly builds up in a blood vessel in the brain.

Another cause of stroke is hemorrhage, which is caused by the rupture of a cerebral artery. This rupture deprives brain cells of oxygenated blood, and accumulating blood forms a hematoma, which compresses the brain and causes more damage. If this bleeding continues without intervention, this condition can be rapidly fatal. Hemorrhagic strokes most commonly are caused by hypertension. Because of the nature of hemorrhagic strokes, the onset and progression of signs and symptoms can be sudden. Unlike the thrombotic strokes, strokes caused by emboli can be abrupt as the clot moves, suddenly blocking a vessel in the brain.

Patients may also experience a **transient ischemic attack (TIA).** These patients have strokelike signs and symptoms. These are temporary because the occlusion of the vessel is incomplete and still allows blood flow to the irritated brain. This is similar to heart patients who have angina pain. The disease narrows the vessel, but there is no cell death since blood still makes it through.

Seizures

Seizures (convulsions) are another cause of altered mental status originating in the brain. Seizure activity occurs when diabetes, fever, infection, hypoxia, or injury interferes with the normal electrical activity in the brain. Seizures can also be caused by compression of brain tissue by a tumor. Irregular, random discharges of electricity in the brain trigger the seizure activity in the part of the body that corresponds with the area of the brain involved. Acute seizure activity may be a one-time response to a specific illness or injury involving the brain. Chronic seizure activity is a pattern of seizure activity that needs to be controlled by medication. **Epilepsy** is a form of chronic seizure activity that is easily controlled by medication.

The most common cause of seizures in children is fever. These are called *febrile seizures*. Seizure activity is generally controlled once the fever is reduced.

Seizure activity can range from staring blankly into space to convulsive uncontrollable muscle twitching through the entire body. This activity is relative to the area and amount of the brain involved. Patients may describe an aura or a sensation of light, smell color, or experience warmth before the onset of the seizure activity.

Generalized seizures.
Generalized seizures include **tonic-clonic**, or **grand mal** seizures, and petit mal seizures. Tonic-clonic seizures may or may not be preceded by an aura and are typified by uncontrolled muscle movement over the entire body. The muscles become rigid during the tonic phase for about 30 seconds before the uncontrolled contractions of the clonic phase begin. This usually lasts for 2 minutes or less. If the seizures last for more than 3 to 5 minutes or the patient experiences multiple seizures without waking up between them, **status epilepticus** results.

Petit mal seizures usually last only a few seconds and can be easily missed. The patient may only stare blankly into space, and there is likely no muscle contraction evident. Children can have several a day and appear to be daydreaming. Petit mal seizures are also known as absence seizures.

Partial seizures.
Partial seizures are described as being simple or complex. Simple seizures are just that. If the EMT looks at the area involved, it is simple for him or her to determine that the area of the brain involved is the part that controls the seizure activity found. For example, a spasm in the right arm traces back to an area on the left side of the brain. Complex seizure activity is, as the name implies, complex. The patient may be wandering around muttering or acting impaired, a more complex set of symptoms than in simple seizure activity. The patient may also stare into space as in petit mal or absence seizures.

After the seizure.
When seizure activity ends, patients typically entire a **postictal state**. This is a rest state in which the patient may appear to be awake but responds only to painful stimuli. The postictal state usually lasts between 5 and 30 minutes and is a "recovery period" for the brain. The EMT should be prepared to lend emotional support to these patients as they come out of this state because they may be confused and embarrassed.

Management of seizure patients.
The first rule in treating seizure patients is "protect, do not restrain." The EMT needs to get everything out of the patient's way to prevent further injury but avoid rigid restraints that may cause injury. The EMT should loosen all restrictive clothing and position the patient in the recovery position (on the side), which will help keep the airway clear.

Although the EMT should be concerned about the patients airway, he or she should not put anything into the seizure patient's mouth. "Bite sticks" and oral airways are contraindicated because they may cause harm or occlude the airway.

If the patient is in status epilepticus or still seizing when the EMT arrives, he or she should protect the patient and hold an oxygen mask near his or her face to prevent the patient from becoming hypoxic.

Organic Brain Syndrome

The organs of the human body lose about 1% of their ability to function with each year of aging. The brain is no exception. Aging and disease can take their toll on the brain and may result in altered mental status. Patients may present with delirium or dementia. Delirium is an abrupt disorientation for time and place, usually with illusions and hallucinations. The mind wanders, speech may be incoherent, and the patient is in a state of mental confusion and excitement. Dementia is slow, progressive loss of awareness of time and place, usually with inability to learn new things or remember recent events. The person may be lost in a time years before the present and remote memories may be intact. Total loss of function and a regression to an infantile state may result. Dementia is often referred to as *senility*.

Organic brain syndrome is a large group of acute and chronic mental disorders with associated brain damage or impaired cerebral function. One such disorder is Alzheimer's disease, a chronic, organic mental disorder caused by atrophy of the frontal and occipital lobes of the brain. It involves progressive, irreversible loss of memory, deterioration of intellectual functions, apathy, speech and gait disturbances, and disorientation. The EMT must take special effort to lend emotional support to and make a thorough assessment of patients with Alzheimer's disease.

Toxicologic Causes of Altered Mental Status

Drugs and alcohol can cause altered mental status. The changes can include unresponsiveness, nervousness, agitation, or hyperactivity. Narcotics cause CNS depression, respiratory depression, and constricted pupils. Cocaine, amphetamines or methamphetamines, which are stimulants, can cause nervousness, agitation, and hyperactivity. Hallucinogens, such as lysergic acid diethylamide (LSD) or phencyclidine hydrochloride (PCP), can cause delusions and alterations of self-awareness, mood, and thought. See Chapter 19 for further information on drug abuse.

Patients who have disease or injury to their renal system (kidneys and liver) may have altered mental status caused by accumulation of toxins in the blood affecting the brain.

Traumatic Causes of Altered Mental Status

Trauma can cause altered mental status by direct injury to the brain or by hypoxia caused by inadequate respirations or circulation. Direct injury to the head can produce bleeding within the skull, which will compress the brain and cause dysfunction. Multisystems trauma can involve the chest, causing inadequate exchange of oxygen and carbon dioxide, causing hypoxia in brain cells and altered cerebral function. Inadequate circulation caused by blood loss secondary to trauma can prevent the brain from getting adequate oxygenated blood, causing altered mental status.

Hypoxia can also occur in the absence of trauma. Patients with respiratory disease may not be able to exchange oxygen and carbon dioxide well, allowing the brain to become hypoxic. Patients suffering from fluid loss resulting from vomiting and diarrhea may lose enough fluid to cause inadequate circulation and hypoxia. Hypoxia will cause ischemia and ultimately death of brain cells and will result in altered mental status.

Assessment of the Patient with Altered Mental Status

Initial Impression

When called to the scene of a patient with altered mental status, after making sure the scene is safe, the EMT should observe the patient to see how he or she is interacting with the environment. The EMT should look for evidence at the scene that may be a clue as to the cause of the patient's altered mental status (e.g., evidence of medications, trauma, or toxic substances). The EMT forms a general impression of the patient's condition, whether immediate life threats exist, and the level of the patient's distress. As the EMT gets nearer to the patient, he or she can tell if the patient is responsive. A talking patient obviously has an open airway, is breathing, and has circulating blood to the brain.

The EMT can see the patient's skin color, his or her condition, and whether he or she is struggling to breathe. The EMT may or may not be able to determine the chief complaint in a patient with altered mental status depending on his or her level of responsiveness and the appropriateness of those responses. The EMT may have history from dispatch personnel or witnesses about injury, pain, respiratory distress, or circulatory or renal problems that may have brought about the change in the patient's mental state. If none of this is available, the patient's chief complaint is the altered mental status.

AVPU

In assessing the patient with altered mental status, the EMT should note and record the patients' baseline mental status as clearly as possible, making note of anything from the scene that may be a clue as to the cause of this change. The EMT can use the acronym AVPU to determine the patients' responsiveness:

A—Alert (spontaneously responds to the environment)
V—Responds to verbal stimuli
P—Responds only to painful stimuli
U—Unresponsive

ABC

The EMT then needs to assess the patient's ABCs (airway, breathing, and circulation):

- *Airway/C-spine.* If there is a chance that the patient has head and neck injuries, the EMT will have to provide manual immobilization of the C-spine while examining the airway. The EMT must pay special attention to the airway in patients with altered mental status because they may have difficulty maintaining an open airway. Depending on the cause and location of the brain dysfunction, the patient may be unable to swallow or clear secretions. The gag reflex may be impaired. In assessing ABCs, the EMT is in a "find it and fix it mode." While determining the problem in the ABCs, the EMT must treat it as it is identified. If the airway is not clear, the EMT must clear it.

- *Breathing.* The patient's breathing may provide clues to the underlying cause of his or her altered mental status. If **Kussmaul's respirations (air hunger)** are present with acetone odor on the breath, diabetes may be the cause. If the patient exhibits Cheyne-Stokes respirations, he or she may have suffered a head injury or hemorrhage within his or her skull. If the patient has bradypnea, or slow ineffective ventilations, drugs may be involved. If the patient's respirations are ineffective, he or she will be hypoxic, which may well be the cause of or a contributing factor to the altered mental status. Respirations of less than 8 or more than 30 per minute will not allow adequate volumes of air to make proper exchanges of carbon dioxide and oxygen, causing the patient to become hypoxic. The EMT should provide supplementary respirations via mouth-to-mask with 100% oxygen.
- *Circulation.* Evaluating the patient's circulation may reveal more clues to the underlying causes of the patient's altered mental status. Weak or absent radial pulses indicate inadequate circulation, which may cause hypoxia and the patient's altered mental status. Cool diaphoretic skin indicates shock and warm flushed skin indicates fever and possible infection, both of which may be behind the change in the LOC. The EMT should control bleeding as it is discovered. While looking at the skin, the EMT may also notice jaundice (liver disease) or cyanosis, which points to respiratory problems. These also may cause altered mental status.

At the end of the assessment the EMT should determine the patient priority. If the EMT judges the patient to be critical, after providing adequate airway and respirations and hemorrhage control as needed, he or she should begin transportation and continue the assessment and management of the patient en route to the hospital. All patients with altered mental status should be considered priority patients.

Focused History and Physical Examination

By this time the EMT probably already has an idea as to the cause of the patient's altered mental status. The EMT should now focus his or her history taking and physical examination on the patient's complaints and physical presentation thus far.

The EMT should continuously monitor the patient's mental function. At this point the EMT should expand this evaluation to include the patient's orientation to time, person, place, and events. If the patient is well oriented, he or she is "oriented × 4." The EMT should note any deficit in orientation. For example, "the patient is oriented to time, person, and place but cannot describe to me the events that led to us being called to care for him."

Further assessment of mental status can be accomplished by use of the **Glasgow Coma Scale** (Table 17.1). The Glasgow Coma Scale measures eye opening, verbal response, and best motor response as a way of determining the level of the patient's mental status. The measurement serves as a baseline in further evaluations made at the hospital.

The EMT should now make further neurologic assessments. The EMT should determine whether the patient can move his or her fingers and toes and whether there is sensation to all of the extremities. One examination that may show which side of the brain has a deficit is the pronator drift test. If the EMT asks the patient to hold his or her hands out with the palms up, the hand on the side of the deficit will turn over and drift downward. This should be done with the patient's eyes closed.

The EMT should also get a full set of baseline vital signs at this point. This information will provide a baseline for comparison later and may lend more to the

TABLE 17.1 Glasgow Coma Scale

Eye Opening	Points
Opens eyes spontaneously	4
Opens eyes on command	3
Opens eyes to painful stimulus	2
Does not open eyes	1
Best Motor Response	
Following command	6
Localizing painful stimuli	5
Shows withdrawal to pain	4
Responding with abnormal flexion to painful stimuli (decorticate)	3
Responding with abnormal extension to pain (decerebrate)	2
Gives no motor response	1
Best Verbal Response	
Answers appropriately (oriented)	5
Gives confused answers	4
Gives inappropriate response	3
Makes unintelligible noises	2
Makes no verbal response	1
Total	

Note: Lowest possible score = 3; highest possible score = 15.

explanation of the altered mental status. **Cushing's triad**, bradycardia, hypertension, and bizarre respiratory patterns may indicate increase intracranial pressure (ICP). Tachycardia and hypotension infer inadequate circulation as the cause of hypoxia and the resulting altered mental status.

The EMT must gather as complete a history as possible. The patient may not be much help if he or she is severely impaired, but there may be family or written information available. Family members may be able to provide medical history or medications found at the scene that will imply medical history that may have precipitated this event. A good guide for assessing the patient is SAMPLE:

S—*Signs and symptoms.* The patient's breathing patterns and ability or inability to communicate or move contribute to determining the cause of his or her difficulty.

A—*Allergies.* If the patient may have been exposed to a substance to which he or she is allergic, this may be the cause of this event.

M—*Medications.* Alcohol, drugs, and prescription medications may have caused the altered mental status. It is important for the EMT to know if the patient is taking medications as prescribed. Seizure and diabetes medications must be maintained or the patient may present with an altered mental status.

P—*Pertinent medical history.* The patient may have history of similar events or medical conditions that may contribute to this event.

L—*Last oral intake.* This is especially important in the case of the diabetic and is relevant to the potential for airway compromise by emesis.

E—*Events leading up to this moment.* The EMT must get the story on how the patient got to this point. If possible, the EMT should try to determine when the patient last felt well, when and how the altered mental status began, whether he or she had other complaints or sensations before this event, and whether the patient has a recent or remote history of injury.

At this point the EMT should be on the way to the hospital with the patient. The EMT must continue with an ongoing assessment during the transportation. This assessment will show whether the patient is improving or deteriorating.

Summary

- Altered mental status is caused by hypoxia or inadequate perfusion of the brain. This poor perfusion can be caused by trauma, respiratory problems, circulatory problems, birth defects, fever, disease, medications, drugs, or alcohol.
- The patient's best chance at getting the best care depends on adequate assessment and support of vital functions until he or she is delivered to definitive care.
- The EMT may not be able determine the precise cause of the patient's altered mental status.
- The focus of the EMT's effort should be toward supporting the patient's ABCs and providing a good report and documentation to the hospital.

Scenario Solution

At this point you have obtained the following vital signs: heart rate 100 beats/min, ventilatory rate 24 breaths/min, and blood pressure 116/80 mm Hg. The patient responds to your questions, but his responses are difficult to understand and inappropriate. You have administered oxygen at 100% via a nonrebreather mask and you have to encourage him to keep it on. On further examination you find a MedicAlert bracelet. It reads "insulin dependant diabetic." He is able to swallow, so you give him oral glucose by mouth. He becomes increasingly coherent while en route to the hospital. He tells you that he has been under a lot of personal and professional stress and probably has not been regulating his diet and medication as well as he should. Once at the hospital, he receives a meal, and after monitoring and counseling he is discharged.

Key Terms

Cushing's triad Phenomenon seen with increased cranial pressure distinguished by a rise in blood pressure, change in respirations, and decrease in pulse.

Diabetes A metabolic disorder that results from inadequate insulin secretion.

Epilepsy A group of neurologic disorders characterized by recurrent episodes of convulsive seizures, sensory disturbances, unusual behavior, loss of consciousness, or all of these; uncontrolled electrical discharge from the nerve cells of the cerebral cortex.

Glasgow Coma Scale Standardized rating system used to evaluate the degree of consciousness impairment based on eye opening, motor response, and verbal response. Points are scored for the patient's best response in each of the three categories.

Glucagon Hormone secreted by the pancreas that stimulates the breakdown of glycogen and the release of glucose by the liver.

Glucose A simple sugar used by the cell for energy; it is derived from the digestion of complex carbohydrates that are eaten, from the breakdown of glycogen in the liver, or by conversion of protein in the liver.

Glycogen A starch that is the major storage form of glucose; it is stored in the liver and can be broken down to glucose when needed.

Grand mal A generalized full tonic-clonic seizure.

Hemiparesis A partial paralysis that affects only one side of the body.

Hemiplegia A total paralysis that affects only one side of the body.

Hyperglycemia Elevated blood glucose level.

Hypoglycemia Low blood glucose level.

Ischemia Inadequate blood flow to a tissue; can cause anginal pain and/or a myocardial infarction.

Insulin Hormone produced in the pancreas needed for proper metabolism of blood sugar.

Insulin-dependent diabetes mellitus An inability to metabolize carbohydrates (sugar) because of a lack of insulin.

Islets of Langerhans Clusters of cells in the pancreas that produce insulin.

Kussmaul's respirations (air hunger) A deep, rapid breathing rate directly attributed to diabetic ketoacidosis.

Non–insulin-dependent diabetes mellitus A diabetic condition that usually occurs in individuals over 40 years of age and usually can be controlled by diet and oral insulin.

Oral hypoglycemics Medication taken orally that stimulates the pancreas to produce insulin.

Pancreas A gland located in the abdomen that makes digestive enzymes and insulin.

Paralysis Loss of muscle function, sensation, or both.

Parasthesia Any subjective sensation experienced as numbness, tingling, or a "pins and needles" feeling that may be a symptom of hyperventilation or a spinal cord injury.

Petit mal Usually refers to a partial seizure that is seen in children.

Polyuria Frequent urination.

Postictal state Period immediately after a seizure.

Status epilepticus Continuous seizure lasting more than 30 minutes or a seizure in which the patient does not regain consciousness.

Tonic-clonic The rhythmic motion of the body and extremities that occurs with a seizure.

Transient ischemic attack (TIA) A temporary disruption in blood flow to the brain, which results in dizziness, imbalance, and generalized weakness.

Review Questions

1. The organ(s) affected by diabetes is (are) the:
   a. Kidneys
   b. Liver
   c. Pancreas
   d. Spleen
2. The diabetic emergency that is apt to have a rapid onset is:
   a. Hyperglycemia
   b. Hypoglycemia
   c. Nonketotic hyperosmolar syndrome
   d. All of the above
3. Patients suffering from hyperglycemia may present with:
   a. Increased thirst and frequent urination
   b. Fruity or acetone odor to breath
   c. Deep, rapid respirations (Kussmaul's)
   d. All of the above

Review Questions (cont'd)

4. Oral glucose:
   a. Can reverse hypoglycemia but should only be used in patients with an active gag reflex
   b. Should be given to any patient with an altered mental status regardless of the status of the gag reflex
   c. Should only be used after a blood glucose test
   d. Can make hyperglycemic patients worse
5. The EMT's biggest concern in a patient with altered mental status is:
   a. Determining the cause
   b. Circulation
   c. Airway and breathing
   d. Looking for signs of injury
6. The most frequent cause of seizures in children is:
   a. Head injury
   b. Drugs
   c. Fever
   d. Allergies
7. Status epilepticus is:
   a. Any seizure activity
   b. Any seizure activity lasting more than 5 minutes
   c. Any time the patient has multiple seizures without regaining consciousness between them
   d. b and c
8. A patient who is said to be "postictal" is:
   a. Unconscious
   b. Actively seizing
   c. Lying on his or her stomach
   d. In a sleeplike or trancelike state
9. A patient who has suffered a "stroke" on the left side of his brain is most likely to suffer:
   a. Paralysis or weakness on the left side of his body
   b. Paralysis or weakness on the right side of his body
   c. Paralysis or weakness from the waist down
   d. Paralysis or weakness above the waist
10. Patients suffering from increasing intracranial pressure resulting from injury or stroke exhibit a specific group of signs and symptoms called Cushing's triad, which includes:
    a. Increased respiratory rate, increased heart rate, elevated blood pressure.
    b. Decreased respiratory rate, decreased heart rate, lower blood pressure.
    c. Bizarre respiratory patterns, decreased heart rate, elevated blood pressure
    d. Bizarre respiratory patterns, increased heart rate, lower blood pressure

Answers to these Review Questions can be found at the end of the book on page 866.

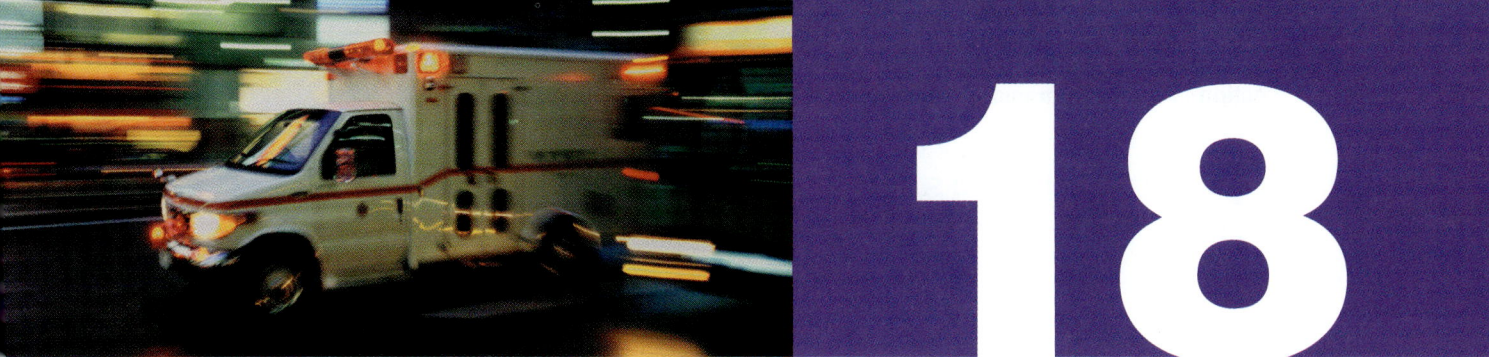

Allergies

Lesson Goal

The goal of this chapter is to familiarize the EMT-Basic with the signs and symptoms of allergic reactions and the body's response. This chapter also explores the role of the immune system.

Scenario

You are called to the scene of a residence for a report of "difficulty breathing." You arrive at a suburban residence where you find a 30-year-old woman lying next to a lawnmower that is still running. A disagreeable buzzing alerts you to angry hornets that are flying about. You secure the scene by turning off the lawnmower and moving the patient a safe distance from the insects.

As you begin your assessment, you note that the patient is having difficulty breathing and you note a "crowing" noise that is worse on inspiration than on expiration. The patient's skin is bright red, and she appears to have facial swelling. Her skin is cool and moist, and her blood pressure is 84/60 mm Hg with a pulse rate of 120 beats per minute. When you attempt to get more medical history, she pushes you away. At that point her husband arrives with her epinephrine and asks for your help in administering it.

 What is your initial impression of the patient? What steps should you take to manage this situation?

Key Terms to Know

Allergic reaction	Antigen	Hives	Vasodilator
Anaphylactic reaction	Epinephrine	Immune system	
Anaphylaxis	Epi-Pen	Stridor	
Antibodies	Histamine	Urticaria	

335

Learning Objectives

As an EMT-Basic, you should be able to do the following:

DOT

- Recognize the patient experiencing an allergic reaction.
- Describe the emergency medical care of the patient with an allergic reaction.
- Establish the relationship between the patient with an allergic reaction and airway management.
- Describe the mechanisms of allergic response and the implications for airway management.
- State the generic and trade names, medication forms, dose, administration, action, and contraindications for the epinephrine autoinjector.
- Evaluate the need for medical direction in the emergency medical care of the patient with an allergic reaction.
- Differentiate between the general category of those patients having an allergic reaction and those patients having an allergic reaction and requiring immediate medical care, including immediate use of the epinephrine autoinjector.
- Demonstrate the emergency medical care of the patient experiencing an allergic reaction.
- Demonstrate the use of the epinephrine autoinjector.
- Demonstrate the assessment and documentation of patient response to an epinephrine injection.
- Demonstrate proper disposal of equipment.
- Demonstrate completing a prehospital care report for patients with allergic emergencies.

Supplemental

- Distinguish an anaphylactic reaction from a simple allergic reaction.
- Define *allergic reaction*.
- Describe and identify urticaria.
- List the antigens that most commonly cause anaphylaxis.
- List the indications for assisting a patient with the administration of epinephrine.
- Describe the use of an epinephrine autoinjector.
- Describe the use of a syringe to administer epinephrine.

An **allergic reaction** is a response of the body's immune system when challenged by a foreign substance such as bee venom, foods, medications, animal dander, or pollen. Allergic reactions range from a minor single-system reaction, such as that caused by poison ivy, to a life-threatening anaphylactic reaction, such as that caused by an insect sting.

Each year in the United States, 400 to 800 deaths are caused by severe allergic reactions. These deaths frequently occur within minutes of the onset of the allergic reaction. If properly assessed and managed in the prehospital setting, some of these deaths may be averted.

Allergic reactions are caused by the activity of the immune system. The body recognizes and protects itself from foreign material (**antigen**) with a complex system of circulating protective proteins (**antibodies**) and immune tissue that includes the liver, spleen, bone marrow, and lymph glands throughout the body.

Additionally, white blood cells (WBCs) are involved in the immune response. Some of these WBCs detect the presence of antigen in the body and signal other cells. These other cells respond by releasing various chemicals that amplify the response and recruit still other cells. The various chemicals and proteins released by these cells then interact with the antigen to kill or neutralize it. An allergic reaction can be thought of as an excessive immune reaction or one that causes discomfort or illness in a patient.

> ✓ Allergic reactions are the body's response to a challenge by foreign materials. These reactions are directed by the immune system, which includes white blood cells, the liver, the spleen, and the lymph nodes.

Anatomy and Physiology

The **immune system** consists of several organs including the liver, spleen, and bone marrow. Immune cells are also scattered throughout the body (e.g., the lymph nodes contain immune cells). The immune system recognizes foreign invaders and eliminates them from the body.

Nearly all immune reactions involve an interaction between an antigen and antibodies. Antibodies are made by lymphocytes and bind to the antigen (Figure 18.1). The antibody-coated antigen stimulates responses by other cells in the immune system that neutralize or destroy the antigen. The liver and spleen may also remove

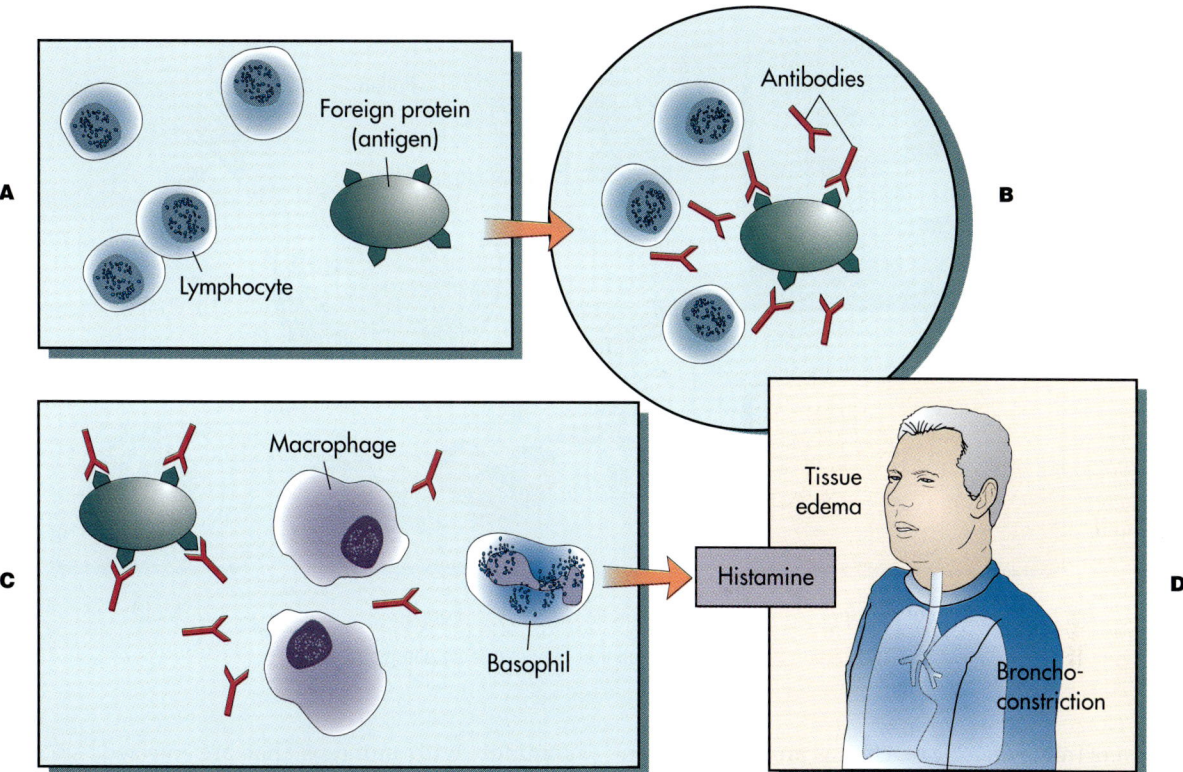

FIGURE 18.1 Antigen-antibody reaction. **A,** Lymphocytes detect the presence of a foreign invader (antigen). **B,** Antibodies are produced. **C,** Antibodies bind to the antigen and stimulate other immune cells (such as basophils). Basophils release histamine. **D,** Histamine causes various effects, such as constriction of the bronchioles and tissue edema.

the antibody-coated antigen. The body makes a distinct antibody for each antigen that it contacts.

> **Physician Notes**
>
> Immunization is the intentional exposure of the body to small amounts of antigen. The lymphocytes that are stimulated to make antibodies also "remember" the antigen so that if the body is reexposed to the same antigen, antibodies can be produced quickly.

Pathophysiology

The most common type of allergic reaction that requires transportation to the hospital is an *immediate hypersensitivity* reaction. Common types of antigens associated with an immediate hypersensitivity reaction include insect venom, antibiotics (especially injected penicillin), plants, and some foods such as nuts, shellfish, and strawberries (Figure 18.2). Hypersensitivity reactions cause the release of a chemical called **histamine** from WBCs. Histamine is a potent **vasodilator** and can cause leaking of blood vessels. Vasodilatation within the skin causes redness of the skin and a characteristic rash called **hives**, or **urticaria**. Hives are raised, blanched, irregularly shaped lesions with surrounding redness (Figure 18.3). Hives cause severe itching. If the tissue swelling occurs in the tongue, lips, oropharynx, or larynx, it can cause upper airway obstruction and result in stridor or progress to airway obstruction and respiratory compromise. Additionally, vasodilatation in the intestinal mucosa can cause stomach cramps and vomiting. Generalized vasodilatation may lead to hypotension and shock. The heart rate will increase in an attempt to counteract the low blood pressure. Chapter 9 provides a more detailed discussion of shock management.

Histamine is also a potent bronchoconstrictor that can result in wheezing and difficulty breathing. Histamine release can also cause itchy, watery eyes and a runny nose. Most patients who have limited signs and symptoms, such as hives without respiratory or cardiac compromise, will not require aggressive treatment.

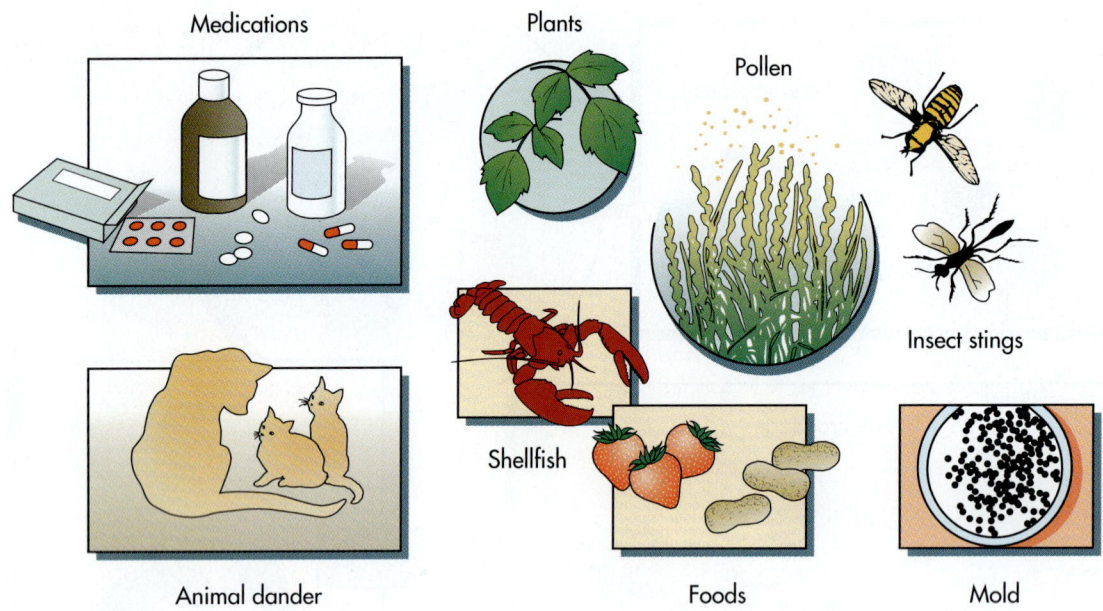

FIGURE 18.2 Substances that may cause an allergic reaction.

The most extreme allergic reaction is **anaphylaxis**. An **anaphylactic reaction** involves several organ systems and may be life threatening (Figure 18.4). Difficulty breathing or shock are the primary signs of a severe reaction. An anaphylactic reaction may develop over the course of seconds to minutes. Patients who have fast progression of symptoms are at the greatest risk. In anaphylaxis, the administration of epinephrine may be life saving.

The three most common antigens that cause anaphylaxis are penicillin, bee stings, and some foods (especially nuts and shellfish). Many other foods and drugs less commonly cause anaphylaxis. Severe reactions are more common with antigens that are injected, such as penicillin shots or bee stings.

Assessment

Initial Assessment

Patients who die from anaphylaxis die from either anaphylactic shock (25%) or from respiratory problems (75%). The emergency medical technician (EMT) should perform initial assessment of a possible allergic reaction, including assessment of the airway, breathing, and circulation, to be certain that the airway is patent and circulation is adequate.

History

The EMT should obtain a focused SAMPLE history that includes the following:

1. Signs and symptoms particularly related to the respiratory, cardiac, and dermatologic systems
2. History of allergies or allergic reaction
3. Substance to which the patient was exposed (if known)
4. Mode of exposure (ingestion, inhalation, absorption, or injection)
5. Progression of the effects and time period; rapid progression of symptoms is a more worrisome history

> ✓ Anaphylaxis is a reaction that is caused by the release of histamine from cells. Histamine causes dilatation and leaking of blood vessels, which causes tissue swelling. It also causes bronchoconstriction, or narrowing of the airways. Tissue swelling and bronchospasm are responsible for the clinical signs of an anaphylactic reaction.

Physician Notes

Anaphylactic reactions from insect exposures occur most commonly from the venom of the order *Hymenoptera*, which includes the honeybee, hornet, wasp, yellowjacket, fire ant, and bumblebee.

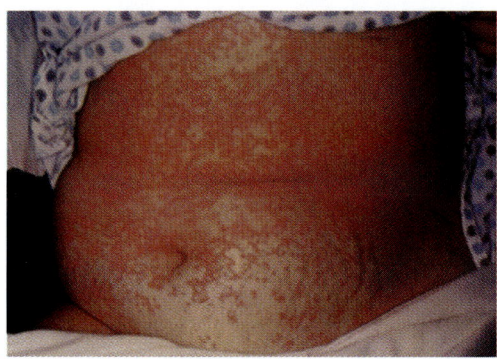

FIGURE 18.3 Hives (urticaria) are raised, blanched, irregularly shaped lesions with surrounding redness.

> **Signs and Symptoms of Anaphylaxis**
> * Hives, urticaria
> * Facial redness/swelling
> * Watery eyes, runny nose
> * Hypotension
> * Laryngeal edema/stridor
> * Tachycardia/thready pulse

FIGURE 18.4 Signs and symptoms of anaphylaxis.

6. Any interventions such as antihistamine or epinephrine already received

Physical Examination

After the EMT obtains the history, he or she should obtain baseline vital signs. The most dangerous complication of a severe allergic reaction is respiratory distress. Therefore specific attention must be directed at airway and breathing assessment. The EMT should administer oxygen to any patient who complains of respiratory distress.

Swelling of the tissues of the oropharynx and larynx can lead to airway obstruction, which is evident by the presence of stridor. **Stridor** is characterized by a high-pitched "crowing" sound often associated with hoarseness. The patient's airway usually is not obstructed by swelling in the mouth or tongue, but such swelling is a warning sign that the vocal cords may also be swollen, which can obstruct the airway.

Swelling and spasm of the smaller airway passages known as *brochospasm* may be manifested by a high-pitched whistling sound (wheezing) over the lungs. Severe brochospasm can limit air flow so much that wheezing actually decreases or is absent.

The EMT then assesses circulation because vasodilatation may result in hypotension. In the ongoing assessment, the EMT must direct special attention toward the skin for hives or generalized redness or swelling, which may be more pronounced in the face. Abdominal cramps and vomiting may occur. Also, the patient often will complain of significant itching.

If the patient has the signs and symptoms of shock or respiratory compromise, the EMT must determine if he or she has a prescription for epinephrine. The signs and symptoms of shock or respiratory compromise are an indication to assist a patient in administering his or her epinephrine. If the patient has the signs and symptoms of shock, respiratory compromise, or rapidly progressing symptoms and does not have epinephrine, the EMT should implement early transportation. If no signs and symptoms of shock or respiratory compromise exist, the EMT can complete a full assessment. However, the EMT must remember that symptoms can progress rapidly.

> ✓ Anaphylaxis can cause respiratory and circulatory problems. Upper airway obstruction results in stridor, whereas lower airway obstruction results in wheezing. Vasodilatation can cause erythema of the skin, hives, or in more severe cases, hypotension.

Management

The management of allergic reactions is aimed at reducing further histamine release and managing present problems. Anaphylaxis may be rapidly fatal, and drug therapy may be life saving. If paramedic intercept is available, the EMT should call for it as early as possible.

Airway Management

The EMT must maintain the airway and deliver high-flow oxygen if any signs of airway compromise are present. In the event that the patient appears to have inadequate ventilation, early use of a bag-valve-mask (BVM) may be appropriate. BVM management is discussed in Chapter 10.

A Combitube may be no more effective than a BVM since it will not pass the obstruction in the trachea. If the EMT is able to use endotracheal intubation for airway control, it may be wise to consider its use early because

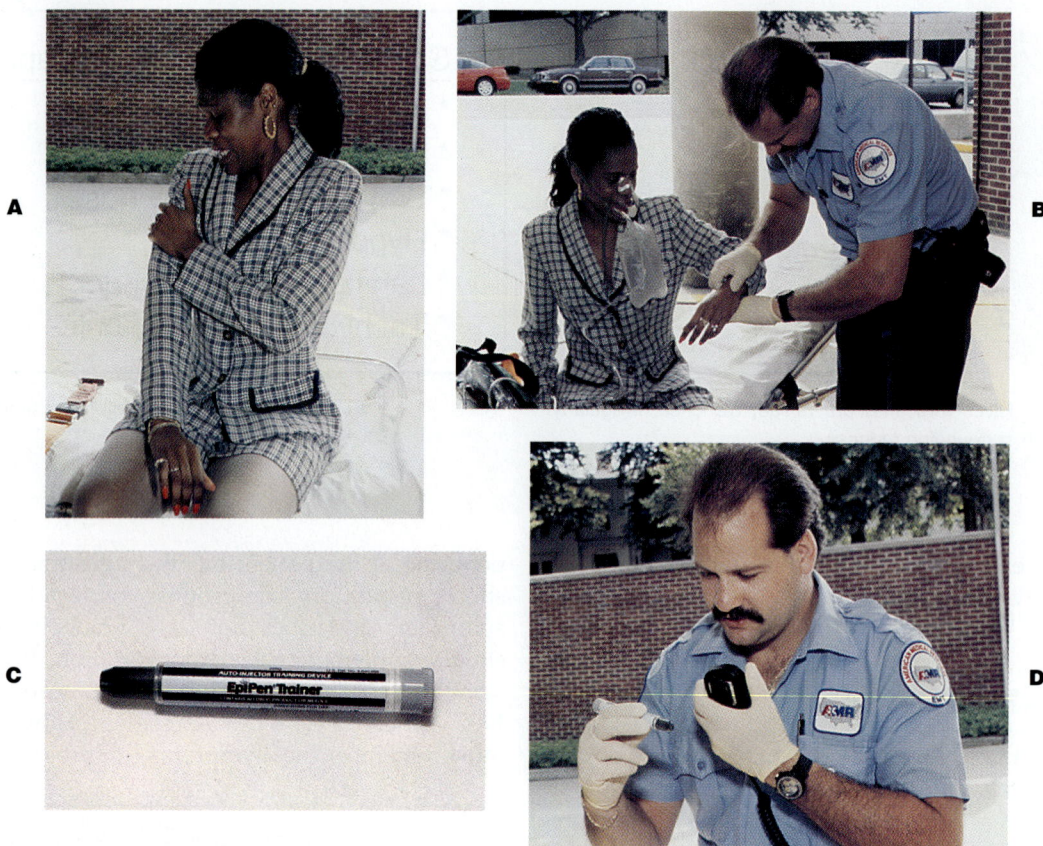

FIGURE 18.5 Epinephrine autoinjector. **A,** Determine that the patient is having a severe allergic reaction. **B,** Perform an initial assessment. Administer oxygen by nonrebreather mask. Obtain a SAMPLE history, and take the patient's vital signs. **C,** Determine if the patient has a prescribed epinephrine autoinjector. Verify that the medication is the patient's and, if medication is visible, is not discolored. **D,** Obtain order from medical direction to administer medication.

the development of laryngeal edema may make it more difficult to accomplish later.

Drug Therapy

High-flow oxygen is the primary drug to be used for any patient suffering from respiratory symptoms. Antihistamines such as diphenhydramine (Benadryl) are useful in mild allergic reactions to reduce progression of symptoms and relieve itch. In more severe cases, epinephrine (adrenalin) may be indicated and can be life saving. Antihistamines are not approved drugs for administration by an EMT. Some EMTs, depending on local protocol, may be permitted to assist a patient in injecting epinephrine when the patient has an epinephrine injector and is unable to use it without assistance.

Epinephrine is a potent vasoconstrictor and bronchodilator that counteracts the effects of histamine. It can cause pronounced side effects including tachycardia, hypertension, angina, and myocardial ischemia, particularly in patients with preexisting heart disease. For this reason, it should be used very cautiously in patients older than 50 years of age and should not be used to treat minor allergic reactions.

Epinephrine for patient use is available in the form of an **Epi-Pen**, which is an autoinjector. The DOT curriculum allows an EMT-Basic, under medical direction, to assist a patient who has been prescribed an Epi-Pen or equivalent.

The autoinjector is a device that contains a preloaded 0.3 mg ampule of epinephrine. A pediatric formulation with 0.15 mg is also available. Epinephrine is injected by a spring-loaded plunger that is automatically activated when the needle of the device is forcefully plunged into the patient's shoulder or thigh. The device is inserted perpendicular (90-degree angle) to the skin and held in place for 10 seconds while the entire dose is given subcutaneously (beneath the skin) (Figure 18.5). Before use, the EMT should confirm that the medication is not discolored and that the expiration date has not passed.

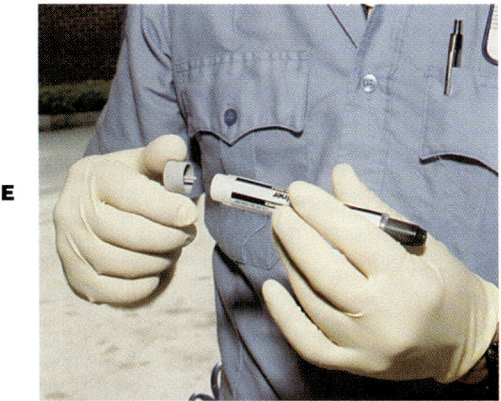
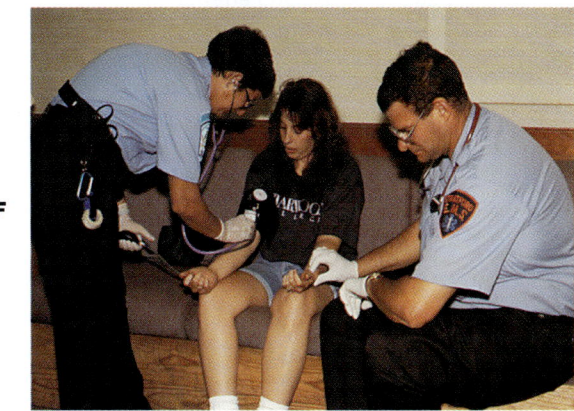
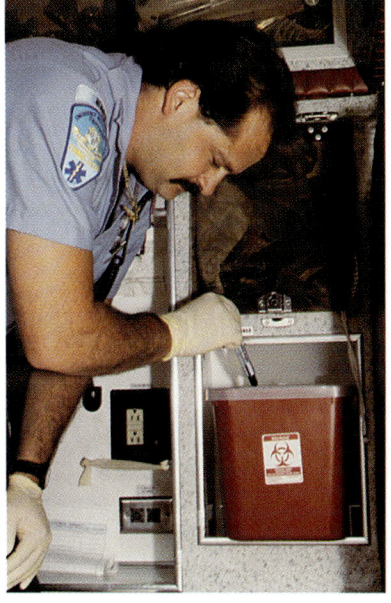

FIGURE 18.5, cont'd **E,** Expose the extremity, and remove the safety cap on the autoinjector. **F,** Place the tip of the autoinjector at a 90-degree angle firmly against the lateral portion of the patient's thigh, midway between the waist and knee, until the injector activates. Hold the injector in place until the medication is injected. Reevaluate vital signs. **G,** Dispose of the injector in an approved biohazard container.

> ✓ Epinephrine is the primary treatment for anaphylaxis. In systems in which it is permitted, an EMT may assist a patient in administering his or her epinephrine. Airway maneuvers, fluids, and the shock position may be of additional benefit to patients experiencing an anaphylactic reaction.

If no medication is available, the EMT should transport the patient in the shock position (legs elevated) with supplemental oxygen. In systems in which there is tiered response, early consideration of ALS intervention is appropriate.

Summary

- Allergic reactions are a result of the interaction of antigen and antibody.
- Allergic reactions can range from simple skin reactions to generalized life-threatening reactions with shock and airway compromise.
- Patients with life-threatening allergic reactions may need epinephrine.
- Epinephrine is available in an autoinjector (Epi-Pen), and patients having severe reactions may need assistance in administration.
- Epinephrine has multiple side effects including tachycardia, hypertension, and myocardial ischemia.
- The patient in anaphylactic shock also may benefit from the other usual modalities for shock, including the shock position and IV fluids.

Scenario Solution

You recognize the constellation of signs and symptoms as consistent with an anaphylactic reaction to a hornet sting, which occurred when the patient ran over a hornet's nest with her lawnmower. The patient's airway is compromised by swelling of the laryngeal tissue, causing stridor. Additionally, the patient has signs and symptoms of shock. Her confusion and combativeness are a result of low blood flow to the brain. Additional signs and symptoms of shock include cool, clammy skin; decreased blood pressure; and tachycardia.

You place the patient in a supine position with her legs elevated and attempt to maximize the airway patency with a jaw thrust. You assist ventilations with a bag-valve-mask and 100% oxygen.

Off-line medical direction protocols exist authorizing you to administer an epinephrine autoinjector, when available, to a patient assessed as exhibiting an anaphylactic reaction. After taking the injector from the patient's husband, you confirm that it is prescribed for the patient. You confirm that the medication is not discolored and that the expiration date has not passed, and then you inject the medication into the patient's thigh.

After you inject the epinephrine and give supplemental oxygen, the patient's stridor and mental status improve. She is hospitalized for a day, and arrangements for allergy shots are made before her discharge.

Key Terms

Allergic reaction A response of the body's immune system when challenged by a foreign substance either on the surface or into the body.

Anaphylactic reaction An extreme allergic reaction that is caused by the release of histamine form the cells.

Anaphylaxis An exaggerated, life-threatening hypersensitivity reaction to a previously encountered antigen.

Antibodies A complex system of circulating protective proteins used to fight off foreign material in the body.

Antigen A substance, usually a protein, that causes the formation of an antibody and reacts specifically with that antibody; antigens are usually found on the surfaces of microorganisms.

Epinephrine Hormone secreted by the adrenal gland; causes tachycardia, vasoconstriction, and release of insulin.

Epi-Pen An autoinjector that contains epinephrine used subcutaneously to counteract the effects of histamine.

Histamine The specific substance produced by the body responsible for the attack.

Hives Raised, blanched, irregularly shaped lesions with surrounding redness. Hives cause severe itching.

Immune system Recognizes foreign invaders and eliminates them from the body.

Stridor An abnormal, high-pitched, musical sound caused by an obstruction in the trachea or larynx; usually heard during inspiration.

Urticaria Medical term for hives.

Vasodilator Expansion of the blood vessels that cause redness of the skin.

Review Questions

1. A foreign material that enters the body is known as a(n) _____.
2. The liver, spleen, lymph glands, and white blood cells are all part of the _____ system.
3. There are _____ deaths annually in the United States as a result of anaphylactic reactions.
4. _____ is the treatment of choice for an anaphylactic reaction.
5. Before administration of epinephrine, the EMT must check:
    a. Patient's name
    b. Expiration date
    c. Clarity and color of medication
    d. All of the above

Answers to these Review Questions can be found at the end of the book on page 866.

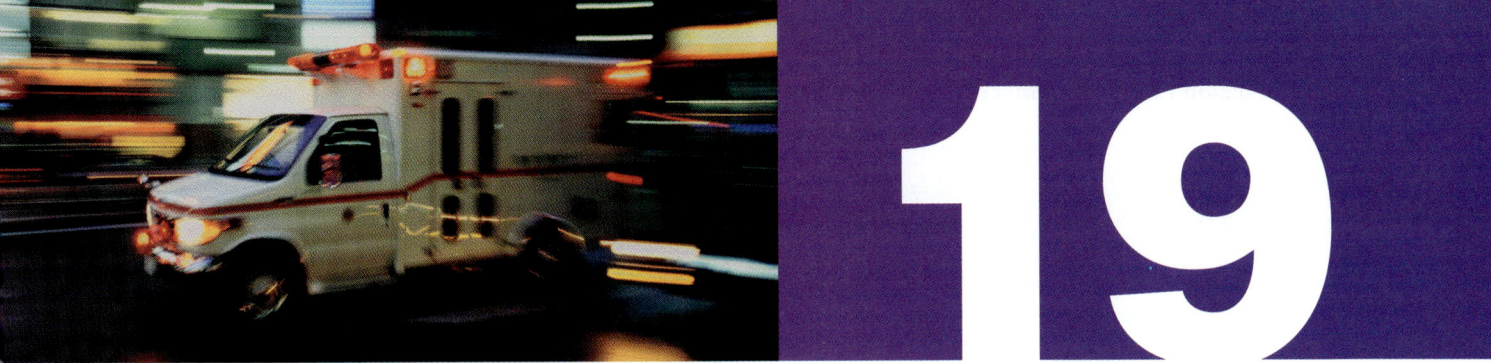

19

Toxic Emergencies: Poisoning and Overdose

Lesson Goal

The goal of this chapter is to review the signs, symptoms, and methods of patient poisoning.

Scenario

You are called to the scene of a possible overdose. You arrive on the scene to find a mother and her 16-year-old daughter supporting each other in the doorway, both in tears. The mother tells you that her daughter was depressed over a relationship and took about ten 5 mg Valium tablets about 10 minutes ago. The daughter says, "Yes I did and I know it was stupid."

 How would your assessment of this patient progress? What can you do for her? What should you do to prepare the hospital for her arrival?

Key Terms to Know

Activated charcoal
Antidotes
Gastric lavage
Material safety data sheet
Poison control centers
Poisoning

Learning Objectives

As an EMT-Basic, you should be able to do the following:

DOT

- List various ways that poisons enter the body.
- List signs and symptoms associated with poisoning.
- Discuss emergency medical care of the patient with possible overdose.
- Describe the steps in emergency medical care of the patient with suspected poisoning.

343

Learning Objectives (cont'd)

- Establish the relationship between the patient suffering from poisoning or overdose and airway management.
- State the generic and trade names, indications, contraindications, medication form, dose, administration, actions, side effects, and reassessment strategies for activated charcoal.
- Recognize the need for medical direction in caring for the patient with poisoning or overdose.
- Demonstrate the steps in emergency medical care of the patient with possible overdose.
- Demonstrate the steps in emergency medical care of the patient with suspected poisoning.
- Perform the necessary steps required to provide a patient with activated charcoal.
- Demonstrate the assessment and documentation of patient response.
- Demonstrate proper disposal of the equipment for the administration of activated charcoal.
- Demonstrate completing a prehospital care report for patients with a poisoning or overdose emergency.

Supplemental

- Define *poison*.
- Describe the appropriate interaction with the poison control center.
- Explain the various effects of poisons on the body.
- List the forms of activated charcoal that are available.
- Identify the appropriate circumstances in which to use activated charcoal.
- List the contraindications of activated charcoal.
- Define *substance abuse*.
- Discuss various types of abused substances and their effects.
- Discuss warning signs of substance abuse.
- Discuss the management of toxic emergencies.

Poisoning is defined as the adverse effects of plants, foods, chemicals, or pharmaceutical agents on the body. Poisoning commonly occurs accidentally but also may occur intentionally, as in suicidal behavior. Approximately 2.5 million human poison exposures were reported to poison control centers in 1993. Poisoning most commonly occurs in two age ranges. The first is in the toddler to preschool age range when children are exploring their environment and will accidentally be exposed to poisons. The most common poisons to which this age group is exposed are household cleaning agents and medications stored in an area that is not child-proofed. The second peak age range is the adolescent to young adult age group, when ingestion as a form of suicidal behavior most commonly occurs.

Most poisoning cases do not require hospital admission. A small percentage result in significant toxicity, and an even smaller percentage result in death (Figure 19.1).

Poisons exert their effects after being absorbed into the body. The management of most poisonings is supportive, but often an attempt is made to limit the absorption of the poison. A few poisons have specific **antidotes** that reverse or block the effect of the poison. Prehospital care of poisoning patients is directed at assessment and stabilization of the airway, breathing, and circulation. Prehospital care may also involve initiating decontamination in an attempt to reduce the poison concentration present at the scene, in the patient, or both.

Poison Control Centers

A centralized facility with access to poison information and toxicologic consultation can result in improved care for the poisoning patient. Centralizing these resources with 24-hour telephone access is the key to poison control. **Poison control centers** benefit patients by allowing earlier, appropriate management and, in many circumstances, avoidance of hospital-level care altogether. Poison control centers also collect statistical information about poisoning. As of 1994, more than 70 poison control centers in 40 states served a population of 200 million people. Now there are nearly 100 in the United States and many more worldwide. Emergency medical technicians (EMTs) should know if their area has a regional poison

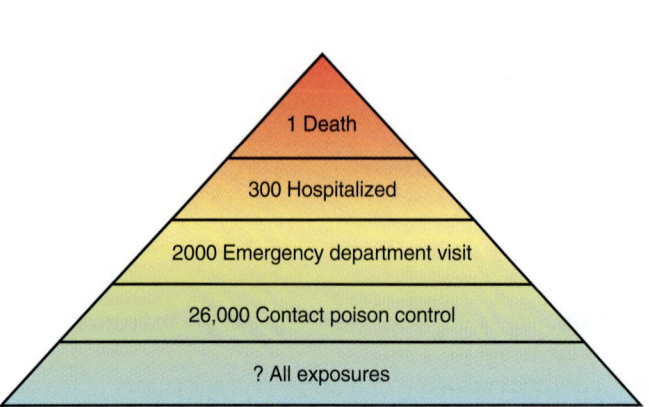

FIGURE 19.1 Injury pyramid for poisoning.

control center and should be familiar with its phone number and hours of operation. The American Association of Poison Control Centers (AAPCC) maintains a database containing information on all of its member poison control centers. A list of local poison control centers is available on the AAPCC website (www.aapcc.org) or by phone at 202-362-7217.

> ✓ Poisoning is the adverse effect of plants, food, chemicals, or pharmaceutical agents on the body. Most poisonings do not result in significant medical problems. Poison control centers may be a resource for poison information for patients and health care providers.

Anatomy and Physiology

Poisons are generally introduced to the body in one of four ways: ingestion, absorption, (dermal [skin] exposure or ocular [eye] exposure), inhalation, or injection (Figure 19.2).

Ingestion

Poisoning by ingestion occurs when a poison is taken into the mouth. Poisoning can occur with or without swallowing because some poisons are irritating or corrosive to the tissue that lines the mouth and esophagus. A person who ingests one of these poisons may experience burning and swelling of the soft tissues of the mouth. The patient usually will attempt to remove the material from his or her mouth. Depending on the concentration of the poison and the speed with which a patient removes the poison, the injury may be limited to discomfort. However, if the concentration of the poison is high or exposure is prolonged, significant swelling and potential compromise to the upper airway may occur.

Not all poisons that injure tissue cause pain on ingestion. Some corrosives such as lye do not cause a significant amount of pain and therefore can be swallowed. These poisons can then significantly damage the lining of the mouth and the esophagus. In the period immediately after such an injury, the patient is at risk for perforation

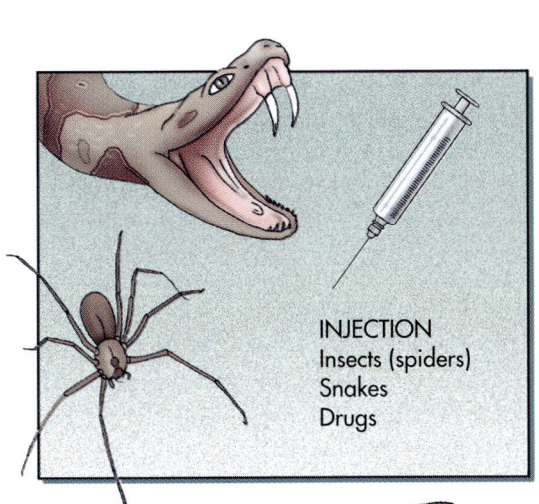

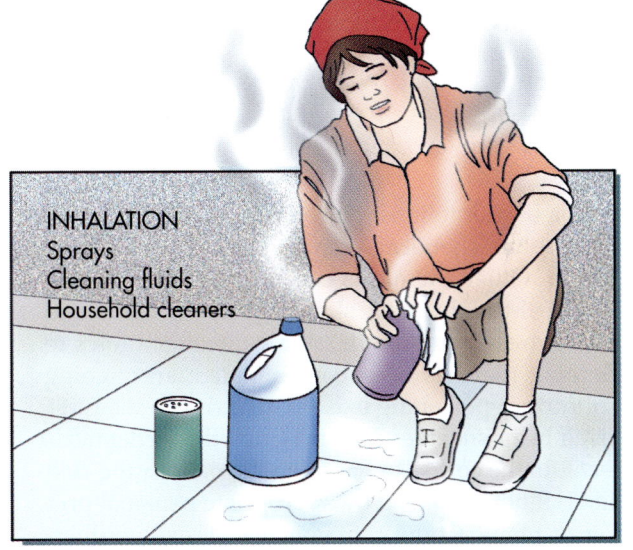

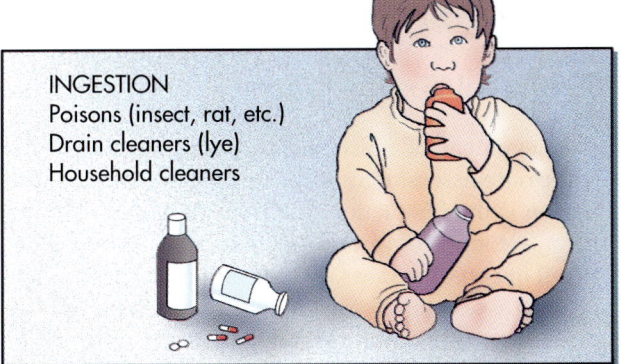

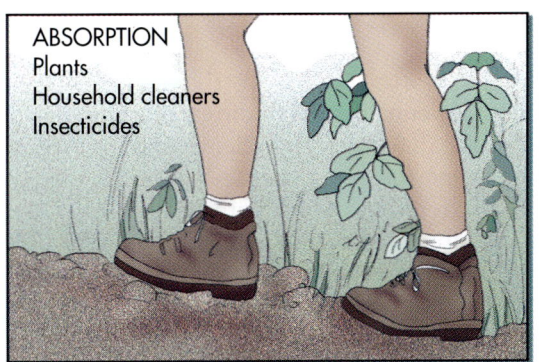

FIGURE 19.2 How poisons enter the body.

Poison Information That May Be Available at the Scene

* Unusual odors
* Containers of medications or chemicals
* Samples
* Material safety data sheet

FIGURE 19.3 Much poison information in available at the scene.

of the esophagus. In the healing phase, the esophagus can scar and strictures (narrowing) can occur, which may cause difficulty swallowing.

Ingested poisons that do not have a direct irritant effect are absorbed from the stomach and small intestine. Most absorption takes place in the small intestine. Administration of activated charcoal will limit the absorption. The use of ipecac in the field is no longer advocated because of limited success and potential complications caused to the airway by induced vomiting.

Absorption

Dermal (Skin) Exposure

The skin is a barrier to most poisons; however, if the skin is broken, some chemicals can be absorbed into the bloodstream. Other chemicals can be absorbed into the bloodstream through intact skin (e.g., insecticides and some heavy metal compounds). If a patient continues to wear clothing that has been contaminated, an ongoing source of further poisoning exists. Great risk to the EMT may exist if he or she does not know that these chemicals are present. In the course of handling the patient, the skin of the EMT, if not protected by appropriate personal protective gear, may become contaminated. Usually adherence to body substance isolation (BSI) precautions and the use of vinyl or latex gloves provide adequate protection to the EMT.

Ocular (Eye) Exposure

Most ocular poisoning results in direct injury to the covering of the eyeball (cornea and sclera) or to the conjunctiva, which is the lubricated tissue beneath the eyelids that partially covers the eyeball. Both acids and alkalis, as well as many other chemicals, can injure the tissue of the eye. Additionally, small amounts of materials that get in the eye can be absorbed into the bloodstream. However, this means of poisoning is uncommon because the surface area of the eye is relatively small.

Inhalation

Poisonous gases are absorbed through the lungs. Some gases, such as carbon monoxide, act as poisons by displacing oxygen from the air and suffocating the victim. Other gases, such as cyanide, are absorbed across the lung tissues and into the bloodstream. EMT safety is again a significant issue in inhalation poisoning because the poisonous gas still may be present. If the EMT does not take appropriate means to protect himself or herself either by appropriately ventilating the area or using a self-contained breathing apparatus, the EMT can be injured in the course of patient care.

Injection

Poisons can be injected, bypassing the skin, and delivered directly into the circulation. Usually poisoning by injection is a result of intravenous (IV) drug abuse. Poisoning can result from an excessive dose of the intended drug or from unintended adulterants that are sometimes used by drug dealers to substitute for or dilute the desired drug.

Poisoning by an excessive dose is also called an *overdose*. EMTs who work in large urban areas may see small epidemics of narcotic overdose if a more pure supply of narcotic drugs suddenly becomes available.

Another source of injected poisons is the venom of various animals, including snakes, bees, spiders, and some sea creatures. For more specific information related to dealing with envenomation, see Chapters 18 and 29.

✓ Poisons can enter the body by absorption through the intestine, eyes, or lungs or by absorption or injection through the skin. The type of exposure affects the risk to the patient and the way the EMT approaches patient care.

Assessment

General Assessment

Management of poisoning is primarily supportive. Appropriate assessment of the airway, breathing, and circulation is the first action. If airway, breathing, and circulation are not compromised, the next assessment is the level of consciousness and the adequacy of the gag reflex. These assessments are necessary for medical direction and/or poison control to determine if other field intervention is appropriate.

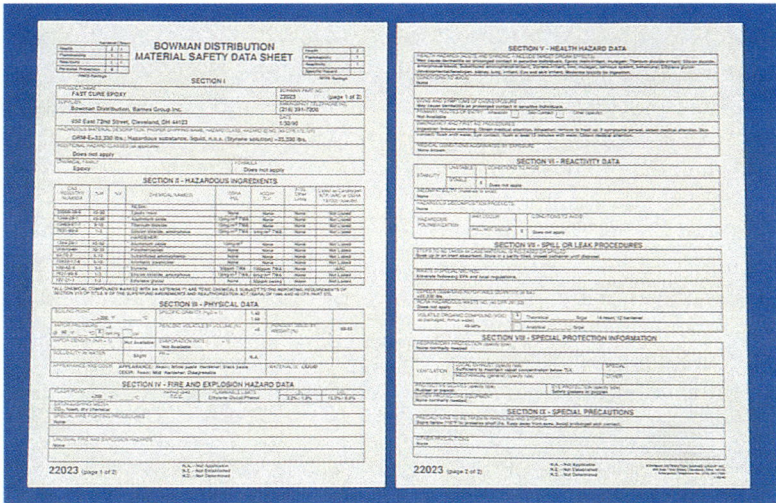

FIGURE 19.4 Sample of material safety data sheet.

Scene Assessment

Assessment of the scene is the EMT's first responsibility. When the route of poisoning is inhalation or absorption, the EMT must be certain that a hazardous materials (HAZMAT) situation does not exist to avoid becoming a secondary casualty (see Chapter 40).

Poisoning is a situation in which scene information may be extremely useful and unavailable to hospital staff if not noted by the EMT (Figure 19.3). Important scene information includes a description of any unusual odors at the scene. It is vital for the EMT to identify the specific medication or chemical to the best of his or her ability. If a container or material is present at the scene that can be safely transported, it generally is helpful to bring it with the patient. At industrial sites, a **material safety data sheet**, which identifies the poison and gives information regarding its toxicity, should be available (Figure 19.4).

The quantity of poisonous material, especially in ingestion, is also important information. Frequently, the EMT is in the best position to make an estimate of the amount of poison ingested by the patient by noting pills or tablets on the floor and taking a moment to collect as many as can be quickly recovered. Emergency physicians or poison control staff will frequently do a pill count on bottles of medication to estimate the number of pills ingested. If a large quantity of spilled tablets is not noted or recovered by the EMT, hospital staff may anticipate a higher risk to the patient and undertake more aggressive treatment than is needed.

Many times children will ingest liquids and simultaneously spill large amounts. Noting that the child was found in a large puddle of the material again is useful information that sometimes only the EMT on the scene is able to report.

SAMPLE History

If the patient is stable, the EMT should obtain a SAMPLE history:

- *Signs and symptoms.* Because the variety of poisons is wide, signs and symptoms of poisoning vary. Central nervous system (CNS) symptoms may include dizziness, headache, and confusion, and physical findings include altered mental status ranging from coma to drowsiness to agitation, with some poisons causing seizures. Cardiac symptoms may include chest pain or palpitations, and physical findings may include fast, slow, or normal heart rate. Respiratory symptoms may include hoarseness, cough, and difficulty breathing, and ventilatory rates may be increased, normal, or decreased. Some poisons may cause abdominal pain, nausea, vomiting, or diarrhea. However, most poison exposures result in no signs or symptoms at all.
- *Allergies.* This part of the history is the same as for any patient.
- *Medications.* The EMT should obtain a history of current medications and assess the specific type, timing, and quantity of poison as well as possible. The EMT must also remember to ask if poison control or the patient's physician has been contacted before the EMT's arrival. Often if poison control or the physician has been contacted, syrup of ipecac, if available, may have already been given before the EMT's arrival. Knowing this information will permit the EMT to be prepared for vomiting by the patient.
- *Pertinent history.* If the EMT suspects an intentional poisoning, he or she should ask questions about previous suicidal behavior.

- *Last meal.* The EMT should note the time of the last meal. In the event of an acute poisoning, the best available estimate of the time of the poison ingestion is valuable, particularly for poisons that can be measured in the bloodstream such as aspirin, acetaminophen, or aminophylline. The time of ingestion may also influence decisions about stomach emptying or the use of antidotes or binding agents. Some poisons cause spontaneous vomiting. If vomiting has occurred, the EMT should note the amount and character of the vomitus, especially information about the presence of pill fragments or other evidence that the poison is in the vomitus. If the vomitus is in a container, the EMT should transport it with the patient and give it to the hospital receiving personnel.
- *Events.* The EMT should note the events surrounding the poisoning, including whether the poisoning was accidental or intentional. If the ingestion was intentional, appropriate assessment of suicidal risk and precautions are important to prevent additional self-destructive behavior during the transportation.

Physical Examination

Airway, Breathing, and Circulation

The first priority in any patient who has been poisoned is the same as in all patients—attention to airway, breathing, and circulation. Only after assessment and stabilization of these areas are complete should further assessment take place.

Central Nervous System

A patient who is oriented, answers questions, and is not drooling generally can be considered to have an adequate gag reflex. If the EMT is uncertain, he or she should insert a tongue blade into the patient's mouth and place it on the back of the tongue or throat. This action should cause the patient to gag. Patients with an impaired gag reflex must be watched more carefully for development of airway problems and may not be appropriate candidates for prehospital use of activated charcoal because of the risk of aspiration of either vomitus or charcoal.

Cardiovascular System

The EMT should assess circulation with special attention to any abnormalities of blood pressure or pulse that may predict further deterioration of the patient.

Skin

The EMT should assess the patient for signs of liquid or powder on the skin or clothing. The patient may report burning or itching of the skin. The EMT should assess the skin for redness or blisters, which are frequent signs of chemical damage, and for cyanosis (blue color), which suggests a lack of oxygen. Patients with carbon monoxide poisoning classically are described as having "cherry-red" skin and mucous membranes, but in clinical practice most patients with carbon monoxide poisoning do not have this finding.

Eyes

The EMT should assess the eyes for tearing or redness. The EMT should assess the patient's vision by asking him or her to note gross vision. The EMT may need to distinguish vision in at least four general categories, which represent progressively better vision:

1. No vision
2. Able to distinguish light and dark
3. Able to count fingers at a distance of several feet
4. Able to read letters or numbers on paperwork or an IV bag

Respiratory System

The EMT should assess the airway and lung sounds for stridor, which is the crowing noise that can signal an obstruction in the upper airway, or wheezing, which signals lower airway narrowing either from swelling, mucous production, or spasm of the muscles around the airway.

> ✓ The assessment of the poisoning patient includes evaluation of scene data, including scene safety, specific information regarding the exact substance involved, and any clues as to the timing and quantity of the poisoning. The EMT should pay special attention to airway, circulation, mental status, and skin findings during the physical examination. If the patient appears stable, the EMT should contact a poison control center or medical direction to get additional information on assessment and management.

Management

Ingestion

The approach to preventing the absorption of ingested poisons is to give a substance that binds to the poison. **Activated charcoal** is a specially prepared form of charcoal that can absorb, or bind to, many chemicals. Chemicals that are absorbed in the charcoal do not cross the intestinal lining into the bloodstream and are excreted in the stool. Activated charcoal is a finely powdered form of charcoal. Each gram of charcoal may have a total surface area of 1000 m^2 or more, allowing a tremendous number of binding sites to attach to the poison molecules. Several forms and brands of activated charcoal are available (Figure 19.5).

Activated charcoal powder must be mixed with juice or water before it is given to the patient. Mixing can be messy and difficult, so most activated charcoal now in use is premixed in a "slurry," or suspension, of charcoal in water or other liquid. Patients with altered mental status who have ingested acids or alkalis, or who cannot or will not swallow the solution, should not be given charcoal.

The EMT must obtain an order for activated charcoal administration from either online or offline medical direction. Dosage is usually 0.5 to 1 g per kilogram of body weight, resulting in a usual adult dose of 25 to 50 g and a pediatric dose of 12.5 to 25 g. Because charcoal generally is considered nontoxic, the dose frequently is rounded up or down to the amount that is available in the packaged form.

Before use, the EMT needs to shake the activated charcoal container well. The patient frequently will be less than enthusiastic about drinking the charcoal because it looks like mud and has a gritty texture. Some flavored forms are now available, which may improve compliance. Additionally, having the patient drink the material through a straw from a covered container so that it cannot be seen may help. If the patient takes a long time to drink, the solution should be intermittently shaken or stirred to resuspend the charcoal.

Activated charcoal causes few side effects. Stools will become black, which can occasionally be mistaken for intestinal bleeding, and some patients, especially those who have ingested poisons that cause nausea, may vomit. If the patient vomits shortly after dosing, the EMT may contact medical direction for an order to repeat the dose.

Absorption

For purposes of management, dermal and ocular poisonings are the same. If a dry powder is on the skin, the EMT should brush it off and remove any contaminated clothing. The EMT should be careful to protect himself or herself from contamination. In a liquid exposure or any ocular exposure, the EMT should pereform large-volume clear water irrigation of the skin or eye for a minimum of 20 minutes and continuously until arrival at the hospital if possible. The EMT can irrigate the eye or skin with tap water, normal saline, or dextrose solutions.

The EMT should gently hold the e eyelid open and pour the stream of water directly into the eye. Patients usually will involuntarily close the eyes, which is a normal protective mechanism. Sterile water is *not* necessary, and the EMT should always decontaminate with clean water if no sterile fluid is available.

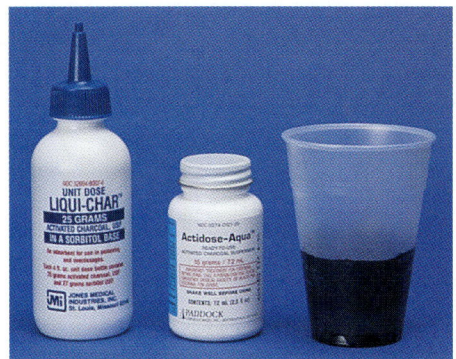

FIGURE 19.5 Activated charcoal.

Inhalation

The primary management of any respiratory poisoning is removal of the patient from further exposure to the toxic gas or fumes. The EMT must be certain that the scene is safe or be specifically trained in the use of respirators before attempting a rescue in an area where toxic fumes or gases are still present (see Chapter 40). The EMT should assess and manage the airway per basic life support (BLS) protocols. The EMT should give high-flow oxygen to any patient suspected of inhaling toxins. The EMT should consider early transportation for any unresponsive patient or any patient with difficulty breathing or abnormal respiratory rate. If the EMT suspects carbon monoxide poisoning, he or she should contact medical direction for consideration of primary transportation to a hyperbaric facility if one is available.

Injection

Narcotic overdose depresses respirations and mental status, which can lead to compromise of the airway. The EMT must remember that the tongue is the most common obstruction in the unresponsive patient, and a jaw lift or thrust may be needed to maintain the airway. If the coma is profound, mechanical adjuncts such as an oropharyngeal or nasopharyngeal airway or even intubation may be needed with bag-valve-mask (BVM) ventilation. A specific antidote for narcotic overdose called naloxone (Narcan®) is available. Naloxone is a paramedic-level drug. In a tiered response system, paramedic access may be appropriate. If injection paraphernalia is present at the scene, the EMT should take extreme care to avoid accidental needle stick and blood or body fluid exposure.

Envenomation is a type of injection poisoning that occurs when a poison is injected through the skin by a venomous animal. For more information on the specific care of the envenomated patient, see Chapter 29.

> ✓ Management of absorption and inhalation poisoning involves removal of the patient from a continued exposure to the poison. Ingestion may be treated with activated charcoal, which binds to the toxins to prevent absorption. Types of poisoning by injection include substance abuse and envenomation by animals.

Substance Abuse

A large part of the EMT's job in prehospital care focuses on substance abuse. Substance abusers are subject to a wide range of illnesses and injuries resulting from their substance abuse. This is further complicated by the hazards they present to others. Although the incidence motor vehicle collisions caused by intoxicated drivers has been steadily declining throughout the 1990s, over 50% of the fatalities from motor vehicle collisions showed alcohol as a major factor as recently as 1987.

Overdose is a common complication of substance abuse. Overdose can be accidental or intentional. The EMT-B must be able to recognize the signs and symptoms associated with overdose and the management of these emergencies.

Substance abuse affects the patient's potential for illness and injury and the EMT's ability to assess the patient. Substance abuse causes changes in the patient's level of consciousness (LOC) that may mask signs and symptoms of life-threatening or potentially life-threatening situations.

EMT-Bs must also be careful to not discriminate against patients because they have a history of substance abuse. Substance abusers are even more likely to have life-threatening illness and injury. Patients who are suffering from internal bleeding or diseases such as diabetes may mimic the signs and symptoms associated with their history of substance abuse.

Abused Substances

This section identifies the major abused substances, the effects they have on patients, and how to manage life-threatening situations brought on by abuse of these substances. Most of these drugs have legitimate medical uses, but because they are so good at what they do, they have become commonly abused substances.

Narcotics

Narcotics can be taken orally or injected. They depress the CNS, which can cause an altered LOC with constricted pupils and respiratory depression. Commonly abused narcotics include morphine, heroin (may also be smoked), codeine, Demerol, Dilaudid, Talwin, Percodan and fentanyl. Street names include Big M, Birdie powder, Dreamer dust, Gunk, Happy medicine, Morph, MS, Piece, Red cross, Sweet morpheus, and Witch. Abusers take these drugs for the euphoric effect that they induce. These patients may appear to be drowsy and calm.

When overdose occurs, the patient exhibits shallow or absent respirations with decreases in pulse rate and blood pressure. The skin may be cool and clammy and the patient will progress toward convulsions, coma, and death without intervention.

Patients who abuse narcotics become physically addicted and are also subject to withdrawals when they stop taking the drugs. Patients in withdrawal may be agitated, restless, anxious, and nauseated. They may complain of stomach cramps, diarrhea, cold sweats, and insomnia. These patients are very uncomfortable and will usually seek care.

Benzodiazepines

This group includes Valium, Librium, Xanax, and Ativan, although on the street any of them may be called "Downs." These drugs, taken orally or by injection, can cause slurred speech and disorientation. The patient may appear drunk without the odor of alcohol. There is occasionally a paradoxic effect in which very young or very old patients can become excited.

In overdose situations the EMT can expect to see depressed respirations, clammy skin, and possibly dilates pupils. The patient's pulse may be weak and rapid as he or she progresses from being sleepy to coma and death if not treated definitively.

These patients may also suffer withdrawal if the drugs are withheld, with symptoms including headaches, insomnia, tension, sweating, difficulty concentrating, fatigue, agitation, and seizures.

Barbiturates

Phenobarbitol and Seconal are examples of barbiturates. They can be taken orally or injected. Street names include Barbs, Blue birds, Blues, Candy, Crosses, Downs, Downers, Drowsy high, Phennies, Purple hearts, and Yellow jackets. Users may appear sleepy with slurred speech, again seeming intoxicated without the smell of alcohol.

Overdose patients may present with lethargy and shallow or absent respirations. The patient's pulse may be weak and rapid. If untreated, the patient may progress to coma and death.

Patients suffering withdrawal from barbiturates may experience anxiety, hallucinations, tremors, nausea, vomiting, diarrhea, abdominal cramps, insomnia, agitation, and convulsions.

Amphetamines

Amphetamine, methylenedioxymethamphetamine (MDMA), methylenedioxyethylamphetamine (MDME), methamphetamine, and Ice methanphetamine are examples of amphetamines. Street names for these drugs include "A," Bennies, Black beauties, Black mollies, Crosses, Jelly beans, Lid poppers, Uppers, Ecstasy, Adam, X, XTC, Hug drug, Clarity, Eve, Crank, Crystal meth, Meth, Speed, Crystal, and Glass. Users take these drugs by snorting, injecting, or swallowing to experience euphoria, increased alertness, and excitation. Ice is the only form that can be smoked. Side effects include depression after several days of using the drug.

In overdose situations the EMT can expect to see restlessness, dizziness, tremor, agitation, irritability, weakness, nausea, dilated pupils, hyperthermia, chest pain, and irregular heart rates. The patients may also be combative and suffer hallucinations. Convulsions may precede coma and death if not treated.

Patients withdrawing from amphetamines experience listlessness and lack of energy, and they seem to be always sleeping.

Cocaine

On the street, cocaine as a powder may be known as Bernie's, Blow, Cadillac, Candy, Coke, Coconut, Dream, Flake, Girl, Happy dust, Leaf, Nose candy, Snow, Toot, White horse, or White powder. When used in freebase form, it may be called "Crack" or "Rock." Cocaine is a popular drug because people report euphoria or feeling "powerful." Cocaine may be snorted, smoked, or injected. Many become addicted to the lifestyle they feel they can only maintain by using the drug, as though the drug makes them more than they are without it (stronger, faster, smarter). Chronic users are usually thin, may have constant nasal drainage (explaining the frequent sniffing), and may have red or raw nostrils. Many even develop perforations of the nasal septum.

Cocaine overdose patients may present with agitation and belligerence. Their pupils may be dilated, and they may be hyperthermic. Overdose patients often have severely elevated blood pressures, which can become lethal. Some of these patients may also develop slurred speech and lethargy, especially after binging. This can be followed by coma and death.

Cocaine users deprived of the drug may suffer withdrawal with depression, listlessness, lack of initiative, and lethargy.

Phencyclidine

"PCP" is also known as Angel dust, Crystal, Dead on arrival (or DOA), Embalming hog, Killer weed, Loveboat, Peace pill, Pop, or Supergrass. PCP can be smoked, taken orally, injected, or snorted. Users like it because it creates illusions and hallucinations and alters their perception of time.

If overdosed, patients can become severely agitated, belligerent, and paranoid. They can become hyperthermic with an increased blood pressure. If left untreated, they can experience convulsions, coma, and death.

Withdrawal from PCP causes depression in many users.

Lysergic Acid Diethylamine

LSD can be taken orally, snorted, or smoked. It is also called Acid, Beast, Haze, Lucy in the sky with diamonds, Mind detergent, Peace, Strawberry fields, Sunshine, or Zen. Users take LSD for the illusions and hallucinations. It can cause wild emotional swings and unpredictable behavior. These patients may even become violent. Some users even commit murder or suicide possibly induced by the drug.

Overdose is usually evidenced by more severe examples of the desired effect. Some users who stop taking the drug become depressed.

Cannabis

Marijuana and hashish can be eaten or smoked. They may also be known as Acapulco gold, Baby flowers, Ganja, Goof butts, Happy cigarettes, Indian boy, Jane, Juan Valdez, Lobo, Mary Jane, MJ, Poke, Pot, Reefer, Salt and pepper, Sinsemilla, Smoke, Tea, Weed, or Yerba. It relaxes and decreases the users inhibitions and may last for 30 to 40 minutes. These patients may appear disoriented.

In overdose fatigue, paranoia and occasionally psychosis are evident. Some users report depression when they stop using these drugs.

Methaqualone

Qualudes or Sopar may also be known as Ludes, Quay, Quad, Soaps, Soapers, 714s. Users may call it "luding out" if taking methaqualone with wine. They are usually taken orally but may be injected. Used as a pain reliever and tranquilizer at one time, users take it for the euphoric, indestructible feeling that it can create.

Inhalants

Vapors of paints, glues, fuels, cleaning products, and beauty products are often inhaled to elevate moods, decrease inhibitions, or create a type of euphoria. This effect is often followed by nausea, drowsiness, and headaches. Users frequently have red and watery eyes.

Overdose can cause muscle weakness, loss of control, and confusion. "Sudden sniffing death" refers to a rapid loss of consciousness. More frequently these patients can suffocate if they are breathing into plastic or paper bags.

These patients also often have faces that are stained by the paint they are "sniffing."

Alcohol

Beer, wine, liqueur, or derivatives are the most commonly abused substances. A significant number of people are chronic alcoholics, but more importantly an even larger number of people only occasionally abuse alcohol. To many people it is socially acceptable to be under the influence of alcohol. While most people may be able to limit the amount of alcohol consumed to levels that will not impair them beyond function, many will abuse alcohol on weekends or special occasion. Alcohol users drink for various reasons. In small amounts, people claim that alcohol "takes the edge off" or helps them relax. Many find it easier to be sociable because alcohol removes inhibitions so that they are less self-conscious in groups.

As the person's blood alcohol level rises, his or her LOC changes. At first the patient may just lose a sense of where they fit into their environment. They may talk too loud, touch others too hard, bump into things, or stumble. At this point, operating vehicles or machinery could be dangerous. Drinkers under the influence of alcohol are at risk because they do not perceive risks well and feel confident that they can overcome any situation. The EMT may find people who will pick a fight with someone twice their size or attempt to perform physically impossible feats. Most people do not realize that they can drink toxic amounts of alcohol. Loss of consciousness is possible, and there is a danger of aspiration because alcohol overdose is frequently accompanied by nausea and vomiting. Seizure, coma, and death may follow in severe cases.

Alcohol withdrawal can be very uncomfortable for alcoholics. Tremors, chills and sweating, and seizures can occur.

Management of Substance Abuse

Although this section has described many poisons and drugs, the management for all of these patients is the same.

Safety

People under the influence of drugs or poisons may be uncooperative or violent. The EMT should protect himself or herself from injury first. The EMT should ensure that he or she, other rescuers, or hospital personnel are not exposed to the poison. In the case of many of the drugs described in this section, needles may be present; therefore the EMT should observe for drug paraphernalia. Drug abusers have an increased incidence of infectious diseases, so the EMT should protect himself or herself from exposure to any body fluids and avoid letting the patients cough or sneeze in his or her face.

Airway

The EMT should pay close attention to the patient's airway. Many substance abuse patients may have depressed respirations and their gag reflex may be unable to protect the airway. Aspiration is a common cause of death in overdose patients. The EMT should have suction ready and be prepared to turn the patient to the side to clear the airway.

Breathing

Since many substance abuse patients have depressed respirations, the EMT should pay close attention to the rate and depth of the patient's ventilations. If they are too slow or fast or if the breathing is too shallow, the EMT should supplement with 100% oxygen and a BVM.

Circulation

The EMT should pay close attention to the patient's vital signs. In significant overdose and poisonings, coma and death are possibilities. The EMT should avoid thinking that the patient will just "sleep it off" because it may be a sleep that the patient will never wake up from. The EMT should be prepared to perform CPR if necessary.

History

The EMT should try to bring samples of the poisons or drugs involved to the hospital. It may be helpful in determining the proper care at the hospital.

Summary

- Toxic emergencies arise from the adverse effects of plants, foods, chemicals, or drugs on the body. The body can be poisoned through oral, inhalation, absorption, or ingestion routes.
- Poisons and drugs can also enter the body by injection through insects, reptiles, sea animals, or needles.
- Poison control centers have resource information on all toxic substances, and the EMT should be familiar with the center in his or her area.

Summary (cont'd)

- General management involves collection of samples of the substance (unless it is dangerous to do so), support of the patient, and expeditious transportation to the nearest medical facility.

- With some poisons the EMT may use activated charcoal but will need to actively monitor and manage the airway in all of these patients.

Scenario Solution

Your partner records the patient's vital signs while you continue the history. You find that she has no physical complaints and she admits to having been depressed over problems with her boyfriend. She is otherwise healthy with no medical problems. She takes no prescription medications, has no allergies, and had dinner about an hour ago. Her vitals signs are as follows: heart rate 84 beats/min, ventilatory rate 20 breaths per minute, and blood pressure 124/80 mm Hg. Your protocol calls for activated charcoal with ingestion overdose and poisonings. She weighs at least 100 lb, so you shake the bottle well and assist her in taking 50 g of activated charcoal by mouth. You continue to monitor her en route to the hospital and notify the hospital about your patient, her history, and her condition.

Key Terms

Activated charcoal A form of charcoal with a high surface area, specially formulated to bind to substances; used to prevent absorption of swallowed substances from the intestine.
Antidotes An agent that directly blocks or reverses the effect of a poison.
Gastric lavage The use of a tube passed through the nose or mouth into the stomach to remove material from the stomach.
Material safety data sheet (MSDS) A government-prescribed form describing the actions and toxicities of substances used in the workplace.
Poison control centers A regional center that provides telephone poison information and advice to patients and health care providers.
Poisoning The method by which a food, plant, chemical, or drug has a toxic effect on the patient's body.

Review Questions

1. True or false: Activated charcoal is useful in any poisoning.
2. True or false: Most victims of poisoning are symptomatic at the time of the EMT's arrival.
3. Peak age incidences of poisoning include (select all correct answers):
   i. Toddlers
   ii. School-age children
   iii. Adolescents
   iv. Adults
   a. i, ii, and iii
   b. ii and iv
   c. i and iii
   d. All of the above
4. The greatest risk to the patient who has had a narcotic overdose is _____.
5. An excellent resource for poison information is a regional _____.
6. A common cause of death in overdose patients is:
   a. Cardiac arrest
   b. Aspiration
   c. Internal bleeding
   d. Cerebral hemorrhage
7. Of the following, which is a hallucinogenic drug?
   a. Amphetamines
   b. LSD
   c. Marijuana
   d. Barbiturates

Review Questions (cont'd)

8. Which of the following drugs can be smoked?
   a. Ice
   b. Crack
   c. Marijuana
   d. Hash
   e. Heroin
   f. All of the above
9. A drug that patients take to feel powerful and more capable to perform is:
   a. Amphetamine
   b. Qualudes
   c. Inhalants
   d. LSD
10. A drug that, in extreme cases, may cause patients to commit murder or suicide is:
    a. Cocaine
    b. Narcotics
    c. Benzodiazepines
    d. LSD

Answers to these Review Questions can be found at the end of the book on page 866.

20

Behavioral Emergencies

Lesson Goal

The goal of this chapter is to provide the EMT-Basic with the knowledge and tools to effectively assess and manage situations involving persons in behavioral crises.

Scenario

You arrive on the scene and find that the patient is a 36-year-old bookkeeper. He states that he has recurrent bouts of extreme fear of sudden onset, accompanied by sweating, shortness of breath, palpitations, chest pain, dizziness, numbness in his fingers and toes, and premonitions of death. He relates that these attacks occur unexpectedly and in a variety of situations many times per week. He refuses to drive because he is fearful that the attacks will reoccur; he also refuses to go to the grocery store for the same reason. He stopped working because the only place he felt comfortable was at home.

The case of the bookkeeper is a mental disorder known as a *panic attack* and in this case is associated with a fear of being in a crowded place. The symptoms that the patient describes are consistent with the condition but could also be related to a heart condition. You should talk calmly and deliberately to patient and convince him to come to the hospital for diagnosis and treatment.

 Is this a behavioral and/or psychiatric emergency? Is there an immediate threat to the patient's life? Is there a threat of violence toward the EMTs? Is suicide a consideration? How will you deal with this scenario? Does this patient need to be restrained?

Key Terms to Know

Activities of daily living
Behavior

Mental disorder

Organic brain syndrome

Psychogenic

355

Learning Objectives

As an EMT-Basic, you should be able to do the following:

DOT

- Demonstrate the assessment and emergency medical care of the patient experiencing a behavioral emergency.
- Demonstrate verious techniques to safely restrain a patient with a behavioral problem.
- Define *behavioral emergency*.
- List risk factors of potential suicide.
- State the medicolegal considerations involved with behaviorally and mentally ill patients including those of consent and restraint.
- Describe assessment of the potentially violent patient, including considerations of history, posture, vocal activity, and physical activity.
- Discuss the general factors that may cause an alteration in a patient's behavior.
- State the various reasons for psychological crisis.
- Discuss the special considerations for assessment of a patient with behavioral problems.
- Discuss methods to calm behavioral emergency patients.
- Describe management and emergency medical care of a patient undergoing a behavioral emergency.

Supplemental

- State the questions to be considered in assessing a behavioral emergency.
- List three major causes of behavioral emergencies.
- Describe the steps to conduct a mental status assessment.
- Describe the steps to conduct an initial assessment of a patient undergoing a behavioral emergency.
- List warning signs of potential suicide.

Current emergency medical technicians (EMTs) are more likely to encounter patients experiencing behavioral emergencies as increasing numbers of individuals, their families, and health care agencies (e.g., Help and Crisis hotlines) call the emergency medical services (EMS) systems. Emergency situations may present either as a psychologic self-perceived crisis or as a disruption of behavior that draws attention, concern, or upheaval in the immediate environment.

The situations that EMTs need to recognize immediately and that require emergency medical care are overdoses, either from drugs (medically prescribed or illicit) or other chemicals, and suicidal, self-destructive, or homicidal behavior.

In view of the often serious outcomes of some behavioral emergencies, EMTs dealing with these problems must have some effective way of responding to them. EMTs are often the first responders to situations involving persons in behavioral crises and must be trained in the management of behavioral crises.

Behavior

Behavior is simply how a person acts. Behavior is usually related to other persons or to the environment. Some behaviors are easy to observe, such as the expression of the emotion of joy on a person's face. Sometimes the behavior is complex, such as how one feels about another person. Love involves many emotions and feelings that are expressed by both outer and inner behaviors. Hugging is but one behavior that expresses the emotion of love; caressing is another.

EMTs encounter a wide variety of behaviors exhibited by patients and others. Some of these behaviors are positive and some are negative. Some indicate pathology of a psychiatric nature, and some are the result of sudden illness or trauma, drug or alcohol intoxication, sudden grief, or acute organic brain syndrome (also known as *organic mental disorder*). **Organic brain syndrome** is caused by a disturbance of physiologic functioning of brain tissue. Still other behaviors result from **psychogenic** causes, which are related to mental or psychic factors.

The causes of human behavior are complex, but they are not so mysterious that the EMT cannot understand them. The EMT must have a basic understanding of human behavior because of its importance in the emergency medical care of patients.

> ✓ *Behavior* is defined as how a person acts. Some behavior alterations are caused by sudden illness or trauma, low blood sugar level, lack of oxygen, excessive cold or heat, drug or alcohol intoxication, or sudden grief. Behaviors can also be caused by organic brain syndrome (or organic mental disorder), a disturbance of the physiologic function of the brain. Others are caused by psychogenic causes, or causes related to mental or psychic factors.

Behavioral Emergencies

Behavior is the outwardly observable action of a person responding to the environment. Most of the time, behavior reflects reasonable responses to what is going on in the environment. People learn to adapt to a variety of situations involving **activities of daily living** (ADL), which are usually accomplished during a normal day (e.g., eating, dressing, and washing). This process of adaptation is called *adjustment*. For the most part, people adjust to various stresses and strains in the environment. However, sometimes the stress is so great that normal adjustment mechanisms do not work. Under enormous stress, behavior is likely to change, even if only for that situation. In some of these instances, the behavior practiced may not be fully appropriate.

A behavioral emergency is any reaction to events that interferes with ADL. For that particular time, and perhaps only for that time, a behavioral emergency exists for that person. If that interruption of daily routine tends to reoccur on a somewhat regular basis, then that behavior may be considered a mental health problem. The behavior exhibited is more than an isolated incident and has now developed into a pattern.

When a behavioral emergency becomes more serious, it is classified as a **mental disorder**. A mental disorder is an illness with psychologic or behavioral manifestations and/or impairment in functioning as a result of social, psychologic, genetic, physical/chemical, or biologic disturbance. A mental disorder is not limited to relationships between the person and society. A mental disorder is characterized by symptoms and/or impairment in functioning.

A behavioral emergency also becomes a cause of concern when the person's response to a situation (e.g., the death of a spouse) causes a major life interruption, such as an act of attempted suicide. The disruption can take many forms, some of which may represent a threat to both the person involved and others in the immediate vicinity (e.g., family, friends, bystanders, and EMTs).

> ✓ A behavioral emergency is any reaction to events that interferes with ADL. A psychiatric emergency is a reaction to events that causes a major life interruption.

Magnitude of Mental Health Problems

According to the National Institute of Mental Health (NIMH), one in five Americans has a mental disorder. A mental health illness or disorder is a disturbance of emotional equilibrium that interferes with ADL. Given the percentage of Americans suffering from mental illness and the higher number that will experience a behavioral crisis, the EMT can expect to deal with these problems in the field on a somewhat regular basis.

Some of these crises may be temporary, such as a person's reaction to a traumatic event, a decrease of oxygen or glucose to the brain, or the pain experienced during a heart attack (myocardial infarction). During a crisis, people react in various ways and behavior is but one reflection of how they adjust. Therefore all abnormal or disturbing behavior is not indicative of mental illness. If an individual displays abnormal behavior for an extended period of time, the behavior is a cause for concern from a mental health standpoint.

Many people experience varying degrees of mental health problems from time to time. Most people have traces of the symptoms and signs described in this chapter. The EMT should not assume that he or she, or for that matter a patient for whom he or she iscaring, is mentally disturbed if some of the behaviors identified here are observed.

The most common misconception about mental illness is that if a person is feeling "blue," the person has a problem. Divorce; death of a spouse, loved one, or friend; and loss of a job are all perfectly justifiable reasons for feeling depressed. For the teenager who just broke up with his girlfriend with whom he had been close for the past 12 months, it is normal to withdraw from his ordinary activities and feel sad. These feelings are normal reactions to crisis situations. However, when the "Monday morning blues" continue, then a mental disorder or behavioral crisis exists. *Monday morning blues* is a term used to describe how some people express their being sad or "down." Sometimes this is also referred to as *the blues, the uglies, the miseries, the black cloud,* or *the fogs*. Many people feel that persons with mental health disorders are dangerous, violent, or otherwise unmanageable. However, only a small percentage of people who have mental health problems fall into these latter categories.

EMTs should be aware that situations calling for intervention in the prehospital environment may expose them to a higher proportion of violent patients. Emergency situations often involve circumstances that have gone beyond the management capability of the family or others involved. In addition, the use or abuse of alcohol or other drugs or a long-term history of mental disorder may contribute to a violent patient reaction. The ability to predict violence is an important assessment tool of the EMT and is discussed later in this chapter.

> ✓ Many misconceptions about mental disorders exist. Although many people have mental disorders, not all disturbing or abnormal behavior is characteristic of a mental disorder. Not all people with mental disorders are violent.

Patient Care Algorithm

Altered Mental Status Patient Assessment

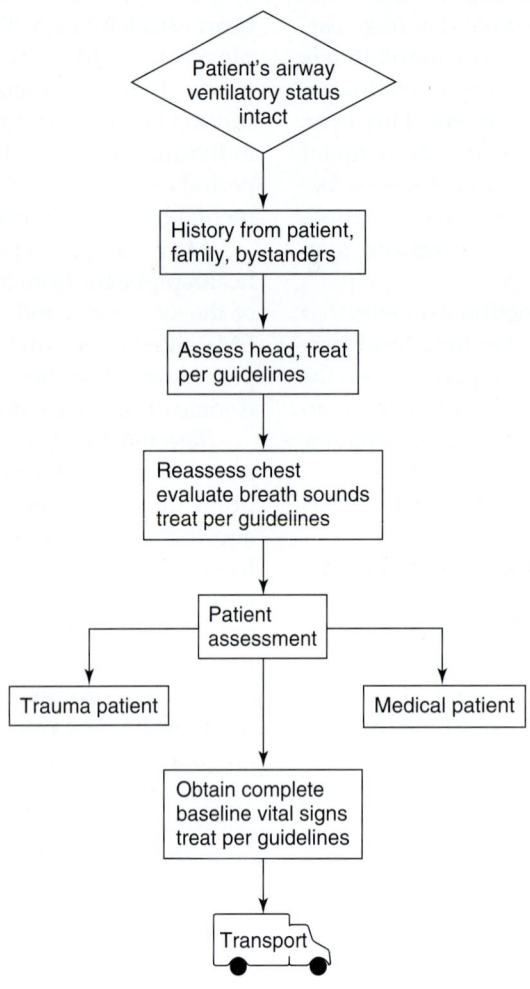

Assessment of Behavioral Emergencies

In assessing a behavioral emergency, the key observation to keep in mind is the patient's sense of reality. Is the patient's perception of reality compromised or distorted? When a behavioral crisis occurs, the patient's capability (innate adequacy, training, and physiologic state) and basic needs are stressed beyond reason. The result, either temporarily in the case of an acute illness or in the long term in more complex mental illness cases, renders the person incapable of making a reasonable response to the current environmental demands.

The EMT next needs to consider possible causative factors. The major areas to consider (or to question) are as follows:

- Is there inadequate cerebral oxygen? Possibilities to consider are diabetic problems (particularly lack of glucose in the body), trauma (including blood loss), and poisoning.
- Are hallucinogens, other drugs, or alcohol involved?
- Are circumstances of a psychogenic nature involved? Examples include major life interruption and death of a loved one.
- Does the patient have a history of mental illness?

- Does the patient show signs of severe depression?
- Does the patient make suicidal threats?

These major indicators, plus other data gathered by the EMT from family, friends, and observers, usually provide the basic information needed to assess these situations. The EMT is not required to determine the exact causes of the current crisis. The EMT's goals are recognizing major life threats and reducing the stress of situations as much as possible.

In assessing a patient involved in a behavioral emergency, the same initial principals apply as for any other patient. The EMT should first assess the ABCs—airway, breathing, and circulation. The signs and symptoms of acute behavioral emergencies are many, and particular syndromes have unique qualities and characteristics. Particular syndromes are discussed later in this chapter. Initially, the EMT should consider how the patient now being cared for is responding to his or her environment. Is the behavior typical or normal for what is going on? If the patient has just been assaulted, good reason exists for that patient to be fearful of those around him or the EMT. On the other hand, if the patient states that he or she is from the planet Venus or is "in heaven" when the EMT asks if the patient knows where he or she is, then the EMT can reasonably conclude that the patient is disoriented, regardless of the cause.

The EMT should consider the following questions while evaluating the patient in terms of a behavioral or psychiatric emergency:

- How does this patient relate to you?
- Are your questions answered appropriately? Is the patient withdrawn or detached?
- Is the patient hostile or friendly? Overly friendly?
- Does the patient understand why you are there?
- How is the patient dressed? Is the dress appropriate for the time of the year and occasion? Are the clothes clean or dirty?
- Are the patient's movements coordinated or jerky and awkward? Is the patient hyperactive?
- Are the patient's movements purposeful (e.g., in putting on his or her clothes)? Are the actions aimless, like sitting and rocking back and forth in a chair?
- Has the patient harmed himself or herself? Is there damage to the surroundings?
- Does the patient present as physically rigid or is there waxy flexibility (often present in catatonic schizophrenics in which the patient's arm or leg remains in the position in which it is placed)? Does the patient appear relaxed, stiff, or guarded?
- What are the patient's facial expressions? Are they bland and flat or expressive? Does the patient show joy, fear, or anger to appropriate stimuli and to what degree?
- Are the patient's vocabulary and expressions what you would expect under the circumstances? Are they related to the patient's social and educational background?

It may not be possible for the EMT to gather all of the information suggested in the questions above. Sometimes a patient undergoing a behavioral emergency will not respond at all. In those cases, observing the patient's emotional state via facial expressions, pulse and respiratory rates, tears, sweating, and blushing may be significant indicators.

Mental Status Assessment

The mental status of a patient undergoing a mental health crisis is usually diagnostically important in assessment. Assessing the mental status of a patient begins with the EMT's observations of the patient. The specific information that is important in assessing a patient's mental status involves two major areas: the patient's behavior during the interview and the patient's sensorium (area of brain responsible for receiving sensory data).

Interview Behavior

Interview behavior includes the following:

- How the patient relates to you. Is the patient friendly or hostile? Are the patient's statements coherent? Is the patient aware that you are questioning him?
- The patient's general appearance and grooming. Is the patient reasonably clean and dressed under the circumstances? Consider this example:

> A patient has several weeks of beard growth, and his body and clothes are dirty. Upon checking records and statements from other people, including his son, you find out that he is president of a successful manufacturing firm in your community. The son informs you that he seemed to be functioning normally until a few weeks ago. A possible diagnosis in this case is severe depression.

Motor Behavior

Motor behavior includes the patient's posture, stride, physical presence (i.e., carriage), and facial expressions. Is the patient moving in a coordinated way? Are the patient's movements jerky or smooth? Is the patient hyperactive? Hypoactive? Do the patient's movements have purpose or are they aimless? Are the patient's facial expressions appropriate to the circumstances? Do the patient's facial expressions change with the subject being discussed? If the patient displays joy or happiness, is it with reason?

Thought Content

What the patient volunteers unprompted best evaluates thought content. Does the patient speak before being asked a question? The EMT should let the patient talk without interruption before he or she begins to ask questions. If the patient appears quiet and does not speak, the EMT should ask some simple questions, such as the following:

- What is bothering you?
- What worries you today?
- What has happened today?
- Do you feel that you are in trouble? Do you want help?

The EMT should note the patient's inability to respond or evade answers; these are as significant as what the patient does say. Questions that are particularly important are those related to suicidal or homicidal thoughts. Preoccupation with such ideas is symptomatic of depression or extremely hostile behavior. Questions asked by the EMT of a patient such as "Do you feel so down that you have thought about killing yourself or someone else?" may provide the EMT with important, even self-saving information.

To determine whether a patient's thinking is OK, the EMT should ask questions such as "What is the difference between apples and oranges?" If the patient says that one is usually red and the other is orange, that both are fruits and can be eaten, or that both grow on trees, the EMT can assume that the patient's higher cerebral functioning is in order. On the other hand, if the patient answers that they are the weapons of the devil and are poisonous, then the EMT can conclude that such statements are bizarre and suggest pathology of some sort.

Words that have no logical connection to one another, such as "The street next year March moon and I love hate the beach," is called *word salad* and typifies mental illness, probably of the schizophrenic variety. If the patient uses other bizarre speech patterns, such as made up words (e.g., pratacataGod) or echolalia, in which the patient echoes your question (e.g., "Name, my name, my name, my name?"), there is a loosening association. Another such pattern is clang (e.g., "Name, my name is Dick, here's the stick, give it a lick.").

The EMT can ask many questions to gauge a patient's thought processes. The EMT does not need to do an extensive test. Checking responses to several simple questions that are appropriate to the situation will give the EMT enough data to determine thought that is within normal boundaries. The EMT should note answers to the questions that suggest abnormality and report the answers to the emergency department. The physician will make definitive or specific causative factors and psychiatric diagnoses. The EMT must be alert to the possibilities that may have caused such disordered thought process (e.g., trauma, drug overdose, alcohol intoxication, diabetic reaction, hyperthermia, electrolyte imbalance, or mental illness). The EMT may not be able to do much to solve the underlying problem, but in some cases the actions of the EMT may be life saving. An example is in recognizing and managing hemorrhagic shock or providing a sugar-enriched juice drink to the conscious diabetic patient who shows signs of hypoglycemia (low blood sugar).

Speech

Observing the patient's speech and voice quality can be revealing evidence of an altered mental state. Consider these characteristics:

- *Intensity*. Is the speech too loud or too soft?
- *Pitch*. Is the voice flat and dreary or does it vary unrestrained?
- *Speed*. Is the speech very slow or very fast?
- *Ease*. Does the patient speak naturally, reluctantly, or as if he or she is under tension?

The EMT does not need to carry out an intensive examination of speech patterns. Observing and noting variations and differences in the voice and speech quality is sufficient.

Orientation

Orientation times three includes orientation to *time* (date or time of day), *place* (where the patient is located), and *person* (who the patient is). These are the important questions used to partially determine the status of the patient's sensorium. These particular questions test the patient's recent memory. Sense of time is the first orientation to diminish, followed by sense of place and a person's ability to remember his or her name. The information derived from an orientation check is important for the emergency department physician.

A patient who thinks that the year is 1910 initially and then 15 minutes later tells the EMT that it is 2000 shows evidence of brain pathology. If the same patient is also disoriented to time and place, something else may be involved (e.g., a space-occupying lesion in the brain). On the other hand, a person who is considered schizophrenic when questioned about place may tell the EMT that he or she lives on the moon, but when pressed will admit where he or she really is.

The following series of questions may help the EMT assess orientation:

- Time: What time of day is it? What day of the week is this? What month? What year?
- Place: Where are you now? What place is this?
- Person: What is your name? Who are you?

Affect

Observations of a patient's affect or emotions are usually apparent. Is the patient attentive, apathetic, or indifferent to what is going on around him or her? Are the patient's emotional reactions appropriate to the subject under discussion? If the patient does not report feelings easily, the EMT should ask questions designed to determine his or her feeling state, such as "Are you mad, in pain, depressed, fearful, or happy?" When there is no response, the EMT should observe such signs as facial expressions, perspiration, pulse and ventilatory rates, tears, eye contact, and so on. Emotions are best described by the patient in his or her own words. The EMT should note inconsistencies.

Proficiency

The ability of the patient to maintain mental status is an important factor in determining the nature of the presenting problem. From the EMT's standpoint, if the patient was speaking reasonably well and then his or her speaking diminishes, something is wrong. That behavior is probably related to an organic problem. If the patient was conscious initially, passes out for 2 minutes, regains consciousness, and then passes out again for 2 minutes, it is likely from another cause. The EMT does not need to determine what is going on with this patient. The EMT must instead recognize any life-threatening conditions that may be involved, manage those in accordance with local protocols, note the behaviors observed, and report them to the emergency department.

Primary and Secondary Psychologic Crises

Although EMTs do not diagnose mental disorders, it may be helpful to identify the basic categories along with illustrative cases. The basic categories are as follows:

- Acute anxiety
- Phobia
- Depression
- Suicide (self-destructive acts)
- Paranoia
- Disorientation
- Disorganization

Acute Anxiety

Case #1

Gerald Anderson brings his wife Mary to the emergency department, reporting that he "cannot take her anymore" (Figure 20.1). This emergency department admission cli-

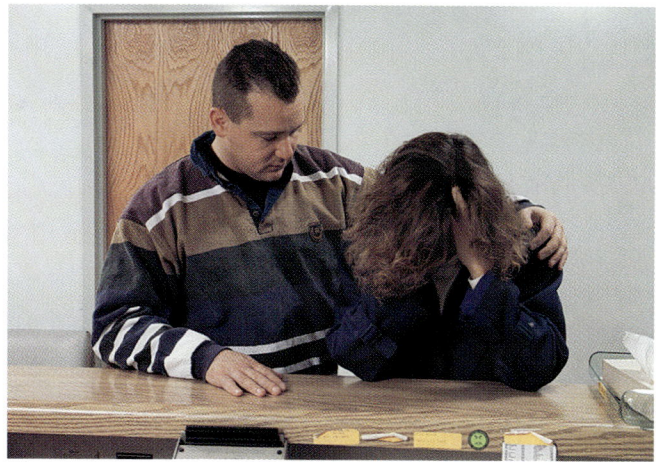

FIGURE 20.1 Seeking medical care is important for a patient who has been under a great deal of anxiety.

maxes a stressful month during which Mrs. Anderson has become progressively more anxious. Although she describes herself as a "tense" person and takes pride in being an immaculate housekeeper, both qualities have dramatically escalated since her last child, Paula, left home for marriage. Since that time she has had trouble sleeping and has demanded that her husband spend all of his time with her. She compulsively and thoroughly cleans the house and worries a great deal. She has been to several physicians for vague physical complaints and concerns. None of the physicians has found anything wrong, although one prescribed a minor tranquilizer. She restricts her activities to the home and "cannot sit still." Mr. Anderson has become increasingly concerned. His wife makes him, their friends, and the children uneasy by her pacing, cleaning, and worrying. Activity brings her no relief. She decides that electricity is in the faucet and commences to touch the faucet continually.

In acute anxiety cases, patients often present as upset, fearful, tense, restless, and tremulous. Anxiety affects physiology. Some patients hyperventilate marked by a decreased level of carbon dioxide (CO_2) in the blood and experienced by the patient as faintness, tingling in the extremities, cardiac palpitations, and dyspnea. The pulse rate increases and blood pressure elevates. Perspiration and muscle tenseness are common clinical signs. The patient may report many bodily ills, be unable to concentrate, and feel overwhelmed. Time for this patient is extended—seconds seem like minutes, and minutes seem like hours. Patients suffering from anxiety find that emotions color all of their activities and severely alter their lives. Anxiety rapidly becomes the focus of their lives, clouding family relationships and work life. Anxiety immediately affects mood, perceptions, and behavior. Anxious patients fear being alone. They often channel their anxiety into a concern about their health. Generally, the

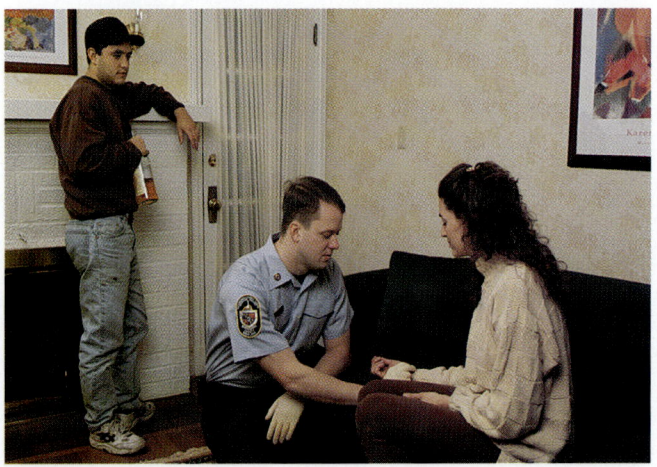

FIGURE 20.2 Being sensitive to a patient's potential fears will help develop trust between the EMT and the patient.

anxiety patient demands immediate care. It is not unusual from the presenting signs and symptoms for others around this patient to become anxious as well.

Emergency medical treatment by the EMT involves the following:

- Appreciating and considering the patient's anxiety
- Maintaining immediate and steady presence
- Offering a structured response that includes physical containment; the ambulance is one of those containments because it provides both boundaries to the patient and the hope of medical treatment (i.e., emergency medical treatment and transportation to the emergency department)
- Continually interacting with the patient, which provides the human contact needed by the patient at this time

Phobia

Case #2

Mrs. Gladys Beaudoin has developed an overwhelming fear of leaving her house. When she even thinks of a trip to the store, she feels anxious; when she finds herself outside, she panics (Figure 20.2). As a result, she now refuses to leave the house and has become a prisoner in her own home. Her family has grown concerned about her behavior and urges her to get help. Mrs. Beaudoin's fears began 3 years ago when this 35-year-old housewife and mother of three experienced an episode of dizziness and nearly fainted while driving alone to a new market. At that moment she thought she was going to die. Despite her family physician's pronouncement of excellent health and his prescription of Valium, she dreads another attack and vows never to drive alone. Her family and friends understand and provide her with traveling companions. Mrs. Beaudoin's fears had been building for some time. At about the time of the episode of dizziness, she and her 44-year-old husband had quarreled about their relationship. Their last child had just entered first grade. Mrs. Beaudoin had participated extensively in the activities of her church. Her widowed mother, who lives in a neighboring community, disapproved of Mrs. Beaudoin's plans to complete college. Around this time Mrs. Beaudoin became uncomfortable in stores and looked for exit signs. She worried about being in the supermarket checkout line and sat by the door in restaurants. She stopped visiting her friends. Then finally she stopped driving.

Phobic patients develop major emotional reactions. These responses include anxiety, depression, and panic. The phobic patient likely will be anxious, reluctant, and suspicious and, depending on the particular phobia, may show unnatural fears of what most people would consider normal activities, such as walking outside. Phobic patients display a variety of reactions depending on the nearness of the feared object (e.g., insects) or situation (e.g., heights). When successful in avoiding the feared thing, the patient feels fine and functions normally. As the patient anticipates the object or situation, he or she becomes anxious, frightened, and sometimes depressed.

> ✓ A phobia is sometimes described as fear looking at itself in the mirror.

Anxiety is the main emotional experience for the phobic patient and is often very intense. When meeting the dreaded object or situation directly, the phobic patient may experience tremendous terror and panic. Sometimes he or she believes that the encounter will result in insanity, loss of control, or death. The phobic patient centers all activities on avoidance of the feared object or situation. Emergency medical treatment by the EMT involves the following:

- Responding to the patient based on the particular presenting features of the phobic incident
- When introducing himself or herself, using his or her formal name and professional title (e.g., My name is Mary Smith and I am an emergency medical technician); this introduction also helps reduce misidentification
- Assuring the patient that he or she will not die or go insane.
- Maintaining a firm, controlled, and confident posture.
- Explaining the purpose of his or her intervention and emergency medical treatment.
- Remaining with the patient at all times.

TABLE 20.1 Some Commonly Prescribed Medications for Psychiatric Disorders

	Trade names
Antianxiety	
Benzodiazepines	Ativan, Klonopin, Librium, Serax, Tanxene, Valium, Xanax
Antidepressants	
Tricyclic (and similar compounds)	Ascendin, Aventyl, Elavil, Wellbutrin
SSRIs	Effexor, Prozac, Serzone
Antipsychotics	
Phenothiazines	Mellaril, Prolixin, Serentil, Stelazine, Thorazine, Trilafon
Thioxanthenes	Navane
Dihydroindolone	Moban
Dibenzoxazepine	Clozaril
Butyrophenone	Haldol
Benzisoxazole	Risperdal
Thienbenzodiazepine	Zyprexa

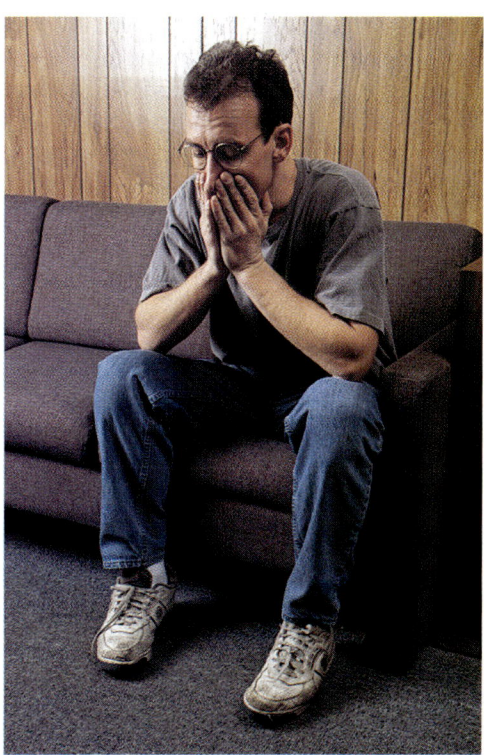

FIGURE 20.3 Depression can affect anyone at any time. In many cases the depressed patient wants to be left alone.

Depression

Case #3

Paul Jacobwitz has noticed something wrong with himself ever since he and his wife separated (Figure 20.3). He experiences difficulty at work because of loss of interest and an inability to concentrate. He cannot fall asleep, and when he does he awakes early without a sense of being refreshed. He worries a great deal, drinks too much, does not eat, has lost 20 pounds, lacks interest in sex, and feels unhappy. He finds his days intolerable, interminable, and oppressive. He views his future with despair and wonders about suicide. He feels guilty for a variety of past and present indiscretions and obsessively reflects on his separation from his wife and two children. He alternately blames himself and his wife. He misses his two children. His mood is sad, his world is empty, and his future is bleak.

The severely depressed patient wants to be left alone; may be huddled in a corner, crying uncontrollably; or may be totally unresponsive. This patient may feel worthless, withdrawn, sad, and guilty. Generally, the depressed patient feels that no one can understand his or her problems and that the problems are not solvable. These patients generate moods of hopelessness and sadness in others.

Many psychiatric conditions may include depression. Depression may be particularly difficult to recognize in the geriatric patient because it may mimic dementia. Any time the EMT encounters a depressed patient, the possibility of suicide must be considered.

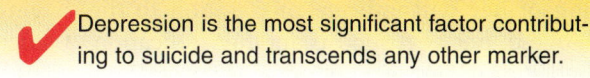
Depression is the most significant factor contributing to suicide and transcends any other marker.

Depression is a disturbance of mood. The person feels down and experiences profound sadness. Lack of color and chronic fatigue dominate his or her life. The depressed patient views his or her world as hopeless and his or her plight as helpless. Perceptual changes in depressed patients include a sense of alienation, pessimism, guilt, loss of the future, and a hazy sense of the future. Sleep disturbances are common. Some patients sleep virtually all the time, but despite a considerable amount of sleep, they still complain about being tired. Others find great difficulty in getting to or staying asleep. Sleep deprivation leads to exhaustion and an inability to concentrate and work effectively. Appetite, sexual activity, and intellectual function are often affected. Abuse of alcohol and drugs is common.

Care of this patient by the EMT involves the following:

- Providing a firm and controlled approach and imposing order on the situation

- Frequently providing personal identification
- Taking clear command of the situation
- Removing dangerous implements, with law enforcement control as necessary
- Stating and repeating the intervention plan
- Remaining with the patient at all times

Suicide

Case #4

Sarah sits alone in her apartment with a bottle of aspirin. She has not been eating or sleeping well, has been drinking more than usual, and has been depressed. Last week she called her closest friend and asked her if she would serve as a witness to her will and as executrix of her estate. She told her friend that if anything ever happened to her, her valuable papers were in a safe depository box at a local savings bank and that she had authorized her friend to have a key. Sarah has just broken up with her boyfriend, Jim, whom she has known for 3 years. She called Jim a few hours ago and said good-bye and that she was leaving. When he called back a half hour later and got no answer, he called the police. The police and the boyfriend arrived at her apartment within minutes of one another and found Sarah on the floor in a state of sluggishness with an empty 500-count bottle of 500 mg aspirin tablets next to her (Figure 20.4). When questioned, Sarah responded weakly and asked them all to leave.

This patient has attempted suicide. Calls made by patient's like Sarah often precede suicide attempts and are referred to as "cries for help." Sarah's arrangements and writing of her will indicate preparation to die. Saying good-bye to her boyfriend is another indication of suicidal behavior. Depression is a major factor in suicide attempts. The EMT should attempt to talk with this patient in a calm manner, try to remove the bottles of pills and aspirin from the patient, and encourage the patient to go to the hospital. If the patient refuses, the EMT should request law enforcement assistance.

 Depression is the most significant factor contributing to suicide.

Suicide threats indicate that a person is in a crisis that he or she cannot handle. Thorough, immediate care is necessary. In many cases suicide threats represent a form of communication, often a cry for help.

The EMT must assess the risk of suicide. The following are risk factors for attempted suicide:

- Depression, any age
- Individuals over 40 years of age, especially males
- Lack of strong emotional bonds
- Recent loss of spouse, significant other, or family member
- Chronic debilitating illness
- Financial setback or loss of job
- Previous suicide attempt
- Family history of suicide
- Substance abuse
- Child of alcoholic parent
- Mental disorder (e.g., paranoia)
- Recent diagnosis of serious illness
- Arrest or imprisonment
- A defined lethal plan of action that has been verbalized

The EMT must assess the risk of suicide to determine the probability of completion of this act. The EMT should be alert to the following warning signs of a suicide attempt:

- Is depression a factor?
- Is there an aura of profound despair, hopelessness, or both?
- Does the patient avoid eye contact, speak slowly or haltingly, and in general project a sense of almost literal "vacancy," as if he or she really is not there?
- Does the patient exhibit an inability to talk about future plans? Patients who are suicidal consider the future so uninteresting that they do not think about it. Asking the patient if he or she has vacation plans may lead to a preliminary assessment. The patient who is seriously depressed will not be able to fantasize about events that far ahead.
- Is there an allusion to suicide? Even vague suggestions should not be taken lightly, even if offered in a joking context. If you think that suicide is a possibility, do not hesitate to bring up the subject out of fear that you may be giving the patient ideas.

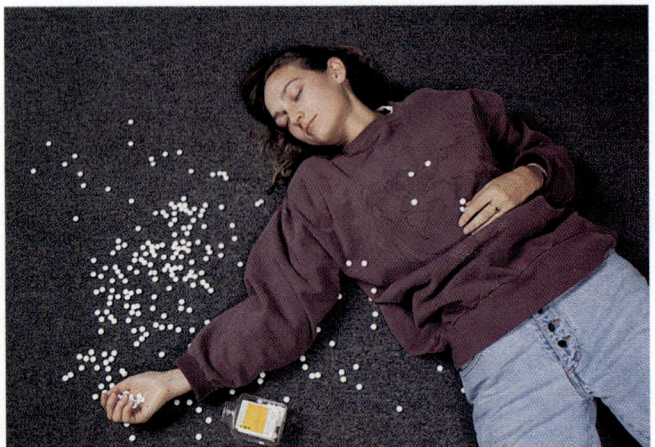

FIGURE 20.4 Overdose of medicine is a common risk factor of attempted suicide.

- Does the patient have a specific suicide plan? Critical warning signs include recently preparing a will, advising close friends what to do with significant possessions, and arranging for funeral services.

The suicidal patient may be homicidal as well. The EMT should do nothing to frighten the patient or arouse suspicion. The EMT should not jeopardize his or her life or members of the emergency unit. In these cases, police intervention is absolutely required.

Paranoia

Case #5

A 911 dispatcher receives a call from a frantic woman who says her husband has threatened to kill her, their children, and his boss. He is reported to be drunk, is shouting obscenities, is looking for his gun, and says that he is also going to commit suicide (Figure 20.5). He states that his mother and father both hated him and that everyone has been against him ever since he can remember. He believes that his boss, family, and friends are conspiring against him. He has said that he thinks his wife is seeing another man. When he heard his wife talking to his boss, he reacted with intense rage, pulled the phone out of the wall, and swung it at his wife. During this outburst he threatened to kill his wife. His wife left the house and went to the neighbor's house to telephone the police. He is known to react with rage when a major conflict comes into his life, and his drinking has increased steadily over the past year. He is worried about being able to support his family and dislikes his job as a janitor, which he considers demeaning and unproductive.

This man is experiencing a major life interruption and is delusional about what is *really* going on. His sense of reality seems to be distorted because he blames others for possible personal inadequacies. This patient is having an acute emotional and mental breakdown, and his behavior is not within the normal range of response.

Assessment of this patient's behavior suggests some form of paranoia. Patients who are paranoid often suffer delusions and believe that people are "out to get them." Their hostility may intensify when EMS personnel intrude on their "personal space." Paranoia is characterized by an intricate and internally logical system of persecutory and/or grandiose delusions. Signs and symptoms of paranoia include the following:

- Distrust
- Jealousy
- Seclusiveness
- Hostile behavior and uncooperativeness

This individual is also stating both self-destructive and homicidal threats and as a result poses additional problems and dangers for all persons coming into contact with him, including EMTs. The EMT in a situation like this should withdraw from the scene and encourage others present to do so and call for law enforcement intervention. In cases of this kind in which no immediate danger or threat to life exists, emergency medical treatment by the EMT involves the following:

- Taking command of the situation and ensuring that there is adequate back-up
- When introducing himself or herself, using his or her formal name and professional title (e.g., My name is Mary Smith and I am an emergency medical technician); this introduction also helps reduce misidentification; it is helpful for the EMTs to remind the patient of their identification during the time that they are rendering treatment
- Approaching the patient in a nonthreatening way and maintaining a safe distance (e.g., 6 to 8 feet)
- Having the proper number of personnel available to control violence (if necessary); a key rule is to display force before it is employed; the greater number of personnel, the faster and more easily the restraint will be achieved

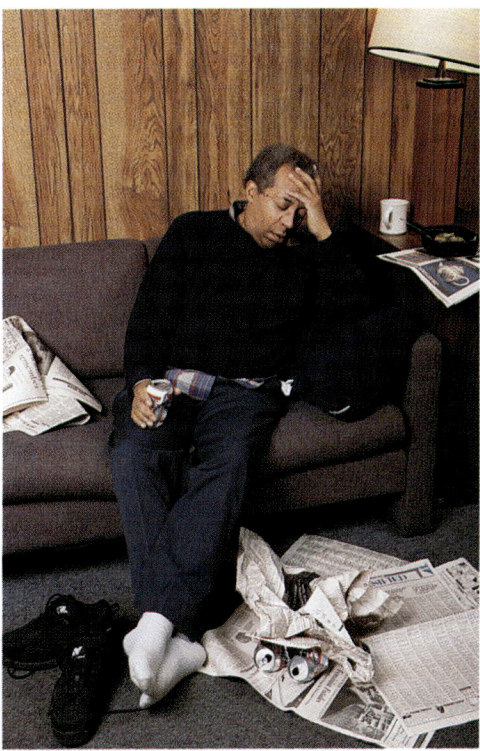

FIGURE 20.5 Patients presenting with self-destructive behavior can pose problems for everyone who comes in contact with them.

- Explaining the purpose of the intervention and emergency medical treatment
- Remaining with the patient at all times

Disorientation and Disorganization

Case #6 (Disorientation)

At 71 years of age, Joe Carluccio feels strangely remote from life (Figure 20.6). He strikes out at his wife for no apparent reason, spontaneously cries for a few minutes, and loses his way while taking a walk in the neighborhood. His speech is rambling, his dress is shabby, and he constantly reminisces about the war. He becomes confused at night, fails to recognize Mrs. Carluccio, occasionally forgets things (e.g., leaves the stove on), and makes up stories. Mr. Carluccio retired as an accountant 6 years ago. At the time he had noticed that he made "stupid" errors. Since then he has had further difficulty in doing even simple calculations. He has also lost interest in many activities such as playing bridge, attending movies, and seeing friends. In his youth he was thrifty; now he has become a miser. His behavior has deteriorated over the past month—he gets lost, stays up all night, hallucinates, and becomes belligerent and agitated.

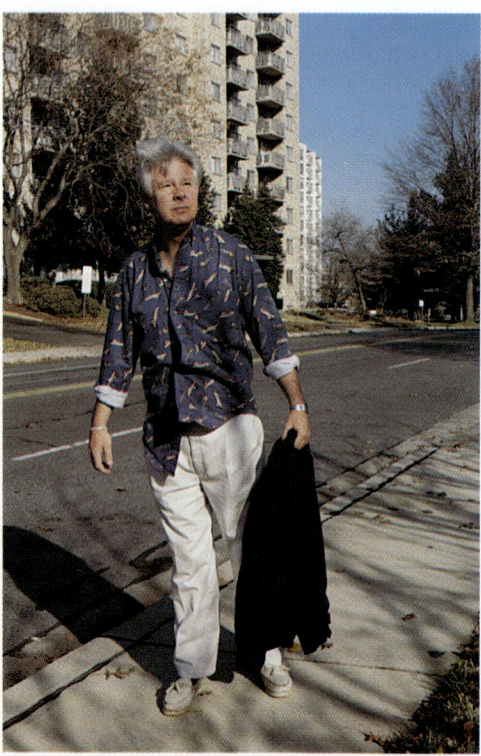

FIGURE 20.6 Patients experiencing disorientation may present with rambling speech, confusion, and shabby dress.

Case #7 (Disorganization)

Jonathan Hatcher is a freshman in college. He is sitting in his dormitory room blankly starring at the wall (Figure 20.7). He barely acknowledges his roommate's presence, responds to questions only in one-word sentences, and does not speak spontaneously. Occasionally he launches into long, illogical discourses about the Devil, acid rain, and department stores. His freshman year is about to end in 1 week. Jonathan graduated from secondary school at the top of his class. Although he was a "loner," people liked him and he had participated in many activities. He experienced a "down" period during his junior year. During his first year in college he became aloof and vague, and his mysterious thinking became apparent to his close associates. He now ponders several levels of thought and attends a variety of religious functions. He says that for the past week he "knows" that a particular professor is "out to get him" and to "control his mind." He spends long hours alone in his room on weekends and even during vacations. He reports hearing voices arguing in his head and later says that thoughts from "level seven clash there." He is convinced that the school newspaper contains messages intended for him. His mood swings have become extreme. He quarrels with his roommate without provocation. At times he thinks he and his roommate are the same person. He has stopped going to classes.

Disorientation and disorganization are characterized by varying degrees of loss with reality. One or more of the normal lines between this person and the world have broken down. This person may not be able to distinguish among voices, noises, sights, smells, and other perceptions, some of which may now exist in the imagination. This person may not be aware of feelings toward other individuals and may be unable to distinguish between the perception carried inside his or her mind and what really exists outside. The disoriented patient often displays a variety of unpredictable emotions. These range from depression to anxiety, from a dulled quality to terrible rage, from anger and suspicion to calmness, and from passion of feeling to shallowness. Disoriented patients often feel depressed.

In Mr. Carluccio's case, the disorientation could be the result of dementia, cerebrovascular disease, or dementia of the Alzheimer's type. In Jonathan's case, more disorganization of the personality is involved.

Jonathan seems to have lost awareness of the position of self in relation to space, time, or other persons. Jonathan's thought processes are inappropriate to his surroundings, and he has been steadily withdrawing from normal day-to-day activities. Some of his thoughts are bizarre and delusional. He also thinks that people are out to get him, indicating some delusional trends. Hearing voices is another sign of detachment.

Jonathan is likely suffering from a *schizophrenia* manifested by thought disorder marked by a deep disturbance of thoughts and their integration. Jonathan's behavior is noticeable by disturbances in his mood, perceptions, and behavior. Schizophrenia saturates all aspects of one's behavior. Patients with this mental illness display some of these mood problems throughout their lives; others have late manifestations. These patients often exhibit flat affect (e.g., no outward display of emotions), inappropriate affect (e.g., inappropriate behavioral responses to the conditions at the time), elements of both depression and anxiety, and detachment. A patient displaying these signs and symptoms who is in a schizophrenic crisis requires a clear, solid, and directed response from the EMTs. The EMT must address the patient's disorganization with a structured approach. An approach to a patient in this condition involves the following:

- Promptly responding
- Unmistakably identifying himself or herself so that the patient does not misidentify the EMT as an agent of others
- Containment, recognizing the patient's reaction
- Orienting the patient to the plan of emergency medical treatment,
- Controlling violence (with law enforcement intervention, if necessary)
- Avoiding excess stimulation, which may be accomplished by limiting the number of responders who deal with the patient
- Staying with the patient at all times

Care of the disoriented patient by the EMT involves the following:

- Providing a firm and controlled approach and imposing order on the situation
- Frequently offering personal identification
- Taking clear command of the situation
- Removing dangerous implements, with law enforcement control as necessary
- Stating and repeating the intervention plan
- Remaining with the patient at all times

Alzheimer's Disease

The incidence of Alzheimer's disease is increasing in the older adult population, and it is believed that 10% of Americans may have the disease. Alzheimer's disease results from an accumulation of plaque around nerves and unusual bundles of cells in the cerebral cortex, the part of the brain responsible for memory and reason. A person with Alzheimer's disease lives an average of 8 years after diagnosis, although many live longer. During this period the patient grows forgetful, suffers personality changes, and loses the ability to perform ADL tasks, such as shopping, preparing meals, or driving a car. In the final stages, patients often become incontinent and mute and are unable to recognize friends and family members.

> ✓ Memory loss, asking repeated questions, trouble using words, confusion, and disorientation are classic indications of Alzheimer's disease.

Patient's with Alzheimer's disease often have behavioral problems that accompany the disease. Agitation, rage, paranoia, and hallucinations are common behavioral problems and often the first signs of the disease. Some patients with Alzheimer's disease become apathetic and do not speak unless spoken to. Others act like unruly children, saying no to every request. Still others exhibit signs of depression (e.g., feelings of sadness or hopelessness or disruptions of eating and sleeping patterns). Some patients become fixated on certain tasks, such as turning off and on lights or washing dishes; some may hide and hoard food. Possibly because of becoming over-tired, patients' behavioral problems may worsen in the evening in what is known as the "sundown syndrome." It seems to occur more frequently with patients who suffer from dementia. Many people with Alzheimer's disease have low sleep efficiency, spend a high percentage of sleep time in "early sleep time," and experience more arousals and awakening. Some of the reversible causes involve drug-related toxicity, infections, dehydration, and drug-drug interactions. Napping during the day may help consolidate the sleep schedule, but a long nap may interfere with nighttime sleep.

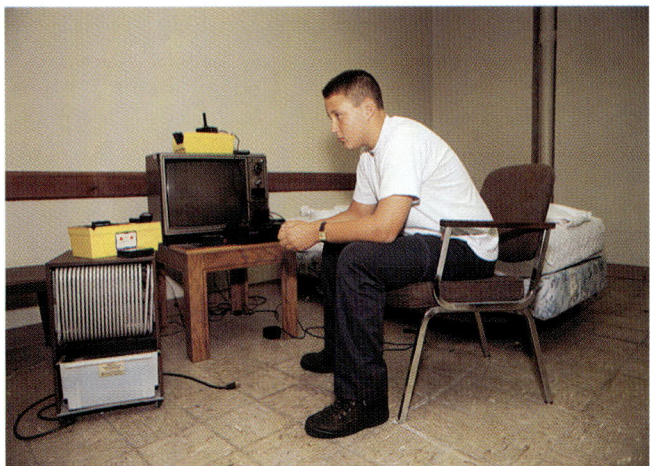

FIGURE 20.7 Disorientation and disorganization are characterized by varying degrees of loss of reality.

Medicolegal Considerations

Standard of Care

The medicolegal considerations involved in managing a patient undergoing a behavioral emergency require careful attention to the EMT's standard of care. The EMT must carefully adhere to a standard of care because the patient experiencing a behavioral emergency does not have the ability to make rational decisions about his or her emergency medical care. In these situations, the law presumes that providers of emergency care will be more diligent in their efforts.

Consent

When a patient is not mentally competent to grant consent for care, implied consent exists. For example, if life or health is at risk in the unresponsive patient, consent is implied. The law refers to this as the *implied consent emergency doctrine*. If no emergency exists, then the situation is a nonemergency and the EMT may delay care or transportation until the proper consent is obtained. In cases involving psychiatric emergencies, it is not always a clear-cut matter that a life-threatening emergency exists. These cases may require the assistance of law enforcement personnel.

Limited Legal Authority

EMTs have limited legal authority to require or force a patient to undergo emergency medical care when no life-threatening emergency exists. Most states have statutory provisions regarding the emergency care of the mentally ill and drug-dependent persons. These statutory provisions provide law enforcement personnel with authority to place such a person in protective custody so that emergency care can be rendered. These provisions, such as those found in the Connecticut General Statutes, generally state that:

> . . . any police officer who has reasonable cause to believe that a person is mentally ill and dangerous to himself, herself, or others or gravely disabled . . . may take such person into custody and take or *cause* such person to be taken to a general hospital for emergency examination . . .

The general rule of law is that as long as the person is an adult and competent, he or she has the right to refuse treatment. If a life is at risk from serious injury or incapacity, emergency medical care may be rendered. In such cases, it is likely that a court of law would decree that the EMT's actions in rendering life-saving care were appropriate.

In emergency situations, the implied consent rule applies to the mentally ill patient. If an emergency exists and the patient is unable to give consent, the EMT is able to provide care because implied consent exists. In some psychiatric emergencies, it is not always clear that a life-threatening emergency exists.

Restraint

Restraint of a person must be ordered by medical direction. Restraining a person without authority, *except* in life-threatening or emergency situations, exposes the EMT to possible litigation and personal danger. The legal actions against the EMT can involve assault, battery, false im-

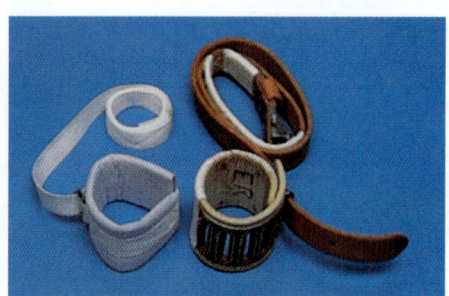

FIGURE 20.8 Examples of restraints.

> ✓ The major basic principal behind restraint is to have the proper number of personnel available to do so; a key rule is to display force before it is employed. The greater the number of personnel, the faster and more easily the restraint will be achieved. The EMT should also do the following:
>
> - Plan activities
> - Estimate range of motion of patient's arms and legs and stay beyond range until ready
> - Once a decision has been made, act quickly
> - Have one EMT-B talk to patient throughout restraining
> - Approach patient with four persons, one assigned to each limb all at the same time
> - Secure patient's limbs together with equipment approved by medical direction
> - Turn patient face down on stretcher
> - Secure patient to stretcher with multiple straps
> - Cover patient's face with surgical mask if he or she is spitting on EMT-Bs
> - Reassess patient's circulation frequently
> - Document indication for restraining patients and technique of restraint
> - Avoid unnecessary force

prisonment, and claims of violation of civil rights. Restraints can be used when the EMT is protecting himself or herself or others from bodily harm or if a potential for self-injury exists. In all restraint, only reasonable force can be used to control the patient. However, the definition of reasonable force is subject to legal interpretation.

A general rule is to apply only the force that is necessary to keep the patient from causing injury or harm to himself or herself or others. The restraint devices used should be consistent with those approved by the regulatory provisions under which the EMS agency operates (Figure 20.8). The EMT should not allow law enforcement personnel to handcuff the patient to the ambulance gurney unless the law enforcement officer accompanies the patient, in the event that the patient requires emergency medical care. Placing the patient on his or her stomach with the hands cuffed behind may be life threatening. Patients so restrained have suffered positional asphyxiation.

Cases involving psychiatric crisis ordinarily should involve police intervention. Police involvement provides the appropriate backup often needed in managing such crisis as well as the necessary legal authority to restrain.

> ✓ EMTs can restrain a patient with medical direction. In a nonemergency situation, restraint can only be used after correct authority is given by a court order, a physician, or law enforcement personnel.

Potentially Violent Patient

The potential for violence by patients undergoing a behavioral or psychiatric episode, although small in comparison with the large number of persons with mental health problems, is nonetheless an important consideration for EMTs.

Prudent emergency management of any patient is a responsibility of all providers, but for a presenting mental disorder, the management requirements have special significance. In the case of potential violence, the EMT must exercise care for the patient and for others in the immediate vicinity.

The following principal determinants of violence, which are not intended to be a complete list, are of value for the EMT:

- *History.* Has this patient previously exhibited hostile, overly aggressive, or violent behavior? This information should be solicited by EMS personnel at the scene or requested from law enforcement personnel, family members, previous EMS records, or hospital information.
- *Posture.* How is this person sitting or standing? Does the patient appear to be tense or rigid or sitting on the edge of the bed or chair? The observation of increased tension by physical posture is often a warning signal for hostility. Sometimes hands will be clenched in a fist.
- *Vocal activity.* What is the nature of the speech being used by the patient? Loud, obscene, erratic, and bizarre speech patterns are usually an indication of emotional distress. The patient conversing in quiet and ordered speech is not as likely to strike out against others as is the patient who is yelling and screaming. Sometimes these patients are verbally abusive to EMTs. They may be "venting their emotions." The EMT should realize that this behavior is not directed against him or her.
- *Physical activity.* Perhaps one of the most demonstrative factors to look for is the motor activity of a person undergoing a behavioral crisis. The patient who is pacing, cannot sit still, or displays protection of his or her boundaries of personal space needs careful watching. Agitation is a prognostic sign to be observed with great care and scrutiny.

Other factors to take into consideration for potential violence are as follows:

- Poor impulse control
- Instability of family structure and inability to keep a steady job
- Tattoos, especially those with gang identification
- Substance abuse (e.g., the smell of alcohol on person's breath)
- Functional disorder; if the patient is "hearing" voices that tell him or her to kill, believe the patient
- Depression; depressed persons account for 20% of violent attacks

> ✓ Being aware of the signs and symptoms of the potentially violent patient may help the EMT protect himself or herself.

Management and Emergency Medical Treatment

Emergency medical management of patients experiencing psychiatric emergencies involves different skills than those applied to a patient in cardiac arrest. In a cardiac arrest case, application of cardiopulmonary resuscitation is the skill used. In the case of a behavioral

> ✓ The EMT should be prepared to spend time. It may take longer to assess, listen to the patient, and prepare for packaging and transportation.

emergency, although basic EMT skills of assessment, patient approach, history taking, and patient communication are used, other management factors are involved. Although this chapter does not permit a full discussion of these factors, the following are general guidelines:

- Have a definite plan of action. Determine who will do what and how restraint will be accomplished if it is needed.
- Calmly identify yourself. If you begin shouting, the patient is likely to shout louder or become more excited. Speaking in a low, calm voice often is a quieting influence.
- Be direct. State your intentions and what you expect of the patient.
- Assess at the scene; do not wait until you are in the ambulance. If the patient is armed, weapons should be removed by law enforcement personnel before you transport.
- Stay with the patient; do not let the patient leave the area. The patient may go to a room and obtain weapons, lock himself or herself in the bathroom, or consume pills.
- Encourage purposeful movement. Help the patient get appropriate items to take to the emergency department and to get dressed.
- Avoid challenging the patient's personal space; provide for a means of getting away. Do not talk down physically to the patient or directly confront him or her. A squatting, 45-degree angle approach is usually the least confrontational.
- Avoid fighting with the patient or getting into a power struggle with him or her. The patient is not responding as a person but rather is responding to internal forces.

The EMT and others stimulate these inner forces. If you can respond to the feeling that the patient is acting out or the emotion he or she is expressing (such as anger, fear, or feelings of desperation), the patient may feel that the EMT understands and be more cooperative. The EMT should plan for adequate resources to handle patients who are experiencing a behavioral crisis or mental disorder.

The EMT should always ensure that the environment is safe for all emergency medical personnel. The EMT's safety comes first. If it is necessary to use force, the EMT should ensure that there is adequate help and move softly, quietly, and with firmness. The EMT should do the following:

- Acknowledge that the patient seems upset and restate that he or she is there to help.
- Inform the patient of what he or she is doing.
- Maintain a comfortable distance.
- Encourage the patient to state what is troubling him or her.
- Avoid quick moves.
- Respond honestly to patient's questions.
- Avoid threatening, challenging, or arguing with disturbed patients.
- Avoid "playing along" with visual or auditory disturbances of the patient.
- Involve trusted family members or friends.
- Avoid unnecessary physical contact and call for additional help if needed.
- Use good eye contact.

> ✓ Management of a patient experiencing a behavioral emergency involves different skills than those applied to other patients. Skills such as taking time, having a plan of action, encouraging purposeful actions, avoiding challenging the patient, and being honest and interested are helpful in managing the patient with a behavioral emergency.

Summary

- Understanding and managing psychiatric emergencies presents EMTs with great difficulties that will often provide enormous challenges to their training and experience.
- The first responsibility in these situations is to reduce potential life-threatening incidents and the influence of the stress condition. The second priority is to use the situation to help those affected to deal with the present problem. The third is to prepare the way for coping with this crisis and reducing the psychologically damaging consequence by rendering appropriate emergency medical care.
- Basic categories of mental disorder include acute anxiety, phobias, depression, suicide, paranoia, and disorientation and disorganization. Suicide attempts or threats constitute a critical and urgent emergency situation.
- A behavioral emergency is a reaction to an event that interferes with the daily activities of living.
- Behavioral emergencies may be caused by organic (physiologic) or psychiatric causes. Organic causes include drug and alcohol abuse, drug withdrawal, trauma, diabetes, infection, and malnutrition.

Summary (cont'd)

- Determining the causative factors of a behavioral emergency may be helpful. These factors may include inadequate cerebral oxygenation, drug abuse, or psychogenic circumstances (e.g., death of a loved one, major life interruption).
- The implied consent concept allows the EMT to give medical care to a patient unable to give consent if an emergency exists. In psychiatric emergencies, the existence of a medical emergency may not be clear-cut. Most states allow a mentally ill patient to be taken into protective custody by law enforcement so that medical care can be given. If restraint is needed, the EMT may restrain a patient only when authorized to do so by medical direction.
- Management of a mentally ill patient requires different skills than management of a patient with a medical emergency. A calm, reassuring manner; taking time; not arousing suspicion or challenging the patient; and being interested and honest are skills an EMT needs to learn to manage patients experiencing a behavioral emergency.
- Emergency medical treatment involves calmness, deliberate actions, and sensitivity to the patient. If dangerous weapons or implements are seen or shown or threats of bodily harm are made, the EMT must withdraw from the scene and seek immediate law enforcement assistance. In all of these cases, transportation to the hospital is necessary.

Scenario Solution

You should talk calmly and deliberately to the patient and convince him to come to the hospital for diagnosis and treatment. Although the psychosomatic responses to this panic attack usually subside when the event that precipitated it is reduced, there are symptoms present that relate to a cardiac event. It may be advisable to place the patient on oxygen, and you should urge the patient to come to the emergency department.

Key Terms

Activities of daily living The activities usually accomplished during a normal day (e.g., eating, dressing, washing).

Behavior How a person functions or acts.

Mental disorder An illness with psychologic or behavioral manifestations and/or impairment in functioning as a result of social, psychologic, genetic, physical/chemical, or biologic disturbance.

Psychogenic Causation of a symptom or illness by mental or psychic factors as opposed to organic ones.

Organic brain syndrome Transient or permanent dysfunction of the brain caused by disturbance of physiologic functioning of brain tissue.

Review Questions

1. List urgent behavioral emergencies that need to be recognized immediately.
2. What are warning signs of potential suicide?
3. What are the steps that the EMT should take if a patient who is undergoing a behavioral emergency threatens violence?
4. What are the medicolegal principles of dealing with a patient who is undergoing a behavioral crisis?
5. What are the principal assessment factors involved with a paranoid patient? Of the disoriented patient? Of the disorganized patient?

Answers to these Review Questions can be found at the end of the book on page 866.

Obstetric and Gynecologic Emergencies

Lesson Goal

This chapter reviews the importance of doing an organized assessment of the pregnant and non-pregnant female patient and prehospital care that the patient needs. The birthing process, complications of pregnancy, care of newborns, and sexual assault are also reviewed.

Scenario

You are dispatched to a woman experiencing abdominal pain. Upon arrival you find a 23-year-old woman lying in bed. The patient states that she is 9 months pregnant and having contractions. As you examine the patient, you find that she is alert and oriented with some difficulty breathing. The patient is having contractions at this time and feels the need to move her bowels. Your examination also shows that with each contraction the infant's head is starting to crown. Her vital signs are stable: blood pressure is 132/80 mm Hg, pulse is 88 beats/min, and ventilations are 24 breaths/min.

 Describe in detail how you should handle this situation and your main concerns.

Key Terms to Know

Abortion	Contraction	Labor	Oviducts
Abruptio placentae	Crowning	Meconium	Ovulation
Amniotic fluid	Eclampsia	Menopause	Para
Amniotic sac	Embryo	Menstrual period	Perineum
APGAR score	Fallopian tubes	Menstruation	Placenta
Birth canal	False contractions	Miscarriage	Placenta previa
Braxton Hicks contractions	Fetus	Mucous plug	Presenting part
Breech birth	Gravida	Obstetrics	Prolapsed cord
Cervix	Gynecology	Ovaries	Trimester

Obstetric and Gynecologic Emergencies | Chapter 21   373

Key Terms to Know

True contractions
Tubal pregnancy
Umbilical arteries

Umbilical cord
Umbilical vein
Umbilicus

Uterine rupture
Uterus
Vagina

Vaginal opening

Learning Objectives

After reading this chapter, the EMT-Basic should be able to do the following:

DOT

- Describe the function of the following structures: uterus, vagina, fetus, placenta, umbilical cord, amniotic sac, amniotic fluid, and perineum.
- Demonstrate the use of personal protection precautions when dealing with the obstetric and gynecologic patient.
- Identify and describe the use of the equipment in an obstetric kit.
- Identify and describe appropriate care for patients with predelivery and gynecologic emergencies.
- Identify indications for imminent delivery and state the steps necessary in the predelivery preparation of the mother.
- Identify and describe the care needed for a normal vaginal delivery, multiple birth delivery, breech delivery, prolapsed cord delivery, limb delivery, meconium delivery, and premature delivery.
- Describe the necessary steps for the care of the infant as the head appears.
- Describe the technique and appropriate time to cut the umbilical cord and the indications and steps necessary for the delivery and transportation of the placenta.
- Differentiate between the emergency medical care provided to a patient with predelivery emergencies and that provided to a patient with a normal delivery.

- Differentiate among the special considerations for multiple births.
- Describe special considerations of meconium.
- Describe special considerations of a premature infant.
- List the steps in the emergency medical care of the mother after delivery.
- Summarize neonatal resuscitation procedures.
- State the steps to assist in the delivery.
- Discuss the emergency medical care of a patient with a gynecologic emergency.
- Demonstrate the steps to assist in the normal cephalic delivery.
- Demonstrate necessary care procedures of the infant as the head appears.
- Demonstrate infant neonatal procedures.
- Demonstrate postdelivery care of the infant.
- Demonstrate how and when to cut the umbilical cord.
- Attend to the steps in the delivery of the placenta.
- Demonstrate postdelivery care of the mother.
- Demonstrate the procedures for the following abnormal deliveries: vaginal bleeding, breech birth, prolapsed cord, limb presentation.
- Demonstrate the steps in the emergency medical care of the mother with excessive bleeding.
- Demonstrate completing a prehospital care report for patients with obstetric-gynecologic emergencies.

One of the most exciting experiences an emergency medical technician (EMT) will encounter is the birth of a child. Assisting with the entrance of life into the world can be a rewarding and memorable experience. However, this chapter is titled "Obstetric and Gynecologic Emergencies" and encompasses more than just the birth of a child. **Obstetrics** is defined as the branch of medicine that deals with the management of women during pregnancy, childbirth, and 42 days after the expulsion of all contents of pregnancy. **Gynecology** is defined as the study of the diseases of the female reproductive organs.

In this chapter, the EMT will learn the importance of doing a detailed and organized assessment of the pregnant and nonpregnant woman and delivering the appropriate prehospital interventions. This chapter explores birth and the birthing process, problems associated with pregnancy, care of newborns, and care necessary for the person who may have been sexually assaulted.

Anatomy and Physiology

The female reproductive anatomy is complex, which may make assessment more difficult. Pregnancy may also complicate assessment. All women of reproductive age (9 to 55 years of age) have the potential for pregnancy. Although rare, even the woman who has had her "tubes tied" could be pregnant. Therefore during an assessment

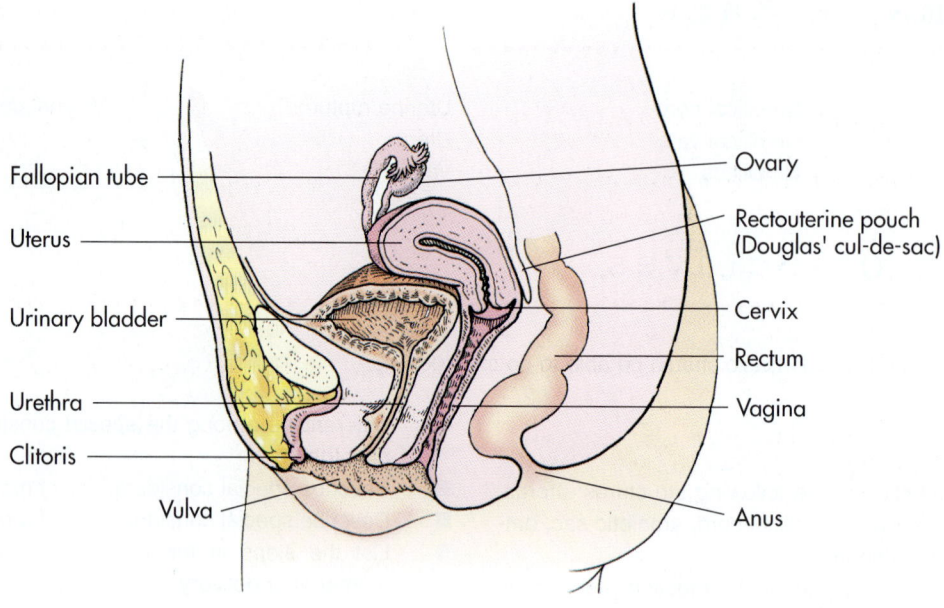
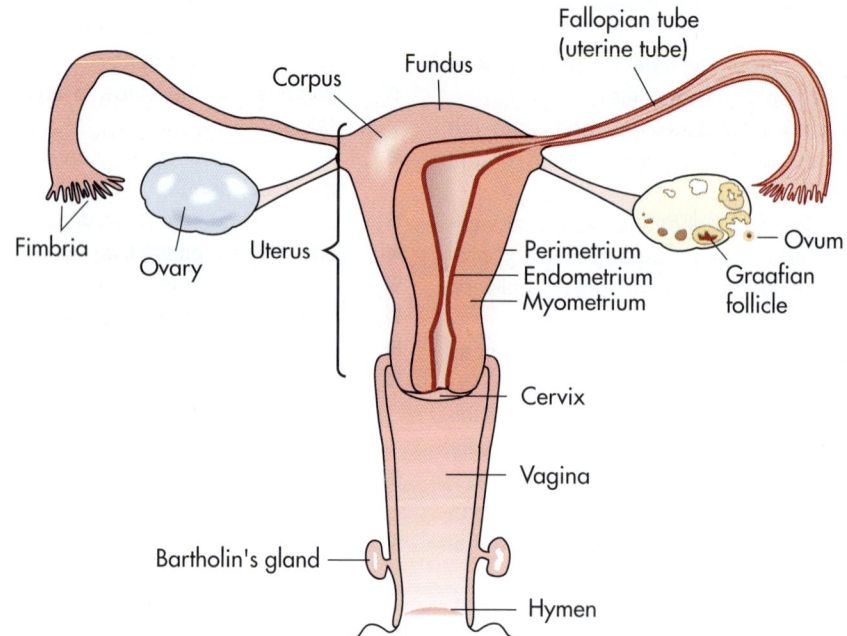

FIGURE 21.1 Organs of the female reproductive system.

of the female patient, the EMT should always fully evaluate the possibility of pregnancy.

Reproductive Anatomy

Female reproductive organs include the ovaries, fallopian tubes or oviducts, uterus, vagina or birth canal, and the perineum (Figure 21.1).

The **ovaries** are paired, almond-shaped organs suspended by ligaments in the left and right lower quadrants of the abdomen (below the level of the **umbilicus**, or navel). A primary function of the ovaries is the release of eggs and hormones. Women are born with a lifetime supply of eggs. Normally, one ovary releases a mature egg once a month in a process known as **ovulation**. Ovulation can begin as early as 9 years of age and continue until about 50 years of age. **Menstruation**, or **menstrual**

period, is the process in which the lining of the uterus is shed when the egg is not fertilized. If both ovaries are damaged, are removed, or have stopped producing matured eggs, a woman will go through **menopause**. During menopause, ovulation and menstruation cease.

The **fallopian tubes**, or **oviducts**, are also paired and provide a pathway from each ovary to the uterus. One end of each fallopian tube surrounds the ovary, and the other end of the fallopian tube acts as a canal to the uterus. These tubes are approximately 4 inches long and very vascular (blood engorged). If a fertilized egg implants in a fallopian tube, that fertilized egg will grow until the fallopian tube ruptures. This condition is known as a **tubal pregnancy** and can threaten the mother's life by causing severe pain and rapid internal hemorrhaging. A tubal pregnancy, if undetected, can be fatal because of the sudden, massive loss of blood from the ruptured fallopian tube.

The **uterus** is a single, pear-shaped, muscular organ located between the rectum and the bladder. In the nonpregnant state, this muscle is approximately 3 inches long and can enlarge to 60 times its nonpregnant size during pregnancy. The narrow portion of the uterus points downward toward the feet and is called the "neck" of the uterus. At the bottom of the neck is the opening of uterus, called the **cervix**. The uterus houses the unborn infant during fetal development. In the last 3 months of pregnancy, the uterus becomes heavy because of the weight of the fetus. Lying on the back at this stage of pregnancy can restrict the circulation of blood to the placenta because the uterus will be resting on the mother's inferior vena cava. This position can also result in the mother experiencing lightheadedness or fainting. To avoid compressing the vena cava, a pregnant woman should lie on her left side instead of her back when sleeping or resting (Figure 21.2).

The **vagina** is a fibromuscular sheath that encloses the lower end of the uterus and extends to the vaginal opening. The **vaginal opening** is located between the anus and the urethral orifice. The vagina is also known as the **birth canal**.

The **perineum** is the area between the vaginal opening and the anal opening (Figure 21.3). During birth, this area may be stretched to the point of tearing and is another potential site for blood loss.

> ✓ Female reproductive organs include the ovaries, fallopian tubes (oviducts), cervix, and birth canal (vagina). The perineum is the area between the vaginal and anal openings.

Specialized Structures of Pregnancy

During pregnancy, several new structures begin to develop and fill the pelvic/abdominal cavity (Figure 21.4).

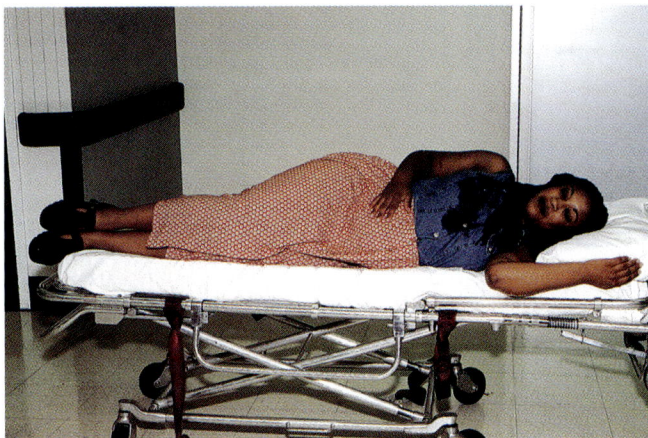

FIGURE 21.2 When transporting a mother in the last 3 months of pregnancy, position her on her left side to facilitate blood flow between the mother and the infant.

These structures include the fetus, placenta, umbilical cord, amniotic sac, and amniotic fluid.

Once fertilization of the egg has occurred, and for the first 8 weeks of pregnancy, the product of conception is known as an **embryo**. After the eighth week and until delivery, the embryo is known as a **fetus**. A fetus is classified as the developing unborn infant. The normal time span for a pregnancy averages about 40 weeks and consists of three 3-month intervals, each of which is known as a **trimester**.

When the fertilized egg implants in the uterus, a dish-shaped structure develops that links the tissue of the mother with that of the fetus. This organ is called the **placenta**. The placenta is attached to the inner portion of the uterus and continues to grow as the fetus grows. This highly vascular organ has many functions. The placenta exchanges oxygen and carbon dioxide between fetus and mother, transports nutrients and waste by-products, and serves as a temporary source for hormone production necessary to sustain the pregnancy. The placenta also serves as a barrier between fetus and mother; however, studies show that this barrier is more of a filter than a barrier. Medications and other substances can cross the placenta from the mother to the infant. Many of these substances can cause fetal harm.

The **umbilical cord** is a fibrous, whitish tube that connects the fetus to the placenta. Within the umbilical cord are three vessels. Two vessels are the **umbilical arteries**, which carry deoxygenated blood from the fetus to the placenta. The remaining vessel, known as the **umbilical vein**, carries oxygenated blood from the placenta to the fetus. The texture and the length of the umbilical cord vary with each pregnancy.

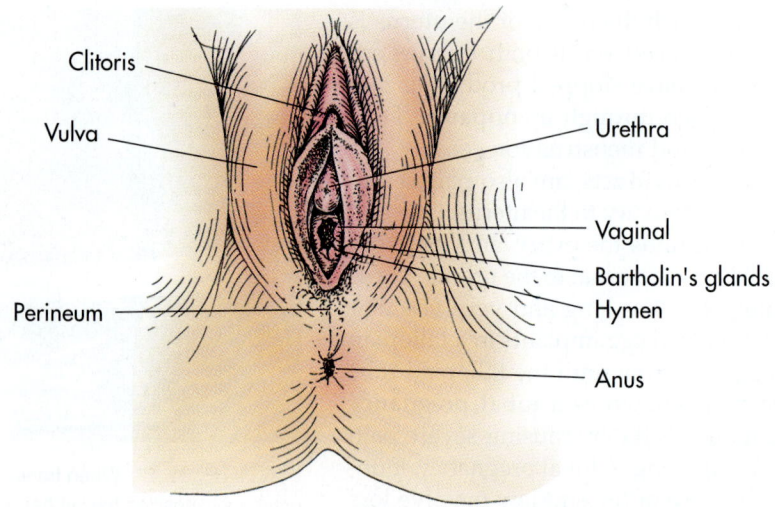

FIGURE 21.3 The perineum is the space between the vaginal and anal openings.

Once the embryo is imbedded in the uterus, a protective covering known as the **amniotic sac** completely surrounds the embryo. This sac is also fibrous and is filled with a clear to straw-colored fluid called the **amniotic fluid**. The amniotic sac acts as a shock absorber, and maintains a uniform pressure and temperature for the fetus. The amniotic sac is also known as the "bag of waters."

At the opening of the cervix, which is part of the uterus, an accumulation of mucus forms and interlocks with the capillaries of the cervix, creating a **mucous plug**. This mucous plug acts as a protective barrier between the cervix and the vagina for the length of the pregnancy. The mucous plug usually stays intact until the preliminary phase of labor. At that point, the cervix starts to dilate, causing the mucous plug to pull away from the cervical capillaries and become blood tinged. This blood-tinged mucous is then deposited in the vagina. The appearance of the bloody mucous is sometimes called the "bloody show" and usually heralds the first stage of labor.

> ✓ Specialized structures of pregnancy include the amniotic sac and fluid, placenta, umbilical cord, and mucous plug.

TABLE 21.1   Stages of Labor

First Stage	Second Stage	Third Stage
From the first contraction until the dilation of the cervix	From dilation of the cervix to the birth of the child	From the birth of the child until the delivery of the placenta

Stages of Labor

The stages of **labor** are time frames whereby the mother's body works to expel the fetus from the uterus. There are three stages of labor (Figure 21.5, *A*; Table 21.1). Labor cannot be controlled by the mother; however, different comfort measures may momentarily ease the discomfort. As the labor progresses, so does the intensity of pain and discomfort.

First Stage

The first stage of labor begins with the onset of the first true contraction and ends with the complete dilation of the cervix (Figure 21.5, *B*). The cervix can dilate to a maximum diameter of 10 cm. Usually the amniotic sac ruptures during this stage. A **contraction** is a tightening and hardening of the uterus. During pregnancy, and especially in the last month of pregnancy, a pregnant woman will experience intermittent contractions of the uterus. These are called **Braxton Hicks contractions**, named for the physician who first noticed them in patients. They occur at irregular intervals but do not increase in pain intensity. Braxton Hicks contractions are also known as **false contractions**.

True contractions are generally regular, with intervals lasting between 5 and 15 minutes. True contractions generally increase in pain and intensity as labor progresses. This pain is a cramplike abdominal pain that may radiate to the lower back. For first-time mothers, the first stage of labor usually lasts 8 to 12 hours. This time frame tends to be shorter in women who have had previous deliveries. The average time for the first stage of labor is approximately 8 hours.

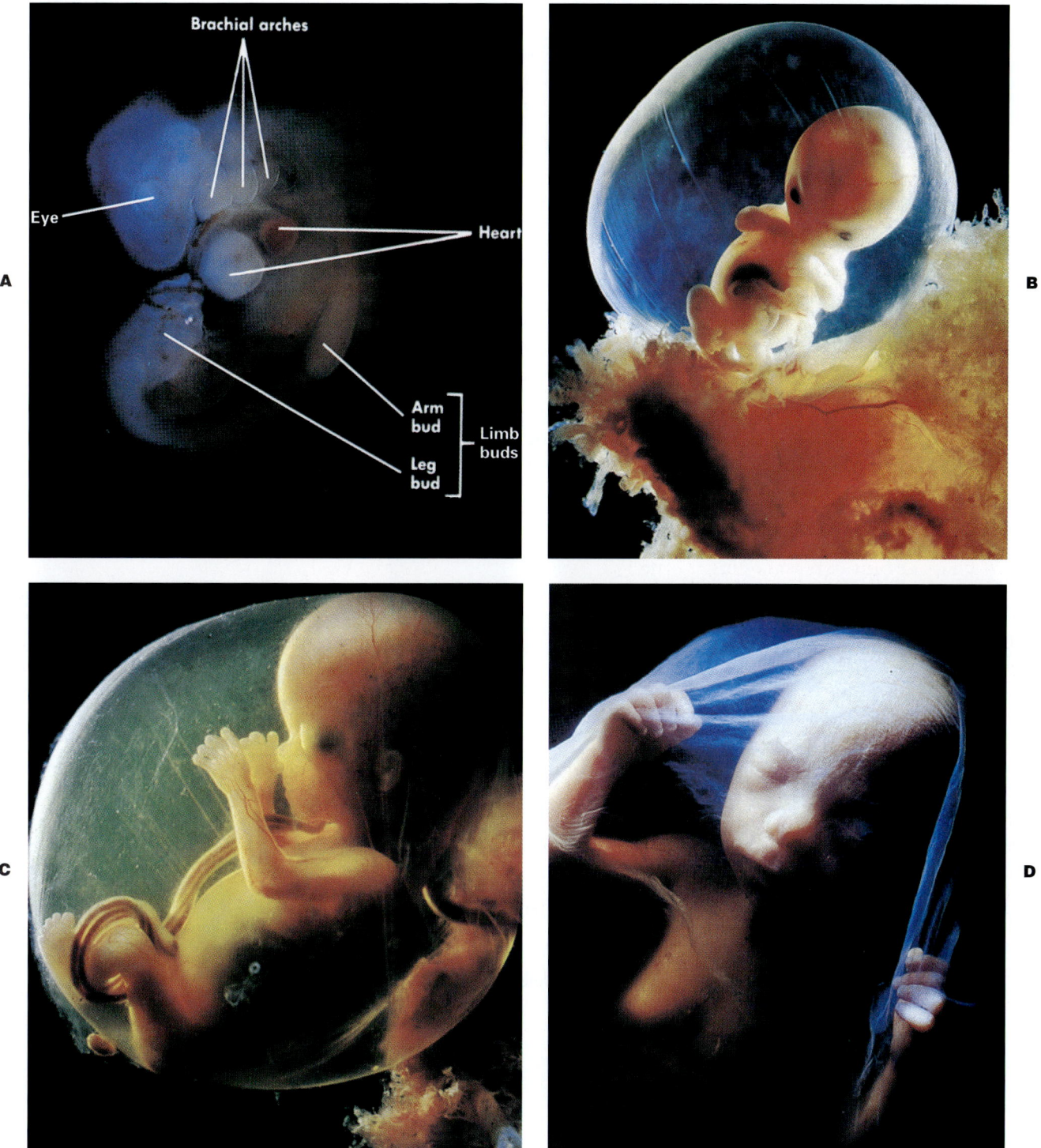

FIGURE 21.4 **A,** Human fetus at 35 days' gestation. **B,** Human fetus at 49 days' gestation. **C,** Human fetus at the end of the first trimester. **D,** Human fetus at 4 months' gestation.

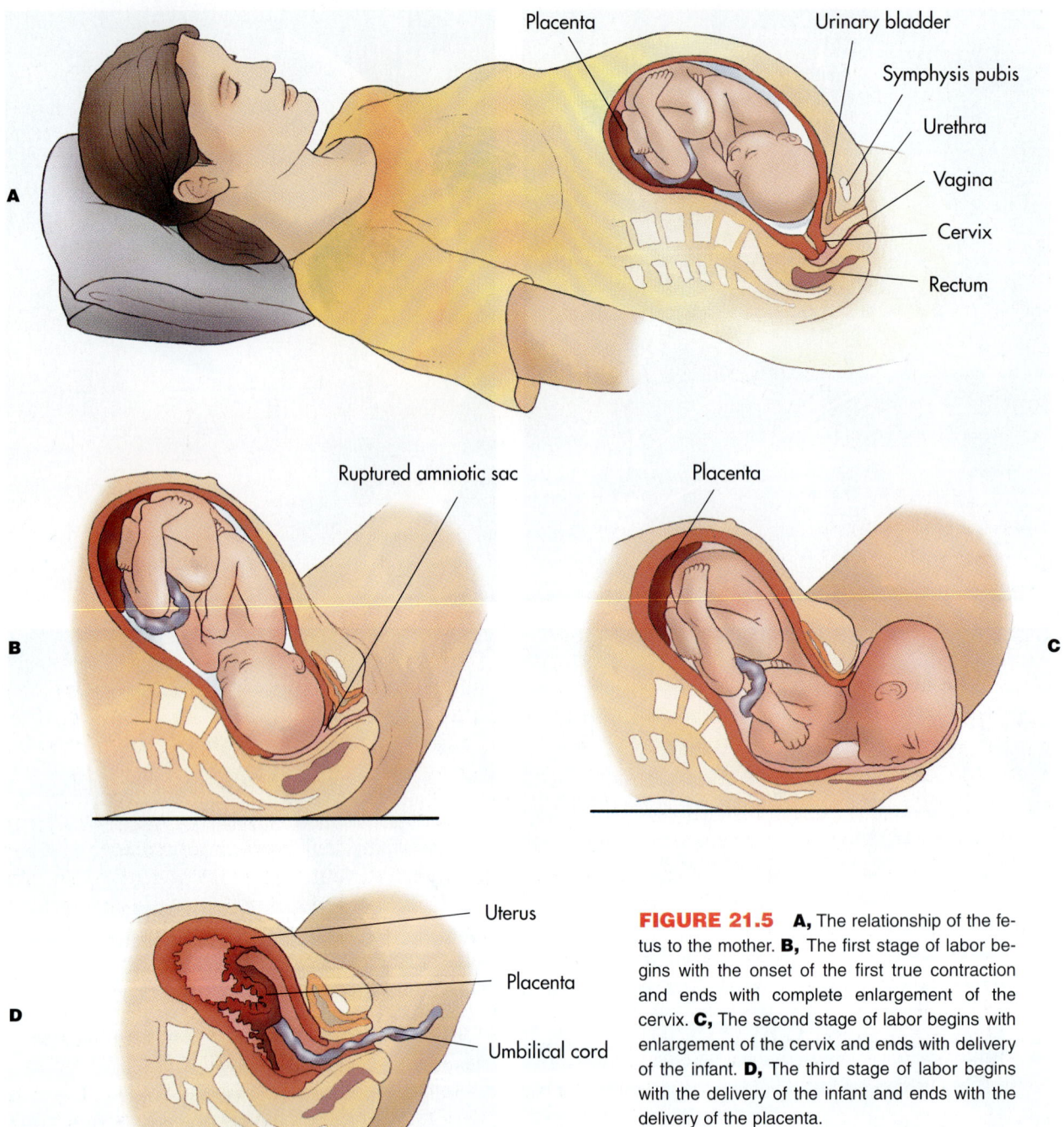

FIGURE 21.5 **A,** The relationship of the fetus to the mother. **B,** The first stage of labor begins with the onset of the first true contraction and ends with complete enlargement of the cervix. **C,** The second stage of labor begins with enlargement of the cervix and ends with delivery of the infant. **D,** The third stage of labor begins with the delivery of the infant and ends with the delivery of the placenta.

Second Stage

The second stage of labor begins with the full dilation of the cervix and ends with the delivery of the infant (Figure 21.5, *C*). During this time the infant's head enters the birth canal, which increases the pain experienced by the mother. The mother also will feel the urge to bear down or feel as though she needs to move her bowels. At this point, contractions are more intense and frequent, about 2 to 4 minutes apart. The part of the infant that protrudes initially is called the **presenting part**. On visualization of the perineum area, the skin over the perineum appears stretched and glistening as the presenting part of the fetus emerges from the vaginal opening. The visualization of the presenting part is commonly referred to as

TABLE 21.2 Vaginal Bleeding

Diagnosis	Pregnancy	Symptoms	Care
Miscarriage, abortion	Early, usually first trimester	Abdominal pain; vaginal bleeding	Assess airway, breathing, and circulation (ABCs and provide oxygen; use sanitary pads; if products of conception passed, bring to hospital
Abruptio placentae	Third trimester	Sudden, severe abdominal pain; vaginal bleeding may or may not be present	Assess ABCs and provide oxygen; treat for signs and symptoms of shock; use sanitary pads; provide rapid transportation
Placenta previa	Third trimester	Painless, bright red vaginal bleeding	Assess ABCs and provide oxygen; treat for signs and symptoms of shock; use sanitary pads; provide rapid transportation
Uterine rupture	Third trimester	Painful tearing sensation; vaginal bleeding may or may not be present	Assess ABCs and provide oxygen; treat for signs and symptoms of shock; provide rapid transportation

crowning. The head is most commonly the presenting part; however, the buttock or a hand or a foot also may be the presenting part. Sometimes it is necessary to delay this stage to facilitate a better contraction or to delay the birth so that the mother and infant do not sustain injury. One such technique to stop the mother from bearing down is to instruct her to breathe out regularly, or to "blow out the candles." By "blow" breathing the mother can temporarily delay the pushing sensation. This stage can progress very rapidly in women who have had many births, but for a new mother the time span is approximately 1 to 2 hours.

Third Stage

The third stage of labor begins after the delivery of the infant and lasts until the delivery of the placenta (Figure 21.5, *D*). This stage varies in duration but generally is finished within an hour after the delivery of the infant. The mother experiences contractions before and after the placenta is delivered. During the delivery of the placenta, the EMT should expect a copious amount of blood. Approximately 300 to 500 ml of blood is normal.

For approximately 2 hours after the delivery of the placenta, the EMT should constantly monitor the mother's vital signs and bleeding. If parts of the placenta are retained in the uterus, the mother could experience increased and constant bleeding and become unstable.

> ✓ The first stage of labor begins with the initial contraction and ends with complete dilation of the cervix. In the second stage of labor the fetus is expelled. In the third stage of labor the placenta is delivered and the mother is monitored for increased vaginal bleeding.

Pathophysiology

Early Pregnancy Vaginal Bleeding: Abortion and Miscarriage

An embryo or fetus that is expelled from the uterus before the twentieth week, whether by nature or choice, is classified as an **abortion** (Table 21.2). A "natural," or spontaneous, abortion is sometimes called a **miscarriage**. Spontaneous abortion usually occurs in the first trimester, or the first 3 months of pregnancy. The major complaints from the patient include vaginal bleeding, which can be mild to profuse, and cramplike pain or pain in the back. In any situation in which miscarriage is suspected, the EMT should constantly monitor the patient's airway, breathing, and circulation. For patients with low blood pressure, the EMT should administer supplemental oxygen and place the patient on a flat surface with her legs elevated. If the patient has had a miscarriage, the EMT should bring the fetal tissue (also known as *products of conception*) to the hospital for analysis in a BSI container (a plastic bag or container). In some situations the patient may not even have known that she was pregnant.

> ✓ Bleeding during the first trimester may be an indication of a spontaneous abortion. The EMT should monitor airway, breathing, and circulation. If the blood pressure is low, the EMT should administer oxygen and elevate the lower extremities. The EMT should collect any fetal tissue that is expelled in a BSI container for transportation to the hospital with the patient.

Late Pregnancy Vaginal Bleeding: Abruptio Placentae, Placenta Previa, and Uterine Rupture

Bleeding in the last 3 months of pregnancy is an unusual situation. If bleeding does occur, the patient needs to be placed on high-concentration oxygen and transported to the hospital as quickly as possible. If the patient is exhibiting the signs and symptoms of shock, the EMT should treat the shock. Vaginal pads should be placed on the perineum to absorb and document blood loss. Also, in many areas use of a pneumatic antishock garment (PASG) beyond the first trimester is contraindicated.

One cause of late vaginal bleeding is known as **abruptio placentae** in which the placenta suddenly separates from the wall of the uterus. Abruptio placentae is characterized by sudden, severe, low abdominal pain with or without vaginal bleeding. Another cause of late pregnancy bleeding is **placenta previa**. In this condition, the placenta implants either on or near the opening of the cervix. When the cervix begins to dilate in the early stages of labor, the highly vascular placenta tears, and profuse bleeding results. The bleeding is painless and bright red.

Management of patients with abruptio placentae and placenta previa consists of maintaining an open airway, administering high-concentration oxygen via a nonrebreather mask with reservoir, managing the signs and symptoms of shock by protecting the patient from heat loss, placing the patient in a supine position and elevating the legs or placing the stretcher in the Trendelenburg position, and transporting rapidly. In true abruptio placentae and placenta previa, the mother needs to have a surgical delivery by cesarean section.

Another cause of late pregnancy vaginal bleeding is a **uterine rupture**. The uterus can rupture in traumatic situations or from previous cesarean scarring. The typical presentation is a female patient who may complain of abdominal pain that feels like tearing. Severe shock usually follows. Vaginal bleeding may or may not be present. Palpation of the abdomen reveals firmness and rigidity. Sometimes the fetus may also be palpated. The EMT should manage for shock and transfer the patient to the hospital as quickly and safely as possible. This patient will probably need a surgical delivery by cesarean section.

Seizures

Two seizure situations may present during pregnancy. The first type is the pregnant woman who has a seizure history. Because of the increased weight gain during pregnancy, the dosage of prescribed seizure medication may not be sufficient to prevent seizure activity. This situation is most common in pregnant women who have not received prenatal care. With proper prenatal care, this type of seizure can be prevented.

The second type of seizure activity is eclampsia. **Eclampsia** is experienced only during pregnancy, has an unknown cause, and is more common in women who are pregnant for the first time. It is characterized by a progressive increase in blood pressure. The increase in blood pressure becomes evident after the twentieth week of pregnancy, and in most cases the patient retains large amounts of fluid, especially in the ankles and face. Other common complaints are persistent headaches, visual disturbances, periods of confusion, and protein found in the urine.

The most important tools available to the EMT in evaluating the pregnant woman for seizures are the ability to gather an informative history (e.g., Has this patient had prenatal care? Has this patient been compliant with her prescribed medications?) and to use this history with a visual evaluation of the patient (e.g., swelling of extremities or face).

As with all patients, evaluating the patency of the airway, monitoring the quality and quantity of ventilations, and checking the circulation status, especially the blood pressure, are imperative. An EMT who suspects the possibility of a seizure should consider the use of supplemental oxygen. Because of the weight of the fetus on the inferior vena cava, the EMT should place the mother on her left side to facilitate blood flow to the infant and mother.

If the EMT arrives at a scene in which a pregnant woman is actively having a seizure, the three most important interventions are protecting the patient from injury, maintaining an airway, and providing high-concentration oxygen. If possible, the EMT should keep the mother on her left side. When the seizure is over, the EMT should clear the mother's airway and ventilate the patient with a bag-valve-mask (BVM) with 100% oxygen (this can be difficult until the seizure activity decreases or stops). Rapid and safe transportation is important; if possible, sirens should be turned off. The elimination of sirens is beneficial for the patient because an increase in stimulation has been shown to cause seizure activity in some people.

> ✓ Bleeding in the third trimester is extremely serious and may indicate abruptio placentae (premature separation of the placenta), placenta previa (a condition in which the placenta implants too low in the uterus and bleeds during labor), or uterine rupture. The EMT should place the patient on high-concentration oxygen and transport her to the hospital as quickly as possible. The EMT should manage for shock if necessary.

> ✓ Care for seizures during pregnancy consists of managing the airway, monitoring the quality and quantity of respirations, and checking circulation. The EMT should use supplemental oxygen and place the patient on her left side to facilitate blood flow to the infant and mother. The EMT should treat actively seizing patients with high-concentration oxygen and transport them quickly to the medical facility.

Assessment

The EMT must use BSI when assessing a pregnant patient. Protective eyewear is essential during delivery (Figure 21.6). If possible, the EMT should transport the patient to a hospital for delivery. However, sometimes prehospital delivery is imminent, and the EMT must be prepared to deliver the infant. The EMT must base the decision on the answers to these questions:

- When was the patient's last menstrual period? This question identifies the possibility of pregnancy and gives an idea about the gestation of the fetus.
- When is the patient's due date? The EMT can assess the gestation of the fetus and whether the mother has had prenatal care.
- How many times has patient been pregnant (**gravida**)?
- How many children does patient have (**para**)?
- Does the patient have back pain or contractions? If the answer is yes, the EMT can assess that the mother may be in labor.
- What is the frequency and duration of the contractions? If the EMT finds that the frequency of contractions is 1 to 2 minutes apart and that the contractions are regular, birth is imminent.
- Is the patient's abdomen rigid and hard? By placing a hand on the mother's abdomen, the EMT can assess the abdomen for rigidity and firmness. If this sign eventually disappears, the patient has had a contraction.
- Have the patient's membranes ruptured? If the membranes have ruptured, the contractions may increase in frequency and the birth process may also proceed at a faster rate. The fetus usually needs to be delivered within 24 hours after the membranes have ruptured even if labor has not started.
- Does the patient have any bleeding or discharges? Vaginal discharge may indicate the onset of labor. If the EMT notes bleeding, the mother may need an operating room for a surgical delivery of the fetus. Additional oxygen and rapid transportation are necessary.

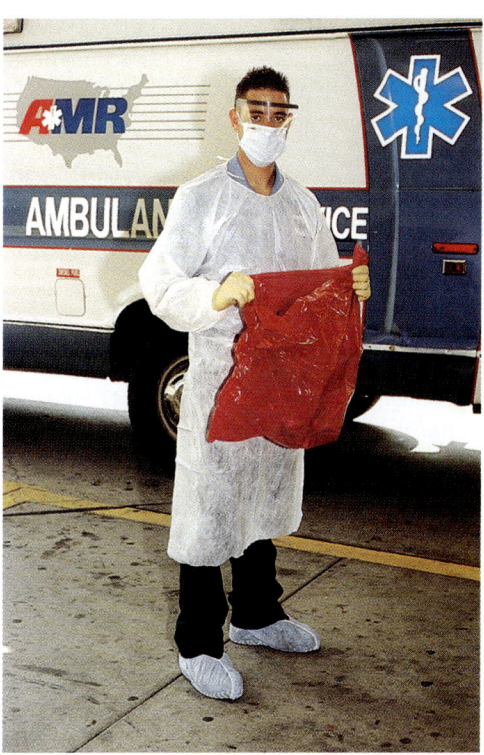

FIGURE 21.6 Personal protective equipment is essential when assisting with a delivery.

- Does the patient feel like she has to move her bowels or bear down? If the EMT finds a woman in late pregnancy who feels like she has to move her bowels or bear down, the EMT should realize that this could be labor and that birth is imminent.

Depending on the answers to these questions, the EMT must decide whether to transport the mother to the hospital or deliver the infant in the prehospital setting. A delivery means that one patient becomes two patients; therefore the EMT must notify dispatch for assistance once he or she decides that birth is imminent. For optimum care each patient (mother and infant) will need at least one EMT.

The following are signs that the EMT must prepare for delivery:

- The length of time between the beginning of one contraction and the beginning of the next contraction is 1 to 2 minutes.
- Contractions are regular and last 45 to 60 seconds.
- The patient in later pregnancy wants to go to the bathroom to move her bowels.
- The patient wants to bear down or push.

- With your partner (this will protect the EMT and the patient from any unnecessary false accusations), visualization of the perineum reveals bulging and crowning with each contraction.

If these signs are present, preparations for delivery are necessary. If possible, the EMT should place the mother on the ambulance stretcher and in the ambulance to expedite transportation if complications or delays in the birthing process arise.

> If a patient is in active labor, the EMT should try to transport her to a hospital as soon as possible. However, if delivery is imminent (contractions are 1 or 2 minutes apart and the patient feels an urge to push), then the EMT should prepare immediately for delivery.

Management

Delivery Kit

Births can be spontaneous. Prepackaged equipment is essential for a successful and organized delivery. The contents of a delivery kit should include the following components (Figure 21.7):

- Surgical scissors for cutting the cord
- Hemostats or cord clamp for clamping the cord
- Umbilical tape or sterilized cord for tying off the placenta side of the umbilical cord
- Bulb syringe for suctioning the mouth and nose of the infant
- Towels for drying and stimulating the infant
- Two 3 × 10 gauze sponges to clear secretions from the infant's mouth and pat the ends of the cut umbilical cord
- Sterile gloves, eye protection, and a skull cap for body substance isolation (BSI) for the EMT
- One baby blanket to keep the infant warm
- Sanitary napkins to absorb the drainage of blood from the vagina
- Plastic bag as a receptacle for transporting the placenta

Ideally, the kit should be packaged in a moisture-resistant receptacle with a date of expiration to prevent deterioration of the contents.

> A prepared delivery kit greatly facilitates management when birth is imminent.

Delivery Procedure

At the time of delivery, the mother is usually very tired and may not be receptive to suggestions. For the first time, the patient is beginning to realize that she has no control over her body. Her body is going to deliver the infant whether she wants to or not. Therefore the EMT must do everything in the patient's best interest even if she is too tired to cooperate. Privacy is important; the EMT should try to protect the patient's privacy by exposing only the perineum. This can be accomplished by draping the mother's lower body with a combination of towels and sheets. If the area is not private, the EMT should try to have the other EMT or police redirect pedestrian traffic.

EMTs must protect themselves before rendering care to the patient. At this point, the EMTs should put on protective eyewear, a double pair of gloves, protective covering for their clothing, and protective shoe guards because the delivery process can be very bloody. Before examination of the perineum, the EMT must make sure that his or her partner is also present. This will serve as protection for the EMT and the patient to prevent any lawsuits for improper conduct.

The EMT should have the mother lie on her back with knees drawn up and spread apart and elevate the patient's buttocks with a blanket. The EMT should create a sterile field around the vaginal opening using sterile towels or sterile packaged paper drapes (Figure 21.8). The EMT should make sure that enough space exists in front of the mother at the end of the stretcher or bed. Infants are very slippery, and having a clear area at the end of the bed will prevent the child from falling to the floor.

The EMT can anticipate imminent delivery by observing for bulging of the perineum and the appearance of the presenting part at the vaginal opening (Figure 21.9). At this point the EMT should make no attempts to delay delivery. The EMT must control the delivery to prevent maternal and fetal injury. With each contraction, the

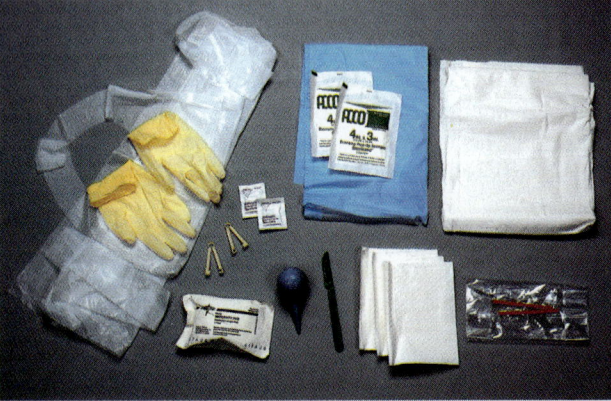

FIGURE 21.7 Contents of a delivery kit.

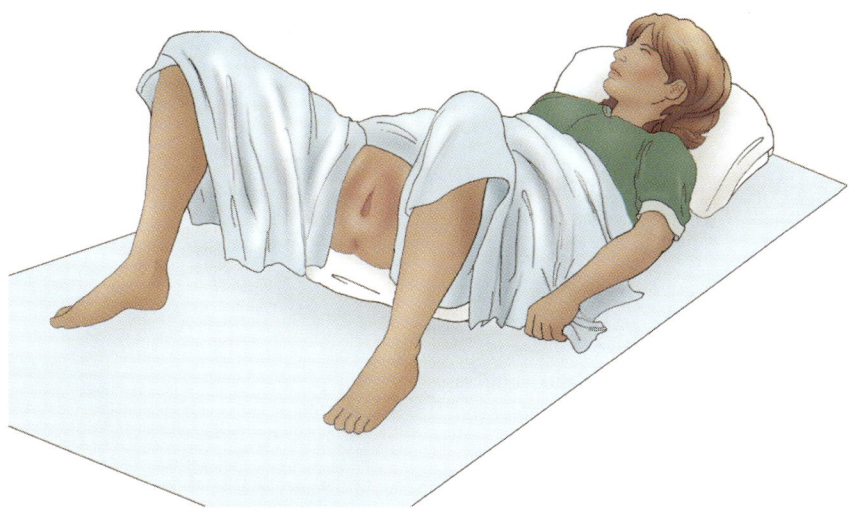

FIGURE 21.8 Have the mother lie on her back with her knees drawn up and spread apart. Elevate the patient's buttocks with a towel or blanket. Create a sterile field around the vaginal opening using sterile towels or sterile packaged paper drapes. Make sure enough space exists in front of the mother, at the end of the stretcher or bed, to accommodate the infant after delivery.

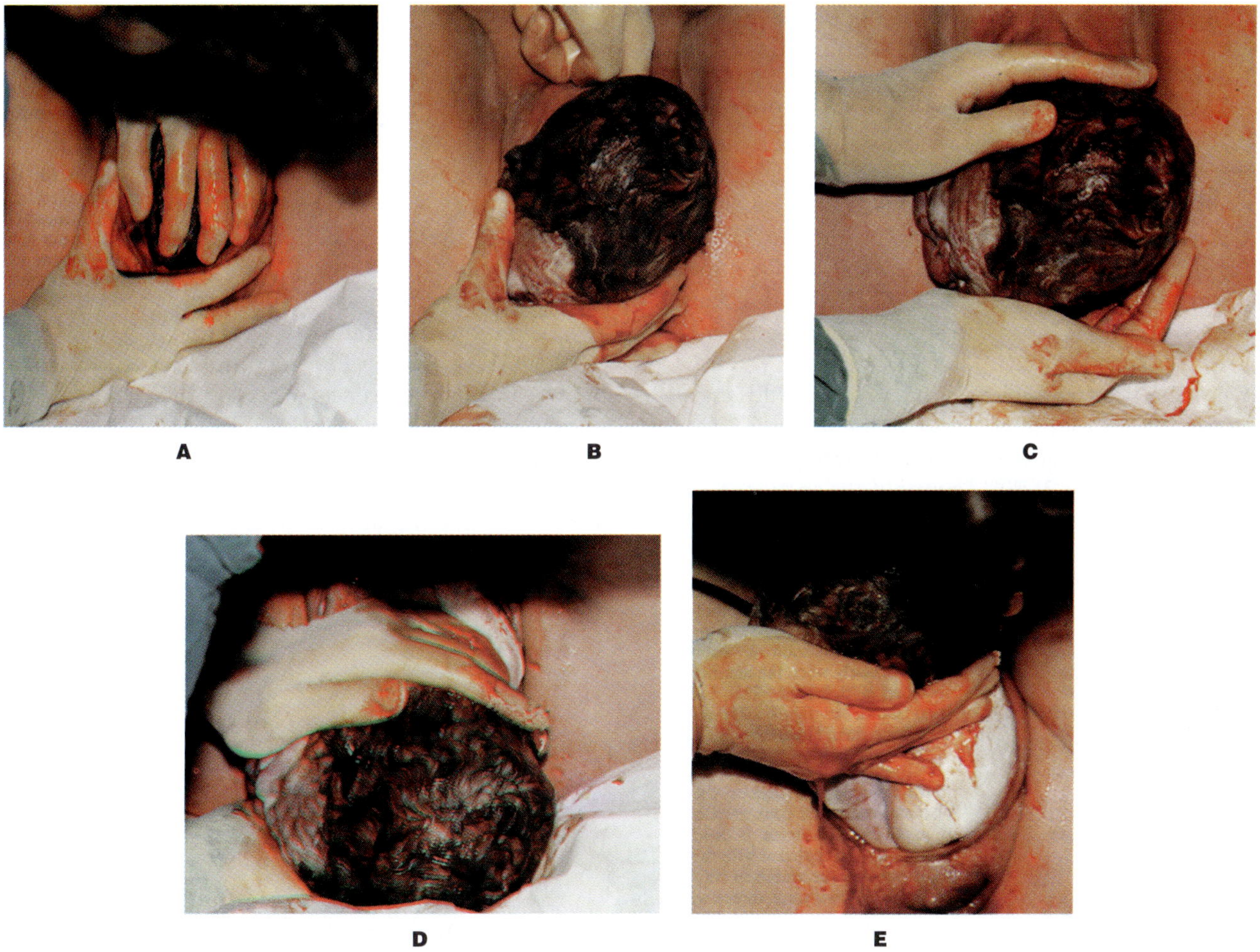

FIGURE 21.9 Normal delivery. **A,** When crowning occurs, apply gentle palm pressure to the infant's head. **B,** Examine the infant's neck for the presence of a looped umbilical cord. **C,** Support the infant's head as it rotates from shoulder presentation. **D,** Guide the infant's head downward to deliver the anterior shoulder. **E,** Guide the infant's head upward to release the posterior shoulder.

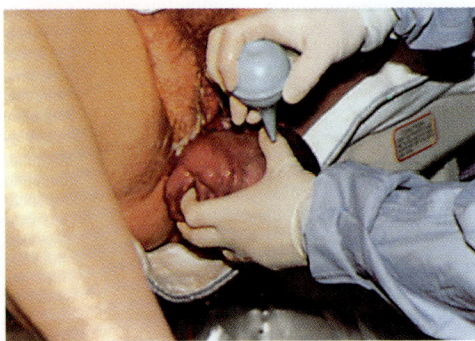

FIGURE 21.10 Once the head is delivered, suction the mouth of the infant first, then the nose. The bulb syringe should be compressed before placing it in the infant's mouth.

vaginal opening bulges to accommodate the delivery of the head. The EMT places a gloved hand on the presenting part and exerts slight pressure to prevent an explosive delivery. If at this point the amniotic sac (bag of water) has not broken, the EMT should use a clamp to puncture a hole in this membrane. With the fingers, the EMT should tear the membrane away from the head and mouth of the infant. Once the head has emerged from the vaginal opening, the EMT should examine the infant's neck for a loop of umbilical cord. If the looped umbilical cord can be gently slipped over the infant's head, then the EMT should do so. If the looped umbilical cord is tight around the infant's head, the EMT should clamp the umbilical cord in two places and cut between the clamps with the surgical scissors. The EMT should then remove the cord from around the infant's neck.

Once the head is delivered, the EMT should aggressively suction the mouth and nose of the infant. The bulb syringe needs to be squeezed before inserting it in the infant's mouth (Figure 21.10). The mouth is suctioned first, followed by the nose. The rationale for this order is that suctioning the nose is more irritating and will stimulate the infant to cry. If the infant cries, the fluid in the back of the infant's throat will be aspirated into the trachea and lungs. After the head is delivered, the shoulders are delivered by placing both hands on either side of the infant's head and, with a gentle downward pressure, gently easing one shoulder out at a time. Some infants will start to cry, which is a normal reaction. The delivery of the rest of the infant progresses very quickly, usually with the next couple of contractions. The infant will be very slippery, so the EMT should plan to support the head, shoulders, and feet. The EMT should keep the infant's head lower than the infant's feet to facilitate drainage of secretions into the mouth. The EMT should wipe the blood and mucus from the mouth and nose with the sterilized gauze and suction the mouth and nose again.

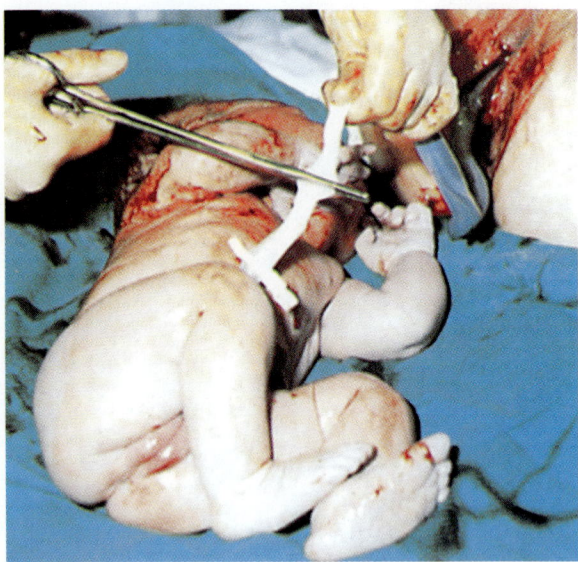

FIGURE 21.11 Cutting the cord. Fasten one clamp approximately 4 inches away from the infant's belly. Fasten the second clamp approximately 2 inches away from the first clamp. With sterile scissors, cut between the two clamps and pat with sterile gauze.

The EMT should dry off the infant, wrap him or her in a warm blanket, and keep the infant at the level of the vagina until the umbilical cord is cut. To cut the umbilical cord, the EMT should fasten one clamp approximately 4 inches away from the infant's belly. The EMT should fasten the second clamp approximately 2 inches away from the first clamp toward the placenta. With the sterilized scissors, the EMT should cut between the two clamps and pat both ends of the umbilical cord with the steriled gauze. He or she should examine both sides of the cut umbilical cord for oozing blood (Figure 21.11). If blood is noted, the EMT should use the umbilical tape to tie off the oozing umbilical cord above the umbilical clamp.

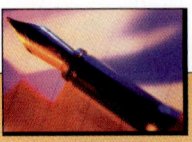 **Tips from the Pros**

- If the umbilical clamps accidentally close shut, the umbilical cord can be tied off with a shoe lace, gauze, or rope. Make sure that there is no bleeding after the cord is cut.
- Newborns are very slippery. Have an area available past the mother's buttocks just in case the infant slips out of your hands. Have plenty of towels and gauze to hold onto the infant.

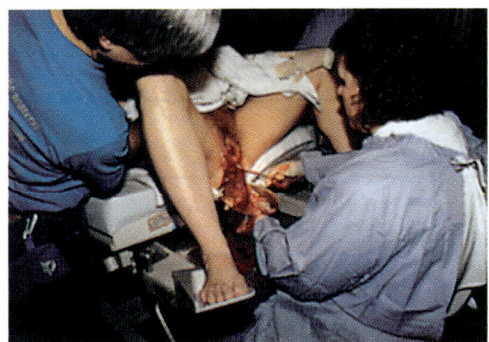

FIGURE 21.12 The placenta should be wrapped in a towel and placed in a plastic bag for transportation to the hospital.

After the delivery of the infant, the mother's contractions will increase in intensity. A large gush of blood usually follows. In a vaginal delivery, up to 500 ml of blood is lost without adverse effects on the mother. The placenta is then expelled from the vagina. The EMT should never pull on the umbilical cord to "help" deliver the placenta because it will cause harm to the mother. The average time for the delivery of the placenta is approximately 20 minutes after the delivery of the infant. The EMT should not delay transportation while waiting for the placenta to be delivered. The EMT should wrap the placenta in a towel and place it in a plastic bag for transportation to the hospital (Figure 21.12). The EMT should place a sterile pad over the vaginal opening and lower the mother's legs on the stretcher. The mother's legs may be very fatigued, and she may need assistance keeping her legs together. The EMT should document the time of day of delivery of the infant and the placenta.

If after delivery of the placenta bleeding is still excessive, the EMT should initiate rapid transportation to the hospital. While en route, the EMT should place his or her hand with fingers fully extended just below the mother's umbilicus and, with a circular motion, massage the uterus to help with contractions, which will slow bleeding (Figure 21.13). Another technique to decrease bleed-

> ✓ The delivery procedure includes observing proper BSI, controlling the delivery of the infant's head, and clamping and cutting the umbilical cord. When the infant's head is delivered, the EMT should suction the mouth first, then the nose. Once the entire infant is delivered, the EMT should dry off the infant and wrap him or her well. The EMT should deliver the placenta and put it into a plastic bag for transportation. If bleeding is excessive, the EMT should administer oxygen and manage for shock if necessary.

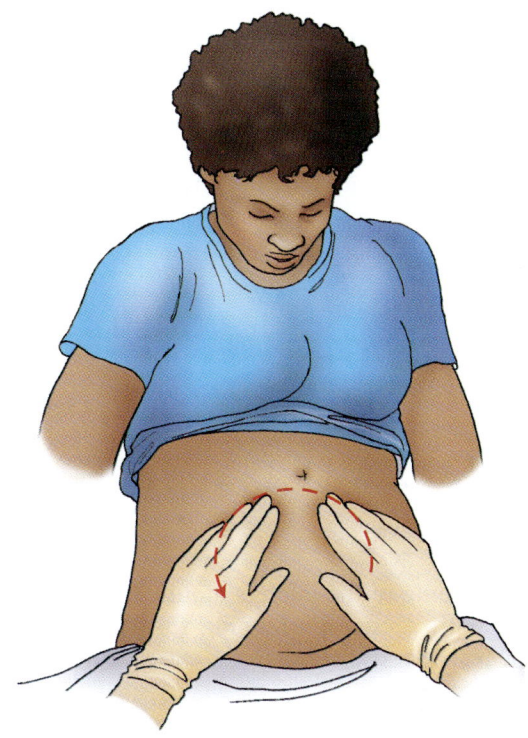

FIGURE 21.13 The EMT should place his or her hand with fingers fully extended just below the mother's umbilicus and, with a circular type motion, massage the uterus to slow bleeding.

ing is to encourage the mother to breastfeed the newborn. Breastfeeding causes the uterus to contract and may slow bleeding. Continuing assessment of the mother is as important as continuing assessment of the newborn. If the mother has the signs and syptoms of shock, regardless of the amount of blood loss, the EMT should manage for shock with supplemental oxygen, proper positioning, and rapid transportation to the hospital.

Initial Care of the Newborn

Over 90% of term infants (an infant who has had the normal 9-months prenatal development period) require little care except for drying, warming, suctioning of the airway, and mild stimulation. A wet infant can lose heat rapidly, so drying the infant quickly is critical. One of the most useful pieces of equipment that should be included in the delivery kit is a piece of stockinet, which emergency departments use as the first layer under a new cast. The EMT can tie a knot at one end of the stockinet and use it as a cap for the newborn. The head of a newborn infant is large and can be a major source of heat loss; therefore it is important to keep the head dry and warm.

During the 9 months of gestation the infant's lungs are not used and the infant's body is floating in amniotic

TABLE 21.3　APGAR Scoring System

Sign	0	1	2
Appearance (skin color)	Blue, pale	Pink body, blue extremities	Completely pink
Pulse rate (heart rate)	Absent	<100/minute	>100/minute
Grimace (irritability)	No response	Grimace	Cough, sneeze, cry
Activity (muscle tone)	Limp	Some flexion	Active motion
Respirations (respiratory effort)	Absent	Slow, irregular	Good, crying

From Aehlert B: *Pediatric advanced life support study guide*, St Louis, 1994, Mosby.

fluid. Suctioning of the infant's mouth and nose in combination with proper positioning (head slightly lower than the rest of body) removes the excess fluid and maintains a clear airway.

The infant should receive the same care as any other patient. If the infant needs oxygen, then the EMT should do so. An infant with a pulse rate less than 100 beats per minute would benefit from the use of supplemental oxygen. This is a short-time treatment until the pulse rate is between 120 to 140 beats per minute. The mode for the delivery of oxygen is slightly different. If the infant has spontaneous respirations, the EMT can administer "blow-by" oxygen. This is accomplished by holding either oxygen tubing or a face mask with the oxygen liter flow sufficient to have oxygen passively flow in front of the nose and mouth of the infant. This procedure will increase the oxygen concentration that is inspired with each breath by the newborn. Oxygen is a cool gas and initially can cause a decrease in the infant's heart rate. This decrease lasts only for a short time (approximately 30 to 60 seconds) and should not deter the use of oxygen.

If possible, the EMT should keep the newborn with the mother. If identification bracelets are available in the prehospital environment, then both mother and newborn should receive the same bracelet. In other systems the mother and newborn will receive their matching bracelets once admitted to the hospital. The goal is to maintain the correct mother with the correct newborn.

A scoring system has been instituted to evaluate the condition of the infant after 1 and 5 minutes of life. This scoring system is called the **APGAR score** (Table 21.3). The APGAR score labels the following characteristics: **A**ppearance, **P**ulse, **G**rimace, **A**ctivity, and **R**espiration. Each of these characteristics is assigned a value of either 0, 1, or 2. On completed assessment of the newborn, the numbers are added for a total APGAR score. The calculation of an APGAR score should not delay resuscitative efforts of a newborn. Most newborns have a calculated APGAR score of 8 to 10 at 1 minute after birth.

During assessment of a normal newborn, the EMT should note the following characteristics. Many newborns will start to cry once suctioning of the airway, drying, and warming have been completed. If the newborn does not cry, additional tactile stimulation is needed. Other techniques to try include flicking the soles of the feet or rubbing the infant's back (Figure 21.14). These techniques should stimulate the infant to cry, and with each cry the EMT can assess the infant's breathing capabilities. The trunk of the infant will be a normal, well-perfused flesh color, but the extremities may be cyanotic. It is not unusual for the extremities to be cyanotic for some time after delivery. The arms and legs should move with each cry.

The newborn's circulation is assessed by evaluating a brachial or apical pulse. The brachial pulse is located on the upper portion of either arm, and the apical pulse is located halfway between the newborn's left nipple and the middle of the chest. The pulse rate of a newborn should be greater than 100 beats per minute. As long as the infant is warm and maintaining the functions of airway, breathing, and circulation, the infant will progress normally (maintaining ventilations, oxygenation, and perfusion). However, a small population of newborns need resuscitation.

> ✓ Care of a newborn includes drying, suctioning, and stimulating. The APGAR score provides a way of assessing the newborn's appearance, pulse, grimace, activity, and respirations. Some infants need oxygen.

Newborn Resuscitation

Newborns who need resuscitation have problems with either airway, breathing, or circulation. The best resuscitation occurs in a controlled environment; therefore the EMT should make every attempt to get the mother to the hospital. Situations in which resuscitation may be likely include the following:

- Multiple births
- A mother who is drug dependent
- A mother who delivers before the seventh month of pregnancy
- Prolonged delivery
- A delivery in which the head is not the presenting part
- Presence of meconium-stained amniotic fluid (to be discussed later in this chapter)

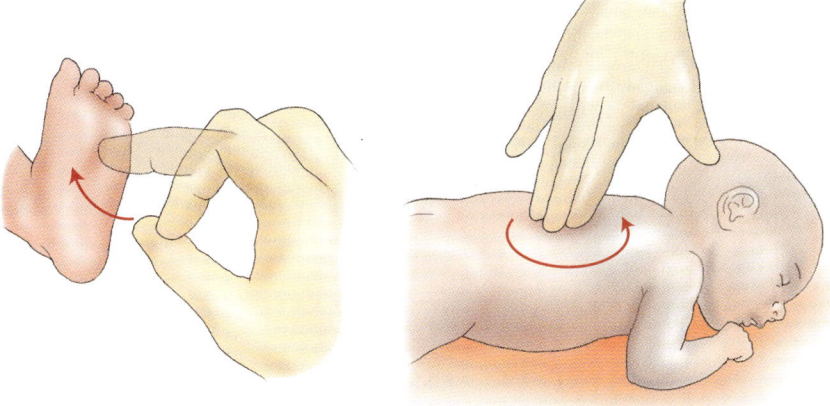

FIGURE 21.14 If the newborn does not cry, flick the soles of the feet and rub the newborn's back as another means of tactile stimulation.

- An infant whose breathing efforts are shallow, slow, or nonexistent
- An infant whose heart rate is 100 beats or less per minute
- An infant whose chest and abdomen are cyanotic

If one of these situations occurs, the EMT should do the following:

1. Warm, dry, position, suction, and stimulate the infant. For infants born with thick meconium, suction the airway until clear. This situation is the only one in which breathing or delivering supplemental oxygen is delayed.
2. Apply oxygen for breathing infants.
3. Apply oxygen by bag-valve-mask (BVM) at 100% oxygen for nonbreathing infants.
4. If no pulse is palpated, perform chest compressions with oxygen by BVM at 100% oxygen.
5. If the infant has spontaneous respirations, has received supplemental oxygen for 30 seconds, and still maintains a heart rate of 80 beats per minute, start chest compressions.
6. If the infant has spontaneous respirations and a heart rate greater than 80 beats per minute but has central cyanosis (cyanosis of the chest and abdomen), administer high-concentration oxygen by the blow-by method.

After initiating one of these interventions, the EMT should reassess the infant after 30 seconds and either continue, change, or stop the intervention.

In resuscitating infants, special care is needed during BVM ventilation to prevent overexpanded lungs. The EMT should judge the correct amount of oxygen given during BVM ventilation by visually looking at the rise and fall of the infant's chest.

Newborn infants, whether they initially are in need of resuscitation or are healthy, do well as long as the inverted pyramid is followed (Figure 21.15). These actions are complemented by constant reassessment of the infant. These steps will help the EMT deliver the highest level of patient care in the worst possible situation.

> ✓ Some infants require resuscitation. Breathing infants with a pulse rate less than 100 beats per minute require high-concentration oxygen, whereas nonbreathing infants need bag-valve-mask ventilation and may require chest compressions. The EMT must continually assess the infant's condition while performing these interventions.

Abnormal Delivery

With every birth the chance exists that delivery will not follow the sequence previously described in this chapter. To help facilitate treatment in these unusual situations, the prolapsed cord and abnormal deliveries are described separately.

Prolapsed Cord

A **prolapsed cord** occurs when the umbilical cord is delivered first (Figure 21.16). The following is a typical scenario for this situation:

> The EMT is called to a home for a patient with abdominal pain. On arrival the EMT finds a 35-year-old woman who is visibly pregnant and says that her due date was last

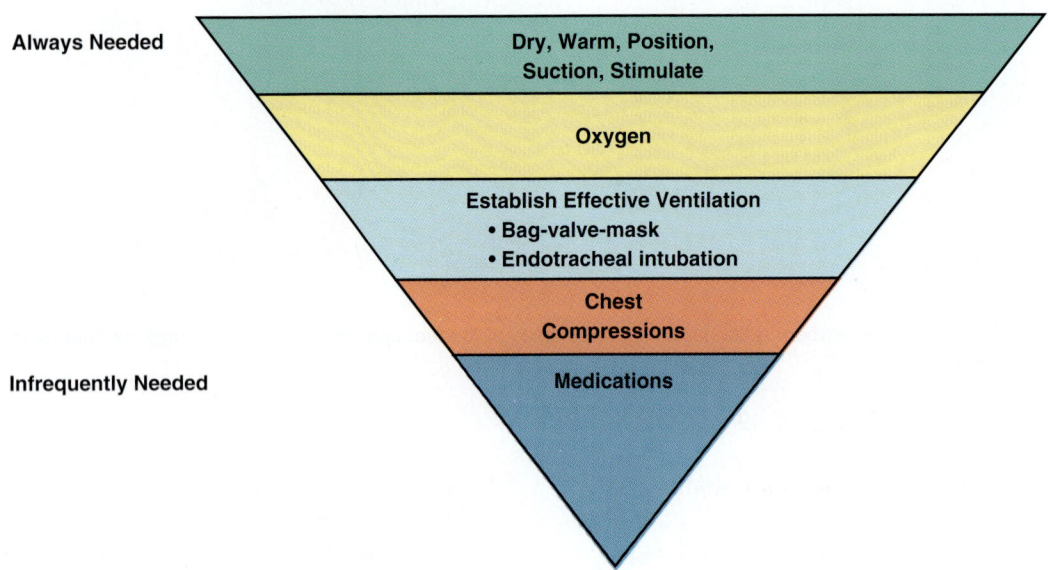

FIGURE 21.15 Inverted pyramid.

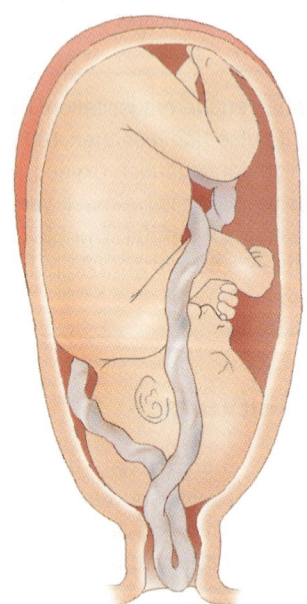

FIGURE 21.16 Prolapsed cord.

week. The patient also admits that she was experiencing regular contractions that were about 15 minutes apart. She is also embarrassed because she thinks she wet the bed.

The EMT institutes BSI precautions including protective eyewear, double gloves, and a protective clothing barrier. The EMT determines that the patient's airway is patent, she is breathing without distress, and her circulation is being maintained because she is able to answer all questions appropriately. Her appropriate response indicates adequate perfusion to the brain.

From the history, the EMT decides that this patient is in labor and that the patient has ruptured her membranes (bag of waters). The EMT proceeds to examine the patient, first making sure that his or her partner is in the room. On examination of the patient's perineum, the EMT sees the whitish-colored umbilical cord protruding from the vaginal opening. Immediately, the EMT instructs his or her partner to place the mother on high-concentration oxygen using a nonrebreather mask with reservoir. The EMT then positions the mother with her head and upper torso lower than her hips and buttocks. The mother will be transported in this manner to a hospital as rapidly and safely as possible.

This patient will need a cesarean delivery. The EMT inserts a sterile gloved hand into the vagina (this is one of the only times that an EMT is ever allowed to touch a woman's perineal area), pushing the presenting part of the fetus off the umbilical cord. If the EMT is able to get the fetus off the umbilical cord, the umbilical cord will have a pulsating sensation that can be felt. The mother is instructed not to bear down and, with the urge of each contraction, to use the breathing technique of "blow" breathing. Once the EMT places his or her hand in the vagina, the patient will be transported in that position directly to the hospital and directly into the operating room until the fetus is delivered by cesarean section.

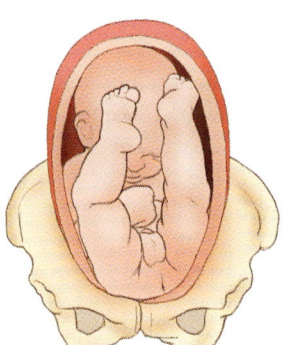 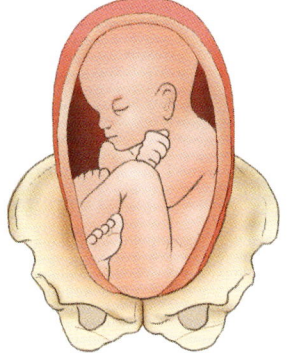 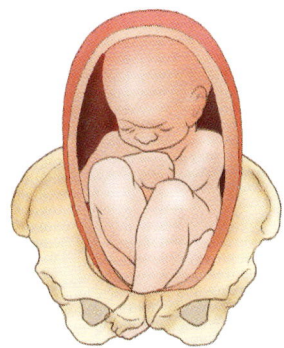

FIGURE 21.17 Types of breech presentations.

Breech Presentation

Another abnormal delivery is called a **breech birth** presentation (Figure 21.17). In this delivery, the presenting part is either the buttocks or the foot or leg of the fetus. The following is a scenario for a breech presentation:

> The EMT is called to a home for a patient with abdominal pain. On arrival, the EMT finds a 35-year-old woman who is visibly pregnant and admits that her due date was last week. The patient also says that she was experiencing regular contractions that were about 3 minutes apart. She is also embarrassed because she feels something between her legs.
>
> The EMT institutes full BSI including protective eyewear, double gloves, and a protective clothing barrier. The EMT determines that the patient's airway is patent, she is breathing without distress, and her circulation is adequately maintained. From the history, the EMT decides that this patient is probably in labor. The EMT proceeds to examine the patient, first making sure that his or her partner is in the room. On examination of the patient's perineum, the EMT sees what appears to be a right foot and leg protruding from the vaginal opening. Immediately, the EMT instructs her partner to place the mother on high-concentration oxygen using a nonrebreather mask with reservoir. If delivery is imminent, the EMT assists the delivery while trying to expedite transportation to the hospital.
>
> The child will probably need resuscitation after delivery, especially if the head is delayed and the umbilical cord is depressed. If the head is not delivered immediately, the EMT should place a sterile gloved hand in the vagina with her palm toward the infant's face (this is a second situation in which an EMT can touch a female patient's perineal area). With the EMT's index finger and middle finger, a "V" is formed around the infant's nose, helping to push the vaginal wall away from the infant's face (Figure 21.18). This technique prevents suffocation of the newborn. The mother will be transported in this manner to a hospital as rapidly and safely as possible for a possible cesarean delivery.

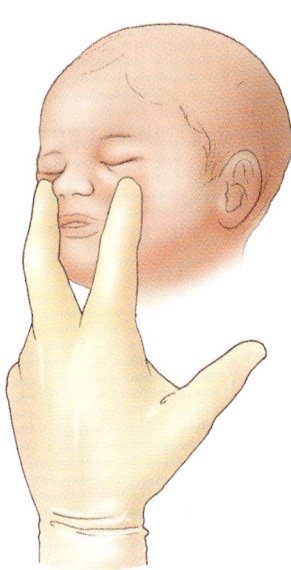

FIGURE 21.18 V-finger position. The EMT's index finger and middle finger form a "V" around the infant's nose, helping to push the vaginal wall away from the infant's face.

In cases in which a hand or shoulder is the presenting part, the EMT should place the mother on her left side. The case is then handled the same way as one involving a prolapsed cord. High-concentration oxygen is given to the mother, and the mother is positioned with her head lower than her buttocks. This scenario is the third and final time an EMT may place a sterile gloved hand into the mother's vagina to lift the infant away from

> ✓ Three situations in which the EMT inserts a gloved hand into the vagina are a prolapsed cord (in which the cord is delivered first), a lower body or leg breech delivery, and a shoulder or hand delivery (the latter two are deliveries in which a part other than the infant's head is the presenting part). The EMT should transport these patients as soon as possible to the medical facility.

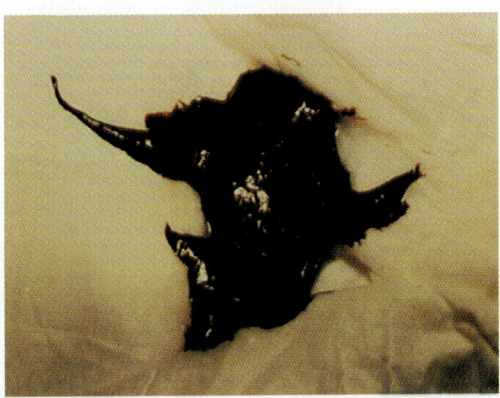

FIGURE 21.19 Meconium.

a possibly compressed umbilical cord. If the mother has a contraction or feels like she has to bear down, the EMT should instruct the mother to breathe forcefully through the contraction. Again, this mother will need a cesarean delivery.

Multiple Births

If an EMT arrives at a scene and finds a mother who is expecting multiple births, the EMT needs to call for assistance. A good rule to follow is one patient for each EMT. Therefore a patient delivering twins should have three EMTs at the scene: one for the mother, one for the first infant, and one for the second infant. Multiple births are at risk for premature deliveries. Premature infants are always at risk for rapid body heat loss. Extra attention is needed to minimize heat loss (e.g., be careful to keep infants out of drafts, especially when they are wet after delivery). Dry blankets and protection from drafts will help maintain the infant's body temperature. The need to resuscitate is greater for the premature infant. The inverted pyramid should be used for this population group (see Figure 21.15).

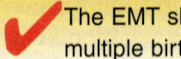 The EMT should call for assistance in the event of multiple births.

Meconium

Greenish or blackish amniotic fluid (known as **meconium**) indicates that the infant has had a bowel movement in the uterus due to some sort of stressful situation (e.g., umbilical cord around the neck) (Figure 21.19). The following scenario discusses how the EMT should manage a delivery in which meconium is in the amniotic fluid:

> An EMT arrives at a house where he finds a 22-year-old woman in active labor. After instituting the appropriate BSI precautions, the EMT sees that the perineum is bulging and the presenting part is the top of the infant's head. According to the patient, her membranes ruptured about 6 hours ago, followed by regular strong contractions that are now about 3 minutes apart. The EMT questions the patient about the color of the amniotic fluid when her membranes ruptured, but the patient cannot remember. The EMT places a clean, white absorbent pad under the patient's buttocks and in a short time notices that the pad has absorbed some of the amniotic fluid. The fluid is greenish in color, and the EMT remembers that the amniotic fluid should be clear or straw colored. The EMT realizes that there may be meconium in the amniotic fluid and the infant is probably in fetal distress. The EMT places the mother on 100% oxygen using the nonrebreather mask with reservoir.

The contractions have now increased and the head is being pushed out by the mother. The infant's head is covered with a thick greenish oily substance, and immediately the EMT suctions the mouth multiple times while waiting for the rest of the infant to be delivered. The EMT assesses the infant's mouth and sees that meconium is still in the mouth. At this time the infant is delivered and the EMT continues to suction the mouth and pharynx until clear. The EMT then proceeds to suction the nose until clear. The EMT dries, warms, and stimulates the infant, causing him to cry. The EMT double clamps the cord approximately 6 inches from the infant's umbilicus and cuts between the clamps. The EMT examines the ends for bleeding. The infant is now pink and forcefully crying. The infant is wrapped, in no distress, and placed in the mother's arms, and the mother places the infant to her breast. (If this had been a depressed infant or if meconium were still present in the child's airway, the child should not have been placed to the mother's breast.)

The first step with a child from a meconium delivery is to clear the infant's airway of all meconium. Aggressive suctioning could prevent this child from having a severe respiratory problem. Rapid and safe transportation to the hospital, preferably one with neonatal capability, is necessary for rapid evaluation.

✓ Meconium in the amniotic fluid indicates fetal distress. The EMT must clear the infant's airway of meconium with suction when the infant is born to avoid a severe respiratory problem.

Trauma During Pregnancy

Pregnancy causes anatomic and physiologic changes in the body systems. These changes affect the potential patterns of injuries. With a pregnant patient, the EMT is treating two patients and must be alert to changes that have occurred throughout the pregnancy.

The mother's heart rate increases throughout pregnancy, rising 15 to 20 beats per minute above normal by the third trimester. Systolic and diastolic blood pressures will drop 5 to 15 mm Hg during the second trimester but will be normal at term. Some women may experience significant hypotension when supine. This condition is caused by compression of the inferior vena cava and is usually relieved if the woman lies on her left side. However, with blunt trauma or suspicion of a cervical spine injury, the EMT should not neglect the backboard. The EMT should immobilize the patient on the backboard quickly and receive high-flow supplemental oxygen. At this point, the backboard, with the patient properly secured to it, should be turned to the patient's left side approximately 10 to 15 degrees (Figure 21.20). After the tenth week of pregnancy, cardiac output is increased by 1.0 to 1.5 L/min. Blood volume increases 48% by term. Because of this significant increase, 30% to 35% of the blood volume can be lost before signs and symptoms of hypovolemia (the loss of circulating blood in the body characterized by a decrease in blood pressure and a rapid pulse) become apparent.

Although a marked protuberance of the abdomen is obvious in late pregnancy, abdominal organs experience slight changes, with the exception of the uterus. The liver is displaced backward, upward, and to the right, and the large intestine is displaced superiorly and is shielded by the uterus in the last two trimesters of pregnancy. The increased size and high blood flow of the uterus make it susceptible to both blunt and penetrating injury (Figure 21.21).

The ventilatory rate is also altered by pregnancy. During the third trimester, the diaphragm is elevated and may cause some dyspnea, especially when the patient is supine. Predelivery increase in blood pressure with resultant seizure activity is a late complication of pregnancy but may mimic a head injury. Careful neurologic assessment and discovery of any pertinent associated medical history are important.

During pregnancy, the activity of the intestine called *peristalsis* is slowed, so food may remain in the stomach for hours after eating. The pregnant patient is therefore at higher risk of vomiting and subsequent aspiration. As with the nonpregnant patient, auscultation (listening with a stethoscope to the abdomen for bowel sounds) of the abdomen is nonproductive. Searching for fetal heart tones on the scene is also nonproductive because their presence or absence is not going to alter the prehospital care. Rapid transportation to the trauma center is the correct management.

Blood loss from abdominal injury may present with anything from minimal signs and symptoms of shock to severe shock. The condition of the fetus depends on the condition of the mother. However, the fetus may be in severe jeopardy while the mother's condition and vital signs appear stable. The goals of management are essentially the same as for any patient experiencing shock, including increased attention to providing high levels of oxygen to meet the needs of the mother and fetus.

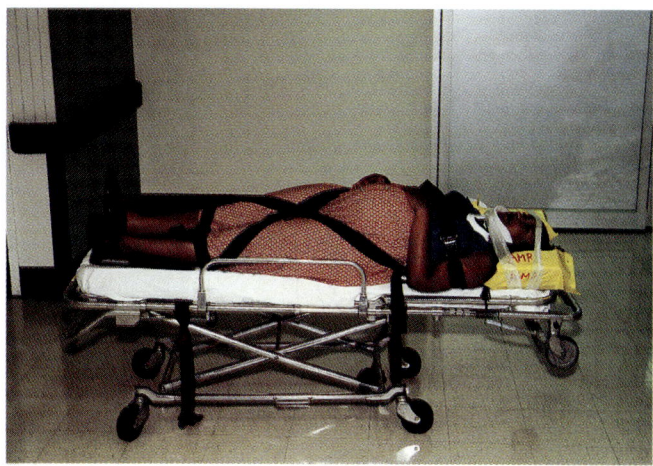

FIGURE 21.20 When spinal injury is suspected, immobilize and transport the pregnant woman in the supine position. To prevent compression of the vena cava, carefully tilt the long board 10 to 15 degrees to the left.

Any evidence of vaginal bleeding or a rigid boardlike abdomen with external bleeding in the last trimester of pregnancy should alert the EMT to possible abruptio placentae or ruptured uterus. The loss of circulating blood volume may occur rapidly. *The EMT should not delay transportation of the pregnant trauma patient.*

The EMT should transport a pregnant trauma victim even though the injury appears to be minor, because any trauma to the abdomen of a pregnant patient should be evaluated by a physician. Adequate resuscitation of the mother is the key to survival of the mother and fetus.

> ✔ Key points in the assessment and management of a pregnant trauma patient include management of shock, immobilization on a backboard if spinal injury is suspected, and resuscitation. The EMT should be alert to the possibility of vomiting. In some situations, the mother's condition may be stable while the infant's condition is distressed. Recognition and appropriate resuscitation may ensure survival of both mother and fetus.

Alleged Sexual Assault

Sexual assault is a crime that is not always reported because of the negative connotations associated with the crime. Until recently, many people would not admit to being raped or sexually assaulted.

When an EMT arrives at the scene of an alleged sexual assault, he or she should keep the retrieval of the

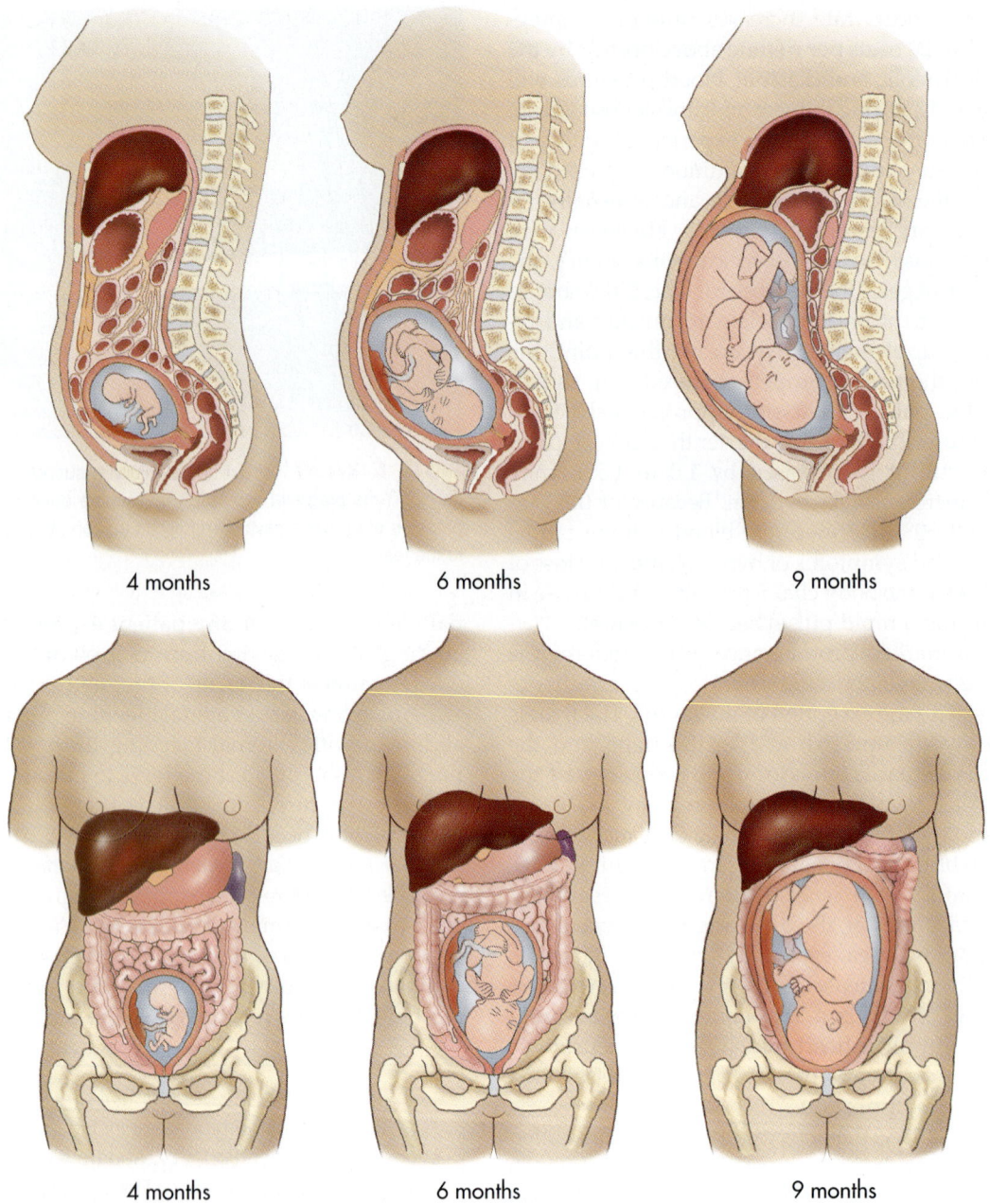

FIGURE 21.21 Displacement of internal abdominal structures and diaphragm by the enlarging uterus.

Tips from the Pros

A male EMT who has to treat a female sexual assault victim needs to remember that the patient may perceive the male EMT as the assailant. Before the EMT does anything, he needs to identify himself and identify everything that he is going to do before he does it. His sentences should be short and easy to understand. He should not do anything that makes the patient uncomfortable unless it is directly related to the airway, breathing, and circulation.

history of events to a minimum unless the patient wants to talk. If the patient is talking, the EMT must listen and document in quotation marks what the patient says. If possible, a female EMT should be with a female patient to render care. The EMT should discourage the patient from bathing, showering, voiding, or cleaning off debris from his or her body. Unfortunately, many patients who have been sexually assaulted have changed their clothing and showered. In these cases, the EMT should encourage the patient to bring the soiled clothing to the hospital. The EMT should place all clothing in a paper bag (a plastic bag will ruin the evidence through spoilage). The EMT must use BSI precautions and refrain from examining the perineum unless profuse bleeding is noted. All documentation should be facts, not opinions.

The assessment of the sexually assaulted victim includes the normal assessment of airway, breathing, and circulation. The EMT should manage any threats to the airway, breathing, or circulation and control bleeding. The EMT should not clean or dress abrasions and superficial wounds because clues or evidence may be obtained from these injuries. The EMT's most valuable service for this situation is emotional support and preservation of evidence.

> ✓ For victims of sexual assault, the EMT should provide emotional support. The EMT should encourage the victim not to shower or change clothes because key evidence may be lost. The EMT should not clean or treat abrasions or superficial wounds.

Summary

- A woman's abdominal cavity also contains the reproductive organs. All women of reproductive age have the possibility of being pregnant.
- Pregnancy averages about 40 weeks and consists of three 3-month intervals known as *trimesters*. There are three stages of labor. A normal delivery can produce a copious amount of blood and may be sudden. Prepackaged equipment is helpful when delivery is imminent.
- Expulsion of the products of conception before the twentieth week is called an *abortion*. All natural or spontaneous abortions are called *miscarriages*. Bleeding in the first trimester can indicate a miscarriage.
- Bleeding in the third trimester can endanger the lives of the mother and fetus. Treatment for bleeding in the third trimester consists of increased oxygen, management of shock, and rapid transportation for a cesarean section.
- Seizures in a pregnant woman could result from a known seizure history or increased blood pressure due to pregnancy.
- For a woman in active labor, and EMT should expedite transportation unless the signs of imminent birth are present.
- If delivery is imminent, the EMT must observe full body substance isolation precautions; protective eyewear is essential.
- Newborns need to have their mouths suctioned first and then the nose. Newborns lose heat rapidly from their head and wet body. The umbilical cord needs to be clamped in two sections and cut between both clamps. Initial care of all newborns consist of drying, warming, and suctioning the airway. The APGAR score should not delay resuscitative efforts.
- Resuscitation is indicated for infants who have problems with their airway, breathing, or circulation. Resuscitation of newborns consists of providing additional oxygen and warmth and doing chest compressions.
- The only times that an EMT can place a gloved hand into the mother's vagina is for a prolapsed cord, a lower body or leg breech delivery, or an upper shoulder or hand breech delivery.
- Ideally, one EMT is needed for each patient (e.g., a mother with twins needs three EMTs). Transportation should not be delayed if EMT backup is not available in a timely fashion.
- Meconium is the infant's first stool in the amniotic fluid and indicates fetal distress. An infant with thick meconium needs to have the meconium suctioned immediately before respirations begin.
- A pregnant woman in a trauma situation will maintain a normal blood pressure until the circulating volume of the infant is depleted. All pregnant women subjected to trauma should be treated in accordance with the mechanism of injury and with a high index of suspicion. Increased oxygen taken in by the mother will also increase the oxygen level of the infant.
- Sexual assault is a crime, and the patient needs physical and emotional support. Sexual assault victims should not bathe, shower, void, or put on clean clothes. The sexual assault victim's body is the source for evidence in this crime.

Scenario Solution

You are wearing gloves and appropriate protective wear, including glasses. Treatment interventions should start with preparing the mother for eminent delivery and placing her on oxygen with a nonrebreather mask at 15 L/min. You note with each contraction a bulging of the perineum. You dress in the body substance isolation precaution outfit, open

Scenario Solution (cont'd)

the delivery kit, put on a second pair of sterile gloves and protective eyewear, and drape the perineum. On visualization of the perineum, you see that the head is crowning. The membranes rupture leaking greenish fluid, and you realize that this infant may need resuscitation. You place the palm of your hand against the presenting infant's head to prevent an explosive delivery, deliver the head, and immediately suction out the infant's mouth until clear. You then proceeds to suction the infant's nose until clear.

You now continue with the delivery, and with a slight downward motion you deliver one shoulder. You proceed with a slight upward motion and deliver the other shoulder. At this point the infant's chest, abdomen, and feet are delivered with the mother's next two pushes.

You immediately cover the newborn with a dry sterile towel and proceed to suction out the mouth and nose until clear, which should stimulate the respirations of the newborn. You should then proceed to clamp the umbilical cord. The first clamp is applied 4 inches from the infant's belly and the second clamp approximately 2 inches from the first. Once cut, you examine the cord for any bleeding. If none is present, you wrap the infant in a warm blanket; the infant can now be held by the mother. You can now prepare for the delivery of the placenta and transport the mother and newborn to the hospital.

Key Terms

Abortion The expulsion of an embryo or fetus from the uterus before the twentieth week; can occur spontaneously or through a medical procedure.

Abruptio placentae Sudden separation of the placenta from the wall of the uterus; signs and symptoms include sudden severe, low abdominal pain with or without vaginal bleeding.

Amniotic fluid Clear to straw-colored fluid in the amniotic sac that acts as a shock absorber and maintains a uniform pressure and temperature for the fetus.

Amniotic sac Fibrous sac filled with a clear to straw-colored fluid called the *amniotic fluid*; protects the fetus; also called *bag of waters*.

APGAR score Scoring system used to evaluate the condition of the infant after 1 minute of life and after 5 minutes of life; scores of 0, 1, or 2 are given for Appearance, Pulse, Grimace, Activity, and Respiration. Most newborns have a calculated APGAR score of 8 to 10 1 minute after birth.

Birth canal Structure located between the anus and the urethral orifice; also known as the *vagina*.

Braxton Hicks contractions Contractions that occur at irregular intervals but do not increase in pain intensity; also known as *false contractions*.

Breech birth A birth in which the presenting part of the fetus is either the buttocks, foot, or leg.

Cervix The opening to the uterus.

Contraction Tightening and hardening of the uterus that expels the fetus.

Crowning Bulging of the perineum when birth is imminent.

Eclampsia In the pregnant patient, predelivery increase in blood pressure with resultant seizure activity.

Embryo Fertilized egg to the first 8 weeks of pregnancy.

Fallopian tubes Paired canals approximately 4 inches long connecting the ovary to the uterus; also called *oviducts*.

False contractions Contractions that occur at irregular intervals but do not increase in pain intensity; also known as *Braxton Hicks contractions*.

Fetus The developing unborn offspring from 8 weeks after conception until birth.

Gravida Refers to number of times the patient has been pregnant.

Gynecology The study of the diseases of women's reproductive organs.

Labor Regular uterine contractions that increase in frequency and intensity that propel the fetus from the uterus.

Meconium Fetal intestinal contents that stain the amniotic fluid green or black; fetus may expel contents of bowels before birth due to stress; indicates a birth complication.

Menopause The permanent absence of menstruation (menses or period).

Menstrual period See *Menstruation*.

Menstruation The periodic sloughing of the uterine lining, which is composed of blood, tissue, and cells.

Miscarriage Natural or spontaneous abortion.

Mucous plug Accumulation of mucus that forms and interlocks with the capillaries of the cervix during pregnancy; acts as a protective barrier between the cervix and the vagina for the duration of pregnancy.

Obstetrics Branch of medicine that deals with the management of women during pregnancy, childbirth, and 42 days after the expulsion of all contents of pregnancy.

Key Terms (cont'd)

Ovaries Paired, almond-shaped organs suspended by ligaments in the left and right lower quadrants of the abdomen that release a mature egg once a month in women.

Oviducts Paired canals approximately 4 inches long connecting the ovary to the uterus; also called *fallopian tubes*.

Ovulation The release of a mature egg from an ovary once a month.

Para Refers to previous number of children delivered.

Perineum Space between the vaginal opening and the anal opening.

Placenta Highly vascular disklike structure that links the tissue of the mother with that of the fetus. The placenta exchanges oxygen and carbon dioxide between fetus and mother, transports nutrients and waste byproducts, and serves as a temporary source for hormone production necessary to sustain pregnancy.

Placenta previa Condition in which the placenta implants itself either on or near the opening of the cervix; severe bleeding in late pregnancy occurs when the cervix begins to dilate in early labor.

Presenting part Part of the fetus that protrudes initially during the birthing process.

Prolapsed cord Premature expulsion of the umbilical cord.

Trimester A 3-month period; there are 3-three month periods, or three trimesters, during a pregnancy.

True contractions Labor contractions; cramplike pain that may radiate to the lower back, generally regular, with intervals lasting between 5 and 15 minutes and increasing in pain intensity as labor progresses.

Tubal pregnancy Pregnancy in which the fertilized egg implants in a fallopian tube.

Umbilical arteries Arteries that carry deoxygenated blood from the fetus to the placenta.

Umbilical cord Fibrous, whitish tube that connects the fetus to the placenta.

Umbilical vein Vein that carries oxygenated blood from the placenta to the fetus.

Umbilicus Navel.

Uterine rupture Rupture of the uterus caused by trauma or previous cesarean scarring.

Uterus Single, pear-shaped, muscular organ located between the rectum and the bladder that houses the fetus during fetal development.

Vagina Fibromuscular sheath that leads from the uterus and extends to the vaginal opening.

Vaginal opening Opening to the vagina located between the anus and the urethral orifice.

Review Questions

1. True or False: Women always know when they are pregnant.
2. In the last 3 months of pregnancy, a woman lying on her back may experience lightheadedness or fainting. What could be done to prevent this from happening?
   a. Position the woman on her right side.
   b. Position the woman on her left side.
   c. Instruct the woman to decrease her salt intake.
   d. Increase the amount of fluids the woman has been taking.
3. As an EMT, you are dispatched to a woman who is 8½ months pregnant who developed vaginal bleeding. You would do which of the following?
   a. Administer high-concentration oxygen, place the woman on the stretcher with her legs elevated, keep the woman warm, and transport rapidly.
   b. Walk the patient to the ambulance and transport.
   c. Prepare the woman for a home delivery.
   d. Put on a body substance isolation outfit and, with a gloved hand, place your fingers in the woman's vaginal area, feeling for the umbilical cord.
4. An infant had been delivered at home and was handed to the EMTs as soon as they walked into the house. There was greenish-black staining all over the infant's body, the infant was not breathing, and the umbilical cord was tied off and cut from the placenta. What action should be taken by the EMT?
   a. The infant should be washed off, dressed, and put to the breast of the mother.
   b. The infant should be presumed dead.
   c. The infant should be kept warm while the airway is aggressively suctioned until clear. The infant would then receive bag-valve-mask ventilations followed by an assessment of the circulation status.
   d. The family should be reported for child abuse.
5. True or False: A sexual assault victim should be encouraged to bathe and change his or her clothing before being transferred to the emergency department.

Answers to these Review Questions can be found at the end of the book on page 866.

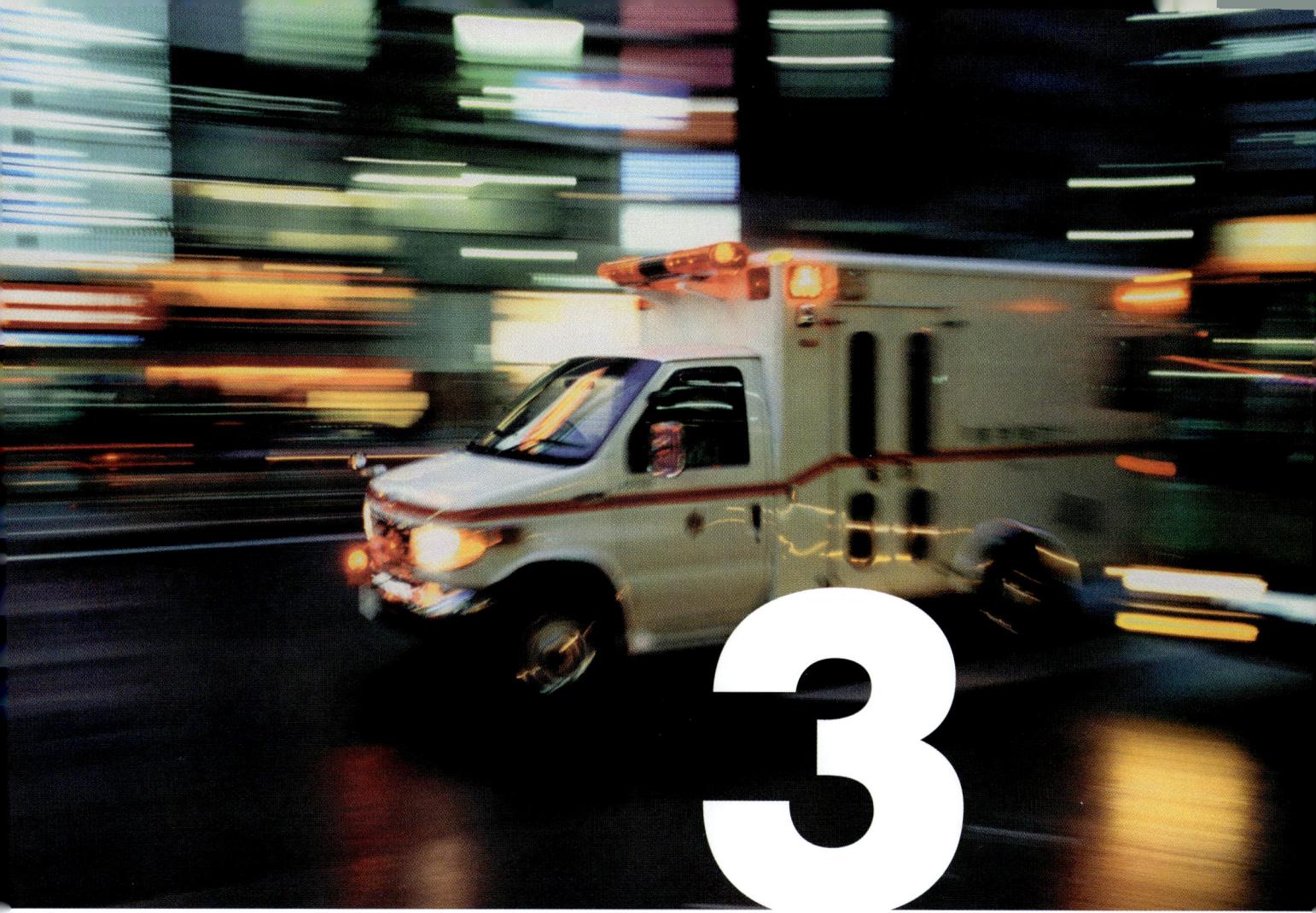

Section Three

Trauma

Kinematics of Trauma

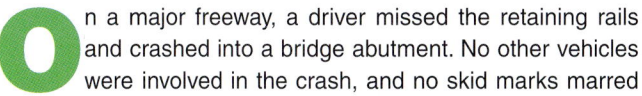

This chapter is designed to allow the emergency medical technician to understand how a crash occurs, the energy exchange involved, and how to use this information to predict (at the time of the scene survey) the injuries that are most likely to be found.

Scenario

On a major freeway, a driver missed the retaining rails and crashed into a bridge abutment. No other vehicles were involved in the crash, and no skid marks marred the road. The call came in at 2115 hours. Arrival at the scene is at 2121 hours. Only one occupant is in the car. The crash scene is depicted in Figure 22.1.

 What injuries should the EMT expect to find on arrival?

Key Terms to Know

Anatomy
Angular-impact collision
Anterior flail chest
Aortic insufficiency
Blunt trauma
Cardiac contusion
Cavitation
Compression
Crash
Descending aorta
Energy
Fragmentation
Great vessels
Head-on collision
High-energy weapons
Kinematics
Kinetic energy
Ligaments
Low-energy weapons
Mass (multiple) casualty incident (MCI)
Medium-energy weapons
Pedicle
Penetrating trauma
Permanent cavity
Pneumothorax
Postcrash
Precrash
Primary injuries
Pulmonary contusion
Ribs
Secondary injuries
Shape
Shear
Stopping distance
Temporary cavity
Tendons
Tertiary injuries
Tumble
Velocity
Vertebral column

399

Learning Objectives

As an EMT-Basic, you should be able to do the following:

Supplemental

- Define *energy* and *force* as they relate to trauma.
- Define the laws governing motion.
- Describe the role increased speed plays in causing injuries.
- Describe each type of automobile impact and its effect on unrestrained victims (e.g., down and under, up and over, compression, shear).
- Describe the injuries produced in the head, spine, thorax, and abdomen that result from the various types of automobile collisions.
- Describe the kinematics of penetrating injuries.
- Describe the mechanism of energy exchange and the factors that affect speed reduction for a moving body.
- List the motion and energy considerations of mechanisms other than motor vehicle crashes.
- Define the role of kinematics as an additional tool for patient assessment.

Each patient who arrives in the emergency center appears to have his or her own unique presentation and set of injuries, despite a mechanism of injury similar to that of previous patients. In truth, many patients have similar patterns of injury, but with varied outcomes depending on the amount of **energy** exchanged in the crash, the force that created the crash, and its direction. These patterns and the alterations that occur in them reflect differences in age or **anatomy**, the influence of disease or substance abuse in the victim, and individual variations in response to the energy transfer of trauma.

Patient Care Algorithm

Patient Assessment

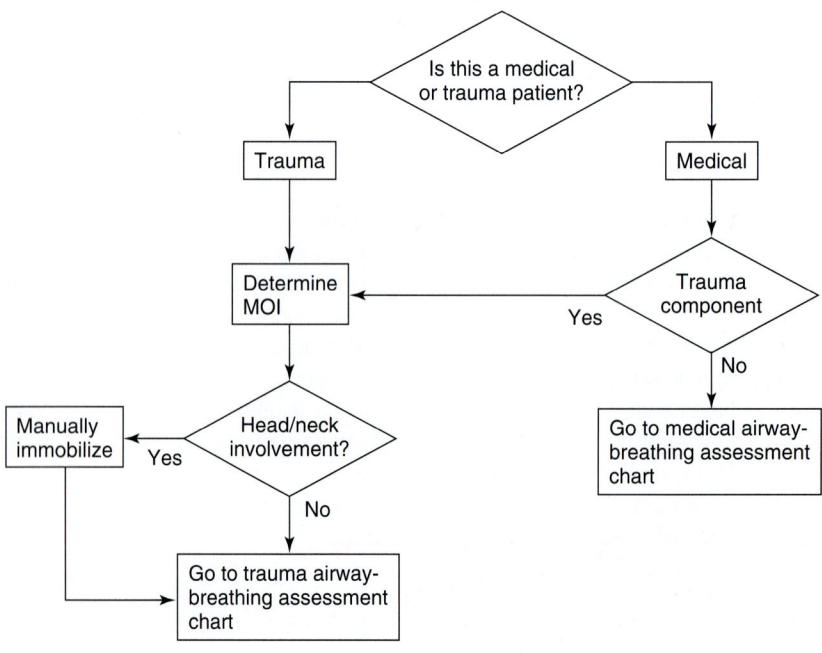

A knowledge of mechanism of energy exchange allows the physician or other caregiver to rapidly assess for the potential injuries, predicting many of them based on the history of the incident and the understanding of the **kinematics** of energy exchange. An understanding of patterns generally produced in each type of traumatic incident allows the attending physician, emergency medical technician (EMT), resident in training, medical student, and nurse to learn about the management of trauma patients at an accelerated pace.

Unexpected traumatic injuries are responsible for more than 140,000 deaths in the United States each year. Automobile collisions alone accounted for approximately 40,000 deaths in 1998 (data from the National Highway Traffic Safety Administration). Penetrating trauma resulted in an almost equal number of deaths in the same period. Injuries by vehicle trauma totaled 3,125,000 in 1993. Management of these patients depends on identifying injuries or potential injuries. Good assessment skills are a necessity. But even with these assessment skills, many injuries can be missed. The EMT may overlook injuries simply because they are not suspected. Injuries that are not obvious can be fatal because they are not recognized in a timely manner. Knowing where to look for injuries is as important as knowing what to do after injuries are found. A complete, accurate history and proper interpretation of this information permits the EMT to predict more than 90% of the patient's injuries before he or she touches the patient.

Part of the job as a member of the medical care team is to become active in injury prevention. Words can have important implications. For example, Webster's dictionary defines an "accident" as "an event occurring by chance or arising from unknown causes," although the second definition is "an unfortunate event resulting from carelessness, unawareness, or ignorance." The EMT should strive to be careful, aware, and informed. Part of the EMT's responsibility is to educate patients and potential victims regarding prevention. The EMT should use the term *collision* or *crash*, not *accident*, to describe this event.

Definitions

Trauma is a wound or injury characterized by a structural alteration or physiologic imbalance resulting from acute exposure to mechanical, thermal, electrical, or chemical energy, or from the absence of such essentials as heat or oxygen. This definition encompasses a wide variety of injuries, many of which require urgent diagnosis and treatment. The study of this process is called *kinematics, biomechanics, mechanisms of injury,* or a variety of other names that in a simplistic or complex way describe what happens when two objects try to occupy the same space at the same time and one of these objects is the human body. The exchange in energy that results is injury to the human body and perhaps damage to the other object as well.

Energy exchange is that circumstance that produces damage to the human body (or other object) when two objects of unequal speed attempt to occupy the same point in space in the same period of time. Two objects cannot do this; one or both objects will absorb the energy and will be damaged by this energy exchange.

Precrash, Crash, Postcrash

Three phases of a traumatic incident require analysis to understand the entire etiology of the death and injury: **precrash, crash,** and **postcrash.** All three are important.

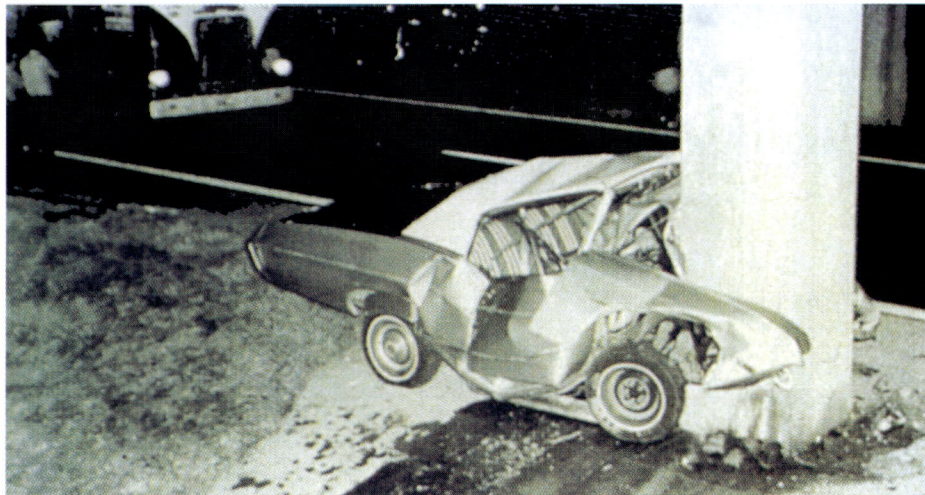

FIGURE 22.1 A motor vehicle collision involving a single occupant. What injuries would you expect to find?

The precrash phase addresses those things that lead up to the incident. These are as varied as mind-altering substances consumed by the patient; the speed of the collision; the condition of the roads; preexisting medical conditions; and so on. All of these factors can affect the outcome of the injuries suffered by the patient. The postcrash phase is equally consequential. It encompasses the prehospital medical care provided to the patient; the type of emergency medical services (EMS) system that exists in the community; the access time of the EMS system; the hospital (trauma center versus non–trauma center) to which the patient is transported; the care available in the emergency department; and so on.

Although all these factors are influential, this chapter focuses on the crash phase. The term *crash* does not necessarily mean *automotive* crash. The crash of an automobile into a pedestrian, the crash of a missile (bullet) into the abdomen, and the crash of a construction worker falling onto asphalt are all crashes. Energy exchange between a moving object and the tissue of the trauma victim or between the moving trauma victim and a stationary object are similar examples of the energy exchange that produces injuries. The history of a traumatic incident begins in the precrash phase with the events that precede the incident, such as the ingestion of alcohol or drugs. Conditions that predate the incident are also part of the precrash phase, such as acute or preexisting medical conditions or the person's state of mind. Although the typical young trauma patient does not have a chronic illness, as the population becomes older, the medical conditions that are present before the accident can produce serious complications in the prehospital management of the patient and can significantly influence the outcome.

The second and perhaps most important phase in the history of a trauma incident is the crash phase, which begins when one moving object collides with another object. The second object can be either stationary or in motion. Either or both of the objects can be a human being. The directions in which the energy exchange occurred, the amount of energy that was exchanged, and the way these forces affected the patient are important considerations for medical providers.

The information gathered about the crash and precrash phases is used by the EMT to manage the patient in the postcrash phase. This phase begins as soon as the energy is absorbed and the patient is traumatized. The onset of the results of life-threatening trauma can be slow or fast, depending in part on the action taken by the EMTs.

Physics of Energy Exchange

Physical Laws

Newton's first law of motion states that *a body at rest will remain at rest and a body in motion will remain in motion unless acted on by some outside force.* The motorcycles in Figure 22.2 were stationary until the energy from the engine started them moving along the dirt track. Once they are in motion, even though they may leave the ground, they remain in motion until some force retards that motion. This force may be some object on the track or in the air or the brakes that are applied to slow the forward motion once the motorcycle returns to the ground. The same laws apply to the person sitting in the front seat of an automobile. Although the car hits a tree and stops, the unrestrained occupant continues in motion until he or she is suddenly stopped by hitting the steering column, the dashboard, or the windshield.

The second important principle of physics that relates to energy exchange states that *energy cannot be created or destroyed but can be changed in form.* The motion of the vehicle is a form of energy, and when the motion starts or stops the energy must be changed to another

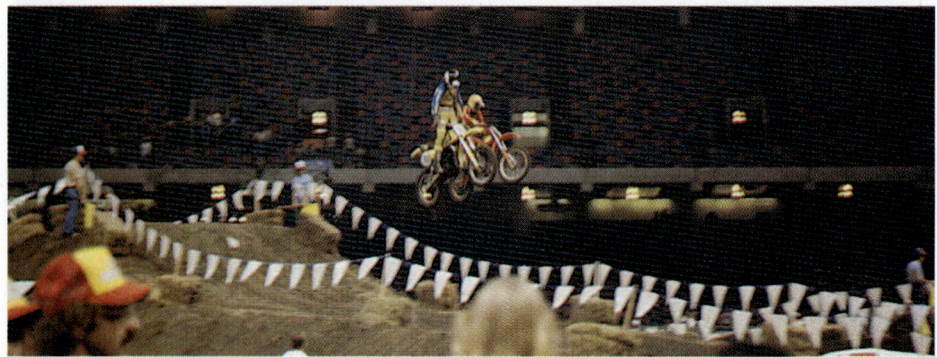

FIGURE 22.2 A motorcycle going over a jump does not suddenly stop when contact is lost with the ground. The momentum of the motorcycle and the previously existing energy carry both the motorcycle and the rider forward unless obstructions stop the motion.

form. It may become a form of mechanical, thermal, electrical, or chemical energy.

When a driver brakes, the car decelerates slowly. The energy of motion is converted into the heat of friction (thermal energy) on the brake drum and on the roadway as rubber is burned onto the asphalt. The energy of motion of a car crashing into a wall is dissipated by the bending of the frame and other parts of the car.

Kinetic energy is the energy of motion and is a function of an object's weight and speed. In humans, the victim's weight and mass are essentially the same thing. Likewise, speed and **velocity** are the same. The relationship between weight and speed as it affects kinetic energy is as follows:

$$\text{Kinetic energy} = \frac{\text{Mass} \times \text{Velocity}^2}{2}$$

This relationship indicates that the velocity is much more important than the mass. An increase in velocity increases the rate of production of kinetic energy more than an increase in the mass. Much greater damage occurs in a high-speed, or high-velocity, collision than in a collision at a slower speed. The speed of a bullet as it emerges from the barrel of a gun has missile velocity. Some bullets travel slowly, whereas others travel much faster. The same rules for kinetic energy also apply. Differences in mass among occupants of the same vehicle have less effect on their vulnerability to injury than does the speed of impact.

For example, a small child and a 200 lb adult are quite different in size and weight, but if they are both in a vehicle that is traveling at 55 miles per hour (mph), the most significant determinant of the amount of force that will be applied to them in a crash is their common speed, not their weight difference.

Imagine that a car traveling at 35 mph hits a brick wall. The wall stops the car, but the 150 lb driver continues to travel at 35 mph until he or she is stopped by impact with the steering wheel. The impact of the steering column against the chest of the driver would be equivalent to standing against a brick wall and having a telephone pole driven into the chest at 35 mph.

The other factor that must be considered in a collision is the **stopping distance.** Before a crash, the driver moves at the same speed as the car. During the split second of the crash, car and driver both decelerate to a speed of zero, but not at the same time. The car stops first against the wall, but the driver does not stop until he or she crashes against the steering column. This deceleration force is transmitted to the driver's body. If the stopping distance of the driver is increased by lap belt or diagonal belt, or both, the force of deceleration is decreased and the resulting damage to the patient's body is proportionately decreased.

This inverse relationship between stopping distance and severity of injury also applies to falls. A person may survive a fall if he or she lands on a compressible surface, such as deep powder snow. The same fall terminating on a hard surface, such as concrete, can produce severe injury. The compressible material increases stopping distance and absorbs at least some of the energy, rather than allowing it all to be absorbed by the body. The result is decreased injury.

This principle also applies to other kinds of collisions. For instance, a car that hits an unyielding bridge abutment will be damaged more seriously than a car that hits another car from behind or a pedestrian. In either of these instances, the car or the pedestrian is thrust forward by the energy from the moving auto. The moving vehicle does not immediately stop; therefore all of its energy is not absorbed.

An unrestrained driver will be more severely injured than a restrained driver because the restraint system, rather than the body, absorbs a significant portion of the energy of deceleration. The stopping distance of a restrained driver is expanded as the lap and diagonal belts stretch. This stretch slows the stopping rate of the driver and absorbs some of the energy. An air bag, if present, will also absorb some of the energy. Both serve to prevent the occupant from reaching the rigid dash and the steering column. All of this prevention can be defeated if the occupant is so close to the dash that the belts do not have a chance to perform adequately or if the occupant is seated next to the air bag. The rapid opening of the air bag will transfer its energy to the occupant and will force him or her rapidly away from the inflation of the bag.

Thus, once an object is in motion and has a specific energy of motion, to come to a complete rest it must lose all of its energy by converting this energy to compression of the body parts or by transferring it to another object. If an automobile strikes a pedestrian, for example, the pedestrian is crushed by the vehicle and knocked away from it (Figure 22.3). The vehicle is slowed by the impact, but this reduced velocity is transferred to the pedestrian, resulting in injury and creating velocity. Loss of motion by a moving object translates into tissue damage to the victim.

Newton's second law of motion (force) states that *force equals mass times acceleration* ($F = M \times A$). Force is required to put an object in motion. Once in motion, according to Newton's first law, the object will continue in the same motion in the same direction and with the same force until a force that is equal to the starting force acts on the object to stop it (Figure 22.4):

Mass $\times$ Acceleration = Force = Mass $\times$ Deceleration

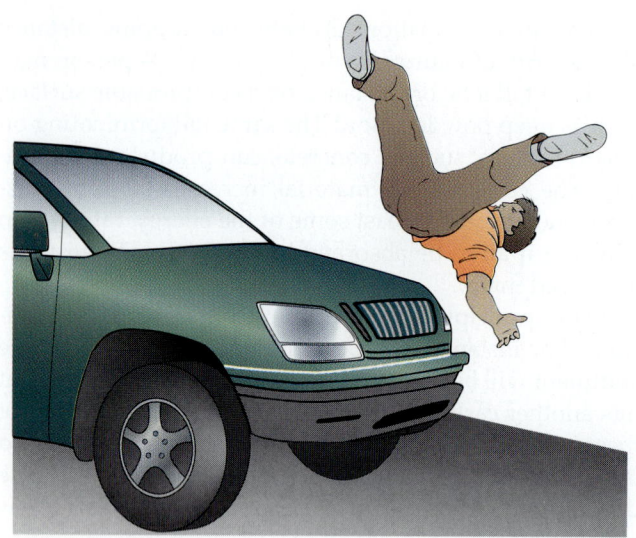

FIGURE 22.3 If an automobile strikes a pedestrian, initially the pedestrian is crushed by the vehicle and then knocked away from it, producing tertiary injuries.

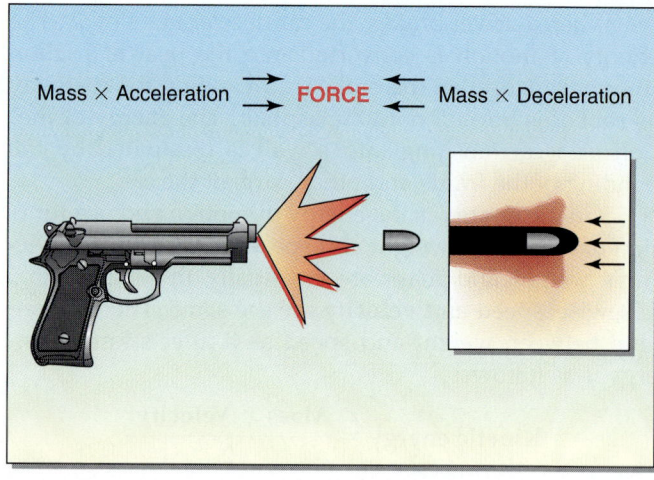

FIGURE 22.4 Once in motion an object will continue until an equal but opposite force acts on it.

> ✓ Knowledge of basic physics is important for the EMT in assessing both mechanism and severity of injury. *Kinetic energy* is the energy of motion and is a function of an object's weight and speed. An increase in velocity (speed) increases the rate of production of kinetic energy more than an increase in the mass. The EMT should find out the speed of the vehicle and the victim at the time of the incident.

Cavitation

In the game of pool, the cue ball is driven down the table into the rack of balls, scattering them away from the point of impact (Figure 22.5). The pool balls are knocked out of their position. The same thing happens when a moving object, such as a bullet or an automobile, strikes the human body or when the human body is in motion and strikes a stationary object. The tissue of the human body is knocked out of its normal position, creating a cavity. This process is called **cavitation.**

Two types of cavities are produced. A **temporary cavity** forms at the time of impact, but the tissue returns to its previous position, and the cavity cannot be seen when the EMT or physician examines the patient later. A temporary cavity is caused by stretch. A **permanent cavity** can be seen when the patient is examined and is caused by impact and compression of tissue, although it may also be caused partly by stretch (Figure 22.6).

The difference between the two cavities is related to the elasticity of the tissue involved. For example, forcefully swinging a baseball bat into a steel drum leaves a dent, or cavity, in its side. Swinging the same baseball bat with the same force into a similarly sized and shaped mass of foam rubber will leave no dent once the bat is removed. The difference is *elasticity*—the foam rubber is more elastic than the steel drum.

Summary of Cavitation and Energy Exchange

With this background information about energy exchange and cavitation, patient injury can be more fully understood. Several kinds of injuries are discussed in the following sections, including automotive trauma, pedestrian trauma, blasts, falls, and penetration wounds caused by knives and guns.

In **blunt trauma,** injuries are produced as the tissues are compressed or sheared (torn), whereas in **penetrating trauma,** injuries are produced as the tissues are crushed and stretched along the path of the penetrating object. Both types create a cavity, forcing the tissues out of their normal position. Energy exchange is directly related to the density and to the size of the frontal area at the point of contact between the object and the victim's body.

A driver who hits the steering column has a large cavity in his or her anterior chest at the time of impact; however, the chest rapidly returns to its original shape as he or she rebounds from the steering wheel. Suppose two EMTs examine the patient separately. One understands kinematics and the other does not. The one without such understanding is concerned only with the bruise visible

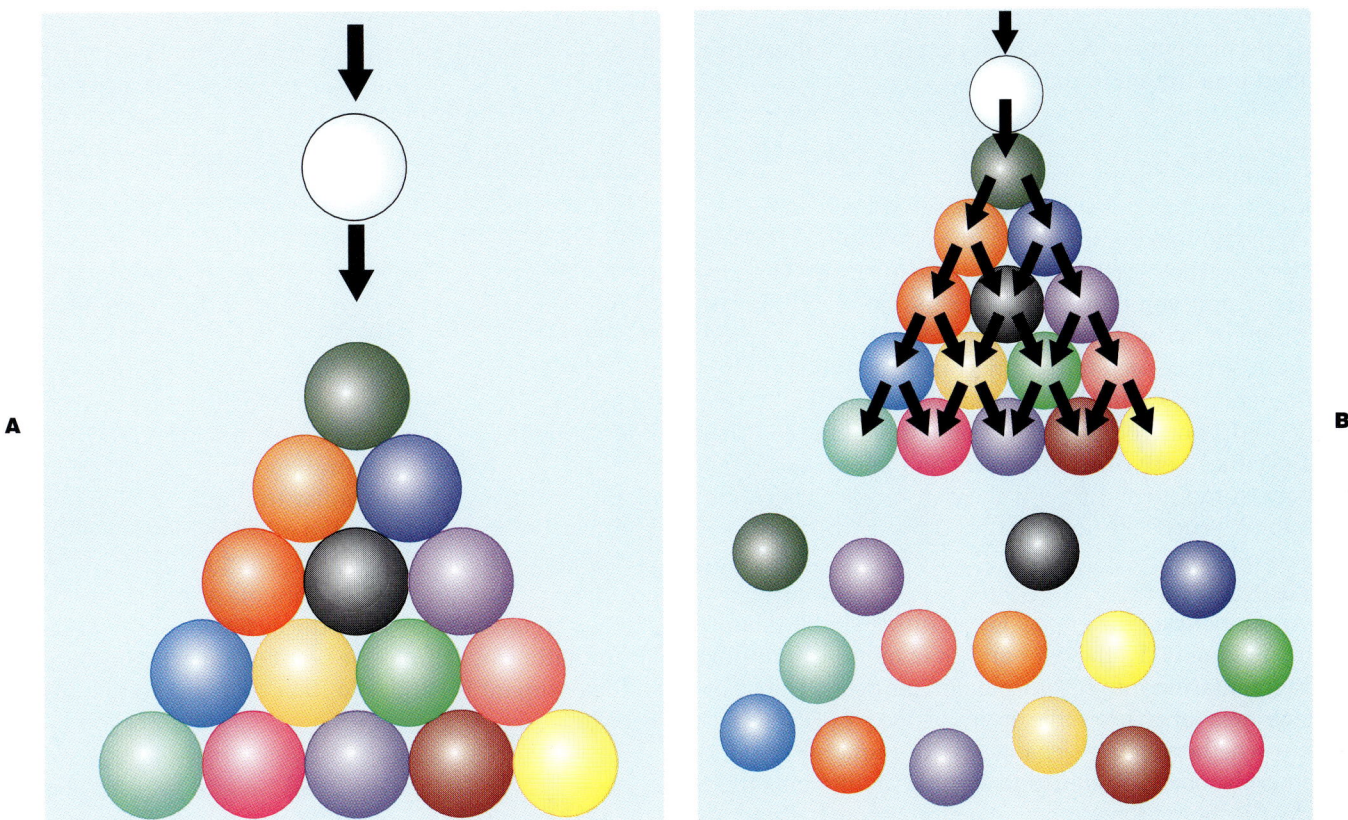

FIGURE 22.5 **A,** The energy of a cue ball is transferred to each of the other balls. **B,** The energy exchange pushes the balls apart or creates a cavity.

on the patient's chest. The EMT who understands kinematics recognizes that a large cavity was created at the time of impact, that the **ribs** had to bend in for it to form, and that the heart and lungs were compressed by the formation of the cavity. Therefore the knowledgeable EMT suspects injuries to the heart, lungs, and chest wall, whereas the other EMT is not aware of these possibilities.

The knowledgeable EMT assesses the injuries, manages the patient, and initiates transport more aggressively because he or she suspects serious chest injuries rather than reacts to what otherwise appears to be only a minor, closed, soft tissue injury. The early identification, adequate understanding, and appropriate management of the underlying injury significantly influences whether the patient lives or dies.

The physical forces, the cavitation phenomena, and the energy exchange are similar in blunt trauma and penetrating trauma. When only a temporary cavity is created, the injury is classified as blunt trauma. The energy of a rapidly moving object with a small frontal projection is concentrated in one area and may exceed the tensile strength of the tissue and penetrate it. The temporary cavity that is created will spread away from the pathway

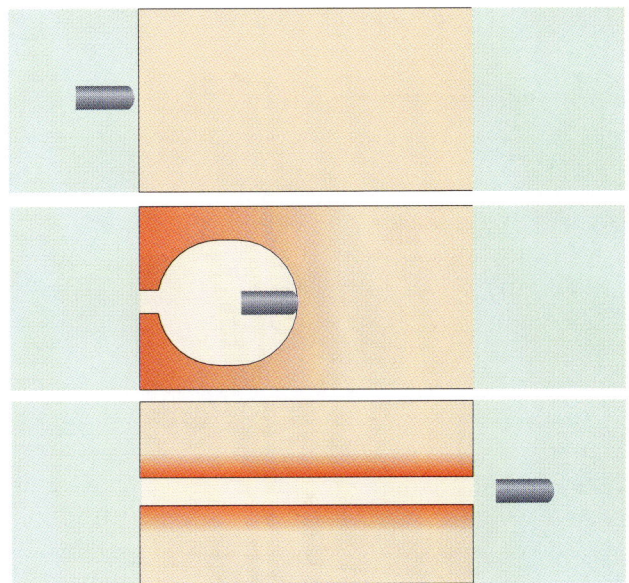

FIGURE 22.6 A permanent cavity is seen as the patient is examined in the emergency department or operating room. However, a temporary cavity is produced as the bullet passes through.

of this missile in both frontal and lateral directions. When both a permanent and a temporary cavity exist, the injury is called penetrating trauma.

Density

The amount of energy that is exchanged when two objects collide depends on how many particles are hit. When the human body is one of the objects, the particles are tissue particles. The denser a tissue (measured in particles per unit volume), the greater the number of particles that are hit by a moving object. Similarly, enlarging the front surface area of the object increases the number of tissue particles hit. Driving your fist into a feather pillow and driving your fist at the same speed into a brick wall produce very different effects on the hand. The fist exchanges more energy with the dense brick wall than with the less dense feather pillow.

Surface Area

The surface area of the impact is determined by the **shape** of the moving body, the over-and-over motion (**tumble**), or **fragmentation** into several smaller particles. The front surface area of a projectile is influenced by its initial shape, whether the size changes at the time of impact, whether the object tumbles and assumes a different angle inside the body than when it entered the body, and whether the object fragments. The energy exchange or potential energy exchange can then be analyzed based on the following considerations.

An example of this interaction is the pressure that wind exerts on a hand when it is extended out of the window of a moving car. When the palm of the hand is parallel to the street and parallel to the direction of the flow through the wind, some backward pressure is exerted on the front of the hand (index finger) as the particles of air strike the hand. Rotating the hand 90° places a larger surface area into the wind; thus more air particles make contact with the hand, increasing the amount of force on it.

As the human body collides with an object, the number of tissue particles affected by the impact determines the amount of energy exchange that will occur and therefore the amount of damage that results. The number of tissue particles affected is determined by the density of the tissue and by the size of its front surface area.

The front surface area of a small object, such as a knife or bullet, can penetrate both the skin and the tissues inside the body. This penetration creates crush damage along a pathway that is similar to the size of the object. The size, however, is related to other factors as well.

Conversely, an object with a larger frontal surface area (such as an automobile) cannot easily penetrate the skin. Therefore the force produces a wider area of damage radiating away from the point of impact. The damage to the occupant is similar in force and area to that of the vehicle.

Blunt Trauma

Vehicular Crash Types

Motor vehicle collisions (MVCs), including motorcycle collisions, are the most common kind of blunt trauma, with pedestrian injuries a close second. MVCs can be divided into five types:

1. Head-on, or frontal, impact
2. Rear impact
3. Lateral, or side, impact
4. Rotational impact
5. Rollover

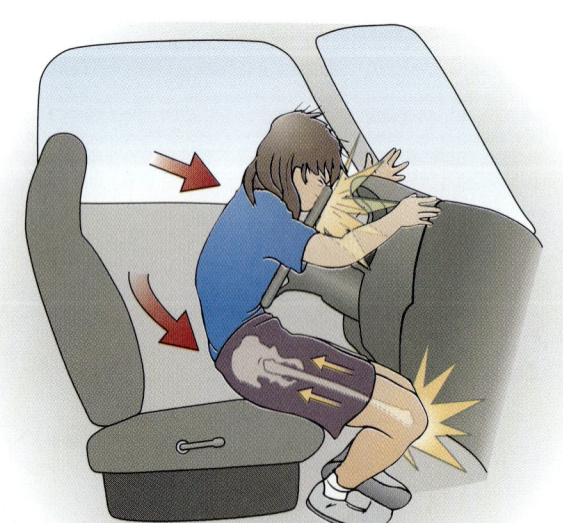

FIGURE 22.7 Down and under: the occupant and vehicle travel forward together. When the vehicle stops, the patient keeps moving forward until something retards that motion.

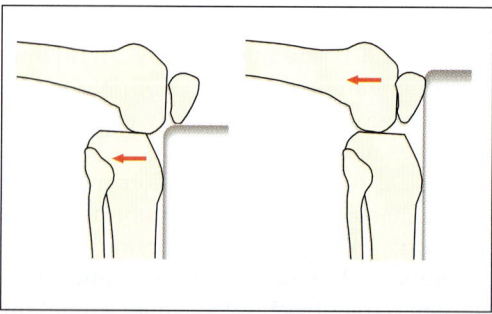

FIGURE 22.8 If the tibia strikes the dashboard, the femur overrides it, tearing the supporting structures of the knee and the popliteal artery. If the femur is the impact point, energy absorption is distributed along the length of the femur and onto the pelvis.

Although variations exist within each pattern, being able to identify the five patterns provides insight into other similar types of crashes.

In MVCs three separate impacts (collisions) occur: (1) the vehicle crashes into an object, (2) the unrestrained occupant collides with the inside of the vehicle, and (3) the occupant's internal organs collide with one another or with the wall of the cavity. An automobile hitting a tree will serve as an example.

When an automobile strikes a tree, the first collision occurs. Although the vehicle stops, the unrestrained driver keeps moving forward. When the driver hits the steering wheel and windshield, the second collision occurs. In the third collision, the driver stops moving forward, but many of his or her internal organs keep moving until they strike another organ or cavity wall or are suddenly stopped by muscle, vessel, or bone attachments.

Each of these collisions causes different kinds of damage, and each must be considered separately to analyze the incident. As a general rule, the occupant receives the force from the same direction as the vehicle; the energy exchange will be similar and will occur in a similar direction. Whether that energy exchange is completely transmitted to the body depends on whether the occupant is using a restraining device.

Head-on, or Frontal, Impact

In a head-on collision, forward motion stops abruptly. In an MVC, such as a car hitting a brick wall, the first collision occurs when the car hits the wall, resulting in damage to the front of the car. The amount of damage to the car can indicate the approximate speed of the car at the time of impact. A severely damaged car, for example, was probably moving at a high speed and will probably contain severely injured victims.

Although the vehicle suddenly ceases to move forward, the occupant, if unrestrained and therefore not slowed with the car, continues to move and will follow one of two possible paths: down and under or up and over.

Down and under.
In a down-and-under path, the occupant continues to move downward into the seat and forward into the dashboard or floor pan with the lower part of the body as the leading portion (Figure 22.7). To understand the importance of good kinematics reporting and comprehension, consider the knee as an example. The knees are most often the lead point of this human missile, which will strike the dashboard.

The knee has two possible impact points against the dash: the femur and the tibia. If the tibia hits the dash and stops first, the femur remains in motion and overrides it, resulting in a dislocated knee with torn **ligaments, tendons**, and other supporting structures (Figure 22.8). Because the major vessels of the leg are so tightly attached to the femur and the tibia, the opening of the joint stretches the vessel at this point, tearing the lining of the artery or causing complete disruption (Figure 22.9).

If such a mechanism of injury is not reported to the hospital personnel and the patient is severely injured, several hours or days may pass before this injury is found and managed. A high frequency of arterial injuries is associated with knee dislocations. For several hours the

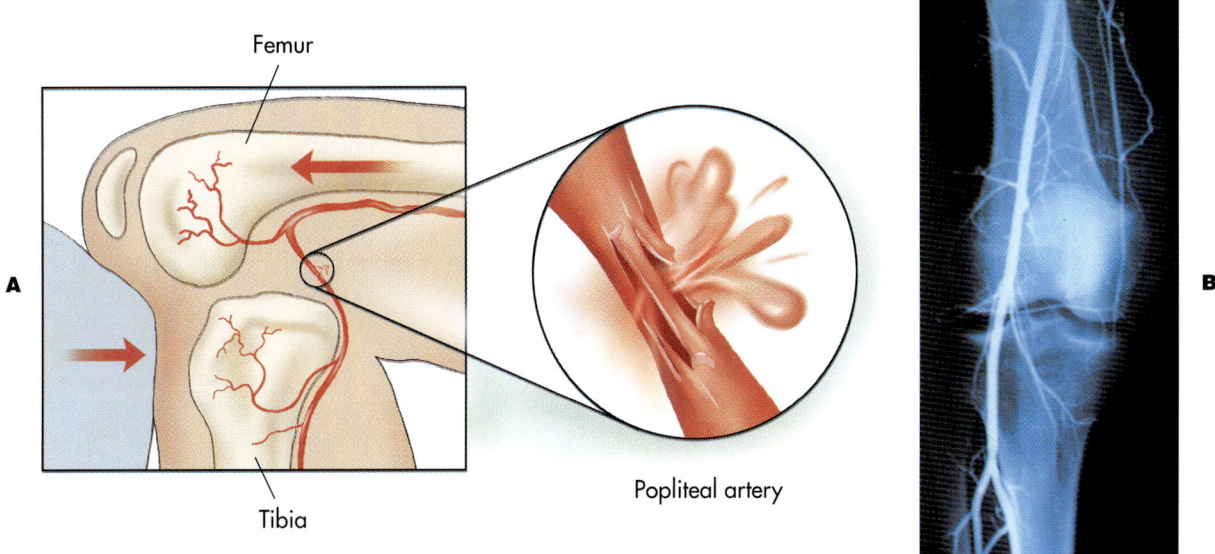

FIGURE 22.9 **A,** The popliteal artery lies in close proximity to the joint, tightly tied to the femur above and the tibia below. Separation of these two bones stretches, kinks, or tears the artery. **B,** This radiograph shows the relationship of the artery and the two bones.

pulse may be palpable; however, a clot may develop later when the patient is in surgery for management of other injuries or in bed with the legs covered up. If the loss of blood flow to the extremity is not detected for several hours, amputation may be necessary. This delay can increase the adverse outcome for the patient.

If recognized, a dislocation with tears of the major supporting ligaments and tendons of the knee can be surgically repaired early, with a good chance that the knee will completely regain its normal function. To determine whether such an injury exists, the knee must be examined within a short time of the trauma to determine accurately whether surgical repair will be necessary. If such an injury is not suspected and several hours pass before the orthopedist sees the patient, so much bleeding and swelling will have occurred in the injured area that an accurate examination cannot be performed. Only after 10 days to 2 weeks does the swelling sufficiently resolve to permit an accurate examination. At that point, the prognosis for full repair is much less favorable, and the patient may be permanently disabled. Such an overlooked injury may have a major effect on the patient's lifestyle.

A knee imprint on the dashboard frequently is the key indicator of this event (Figure 22.10). The EMT must look for this imprint and other impact points on the inside of the automobile, as well as on the outside. These imprints often shrink spontaneously either shortly after impact or during extrication. Unless the dents in the dashboard caused by the knee impact are observed and recognized, this injury may not be suspected and thus not reported to the emergency physicians.

When the femur is the point of impact, the energy must be absorbed on the bone's shaft, which can break. In addition, the continued forward motion of the pelvis onto the femur can override the femoral head, resulting in a posterior dislocation of the hip joint. This dislocation is frequently associated with a fracture of the posterior lip of this joint (Figure 22.11).

After the knees smash into the dash, the upper body rotates forward into the steering column or dashboard (Figure 22.12). The chest or abdomen may hit the steering wheel or dash.

Up and over. In the up-and-over sequence, the body's forward motion carries it up and over the steering wheel (Figure 22.13). The head is usually the lead body portion striking the windshield or windshield frame. The chest or abdomen collides with the steering wheel. If the abdomen hits it, compression injuries can occur, most often to the solid abdominal organs (kidneys, liver, pancreas, and spleen). Hollow organs can also be injured.

The kidneys, spleen, and liver are also subject to shear injury as the torso strikes the steering wheel and stops abruptly. An organ may be torn from its normal anatomic restraints and supporting tissues. The continued forward motion of the kidneys after the **vertebral column** has stopped moving may cause tears in the renal

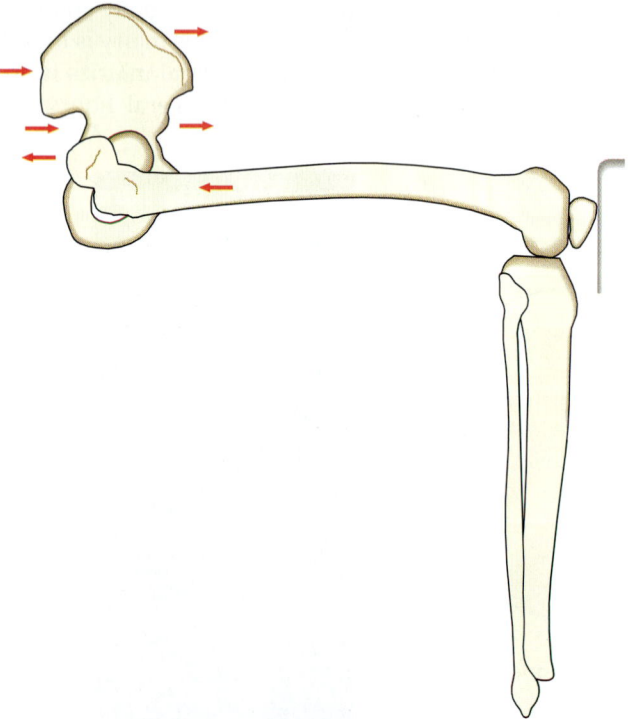

FIGURE 22.10 If the femur stops its forward motion because of impact on the dash, the continued forward motion of the pelvis stretches the supporting ligaments at the joints and surrounding muscle, resulting in a posterior dislocation of this joint.

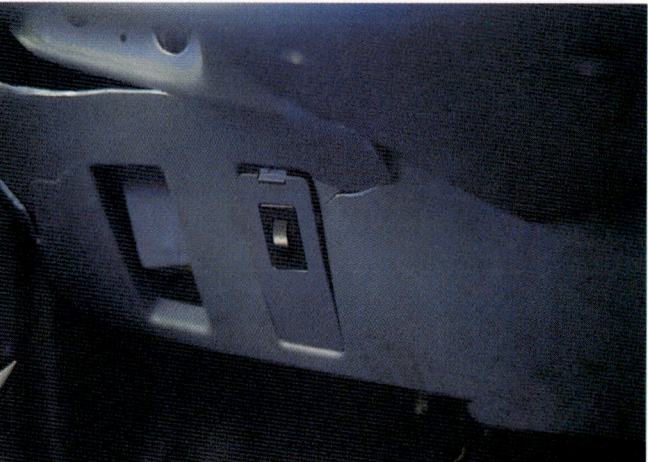

FIGURE 22.11 The impact point of the knee on the dashboard indicates both a down-and-under pathway and significant absorption energy along the lower extremity.

vessels near the points at which they join the inferior vena cava and the **descending aorta.** These **great vessels** adhere so tightly to the vertebral column that the continued forward motion of the kidneys can stretch the renal vessels to the point of rupture.

As the body continues to rotate forward and upward, the chest strikes the steering wheel or dashboard. The victim will have compression injuries to the anterior chest, which may include broken ribs, an **anterior flail chest**, pulmonary contusion, cardiac contusion, or, if the impact is low on the chest wall, rupture of the higher solid abdominal organs (liver and spleen).

The head is also a point of impact. When its forward motion stops, the momentum of the still-moving torso following it must be absorbed. One of the most easily bent or fractured parts of the body lies between the head and the torso—the cervical spine.

Rear Impact

Rear-impact collisions occur when a slow-moving or stationary object is struck from behind. In such cases, the energy of the impact is converted to acceleration. The greater the difference in the speed of the two vehicles, the greater the force of the initial impact and therefore the more energy that can create damage. For example, when a stopped vehicle is struck from behind by a second vehicle traveling at 55 mph (55 − 0 = 55), the impact and the energy exchange will be far greater than that produced when a vehicle going 30 mph is struck by another vehicle traveling at 55 mph (55 − 30 = 25). In frontal collisions, the sum of both vehicles' speeds becomes the velocity at which damage is produced. In rear-impact collisions, the velocity is the difference between these speeds.

On impact, the vehicle in front is driven forward, like a bullet discharged from a gun, as does everything in contact with the car. If the headrest is not positioned to prevent hyperextension of the neck over the top of the seat, tearing of the ligaments and anterior supporting structures of the neck often occurs (Figure 22.14). If the victim's headrest was not properly positioned when the neck injury occurred, some courts reduce the liability of the party at fault in the collision on the grounds that the victim's negligence contributed to the injuries. Similar measures have been considered in cases of failure to use occupant restraints.

If the headrest is up, the head moves with the seat (Figure 22.15). If the car is allowed to move forward without interference until it slows to a stop, the occupant

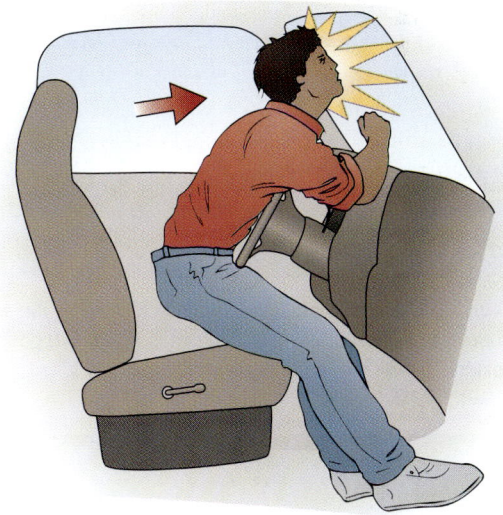

FIGURE 22.13 Up and over: the configuration of the seat and the position of the occupant can direct the initial force on the upper torso with the head as the lead point.

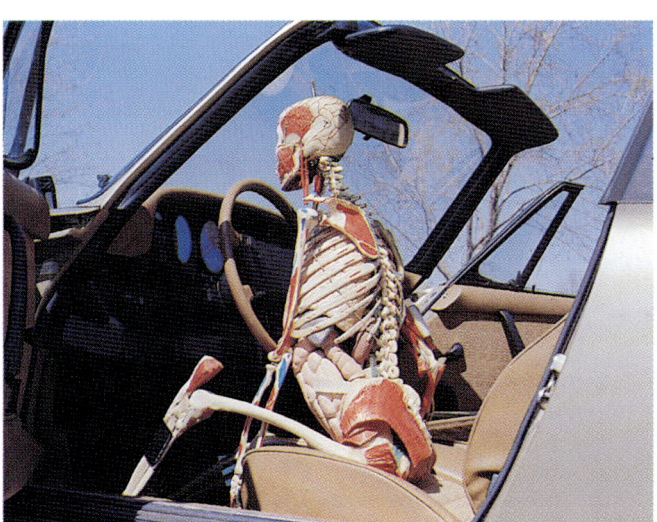

FIGURE 22.12 In a down-and-under pathway, the feet or knees are the lead point. The knees crash into the dashboard, absorbing most of the forward energy.

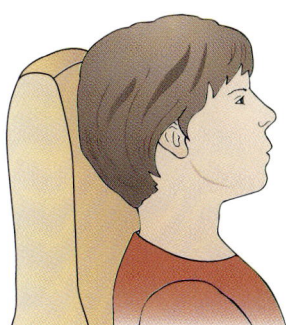

FIGURE 22.14 If the head restraint is up, the head moves forward with the torso, and neck injury is prevented.

probably will not be injured. However, if the car strikes another car or object or if the driver slams on the brakes and stops suddenly, the occupants are thrown forward, following the characteristic pattern of a front-impact collision. The collision then involves two impacts—rear and frontal. The double impact increases the likelihood of injury. The EMT should consider this possibility when dealing with this kind of collision and should look for two sets of injuries—those caused by the rear impact and those caused by the (secondary) frontal impact.

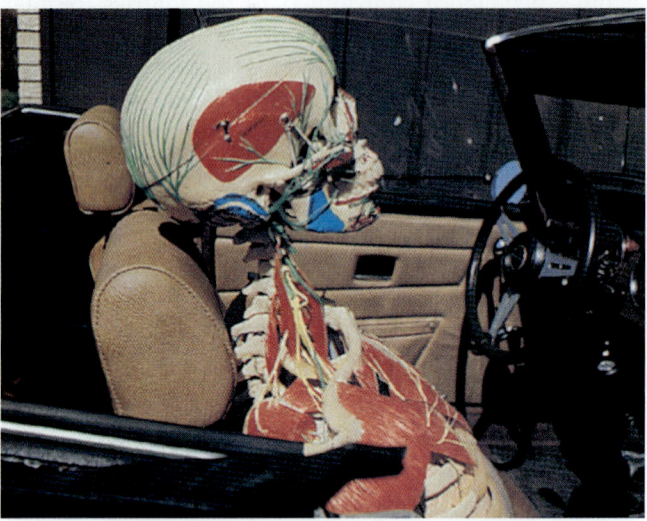

FIGURE 22.15 Rear-impact collision forces the car, the seat, and then the driver forward. If the head restraint is in a down position, the neck is extended over the top of the seat.

Lateral, or Side, Impact

Lateral-impact collisions occur when a vehicle is struck from the side. The vehicle that is hit is propelled away from the impact in the direction of the impact. The entire side of the vehicle is thrust against the side of the occupant. The occupant, then, may be injured in two ways: (1) by the movement of the car (Figure 22.16, *A*); and (2) by the door's encroachment into the passenger compartment (Figure 22.16, *B*). Injury caused by the car's movement is less severe if the occupant is belted and moves away from the impact along with the car.

This lateral impact affects three parts of the body: the chest, the pelvis, and the cervical spine. As the chest receives the impact, lateral compression and shear injuries result. Compression fractures the ribs on the side of the impact and can produce a flail chest with its associated **pulmonary contusion** and possible **pneumothorax**. Other injuries may include a ruptured liver or spleen (Figure 22.17). Occupants on the driver's side are vulnerable to spleen injuries, because the spleen is a left-sided organ, whereas those on the passenger side are more likely to receive an injury to the liver.

If the victim's arm is at his or her side, it can rotate posteriorly out of the way. If the arm is pinned between the chest and the door, it absorbs the impact and transfers much of the force to both the clavicle and the chest wall. When this transfer occurs, the clavicle is usually fractured outward along the curve of the central one third (Figure 22.18).

The pelvis and femur are also frequently struck by the door, forcing the head of the femur to move medially through the pelvis at the hip joint (Figure 22.19). The

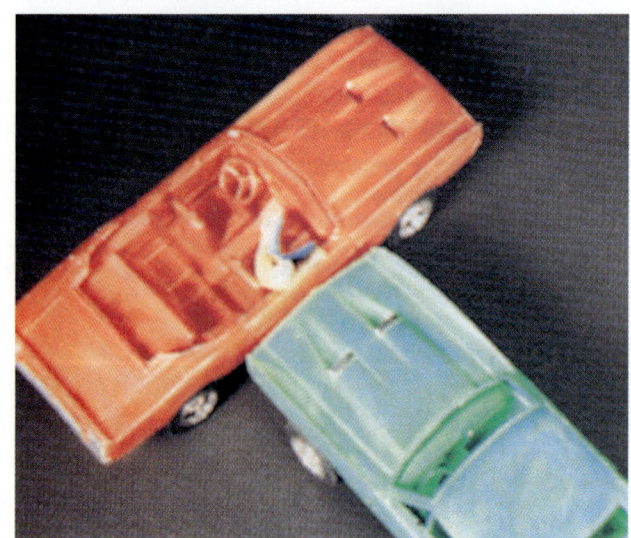

A

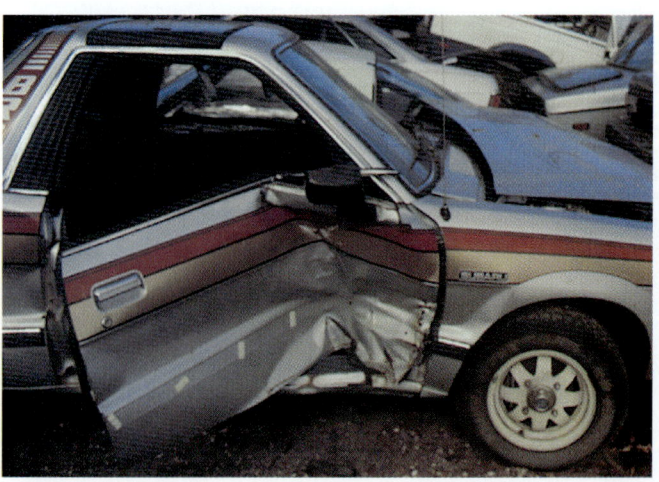

B

FIGURE 22.16 **A,** Lateral impact of the vehicle pushes the entire automobile into the unrestrained passenger. The restrained passenger is moved laterally with the vehicle. **B,** Intrusion of the side panels into the passenger compartment provides another source of injury.

wing of the pelvis can be pushed in, fracturing the pelvis both anteriorly and posteriorly.

The head is supported by the spine, but in an off-center position. The center of gravity is forward and superior to the point of support. As the trunk is pushed laterally by the side impact, the tendency of the head to remain in its original position until pulled by the neck will produce both lateral flexion and rotation of the cervical spine (Figure 22.20). The combination of these movements produces more frequent and more severe cervical injuries than either of the two alone. The result is tears or strains of the ligaments and supporting structures of the neck. Fractures of the spine are more common with lateral collisions than with rear collisions. Injury to the spinal cord caused by this kind of impact may result in a neurologic deficit.

Head or scalp injuries can occur as the door, side window, or door post strikes the side of the head. These injuries range from simple facial lacerations to cerebral contusions and hemorrhage (Figure 22.21).

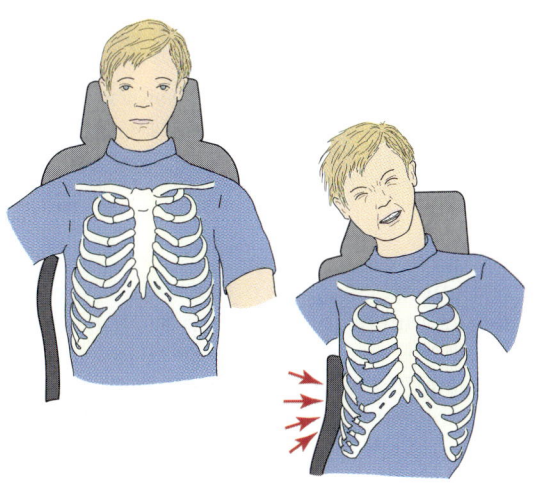

FIGURE 22.17 Compression against the lateral chest and abdominal wall injures the underlying spleen, liver, and kidney, resulting in retroperitoneal hemorrhage. Compression of the upper leg and femur through the acetabulum fractures this joint, resulting in retroperitoneal hemorrhage.

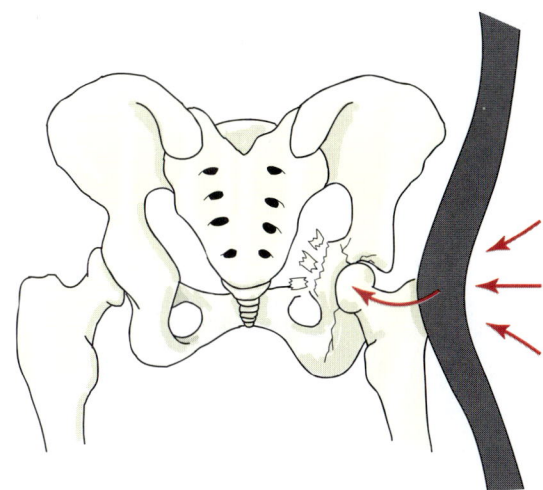

FIGURE 22.19 Lateral impact on the femur pushes the head through the acetabulum and can fracture the pelvis.

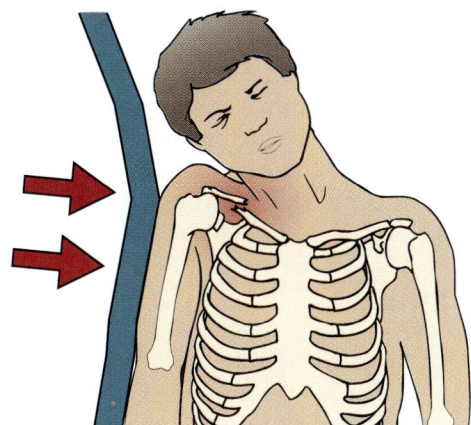

FIGURE 22.18 Compression of the shoulder against the clavicle produces midshelf fractures of this bone.

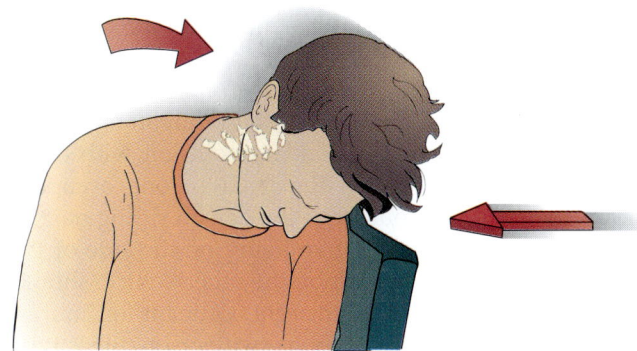

FIGURE 22.20 During a lateral impact when the torso is rapidly accelerated out from under the head, the head turns toward the point of impact, both in the lateral and anterior-posterior angles. Such motion separates the vertebral bodies from the side opposite impact and rotates them apart. Offset facets, ligament tears, and lateral compression fractures result.

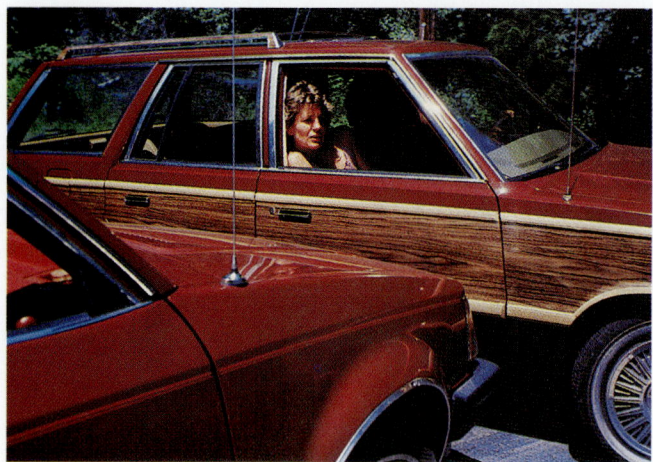

FIGURE 22.21 The head can strike the door post, side window, or other component of the door, producing contusions and fractures.

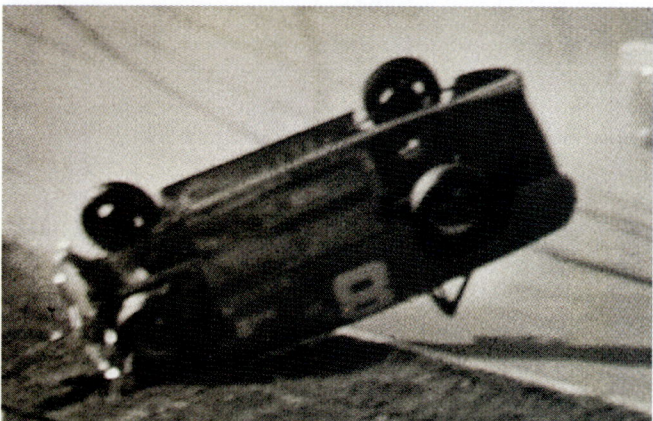

FIGURE 22.23 During a rollover, the unrestrained occupant can be completely or partially ejected out of the car or can bounce around inside the car. This action produces multiple and somewhat unpredictable injuries, but they are always severe.

Rotational Impact

Rotational-impact collisions occur when one corner of a car strikes an immovable object, or a slower-moving vehicle is hit in this area by a faster-moving vehicle or a vehicle traveling in the opposite direction of the automobile. Following Newton's first law of motion, this part of the car will stop while the rest of the car continues its forward motion until its energy is completely transformed.

Rotational-impact collisions result in injuries that are a combination of those seen in head-on and lateral-impact collisions. The victim continues to move forward and then is hit by the side of the car (as in a lateral-impact collision) as the car rotates around the point of impact.

Rollover

During a rollover, the car may undergo several impacts at many different angles, as may the occupant's body and internal organs (Figure 22.23). Injury and damage occur with each one of these impacts. It is almost impossible to predict the injuries these victims may receive, although, as in other types of collisions, the occupant frequently will be hit on the same body areas as the automobile.

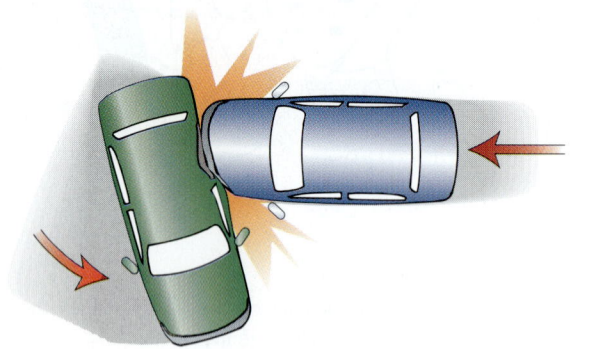

FIGURE 22.22 Even lateral impacts can result in severe occupant injuries.

When the vehicle is moved by the force of the impact, it is as if the car is suddenly moved out from under its occupants. In this case, the use of seat belts reduces the severity of injury. Because of the lap belt, the occupant begins lateral motion with the car and is "pulled" away from the impact point.

During a side-impact crash, the occupants are also subject to injury from a secondary collision with other passengers, such as when the head of one occupant strikes the head or shoulder of the person sitting next to him or her. The presence of an injury on the side of the patient opposite the side hit by the other vehicle should alert the EMT to check the adjacent occupant for injuries resulting from the collision of the two persons. This type of injury is also prevented or significantly reduced when both occupants are restrained, which is yet another reason that the EMTs should always wear their belts. It also protects them from injury in a lateral-impact collision (Figure 22.22).

Organ Injury

As noted previously, the difference between blunt and penetrating trauma is whether the skin is actually penetrated by the object or not. If it is penetrated, the cavity will be directed laterally away from the point of impact. If not, the cavity is directed away from the point of impact (Figure 22.24). Additionally, in blunt trauma, two forces are involved in the impact: change of speed (**shear**) and **compression.** Change-of-speed and change-of-direction

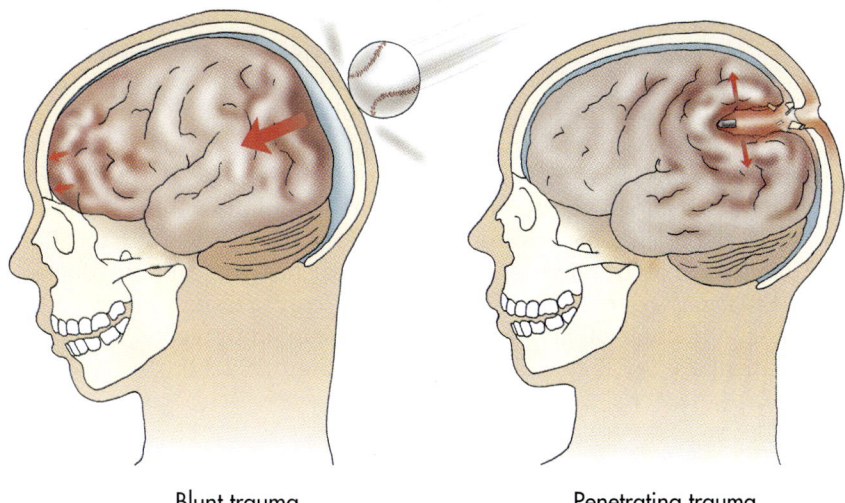

FIGURE 22.24 The difference between blunt and penetrating trauma is the direction of the forces inside the body. Blunt trauma occurs when the forces are directly away from the point of impact. Penetrating trauma occurs when the forces are directed laterally away from the point of impact.

injuries are associated with deceleration- or acceleration-type injuries. Injury can result from any type of impact, such as a collision on the athletic field, a fall, a motorcycle or automobile crash, or a pedestrian collision. Compression injuries occur as a result of the organ being trapped between the continuing movement of the posterior abdominal or thoracic wall and the anterior abdominal or thoracic wall that has been stopped against the steering column or the dash.

When two parts of an organ are suddenly traveling at two different rates of speed, the parts are sheared apart. As an automobile gains speed gradually, the occupant gains speed at the same rate. If the change of speed, either in deceleration or acceleration, is rapid (such as in a collision), the occupant may change speed at a different rate from that of the automobile. The occupant will become separated from the seat, causing the occupant to hit objects inside the passenger compartment. If the occupant is partially restrained, one part of the body will remain in place and another will move. For example, during a frontal crash, the hips remain in place if restrained by a lap belt, but if no diagonal strap is used, the head and thorax freely move toward the steering column of the dash. This movement stretches the attachments of the thorax to the hips. If the force is great enough the thorax "shears" away from the hips. This type of separation is seen in children with poorly developed bones.

These shear forces tearing organs or their supporting structures come into play with deceleration, such as a vehicle suddenly stopping against a bridge abutment, or acceleration, such as when a vehicle is hit from the side in an intersection "T-bone" crash. The bony skeleton and

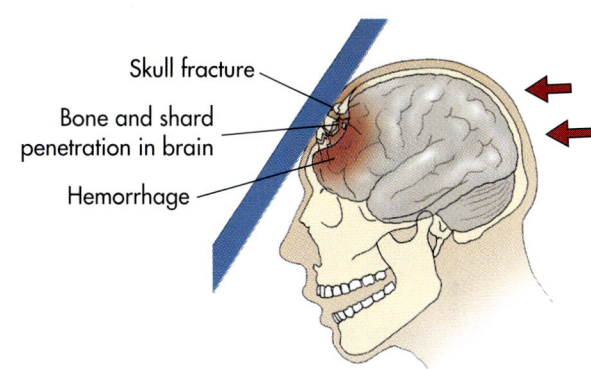

FIGURE 22.25 As the skull strikes an immovable object, pieces of bone are fractured and pushed into the brain tissue.

other rigid parts of the body stop or rapidly accelerate, whereas the more mobile organs, such as the kidney, spleen, and liver, move at a different rate of speed.

The various body parts can be subjected to both shear and compression forces. Because these forces produce different injuries based on the construction of the various regions and the organs that are contained within, these regions are each discussed separately.

Head

Compression. When the body is traveling forward, such as in a frontal vehicular collision or a head-first fall, and the head is the lead point of the "human missile," the initial energy exchange occurs on the scalp and the skull. The skull can be compressed and fractured, pushing the broken bones of the skull into the brain (Figure 22.25).

The brain continues to move forward and becomes compressed against the intact or fractured skull, producing a concussion, contusions, or lacerations.

Shear. The brain is soft and compressible; therefore its length will be shortened, separating the posterior part of the brain from the skull and stretching or breaking any vessels in the area (Figure 22.26). Hemorrhage into the epidural or subarachnoid space can result. If the brain separates from the spinal cord, it will most likely occur at the brainstem.

The only indication the EMT may have that this injury has occurred is a bull's-eye fracture of the windshield or a contusion of the patient's scalp (Figure 22.27).

Neck

Compression. The dome of the skull is fairly strong and can absorb the impact of a collision quite well. The cervical spine, however, is much more flexible and cannot tolerate the pressure of the impact without significant angulation or compression (Figure 22.28). Hyperextension or hyperflexion of the neck produces severe angulation, often resulting in fracture or dislocation of the vertebrae. Direct in-line compression crushes these bony blocks. Either angulation or in-line compression can result in an unstable spine, which can impinge on the spinal cord in the spinal canal (Figure 22.29).

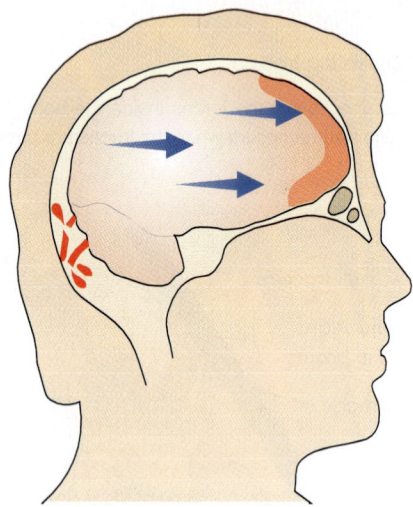

FIGURE 22.26 As the skull stops its forward motion, the brain does not. The brain continues to move forward. The part of the brain nearest the impact is compressed, bruised, and possibly lacerated; the portion furthest away from the impact is separated from the skull with tearing and lacerations of the vessels involved.

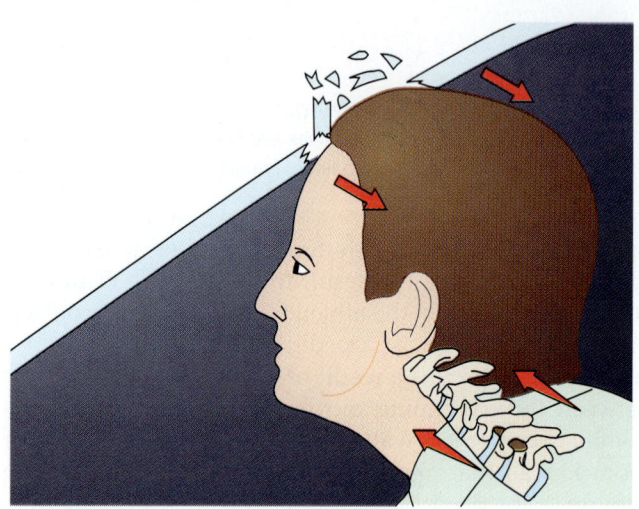

FIGURE 22.28 The skull frequently stops its forward motion, but the torso does not. Just as the brain compresses within the skull, the torso continues its forward motion until its energy is absorbed. The weakest point of this forward motion is the cervical spine.

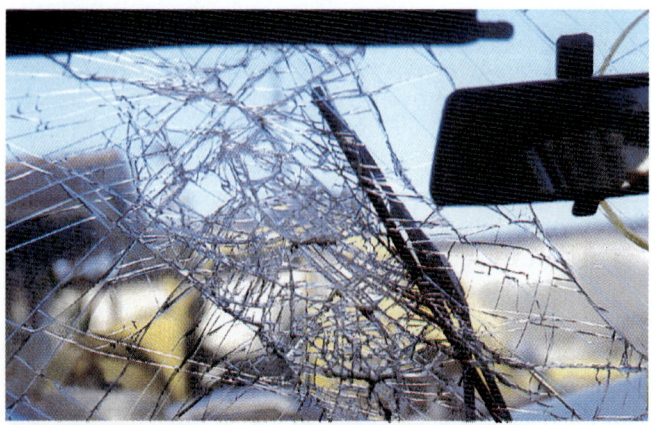

FIGURE 22.27 A bull's-eye fracture of the windshield is the EMT's major indication that the skull has struck the windshield and energy has been exchanged between the windshield and the skull and cervical spine.

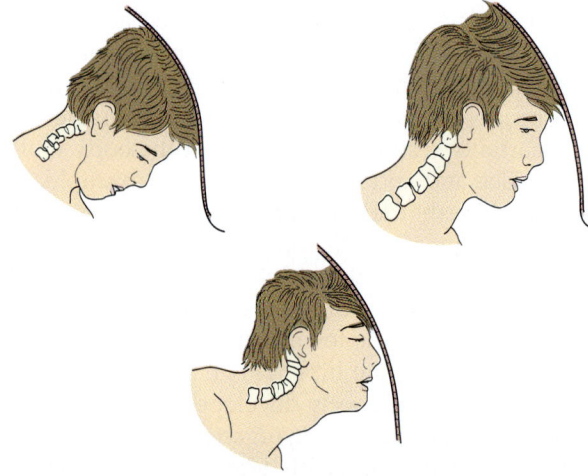

FIGURE 22.29 The spine can be compressed directly along its own axis or angled into either hyperextension or hyperflexion.

Shear. The skull's center of gravity is anterior to and on top of the point at which the skull attaches to the bony spine. Therefore a lateral impact on the torso produces lateral flexion and rotation of the neck (Figures 22.30 and 22.20). Cervical flexion or hyperextension, such as may occur in a rear-impact collision or around a lap belt, may also cause significant damage to the soft tissues of the neck.

Thorax

Compression. If the impact of a collision is centered on the anterior part of the chest, the sternum receives the initial energy exchange. The sternum stops its forward motion, but the posterior thorax continues to move forward until the energy is absorbed.

Compression injuries of the external thorax may produce fractured ribs, leading to a flail chest (Figure 22.31). The frame of the automobile bends when the front of the car stops suddenly against a dirt embankment; however, the rear of the car continues to move forward until all the energy is absorbed by the embankment (Figure 22.32). The posterior thoracic wall also continues to move until all the energy is absorbed by the ribs, resulting in multiple fractures or even a flail chest (Figure 22.33).

Compression injuries to the internal structures of the thorax may include a **cardiac contusion,** which occurs as

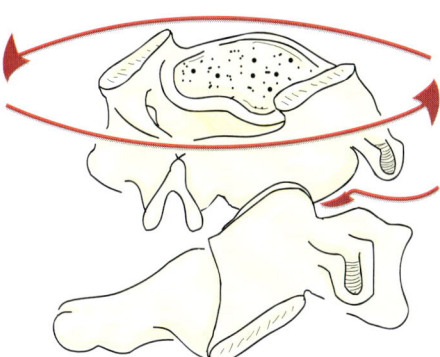

FIGURE 22.30 The skull's center of gravity is anterior and superior to its pivot point between the skull and cervical spine.

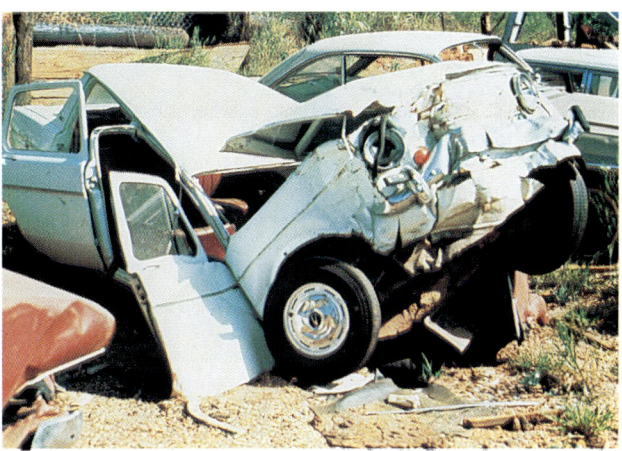

FIGURE 22.32 The front of the car stopped against a dirt wall but the rear continued in the original direction of travel until the energy was absorbed by the bending of the frame. The chest wall reacts in a similar way.

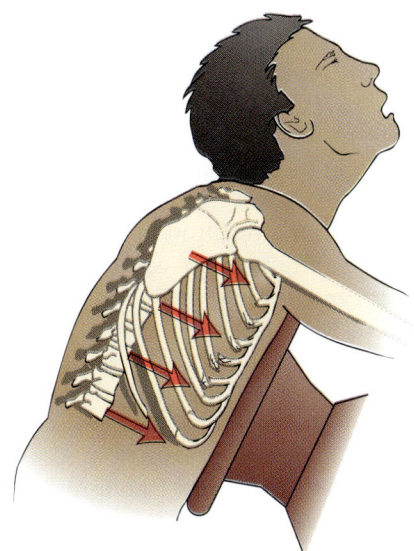

FIGURE 22.31 The posterior thoracic wall continues to move forward until the energy is absorbed by the steering wheel.

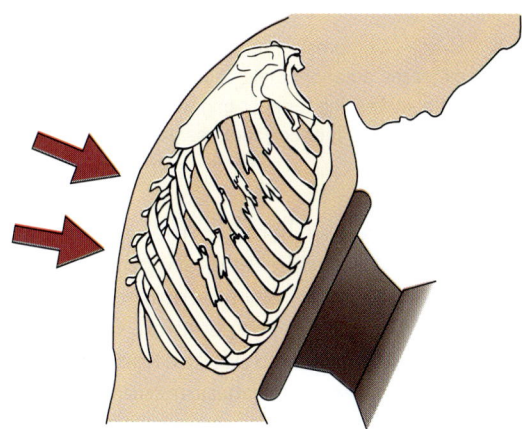

FIGURE 22.33 Ribs forced into the thoracic cavity by external compression usually fracture in multiple places, producing the clinical condition known as flail chest.

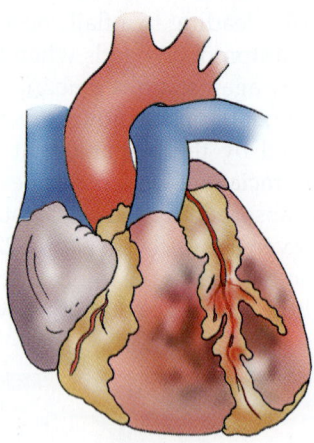

FIGURE 22.34 The heart muscle can be bruised as a result of blunt trauma to the chest.

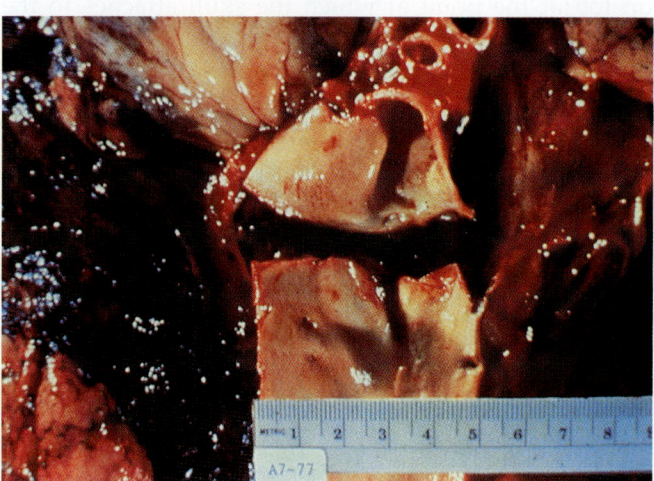

FIGURE 22.36 Tears at the junction of the arch and descending aorta frequently result from shear forces.

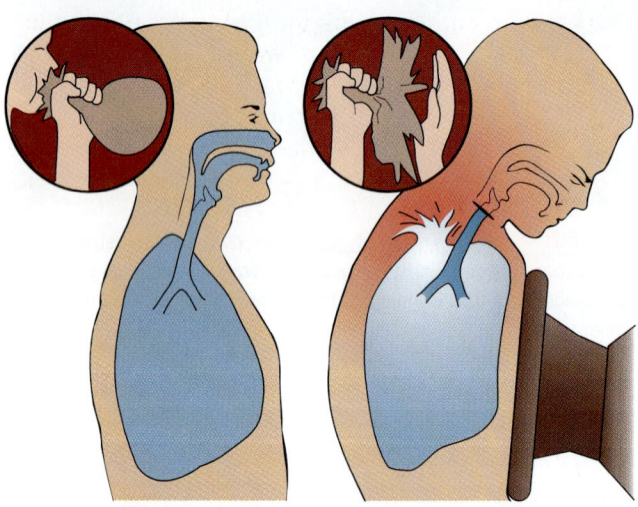

FIGURE 22.35 Compression of the lung against a closed glottis, by impact on either the anterior or lateral chest wall, produces an effect similar to that of compressing a paper bag when the opening is closed tightly by the hands. The paper bag ruptures, and so does the lung.

the heart is compressed between the sternum and the spine (Figure 22.34). Significant dysrythmia can result.

The lungs also can become compressed and contused, which compromises oxygenation. Compression of the chest wall is common with frontal and lateral impacts and produces an interesting phenomenon called the paper bag effect, which results in a pneumothorax (air in the thoracic cavity). As the victim sees the collision coming, he or she instinctively takes a deep breath and holds it. In doing so, the glottis closes, sealing off the lungs. When the impact occurs, the lungs burst like a paper bag full of air that is popped (Figure 22.35).

Shear. When the sternum stops moving, the posterior thoracic wall (muscles and thoracic spine) and all the organs in the thoracic cavity will continue to move toward the anterior chest wall.

The heart and ascending aorta and arch are relatively unrestrained within the thorax. The descending aorta is tightly attached to the posterior thoracic wall and the vertebral column. The resultant motion is analogous to holding the flexible tubes of a stethoscope just below the point where the head attaches and swinging the acoustic head from side to side. As the skeletal frame stops abruptly in a collision, the heart and the initial segment of the aorta continue their forward motion. The shear forces produced may tear off the aorta at the point where these two forces meet (Figure 22.36).

An aortic tear may result in an immediate complete disruption of the aorta or, more commonly, may produce only a partial tear with one or more layers of tissue remaining intact. The remaining layers are under great pressure, however, and a bubble (pseudoaneurysm) can form on a weak part of the artery (Figure 22.37). The bubble eventually ruptures within minutes, hours, or days after the original injury. Approximately 80% of these victims die on the scene or within 1 hour of the time of initial impact. Of the remaining 20%, one third die within 6 hours, one third within 24 hours, and one third live 3 days or longer. The EMT must recognize the potential for such injuries and relay this information to the hospital personnel so that they can investigate this possibility.

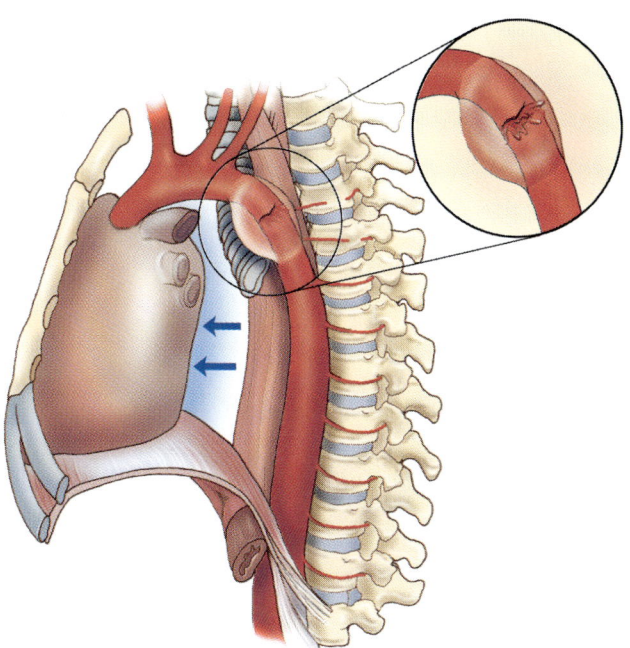

FIGURE 22.37 The descending aorta is a fixed structure against the thoracic spine. The arch, aorta, and heart are freely movable. Acceleration of the torso in a lateral-impact collision or rapid deceleration of the torso in a frontal collision produces a different rate of motion between the arch-heart complex and the descending aorta.

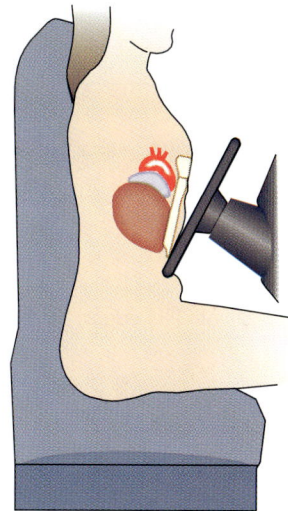

FIGURE 22.38 The upper torso rotates forward onto the steering column as the lower extremity stops its forward motion.

Abdomen

Compression. Organs compressed against the vertebral column by the steering column or the dash during a frontal-impact collision may rupture. The effect of this pressure is similar to the effect of placing the organ on an anvil and striking it with a hammer. Organs frequently injured in this manner are the pancreas, spleen, liver, and kidneys (Figure 22.38).

Injury may also result from a buildup of pressure in the abdomen. The diaphragm is a 5 mm–thick muscle located across the top of the abdomen, separating the abdominal cavity from the thoracic cavity (Figure 22.39). The diaphragm is the weakest of all the walls surrounding the abdominal cavity. It may be torn or ruptured as the pressure increases (Figure 22.40). This injury has four common consequences: (1) the "bellows" effect normally created by the diaphragm as an integral part of breathing is lost; (2) the abdominal organs can enter the thoracic cavity and reduce the space available for lung expansion; (3) the displaced organs can become oxygen starved from compression of their blood supply; and (4) if there is any intraabdominal hemorrhage, this blood also can cause a hemothorax (blood in the thoracic cavity). The intraabdominal pressure increase can result from an impact on any body part, but most commonly it occurs from an impact on the anterior abdominal wall.

Another injury caused by increased abdominal pressure is a rupture of the aortic valve as a result of reverse blood flow (Figure 22.41). This injury is rare, but the EMT should be aware of such a possibility when the victim has collided with the steering column or was involved in another kind of collision (e.g., ditch or tunnel cave-in). This injury is detected by a loud murmur of **aortic insufficiency.**

Shear. Shear injury to the abdominal organs occurs at their points of attachment to the mesentery. During a collision, the forward motion of the body stops, but the organs continue to move forward, causing tears at the points of attachment of the organ to the abdominal wall. These tears can occur where the organ attaches directly to the wall. If the organ is attached by a vascular connection, the tear can occur where the **pedicle** attaches to the organ, where it attaches to the wall, or anywhere along the length of this connection (Figure 22.42). Organs that can shear this way are the kidneys, small intestine, large intestine, and spleen.

Another kind of injury that often occurs during deceleration is laceration of the liver on its impact with the ligament that connects the liver to the umbilicus. The liver is mainly supported by its attachments to the diaphragm. The down-and-under pathway in the frontal-impact collision or feet-first fall causes the liver to bring the diaphragm with it as it is forced into this ligament (Figure 22.43). It will fracture or cut into the liver, like a cheese slicer slices cheese.

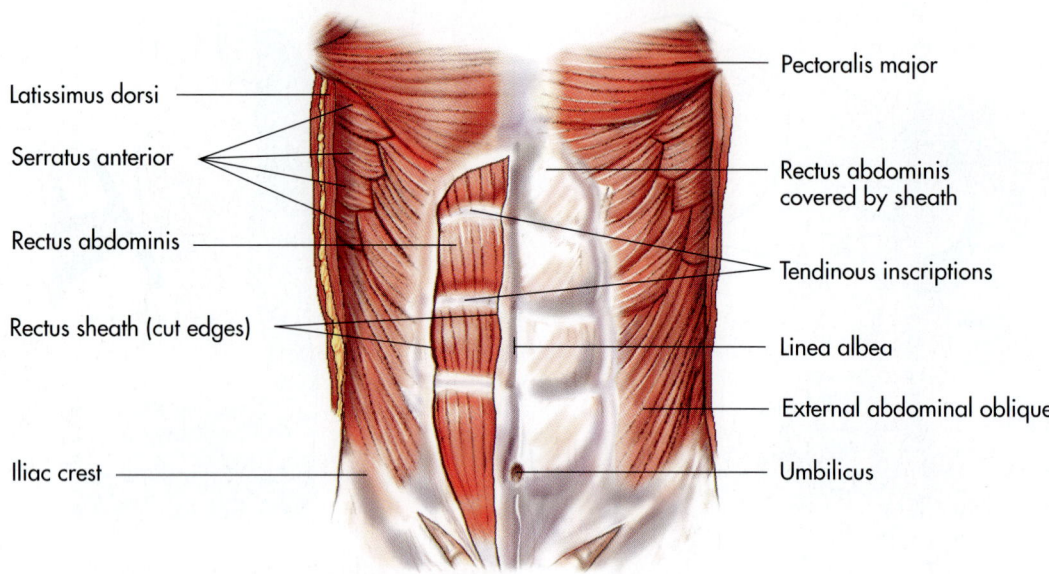

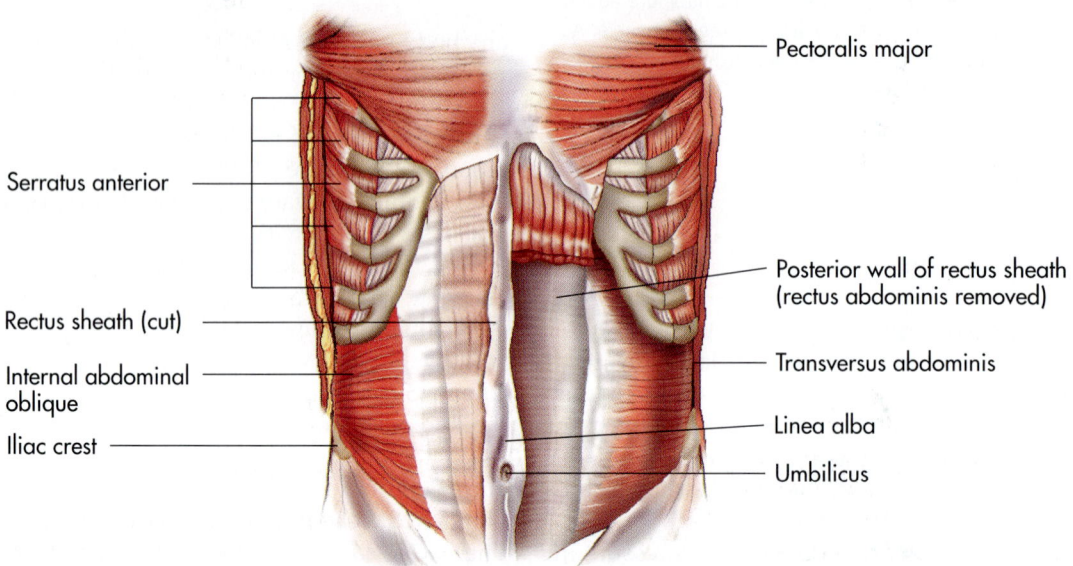

FIGURE 22.39 The anterior, lateral, posterior, and inferior walls of the abdomen are extremely strong, with multiple layers of fascia and muscle. The superior component of the abdominal cavity (the diaphragm) is only a 5 mm–thick muscle and the weakest part of the abdominal cavity.

Pelvis

Pelvic fractures are the result of damage to the external abdomen and may cause injury to the bladder or lacerations of the blood vessels in the pelvic cavity. Approximately 10% of patients with pelvic fractures also have a genitourinary injury. These injuries occur as a result of impact of the pelvis into a rigid structure such as the door in a lateral impact or a fall onto the side or the front of the abdomen, with the impact points on the symphysis or onto the front of the ileum.

Restraints

In the injury patterns previously described, the victims were assumed to be unrestrained, as are many automobile occupants in the United States (30% to 40% in 1999). The effectiveness of occupant protection laws in the various states is significant; the seat belt usage rate increased from 11% in 1982 to 45% in 1988 and to 60% to 70% in 1999. Ejection from vehicles accounts for 27% of the 40,000 automobile trauma deaths that occur each year.

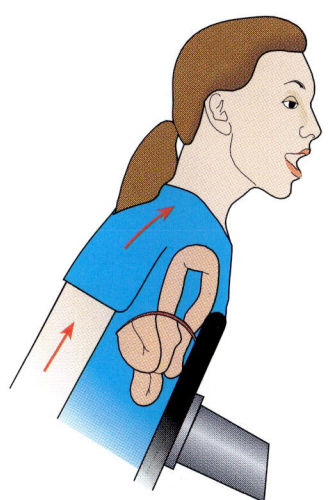

FIGURE 22.40 With increased pressure inside the abdomen, the diaphragm can rupture.

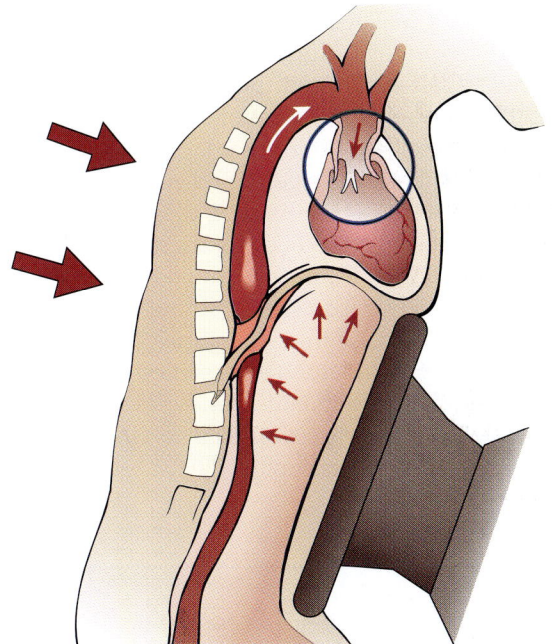

FIGURE 22.41 Increased intraabdominal pressure can force blood in a retrograde fashion up the aorta and against the aortic valve. The aortic valve is torn.

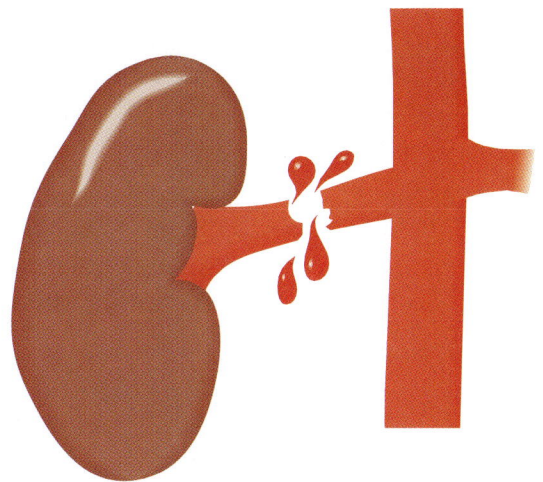

FIGURE 22.42 Just as the heart and arch of the aorta can tear away from the fixed descending aorta during thoracic acceleration-deceleration injury, so do other organs whose fixation is less tight than that of the aorta. The spleen, kidney, and small intestine are particularly susceptible to these types of shear forces.

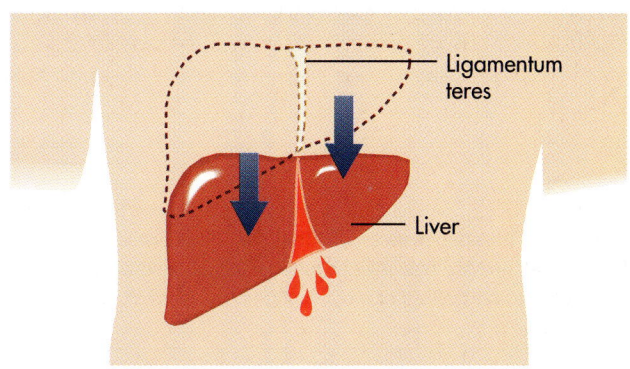

FIGURE 22.43 The liver is not supported by any fixed structure. Its major support comes from the diaphragm. The diaphragm is freely movable. As the body travels in a down-and-under pathway, so does the liver. When the torso stops but the liver does not, the liver continues downward onto the ligamentum teres (a remnant of the uterine vessels), tearing the liver. This is much like pushing a piece of cheese into a tight cheese-cutting wire.

One out of 13 ejection victims suffers a spine fracture. Most injuries occur before the victim is ejected from the vehicle. After ejection from the automobile, the body is subjected to a second impact as the body strikes the ground (or another object) outside the car. This second impact can result in injuries that are even more severe than the initial impact. This is one way that seat belts save lives. The EMT should evaluate the ejected victim carefully, remembering that the distance between the victim and the automobile indicates the rate of speed at which the vehicle had been traveling and therefore the amount of energy absorbed by the patient.

What occurs when the victims are restrained? If the seat belts (lap and diagonal belts) are positioned properly, the pressure of the impact will be absorbed by the pelvis and the chest, resulting in few or no serious injuries. The proper use of restraints transfers the force of the impact from the patient's body to the restraint belts and restraint system so that the injuries received are not life threatening, or at least the chance of receiving life-threatening injuries is greatly reduced. If the belts are positioned improperly, with the lap belt above the pelvis, the pressure is absorbed by the soft tissues of the abdominal cavity and posterior abdominal wall, and injury can result. Although the injury may be significant, it will be less severe than if no restraint had been used.

An often-used example of the significance of restraint usage is a 30 mph crash into a brick wall producing a 2 ft deformity to the front of the car. An unrestrained occupant will decelerate against the front of the passenger compartment with a force of 180 G (force of gravity), whereas a restrained occupant in the same crash will undergo only 16 G of deceleration. He or she will mostly likely survive with minor injuries. The unrestrained occupant, if he or she survives, will have major injuries.

When lap belts are worn loosely or are strapped above the top of the pelvis, compression injuries of the soft abdominal organs can occur. Compression injuries of the soft intraabdominal organs (spleen, liver, and pancreas) result from compression between the seat belt and the posterior abdominal wall (Figure 22.44). Increased intraabdominal pressure can cause diaphragmatic rupture and herniation of abdominal organs. Anterior compression fractures of the lumbar spine can also occur as the upper and lower parts of the torso pivot over the restrained T12, L1, and L2 vertebrae.

As mandatory seat belt usage laws are passed in the United States, injuries caused by improperly positioned or loose lap belts will become more frequent. However, the overall severity of the injuries will be lessened, and the number of fatal collisions will be significantly reduced.

Even when worn properly, lap belts ideally should not be worn alone. Without the diagonal shoulder strap to stop the forward movement of the upper body, severe facial, head, and neck injuries may occur as the head strikes the dashboard or steering wheel (Figure 22.45, *A*). As was initially shown in Europe, diagonal straps worn alone can produce severe neck injuries, including decapitation (Figure 22.45, *B*). In the United States in 1994, automatic diagonal straps worn without the manual lap strap led to an increase in neck injuries. One suit against an automobile manufacturer was settled for $1.6 million when the automatic diagonal strap was worn alone.

Forward air bags are designed to cushion only the forward motion of the occupant. They absorb the energy

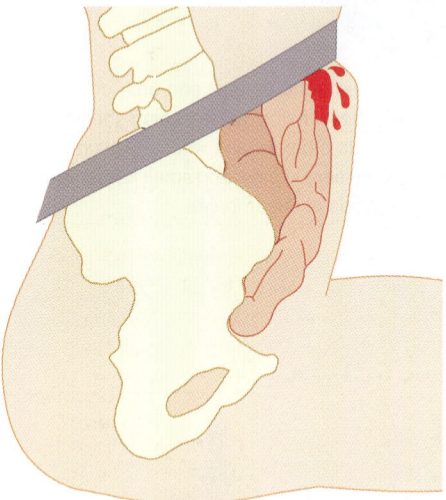

FIGURE 22.44 A seat belt that is positioned above the brim of the pelvis allows the abdominal organs to be trapped between the moving posterior wall and the belt. Injuries to the pancreas and other retroperitoneal organs, as well as blowout ruptures of the small intestine and colon, result.

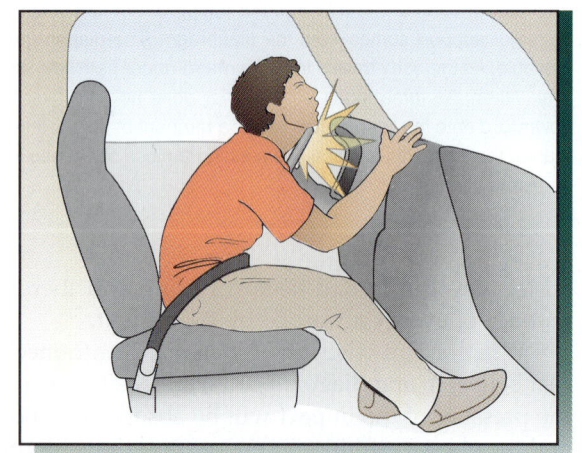 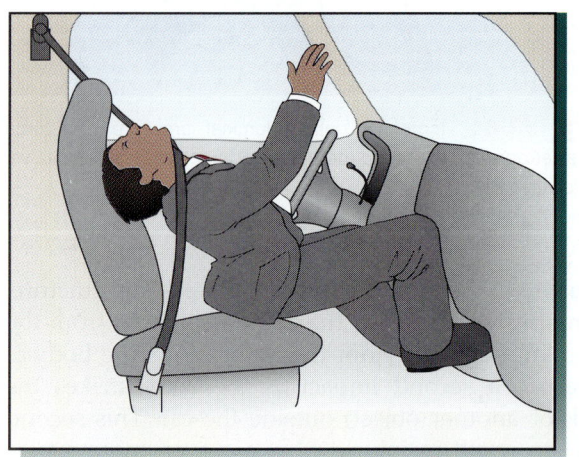

FIGURE 22.45 **A,** Without the diagonal strap the forward motion of the upper body can cause severe injuries to the face, head, and neck. **B,** When worn alone, the diagonal strap retards forward motion, but produces an excessive force on the neck. Neck injuries as severe as decapitation have been reported.

slowly by increasing the body's stopping distance. They are extremely effective in the first collision of head-on impacts, but they are not effective in multiple-impact collisions, nor are they effective in lateral- or rear-impact collisions. Thus they are useful in only the 65% to 70% of collisions that are frontal impacts. After the air bag has deployed and deflated (greater than 0.5 sec), if the car veers into the path of an oncoming car or off the road into a tree, the deflated air bag offers no protection. Air bags should always be used in combination with seat belts for maximum protection.

When air bags deploy, they can produce minor but noticeable injuries that should be identified by the EMT. These include abrasions of the arms, chest, and face and injuries caused by the occupant's eyeglasses (Figure 22.46).

Part of the EMT's responsibility is prevention. Restraints can significantly reduce the energy transfer at the time of an impact and along with it produce a significant reduction in the injury and death rate. The EMT should take every opportunity to talk to patients, friends, and co-workers to increase the use of these valuable safety devices.

Motorcycle Collisions

Motorcycle collisions account for a significant number of the motor vehicle deaths that occur in the United States each year (Figure 22.47). Helmet usage is extremely important for injury prevention. The laws of physics are the same as in other kinds of collisions, but the mechanism of injury varies slightly from automobile and truck collisions. This variance occurs in head-on, angular, and ejection impacts.

A **head-on collision** into a solid object stops the forward motion of the motorcycle. Because the motorcycle's center of gravity is above and behind the front axle (Figure 22.48), the axle is the pivot point in such a collision. The motorcycle tips forward, propelling the rider into the handlebars. The rider may receive injuries to the head, chest, or abdomen, depending on what part of the anatomy strikes the handlebars. If the rider's feet remain on the pegs of the motorcycle and the thighs hit the handlebars, the forward motion will be absorbed by the midshaft femur, commonly resulting in bilateral femur fractures (Figure 22.49).

In an **angular-impact collision,** the motorcycle hits an object at an angle. The motorcycle collapses on the rider, crushing the lower leg and causing fractures of the tibia or fibula and dislocations of the ankle. These injuries are frequently open (Figure 22.50).

In an ejection-impact collision, the rider travels from the motorcycle like a missile. The rider continues in flight

> ✓ In MVCs, the type of collision that occurs (vehicle, occupant, and organ), the direction of travel, the speed of the vehicle just before the time of the impact, and the types of restraints used by the patient are the major determinants of both the type and extent of injuries that occur. In the management of trauma patients, one of the most critical determinants of the outcome is the time from the onset of the injury to the time of definitive care. The patient cared for by the thinking EMT has a better chance for survival than the patient cared for by the EMT who does not understand the exchange of energy.

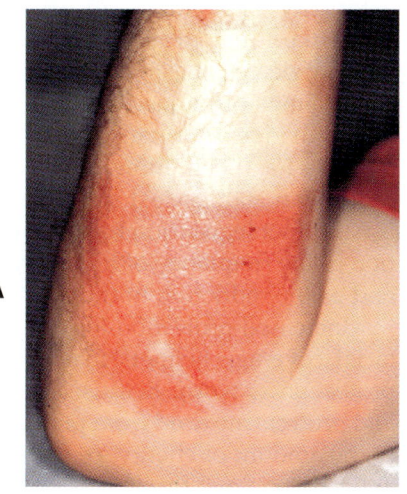
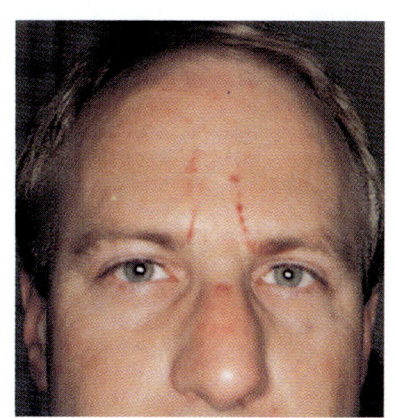

FIGURE 22.46 **A,** Abrasions of the forearm are secondary to rapid expansion of the air bag when the hands are tight against the steering column. **B,** Expansion of the air bag into eyeglasses produces abrasions.

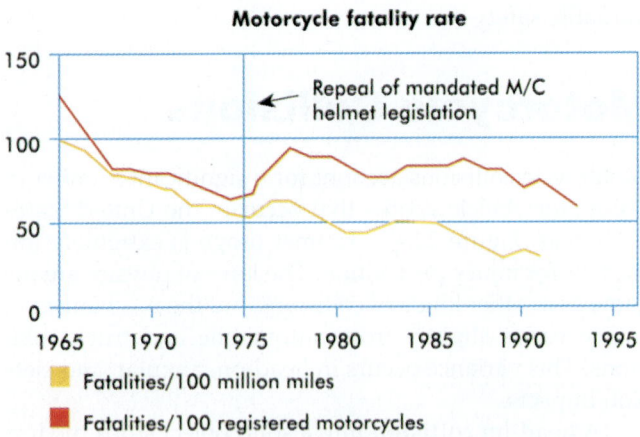

FIGURE 22.47 Motorcycle helmet legislation has significantly reduced the motorcycle fatality rate. Repeal of this law in 1975 produced a marked increase in the numbers of fatalities. The number of fatalities for registered motorcyclists has recently dropped because many states have reinstated their own laws.

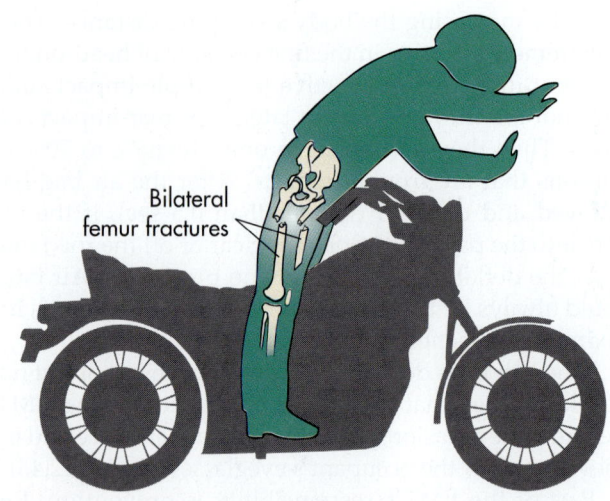

FIGURE 22.49 The body travels forward and over the motorcycle, and the thighs and femurs strike the handlebars. The driver can also be ejected.

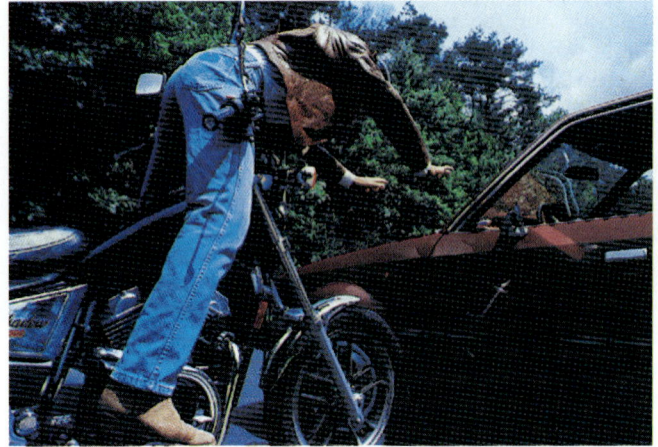

FIGURE 22.48 The position of the driver of a motorcycle is above the pivot point of the front wheel as the motorcycle strikes an object head-on.

until the head, arm, chest, or leg strikes another object, such as a motor vehicle, a telephone pole, or the road. Injury occurs at the point of impact and radiates to the rest of the body as the energy is absorbed. As with the occupant ejected from an automobile, the potential for serious injury is very high for this essentially unprotected rider.

"Laying the bike down" is a protective maneuver used by professional racers and some street bikers to separate themselves from the motorcycle in an impending collision. To perform this maneuver, the rider turns the motorcycle sideways and drags his or her inside leg on the pavement or grass. This maneuver slows the rider more than the motorcycle so that the motorcycle moves out from under the rider. The rider then slides along on the pavement but is not trapped between the motorcycle and the object it hits. These riders usually end up with abrasions and minor fractures but avoid the severe injuries associated with the other kinds of impacts (Figure 22.51).

Protection for motorcyclists includes boots, leather clothing, and helmets (when they are worn) (Figure 22.52). Of the three, the helmet offers the best protection. It is built like the skull—strong and supportive externally and energy-absorbent internally. The helmet's skull-like structure absorbs much of the impact, thereby decreasing injury to the face, skull, and brain. The helmet provides only minimal protection for the neck but does not cause neck injuries. Failure to use helmets has been shown to increase head injuries by more than 300%. Most states that have passed mandatory helmet legislation have found an associated reduction in the frequency of motorcycle collisions. Louisiana had a 60% reduction in the first 6 years after passage.

Increased protection to the face is provided with full facial coverage helmets than when partial or no facial protection is worn. Because the helmet absorbs energy and protects the head from penetration, to get an estimate of the amount of energy exchanged, the EMT should examine the helmet for defects produced by the collision.

The factors that affect the motorcyclist at the time of impact are the direction of the impact (frontal, side collapse,

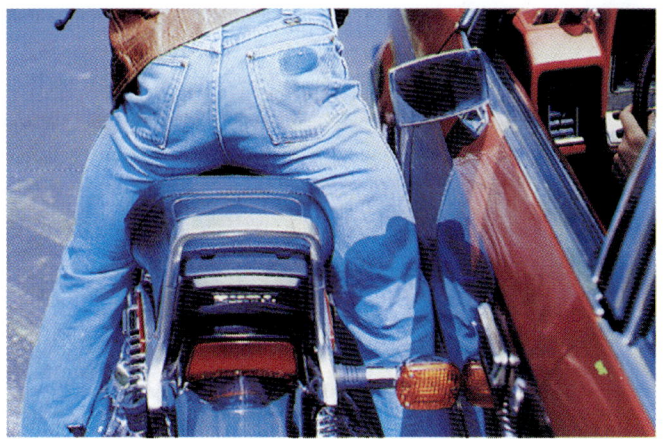

FIGURE 22.50 If the motorcycle does not hit an object head-on, it collapses like a scissors, trapping the rider's lower extremity between the object and the motorcycle.

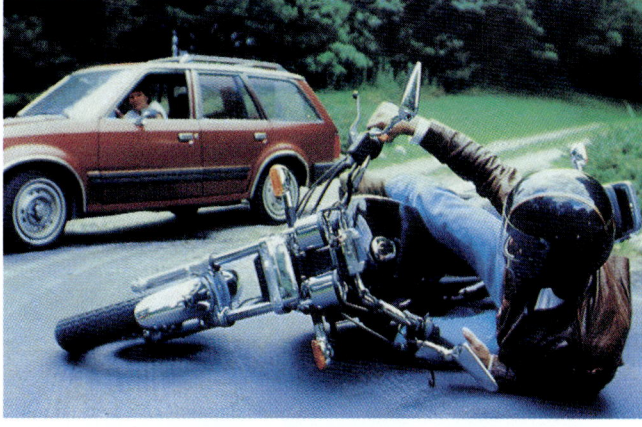

FIGURE 22.51 To prevent being trapped between two pieces of steel (motorcycle and automobile), the rider can lay the motorcycle down to dissipate injury. This maneuver usually causes abrasions (road burns) as the rider's speed is slowed on the asphalt.

ejection), objects the flying motorcycle may hit at the end of the flight, the use or nonuse of a good helmet, the ability of the rider to remove himself or herself from the bike (lay the bike down), and the speed of the impact.

Pedestrian Injury

Two injury patterns are commonly seen in pedestrians struck by motor vehicles: the adult injury pattern and the child injury pattern. The patterns are based on the ages and the heights of the victims. When adults see an oncoming vehicle, they try to protect themselves by turning away; therefore the injuries are frequently lateral or even posterior on the body. Children, on the other hand, face the oncoming vehicle, perhaps out of curiosity. Because of the different heights of a child and an adult relative to the bumper and hood of a car, the striking patterns are also different.

A pedestrian MVC can be divided into three phases. Each phase has its own injury pattern:

1. Initial impact is to the legs of an adult and sometimes to the hips, abdomen, or chest of a child (Figure 22.53).
2. The torso rolls onto the hood of the automobile (Figure 22.54).
3. The victim falls off the automobile and onto the asphalt, usually head first, with possible cervical spine trauma (Figure 22.55).

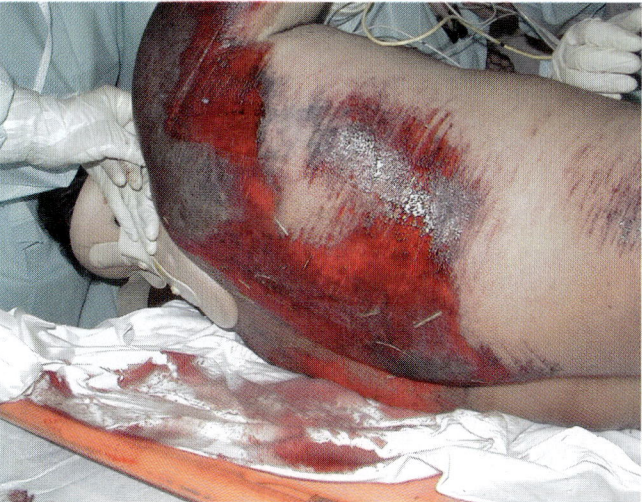

FIGURE 22.52 Road burns after a motorcycle crash without protective clothing.

Both adults and children can be run over by the vehicle after they fall to the ground. Adults are usually struck first by the bumper in the lower legs, fracturing the tibia and fibula and driving the legs out from under the pelvis and torso. As the victim folds forward, the pelvis and upper femur are struck by the front of the vehicle's hood. As the abdomen and thorax fall forward, they strike the top of the hood. This substantial second strike can result in fractures of the upper femur, pelvis, ribs, and spine and produce serious intraabdominal or intrathoracic damage. Injury to the head and face at this point depends on the victim's ability to use the arms for protection. If the head

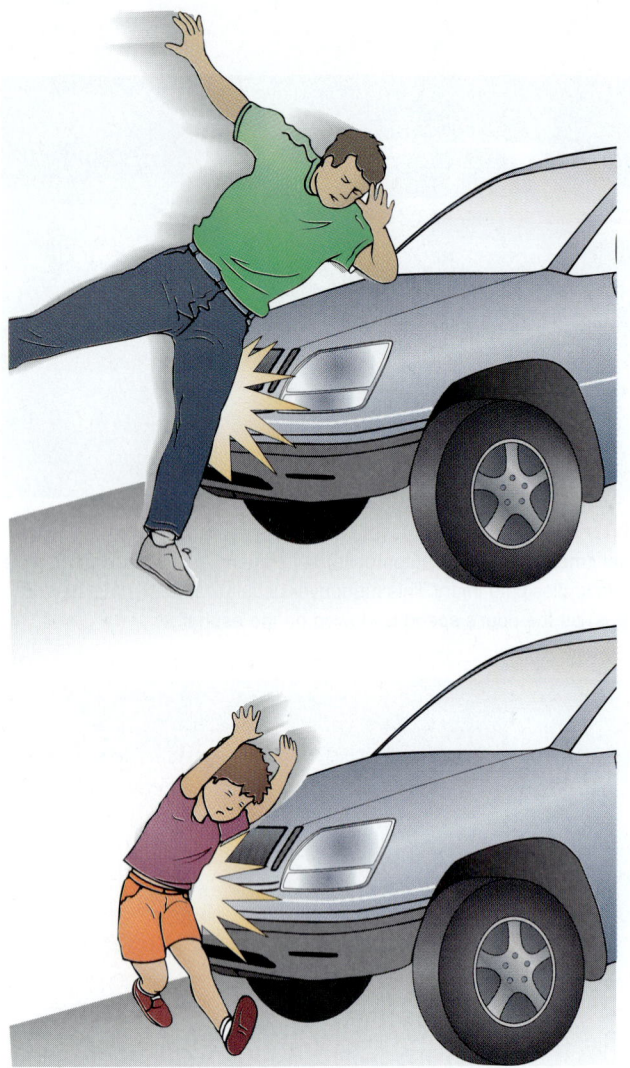

FIGURE 22.53 Initial impact is to the legs of an adult and sometimes to the hips, abdomen, or chest of a child.

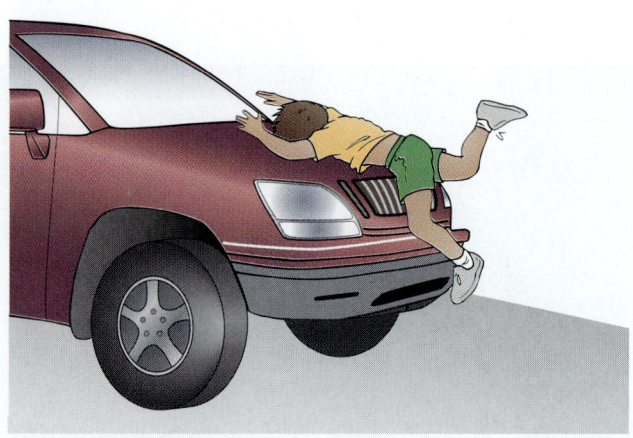

FIGURE 22.54 The torso then rolls on top of the vehicle, striking the hood, windscreen, or roof of the car.

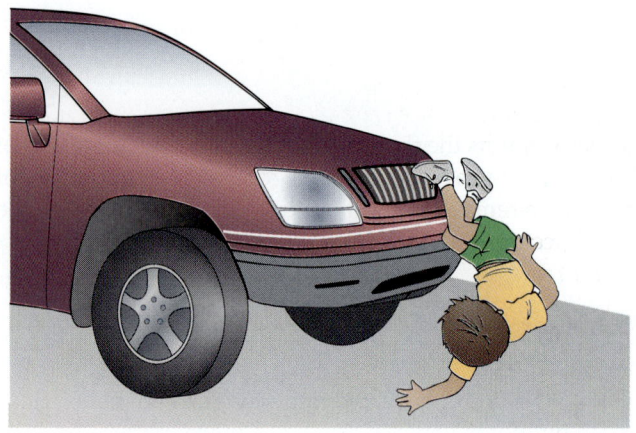

FIGURE 22.55 The torso falls off the car onto the asphalt, producing compression injuries to the head, cervical spine, and torso. A child, being closer to the ground, is struck higher on the body by the bumper or hood of the car.

strikes the hood, or if the body continues to move up the hood so that the head strikes the windshield, injury to the face, head, and spine can occur.

The third impact occurs as the victim falls off the automobile and strikes the pavement. The victim can generally receive a significant blow on one side of the body to the hip, shoulder, and head. Head injury commonly occurs when the head strikes either the car or the pavement and must always be considered. Similarly, because all three impacts produce sudden, violent movement of the torso, neck, and head, an unstable spine must always be assumed to be present.

An evaluation of the mechanism of injury should include a determination if, after the victim hit the roadway, he or she was struck again by a second vehicle traveling next to or behind the first.

Children, because they are shorter, are initially struck higher on the body than adults. The first impact generally occurs when the bumper strikes the child's legs (above the knees) or pelvis, damaging the femur or pelvic girdle.

The second impact occurs almost instantly afterward; the front of the vehicle's hood continues forward and strikes the child's thorax. The head and face strike the front or top of the vehicle's hood.

Because of smaller size and weight, the child may not be thrown clear of the vehicle. Instead, the child can be dragged by the car while partially under its front end. If the child falls to the side, the lower limbs may also be run

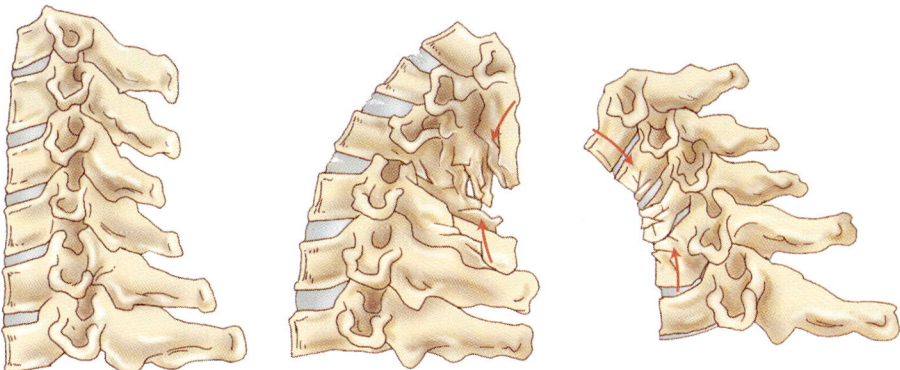

FIGURE 22.56 Hyperflexion (forward bending) changes the spinal vertebrae relationship from the left to the center drawing. Hyperextension changes the relationship from the left to the right drawing. Both produce compression with the bones of the concave side and shear tears on the convex side.

over by a front wheel. If the child falls backward, ending up completely under the car, almost any injury can occur from being dragged, struck by projections, or run over by a wheel.

As in an adult, any child struck by a car usually receives some head injury, and, because of the sudden, violent forces acting on the head, neck, and torso, the child must be assumed to have an unstable spine. Additionally, the force of the impact, which is usually midthoracic, should cause the EMT to be highly suspicious of significant intrathoracic injury even in children who initially appear asymptomatic. Any child who is struck by a car should be suspected of multisystem trauma, requiring rapid transport to the closest appropriate hospital or trauma center.

Knowledge of the specific sequence of multiple impacts and understanding the multiple underlying injuries they could produce are the keys to making the initial assessment and to determining the appropriate management of the patient.

> ✓ The three phases of the impact between the vehicle and the patient (initial impact with the bumper or front of the vehicle, impact with the hood, and falling off onto the roadway) determine to a major extent the injuries that the patient will receive. The height of the patient will determine the parts of the body that are struck first. The speed of the vehicle at the time of the impact will be the major determinant of the extent of the injuries.

Falls

Victims of falls may also suffer injury from multiple impacts. To properly assess a fall victim, the EMT should estimate the height of the fall, evaluate the surface on which the victim landed, and determine which part of the body struck first. Victims who fall from greater heights have a higher incidence of injury because their velocity increases as they fall. In general, falls from greater than three times the height of the victim are severe.

The kind of surface on which the victim lands, and particularly its degree of compressibility (ability to be deformed by the transfer of energy), also has an effect on stopping distance.

Determining which part of the body is hit first is important because it will help the EMT predict the injury pattern. The pattern that often occurs when victims fall or jump from a height and land on their feet is called the Don Juan syndrome. Only in the movies can the character Don Juan jump from a balcony, land on his feet, and walk away. In real life, heel-bone fractures are often associated with this syndrome. After the feet land and stop moving, the legs are the next body part to absorb injury. Knee fractures, long-bone fractures, and hip fractures can result. The body is forced into flexion by the weight of the still-moving head and torso, causing compression fractures of the spinal column in the thoracic and lumbar areas (Figure 22.56). Hyperflexion occurs at each bend of the S-shaped spine, producing flexion injuries (Figure 22.57).

If the victim falls forward onto outstretched hands, the result can be bilateral Colles' fractures of the wrists (see Chapter 28). If the victim did not land on his or her feet, the part of the body that struck first should be assessed, the pathway of energy displacement evaluated, and the injury pattern determined.

If the falling victim lands on the head with the body almost in line, such as commonly occurs in shallow-water diving injuries, the entire weight and force of the

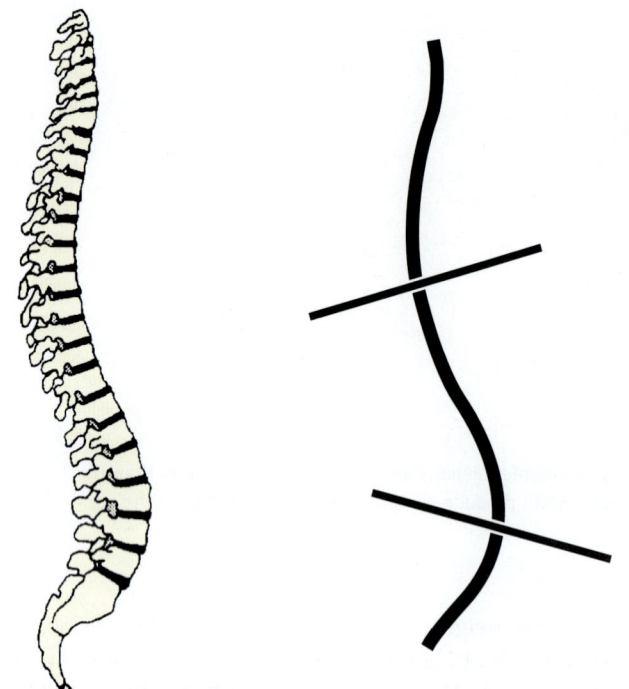

FIGURE 22.57 As the lower part of the spine stops its forward motion, the continued motion of the upper torso and head compresses the spine. This motion tends to produce compression injuries on the side of the concavity and extraction injuries on the side of the convexity.

moving torso, pelvis, and legs are brought to bear on the head and cervical spine.

> ✓ Victims of falls may suffer injury from multiple impacts. Knowledge of the kinetics of falls can help the EMT assess for life-threatening and bodily injuries. The EMT must be aware that a minimal fall may be critical to the geriatric patient.

Sports Injuries

Many sports or recreational activities such as skiing, diving, baseball, and football are capable of causing severe injury (Figure 22.58). These injuries may be caused by sudden deceleration forces or by excessive compression, twisting, hyperextension, or hyperflexion.

In recent years, a variety of sports activities have become available to a wide spectrum of occasional, recreational participants who often lack the necessary training and conditioning or the proper protective equipment. Recreational sports and sportlike activities today include participants of all ages. Some of these sports, such as downhill skiing, waterskiing, bicycling, and skateboarding, involve potentially high-velocity activities. Others, such as trail biking, all-terrain vehicle riding, in-line skating, and snowmobiling, may produce velocity, deceleration, collisions, and impacts similar to motorcycle or motor vehicle collisions. The potential injuries of a victim who is in a high-speed collision and is then ejected from a skateboard, snowmobile, or bicycle are similar to those sustained when a person is ejected from an automobile at the same speed because the amount of energy is the same. The specific mechanisms of car and motorcycle collisions have been described earlier in this chapter.

The potential mechanisms commonly associated with each sport are too numerous to list in detail. The general principles, however, are the same:

- What forces acted on the victim and how?
- What are the apparent injuries?
- To what object or part of the body was the energy transmitted?
- What other injuries are likely to have been produced by this energy transfer?
- What was compressed (by either cavitation or the "second collision" of internal organs)?
- How sudden was the deceleration or acceleration?
- What injury-producing movements occurred (e.g., hyperflexion, hyperextension, or excessive lateral bending)?

If the mechanism of injury involves a high-speed collision between two participants, such as in a collision between two skiers, it is often difficult to reconstruct the exact sequence of events from witnesses. In such collisions, the injuries sustained by one skier are often guidelines for examining the other. For example, if one victim sustains an impact fracture of the hip, a part of the other skier's body must have struck with substantial force and therefore must have suffered a similar high impact. What part struck what, and what injury resulted from the energy transfer? If the second skier's head struck the first skier's hip, the EMT should suspect potentially serious head injury and an unstable cervical spine (Figure 22.59). In such collisions, the importance of relating the injuries of one victim to the area struck on the second participant and of recognizing the potential underlying injuries to both cannot be overemphasized.

Broken or damaged equipment may also be an important indicator of injury and must be included in the evaluation of the mechanism of injury. A broken sports helmet is evidence of the violence with which it was struck. Because today's skis are made of highly durable materials, a broken ski indicates that extreme localized force came to bear even when the mechanism of injury may appear unimpressive. The severely dented front of a snowmobile indicates the force with which the tree was struck. The presence of a broken stick after an ice hockey skirmish raises the question of whose body broke it, how, and specifically what part of the victim's body was struck by it or fell on it.

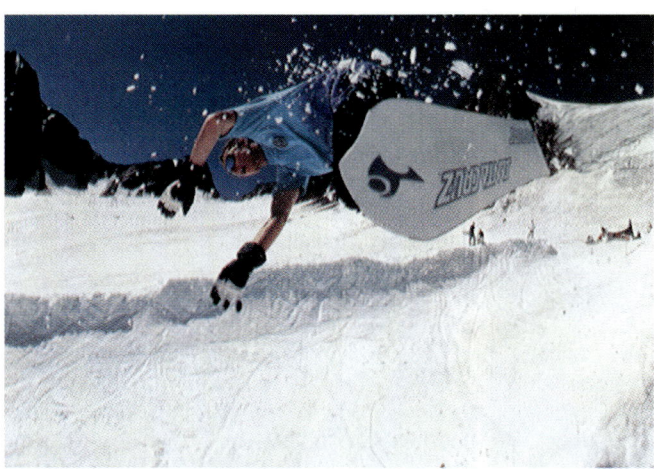

FIGURE 22.58 Many recreation activities can result in severe injury.

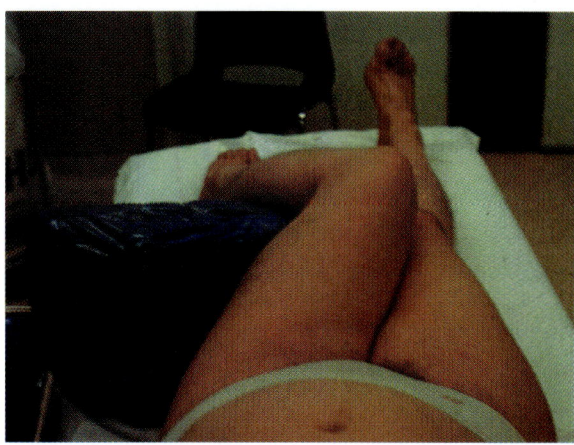

FIGURE 22.59 Dislocated hip in a cross-country skier.

The injuries caused by these forces must be taken seriously, and the victim must be evaluated thoroughly before he or she is moved from the scene. The patient must be evaluated as follows:

- For life-threatening injury
- For mechanism of injury (what happened and exactly how?)
- To determine whether protective gear was worn
- To determine how the forces that produced injury in one victim affected any other person involved in the collision
- To determine injury by assessing damage to equipment (what are the implications of this damage relative to the body?)
- For possible associated injuries

The common occurrence in many sports of violent contact, high-speed falls, and falls from heights without serious injury often clouds the EMT's assessment. Athletes frequently sustain incredible collisions and falls with only minor injury. Applying the principles of kinematics and carefully considering the exact sequence and mechanism of injury can be important additions to the EMT's assessment skills, helping him or her recognize those sports collisions in which greater forces than usual came to bear. Kinematics can be an essential tool in identifying possible underlying injuries and in determining which patients require further evaluation and treatment at the hospital.

Blast Injuries

Incidence of blast injuries increases during warfare, but these injuries are also becoming more common in the civilian world as terrorist activities and hazardous material incidents increase. Blasts may injure 70% of the people in the vicinity, whereas an automatic weapon used against the same size group may injure only 30%. Mines, shipyards, chemical plants, refineries, fireworks firms, factories, and grain elevators are some of the areas in which explosions are a particular hazard. However, many volatile materials are transported by truck or rail, and domestic and bottled gas are common household items, so an explosion can occur almost anywhere.

Different types of injuries occur during the three phases of explosions: primary, secondary, and tertiary (Figure 22.60). **Primary injuries** are caused by the pressure wave of the blast. They usually occur in the gas-containing organs, such as the lungs and the gastrointestinal system. Primary injuries include pulmonary bleeding, pneumothorax, air emboli, or perforation of the gastrointestinal organs. Pressure waves rupture and tear the small vessels and membranes of the gas-containing organs (cavitation) and may also injure the central nervous system. These waves may cause severe damage or death without any external signs of injury. Burns from the heat wave are also a common primary injury. Burns occur on unprotected body areas that are facing the source of the explosion.

> ✓ The type of energy exchange that occurs in sports injuries is similar to the exchange that occurs in other types of blunt trauma. The energy exchange must be transposed to the correct body position at the time of the impact to correctly understand the potential injuries.

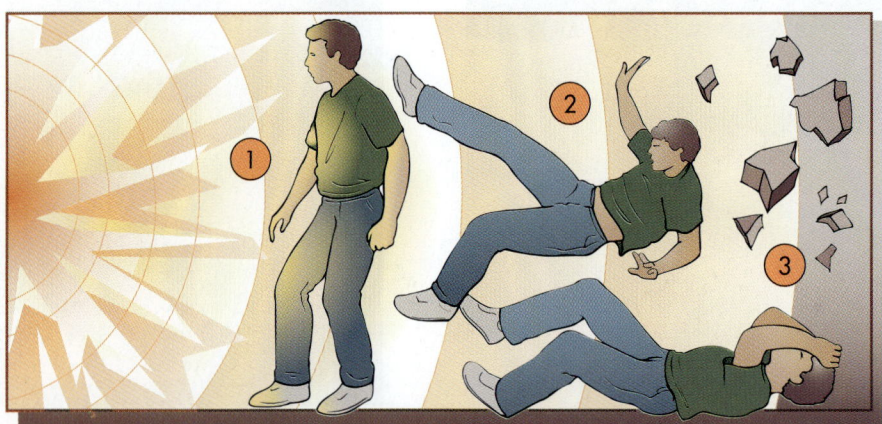

FIGURE 22.60 In a blast there are three phases of injury: (1) the blast wave hits first to produce overpressure; (2) projectiles from the blast hit the victim; (3) victim becomes a projectile and is knocked to the ground.

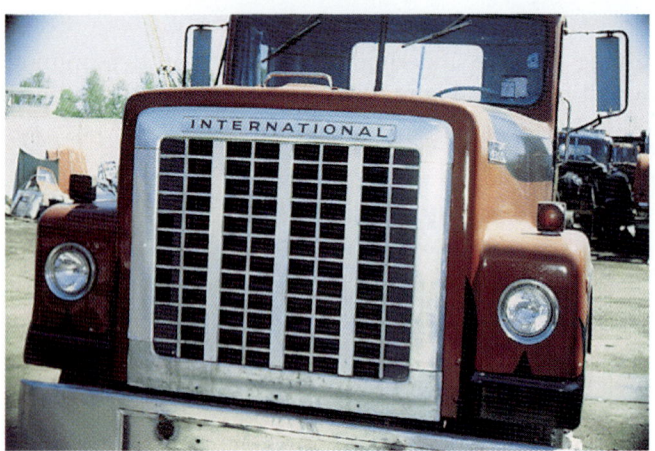

FIGURE 22.61 The profile or frontal area of an ice pick produces a much smaller impact point than a truck. A bullet that flattens or spreads out on impact has a larger frontal area than one that remains intact.

Secondary injuries occur when the victim is struck by flying glass, falling mortar, or other debris from the blast. Lacerations, fractures, and burns are the obvious injuries.

Tertiary injuries occur when the victim becomes a missile and is thrown against some object. Injury occurs at the point of impact, and the force of the blast is transferred to other organs of the body as the energy from the impact is absorbed. Tertiary injuries are usually apparent, but the EMT must look for associated injuries according to the type of impact that the victim suffered. The injuries that occur in the tertiary phase are similar to those sustained in ejections from automobiles and falls from significant heights.

Secondary and tertiary injuries are the most obvious and are usually the most aggressively treated. Primary injuries are the most severe, but they are often overlooked and sometimes never suspected. Adequate assessment of the various kinds of injuries is vital if the EMT is to manage the patient properly. Blast injuries often cause severe complications that may result in death if they are overlooked or ignored. Blasts produce many casualties and may result in a **mass (multiple) casualty incident (MCI)**.

> ✓ The distance from the blast and the amount of energy of the blast affects the patient in three ways: pressure, flying objects, and movement of the patient by the blast. Knowing the various types of energy exchange that occur in these areas assists the EMT in predicting the injuries that the patient may have. The EMT will therefore be better able to treat the patient and transport him or her to the correct medical facilty.

Penetrating Injuries

The principle of physics illustrated in the introduction to this chapter, the kinetic energy of a striking object transferring to body tissue, is important when dealing with penetrating injuries. Energy can neither be created nor destroyed, but it can be changed in form. For example, while a lead bullet is in the brass cartridge casing, which is filled with explosive powder, the bullet has no force. But when the primer explodes, the powder burns, producing rapidly expanding gases that are transformed into force. The bullet then moves out of the gun and toward its target.

According to Newton's first law of motion, after this force has acted on the missile, the bullet remains at that speed and force until it is acted on by some outside force. When the bullet hits a human body, it strikes the individ-

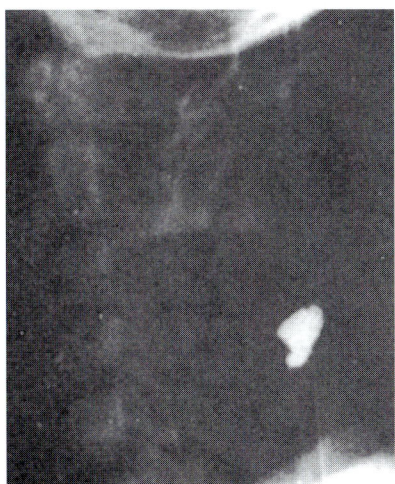

FIGURE 22.62 Changes in the profile or projection increase the particles hit and therefore the amount of energy dispersal.

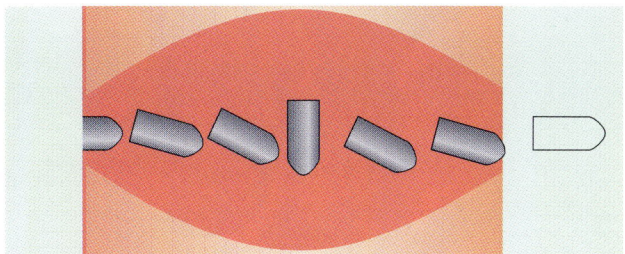

FIGURE 22.63 The tumble motion of a missile maximizes its damage at 90 degrees.

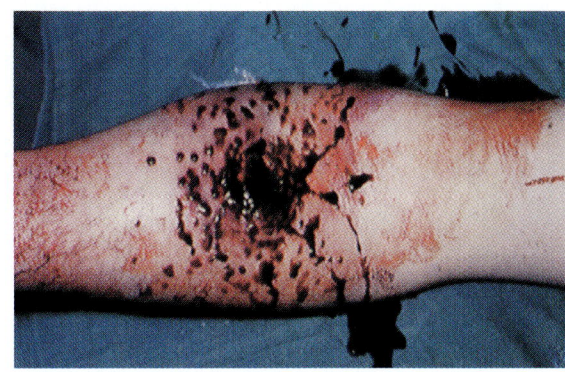

FIGURE 22.64 Shotgun wound.

ual tissue cells. The energy (speed and mass) of the bullet's motion is exchanged for the energy that crushes these cells and moves them away from the path of the bullet.

Frontal Area

The larger the frontal area of the moving missile, the greater the number of particles that will be hit, and therefore the greater the energy exchange that occurs and the larger the cavity that is created. Three factors affect the size of the frontal area: size and shape, tumble, and fragmentation.

Size and Shape
The profile or frontal area of an ice pick is much smaller than that of a baseball bat, which in turn is much smaller than that of a truck (Figure 22.61). A pointed missile, if crushed and deformed as a result of striking the body, has a much larger frontal area than before its shape was changed. A hollow-point bullet flattens and spreads on impact. This spreading enlarges the frontal area, allowing more tissue particles to be hit and producing greater energy exchange, which in turn leads to a larger cavity being formed and more injury produced (Figure 22.62).

Tumble
A wedge- or cone-shaped bullet's center of gravity is located nearer to the base than to the nose of the bullet. When the nose of the bullet strikes something, it slows rapidly. Momentum continues to carry the base of the bullet forward; in other words, the center of gravity seeks to become the leading point of the bullet. This movement causes an end-over-end motion, or tumble. As the bullet tumbles, the normally horizontal sides of the bullet become its leading edge from time to time, thus striking far more particles than when the nose was the leading edge, which in turn produces far more energy exchange and therefore greater tissue damage (Figure 22.63).

Fragmentation
Bullets such as those with soft noses or vertical cuts in the nose increase body damage by breaking apart on impact. The fragments produced create a larger frontal area than the single solid bullet, and energy is dispersed rapidly into the tissue. The multiple pieces of shot from a shotgun blast produce similar results. Shotgun wounds are an excellent example of the fragmentation injury pattern (Figure 22.64).

Damage

Damage caused by a penetrating injury can be estimated by classifying penetrating objects into three categories according to their energy capacity. **Low-energy weapons** include hand-driven weapons, such as a knife, a needle, and an ice pick. These missiles produce damage only with their sharp cutting edges. Because these are low-velocity injuries, less secondary trauma is usually associated with them. Injury in these victims can be predicted by tracing the path of the weapon into the body. If the

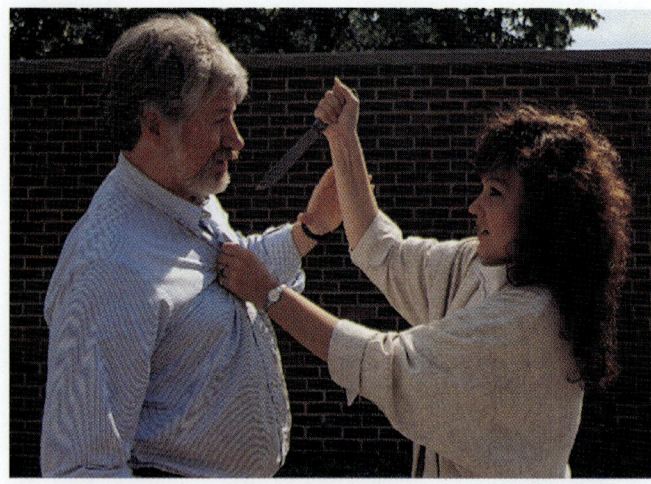

FIGURE 22.65 Women tend to stab down, with the knife held on the little-finger side of the hand.

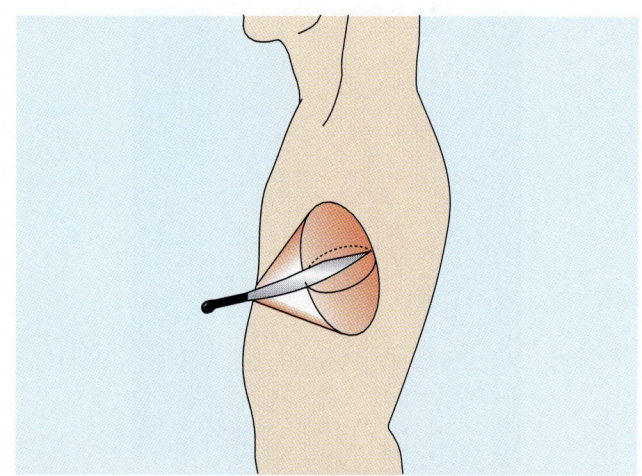

FIGURE 22.66 The damage produced by a knife depends on the movement of the blade inside the victim.

weapon has been removed, the EMT should identify the type of weapon used and the sex of the attacker whenever possible; men tend to stab with the blade on the thumb side of the hand and with an upward thrust, whereas women tend to stab downward and hold the blade on the little-finger side (Figure 22.65).

When evaluating a patient with a stab wound, it is important to look for more than one wound. Multiple stab wounds are possible and should not be ruled out until the patient is completely exposed and closely examined. This close inspection may take place at the scene or en route to or at the hospital, depending on the circumstances surrounding the incident and the condition of the patient.

The attacker may stab the victim and then move the knife around inside the body. A simple entrance wound may therefore give the EMT a false sense of security. The entrance wound may be small, but the damage inside may be extensive. This internal damage cannot be determined in the field, but the possibility must always be suspected, even in seemingly minor injuries. The potential scope of the movement of the inserted blade is an area of possible damage (Figure 22.66).

Evaluation of the patient for associated injury is important. For example, the diaphragm can reach as high as the nipple line on deep expiration. A stab wound to the lower chest can injure intrathoracic and intraabdominal structures as well. Therefore, when evaluating the victim of a penetrating trauma, the EMT should evaluate entrance and exit wounds. The EMT should be aware that tissue damage occurs in the path of the weapon's entrance and exit from the body. Knowledge of the victim's position, the attacker's position, and the weapon used is essential in determining the path of injury.

Firearms fall into two groups: medium energy and high energy. **Medium-energy weapons** include handguns and some rifles. As the amount of gunpowder in the cartridge increases, the speed of the bullet, and therefore its kinetic energy, increases (Figure 22.67).

The difference between these two groups is in the size of the temporary cavity and of the residual permanent cavity. These weapons, in general, damage not only the tissue directly in the path of the missile but also the tissue on each side of the missile's path. The variables of tumble, fragmentation, and size and shape influence the extent and direction of the injury. The pressure of tissue particles, which are moved out of the direct path of the missile, compresses and stretches the surrounding tissue. A temporary cavity is always associated with weapons in the medium-energy classification. This cavity is usually three to six times the size of the missile's frontal surface area (Figure 22.68).

High-energy weapons include assault weapons, hunting rifles, and other weapons that discharge high-velocity missiles (Figure 22.69). These missiles not only create a permanent track but produce a much larger temporary cavity than lower-velocity missiles. This temporary cavity expands well beyond the limits of the actual bullet track and damages a wider area than is apparent during the initial assessment. The obvious tissue damage is far more extensive with a high-energy penetrating object than with one of medium energy. The vacuum created by this cavity pulls clothing, bacteria, and other debris from the surrounding area into the wound.

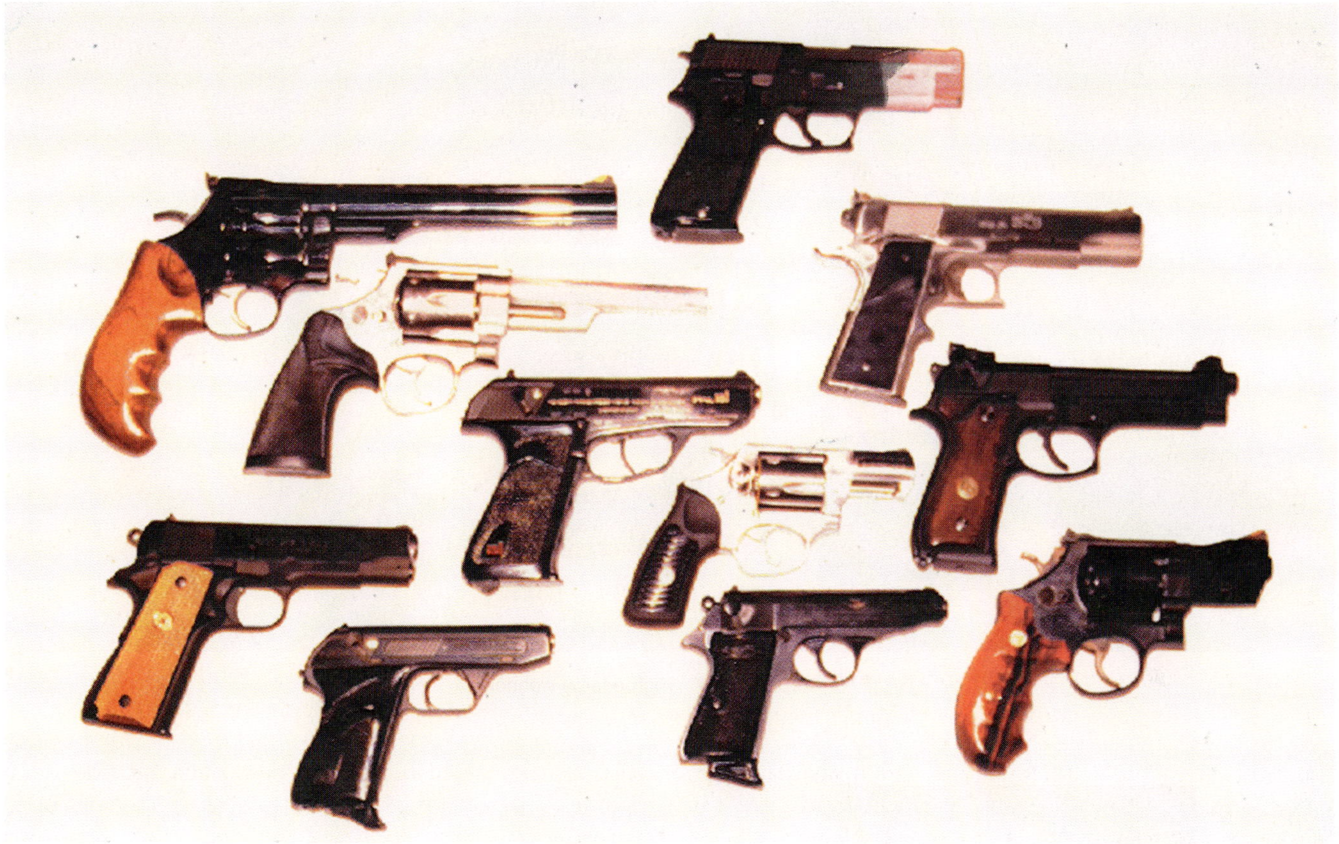

FIGURE 22.67 Handguns.

Distance

The range or distance from which the gun is fired is also important in evaluating the severity of injury to the victim. In certain instances the EMT may be called into court to testify as to the direction and possible distance from which a weapon was fired.

Air resistance slows the bullet; therefore increasing the distance decreases the velocity at the time of impact and results in less injury. Most shootings are carried out at close range with handguns, so the probability of serious injury is high. If the muzzle is directly against the skin at the time of discharge, the expanding gases enter the tissue and produce crepitus on examination. Within 5 to 7 cm the burning gases burn the skin (Figure 22.70); at 5 to 15 cm the smoke adheres to the skin; and inside 25 cm the burning cordite particles tattoo the skin with small (1 to 2 mm) burned areas.

Entrance and Exit Wounds

Evaluating wound sites can provide the EMT with valuable information to direct his or her own management

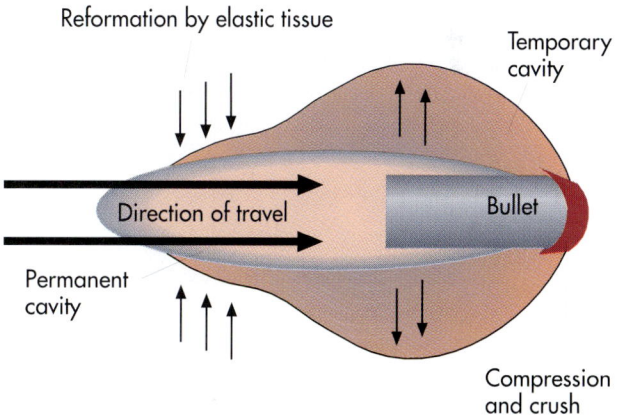

FIGURE 22.68 A bullet crushes tissues directly in its path. A cavity is created in the wake of the bullet. The crushed part is permanent. The temporary expansion can also produce injury.

of the patient and to relay to the receiving hospital, which is in turn helpful to the surgeons who will operate on the patient. Do two holes in the victim's abdomen indicate that a single missile entered and exited or that two missiles are both still inside the patient? Did the

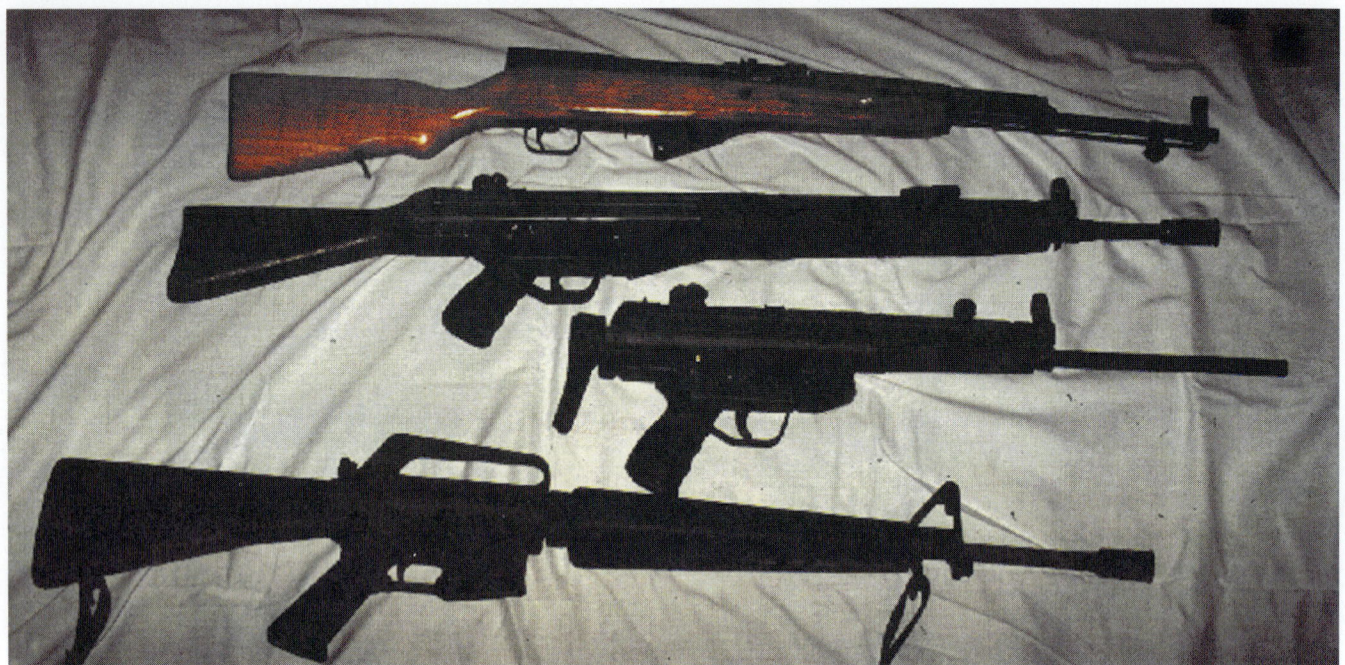

FIGURE 22.69 High-energy weapons.

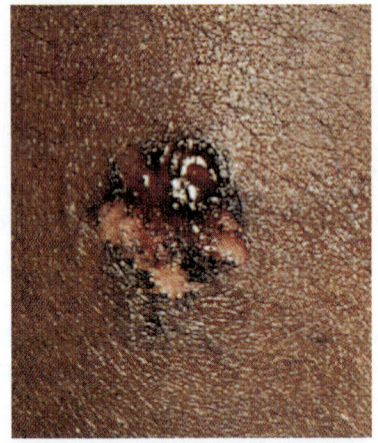

FIGURE 22.70 Gases coming from the end of a muzzle held in close proximity to the skin produce partial- and full-thickness burns on the skin.

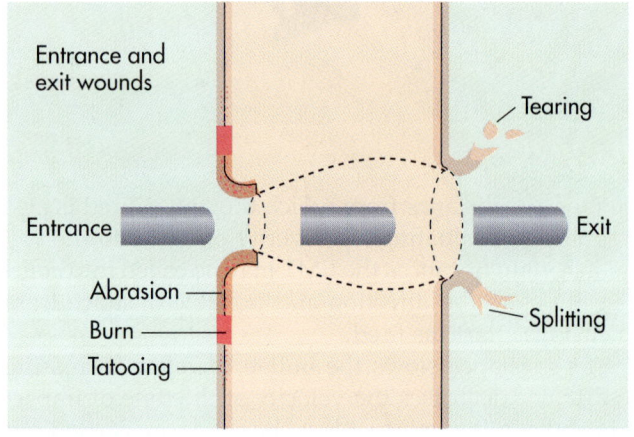

FIGURE 22.71 Spin and compression on entrance produce round or oval holes. On exit the wound is pressed open.

missile cross the midline (usually causing more severe injury) or remain on the same side? In what direction did the missile travel? What organs are likely to have been in its path?

As a bullet enters the body the skin is pressed against the underlying tissue, but as the bullet exits, the skin has no support (Figure 22.71). The entrance wound is a round wound if the bullet pushes straight against the skin (Figure 22.72) or an oval wound if it hits the skin at an angle (Figure 22.73). Without the backing of the underlying tissue the bullet tears the skin as it exits and produces a stellate (starburst) wound (Figure 22.74).

The missile is spinning as it enters the skin, leaving a small area of abrasion (1 to 2 mm in size) that is pink or black from debris from the sides of the bullet. There is no discoloration on the exit side (Figure 22.75).

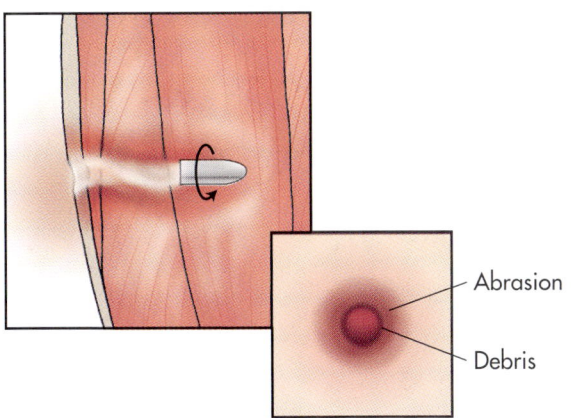

FIGURE 22.72 A round wound results when a bullet pushes straight against the skin.

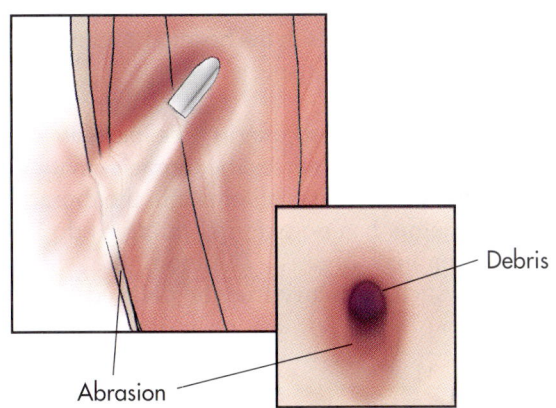

FIGURE 22.73 If the missile enters at an angle, the abraded side is on the bottom of the missile, where there is more contact with the skin, and covers a wider area.

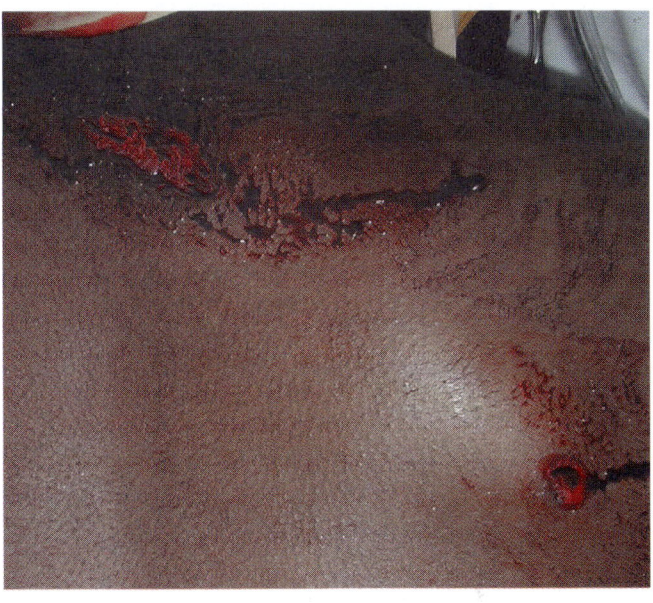

FIGURE 22.74 The entrance wound is round or oval in shape, and the exit wound is stellate or linear.

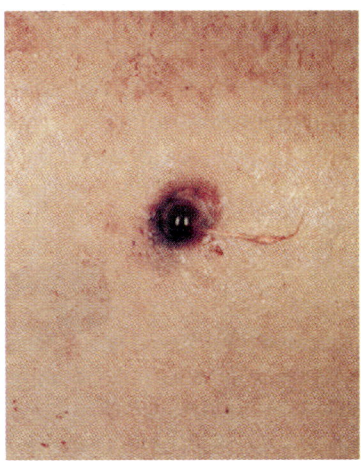

FIGURE 22.75 The abraded edge indicates that the bullet traveled from top right to bottom left.

Specific Regional Injuries

All of these phenomena cause specific injuries to the head, thorax, abdomen, and extremities.

Head

After the projectile penetrates the skull, its energy must be distributed within this closed space. Particles accelerating away from the missile are forced against the unyielding skull, which cannot expand as does the skin when subjected to similar pressures (Figure 22.76). Thus brain tissue is compressed against the inside of the skull, producing more injury than if it could expand freely. If the forces are strong enough, the skull may explode from the inside out.

A bullet may follow the curvature of the interior of the skull if it enters at an angle and has insufficient force to exit the skull, producing significant damage (Figure 22.77). This damage is characteristic of lower- and medium-velocity weapons, such as the .22-caliber

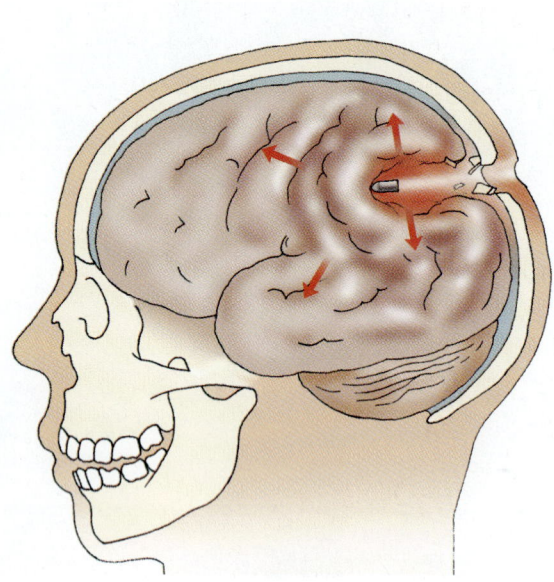

FIGURE 22.76 When a projectile penetrates the skull, the energy is dissipated inside the cranial cavity.

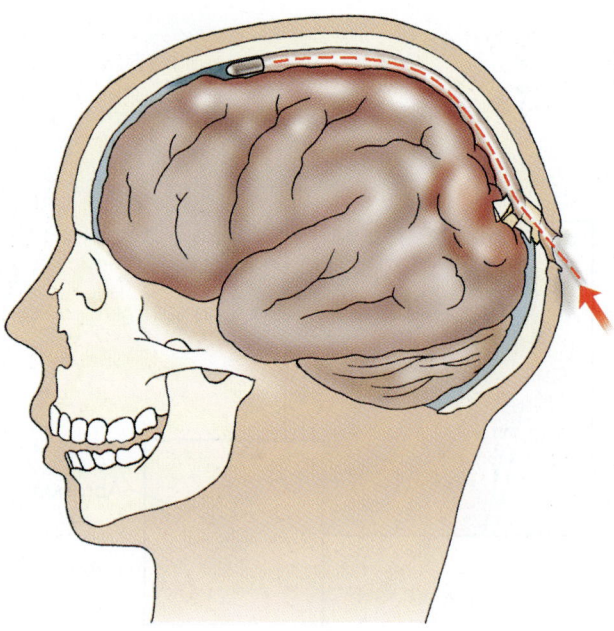

FIGURE 22.77 The bullet may follow the curve of the skull.

or .25-caliber pistol, which has, for this reason, been called the "assassin's weapon."

Thorax

Three major groups of structures inside the thoracic cavity must be considered: the pulmonary, vascular, and gastrointestinal tracts.

Pulmonary. Because lung tissue is less dense and much of the area traversed by the missile is air, fewer particles are hit and less energy is transferred. However, the damage to the lung can be clinically important (Figure 22.78).

Vascular. Smaller vessels that are not attached to the chest wall may be pushed aside without significant damage. However, if larger vessels such as the aorta and vena cava are hit, they cannot move aside easily and are more susceptible to damage.

The myocardium stretches as the bullet passes through and then contracts, leaving a smaller defect. The thickness of the muscle may control a low-energy penetration such as a knife or .22-caliber bullet, preventing life-threatening bleeding and allowing time to get the victim to a hospital. This type of penetration can produce a pericardial tamponade that may allow survival of the patient until he or she arrives at the hospital. If the tamponade is quickly relieved and the associated hemorrhage is controlled, the patient has a chance for survival. The only place where this procedure can be done quickly is in the hospital; therefore the patient should be rapidly transported.

Gastrointestinal. The esophagus, the part of the gastrointestinal tract that traverses the thoracic cavity, can be penetrated and can leak its contents into the thoracic cavity. The esophagus has no external lining as do most of the intraabdominal organs. Therefore the signs and symptoms of such an injury may be delayed for several hours or days.

Abdomen

The abdomen contains three types of structures: air filled, solid, and bony. Penetration by a low-energy missile may not cause significant damage. Only 30% of knife wounds penetrating the abdominal cavity require surgical exploration to repair damage. A medium-energy injury (handgun wound) is more damaging; 85% to 95% require surgical repair. However, even with injuries caused by medium-energy missiles, the damage to solid and vascular structures may not produce immediate exsanguination. Often the hemorrhage can be temporarily controlled and the patient resuscitated by EMTs using the pneumatic antishock garment while the patient is brought to the hospital in time for effective surgical intervention. Although the hemorrhage can be somewhat controlled in the field, it is critical for survival for the patient to get into the operating room as quickly as possible. Therefore the

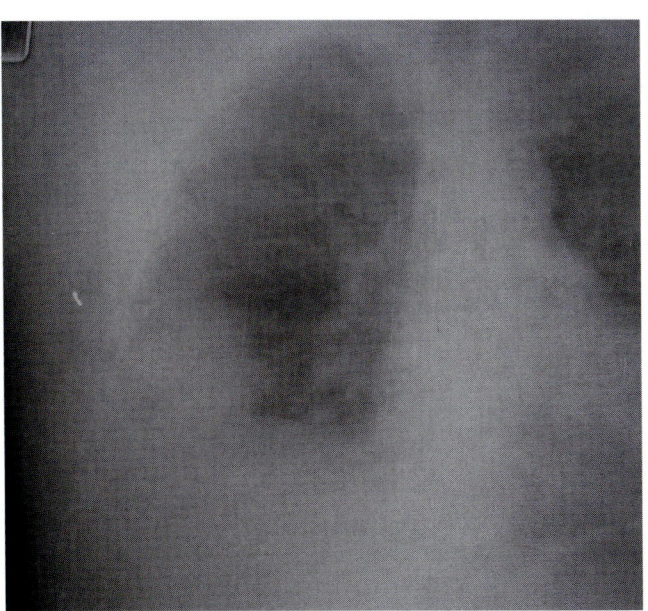

FIGURE 22.78 Lung damage produced by the cavity at a distance from the point of impact is easily appreciated from this radiograph.

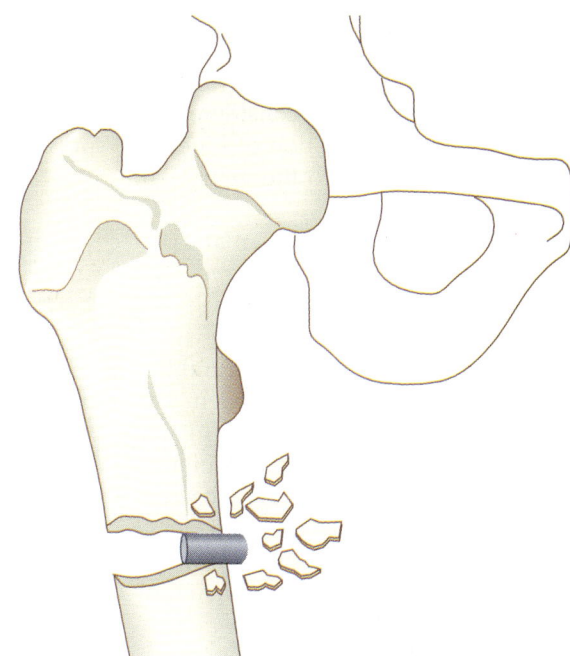

FIGURE 22.79 Bone fragments become secondary missiles themselves, producing damage by the same mechanism as the original penetrating object.

patient must be transported, if possible, to a hospital that has an operating crew and a surgeon in house who are awaiting the arrival of the patient.

Extremities

Penetrating injuries to the extremities can include damage to bones, muscles, or vessels.

Bones. When bones are hit, bony fragments become secondary missiles, lacerating surrounding tissue (Figure 22.79).

Muscles. Muscles often expand away from the path of the missile. This stretching causes hemorrhage (Figure 22.80).

Vessels. Vessels can be penetrated by the missile, or a near miss can damage the lining of a blood vessel, causing clotting and obstruction of the vessel within minutes or hours.

Summary of Penetrating Trauma

Questions to ask when evaluating an injury created by penetrating trauma include the following: What was the potential energy of the penetrating object—low, medium, or high? What pathway did it travel through the body (entrance and exit wounds), and therefore what anatomic

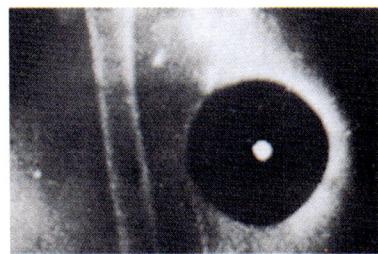

FIGURE 22.80 The more energy that the penetrating object has, the greater the energy exchange and therefore the greater the size of the temporary cavity.

structures would have been in that pathway? What changes potentially occurred to the missile as it passed through the body that would affect the amount of energy that it left behind?

> ✔ Penetrating injuries may occur from objects entering the body at low, medium, and high rates of velocity. A variety of injury patterns may occur depending on the region or regions of the body affected. Evaluate the entrance and exit wound sites to gain valuable information to direct management of the patient. In most situations, transportation to a trauma center is imperative.

Summary

- Kinematics must be considered at every collision scene. Proper evaluation of kinematics provides the EMT with a guide to the injury patterns to suspect, assess, and manage.
- An understanding of kinematics (mechanism of injury) will allow the EMT to predict 90% of the possible injuries before begining the physical examination of the patient. This prediction will assist the EMT in looking for potential injuries and therefore being better able to manage the patient for packaging and transportation to the hosptial. It will also assist the EMT in deciding to which hospital to take the patient when several hospitals are close or a disaster situation exists.
- Energy manifested as motion must be transformed into something else when the motion stops, and that is when the EMT's job begins.
- Asking the following questions helps guide the assessment and ultimately improve the quality of patient care. Answers to these questions are essential to locating the hidden effect of trauma on the body. Proper evaluation of the kinematics of injury can help the EMT to predict and suspect injury patterns and to examine specifically to find or rule out the hidden injuries.
  - *Impacts.* What type of impact occurred—frontal, lateral, rear, rotational, rollover, angular, or ejection? At what speed or velocity did the collision occur? Were the victims using protective devices? Where are the most severely injured victims likely to be? What forces were involved (blunt versus penetrating; compression versus shear)? What path did the energy follow and what organs have been injured on that path? Is the victim a child or an adult?
  - *Falls.* How long was the fall? What was the stopping distance? What part of the body struck first?
  - *Blasts.* How close to the explosion was the patient? What primary blast injuries are likely? What secondary blast injuries are likely? What tertiary blast injuries are likely?
  - Penetrating injuries. Where is the assailant? Who was the assailant? (Male or female? How tall?) What weapon was used? If a gun was used, what type? What type of bullet struck the victim? What was the range? What was the angle?

Scenario Solution

The damage to the vehicle is frontal and severe; therefore one would expect the damage to the occupants to be similar. The automobile is an older model without air bags, but the belt restraint system was available. However, it becomes clear on evaluation of the patient that this person was not wearing the seat belt.

The injuries that one would suspect include the following:

- Head: frontal skull fracture with cerebral contusion and perhaps an intracranial hematoma beneath or posteriorly.
- Chest: steering column impact to the anterior chest producing a flail chest and cardiac contusion. Although the impact was most likely central, one should also consider the possibility of a pneumothorax (even bilateral) and underlying pulmonary contusion.
- Abdomen: the lower part of the steering wheel could have struck the lower abdomen and the steering column could have hit the upper abdomen, resulting in fracture of the liver and spleen with an associated injury to the pancreas.
- Extremities: look for impact points on the dash produced by the knees. If present, consider the possibility of a dislocation of the knee, fracture of the femur, or dislocation of the hip.

Key Terms

Anatomy The structure of the body and the relationship of its parts to one another.
Angular-impact collision Off-center impact.
Anterior flail chest Two or more adjacent ribs fractured in two or more places, resulting in an unstable or potentially unstable segment of the chest wall.
Aortic insufficiency Incompetent aortic valve.
Blunt trauma Injury that is not immediately evident to the human eye.
Cardiac contusion Bruise to the heart.
Cavitation Open area in an organ or tissue.
Compression Squeezed together.

Key Terms (cont'd)

Crash Impact between vehicles or people.
Descending aorta Part of the aorta between the arch and the iliac bifurcation.
Energy Molecular activity.
Fragmentation Breaking apart.
Great vessels Major vessels in the chest.
Head-on collision A frontal impact in which forward motion stops abruptly.
High-energy weapons Weapons with a muzzle velocity between 1500 and 2000 feet per second.
Kinematics Mechanism of injury or biomechanics.
Kinetic energy The energy of motion and a function of an object's weight and speed.
Ligaments Connective tissue that holds bones together at a joint.
Low-energy weapons Weapons that fire a missile that produces damage only with its sharp cutting edge.
Mass (multiple) casualty incident (MCI) Any incident involving one or more patients that cannot be handled by the first responding unit(s) to a scene (e.g., the 1995 bombing of the Murrah Federal Building in Oklahoma City).
Medium-energy weapons Weapons with a muzzle velocity of less than 1500 feet per second.
Pedicle Supporting part of the bone.
Penetrating trauma Injury resulting in an opening in the skin.

Permanent cavity Cavity that remains in the tissue after the complete dissipation of energy.
Pneumothorax A collection of air in the pleural space; always abnormal and may cause collapse of the underlying lung.
Postcrash After the impact.
Precrash Before the impact.
Primary injuries Injuries that result from a blast wave.
Pulmonary contusion Bruise of the lung.
Ribs Twelve pairs of bones that line the wall of the thorax.
Secondary injuries Injuries that result from the victim being knocked down or into an object.
Shape Configuration.
Shear Tearing apart.
Stopping distance Distance required for an object to stop.
Temporary cavity Cavity that results from maximum energy exchange; present only for microseconds and depletes rapidly.
Tendons Straps of tissue that attach voluntary muscles to bone.
Tertiary injuries Injuries that result from flying debris.
Tumble Over and over motion.
Velocity Speed.
Vertebral column Made up of circular bones, called *vertebrae*, which protect the spinal column.

Review Questions

1. All of the following are phases of kinematics *except*:
   a. Assessment
   b. Precrash
   c. Crash
   d. Postcrash

2. The process of surveying or studying the scene of a traumatic injury to determine what injuries might conceivably have resulted from the forces and motions involved is called:
   a. Scene survey
   b. Scene management
   c. Patient care
   d. Precrash

3. In evaluating the forces involved in an motor vehicle collision, which of the following is true?
   a. Velocity is much more important than mass.
   b. Velocity is much less important than mass.
   c. Neither velocity nor mass is important; the frontal area of the car is what counts.
   d. The air bag deployment is the most important factor.

4. In trauma, a cavity is created and tissues are forced out of their normal positions in:
   a. Blunt trauma only
   b. Penetrating trauma only
   c. Both
   d. Neither

5. All of the following are descriptive terms for motorcycle crashes *except*:
   a. Head-on collision
   b. Laying the bike down
   c. Angular-impact collision
   d. Ejection-impact collision

Answers to these Review Questions can be found at the end of the book on page 866.

23

Soft Tissue Injury and Bleeding Control

Lesson Goal

Oxygenation is the most important step that the EMT can take to preserve the life of a trauma patient. The second most important step is hemorrhage control. Some hemorrhage control cannot be accomplished outside the hospital because it is in an area that is unreachable by the EMT. These patients have the greatest chance for survival by rapid transportation to a hospital equipped and staffed to manage such patients (a trauma center if available). Other hemorrhage is reachable and should be controlled quickly. This chapter addresses those injuries and the soft tissue injuries that are usually associated with such hemorrhage.

Scenario

A call is received to dispatch a unit to the scene of an automobile crash. The patient is a 32-year-old man involved in a single-car collision with a bridge abutment. The man is trapped in the car secondary to damage and must be extricated by the responding unit. His legs are caught under the dashboard and there is a large pool of blood on the driver's-side floor. Extrication is prolonged because of the severity of vehicle damage and takes more than an hour to accomplish. The man is lethargic and complains of difficulty breathing and has a wound on the left side of his chest. He also complains of pain in his left forearm and has obvious bruising and an abnormal bend in the forearm. The man is removed from the car. His right leg is bruised over the thigh, the calf is swollen and tender, and the foot is cool to the touch. There is an obvious angulation of the left thigh, with an open wound and bone protruding. There is active bleeding from the left thigh wound.

 What steps should the EMT take in assessing and managing the multiple injuries this patient has sustained? Explain the factors that you would use to decide if transport via helicopter would improve patient care in this situation.

Key Terms to Know

Abrasion	Avulsion	Body surface area	Compartment syndrome
Amputation	Bandages	Closed injuries	Contusion

Key Terms to Know (cont'd)

Crush injury
Dermis
Direct pressure
Dressings
Edema
Elevation
Epidermis
Evisceration
Hematoma
Hemorrhage
Laceration
Open injuries
Palm rule
Penetrating or puncture wounds
Pneumatic antishock garment
Rule of nines
Subcutaneous tissue
Tourniquet

Learning Objectives

As an EMT-Basic, you should be able to do the following:

DOT

- Describe the anatomy and physiology of the skin.
- List the types and describe the emergency medical care of closed and open soft tissue injuries, including control of hemorrhage.
- Describe and contrast the emergency medical care considerations for a penetrating chest injury and an open abdominal wound.
- Describe the purpose and function of dressings and bandages, and outline the steps in the application of a pressure dressing.
- Describe the effects of improperly applied dressings, splints, and tourniquets.
- Describe the emergency medical care of a patient with an impaled object or a traumatic amputation.
- Establish the relationship between body substance isolation (BSI) and soft tissue injuries.
- State the types of open soft tissue injuries.
- Differentiate the care of an open wound to the chest from an open wound to the abdomen.
- List the classifications of burns.
- Define *superficial burn*.
- List the characteristics of a superficial burn.
- Define *partial-thickness burn*.
- List the characteristics of a partial-thickness burn.
- Define *full-thickness burn*.
- List the characteristics of a full-thickness burn.
- Describe the emergency medical care of the patient with a superficial burn.
- Describe the emergency medical care of the patient with a partial-thickness burn.
- Describe the emergency medical care of the patient with a full-thickness burn.
- Establish the relationship between airway management and the patient with chest injury, burns, and blunt and penetrating injuries.
- Describe the emergency care for a chemical burn.
- Describe the emergency care for an electrical burn.
- Demonstrate the steps in the emergency medical care of closed soft tissue injuries.
- Demonstrate the steps in the emergency medical care of open soft tissue injuries.
- Demonstrate the steps in the emergency medical care of a patient with an impaled object.
- Demonstrate the steps in the emergency medical care of a patient with an amputation.
- Demonstrate the steps in the emergency medical care of an amputated part.
- Demonstrate completing a prehospital care report for patients with soft tissue injuries.

Supplemental

- Describe compartment syndrome and its complications.
- Describe estimation of blood loss at the scene.

Soft tissue injuries are among the most common injuries that the emergency medical technician (EMT) encounters. These injuries range from simple bruises (contusions) to large wounds with extensive loss of skin and muscle. Soft tissue injuries are often found with broken bones (fractures). Soft tissue injuries may also result in bleeding (hemorrhage), which must be controlled by the EMT.

Some injuries are more obvious than others. For example, in a crush injury the skin is often intact and no visible bruising is evident. Assessment in this situation includes a careful history of the event. With careful questioning, a mechanism of injury that causes crushing-type damage can be revealed and the appropriate treatment initiated.

Injuries may involve not only the soft tissues but also the body cavity underneath. Penetrating wounds of the

Patient Care Algorithm

Trauma Patient Assessment

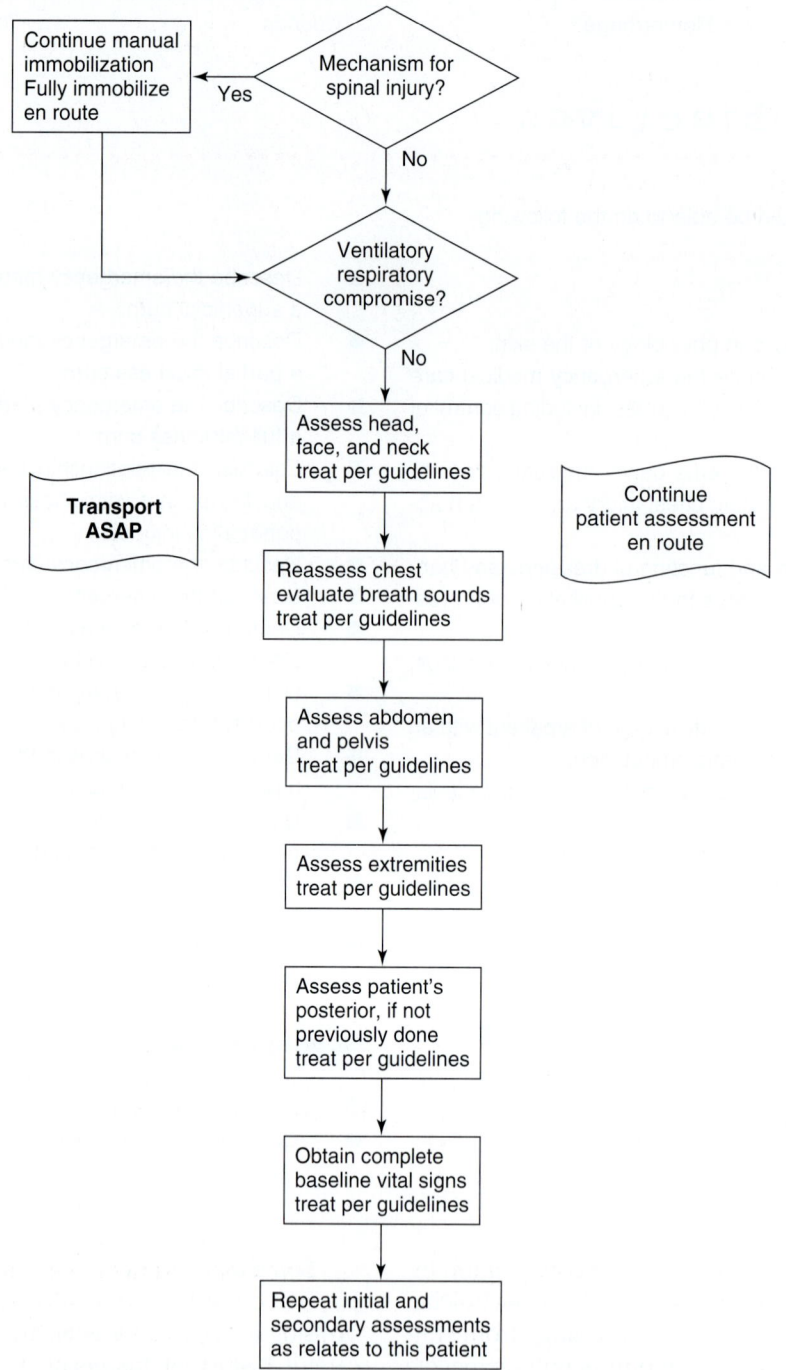

Patient Care Algorithm

Circulatory Assessment

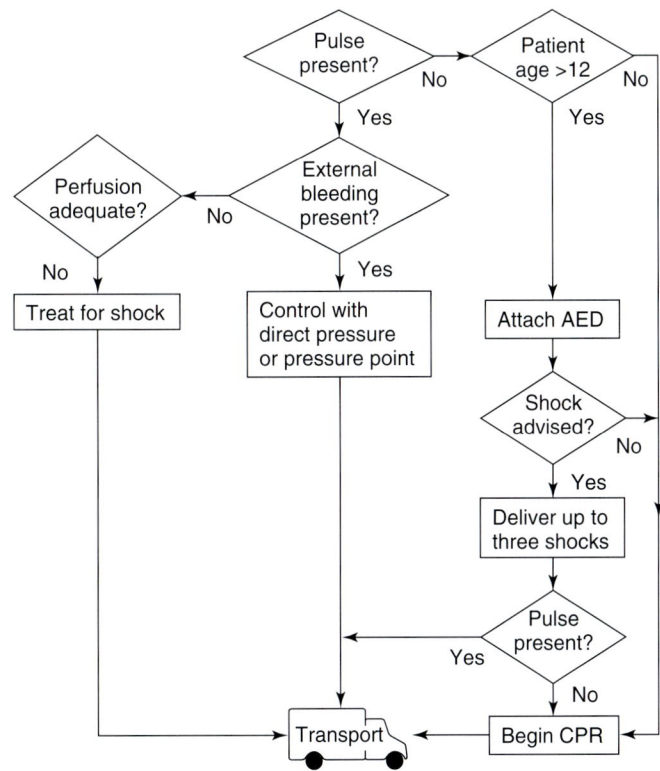

chest affect the patient's ability to breathe properly. Open wounds of the abdomen may expose the intestines and other organs within the abdominal cavity. The treatment of the soft tissue wounds may directly affect the amount and type of damage that is received by the underlying organs. Improper management may result in additional injuries to the exposed organs.

The assessment and management of burn injuries may be found in Chapter 29.

Physician Notes

Soft tissue injuries are often indicators of underlying injuries to other body structures (e.g., bones, organs within body cavities). Their presence should alert the EMT to the potential of more serious, hidden injuries.

Anatomy and Physiology

The skin is the largest organ of the body. It is composed of three layers of tissue: the **epidermis**, **dermis**, and **subcutaneous tissue**. The outermost layer of skin is the epidermis, which contains only cells, no blood vessels. The cells are termed *epithelial cells*, and the most superficial ones are dead. Immediately beneath the epidermis is the dermis. This layer is much thicker than the epidermis and contains a framework of connective tissue. Within this framework are blood vessels, lymphatic vessels, and nerve endings. The dermis also contains the dermal appendages: hair follicles, sweat glands, and sebaceous glands. The cells that make up the epidermis are supplied by these dermal appendages. The deepest layer of the skin is the subcutaneous tissue. This layer is composed of fatty tissue and fibrous and elastic connective tissue. Sweat glands are the deepest of the dermal appendages and may extend down into the connective tissue of the subcutaneous layer (Figure 23.1).

> ✓ The skin is the largest organ of the body and consists of three layers: the epidermis, dermis, and subcutaneous tissue.

From the outside, the skin may appear to be simple, but the functions it performs are complex. The most important function is the formation of a protective barrier between the body and the outside environment. Although the skin is covered with bacteria, it prevents these bacteria from invading the body. The skin is one of the body's most important defenses against infection. The skin also prevents fluid loss from the body and is essential for maintaining normal body temperature. Another function of the skin is to detect environmental dangers. The dermis contains nerve endings that provide signals to the brain. When dangerous conditions exist for the skin and body (e.g., heat), the nerves alert the brain and

Patient Care Algorithm

Expose and Environment

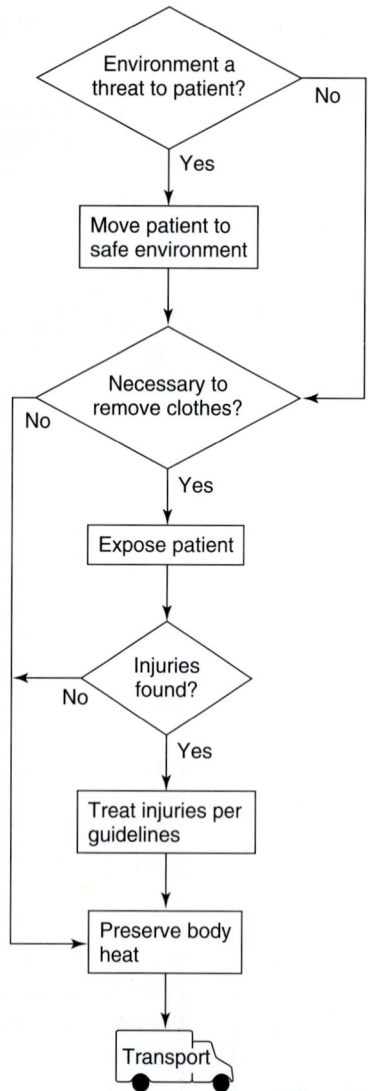

Soft Tissue Injury and Bleeding Control | Chapter 23

the person moves away from the harmful conditions. When the skin is damaged by abrasions, contusions, lacerations, avulsions, or thermal injuries, some or all of these functions may be severely affected or destroyed.

> ✓ Functions of the skin include protection from invading microorganisms such as bacteria, prevention of fluid loss, and maintenance of normal body temperature.

A method to determine the amount of skin that may have been damaged is helpful in determining how much skin function is lost. This estimation is especially important in burn patients, but extensive abrasions must also be estimated. The size of the skin is expressed as **body surface area** (BSA). The BSA varies from person to person and is determined by the individual's height and weight. Mathematical formulas are used to calculate the BSA, but formulas are difficult to use in the field. Therefore an easier method to estimate the BSA has been developed. This method is called the **rule of nines** (Figure 23.2). The rule of nines is not completely accurate but allows an estimation that is close enough to guide fluid replacement needs and estimate risk of death in major skin injuries such as burns. Another rule of thumb that allows an estimate of BSA is that the palm of the patient's hand is equal to about 1% of the BSA (the **palm rule**).

> ✓ The rule of nines is used to estimate the amount of tissue damage that has occurred and guides fluid replacement needs.

Pathophysiology

Soft tissue injuries are broadly classified into closed and open types. **Closed injuries**, in which the skin remains intact, include contusions (bruises), hematomas, and crush injuries. **Open injuries**, in which the integrity of the skin is broken, include abrasions, lacerations, avulsions, penetrating (puncture) wounds, and amputations.

Types of Closed Soft Tissue Injuries

A **contusion** is commonly termed a *bruise* (Figure 23.3). The epidermal layer of the skin remains intact, but cells and blood vessels in the underlying dermis are damaged. This damage causes blood to collect in the dermis and results in the characteristic discoloration. Swelling and pain are commonly present. The contusion itself is rarely

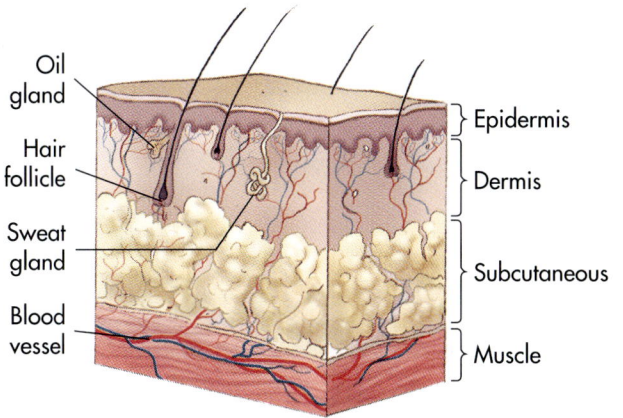

FIGURE 23.1 The layers of the skin.

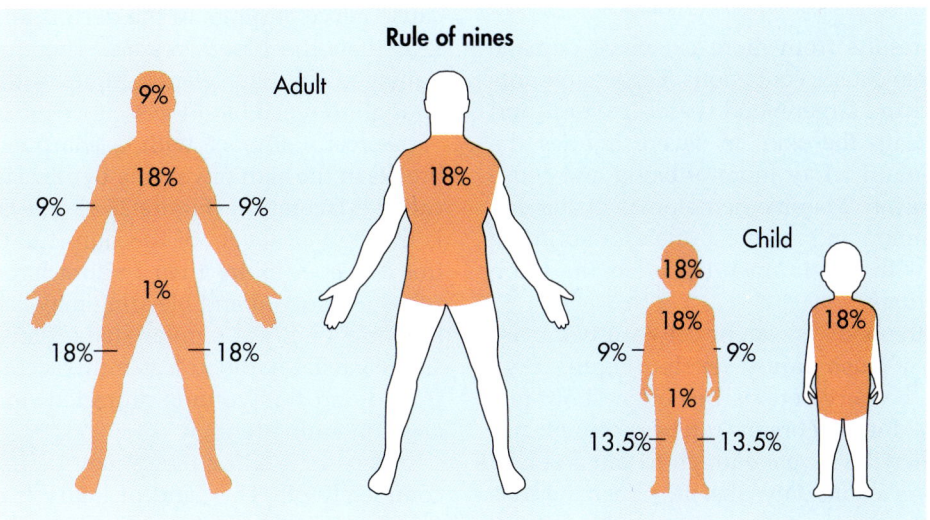

FIGURE 23.2 The rule of nines is one method used to estimate the amount of body surface area burned.

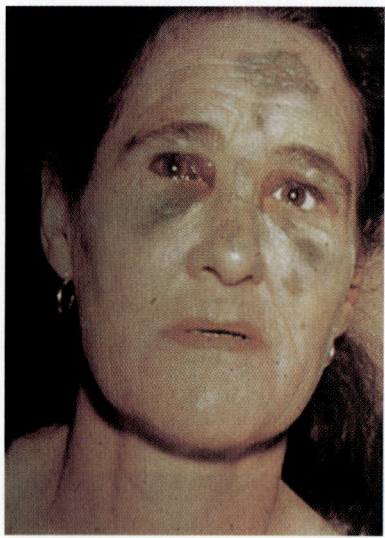

FIGURE 23.3 Bruises caused by blows to the face.

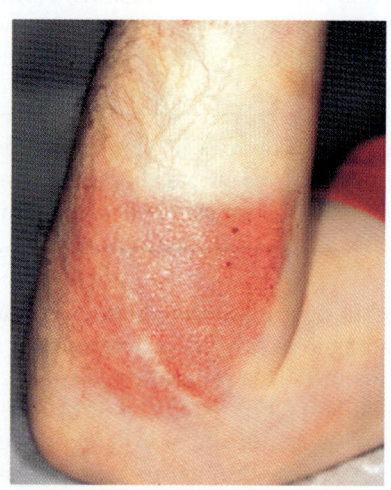

FIGURE 23.5 An abrasion of the forearm.

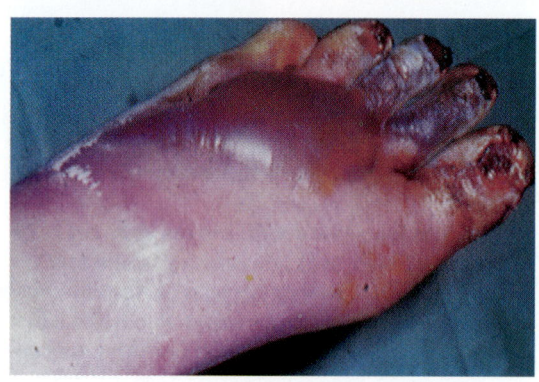

FIGURE 23.4 Severe and extensive crush injury with multiple fractures of the toes, some of which had to be amputated.

> **Physician Notes**
>
> Femur fractures may result in extensive soft tissue injuries and cause large blood loss into the thigh. The EMT must bear this potential blood loss in mind when evaluating the patient with a possible femur fracture.

serious but may be an indicator of more serious injury in deeper tissues.

A **hematoma** results from more extensive damage than the damage that causes contusions. Larger amounts of tissue are injured and larger blood vessels are torn, and blood collects beneath the skin. In severe injuries the hematoma may contain 1 L or more of blood and cause shock and hypotension. Massive hematomas of this nature are not uncommon and are most often found in the pelvis associated with pelvic fractures or in the thigh around femur fractures.

When part of the body is caught between two compressing surfaces, a **crush injury** results (Figure 23.4). These injuries can be very serious but often show few signs on the surface. Internal organs can be ruptured, and internal bleeding may be severe enough to cause shock. External bleeding is commonly absent. Crush injuries may cause painful, swollen, deformed extremities.

Types of Open Soft Tissue Injuries

An **abrasion** results from shearing forces that damage the epidermal layer and may extend into the dermis (Figure 23.5). Bleeding is minimal or absent, but pain is always present, even though the injury is superficial, because nerve endings in the dermis are closer to the surface than the blood vessels. Therefore the nerves are damaged by superficial injuries that are not deep enough to reach blood vessels.

Forceful impact with a sharp object can produce breaks in the skin of varying depth. This type of injury is called a **laceration** (Figure 23.6). The damage to the skin is through all layers of the skin (full thickness), making this a deeper injury than an abrasion. Larger blood vessels are involved and bleeding may be extensive. Lacerations may be of a regular shape (linear) or an irregular shape (stellate). Blood loss from lacerations must be controlled and the wounds protected from further damage and contamination.

Flaps of skin or tissue may be torn loose or pulled completely off. This kind of injury is called an **avulsion** (Figure 23.7). These injuries are often serious and com-

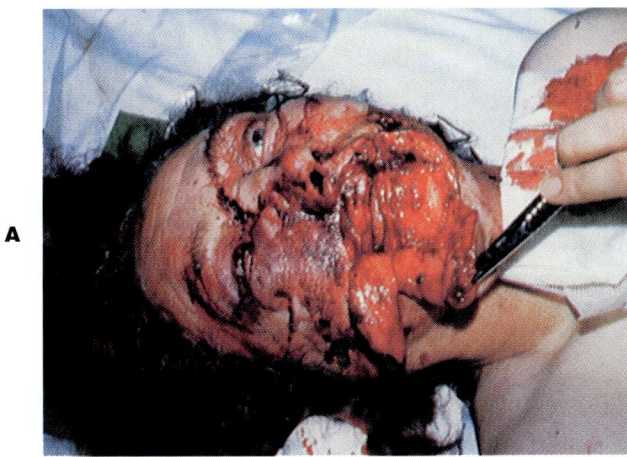
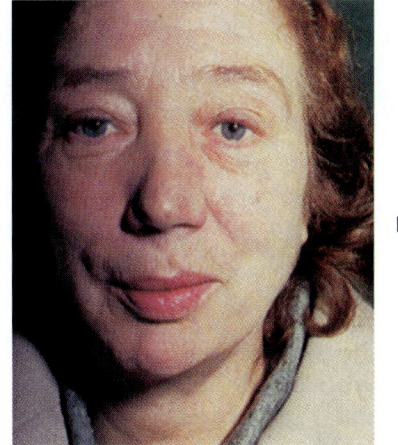

FIGURE 23.6 **A,** Laceration. This patient's lips have been sliced through and turned back. **B,** The same patient 1 year later.

monly are caused by large amounts of force being transferred to the patient's body. The separated tissue is cut off from oxygen and nutrients and will rapidly die. If possible, the separated tissue should be cooled (not frozen) and transported with the patient as rapidly as possible to an appropriate facility, as is done with amputated body parts.

Penetrating or puncture wounds are caused by sharp, pointed objects that puncture the skin (Figure 23.8). The most common penetrating injuries are caused by gunshots and knife stabs. Penetrating wounds may also occur during blunt trauma (car crashes) if a piece of the vehicle punctures the body. Little or no external bleeding may occur, but the internal bleeding can be severe. Secondary exit wounds may be present, especially with gunshot wounds. It is important to perform a careful head-to-toe survey to identify all injuries. The EMT must guard against focusing in on a single penetrating injury and missing possible multiple injuries.

An **amputation** may involve extremities or other body parts (Figure 23.9). The limb or tissue is completely severed from its attachments to the body. Bleeding may be severe, but often the divided blood vessels will constrict and limit the amount of blood loss. The severed body part must be cared for carefully and kept cool during transport. The patient and body part must be transferred as quickly as possible to an appropriate facility.

> ✓ Closed soft tissue injuries include contusions, hematomas, and crush injuries. Open soft tissue injuries include abrasions, lacerations, avulsions, penetrating puncture wounds, and amputations.

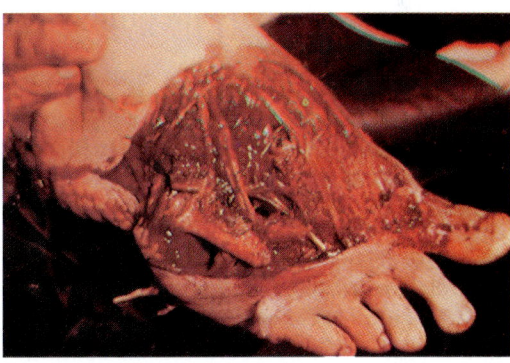

FIGURE 23.7 This avulsion injury was caused when the foot was smashed over the footrest of a motorcycle.

Hemorrhage

Bleeding (**hemorrhage**) is the loss of blood from within the vessels of the body. The amount of blood that is lost is a function of the size of the hole in the vessel and the difference between the pressures inside the vessel (blood pressure) and surrounding the vessel. The first step in controlling bleeding is to increase the pressure surrounding the vessel. Increasing pressure outside the vessel decreases the pressure difference and decreases the amount of blood that leaks out of the hole. Direct pressure applied to the wound is the best method to accomplish this goal. Hemorrhage in any blood vessel in the body can be controlled by direct pressure.

Blood lost into deep tissues from fractures and torn blood vessels can result in shock if the blood loss is severe. Hemorrhage from femur fractures can be massive, with 500 to 3000 ml of blood being lost into each thigh.

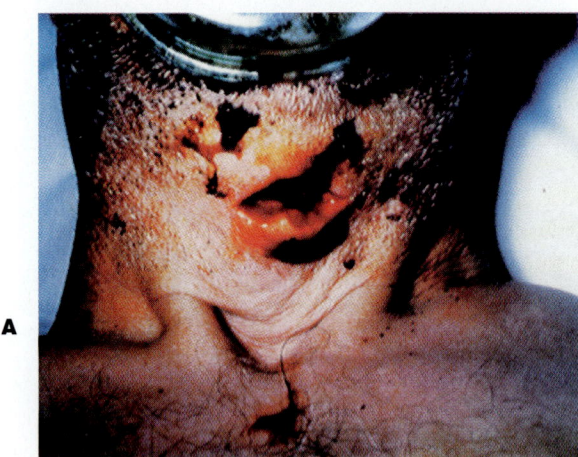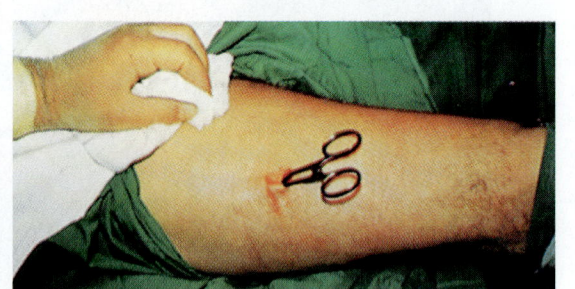

FIGURE 23.8 **A,** A self-inflicted stab wound. This wound was more than 12 hours old and had entered the pharynx. **B,** An accidental stab wound of the thigh.

Pelvic fractures may result in even larger hematomas and resultant hypovolemic shock.

Other Consequences of Soft Tissue Injuries

Avulsion injuries and amputations result in body parts being separated from their oxygen and nutrient supply. These tissues will quickly die. The requirements for nutrients and oxygen may be decreased by cooling the tissue. The tissue should *not* be frozen.

Whenever the integrity of the skin has been breached, bacteria can gain access to the underlying layers. Infections may result if the wound is contaminated by enough bacteria. Limiting the amount of contamination helps prevent infection in open wounds. Proper dressing and protection of wounds helps prevent further contamination.

The skin is essential for the maintenance of proper fluid balance in the body. When the skin is damaged, it can no longer contain fluids, and they leak out through the injured tissues. When the area of skin loss is extensive, the amount of fluids lost can be severe. Enough fluid may be lost to cause hypovolemic shock. Deeper tissues may also be the source of fluid loss in the body. When muscle is damaged by lacerations and crush injuries, the tissue responds by swelling (**edema**). The edema causes an increase in pressure in the surrounding tissues. As this pressure builds, the flow to the area is impaired and additional tissue is damaged by lack of oxygen and nutrients. This additional tissue damage creates more edema, and a vicious cycle is created. This cycle must be broken with surgical relief of the pressure. This condition is called **compartment syndrome**. The EMT can help the patient by recognizing the possibility of such a condition and transporting the patient as rapidly as possible to an appropriate facility.

The last major function the skin performs that can be affected by injury is temperature maintenance. The skin helps control body temperature. The blood vessels in the skin dilate and constrict to regulate blood flow to the surface of the body. To cool the body the vessels dilate and more blood flows near the body surface, where heat is given off to the atmosphere. To conserve body heat these vessels constrict and blood is carried away from the surface to the body's core. When the skin and underlying layers are damaged, the body's ability to control temperature is impaired. The larger the area of skin damaged, the more the body's autoregulatory system for temperature control is affected. The fluids lost through the damaged skin also evaporate on the surface and cause more heat loss.

Infection, shock from fluid loss, and hypothermia (loss of body heat resulting in an abnormally low temperature) are all possible complications of soft tissue injuries. The EMT can decrease the number of these complications through proper initial assessment and treatment of the patient in the field. Traumatic soft tissue injuries are always considered to be contaminated with bacteria. Application of a sterile dressing can decrease further contamination and help prevent additional injury to the damaged tissues. Immediate control of severe external hemorrhage can minimize blood loss and help slow the development of shock. Sterile dressings should be applied when possible to open wounds to help decrease fluid loss. Do not use wet dressings. Wet dressings cause evaporative heat loss from damaged tissues that are no longer able to regulate their own temperature. Attempts should be made to provide cover for patients to minimize heat loss and help prevent hypothermia.

> Infection, shock caused by hemorrhage and fluid loss, and hypothermia are complications of soft tissue injuries.

Assessment

When assessing and managing soft tissue injuries, the EMT must follow procedures for body substance isolation (see Chapter 6). Soft tissue injuries are almost always accompanied by blood loss, and this constitutes a danger to the EMT. Gloves and eye protection should be worn when the possibility exists for exposure to patient blood or body fluids. Hand washing should be strictly observed between patient contacts. These precautions are for the protection of both the patient and the EMT.

> Because soft tissue injuries are often accompanied by blood loss, EMTs must employ body substance isolation precautions to protect themselves against infectious diseases transmitted through body fluids.

Initial Assessment

The initial assessment of any trauma patient begins with airway and breathing. Damaged tissues suffer from lack of oxygen and nutrients. Little can be done in the field to improve the availability of nutrients, but the EMT can help with providing oxygen. The goal of resuscitation is to maximize oxygen delivery to tissues. Resuscitation is accomplished by providing the patient with as close to 100% oxygen ($FiO_2 \approx 1.0$) as possible. The first step in delivering this oxygen is to ensure an adequate airway. If oxygen cannot reach the lungs because of an obstructed airway, it cannot be transferred to the blood for circulation to the tissues (see Chapter 15).

> For any soft tissue injury, assessment begins with assessing airway and breathing.

Hemorrhage

Life-threatening external hemorrhage from open soft tissue injuries should be immediately recognized by the EMT and managed with direct pressure. This assessment should be done immediately after ensuring adequate airway and breathing. The EMT must take care not to miss bleeding that may be hidden by clothing. Previous blood loss that occurred before the arrival of the EMT should be estimated by a quick survey of the area surrounding the patient. The amount of blood present in the area should be visualized so the scene can be described to the physicians accepting the patient at the hospital. The signs of blood loss may be hidden by multiple factors, including dark clothing, being absorbed into the ground, or being washed away by running water or rain.

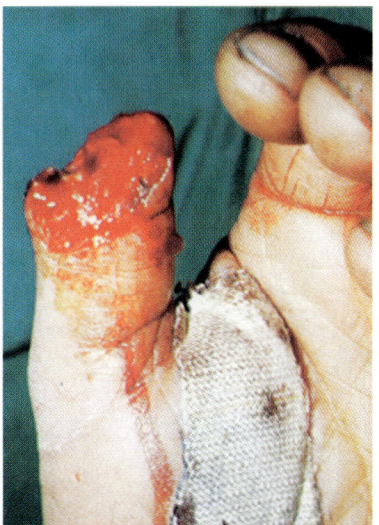

FIGURE 23.9 Amputation of the tip of the thumb.

Major internal hemorrhage can be caused by fractures of long bones (e.g., the thigh [femur] or upper arm [humerus] bones). If these fractures have intact overlying skin, no external bleeding may be present. The absence of obvious hemorrhage does not rule out possible life-threatening bleeding. Assessment of the patient includes a search for painful, deformed extremities and contusions, which may indicate underlying soft tissue injuries. A fractured femur can cause up to 2 L of blood loss into the thigh, and a broken humerus can bleed 1 L of blood into the upper arm (Figure 23.10).

> Assessment of soft tissue injuries should include a thorough assessment for hemorrhage.

Assessing Types of Soft Tissue Injuries

Most closed soft tissue injuries do not require treatment in the field by the EMT. However, contusions and large hematomas may indicate more serious injuries to deeper

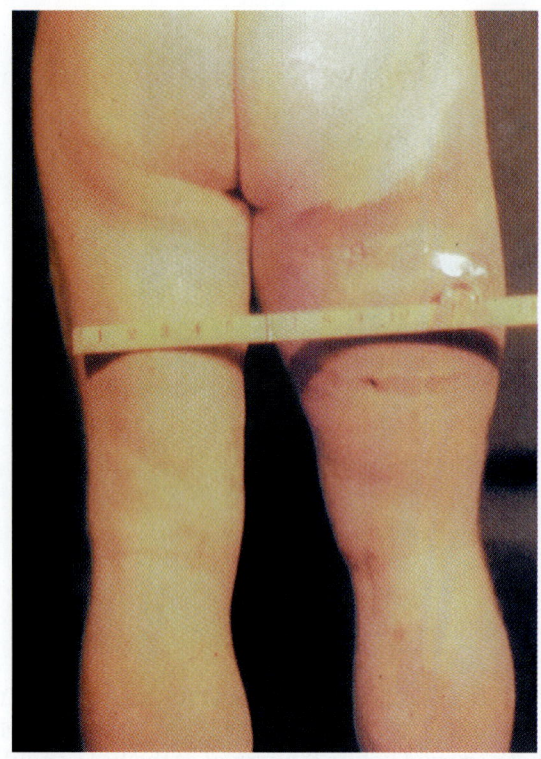

FIGURE 23.10 Blood loss into deep tissues from fractures and torn blood vessels can result in shock if severe. Extensive bruising is evident in this illustration. The right thigh is at least 1 inch bigger in diameter, which represents an increase in volume of between 2 and 3 L of blood.

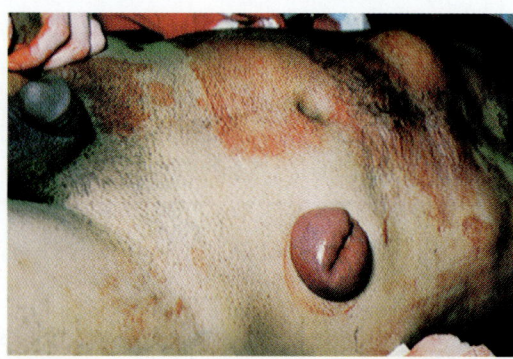

FIGURE 23.11 Evisceration. A loop of bowel emerged through a stab wound.

tissues. Crush injuries often can cause major bleeding into the damaged tissues. The mechanism of injury is the key to this assessment. A careful evaluation of how the victim was injured should lead to a high degree of suspicion for the presence of a crush injury. The presence of a painful, swollen, deformed extremity should alert the EMT to the possibility of a crush injury. Signs and symptoms of shock (hypoperfusion) should be assessed and managed when found or suspected.

Amputations and avulsion injuries are usually readily apparent during the initial assessment. The detached body part should be searched for if it is not in the immediate area of the patient. It is necessary to package and transport the amputated or avulsed body part with the patient if there is to be any hope for successful reattachment.

Certain soft tissue injuries require early identification and treatment. These include chest wounds that penetrate into the thoracic cavity, abdominal injuries with evisceration (Figure 23.11), large open neck wounds, and impaled objects. The last three situations are easily recognized because they tend to be spectacular injuries. A large wound with organs protruding from the abdomen (**evisceration**) requires special treatment and rapid transport to an appropriate facility. Large wounds to the neck may involve injuries to the major vessels in the neck. If left open, air can be sucked into the vessels, which can lead to air embolism. These injuries also may produce massive bleeding. Patients with foreign objects protruding from their bodies also need rapid assessment and transport (Figure 23.12).

Penetrating chest injuries are not always so readily apparent. Signs of a penetrating chest wound include wounds in which air bubbles out of them or a sucking sound heard when the patient breathes. These injuries can compromise breathing and require immediate management. Any patient with a wound to the chest and difficulty breathing should be assumed to have an open chest wound until evaluated by a physician.

> ✓ Determining the mechanism of injury helps the EMT determine the type of injury the patient has sustained. Amputations and avulsions are more obvious injuries, whereas chest injuries may not be so apparent.

Management

Bandages and Dressings

The mainstay of management of soft tissue wounds is the application of a dressing and bandage. The vast majority of these wounds require only this simple maneuver. Dressings and bandages help stop bleeding, protect the wound from further injury, and decrease additional contamination and later infection. **Dressings** are the sterile materials that are placed directly on the wound. They can be gauze pads of various sizes or a standard "universal" dressing that can be used in any situation (Figure 23.13).

Bandages are the materials that are placed over the dressings to hold them in place. There are several differ-

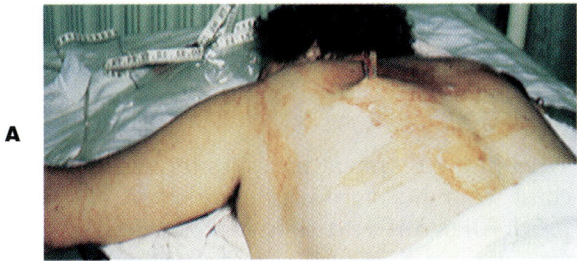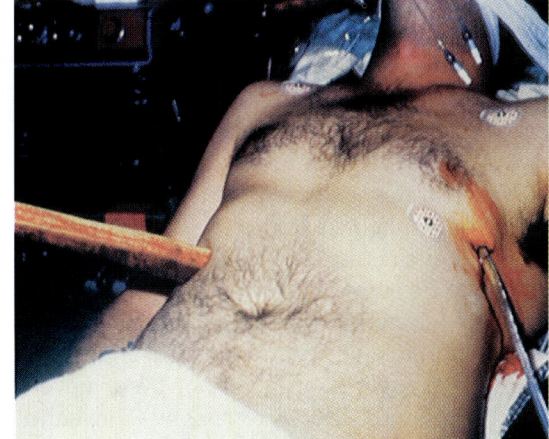

FIGURE 23.12 Patients with foreign objects protruding from their bodies need rapid assessment and transport. **A,** A stab wound in the back. **B,** A shaft of wood entered the right side of the abdomen, pierced the diaphragm, and tore the spleen, stomach, and liver. This patient made a good recovery.

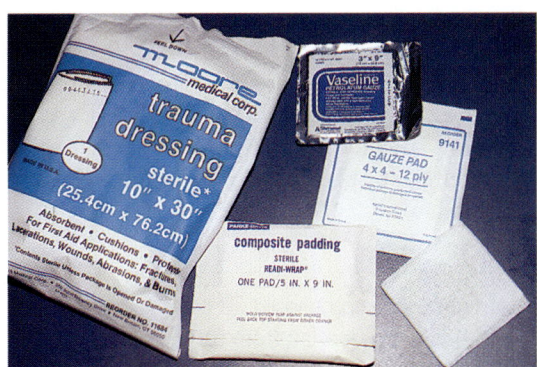

FIGURE 23.13 Dressings are the sterile materials placed directly on a wound. They may be gauze pads of various sizes or a standard "universal" dressing that can be used in any situation.

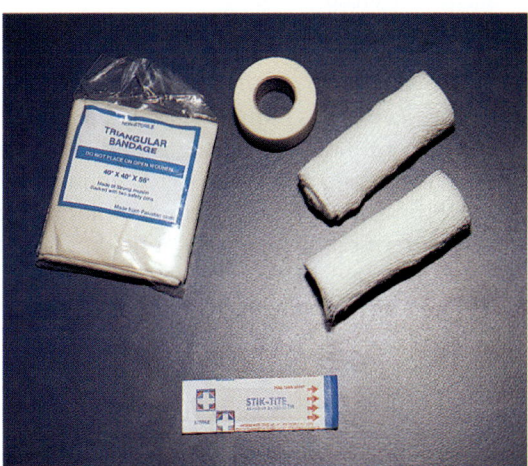

FIGURE 23.14 Bandages are the materials that are placed over dressings to hold them in place.

ent types of bandages (Figure 23.14). Self-adherent bandages are held in place by adhesive, which is part of the bandage. Other types involve material that can be wrapped around the injured area, such as gauze rolls, elastic bandages, triangular bandages, and adhesive tape. Air splints may also be used to hold dressings in place, as well as provide support for the injured extremity. A dressing is considered occlusive if the bandage that is applied over the top to hold it in place also forms an airtight seal.

Dressings must be applied properly to be effective. They should cover all the damaged skin areas to minimize further contamination and protect the wound from additional damage. When an occlusive dressing is required (e.g., to cover an open chest wound to prevent air from entering the chest cavity), care must be taken to ensure that the dressing is completely sealed to prevent air leakage through the dressing. Pressure dressings should be applied tightly enough to control blood loss but must not be so tight that a body part has no blood flow past the pressure dressing. To control arterial hemorrhage, the pressure does not have to exceed arterial pressure; it only must exceed the difference between the intraluminal arterial pressure and the extraluminal tissue pressure. A pressure dressing wrapped too tightly becomes a tourniquet and places the body part in jeopardy. Improperly applied dressings, splints, and tourniquets can lead to further damage to injured areas, continued contamination, and possible limb loss from compromised blood flow.

> ✓ Bandages and dressings are the mainstay of treatment of soft tissue injuries. However, the EMT must apply bandages and dressings properly to avoid further injury to the patient.

Initial Management

The initial management of patients with soft tissue injuries does not vary from the care rendered to any trauma patient. Proper airway management is the first priority, followed by ensuring adequate breathing. When initial assessment demonstrates external hemorrhage, direct pressure should be applied. A sterile dressing is placed over the wound, and pressure is applied directly to the wound with the EMT's hand. A pressure dressing may be applied by tightly wrapping a bandage around the injured body part. The bandage is wrapped tight enough to control bleeding. If proper control cannot be achieved with a pressure dressing, direct pressure with a hand should be continued.

> ✓ Management of the patient with soft tissue injuries begins with management of the airway and ensuring adequate breathing.

Closed Soft Tissue Injuries

Closed soft tissue injuries require little specific care in the field. If assessment indicates the signs and symptoms of shock or if internal bleeding is suspected, management of shock should be started. Any extremity that is painful, swollen, or deformed should be splinted. The patient should be transported to an appropriate facility as dictated by the severity of other injuries.

> ✓ A patient with a closed soft tissue injury should have the extremity splinted, if necessary, and should be transported to the appropriate medical facility.

Open Soft Tissue Injuries

Open soft tissue injuries involve wounds that damage the function of the skin. These wounds should be exposed, and bleeding should be controlled as previously outlined. A sterile dressing should be applied and held in place with an appropriate bandage. This prevents further contamination, protects from additional injury, and decreases fluid loss from the disrupted skin.

Open Chest Wounds

When the assessment indicates the presence of an open chest wound, a sterile occlusive dressing should be applied. An occlusive dressing is one that is securely taped around three sides of the dressing to form an airtight seal but allows for venting from the chest through the fourth side. A completely occlusive dressing may lead to continued air accumulation in the chest cavity and formation of a tension pneumothorax. An excellent dressing may be applied by using a petroleum jelly gauze foil package over the wound and taping it on three sides (Figure 23.15). If the patient's respiratory status deteriorates, the occlusive dressing should be temporarily removed to allow air to escape from the chest. The dressing is then quickly reapplied. This process is repeated as often as necessary. These bandages prevent any further air from being sucked into the thoracic cavity. As with all trauma patients, supplemental oxygen must be supplied to the patient.

> ✓ Airtight dressings should be used for open chest wounds to prevent air from being sucked into the chest cavity.

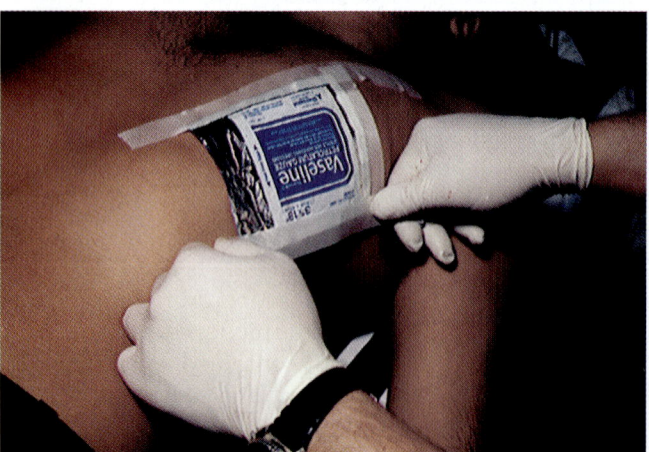

FIGURE 23.15 When the assessment indicates the presence of an open chest wound, a sterile occlusive dressing should be applied.

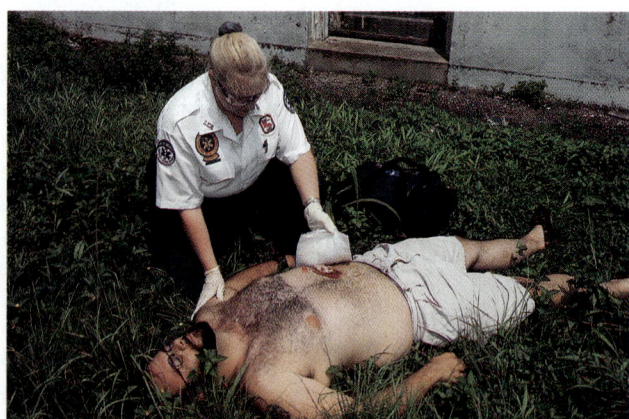

FIGURE 23.16 Abdominal organs protruding through a wound (evisceration) should be covered with a sterile dressing moistened with sterile saline and secured in place.

Evisceration

The EMT may be faced with a patient with an abdominal wound in which organs protrude through the wound (evisceration). The organs should be covered by a sterile dressing as soon as possible (Figure 23.16). This injury is one case in which the dressings should be moistened with sterile saline to prevent drying, to reduce evaporation and heat loss, and to prevent further injury to the exposed organs. The dressing is then secured in place. The EMT should not touch the organs and should not try to push the organs back into the abdomen. If spinal injuries are not suspected, it is appropriate to flex the hips and knees for the comfort of the patient.

> ✓ For eviscerations, a moist dressing should be placed over the injury. The EMT should not attempt to push eviscerated organs back into the body cavity.

Impaled Objects

Impaled objects should never be removed in the field unless the object interferes with necessary chest compressions, establishment of an airway, or the transport of the patient. The object should be secured in the position in which it is found (Figure 23.17). The wound should be exposed as much as possible and the bleeding controlled. A bulky dressing can be "built" around the object to help stabilize it. Transport to an appropriate hospital should be carried out as quickly as possible.

> ✓ Do not remove an impaled object at the scene. Support the object with a bulky dressing, and transport the patient to a medical facility.

Amputations

Amputations present unique management problems. The patient must be managed for the injury, but the amputated body part must also be properly cared for. The care given to the severed part may mean the difference between successful reattachment and failure. The patient is managed for the open soft tissue wound just as any other wound. Hemorrhage must be rapidly controlled and the stump protected with a sterile dressing. The amputated part should be wrapped in a sterile dressing and placed inside a plastic bag or wrapped in plastic. The packaged body part should then be kept cool during transport. It is important not to soak the amputated part in saline or water. Do not place the part directly on ice or ice packs, and do not cool with dry ice. It is important that the part be kept cool, but it must not be frozen. Always transport the severed part with the patient unless it delays the necessary transport of the patient to an appropriate facility.

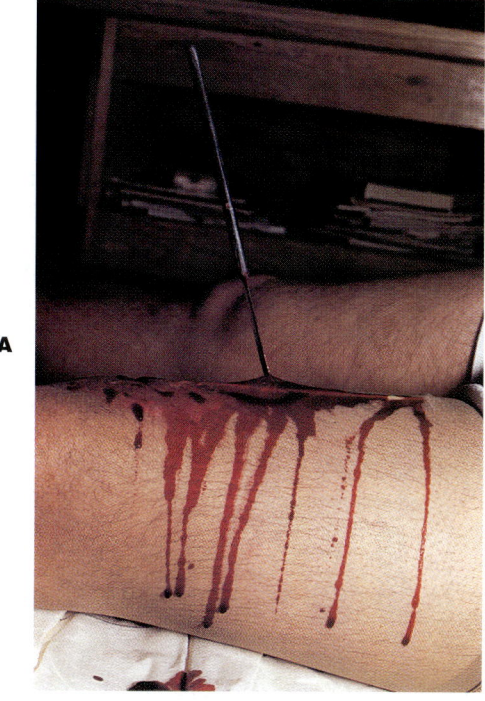
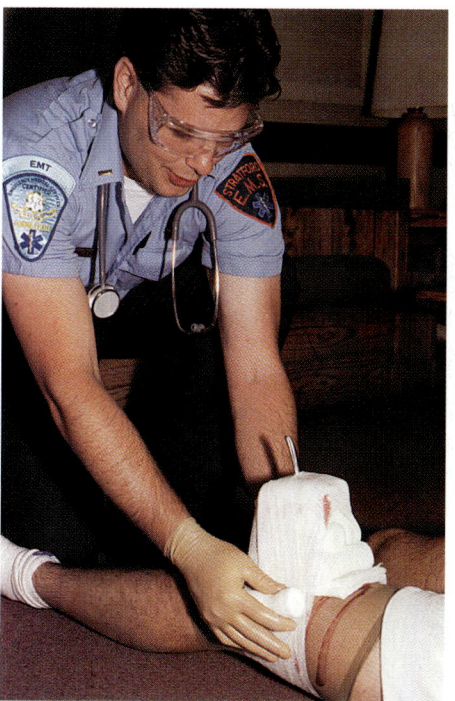

FIGURE 23.17 Management of an impaled object. **A,** The wound should be exposed as much as possible, and bleeding should be controlled. **B,** A bulky dressing can be "built" around the object to help immobilize it. Transport should be carried out as quickly as possible to an appropriate hospital.

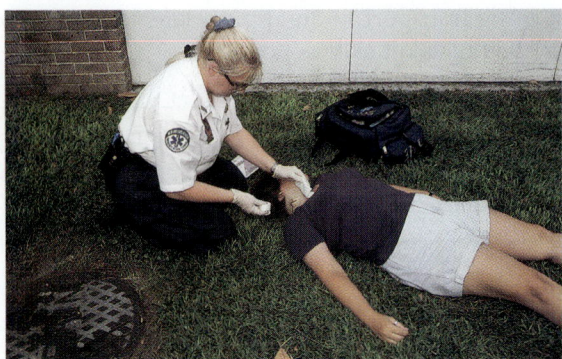

FIGURE 23.18 Open neck wounds may bleed massively. A sterile occlusive dressing should be applied to prevent air from entering the circulation. Direct pressure should be applied to control bleeding.

> ✓ For amputations, manage hemorrhage and protect the stump with a sterile dressing. If possible, locate the amputated part and place it in a plastic bag or wrap it in plastic. Keep the part cool, and transport it with the patient.

Neck Wounds

Open wounds to the neck may bleed massively. With neck wounds, injury to a major vessel in the neck must be assumed. The patient is in danger from two possible complications: bleeding to death from uncontrolled hemorrhage, and air embolism from air being sucked into the blood vessels. A sterile occlusive dressing should be applied to prevent air from entering the circulation (Figure 23.18). Direct pressure should be applied to control bleeding. Compress the carotid artery only if it is necessary to control the bleeding. Bilateral carotid artery compression must be avoided because this stops all blood flow to the brain and can result in death.

> ✓ Neck wounds bleed heavily. Manage the patient for hemorrhage, and apply an airtight dressing to prevent air embolism.

Controlling Bleeding

The control of bleeding is critical for the patient who has experienced a blood loss for any reason. Methods that are useful to prevent further blood loss in patients who have suffered trauma include the following:

- **Elevation** of the injured part. When bleeding is evident in an extremity, simple gravity may work to slow blood flow to the area and therefore reduce the amount of blood lost (Figure 23.19, *A*). Gravity will not work when core organs are involved or when the extremity has multiple breaks in bones and raising the limb would result in more injury to the patient. Elevation should not be used if the patient has a serious injury to the pelvis or spine.
- **Direct pressure**. A gauze dressing or thick pad placed over the wound and tight pressure applied over the dressing will decrease blood loss at the site. Direct pressure is not possible when objects are in the wound or when bone fragments are visible in the wound. A dressing should be placed over every visible wound to protect it from further injury and further contamination. Once a dressing is placed on a wound, it should not be removed; blood that accumulates in the gauze or pad congeals and begins to clot. This process of clotting assists in slowing blood loss and sealing the area. If the dressing becomes saturated with blood, a new dressing should be placed on top of it. Pressure may be applied to a dressing to reduce blood loss by applying a gauze or elastic wrap around the dressing and securing it snugly over the area. The wrapped dressing should not be so tight that it stops blood flow distal to the area of injury (tourniquet). If this type of pressure does not slow bleeding, apply pressure using the hands. The EMT should place a large absorbent dressing over the area and, with one gloved hand behind the injured site and one gloved hand over the site, apply a squeezing, consistent pressure over the injury (Figure 23.19, *B*). If it is not possible to hold the site from behind, the EMT should apply pressure with one gloved hand over the site to reduce bleeding. Pressure is being applied to the ends of the torn vessels to allow them to clot or close and stop blood loss. Direct pressure will work over large, gaping wounds but will require pressure over the entire area of the wound. These open wounds should be packed with dressings and secured in place with a gauze or elastic wrap. The EMT can apply air splints over a dressing for the purpose of applying pressure to the wound to slow bleeding. Air splints are an excellent method of applying consistent uniform pressure over the area, and they leave the EMT free to render other treatments. The **pneumatic antishock garment** (PASG) is useful as an air splint for the lower extremities and abdomen in this manner. Cardboard splints or metal splints may be applied to an extremity to provide support for pressure as well.

> **Physician Notes**
>
> Direct pressure is the key to controlling any type of bleeding. Every EMT was blessed with 10 instruments placed on his or her hands to control blood loss: they are called fingers. The EMT should use them appropriately and in a timely fashion, just as the surgeon uses these 10 instruments to control hemorrhage in the operating room.

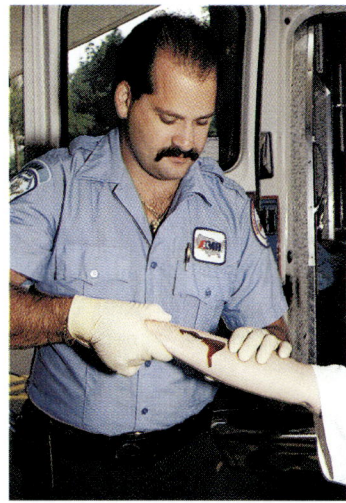
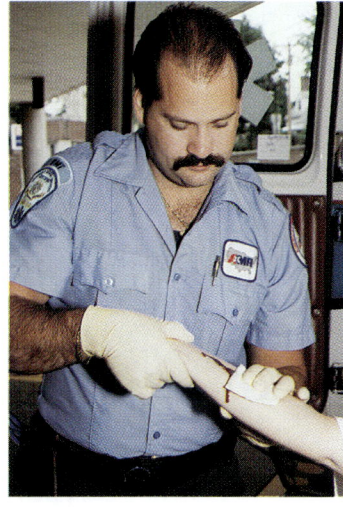
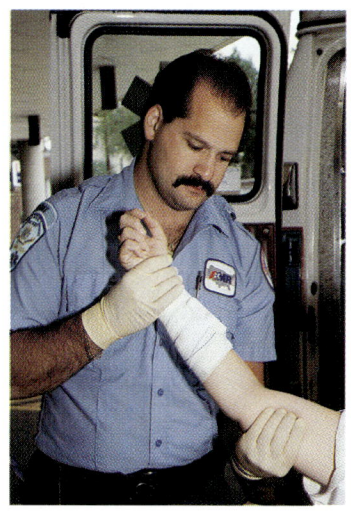
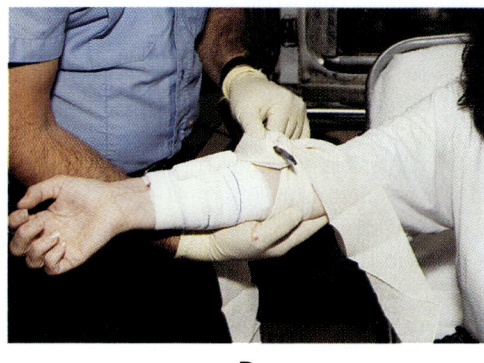

FIGURE 23.19 **A,** Elevate the extremity to slow external bleeding. **B,** A gauze pad or thick pad placed over the wound and tight pressure applied over the dressing will decrease blood loss at the site. **C,** Pulse point pressure. Locate the strongest pulse point above the point of injury and place pressure over the artery to reduce blood flow. **D,** Application of a tourniquet. The tourniquet should be placed as close as possible to the point of injury and tightened only until blood loss is reduced to a controllable state with application of dressings.

- Pulse point pressure. Pulse point pressure should be done only when direct pressure and elevation have not been effective in controlling blood loss in an extremity injury. This method of treatment should be used when the blood coming from a wound is bright red and spurting, indicating that an artery is injured. The EMT should locate the strongest pulse point above the point of injury and place pressure over the artery to reduce blood flow (Figure 23.19, C). The pressure at the pulse point is applied for 5 minutes and then released to see if blood loss has slowed or stopped. Blood flow to the extremity should not be interrupted for more than 5 minutes. If bleeding continues when the pulse point has been released, the pulse point should be compressed again.
- **Tourniquet**. The use of a tourniquet (restricting band) is a last resort treatment for control of bleeding or hemorrhage. Few civilian indications exist for use of a tourniquet to adequately control blood loss. For instance, if a limb is completely severed and all blood flow to the extremity is interrupted, the only method of controlling further loss may be a tourniquet. The tourniquet should be placed as close as possible to the point of injury and tightened only until blood loss is reduced to a controllable state with application of dressings. A triangular bandage or strip of cloth may be used as the tourniquet. It is tied around the extremity using a double knot. A small stick, pencil, or pen is then placed between the two knots, and the band is tightened (Figure 23.19, D). It should be tightened until the blood flow is slowed to an ooze. In the majority of situations when a tourniquet is used, the extremity below the tourniquet will be permanently lost. Therefore the use of a tourniquet to control bleeding should be initiated only after the EMT has given serious thought to the potential outcome for the patient. Tourniquets are seldom used unless the limb or extremity has already been traumatically severed. The potential for successful reattachment of a traumatic amputation is significantly reduced when a tourniquet is applied.

Physician Notes

Tourniquets are used when the choice is between losing the patient's life or losing the patient's limb. Their use should not be taken lightly. (See Chapter 42 for important exceptions.)

Summary

- When treating soft tissue injuries, body substance isolation precautions must be used.
- Airway and breathing must be assessed first and supplemental oxygen provided.
- External bleeding must be identified and controlled; estimate of prior blood loss should be made and reported to the receiving physician.
- Closed soft tissue injuries, such as contusions, may be an indicator of more severe injuries in deeper tissues. A careful assessment for the more major injuries must be made. Evaluation of the mechanism of injury should lead to the suspicion of crush injuries and a careful assessment for signs of compartment syndrome.
- Certain soft tissue injuries, such as the penetrating chest wound, require specific assessment and treatment.

Scenario Solution

The victim of the car crash in the opening scenario has several problems that require assessment and management by the EMT. Body substance isolation precautions must be observed. The EMT should have on gloves, eye protection, and a protective gown. Cervical spine control must always be maintained in this patient. The man is complaining of difficulty breathing and pain, so he has an open airway. Oxygen should be provided with a high-flow face mask.

The breathing problems may be caused by air inside the chest between the chest wall and lung (pneumothorax), and the patient has an open wound in his chest. The open chest wound should be assumed to penetrate into the thoracic cavity. It should be managed with an occlusive dressing.

The large pool of blood on the driver's-side floor indicates that significant external hemorrhage has occurred. This blood loss should be quickly estimated by the EMT for reporting to the accepting facility. This patient also has the potential for significant blood loss into internal parts of the body. The assessment in this patient should demonstrate the possibility of both femurs being fractured; the left one is an open fracture, and the right closed. The mechanism of injury also brings about the possibility of abdominal bleeding or a pelvic fracture with hemorrhage. The patient is noted to be lethargic, which may be secondary to hypoxia, blood loss, and shock. The external bleeding from the open left femur fracture must be controlled. This is best accomplished by placing the leg in a normal position to reduce the fracture and then applying direct pressure over the bleeding site.

The other extremity injuries are assessed and managed only if the patient is stable and does not require rapid transport to the hospital. The pain, bruising, and angulation of the forearm indicate a possible fracture. The arm should be placed in a splint. Assessment of the patient's lower extremity injuries includes an evaluation of the incident history. The patient has been trapped by his legs for more than an hour, and with the physical findings the EMT should suspect the presence of a crush injury to the right lower leg. The calf is swollen and tender, and the foot is cool to the touch. Blood flow may be compromised to the lower leg, and compartment syndrome may be present. The EMT can do very little for compartment syndrome in the field. The important thing is to properly assess the patient and determine the possible existence of compartment syndrome. The patient must be rapidly transported to an appropriate hospital. Surgical evaluation and possible intervention are required to break the cycle and save the leg.

In situations in which the patient is severely injured and the travel time to a hospital capable of managing major trauma is greater than the time to mobilize the helicopter, fly to the scene, load the patient, and fly back to the trauma center, transport via helicopter should be considered.

Key Terms

Abrasion Damage to the epidermis and dermis from shearing forces; commonly referred to as a *scrape*.

Amputation Injury in which a limb or other body part is torn completely from the body.

Avulsion Injury in which flaps of skin or tissue are torn loose or pulled completely off.

Bandages Material that holds a dressing in place over a wound.

Body surface area The measured area of the body involved, usually dealing with thermal injuries.

Closed injuries Blunt trauma that has no break in the integrity of the skin.

Key Terms (cont'd)

Compartment syndrome A condition commonly caused by crush injuries or prolonged lack of blood flow to an extremity. Muscle tissue dies, causing swelling, which increases pressure in the muscle compartment, which decreases blood flow, which kills more muscle, leading to more swelling, and so on. It can result in complete death of the extremity if not stopped by surgical intervention.

Contusion Minor damage in the dermal layer of the skin causing discoloration from blood leaking into surrounding tissue; a bruise.

Crush injury Damage that results from a body part being compressed between two surfaces; deep damage to muscle may result; compartment syndrome may result.

Dermis Middle layer of the skin that contains the blood vessels, glands, hair follicles, and nerve endings.

Direct pressure Controlled pressure applied over a wound with the hands or with bandages; first-resort measure to control bleeding.

Dressings Sterile materials that are placed directly on a wound.

Edema Abnormal accumulation of fluid in tissues in response to injury.

Elevation To raise an extremity or injured part above the level of the heart; measure used to control severe bleeding.

Epidermis Outermost layer of the skin; consists of cells only.

Evisceration Injury in which organs protrude from the abdominal cavity through a wound in the abdominal wall.

Hematoma Damage similar to a contusion but more extensive with larger blood vessels torn and more blood collected in deep tissues.

Hemorrhage Severe loss of blood.

Laceration A break in the skin of varying depth resulting from a forceful impact with a sharp object; deeper injury than is seen with abrasions, with larger blood vessels involved and more bleeding.

Open injuries Blunt or penetrating trauma that is potentially associated with a bony injury.

Palm rule The size of the palm is equal to 1% of the total body skin surface area.

Penetrating or puncture wounds Injuries that result when the skin is pierced by a sharp object (e.g., knife stabs, gunshots).

Pneumatic antishock garment Device used to externally vasoconstrict blood vessels for the purpose of moving blood from periphery to the core of the body.

Rule of nines A system for measuring the percentage of body surface area involved in a burn.

Subcutaneous tissue Deepest layer of the skin; made up of fatty and connective tissue.

Tourniquet Band of cloth placed around an extremity and twisted to increase pressure so that blood flow below the band is interrupted or stopped; last-resort measure used to control severe bleeding

Review Questions

1. Physiologic functions of the skin include all of the following *except*:
   a. Protect against infection
   b. Maintain body temperature
   c. Regulate electrolyte balance in the body
   d. Prevent excess fluid loss
2. When determining a patient's body surface area (BSA), which of the following is true?
   a. Apply the rule of elevens.
   b. The palm of the patient's hand equals approximately 1% BSA.
   c. Children have smaller heads in proportion to the rest of their bodies than adults.
   d. The sole of the patient's foot equals approximately 1% BSA.
3. True or False: The amount of blood that is lost in hemorrhage is a function of the size of the hole in the blood vessel and the difference in the pressure between the inside of the vessel and the outside.
4. True or False: When applying a pressure dressing, it should be placed tight enough to ensure that no blood flow goes past the dressing.
5. True or False: In treating a traumatic amputation, the severed body part should be placed on ice and kept as cold as possible.

Answers to these Review Questions can be found at the end of the book on page 866.

24

Head Trauma

Lesson Goal

The head is a confusing and complex part of trauma management, yet the anatomic and physiologic components are straightforward on the surface. The goal of this chapter is to remove some of the mystery from head injuries and make them understandable to the EMT-Basic. The EMT-B will understand the difference between hemorrhage to the outside of the head and that contained within the skull, brain swelling contained within the skull and the resultant reduction of blood vessel size and its consequences, and how these injuries occur and their delayed signs and symptoms.

Scenario

At 1500 hours on a summer afternoon, the tone goes off on your radio, and you hear dispatch calling your unit number. The operator tells you to respond to a motor vehicle collision (MVC), vehicle versus tree. On arrival at the scene, you find the man walking around and his wife, who was not involved in the MVC but has just arrived on scene. On brief observation, you note a front-end collision with the tree, resulting in an approximately 2-foot indentation to the vehicle and a bull's-eye noted to the windshield. When questioned about restraints, the patient states that he does not remember, but he "usually wears it." He says his name is Hunter Scott and adds, "I'm fine, I just have a small headache. I don't need an ambulance." You ask the patient to let you check him out, "since I'm here anyway," and he agrees. You do not observe any obvious trauma. The patient is alert and oriented $\times$ 4; however, he seems a little slow to respond. Mr. Scott does not remember if he lost consciousness.

You take the patient's vital signs. The patient's blood pressure is 120/80; heart rate is 110; respirations are 28; and the skin is warm, dry, and slightly pale. Mr. Scott tells you, "Thank you for your time, but really, I'm OK." When you question the wife, she states, "He seems OK, but something is just not right."

 How would you handle this situation?

Key Terms to Know

Arachnoid membrane	Brainstem	Cerebrum	Cranial cavity
Battle's sign	Cerebellum	Cheyne-Stokes breathing	Cushing's triad
Brain edema	Cerebrospinal fluid	Closed head injury	Decerebrate posturing

Head Trauma | Chapter 24   **457**

Key Terms to Know (cont'd)

Decorticate posturing
Dura mater
Epidural hematoma
Epidural space

Foramen magnum
Glasgow Coma Scale
Intracranial pressure
Level of consciousness

Meninges
Open head injury
Pia mater
Raccoon's eyes

Subdural hematoma
Sutures

Learning Objectives

As an EMT-Basic, you should be able to do the following:

DOT

- Describe the relationship of mechanism of injury to potential injuries of the head.
- Define the structure of the skeletal system as it relates to the nervous system.
- Describe the implications of not properly caring for potential spinal injuries.
- State the signs and symptoms of a potential spinal injury.
- Describe the method of determining if a responsive patient may have a spinal injury.
- Relate the airway emergency medical care techniques to the patient with a suspected spinal injury.
- Describe how to stabilize the cervical spine.
- Discuss indications for sizing and using a cervical spine immobilization device.
- Establish the relationship between airway management and the patient with head and spinal injuries.
- Describe a method of sizing a cervical spine immobilization device.
- Describe how to logroll a patient with a suspected spinal injury.
- Describe how to secure a patient to a long spine board.
- List instances when a short spine board should be used.
- Describe how to immobilize a patient using a short spine board.
- Describe the indications for the use of rapid extrication.
- List steps in performing rapid extrication.
- State the circumstances when a helmet should be left on the patient.
- Discuss the circumstances when a helmet should be removed.
- Identify different types of helmets.
- Describe the unique characteristics of sports helmets.
- Explain the preferred methods for removal of a helmet.
- Discuss alternative methods for removal of a helmet.
- Describe how the patient's head is stabilized to remove the helmet.
- Differentiate how the head is stabilized with a helmet compared with without a helmet.
- Demonstrate opening the airway in a patient with suspected spinal cord injury.
- Demonstrate evaluating a responsive patient with a suspected spinal cord injury.
- Demonstrate stabilization of the cervical spine.
- Demonstrate the four-person logroll for a patient with a suspected spinal cord injury.
- Demonstrate how to logroll a patient with a suspected spinal cord injury using two people.
- Demonstrate securing a patient to a long spine board.
- Demonstrate using the short board immobilization technique.
- Demonstrate the procedure for rapid extrication.
- Demonstrate preferred methods for stabilization of a helmet.
- Demonstrate helmet removal techniques.
- Demonstrate alternative methods for stabilization of a helmet.
- Demonstrate completing a prehospital care report for patients with head and spinal injuries.

Supplemental

- List the structures of the head and describe the function of each structure.
- Discuss the importance of the meninges.
- Define and draw a "potential space."
- Name the three divisions of the brain and briefly list their functions.
- Discuss the importance of cerebrospinal fluid.
- Discuss why the scalp is more prone to blood loss.
- Discuss bleeding control for open and closed head injuries.
- Discuss brain edema and its consequences.
- Discuss intracranial pressure.
- Discuss the importance of frequent assessments of level of consciousness.

An emergency medical technician (EMT) is called on to perform a diverse range of skills. One of the most important skills is the proper identification of signs and symptoms of head injuries and proper treatment. The EMT must be able to understand the mechanism of injury, how to apply the information, and how it relates to the patient, assessment, and treatment. If one notes that a car involved in a motor vehicle accident (MVC) has a bull's-eye to the windshield, one must be able to focus part of the assessment on level of consciousness (LOC) and possible head injuries. If the patient is unresponsive and also has a fractured tibia-fibula, the EMT's main focus should be the LOC and not the fracture. Sometimes this is difficult because one wants to immediately focus on the most obvious injury. However, the skilled EMT will recognize that unresponsiveness is a sign of the more critical injury.

Head injuries can be one of the most deceptive and subtle injuries the EMT will come across. The EMT must understand the levels of consciousness and be able to detect even the slightest changes. Detection of small changes early can prevent progress to major neurologic impairment later. This is the most important assessment skill for the detection of head injuries. In the continuum of patient care, the time that the EMT spends with the patient may be the least amount of time that anyone in the health care chain spends with the patient; however, this time may be the most critical for assessment of LOC. It is not uncommon for the the patient to be completely alert and oriented when the EMT arrives on scene, but by the time the ambulance reaches the hospital the patient is unresponsive to painful stimuli or has had several seizures en route. It is at these times that the emergency department (ED) physician may question the EMT's ability to assess appropriately; therefore it is extremely important to be able to recognize and document even the slightest change of LOC.

This chapter discusses the anatomy of the head; the physiology of the head as it pertains to the EMT assessment and the ability to recognize even the early changes in LOC; and assessment and management of head injuries.

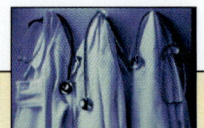 Physician Notes

Much of the material in this chapter is not in the National Standard Curriculum. However, an understanding of the complexities of the brain provides a strong foundation for the EMT-B to expand his or her knowledge and improve patient care.

Anatomy of the Head

The head houses one of the most important organs of the body—the brain. The brain is susceptible to traumatic in-

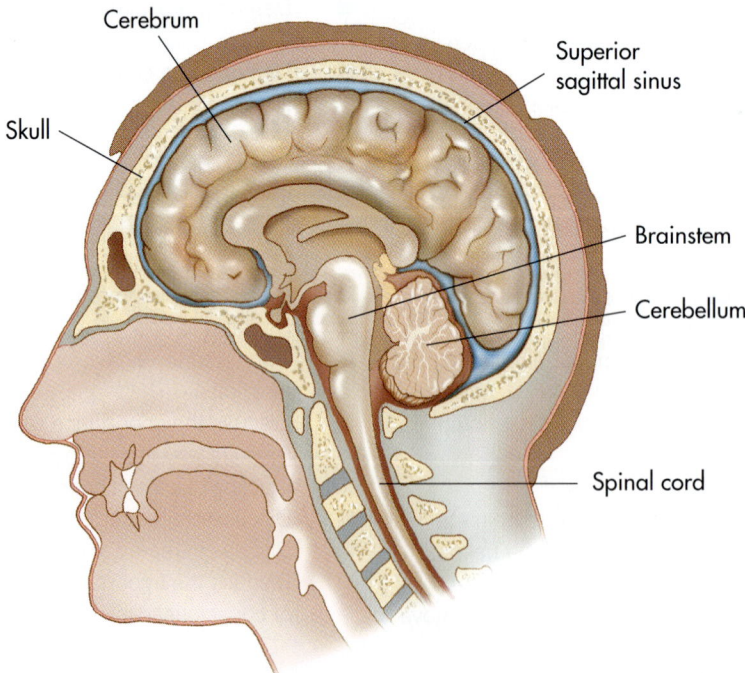

FIGURE 24.1 The head is susceptible to traumatic injury because the skull is its only protection.

jury because it is soft and easily damaged. The brain has only the cranium (skull) and its fluid suspension to shield it from outside forces (Figure 24.1).

Scalp

The scalp is the outermost part of the head and contains numerous tissues, including the hair follicles, the sweat glands, the sebaceous glands, and a great number of blood vessels and capillaries. Because the scalp is highly vascular, it tends to lose more blood and at a faster rate than other portions of the skin and fatty tissue and therefore bleeds more freely. This bleeding can be difficult to control. Usually, however, direct pressure and patience can manage scalp bleeding.

Bones

The cranium is essentially a closed box that houses and protects the brain tissue. It comprises eight cranial bones: frontal, occipital, sphenoid, ethmoid, and two temporal and two parietal bones (Figure 24.2). These bones are joined by immobile interlocking joints called **sutures**. The large opening located at the base of the skull is the **foramen magnum**, through which the brainstem and the spinal cord pass (Figure 24.3).

If the skull is damaged, the brain tissue beneath may also be injured. The ethmoid bone and parts of the temporal bones are much thinner than the rest of the skull and are more easily fractured or penetrated. Injuries to these areas can be serious.

Meninges

Three highly vascular membranes separate the cranium and the brain: the **dura mater** (tough mother), the **arachnoid membrane** (spider membrane), and the **pia mater** (small mother); collectively these membranes are known as the **meninges**. The dura mater is a tough, thick, fibrous tissue. Its name, *tough mother*, describes its structure well. Located between the dura mater and the skull is a "potential space" called the **epidural space**. It is a potential space because although normally the layers are separated, they are flush against each other, separated by only a thin layer of fluid. If blood or other fluid accumulates in this potential space, it becomes an actual filled area (Figure 24.4). When this occurs it can become a mass pressing on the brain.

Hematoma is a condition in which blood leaks into the epidural space. Examples are epidural hematoma and subdural hematoma (Figure 24.5). An **epidural hematoma** is a condition in which blood leaks into the epidural space. This blood usually originates from the meningeal arteries

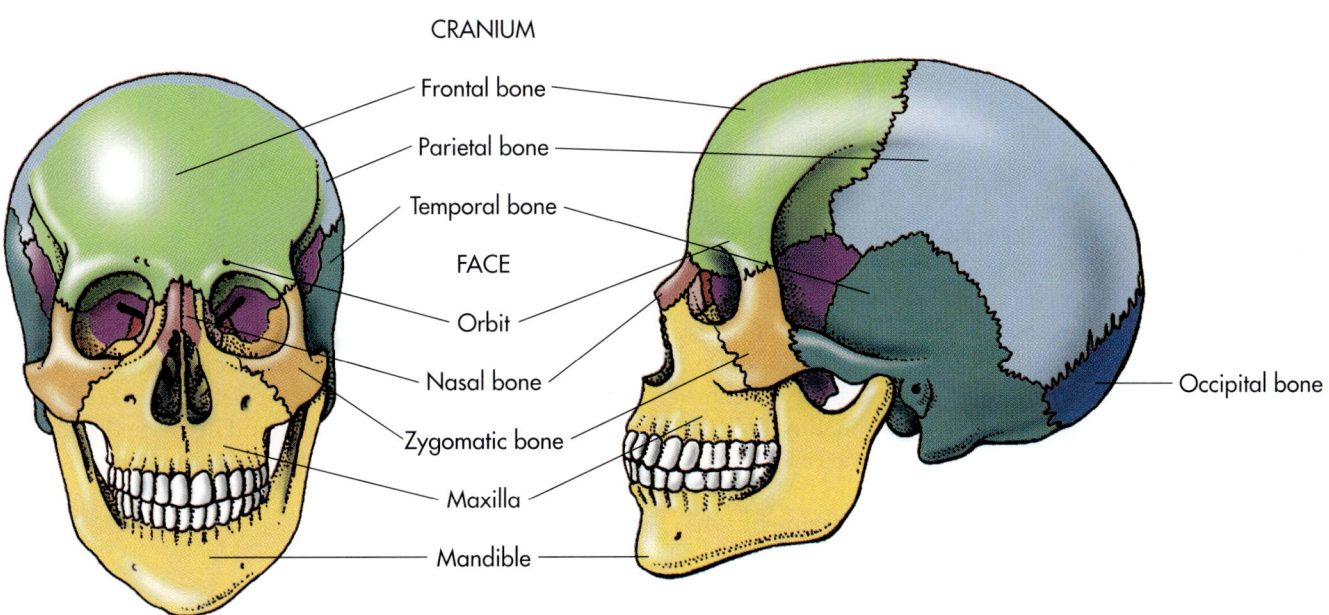

FIGURE 24.2 The brain is encased within the bones of the cranium.

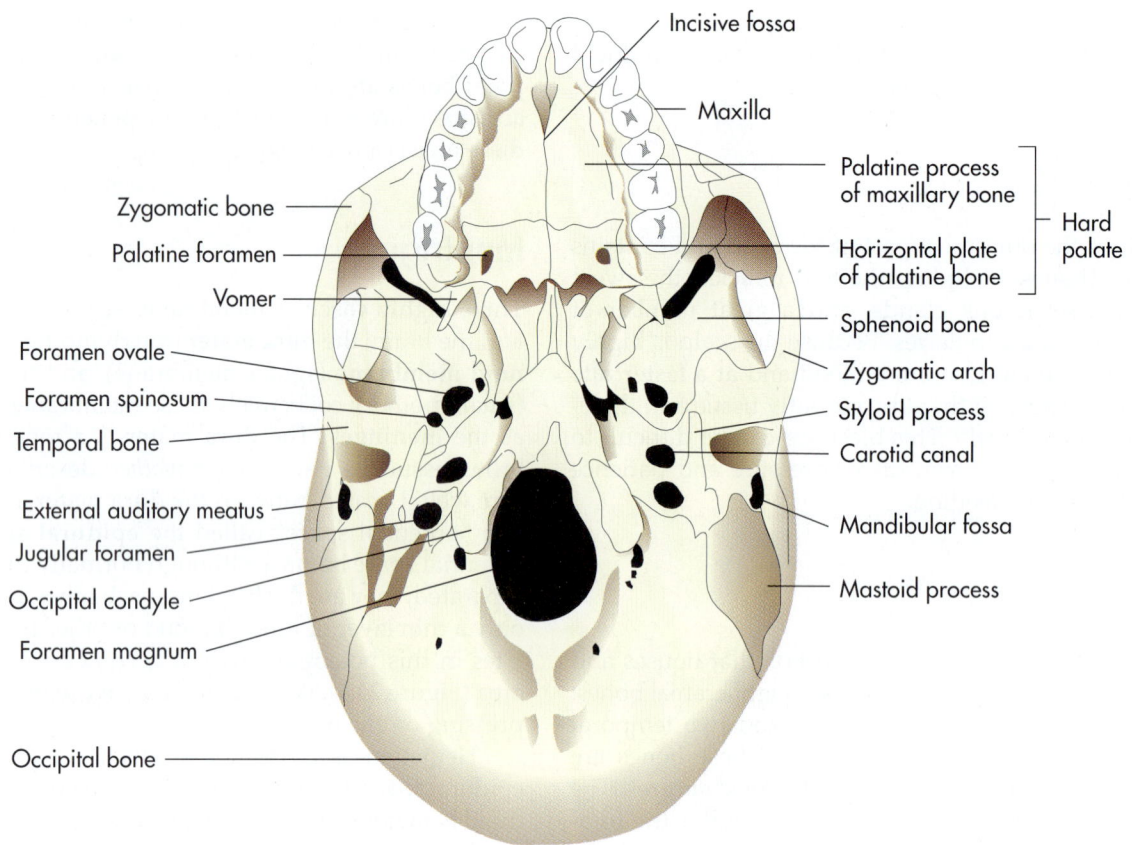

FIGURE 24.3 The large opening at the base of the skull is the foramen magnum, through which the brainstem and the spinal cord pass.

that lie under the cranium. Epidural hematomas usually are caused by low-impact head trauma, such as injury by a baseball bat or from a fall. These hematomas usually involve arterial bleeding, but signs and symptoms may not manifest for several hours.

The patient is awake without symptoms. Blood accumulates in the epidural space. As the volume of blood grows, the expansion squeezes out the liquid components that make up the intracerebral area. **Cerebrospinal fluid** (CSF) is forced out first, and expanding pressure then begins to encroach on the vascular space through which blood flows. Therefore the volume of blood flow is reduced. When this pressure has reduced the volume of the capillaries to the point that oxygen delivery is compromised, anaerobic metabolism occurs in the affected brain cells and the patient loses consciousness. This phenomenon is called the Monro-Kellie doctrine and applies to any closed space and the associated compartment syndrome (Figure 24.6).

The arachnoid membrane is the second membrane. It is named for its spider-like (arachnoid) interlacing fibers. It is transparent and can look like a loosely woven piece of linen.

Another potential space is between the dura mater and the arachnoid membrane. Accumulation of blood in this space is called a **subdural hematoma**. Subdural hematomas are usually caused by traumatic injury and involve venous bleeding. Because the bleeding is venous in nature, it takes more time for the blood to accumulate; therefore signs and symptoms may not manifest for several hours or days after the incident. The survival rate is worse with a subdural hematoma than with an epidural hematoma. This is mainly due to the higher frequency of brain substance trauma with a subdural injury.

The innermost layer of the meninges is the pia mater. Another potential space exists between the pia mater and the arachnoid membrane, appropriately termed the *subarachnoid space*. CSF should be found in this space. In general this type of hematoma is caused by an aneurysm and not trauma.

Brain

The brain is housed within the **cranial cavity** and is divided into the **cerebrum**, **cerebellum**, and **brainstem**.

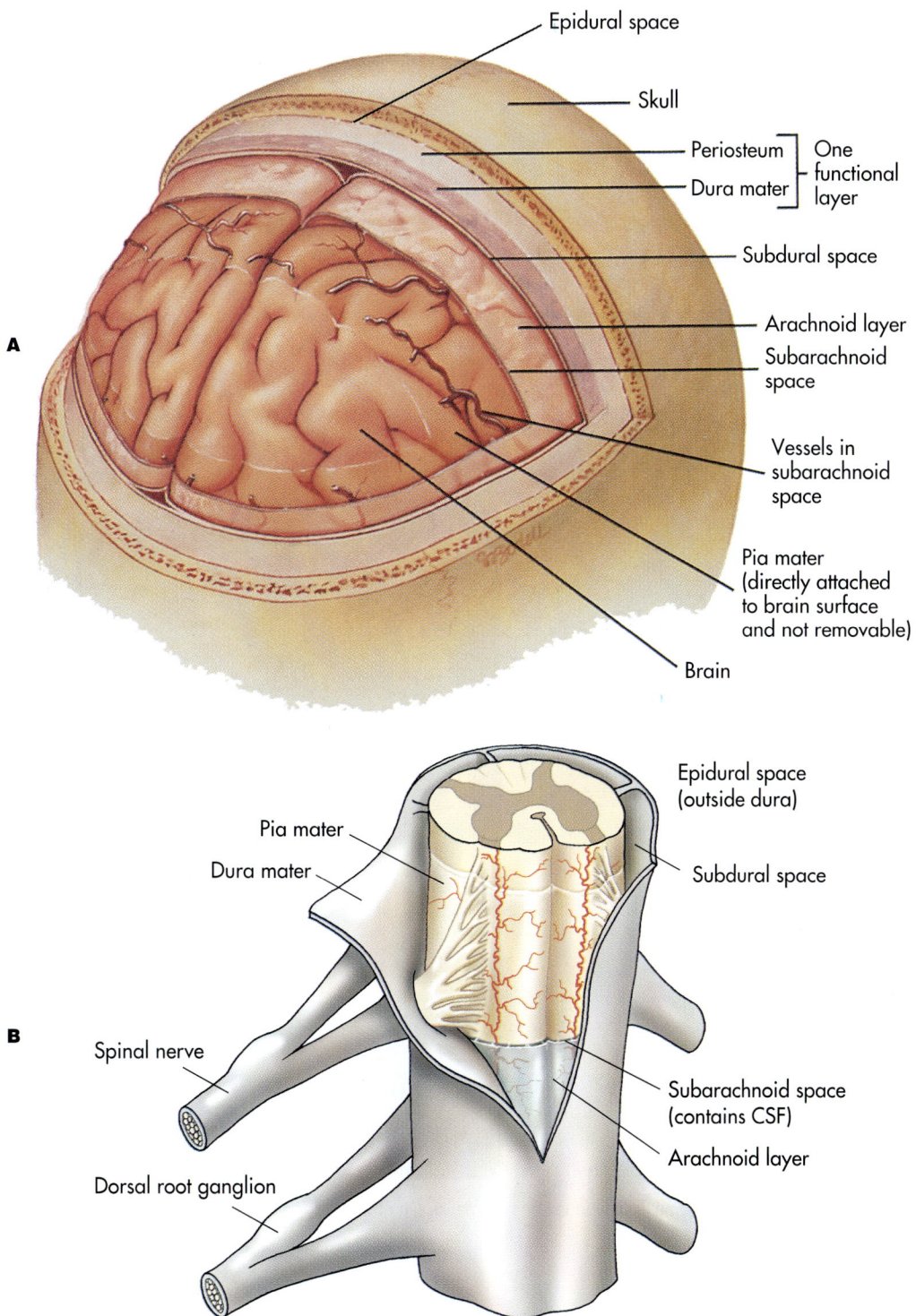

FIGURE 24.4 **A,** Meningeal coverings of the brain. **B,** Meningeal coverings of the spinal cord.

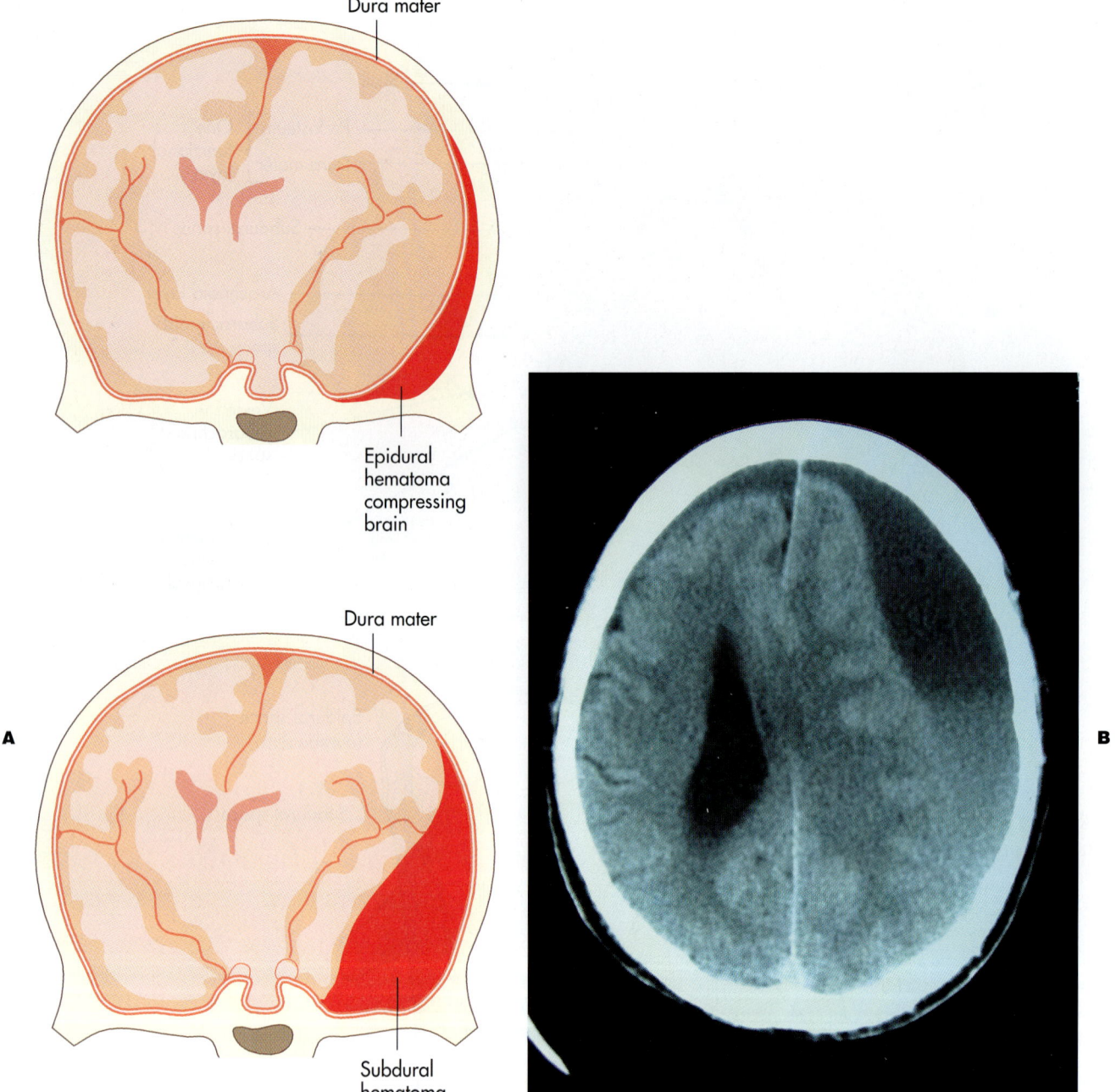

FIGURE 24.5 **A,** Epidural hematoma and subdural hematoma. **B,** Computed tomography (CT) scan of a subdural hematoma.

The cerebrum is divided into the right and left hemispheres. Each hemisphere is further separated into several lobes, each of which has a unique responsibility in the control of specific intellectual, sensory, or motor functions (Figure 24.7).

The cerebellum is located beneath the cerebrum and also surrounds the brainstem. This section of the brain coordinates movement. The brainstem is responsible for responsiveness. The medulla is located in the brainstem and is responsible for vital functions of the body, such as heart rate, respiratory rate, and blood pressure.

Cerebrospinal fluid is produced in the brain and is found within the subarachnoid space. CSF surrounds the brain and acts as a shock absorber, and the brain literally floats within the CSF. Because the dura holds the CSF inside of the skull, damage to the dura can cause CSF to leak to the outside (open head injury). Bacteria can enter the brain through this defect, leading to infection.

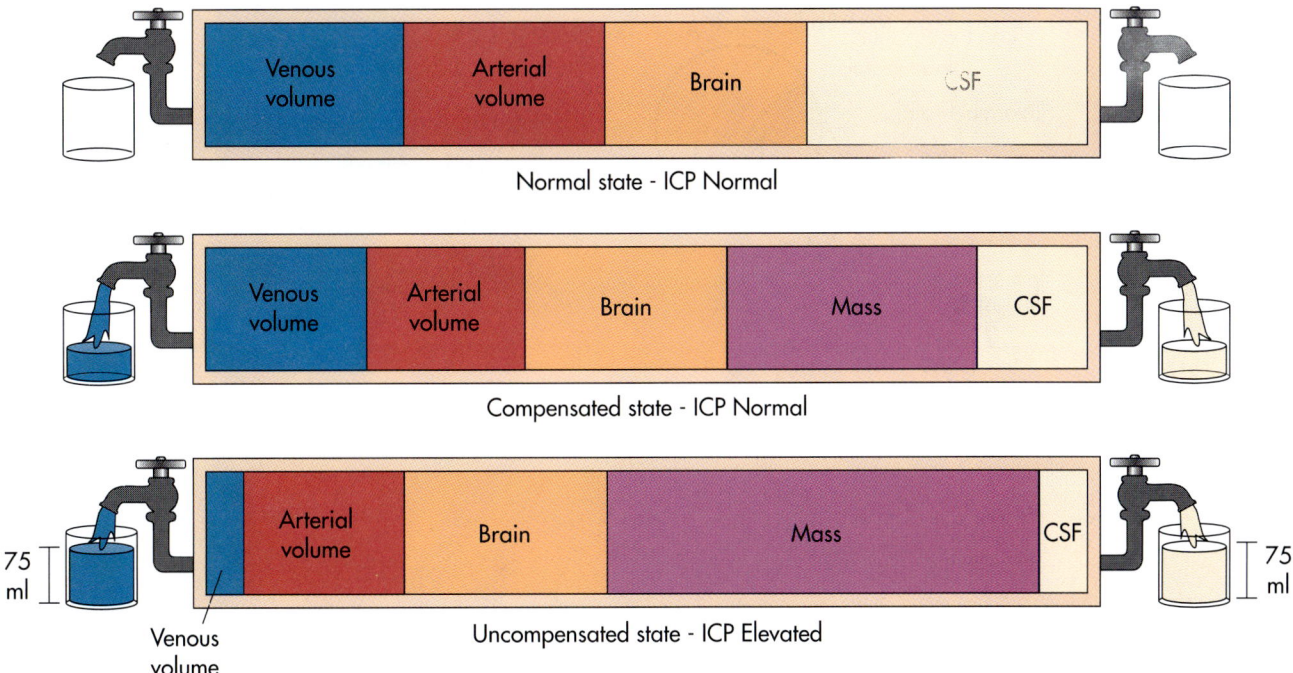

FIGURE 24.6 Monro-Kellie doctrine: intracranial compensation for expanding mass. The volume of the intracranial contents remains constant. If the addition of a mass such as hematoma results in the squeezing out of an equal volume of cerebrospinal fluid and venous blood, the intracranial pressure remains normal. However, when this compensatory mechanism is exhausted, there is an exponential increase in intracranial pressure for even a small additional increase in the volume of the hematoma.

> ✓ The brain is protected by the skull (cranium). The skull is made up of eight bones, which are interlocked by sutures. The scalp covers the cranium, which is extremely vascular. The brain is covered by the meninges, which act as a protectant. Between these membranes is a potential space where blood can accumulate and create pressure on the brain.

Pathophysiology of the Head

The head is divided into three areas, each of which responds differently to trauma. These areas are the scalp, the skull, and the brain. Their anatomic features were previously noted.

Scalp

Hemorrhage and hematomas are the most common prehospital considerations associated with scalp injuries. The head is one of the most vascular areas of the body. Forty percent of the heat loss from the body is from the head and neck, indicating the vastness of the capillary system in this area. Even small injuries to the scalp tend to bleed more than in other areas. Tourniquets are contraindicated,

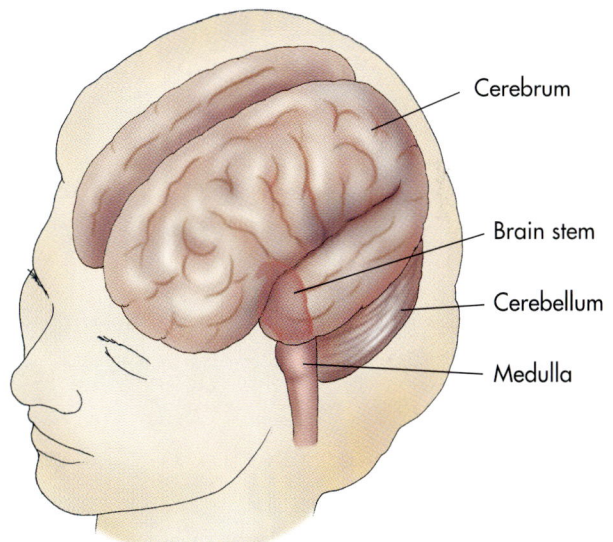

FIGURE 24.7 The major portions of the brain are the cerebrum, cerebellum, and brainstem.

and compression bandages must be used with caution. If the skull is fractured, too much pressure on the injury will transfer this pressure to the brain, further complicating the brain injury beneath it. Additionally, pressure that prevents the escape of blood but is not enough to actually

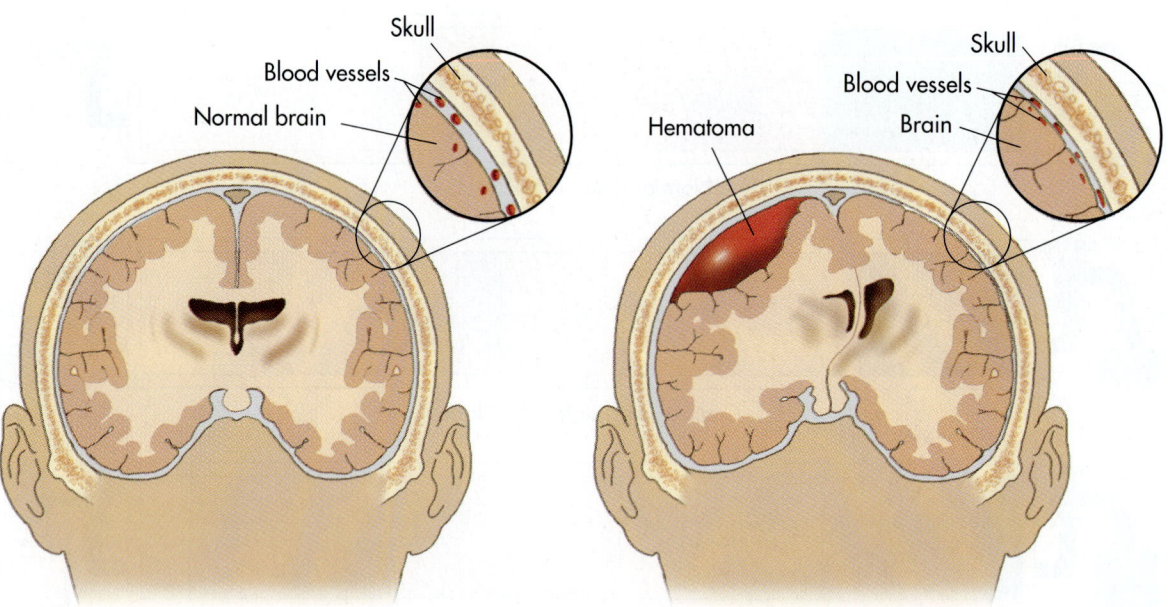

FIGURE 24.8 Subdural hematoma produces pressure on the brain and squeezes vessels into a much smaller size.

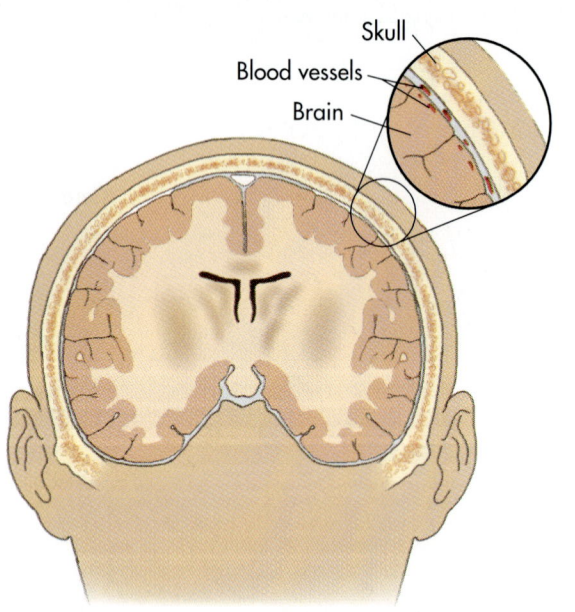

FIGURE 24.9 Swollen brain (edema) squeezes vessels into a much smaller size.

stop it will produce the same effect as bleeding into the intact skull. It then becomes an expanding intracranial mass. The balancing act that the EMT must accomplish is enough pressure to control the hemorrhage but not enough pressure to further injure the brain.

Brain

The parts of the brain subject to injury are the dura, arachnoid vessels, brain tissue itself, and blood vessels that are located inside the brain.

Increased Intracranial Pressure

Increased intracranial pressure comes from two sources: space-occupying or mass lesions, such as a blood clot or tumor, and increased fluid accumulation in and around the brain cells. This increased fluid within the cells is a result of the cellular response to ischemia or accumulation of fluid in the interstitial space.

Space-occupying lesions. If blood vessels inside of the dura in the arachnoid area are torn, bleeding occurs into the closed space of the skull, beneath the dura (subdural) or beneath the arachnoid membrane (subarachnoid). Accumulation of blood in either of these areas compresses the brain directly and occupies some or all of the volume used by the CSF and blood. This can lead to generalized increase in the **intracranial pressure** (ICP).

Brain edema. When injured, the cells of the brain swell (**brain edema**). Two types of damage cause this swelling: direct trauma (compression) of the brain cells themselves at the time of the injury and anoxia from lack of perfusion with oxygenated red blood cells. These changes are not unlike the reaction of other cells in the body to the same kind of injury. The difference, however, is that brain cells

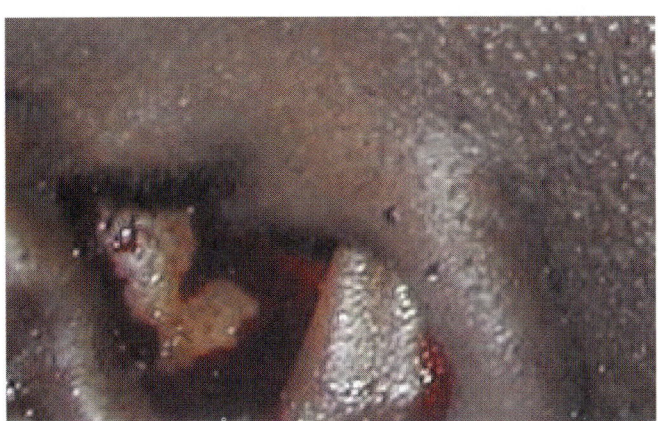

FIGURE 24.10 Blood leaking from the ears.

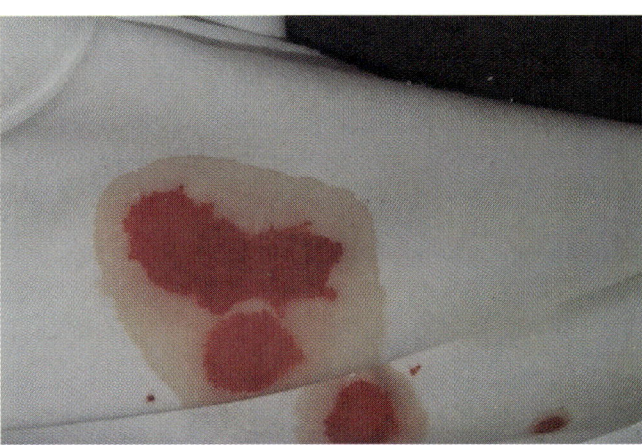

FIGURE 24.11 Halo sign.

are enclosed in a tight box, the skull, and the cells can only expand so far until they meet with resistance.

When the cells swell, they need room to expand. Swollen cells expand into three places: (1) into the space around the cell itself, thus causing the lumen of the blood vessels to be compromised and blood to be unable to supply the brain cells with oxygen; (2) out of the cranium into the spinal cord through the foramen magnum; and (3) out of an open fracture of the skull.

Figures 24.8 and 24.9 demonstrate what happens when the brain swells or hemorrhage occurs into this closed space. Both situations have the same result. The lumen of the blood vessels are reduced. This diminishes the blood flow to the brain cells, and ischemic injury to the brain develops.

The blood flow to the brain is determined by the following formula: blood flow is equal to the systemic blood pressure minus the intracranial pressure. Although the EMT has no method of measuring intracranial pressure, the relationship is important.

Cerebrospinal Fluid Leakage

Blood or fluid leaking from the ears or nose after a suspected head injury indicates an open fracture (Figure 24.10). This produces complications of hospital management such as infection of the brain. It is important to note if the liquid is simply blood or if it has CSF mixed in with it. CSF is usually associated with blood. This can be the result of hemorrhage from the brain itself that is mixed with CSF or CSF leakage with brain injury and injury to nearby structures, such as muscle, bone, or nasal mucosa. Blood leaks out of the nose or ears if the bones are damaged at the base of the skull, cribiform plate, or temporal bones. Blood leaks from one of these areas when the skin is intact and the blood has no other outlet. This phenomenon can be illustrated by placing one box inside another box. The outside box contains cherry Kool-Aid (blood vessels), and the inside box contains clear water (brain floating in CSF). If a hole is punched in the outside box, but not the inside box, only the cherry Kool-Aid escapes (hemorrhage). The box with water is still intact. This example illustrates what happens when only the skin around the nose or in the ear canal or mucous membrane of the nose or mouth is injured. No hole is punched in the dura and therefore no CSF leaks, only blood. If the cribiform plate or the temporal bones are fractured and this fracture tears the dura, a hole is torn in both boxes. The cherry Kool-Aid mixes with the water in the inside box. This mixture leaks from the outside box. Because the two fluids are mixed, the liquid appears much like pure blood.

> **Tips from the Pros**
>
> Frequently there will be drainage from the nose or ear onto the sheet. If the blood appears to be surrounded by a halo or the spot looks like a target, this indicates that the two fluids separated on the sheet. The outer ring of clear, yellowish fluid is CSF. The blood is at the center of the CSF ring (Figure 24.11). This can be also be determined by placing a drop of the blood onto a 4 × 4 gauze pad or paper towel, filter paper, bedsheet, or other similar substance. Fold the absorbent material in half, and then fold it in half again. Dip the corner in the blood. The two fluids will separate on the paper. The outer ring of clear yellowish fluid is CSF. If blood is present, it will be at the center of the CSF ring. This procedure is termed *targeting*.

Intracranial Hematoma

Hemorrhage into the closed space of the cranial cavity increases the pressure in this area. Refer again to the boxes.

The inside box is filled with water, the outside box with cherry Kool-Aid. The inside box, however, is made of flexible plastic and the outside box is made of metal. If more cherry Kool-Aid is added to the outside box (hemorrhage), the pressure exerted on the inside box increases. The water is contained in a smaller space. The increased pressure is caused from a hematoma forming between the brain and the skull (subdural hematoma). The problem is that the outer shell of the skull is very hard and does not stretch as the pressure increases. Therefore the pressure is transmitted inward.

The same increased pressure can result from adding more fluid to the inside box (edema). Increased water pressure in the inside box results in increased pressure throughout both boxes. When either of these situations occurs, CSF is pushed out of the intracranial space into the spinal canal. The blood vessel size is reduced, and this decrease, in turn, reduces the blood volume within the skull. Poor blood flow, poor cerebral oxygenation, and increased anaerobic metabolism are the end results of increased ICP. Cellular anoxia produces more edema, which increases the pressure in the closed box, which compresses the capillaries and other vessels more, increasing the anoxia, increasing the pressure, over and over again as the cycle repeats itself.

The brain detects the decrease in oxygenation and signals the cardiovascular system to increase the blood pressure. It also signals the respiratory system to increase the breathing effort. These responses increase the blood flow to the brain and decrease the amount of carbon dioxide in the blood. When ICP increases, the vagus nerve (one of the cranial nerves) is stimulated and reduces the pulse rate. These signs are known as **Cushing's triad**, an increase in blood pressure, change in respiratory effort, and decrease in pulse. All are classic, but late, signs of a head injury. It is the body's attempt to compensate for the brain's lack of oxygen, not unlike other types of shock.

Intracranial Edema

As the brain swelling worsens without treatment, there is an associated increase in pressure and damage to the brain, leading to an increase in severity of the signs and symptoms. This begins a vicious cycle. As the pressure increases, less blood can flow through the reduced size of the lumen of the vessels, especially the capillaries, because the pressure inside the capillaries is the lowest of the entire system. Reduced blood flow reduces the oxygenation of the brain cells. These cells swell more, producing more intracranial pressure, reducing the blood flow more, producing more ischemia, increasing the swelling, reducing the flow, and so on until the brain is dead. This is termed a *compartment syndrome.*

As the pressure is increased, more pressure is transmitted to the cerebellum and the brainstem. Other signs indicating increased ICP are changes in pupillary size, equality, and reaction. As the hemorrhage or edema affects more and more of the brainstem, the reactions of the pupils are slower because of the increased pressure on the optic nerve.

It is extremely important to document such changes on the patient care report, both in the narrative format and as part of the trauma score (defined later in this chapter). Not only will this documentation track the patient's progress, it will also show the patient's prognosis. As damage continues into lower areas of the brainstem, chances for survival decrease.

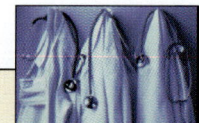

Physician Notes

Compartment syndrome can occur in any closed compartment such as the skull, abdomen, pericardium, chest cavity, kidneys, and muscles of the leg or arm. The term *compartment syndrome* has in the past usually referred to the process that occurs because of anoxia or bleeding in the muscles of the lower leg. However, because it is the same process in other compartments, the term is now commonly used to describe increased pressure producing vessel compression and ischemia in those compartments as well. For example, the term *abdominal compartment syndrome* refers to increased intraabdominal pressure that requires release by opening the abdomen and covering the defect, which cannot be closed by the swollen small and large bowel.

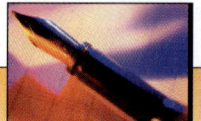

Tips from the Pros

Unequal pupils may be normal for some patients. If the patient is awake and unequal pupils are noted, ask the patient if his or her pupils are normally unequal. Unequal pupils can be the result of previous trauma, cataracts, or some other cause.

✓ Hemorrhage is the most common complication of scalp injuries. The EMT must be careful to assess the scalp completely for injuries. CSF leakage indicates an open head injury, and this can be a life-threatening injury. CSF usually is mixed with blood and therefore can be difficult to assess. Intracranial hematomas and cerebral edema produce pressure to the brain. With closed head injuries, obvious signs of trauma may be absent or late. Signs and symptoms of increased ICP include increase in blood pressure, decrease in pulse, change in respiratory pattern, pupillary change, and change in mental status.

The presence or absence of lacerations in the scalp overlying a fracture determines the classification of open or closed head injury. To be an open head injury, the injury must extend down through the skull (fracture).

An **open head injury** (an injury in which the skin is broken, bone is fractured, and the brain has access to the outside air) can have three complications that are not associated with a **closed head injury** (an injury in which the skin is not open and the skull is not broken):

1. *Leakage of CSF outside of the body.* CSF is produced inside the brain; however, much like a hemorrhage, the leakage must be controlled. This leakage is difficult to control if integrity of the brain is lost, because unlike blood, CSF does not have clotting factors.
2. *Possible bacterial contamination of the brain from the outside.* As with all trauma, one of the main complications after the first 24 hours is infection. This complication is not one that is identified prehospital, but it should always be in the back of a skilled EMT's mind, because prehospital contamination of the wound may be the source of the infection.
3. *Herniation of the brain through the defect in the skull and skin.* Brain tissue swelling through an open area of the scalp and skull is not an encouraging sign (Figure 24.12). This herniation indicates that the swelling (pressure) is so overwhelming that the body is not able to compensate. The main difficulties with this type of herniation are hemorrhage, infection, and loss of consciousness.

Skull

As previously mentioned, the skull is a composite of eight bones, most of which are flat. Some bones are thick, whereas others are very thin. Three major complications are associated with fractures of the skull:

1. *Injury to the brain beneath the fracture (lacerations or compression).* The bone ends may have lacerated the brain tissue; a foreign object or an outside force has compressed the brain tissue; or the brain is being compressed from the inside because of increased ICP.
2. *Hemorrhage from the open ends of the bone.* Hemorrhage from lacerations to the brain and meninges can result from bone ends.
3. *Leakage of CSF to the outside of the body, if the fracture is open.* Loss of CSF is more difficult to control because of the lack of clotting factors.

Any part of a fractured skull that is open to the outside can also be associated with a CSF leak. The two most difficult fractures to treat are the cribriform plate in the bottom of the nasal cavity and the temporal bone in the

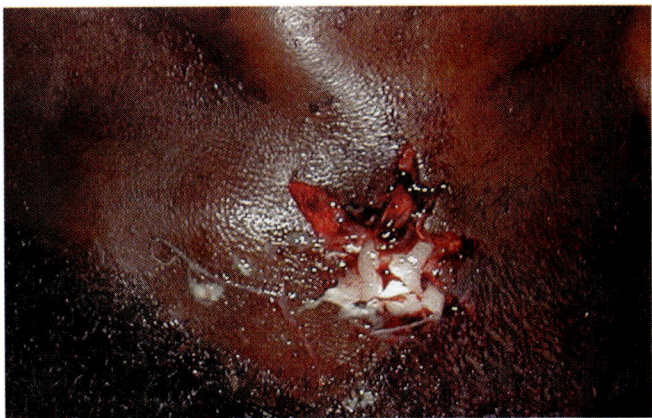

FIGURE 24.12 Brain tissue visible through an open area of the scalp and skull. This is a bad sign.

external ear canal. These fractures are difficult to treat because of their location and complex nature, which make it hard to reach them and control bleeding.

Assessment of Head Injuries

Head trauma is the leading cause of blunt trauma deaths, and the majority of these injuries result from motor vehicle crashes. In most of these situations, the patient is either unresponsive or combative and anxious, resulting from hypoxia, brain injury, or an overdose of alcohol or drugs, or any combination of these causes. In either instance the patient is not helpful in providing information about the mechanism of injury. A skilled EMT properly uses bystanders as a source of information, as well as the evidence on the scene. The EMT must quickly and thoroughly investigate the scene as a priority in patient care. For example, the EMT must look at the vehicle, examine entrance and exit wounds, determine length of fall, or note damage of the assault weapon, all in a matter of seconds. The physician has no eyes and ears at the scene other than those of the EMT. All this information is critical for the physician to know. The EMT should do a complete and thorough observation of the scene and relay this to the physician on arrival at the ED.

Scalp

Injuries to the scalp frequently bleed heavily, due to the large number and volume of vessels in the head and neck (Figure 24.13). This can lead to difficulty in hemorrhage control. Even small lacerations that require only a few sutures may bleed vigorously. Thus the EMT can be confronted with a gross hemorrhage that he or she will not

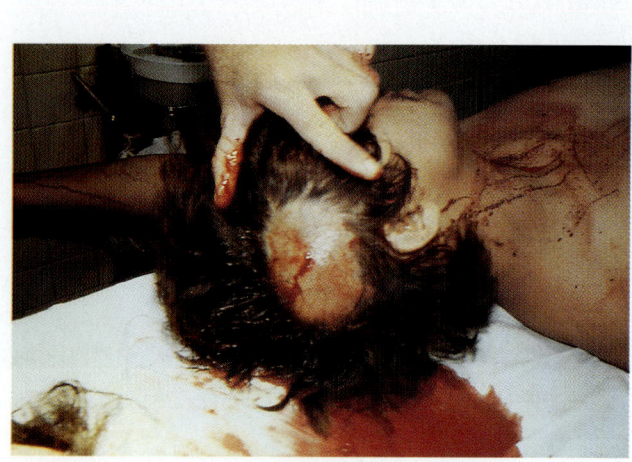

FIGURE 24.13 The vascularity of the scalp produces more blood loss than other areas of the body.

be able to treat any further than to control the bleeding. As in any hemorrhage, the first step is to attempt hemorrhage control with direct pressure. Pressure should be applied over a wide area to compress the vessels in the bleeding area, being careful not to compress the brain if the skull is fractured. Once bandages are in place; simply position more bandages on top of blood-soaked gauze. Do not remove those already soaked with blood. The gauze helps the body's own clotting process by providing a matrix on which the clot can form. If the clot is removed with the gauze, the body must start the whole process again.

The EMT should note whether the blood appears to be arterial (bright red) or venous (darker red). He or she should report this to the medical personnel in the ED.

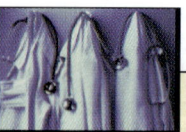

Physician Notes

Elevation of the backboard to 30 degrees (head up) has been advocated to reduce the venous pressure in the scalp and brain, reducing the bleeding of the scalp and assisting in the reduction of the ICP. Many neurosurgeons use this technique; however, others do not, believing that while accomplishing these goals, it also reduces the blood flow to the brain and is of greater harm than benefit. Studies are unclear, and further research is required. Use of this technique must be tempered by the presence of hypotension and other conditions and *must* fit into the protocols used by the neurosurgeons and trauma surgeons in the community where the EMT is working.

Skull

The mechanism of injury provides the EMT with important information as to what injuries to look for (see Chapter 22). The mechanism of injury gives the EMT a starting point and alerts him or her to main areas of concentration during the initial and focused assessments. With any skull injury, it should be assumed that the patient has a spinal injury. Therefore spinal precautions must be taken.

Examine the patient carefully for contusions, lacerations, and hematomas to the scalp; deformity to the skull; blood or fluid leakage from the ears or nose; and bruising around the eyes or behind the ears. Elderly people, in particular, form large hematomas on the scalp. This is due in part to their fragile capillary system and decreased tissue elasticity. They may also be taking medication that affects the clotting system (many elderly persons take nonsteroidal antiinflammatory drugs or aspirin for arthritis or heart conditions). Fragile vessels are easily broken, have little support to contain clots, and have a decreased clotting ability.

Ecchymosis around both eyes is associated with fractures of the base of the skull (**raccoon's eyes**). It is not usually visible on the scene because it develops later, from 6 to 12 hours after the incident.

Periorbital ecchymosis, or "black eye," is caused by blood accumulating in the tissue around the eye. It is caused by local trauma from a blow such as a fist and not a fracture at the base of the skull. This sign may also be seen with direct trauma to the eye (Figure 24.14).

Battle's sign is a discoloration behind the ears (Figure 24.15). Occipital and basilar skull fractures cause this condition. Battle's sign may not develop until 24 to 36 hours after the incident. Therefore if the EMT sees discoloration behind the ears while on scene, it is most probably due to direct trauma to this area and not a basilar skull fracture.

Skull fractures, when not depressed or accompanied by hematomas, brain injury, or leakage of CSF, may not be an immediate danger to the patient. Although this injury may not be life threatening, these patients should be transported to the hospital. Close monitoring is necessary while en route to the hospital. Although many of these patients seem to be uninjured and may want to go home, every effort should be taken to convince them that medical evaluation is important.

Level of Consciousness

Level of consciousness (LOC) is an indirect measurement of cerebral oxygenation. Although other etiologies can produce such a change (brain injury, overdose of alcohol or drugs, and metabolic conditions), the most easily treated and the one that can cause the most immedi-

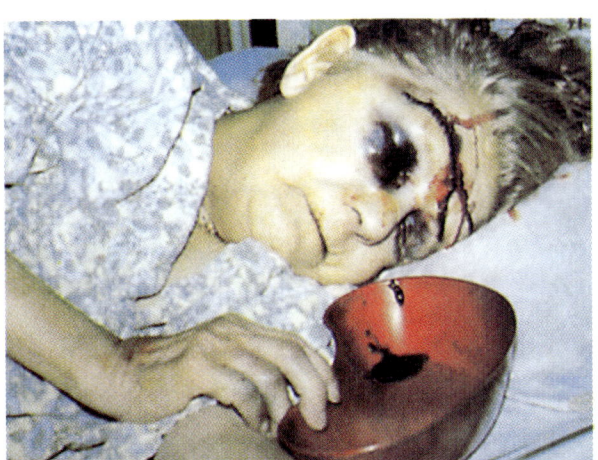

FIGURE 24.14 Bruising around the eyes (raccoon's eyes) is associated with fractures of the base of the skull.

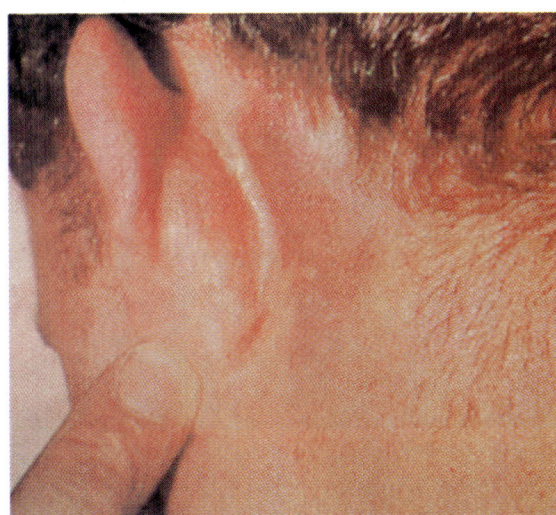

FIGURE 24.15 Battle's sign is a discoloration behind the ear caused by an occipital or basilar skull fracture.

ately life-threatening situation is hypoxia. A number of words commonly used to describe the LOC can be misleading. For example, ask several students to define the terms *semiconscious* and *stuporous*. Most definitions will differ. It is much better to use words that everyone understands; therefore the AVPU system was developed. It is a qualitative rather than quantitative method, but it is helpful until a Glasgow Coma Scale is done. LOC is described by using the acronym AVPU:

A—**A**lert
V—responds to **V**erbal stimuli
P—responds to **P**ainful stimuli
U—**U**nresponsive

The universal definition of being alert is knowing person, place, situation, and time. If a patient knows his name, where he is, what happened, and the date and time, he is considered to be "alert and oriented times four" (A and O × 4). Documentation is an important aspect of the EMT's responsibility. If a patient is A and O × 4, but is slow to respond or appears to be initially confused, this information should be documented. Documentation of LOC on occasion can be difficult and may require a lengthy narrative; detail is extremely useful to the ED personnel. If the patient changes LOC frequently during time on the scene and en route to the hospital, this is important and should be documented correctly and chronologically.

To say a patient is responsive to verbal stimuli means the patient may seem unresponsive or confused, but simply stating the patient's name is enough to arouse or re-orient the patient. Another component to this response is whether the patient is arousable to *tactile* stimulation. Tactile stimulation is different from painful stimulation in that tactile simply means the patient will respond to being touched. Documentation also includes how the patient reacts once aroused. Does the patient moan and groan with no apparent lucid interval, or is the patient A and O × 4? Is the patient awake but confused, and if so, confused to what—place, surroundings, events, time, or a combination of all?

Being responsive to painful stimuli is just that—the patient responds to pain, such as a pinch or sternal rub. The EMT must assess the reaction the patient exhibits to this type of stimulus. Does the patient move the extremities as in withdrawing from pain, localize or move toward the pain as if to stop the stimulation, or fully awaken to be alert and oriented? It is important to document the exact responses to pain.

Unresponsive is no response whatsoever to painful stimulation. When a patient is totally unresponsive, the EMT should look for other signs of head injury, initiate oxygenation as close to an FiO_2 of 1.0 as possible, and transport immediately after immobilization.

Eliciting a response using the AVPU scale is done on an increasing level of stimuli. The EMT must first start with a verbal arousal and then increase in stimulation; do not start immediately with the painful stimulation.

Tips from the Pros

Be careful when eliciting a response from a patient who may be under the influence of drugs or alcohol. These patients tend to be combative when their state of high is compromised. They may try to hurt you or anyone in the area.

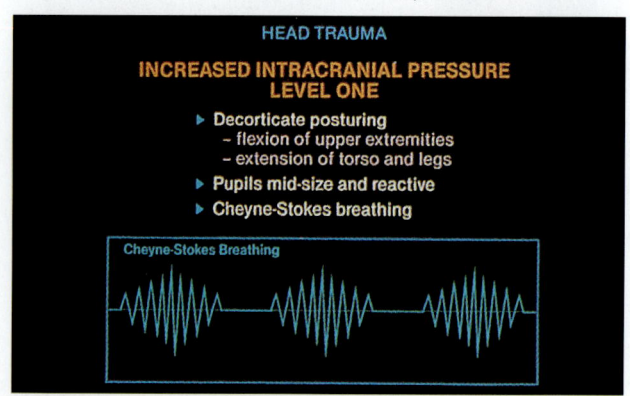

FIGURE 24.16 The pattern of change in breathing (Cheyne-Stokes respiration) is classic and indicates the changing PaO_2 and $PaCO_2$ levels in the patient.

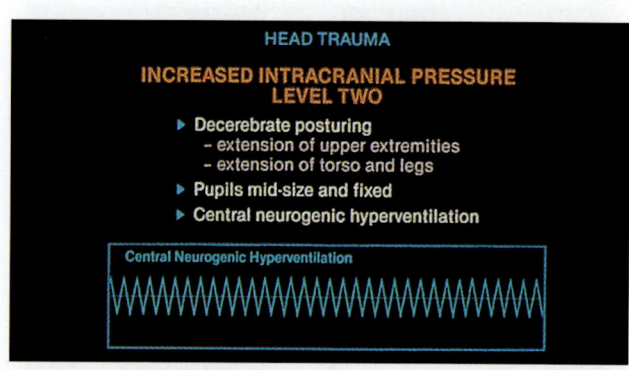

FIGURE 24.17 A fast, shallow respiratory pattern is associated with brainstem involvement and is termed *central neurogenic hyperventilation*.

Pinching the patient before speaking to him or her does not create good rapport.

Glasgow Coma Scale

The **Glasgow Coma Scale** (GCS) is used to determine a patient's LOC by assigning numbers to eye-opening ability, motor response, and verbal response (Table 24.1). This scale is divided into three sections, and the sections are graded individually and then together. This is a much more accurate method of assessing the patient's LOC and carries a more important prognosis.

This scale is to be used in conjunction with, and is a part of, the trauma score. The trauma score and the revised trauma score measure the physiologic response of the patient to the injury. The trauma score is divided into categories, including respiratory rate, respiratory expansion, systolic blood pressure, and capillary refill. The patient is graded by his or her *best* response. Like the GCS, the categories are graded individually and then together. Both the GCS and the trauma score have been used with limited success as a method of triage of patients to be transported to the trauma center. The scales are also used to determine the patient's prognosis.

Pupils

The eyes are actually extensions of the brain to the surface, by way of the optic nerve. As such, the eyes can in many ways reflect the condition of the brain. As an example of this, by examination of the retina using an ophthalmoscope when the patient arrives at the hospital, the physician can see findings that indicate brain swelling and pressure. Pressure that is greater on one side of the brain than the other can be recognized by noting the size and reaction of the pupils on either side. One of the signs of brain death is pupils that are dilated and fixed (do not respond to light). Drug usage can be indicated when the pupils are unusually dilated or constricted.

Because the eyes are a "window to the brain," changes that occur in the eyes are important indicators to the physician. Although the change in size and reaction of the pupils do not alter the field treatment, the change of size and reaction to light from the field to the ED is of tremendous importance and can significantly change the management of the patient in the ED.

Baseline pupil assessment in the field is necessary. Rapidly changing pupil size in the field is one of the signs the EMT should use to indicate rapid transportation to a trauma center.

Other Signs of Head Injuries

Unresponsiveness and altered mental ability are common indicators of head injuries; if no trauma exists, they may be signs of intracranial hemorrhage or stroke. The patient is unresponsive or combative or answers questions inappropriately. This altered LOC may be caused by an increase in cerebral pressure, anoxia, or both. The mechanism and the signs and symptoms indicate that a head injury is present, but no obvious trauma is noted, and the integrity of the skin is not compromised. The mechanism of injury is important to relay to the physician receiving the patient because it may be a major consideration in patient care.

Three levels of signs and symptoms occur as pressure intensifies and lower areas of the brain are involved. Each of these three levels lists characteristic changes in vital signs, pupil reaction, and response to stimuli. In level one, the blood pressure rises, the pulse rate slows, and the

TABLE 24.1 Glasgow Coma Scale

Category	Points
Eye Opening	
Exhibits spontaneous eye opening	4
Exhibits eye opening on command	3
Exhibits eye opening to painful stimulus	2
Exhibits no eye opening	1
Best Motor Response	
Follows command	6
Localizes painful stimuli	5
Exhibits withdrawal to pain	4
Responds with abnormal flexion to pain (decorticate)	3
Responds with abnormal extension to pain (decerebrate)	2
Exhibits no motor response	1
Best Verbal Response	
Answers appropriately (oriented)	5
Gives confused answers	4
Gives inappropriate response	3
Makes unintelligible noises	2
Gives no verbal response	1
	Total

NOTE: Lowest possible score = 3; highest possible score = 15.

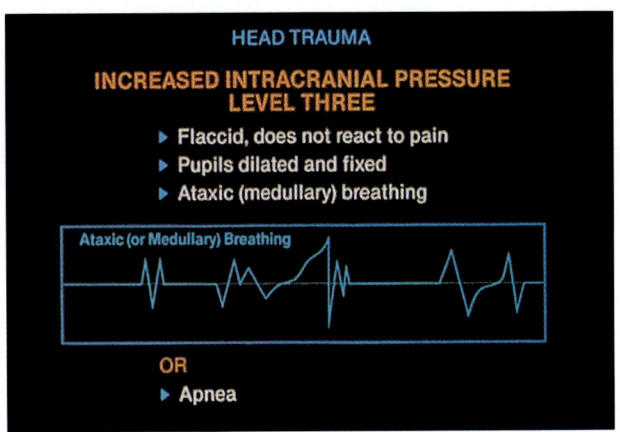

FIGURE 24.18 Medullary-type breathing has no pattern and is highly erratic. Patients commonly become apneic at this stage.

pupils may be constricted but remain reactive. The ventilatory effort is characterized by a condition known as **Cheyne-Stokes breathing**. In this condition, the patient exhibits a breathing pattern that is slow and shallow to rapid, deep ventilation and then back to slow and shallow, with regulary recurring periods of apnea (Figure 24.16).

At this point the patient does not respond to verbal stimuli; however, he or she may initially try to localize and remove painful stimuli. Later, the patient only withdraws from pain and eventually has **decorticate posturing** (flexion of the upper extremities with the lower extremities rigid and extended). This stage is usually reversible with prompt surgical intervention to remove the cause of the increased ICP. Rapid transportation to a trauma center with hyperventilation en route is necessary.

At level two, the blood pressure continues to rise, the pulse becomes slower, and the pupils may become fixed and nonreactive or sluggish in reacting to light. Respiratory effort becomes increasingly difficult, and a pattern of fast, shallow panting will be evident (Figure 24.17). The patient may exhibit a kind of posturing called **decerebrate posturing** (extension of the upper extremities with the lower extremities rigid and extended). These patients will probably not function normally again.

At level three, the patient does not respond to painful stimuli. The patient becomes flaccid, the pulse becomes rapid and irregular, and the blood pressure drops. A "blown" pupil will usually be seen on the same side of the brain as the hematoma or swelling that is causing the symptoms. The pupil that dilates first is a clue as to which side of the brain has the hematoma. Breathing may become erratic or may be absent at this stage (Figure 24.18).

Combinations of these levels may be seen. It is important to recognize and document each change in the patient's condition and relay these change to the attending physician.

> ✓ When a patient is posturing and the patient's arms draw toward the core of the body, the posturing is decorticate.

Open versus Closed Head Injuries

Open head injuries demonstrate the same signs and symptoms as closed head injuries, with the exception of obvious trauma to the head. As with every situation, consider the mechanism of injury. Was the windshield deformed? Is the helmet damaged? Are there other indications of head trauma? Look for contusions, lacerations, and hematomas to the scalp. Pay close attention to the skull. Are there any deformities or depressions? Do not remove impaled objects unless they penetrate the cheek and obstruct the airway. Look for exposed brain tissue if possible. Bleeding is a common occurrence and can be difficult to control because of the increased vasculature of the scalp. Blood or fluid may be leaking from the ears or nose. Bruising around the eyes or behind the ears may indicate further injuries. Increased CSF pressure or simply swallowing blood may cause nausea or vomiting. The EMT must be able to differentiate the reasons a person may exhibit the signs and symptoms of head injuries. Always encourage a patient who is swallowing blood to spit it out and not to swallow it. Blood is irritating to the stomach lining and will cause the patient to vomit. Signs and symptoms of a closed head injury may exist if brain injury has occurred.

Related Medical Conditions

Sometimes the EMT will encounter a patient who has signs and symptoms of head injury without evidence of trauma. These injuries may be the result of clots or hemorrhaging, which can be caused by numerous conditions such as cerebrovascular accident (stroke), subdural and epidural hemorrhage, hypertension (high blood pressure), and any incident that causes an increase in cerebral pressure. Signs and symptoms of medical conditions involving the brain parallel those of traumatic injuries with the exception of evidence of trauma and lack of mechanism of injury. These conditions are just as serious as traumatic head injuries and should be treated with the same urgency. Signs and symptoms usually include headache for a few hours or a few days, confusion, altered mental status, unequal pupils, and posturing. Maintain airway patency, apply oxygen, and monitor for changes in LOC and seizures. Transport immediately.

Management of Head Injuries

As with all patients, body substance isolation precautions must be taken before assessment of the patient (see Chapter 6).

Initial Assessment

While performing the initial assessment, spinal in-line immobilization should be initiated and maintained. With any head injury, the EMT must suspect spinal injury and immobilize the spine. When it has been determined during the initial assessments that the patient has a life-threatening condition, spinal immobilization should be done on the scene with a complete, detailed physical examination performed en route, if possible.

Airway

The EMT must maintain the patient's airway. Mechanical means of maintaining airway may be necessary by means of jaw-thrust, oropharyngeal, or nasopharyngeal airway. Oxygenation is always necessary; 15 L via nonrebreather mask is recommended in cases of emergency. If the patient is unable to breathe, the rest of the assessment is put on hold until the airway can be maintained.

Breathing

If the patient's ventilation rate is below 12 or above 30 breaths per minute, the patient is not oxygenating adequately to supply the body's need for oxygen, or shock exists. Assisted ventilation should be provided for the patient. Lack of oxygen will further exacerbate the problem and thus injury. A ventilation rate between 20 and 30 breaths per minute is borderline and requires at least high FiO_2 if not assisted ventilation as well. In the past, hyperventilation was the standard of care. It has now become controversial as to its true benefit. Adequate oxygenation is one of the most important responsibilities of the EMT. Closely and continually monitor the airway and breathing for deterioration and change. Intervene when necessary.

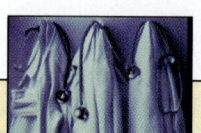

Physician Notes

When the CART race medical team began working and responding rapidly to crashes on the racetrack with well-trained medical personnel, they noted a brief period of apnea or slow, shallow ventilations lasting up to 1 to 2 minutes following head injuries. They found that treating the associated hypoxia with assisted ventilations and high FiO_2 reduced the severe head injury morbidity and mortality rates of the injured drivers.

The important lesson to learn and to use in the field is that all head-injured patients probably have a similar condition in the first 10 to 15 minutes following severe head trauma. Close observation with assisted ventilation using high FiO_2 will work on the street as well as it works on the racetrack to reduce head injury disability and death.

✓ Head trauma is a leading cause of death; therefore assessment of the head must be done quickly and accurately. Because of the heavy vasculature of the head, bleeding can be heavy and can require some time to control. Spinal precautions should be taken for any injury above the clavicle. The Glasgow Coma Scale is used to determine the patient's LOC, and the trauma score is used to determine physiologic response of the patient to the injury. Head injuries can be open or closed with similar signs and symptoms. Medical conditions can also cause increased ICP. These patients are treated with the same precautions, excluding spinal immobilization.

Circulation

Controlling bleeding from the head is essentially the same as with the rest of the body, with one exception: excessive pressure is not applied to an open or depressed skull injury. As mentioned earlier, place dressing to site and exert firm but not too much pressure, because the pressure could do more damage to the structures underneath the visible injury. If necessary, place bulky dressings to site without removing previously applied dressings to absorb and try to control bleeding. In some instances, circulation will be as far as one can proceed in the assessment if the bleeding cannot be controlled. Also remember to look for CSF mixed in with the blood. Dress and bandage open wounds as indicated in the management of soft tissue injuries (see Chapter 23).

> ✓ Be prepared for and anticipate changes in these patients. Document appropriately. Be able to recognize life-threatening injuries, and transport the patient immediately.

Ongoing Assessment

Perform the ongoing assessment as you would for any other patient. Remember to check the patient's back as he or she is rolled onto the backboard. This may be your only opportunity to check this region for injuries. Document thoroughly. This documentation may be lengthy and require a considerable amount of time and thought, but the continuum of care requires it.

> ✓ Assessment of airway, breathing, and circulation (ABCs) in a head-injured patient is done while maintaining in-line immobilization. Oxygen must be initiated, with or without ventilatory support. Bleeding must be controlled and ongoing assessment performed.

Summary

- The cranium is a closed box that houses and protects the brain tissue. It is composed of eight bones: frontal, occipital, sphenoid, ethmoid, two parietal, and two temporal bones.
- Three highly vascular membranes cover the brain: dura mater, arachnoid membrane, and pia mater. A potential space is located between each of these membranes in which hematomas can form.
- The brain is divided into the cerebrum, cerebellum, and brainstem. CSF is produced in the brain and is found within the subarachnoid space. CSF surrounds the brain and acts a shock absorber.
- Accumulation of blood in any of the potential spaces causes compression of the brain directly and a generalized increased intracranial pressure.
- Brain edema is the expansion of brain cells due to traumatic injury or a medical condition. Swollen cells expand into three places: the blood vessels surrounding them, out of the cranium into the spinal cord through the foramen magnum, and out of an open fracture of the skull. All of the edema results in decreased cerebral perfusion and thus decrease in oxygenation of the brain cells.
- CSF leakage can be life threatening.
- Cushing's triad is a sign of increased ICP and is characterized as an increase in systolic blood pressure, a decrease in pulse, and changes in respiratory patterns. Changes in mental status and pupillary changes are also signs of increased ICP.
- The mechanism of injury is extremely important when assessing a head-injured patient.
- Level of consciousness is described by using the acronym AVPU: alert, verbal, painful, and unresponsive.
- Closed head injuries are so called because the brain is injured inside the skull, but the injury does not compromise the integrity of the skin. Open head injuries are injuries in which the integrity of the skin is broken.
- Signs and symptoms of medical conditions involving the brain parallel those of traumatic injuries, with the exception of evidence of trauma and lack of mechanism of injury. These patients usually have headache or seizures. Medical conditions are just as serious as traumatic head injuries and should be treated with the same urgency.
- Management of head injuries begins with ABCs and spinal immobilization (until mechanism of injury can rule out spinal involvement). Perform focused assessment as you would for any other patient.

Scenario Solution

As you arrive on scene you must start looking for mechanisms of injury—for example, how far is the indentation of the hood, is there a bull's eye fracture to the windshield, damage to the interior of the car, damage to the tree, and other persons involved (if any)? You can see that there is a 2-foot indentation to the hood and a bull's-eye to the windshield. Thoughts should also enter your mind about LOC and orientation. Mr. Scott tells you that he is all right, but your assessment should not stop there. He is complaining of a headache, does not remember if he had his seatbelt on, and seems a little slow to respond. His vital signs are OK, and he is stating that he does not want to go to the hospital.

One of the most important things you were told about this man has not yet been mentioned. What is it? His wife tells you that he "seems OK, but something is not right." That statement alone tells you that this patient needs to be transported to and evaluated at a medical facility. Never underestimate the perceptiveness of family and friends. Mrs. Scott may not be able to tell you what is wrong with Mr. Scott, but if she says there is something not right, there is something not right, and he should be evaluated further. It may only be that he is shaken up from the MVC, but that is not your decision to make. Every effort should be made to get Mr. Scott to the hospital. He should be placed on a spine board with cervical spine precautions taken, and his LOC should be constantly assessed for changes.

Key Terms

Arachnoid membrane Second membrane of the meninges; a transparent, spider-like membrane interlaced with fibers.

Battle's sign Discoloration behind the ears, found in basilar or skull fractures; develops 24 to 36 hours after injury.

Brain edema Swelling of the brain.

Brainstem Portion of the brain responsible for consciousness; contains the medulla oblongata, the pons, and the mesencephalon.

Cerebellum Portion of the brain located beneath the cerebrum and surrounding the brainstem; coordinates movement.

Cerebrospinal fluid Fluid that circulates around the brain and spinal cord; acts as a cushion to protect the brain, allowing the brain to literally float; also helps remove by-products of brain metabolism.

Cerebrum Portion of the brain divided into left and right hemispheres, and further divided into several lobes, each of which has a unique responsibility in the control of specific intellectual, sensory, or motor functions.

Cheyne-Stokes breathing Specific type of breathing pattern characterized by a period of slow and shallow breathing, followed by a period of deep ventilation, and then back to slow, shallow breathing, with regular periods of apnea.

Closed head injury Injury to the skull or brain in which the integrity of the skin has not been compromised.

Cranial cavity Bony structure that houses the brain.

Cushing's triad Phenomenon seen with increased cranial pressure, distinguished by a rise in blood pressure, change in respirations, and decrease in pulse.

Decerebrate posturing Extension of the upper extremities with the lower extremities rigid and extended.

Decorticate posturing Flexion of the upper extremities with the lower extremities rigid and extended.

Dura mater Outermost layer of the meninges.

Epidural hematoma A condition in which blood leaks into the epidural space.

Epidural space A potential space located between the skull and the dura mater.

Foramen magnum The opening at the base of the skull.

Glasgow Coma Scale Standardized rating system used to evaluate the degree of consciousness impairment based on eye opening, motor response, and verbal response. Points are scored for the patient's best response in each of the three categories, and then added for a total score.

Intracranial pressure The pressure that builds up inside the cranial cavity due to fluid accumulation.

Level of consciousness This is an indirect evaluation of the cerebral oxygenation, brain injury, and alcohol/drug intoxication. (NOTE: The acronym LOC is frequently misused to mean "loss of consciousness." As you use the term, use it correctly; however, you must recognize what someone means when he or she uses it incorrectly.)

Key Terms (cont'd)

Meninges The three highly vascular membranes that separate the cranium from the brain; includes dura mater, arachnoid membrane, and pia mater.
Open head injury Injury to the skull or brain in which the integrity of the skin has been interrupted.
Pia mater Innermost layer of the meninges.

Raccoon's eyes Bruising around the eyes associated with fractures of the base of the skull; develops 6 to 12 hours after injury.
Subdural hematoma An accumulation of blood in the subdural space.
Sutures Immobile interlocking joints that connect the cranial bones.

Review Questions

1. The general function of the cranium is to
    a. Protect the brain from injury
    b. Keep the brain warm
    c. Protect the brain from swelling
    d. Reduce the need for motorcycle helmets
2. Understanding the mechanism of injury allows the EMT-B to
    a. Predict the movement of the brain inside the skull
    b. Clear patients with potential head injures in the field
    c. Provide better testimony for the plaintiff in court
    d. Reassure the patient that no injury is present so that the patient does not have to be transported
3. Which of the following are meninges?
    a. Dura mater
    b. Plasta mater
    c. Spider mater
    d. Pia mater
4. Which of the following are signs and symptoms of a subdural hematoma?
    a. Reduced level of consciousness
    b. Hypotension and tachycardia
    c. Unequal pupils
    d. Paraplegia
5. Where is CSF produced?
    a. Spinal cord
    b. Subarachnoid space
    c. Dura mater
    d. Cerebellum
6. What does the halo sign indicate?
    a. Hemorrhage into the brain
    b. Contusion of the brain
    c. Impending death
    d. CSF leak to the outside
7. Why is the scalp more prone to blood loss?
    a. Heat produced by the brain
    b. Vascularity of the scalp
    c. Torn easily in trauma
    d. Nearness to the carotid artery
8. What is the correct procedure for trying to control blood loss of an open head injury that is bright red in color?
    a. Firm pressure
    b. Light fluffy dressing on the wound
    c. Carotid pressure point on the side of the hemorrhage
    d. Pneumatic antishock garment

Answers to these Review Questions can be found at the end of the book on page 866.

25

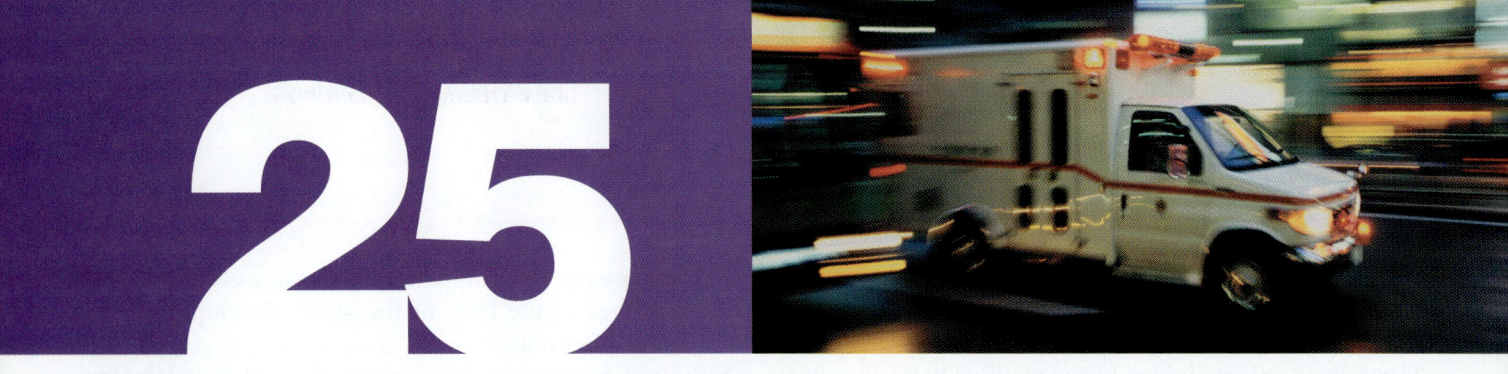

Chest Trauma

Lesson Goal

At the completion of this chapter the student will understand the basic physiology of chest disease and how this physiology is adversely influenced by trauma. The student will also understand the steps to take to manage that trauma situation and the reasons for delivery of such a patient to a properly staffed and equipped hospital (trauma center).

Scenario

Dispatch sends you and your partner to a collision involving at least three people. On arrival at the scene you find two vehicles involved in a classic T-bone intersectional collision, one vehicle with a side impact on the driver side, the other vehicle with a frontal impact. You note that the deformation in the passenger compartment of the side-impact collision is approximately 15 inches and the deformation of the frontal-impact vehicle is approximately 20 inches. Both sides of the windshield of the vehicles with the frontal impact have bull's-eye fractures. There was no air bag deployment in either vehicle (none may have been present). There are two occupants in the frontal-impact vehicle and one occupant in the lateral-impact vehicle when you arrive. The occupant of the lateral-impact vehicle was wearing a seatbelt. No one in the frontal-impact vehicle was wearing a seatbelt.

The driver of the vehicle with lateral impact is angrily screaming at the occupants of the other vehicle, both of whom, to your experienced eye, seem to have the potential of more significant injuries. The vehicle with side impact has the driver-side door crushed and significant deformation of the B-pillar. As the senior emergency medical technician (EMT) on the unit, you assign your partner to the vehicle with one occupant; you take the frontal-impact vehicle with two occupants. Neither the driver nor the occupant of the vehicle you approach is restrained, and the vehicle is not equipped with air bags. There is deformity of the steering wheel on the driver's side and a bull's-eye fracture of the windshield on the passenger side. The driver tells you that the stupid so-and-so driving the other car tried to run a yellow light and pulled out in front of him. He tells you that he is sore from hitting the steering wheel, but he is otherwise okay. The passenger tells you that she is okay but that her head hurts. You notice several lacerations on her forehead with moderate hemorrhage down the side of her face.

You note that the driver's ventilatory rate is fast, but he is exchanging air and talking. A quick pulse check indicates a rapid but palpable pulse at the radial artery, and there is no obvious external hemorrhage. Your partner hollers across from the other car that this patient is complaining of pain in his right side near where the seatbelt attaches. You can tell that he has an open airway from his loud voice screaming at the other driver. He is also complaining of neck pain.

? What are the kinematics of this incident? What injuries do you suspect on each of the occupants? What would be your steps of management?

476

Key Terms to Know

Alveolar/capillary membrane
Alveoli
Atelectasis
Contusion
Diaphragm
Hemothorax
Hypopharynx
Hypoxia
Intercostal muscles
Intrathoracic pressure
Midclavicular line
Open pneumothorax
Oropharynx
Oxygenation
Paradoxic motion
Pneumothorax
Sternum
Tension pneumothorax
Ventilation

Learning Objectives

As an EMT-Basic, you should be able to do the following:

DOT

- Demonstrate the steps in the emergency medical care of a patient with an open chest wound.

Supplemental

- Describe the physiology associated with breathing.
- Describe the anatomy of the chest cavity.
- Describe the relationship of the anatomy of the chest cavity to the ventilatory process.
- Describe why ventilation (breathing) is not respiration.
- Describe the adverse outcome of pulmonary contusion, pneumothorax, hemothorax, and flail chest.
- Describe pneumothorax (simple and tension), hemothorax, flail chest, fractured ribs, and sources of blood contributing to the hemothorax.
- Describe shear injury to the aorta.
- Describe pulmonary contusion.
- Describe the breathing process.
- Describe the prehospital assessment and management of chest injuries.
- Describe the trauma center and the benefit of taking patients to a properly staffed and equipped hospital for the management of these injuries.

The major cause of death following blunt trauma is head injury. The second cause of death following blunt trauma is injury to or malfunction of the ventilatory system. However, death secondary to head injuries may more often be due to airway malfunction secondary to cerebral malfunction than to the brain injury itself. Therefore injuries to that component of the physiology of respiration as it pertains to **ventilation** and **oxygenation** should be the number-one priority in the field regardless of the level of training that has been obtained by the prehospital provider. The lessons learned in this chapter and the airway chapter will be used more often by the emergency medical technician (EMT) than any other lifesaving skill. If applied correctly, this skill and knowledge will contribute to more lives saved than any other skill that the EMT has. Airway techniques are covered in Chapters 10 and 11, and it will be assumed that the student is extremely knowledgeable and will become skilled in those techniques; therefore they are not included in this chapter. This chapter discusses the anatomy of the thorax and the physiology of ventilation.

Anatomy

The thorax is a bony cage that can expand and contract. This enlarging and compressing is achieved by 12 pairs of ribs. The **intercostal muscles** are arranged in a crisscross fashion that spreads the ribs apart then pulls them back together. Assisting in this in-and-out motion that enlarges and reduces the volume of the thoracic cavity is the diaphragm. The **diaphragm** is a muscle 5 mm in thickness that separates the abdominal and thoracic cavities. In its relaxed state it is a dome rising as high as a straight line drawn between the forth intercostal space anteriorly, the sixth intercostal space laterally, and the eighth intercostal space posteriorly. When the muscle contracts, it shortens and flattens, with the top almost reaching the lower end of the **sternum.** The ribs are attached to the

Patient Care Algorithm

Trauma Patient Airway Breathing Assessment

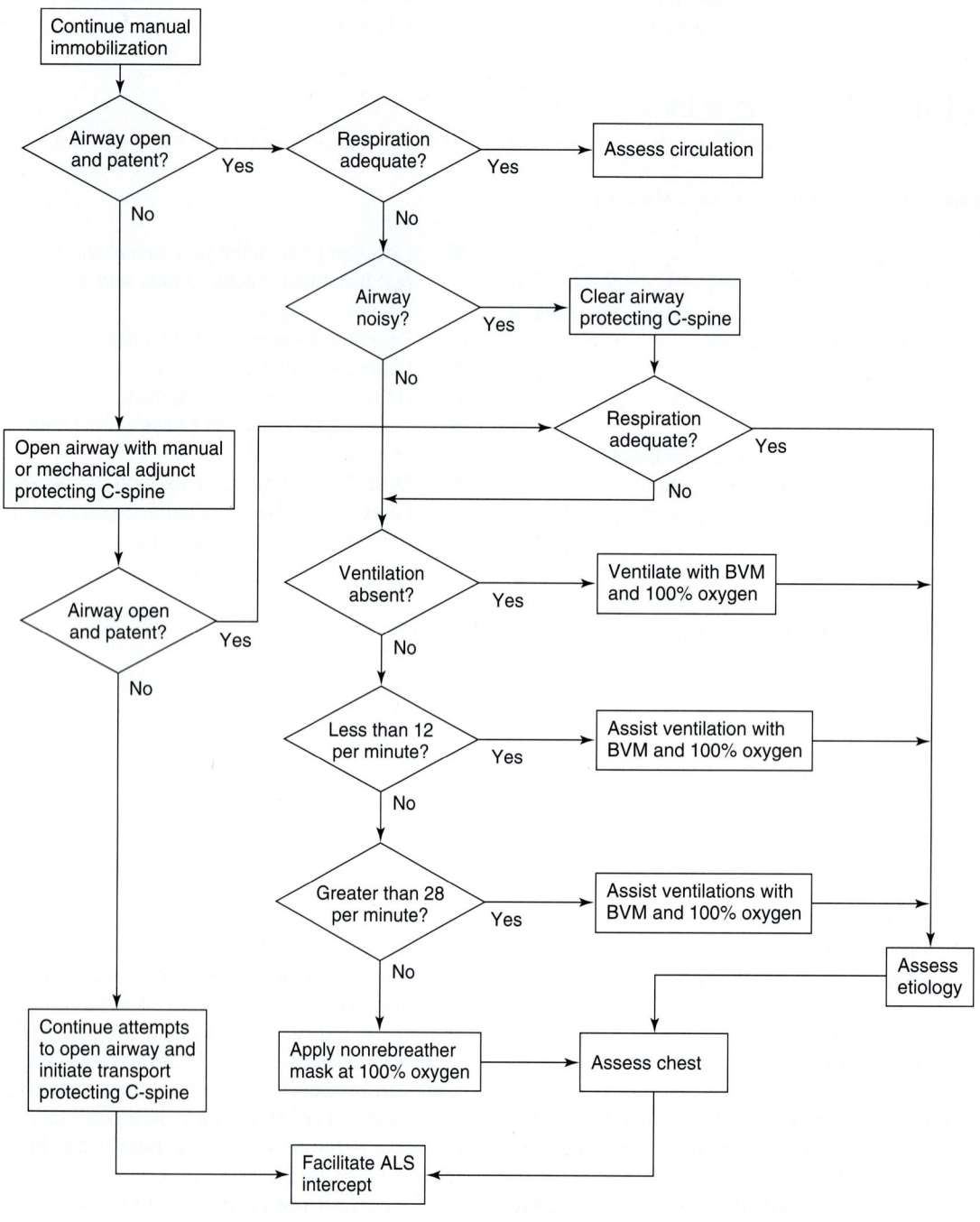

Patient Care Algorithm

Chest Wall Assessment and Management

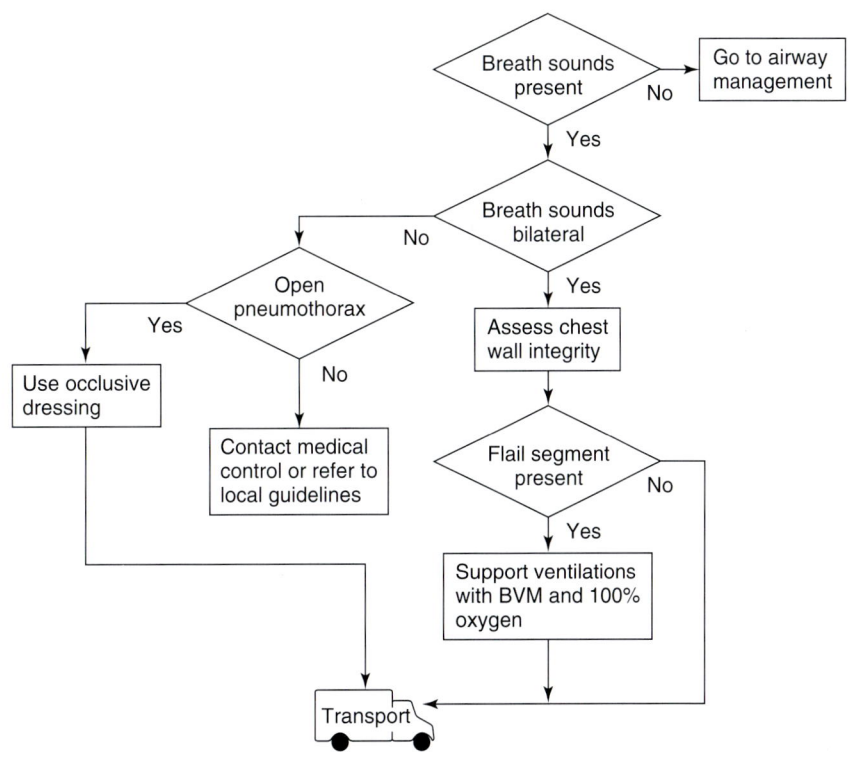

individual vertebrae posteriorly, and the upper sixth attaches directly to the sternum in front. The seventh through the tenth ribs attach to the sternum together as a single cartilage, with the twelfth and sometimes the eleventh rib unattached (Figure 25.1).

The cross section of the ribs and interspace reveals a notch in the inner, lower aspect of each rib that contains the intercostal artery, nerve, and vein. The muscle crisscrosses between the ribs in two layers, one from front to back, the other from back to front.

The lungs consist of a multitude of extremely small air sacks, which connect to tubes; these tubes connect to other tubes, gradually enlarging to come together at the center of the chest, forming one large tube, the trachea, which connects through the larynx to the **hypopharynx,** nasal pharynx, and **oropharynx** (Figure 25.2). This airway's passage is well described in the airway chapter and will not be repeated here.

Blood leaves the right side of the heart through two pulmonary arteries, one to the left and one to the right. These divide and redivide until each capillary is in close contact with each of the alveolar sacks. The exchange of oxygen and carbon dioxide occurs across the **alveolar/capillary membrane** (Figure 25.3). The capillaries merge to form larger and larger vessels, eventually forming the left and right pulmonary veins, which deliver oxygenated blood into the left atrium so that the left ventricle can pump it throughout the body.

The heart lies directly between the lungs and is connected to the systemic circulation by the inferior vena cava and the superior vena cava, which bring blood into the right side of the heart. The aorta exits the top of the heart and arches posteriorly along the spine, giving off the arteries to the head and arms (subclavian and carotid) before traveling down the spine into the abdominal cavity (Figure 25.4). It enters the abdomen through a hole in the diaphragm through which both the aorta and the esophagus pass. Along its pathway the descending thoracic aorta gives off branches of intercostal arteries that supply nutrients to the intercostal muscles and to the spinal cord itself.

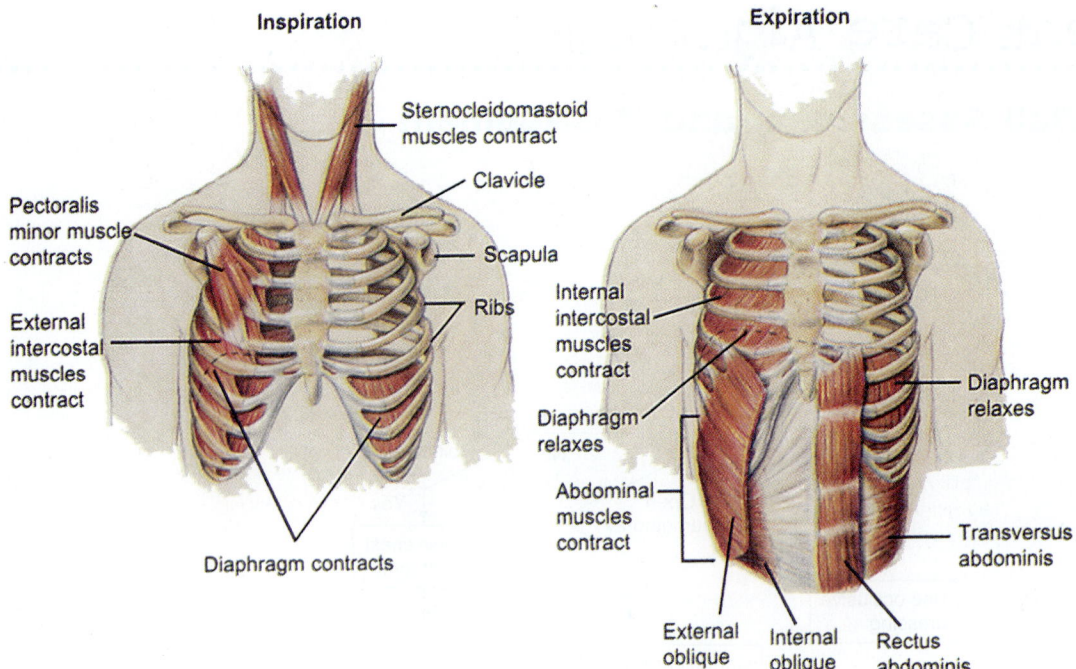

FIGURE 25.1 During inspiration, the diaphragm contracts and flattens. Muscles of inspiration, such as the external intercostal, pectoralis minor, and sternocleidomastoid muscles, lift the ribs and sternum, which increases the diameter and volume of the thoracic cavity. In expiration during quiet breathing, the elasticity of the thoracic cavity causes the diaphragm and ribs to assume their resting positions, which decreases the volume of the thoracic cavity. In expiration during labored breathing, muscles of expiration such as the internal intercostal and abdominal muscles contract, causing the volume of the thoracic cavity to decrease more rapidly.

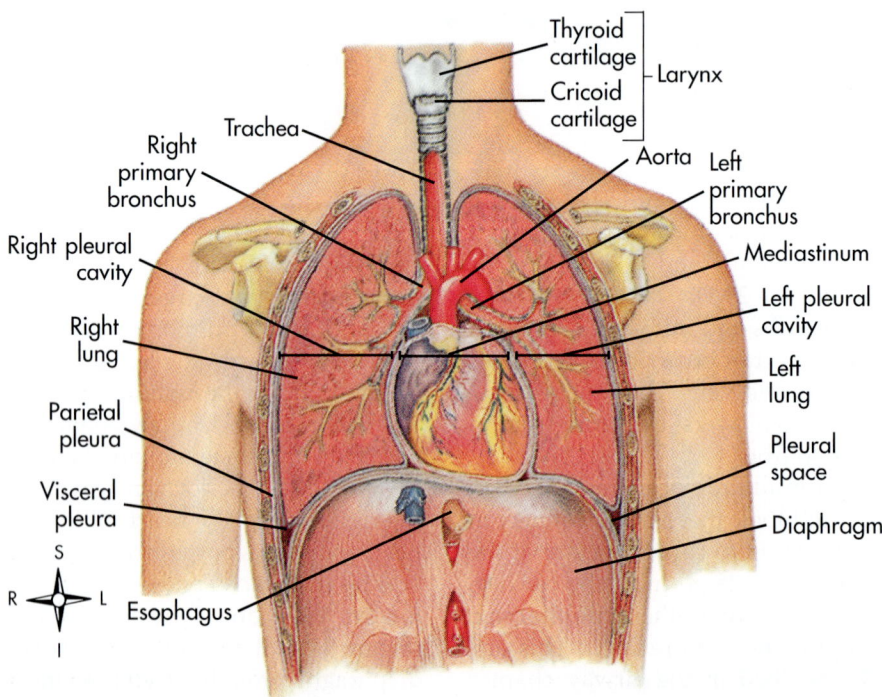

FIGURE 25.2 The thoracic cavity, including ribs, intercostal muscles, diaphragm, mediastinum, lungs, heart, great vessels, bronchi, trachea, and esophagus.

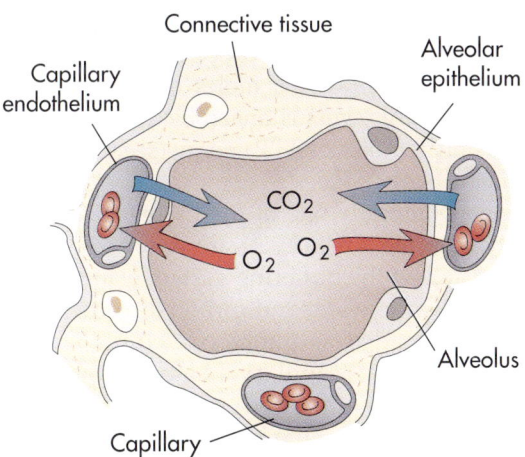

FIGURE 25.3 The capillaries and alveoli lie in close proximity; therefore oxygen can easily diffuse through the capillary, the alveolar walls, the capillary walls, and the red blood cells. Carbon dioxide diffuses back from the plasma to the alveoli.

The thoracic part of the gastrointestinal tract is connected to the lower gastrointestinal tract through a single tube that traverses the thoracic cavity from the hypopharynx to the abdomen. The esophagus lies behind the trachea and above the aorta.

Just as occurs in the abdominal cavity, the organs and the walls are lined with a thin, liquid-secreting membrane. In the abdomen, this membrane is termed the *serosa*; in the chest, it is termed the *pleura*. In both cavities it performs the same function of allowing free movement of the organs and the wall of the cavity in relationship with each other. The potential space between these two membranes in the thoracic cavity is termed the *pleural space*.

The heart is not located in the pleural cavity; it has its own separate cavity within the mediastinum. The sac that surrounds the heart is termed the *pericardial sac*. It, too, is lined with a liquid-secreting membrane; the heart itself does not attach, but has the freedom of movement inside this sac. The walls of the pericardial sac are thick and fibrous; they do not stretch acutely, but can stretch with increased pressure over a period of time.

The heart and the arch of the aorta have no true firm attachments to the supporting framework of the body. The heart is supported in the center of the chest by the pericardial sac. The arch of the aorta is outside of this sac and is freely movable. The descending aorta becomes tightly attached to the vertebral bodies as the arch ends. The shear forces of acceleration and deceleration affect the aorta in three places: (1) at the junction of the aorta and the heart as the aorta leaves the pericardial sac, (2) at the junction between the arch and descending aorta as the movable arch becomes firmly attached to the vertebral bodies, and (3) as the aorta courses through the diaphragm into the abdominal cavity. Shear injuries most

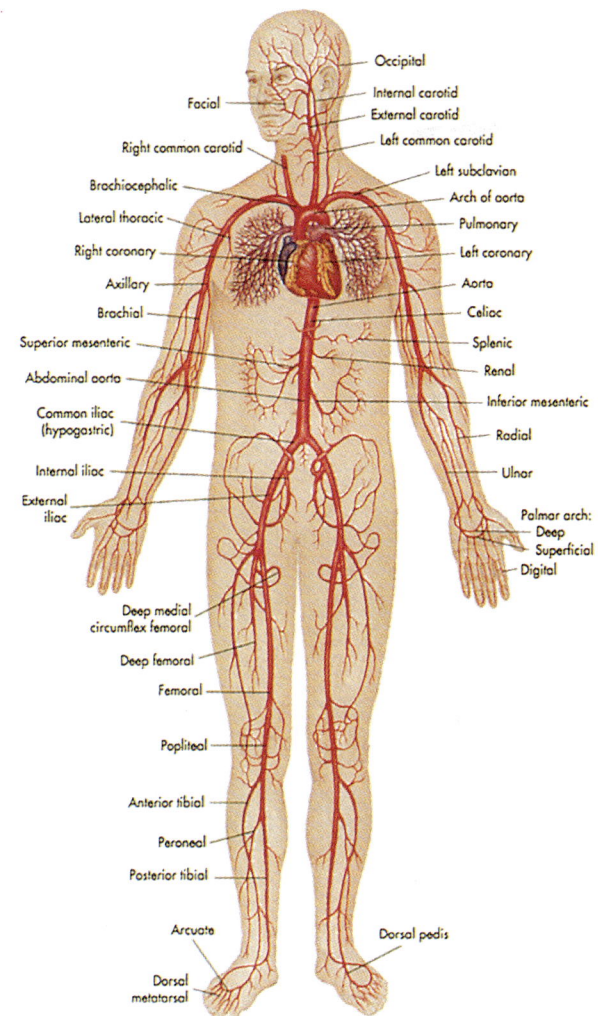

FIGURE 25.4 Principal arteries of the body.

commonly occur as the movable aortic sac joins the fixed descending aorta. More than 90% of blunt aortic injuries occur at this junction (Figure 25.5).

An understanding of the relationships between the lung and pleura and between the heart and pericardium is critical in the understanding of one of the more severe types of pathophysiology that affects the lung and one of the more severe types of traumatic pathophysiology that affects the heart.

Physiology

The contraction of the muscles of the diaphragm shorten the muscles to make them much more flat than in their relaxed dome state. This, along with the contraction of one half of the intercostal muscles that spread the ribs, significantly enlarges the thoracic cavity. The **intrathoracic pressure** then becomes less than the environmental

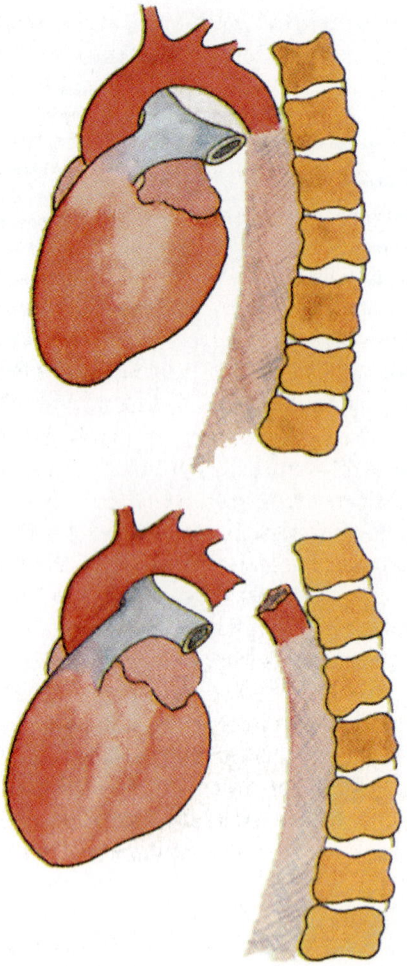

FIGURE 25.5 The descending aorta is tightly affixed to the thoracic vertebrae. The arch of the aorta and the heart are not attached to the vertebrae. Disruption from shear force usually occurs at the junction of the arch and the descending aorta.

into the cell. Respiration is carried on by oxygen and glucose entering into a multistep process called the *Krebs cycle*. This operation produces 36 moles of adenosine triphosphate (ATP) energy, versus anaerobic metabolism, which produces only 2 moles of ATP energy (see Chapter 9). This energy is the basis of life.

The acids that are one of the by-products of cellular metabolism in the Krebs cycle are returned to the blood and converted by the buffering system using agents such as bicarbonate into water and carbon dioxide. The carbon dioxide is off-loaded as the blood returns to the lungs through the alveolar/capillary membrane into the alveolar sac and then out of the body with exhalation. Some of the water is excreted by the kidneys in the form of urine.

The often-used term *respiratory rate* is a misnomer because the ventilation of the lungs and the movement of air in and out is only part of the respiratory process, as noted previously. The rate of chest motion to create this air movement is driven by a multitude of factors, most of which cannot be measured by the EMT. It is far more attuned to the metabolic process and metabolic rate. The inhalation and exhalation process is critically important in the evaluation of a patient's airway and pulmonary status. It is correctly termed *ventilatory rate*. The correct term, *ventilatory rate,* is used throughout this textbook, although *respiratory rate* is used commonly in patient care. Although this might seem nitpicking and simply a matter of semantics, it is not. Use of the correct term by the EMT continually reminds him or her of the physiology involved. This understanding of physiology and pathophysiology is required when the EMT must make decisions that affect the outcome of the patient. It emphasizes the importance of the job that the EMT does in the field for patient survival.

> ✓ Correctness in any scientific endeavor promotes understanding, and understanding promotes better patient care. Good judgments are based on a proper knowledge base. EMTs should not be robots doing strictly what they are told without thinking. They should understand what is happening to the patient and make decisions based on this understanding.

Physician Notes

Correct use of the terms *respiratory rate* and *ventilatory rate* in this text will not change the common use (*respiratory rate*) by most providers. However, it will help the EMT understand the physiology.

atmospheric pressure. Air is forced (or sucked, depending on one's perspective) into the alveolar sac through the mouth, nose, trachea, and bronchi. As the diaphragm relaxes and the ribs return to their previous position, either by relaxation of the intercostal muscles or active contraction of the intercostal muscles, there is an increase in intrathoracic pressure, which forces air out of the alveolar sac and up through the bronchi, trachea, hypopharynx, mouth, and nose back into the environment surrounding the patient. This is the component of respiration termed *ventilation*. *Respiration* is the entire physiologic process in which oxygen is exchanged through the alveolar/capillary membrane into the bloodstream and picked up by the hemoglobin molecules in the red cells, carried to the tissue cells, and off-loaded from the hemoglobin molecule through the liquid part of the blood and

The circulation of blood through the lungs and heart is a critical part of this process (see Chapter 9). The important physiologic aspect that relates to thoracic trauma from the EMT's perspective is that the entire blood volume of the patient moves through the heart and lungs in less than 1 minute. Injuries to the vascular structures of the chest can rapidly lead to exsanguination if not controlled. Hemorrhage control inside the thoracic cavity is not possible prehospital; therefore the patient must be transported as quickly as possible to an appropriate facility.

Pathophysiology

Critical thoracic injuries in the thorax are in many ways organ specific and are so discussed based on physiology.

Ventilation

The movement of air in and out of the lungs is dependent on the intactness and function of three structures: the chest wall, the relationship of the chest walls and the lungs, and the alveolar sac.

Chest Wall

Three major conditions affect the expansion of the chest wall.

Nerve supply. The ability of the ribs to separate and return depends on contraction and relaxation of the intercostal muscles. This in turn is driven by stimuli from the brain through the intercostal nerves to the individual muscles. If an injury or other pathology interrupts this pathway, the intercostal muscles will not work. An example of such interruption would be an injury to the spinal cord cephalad (or proximal) to the takeoff of the particular intercostal nerve involved.

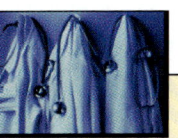

Physician Notes

Although *cephalad* and *proximal* do not mean the same thing, they indicate the same direction *in this situation*. *Cephalad* means toward the head. *Proximal* means toward the point of reference. The point of reference here would be the brain. The same relationship exists in the following paragraph with *caudad* and *distal*. This would be a good learning discussion to have with your instructor and your classmates. Think of situations in which these terms have the same meaning and situations in which they do not.

As examples, a gunshot wound through the spine between the fourth and fifth thoracic vertebrae would result in lack of innervation and therefore paralysis of all of the intercostal muscles caudad (distal) to the point of injury. Therefore the lower half of the intercostal muscles would not expand and contract, and the ventilatory process would be significantly affected. However, unless the thoracic cage were closely examined, such disparity might not be identified early.

A cervical spine fracture at the site of the most common fracture (C5, C6) would paralyze all of the intercostal muscles. This would leave only the accessory muscles of the back and neck and the diaphragm innervated by the phrenic nerve, which comes out of the spine at C2 and C3, to provide ventilation.

A spinal cord injury above C2 (cord injury, not merely fractured spine) would paralyze the diaphragm and accessory muscles, leaving the patient almost totally dependent on assisted ventilation by the EMT to move air in and out.

Bony stability of the thoracic cage. The ability of the ribs to separate and return, and therefore to expand the thoracic cavity, depends on the ribs maintaining their stability to the spine and to the sternum. If several ribs are fractured in several places, this continuity is lost. That portion would not expand with the rest of the chest cavity but would move in the opposite direction. When the intrathoracic pressure becomes less than the environmental pressure outside of the thoracic cavity, this segment moves inward. This loss of expansion and contraction would decrease the volume of air moving in and out of the lung (Figure 25.6).

This abnormal movement of the thoracic wall is called **paradoxic motion** because the affected segment moves inward when the rest of the chest is moving outward. For this problem to be apparent and actually affect the volume of ventilation, two or more ribs must be fractured in two or more places. A single fracture will not affect ventilation from a mechanical standpoint.

Pain. Any condition that produces perceptible pain to the patient when the ribs are moved will naturally result in the patient protecting himself or herself from this pain. The most effective method that the patient has to reduce pain is to not move the broken bone. The end result would be lack of movement of the chest wall and decreased ventilatory effort on the part of the patient and therefore less air moved in and out.

Relationship Between the Lungs and the Thoracic Wall

The two secretory membranes lining the thoracic cavity and the lungs described earlier and the potential space between the two must remain intact for the expanding

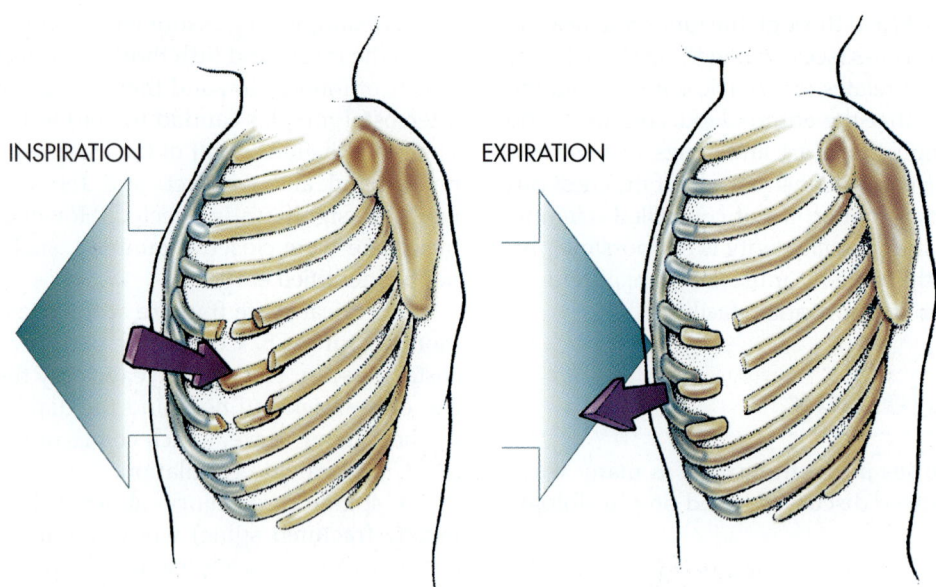

FIGURE 25.6 Paradoxic motion. If stability of the chest wall has been lost by ribs fractured in two or more places, when intrathoracic pressure decreases during inspiration, the external air pressure forces the chest wall in. When intrathoracic pressure increases during expiration, the chest wall is forced out.

chest wall to pull out the lungs. If an injury has occurred that allows air to separate the two membranes, the lungs will not be pulled out or will be pulled out a lesser distance because of the space-occupying mass (air) in the pleural space. This condition is called a **pneumothorax**. The space-occupying mass prevents the lung from fully expanding (Figure 25.7).

Several situations can lead to air accumulating in the pleural space: a penetrating injury from the outside going through the skin, intercostal muscles, and pleura into this space; a rupture of the lung itself, as can occur in blunt trauma (see paper bag effect in Chapter 22,); a spicule of bone from a fractured rib lacerating the lung; an injury to the lung itself; or a combination of these. The most common cause in blunt trauma is rupture of the lung as a result of overpressure (paper bag effect).

A penetrating injury to the chest wall will frequently suck air in during inspiration and blow air out during exhalation. Although the air cannot be seen moving in and out, the sound of this movement can be heard. This volume of air is that which would usually move in and out of the lungs and the alveolar sac to provide oxygenation and off-loading of CO_2. One would correctly assume that air moves in and out of the pleural space more easily than through the usual air passages. There is less resistance to the passage of air through a hole in the wall rather than the tortuous pathway through the nose, pharynx, larynx, trachea, bronchi, and bronchioles. This will reduce the amount of air available for oxygen and carbon dioxide exchange. If the injury is to the lung and not to the chest wall, expansion of the thoracic cage will suck air through the bronchi and out through the lung tissue in the pleural space. The result will be the same.

It is frequently easier for air to be sucked into the pleural space during inspiration rather than blown back out during expiration. It is trapped in the lung by the flaplike action of the chest wall injury. After a few breaths, this can result in enough pleural cavity air that the lung is entirely collapsed. This prevents oxygenation of red cells from occurring in the lung involved. As pressure tends to increase in the one pleural cavity, the heart and mediastinum are shifted into the opposite pleural cavity. The result is partial collapse of the opposite lung, which further reduces the ability of the lungs to oxygenate red cells and kinks the vena cava. The increased intrathoracic pressure and kinking of the vena cava reduce blood return to the right side of the heart. This is manifested by increasing preload pressure and is visualized by distended neck veins.

Lung Injury

Damage to the lungs that reduces the size of the **alveoli** and the bronchioles and therefore reduces the gas exchange to the blood is a mechanical situation associated with trauma to the chest. Just as trauma to the thumb when it is caught between the head of the nail and the downward motion of a hammer will rupture blood vessels in the thumb and cause an accumulation of blood and edema fluid in a closed space, so will **contusion** of the lungs cause hemorrhage and edema into the affected area, filling the alveolar sacs with blood. Any condition that causes accumulation of blood or fluid in the lung (e.g., gunshot wound to one part of the lung that results in blood running from the injured area throughout the bronchial system, filling alveoli; or the loss of ventilation areas destroyed by the penetrating injury) decreases air movement and ventilation.

Vascular injury can deprive a portion of the lungs of the flow of blood to exchange oxygen from carbon dioxide. This loss of flow results in reduction of the effective ventilatory lung space.

Combination Injuries

Several conditions resulting from injury are a combination of the aforementioned conditions. The most notable of these is a flail chest. A *flail chest* is so called because of the paradoxic motion of the chest wall. The paradoxic motion of the chest wall is an important part in reduction of ventilation because of lack of lung expansion; however, the pain associated with the fractured ribs will also reduce the ventilatory effort on the part of the patient. Finally, and most important, the contusion of the lung underlying the area where the trauma forced the chest wall onto the lungs will reduce the effective area of ventilation and reduce the volume of air moving in and out.

Another combination injury results from a gunshot wound to the chest wall and lung. There will be a sucking wound in the thoracic wall, another in the lung, contusion to the alveolar sacs, and hemorrhage into the alveolar sacs.

Hemorrhage

Bleeding into the chest cavity that produces a **hemothorax** can come from three sources. The most common site of intrathoracic blood loss is the intercostal arteries. These arteries are relatively large and are surrounded by minimal connective tissue that would retain hemorrhage. The high pressure, because of its proximity to the aorta and a large potential cavity (the hemithorax) that can hold 2 L or more of blood without difficulty, adds to the potential of developing a hemothorax. This is 40% to 50% of the patient's total blood volume. It is more than enough to place the patient in a condition of decreased tissue perfusion and decreased energy production (i.e., shock). The decreased available gas exchange surface from the compressed lung will add the additional burden of reduced oxygen absorption by the blood in the lung.

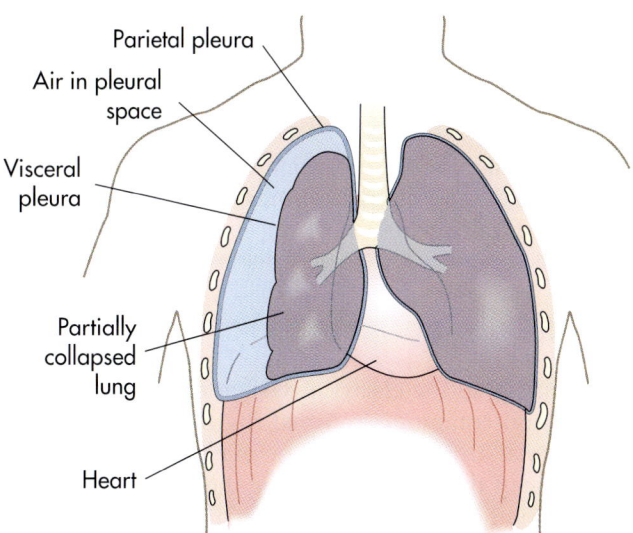

FIGURE 25.7 Air in the pleural space forces the lung in, decreasing the amount that can be ventilated and therefore decreasing oxygenation of the blood leaving the lung.

The second source of blood loss is the lung and the bronchial vessels. Although the pulmonary vascular system is at low pressure in comparison with the systemic system, nonetheless, because of the drop in thoracic pressure with each inhalation and the small amount of connective tissue to retain blood in the vessels, there is little to restrict blood flow once the larger vessels have been injured. The smaller vessels are multiple throughout the lung tissue and capillaries, and therefore injury to the pulmonary parachyma by some penetrating object can injure a number of vessels simultaneously, resulting in large volumes of blood loss.

The third source of potential blood loss, which may not lead to a large pneumothorax but could lead to rapid demise through exsanguination, is the aorta. The shear injury described previously and in Chapter 22 has a high mortality rate. Approximately 80% of such patients die from exsanguinating hemorrhage within the first hour of a traumatic situation. Of the remaining 20%, approximately one third will die within the first 6 hours and another one third within 24 hours; the final one third will live longer than 24 hours. It is in this group of 20% of patients that rapid identification of the injury in the emergency department and the hospital equipped and staffed to provide appropriate, quick intervention can result in survival.

The hemorrhaging trauma patient does not die of a "tension hemothorax" because the volume within each hemothorax is such that half or greater of the patient's blood volume can be lost into the thoracic cavity. This will cause death from hypovolemia before the development of a tension hemothorax.

Heart

As with most injuries, separation into the large categories of blunt and penetrating will provide initial insight into the type of damage to expect.

Blunt Cardiac Trauma

1. Damage to the electrical system of the heart causes several common abnormal rhythms. The EMT can have a suspicion that these may exist by detecting some of them when checking the pulse. This would be another indication that rapid transportation to a trauma center, if available, if not to the closest appropriate hospital, is important.
2. Damage to the wall of the heart. Contusion, bruising intramuscular hemorrhage, traumatic edema, and vascular damage can result from trauma to the heart, just as it can from compression of any other muscle in the body.
3. Rupture of the wall usually ends in immediate death, although some patients have arrived at the hospital alive. Quick response by the trauma team can save a few of these patients.

Penetrating Cardiac Trauma

Penetrating cardiac injuries generally fall into two categories:

1. Injuries in which the hole in the myocardium is large enough to allow such a rapid loss of blood volume that the patient's death is almost instantaneous. The entire blood volume passes through the heart each minute.
2. If the blood is contained within the pericardial sac, it reduces the ability of the heart to expand and fill during diastole and therefore reduces the cardiac output. Blood leaking from the hole in the heart occupies some of the space in the pericardial sac, preventing the full expansion of the heart and complete filling. After a few contractions the amount of volume flowing into the ventricle is so restricted that each systolic thrust contains very little blood. The result is significant drop in blood pressure.

Assessment

Assessment of thoracic injuries begins with a high index of suspicion based on the kinematics of the incident. The next step is airway assessment (see Chapter 10). The third step is analysis of the condition of the thoracic cavity and its contained organs. The ability to achieve such analysis and assessment in the prehospital period and the field is limited to the following:

- Visually examining the chest wall for deformities, paradoxic chest wall motion, rapid breathing pattern, asymmetry of the chest wall, asymmetry of chest wall expansion, and abdominal breathing.
- Palpation of the chest wall identifies abnormal movements of the ribs; pain produced by pressure on the ribs, either globally or individually; the broken bones moving across each other; or subcutaneous air in the tissues.
- Listening to the breath sounds using the stethoscope can identify unilateral absent breath sounds indicative of a large pneumothorax or **tension pneumothorax.** Bronchial sounds transmitted into the lung fields in a patient with a large pneumothorax or tension pneumothorax is frequently confusing. The EMT may require years of experience listening to normal breath sounds and assessing chest injuries before being able to identify the subtleties of a pneumothorax.

Although the following signs are frequently discussed, many are not present or are difficult to identify in the field:

- Tracheal deviation is usually a late sign. In the neck, the trachea is bound to the cervical spine by fascial and other supporting structures; thus the deviation of the trachea is more of an intrathoracic phenomenon, although if severe, it may be felt. It is not often seen in the prehospital environment. Even when it is present, it can be difficult to diagnose by physical examination.

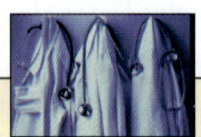

Physician Notes

The part of blood pressure that drops is the systolic pressure. The diastolic pressure remains the same because the difficulty is not a volume loss such as in hypovolemia but a cardiac output loss. This pulse pressure decrease limits the volume of blood available for delivery of oxygen and nutrients to cells. Anaerobic metabolism and decreased energy production result.

An astute, knowledgeable EMT who detects a drop in systolic pressure that is not associated with a drop in diastolic pressure can initiate rapid transportation to the trauma center, where the tamponade can be decompressed.

- Distended neck veins are described as a classic sign of tension pneumothorax. However, because the patient with a tension pneumothorax may also have lost a considerable amount of blood, distended neck veins may not be prominent. If the patient has a pneumatic antishock garment applied, the neck veins may be distended by the device and not by a tension pneumothorax (Figure 25.8).
- Cyanosis is difficult to see in the poor lighting that frequently exists in the field. Poor lighting, variation in skin color, and dirt and blood associated with trauma often render this sign unreliable.
- The most helpful part of the physical examination is checking for decreased breath sounds on the side of the injury. To use this sign, however, one must be able to distinguish between normal and decreased sounds. Such differentiation cannot be done without a great deal of practice. Listening to breath sounds during every patient contact will help.
- Percussion of the chest is an excellent method for determining the status of the chest cavity in the relative quiet of the hospital. In the noisy prehospital environment, this sound is much more difficult to detect. Given the difficulty in obtaining this sign and the time and environment it requires, it is not recommended for field diagnosis of tension pneumothorax.

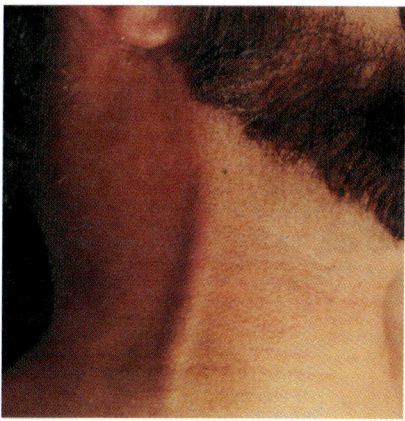

FIGURE 25.8 Distended neck veins are one of the indications of an increase in thoracic pressure.

The potential for any patient with a simple pneumothorax or hemopneumothorax to develop a tension pneumothorax is very real. The development of a tension pneumothorax is an important concern for any patient who has sustained chest trauma, has been intubated, and requires positive-pressure ventilation. In these cases, it is possible to convert a simple pneumothorax to a tension pneumothorax because air is being pushed into the chest with each ventilation. The patient must be constantly monitored for this possibility, and the EMT must be prepared to rapidly intervene.

The usual signs and symptoms of a developing tension pneumothorax are as follows:

- Early signs: unilateral decreased or absent breath sounds; continued increased dyspnea and tachypnea
- Progressive signs: increasing tachypnea and dyspnea, tachycardia, and subcutaneous emphysema; increasing difficulty ventilating the patient (assisted ventilation with bag-valve-mask [BVM] or BVET)
- Late signs: jugular vein distention, tracheal deviation, tympany, signs of acute **hypoxia,** narrowing pulse pressure, and other signs of shock

In many cases, the only signs of a developing tension pneumothorax are compromised oxygenation, tachycardia, tachypnea, and unilateral decreased or absent breath sounds.

Management

Management of a thoracic injury for the prehospital provider is limited to airway, assisted ventilation, decompression of the tension pneumothorax, volume replacement, and rapid transport to an appropriate facility. In a large community with more than one hospital, one of the hospitals is usually dedicated to management of trauma patients. Other hospitals should be bypassed and the patient transported to this facility.

The techniques of airway and assisted ventilation in a patient with thoracic injuries do not vary from these techniques carried out for most other situations. The only skill unique to thoracic trauma is decompression of a tension pneumothorax. Although this is most often an EMT-Paramedic–level skill, some communities may have trained and empowered the EMT-Basic to carry it out, and in other communities the EMT-Basic may assist the EMT-Paramedic. Therefore this skill is included as enrichment or enhancement information.

Rib Fractures

The prehospital management of patients with simple rib fractures is splinting to reduce pain. This can easily and simply done by placing the patient's arm in a sling and then tying a swath around it. Prolonged use of this technique will reduce the expansion of the lung under the affected area. However, it will work during the transportation of the patient to the hospital.

Management should also include patient reassurance and an anticipation of potential complications such as open or closed pneumothorax and hypovolemia. Care must be taken to evaluate tidal volume and the presence of hypoxemia; should ventilation be significantly encumbered, ventilatory assistance is indicated. Deep, full ventilations and coughing should be encouraged despite the associated pain. Such actions prevent **atelectasis** (collapse of alveoli or part of the lung) leading to pneumonia. Fractured ribs should *not* be stabilized by taping or any other firm bandaging or binding that encircles the chest. Such attempts at management can inhibit chest movement and limit ventilation and can lead to atelectasis and pneumonia.

Providing an increased FiO_2 during transportation is important. This is best done with a nonrebreathing mask that delivers an FiO_2 in the range of 0.85 or more.

Flail Chest

There are four consequences of flail chest: (1) a decrease in the vital capacity proportional to the size of the flail segment; (2) an increase in the labor of breathing; (3) pain produced by the fractured ribs, limiting the amount of thoracic cage expansion; and (4) most significant clinically, contusion of the lung beneath the flail segment. Several considerations are important in the management of this injury.

The key step in management is to assist the patient's ventilation with positive-pressure ventilation by the BVM method. Assisted ventilation expands the collapsed alveoli, both in the area of the flail segment and in the area involved when the patient splints. Blood passing through the capillaries lining the collapsed (nonventilated) alveoli leaves the lung still unoxygenated. Providing additional oxygen to the unaffected alveoli, combined with forced expansion of the collapsed alveoli, decreases the amount of oxygen-deprived blood entering the left side of the heart and the aorta.

A large percentage of patients with significant flail chest will progress to respiratory failure and require eventual and often prolonged ventilatory support in the hospital. Hospital management of a severe flail injury includes intubation and positive-pressure ventilation. Some patients may require intubation in the field if emergency medical services personnel are available who have been so trained. If not, vigorous assisted ventilation with BVM is required.

The use of sandbags to prevent movement in patients with a flail chest (described in earlier textbooks) has been found to decrease aeration of the lungs and to promote alveolar collapse. This method should no longer be used. Taping or strapping the chest wall should not be used for the same reason.

Patients with contused lungs do not tolerate excess fluid well. The extra fluid increases the amount of interstitial fluid and decreases oxygen transport even more. Therefore these patients should be closely monitored. If they are hemodynamically normal, intravenous fluid administration should be limited to that needed for maintenance only. Hypotensive or tachycardic patients with multiple injuries should not have fluids restricted.

As with other traumatic conditions involving the lungs, appropriate management includes ensuring adequate ventilation and enriched oxygen administration. If pulse oximetry is available, it can help guide management. Supplemental oxygen should be provided to maintain oxygen saturation at approximately 90%. If the patient cannot maintain adequate ventilation or is suffering from preexisting chronic pulmonary disease, an altered level of consciousness, or other major injuries, the EMT should use BVM ventilation and, if required, endotracheal intubation.

Pneumothorax

As noted previously, the signs and symptoms of a pneumothorax may include pleuritic chest pain and difficult and rapid breathing. Decreased or absent breath sounds on the involved side is the classic sign.

In trauma patients in the prehospital setting, absent or decreased breath sounds plus ventilatory distress equals aggressive management of these symptoms because the pathology may be a pneumothorax. Although this diagnosis is not a prehospital one, the patient must be provided supportive treatment of the ventilatory condition with an understanding of the potential pathophysiology. When the lung collapse is partial, reduced or absent breath sounds may be heard over the apices and bases of the lung earlier than over the midlung fields. These patients require constant monitoring in anticipation of the development of a tension pneumothorax.

The patient is placed in the position of comfort (usually a semi-sitting position) unless contraindicated by a possible spine injury, hypovolemia, or another injury. High-concentration oxygen (FiO_2 of 0.85 to 1.0) should be administered. BVM-assisted breathing may be necessary for patients whose respiratory rate is less than 12 or greater than 20 breaths per minute or who display signs of hypoxia. However, positive-pressure ventilation may increase the possibility of a tension pneumothorax. The patient must be transported rapidly and carefully monitored for signs of a tension pneumothorax while en route. Steps must be taken to alleviate the tension pneumothorax as early as possible.

At the EMT-Basic level, it is especially important that rapid transportation occur as soon as practical in anticipation of the possibility of a developing tension pneumothorax in the patient.

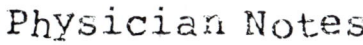

Physician Notes

Each community will have local protocols as to how the patient with potential tension pneumothorax is handled based on local resources.

Open Pneumothorax

Management of an **open pneumothorax** is directed first toward closing the hole in the chest, after which pressure-assisted ventilation will provide benefit to the patient. Closing the wound can be done with Vaseline gauze covered with sterile gauze, or any other type of occlusive dressing secured with tape. Blocking airflow completely with an airtight dressing can lead to a tension pneumothorax if there is a continued air leak from the lung. If only three sides of the plastic or aluminum foil dressing are taped, an effective vent is created that might permit spontaneous decompression of a developing tension pneumothorax (Figure 25.9). Even if a self-venting dressing is applied, any patient who has had an open chest wound sealed by the EMT must be carefully and continually monitored for the onset of a tension pneumothorax until the patient's care can be directly transferred to the hospital emergency department staff. Removal of the dressing may be required if a tension pneumothorax develops.

As for any trauma patient, high-concentration oxygen, ventilatory support, and treatment for hypovolemia must be the EMT's first priorities after closure of the chest wound.

Tension Pneumothorax

The management of a patient with a tension pneumothorax involves reducing the pressure in the pleural space.

Penetrating injury. When there is a wound in the chest wall with signs of a tension pneumothorax, the first step in relieving the increased pressure is to remove the dressing over the wound for a few seconds. If the wound in the chest wall has not sealed under the dressing, air will rush out of the wound. Once the pressure has been released, the wound should be resealed with the occlusive dressing. This short release may need to be repeated periodically if pressure again builds up within the chest. In the rare case that it becomes necessary to keep the defect open to prevent reaccumulation of air in the thoracic cavity, assisted ventilation with an FiO$_2$ of 0.85 to 1.0 is necessary.

Closed tension pneumothorax. If reopening the wound does not immediately solve the condition, or if the pneu-

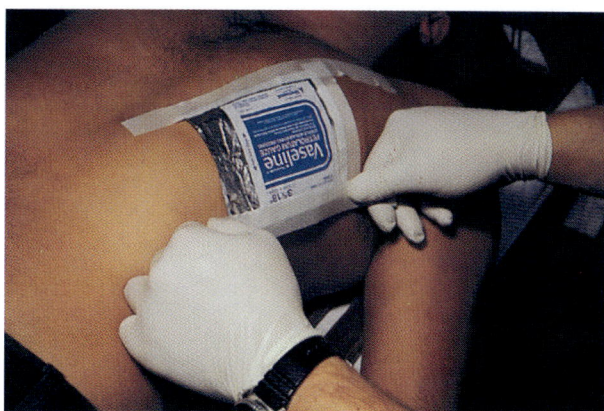

FIGURE 25.9 Taping a piece of foil or plastic on the chest wall on three sides creates a flutter-valve effect, allowing air to escape from the pleural space but not enter into it.

mothorax developed without a wound in the chest wall, decompression is accomplished by insertion of a large-bore needle into the pleural space of the affected side. This procedure can be carried out in the field by an advanced life support (ALS) provider. If ALS personnel are not available, the patient must be transported as rapidly as possible to the appropriate hospital while administering oxygen at a high FiO$_2$ while en route. A tension pneumothorax or a potential tension pneumothorax is a life-threatening condition. It requires rapid transport to an appropriate hospital, because needle insertion or dressing removal is only a temporary solution until more definitive care can be provided.

Needle decompression, if carefully done, carries minimal risk and can greatly benefit the patient by improving oxygenation and circulation. A 14- or 16-gauge hollow needle is inserted into the affected pleural space at the second intercostal space in the **midclavicular line.** The landmark for insertion is the angle of Lewie on the sternum, which marks the space between the second and third ribs (Figure 25.10). The midclavicular line is at the midpoint of the clavicle. This area lacks anatomic structures that could be injured during needle decompression. The internal mammary artery is just lateral to the sternal border (1 cm), hence the use of the midclavicular line. Because the lung is compressed toward the mediastinum, it will be out of the way if the needle is placed high into the second intercostal space. The nerve, artery, and vein pass just beneath each rib, so the needle should pass just over the third or fourth rib. The midclavicular site is better than the midaxillary line, where chest tubes are inserted in the emergency department. The anterior chest allows better visualization of the needle at the midclavicular line while en route to the hospital. Also, the patient's arm is not strapped down across this area as would be the case

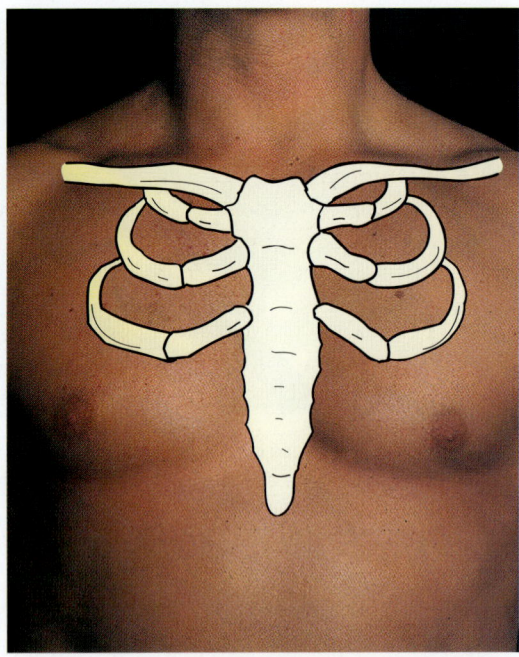

FIGURE 25.10 Needle decompression of the thoracic cavity is most easily accomplished and has the least chance for complication if it is done at the midclavicular line through the second intercostal space.

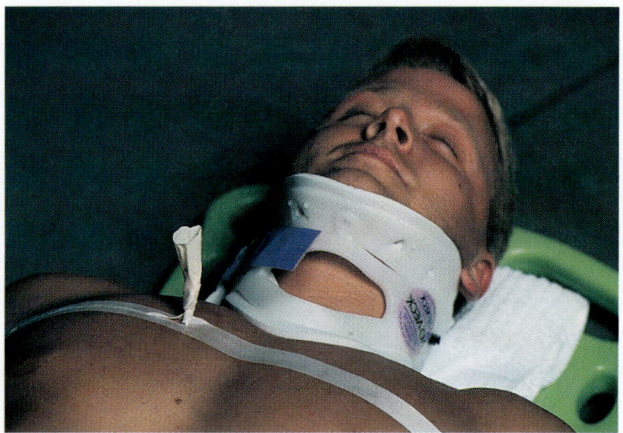

FIGURE 25.11 Once the needle has been inserted, a one-way valve made with the finger cut from the end of a glove will allow air pressure to flow from within the pleural cavity to an outside wall but not in the opposite direction.

if the midaxillary line were chosen. Special situations may require other approaches under the direction of appropriate medical control.

Initially after insertion, air will rush from the needle as the pressure in the chest is relieved. A one-way valve can then be attached to the needle to allow air to escape from the pleural space but not enter it. Such a valve can easily be made by cutting a finger from a sterile glove. Rinse the inside of the glove finger with sterile water or normal saline before using it. Rinsing removes the talcum powder and results in a better seal when the valve is closed. Pass the needle and catheter through the length of the glove finger and puncture the fingertip with it.

If the needle has been inserted in the patient's chest without a one-way valve, the sterile glove finger can be added. Simply cut the finger from the glove, cut a small hole at the fingertip, spread the tip over the catheter hub, and fasten with a rubber band. If available, tubing and a flutter valve can be added to the hub of the needle instead of a glove finger (Figure 25.11).

Summary

- Injuries to the chest resulting from either blunt or penetrating trauma produce two common major problems for the EMT and one uncommon major problem: ventilation compromise, hemorrhage, and cardiac dysrhythmias.
- The definitive management of these conditions occurs at the hands of a physician experienced in trauma care. This is most often available in a trauma center. The patient must be transported to such a center if one is available.
- The field management of thoracic injuries begins, as always, with identification (assessment and diagnosis) of the problem. This diagnosis is not, for example, the presence of a pneumothorax, but the presence of hypoxia, the treatment of which is increased percentage of inhaled oxygen (FiO_2) and assisted ventilation. In the field, the EMT may not be able to determine the exact cause of the hypoxia. The goal of the EMT in this situation is to package the patient, support the hypoxia, and provide rapid transportation to the hospital that can best care for the patient.

Scenario Solution

The driver of the vehicle that underwent the frontal impact would continue his forward motion, striking the steering column with his chest, thus stopping the forward motion of the sternum. The continued motion of the posterior thoracic wall would compress the heart against the sternum, potentially producing dysrhythmias, contusion, or rupture. The volume of the thoracic cavity would be reduced, potentially producing a pneumothorax on one or both sides.

The driver in the vehicle undergoing the side impact received energy exchange to his lateral chest wall. The potential of this impact would be to produce pneumothorax to the lung on the side of the impact and to the intraabdominal organs under the diaphragm on that side. A major pelvic fracture must also be considered. The driver indicates injury from the seatbelt attachment by the history of pain in his left hip. Intraabdominal and retroperitoneal hemorrhage would be a major consideration.

A rapid ventilation rate would indicate either decreased oxygenation of the RBCs or increased CO_2 production secondary to anaerobic metabolism within the tissue cells. Blood loss or pneumothorax could cause these conditions. Some of the mental state of the patients could come from hypoxia. Although they tell you they are all right, there are multiple indications that this may not be so. These patients should be transported to a trauma center, if available. If a trauma center is not available, they should be transported to the closest facility that can manage trauma patients quickly. Rapid transportation does no good if the staff of the hospital cannot respond quickly.

Key Terms

Alveolar/capillary membrane Gas exchange that occurs in the lungs; oxygen enters the capillaries and is transported by the blood, and carbon dioxide enters the alveoli and is exhaled.

Alveoli Small air sacs in the lungs where the exchange of gas takes place.

Atelectasis Collapsed alveoli in the lung. These sections are not ventilated and contribute to lack of oxygenation of the RBCs and can lead to pneumonia.

Contusion Minor damage in the dermal layer of the skin causing discoloration from blood leaking into surrounding tissue; a bruise.

Diaphragm The dome-shaped muscle that separates the thoracic cavity from the abdominal cavity. When it contracts, the thoracic cavity enlarges, allowing air to enter the lungs.

Hemothorax Accumulation of blood and fluid in the pleural cavity usually caused by trauma.

Hypopharynx Lower one third of the pharynx.

Hypoxia Shortage of oxygen at the cellular level. Signs and symptoms include dyspnea, restlessness, confusion, lethargy, and poor skin color.

Intercostal muscles Muscles located between the ribs that lift the ribs upward and outward during inhalation, increasing tidal volume.

Intrathoracic pressure The pressure inside the thorax that changes with ventilation.

Midclavicular line A vertical line on a standing patient that runs caudad from the center of the clavicle on either side.

Open pneumothorax Injury that penetrates through the skin, subcutaneous tissue, and intercostal muscles and into the thoracic cavity.

Oropharynx The portion of the pharynx that is inside the mouth.

Oxygenation Transporting of oxygen to the red blood cells and tissue cells.

Paradoxic motion Movement of the chest during respiration when one section of the bony rib cage moves in an opposite direction from the rest of the rib cage, indicating that a section of the rib cage has broken loose.

Pneumothorax A collection of air in the pleural space; always abnormal and may cause collapse of the underlying lung.

Sternum Flat bone lying in the anterior center of the thorax.

Tension pneumothorax Pneumothorax that has increased pressure in one hemithorax, collapsed the lung on the affected side, and pushed the organs of the mediastinum into the opposite side of the chest, restricting the ventilation of that lung.

Ventilation Movement of air into and out of the lung.

Review Questions

1. The most common cause of death in a patient with a hemothorax is:
   a. Airway compromise
   b. Ventilation compromise
   c. Hypoxia
   d. Hemorrhage
2. Blunt cardiac injuries cause three types of injures. One of these is:
   a. Airway compromise
   b. Ventilation compromise
   c. Hypoxia
   d. Hemorrhage
3. Blunt trauma to the chest can produce all but which one of the following?
   a. Airway compromise
   b. Ventilation compromise
   c. Hypoxia
   d. Hemorrhage
4. Which of the following should be the first priority of patient management?
   a. Airway compromise
   b. Ventilation compromise
   c. Hypoxia
   d. Hemorrhage
5. The most common cause of death in a flail chest is:
   a. Airway compromise
   b. Ventilation compromise
   c. Hypoxia
   d. Hemorrhage

Answers to these Review Questions can be found at the end of the book on page 866.

Abdominal Emergencies

Lesson Goal

Examination of the abdomen in the field is complicated by several factors, including time; lack of significant signs and symptoms early; subtlety of abdominal findings; lack of specialized equipment such as computed tomography (CT), ultrasound (U/S), and radiography (x-ray) equipment; and perhaps the most important, the inability to treat most ongoing problems. The bottom line for field care of the patient with abdominal trauma is rapid transportation to a medical facility. On the other hand, the identification of nontrauma conditions of the abdomen and correct field management require that the EMT-B has an understanding of the anatomy and physiology of the abdominal and retroperitoneal organs so that he or she can identify the pathologic and potentially pathologic conditions and institute proper management. This chapter addresses the field care of the trauma and nontrauma conditions.

Scenario

You just received a call from the dispatcher that a 17-year-old male was hit in the side with a baseball bat during a game. On arrival at the scene, you discover that the patient was pitching in a high school baseball game. His inside pitch was too close and hit the batter on the helmet. The batter ran to the mound and hit the pitcher in the side with the bat. With the notification time and your response time, you and your partner arrived on the scene approximately 15 minutes after the incident occurred. You are the senior EMT-B on the unit. The pitcher is obviously very agitated and mad, but he is in the top of the seventh inning and pitching a perfect game. You find out that he is trying to get a baseball scholarship to State University, a scout from the university is in the stands, and this is near the end of the baseball season. An outstanding game at this point may get him the scholarship. He tells you the he feels fine and just has some sore muscles, but he refuses to leave the game and give up the chance for a big game and possibly a scholarship.

On examination you find moderate tenderness overlying the lateral aspect of the left ninth, tenth, and eleventh ribs. He tells you that he has had broken ribs before when he played football and that he played an entire game like this. You know this to be true because you were in the EMS unit assigned to that game. You watched the game from the sidelines and heard the discussions about the broken ribs from the coach, the trainer, and the player. He tells you that simply having them taped will allow him to continue the game. His coach assures you that he knows how to tape ribs and that they will bring him to the hospital after the game. The coach calls you aside and tells you that this is a poor kid from the country and that his parents have no money to send him to college. With the scout in the stands, this may be his best or perhaps only chance to go to college.

He is obviously splinting this area. At rest his ventilatory rate is 30 breaths/min, his pulse rate is elevated to 110 beats/min, his capillary refilling time is approximately 2 seconds, and his blood pressure is 100/85 mm Hg.

493

> How would you manage this situation? Are there any risks in allowing him to finish the baseball game? If so, list some of these risks. If you decide that he should not finish the baseball game and should go to the hospital, what would you use to convince the patient and the coach of your decision? If your decision is that it is safe for him to finish the ball game, what follow-up advice would you give him?

Key Terms to Know

- Abscess
- Amylase
- Appendicitis
- Cholecystitis
- Colon
- Common duct
- Costovertebral angle
- Duodenum
- Endocrine
- Fistula
- Gallbladder
- Gastrointestinal (GI) tract
- Gynecologic
- Inflammation
- Liver
- Lipase
- Pancreas
- Paraspinal muscles
- Peritoneum
- Peritonitis
- Rectus abdominis
- Renal (kidney) stones
- Retroperitoneal space
- Small intestine
- Stomach
- Ulcers

Learning Objectives

As an EMT-Basic, you should be able to do the following:

DOT

- Demonstrate the steps in the emergency medical care of a patient with open abdominal wounds.

Supplemental

- Describe the anatomy of the abdominal cavity and the retroperitoneal space.
- Describe the physiology of the major abdominal organs.
- Describe the pathophysiology or traumatic injuries to the abdominal organs.
- Describe the pathophysiology of significant conditions seen in the prehospital period that require assessment and management from the field.

Prehospital personnel must address two significant injuries in the management of intraabdominal trauma: (1) hemorrhage and (2) injury to the **gastrointestinal (GI) tract**. Signs of intraabdominal trauma are rarely evident, but one possible indication of intraabdominal trauma is a compromised airway. To appropriately evaluate and manage intraabdominal trauma, the emergency medical technician (EMT) must recognize the extent and severity of the injury or potential injury and transport the patient rapidly to a medical facility that is equipped and staffed to manage those injuries. Because of the lack of evident signs of intraabdominal trauma, it is difficult for the surgeon to decide whether to operate.

The EMT can make active or passive decisions regarding a patient with intraabdominal injuries. An example of an active decision is when the EMT takes positive actions in patient care based on experience and the ability to assume responsibility for his or her actions for the benefit of the patient. An example of a passive decision is when the EMT refuses to make a decision about taking the patient to an appropriate medical facility (unless no trauma centers exist in the community). He or she transports the patient to a nontrauma center and waits for someone else to decide that the patient is injured enough to be transported to a trauma center. Such inaction or passivity is an error that is as inappropriate as entirely missing the injury.

Anatomy

The abdominal cavity (Figure 26.1) is bounded superiorly by the diaphragm, laterally on each side by three strong muscles and their fascia, posteriorly by the **paraspinal muscles** and the vertebrae, anteriorly by the **rectus abdominis** muscle and its fascia compartments, and inferiorly by the perineum (see Chapter 7). The human body

Patient Care Algorithm

Trauma Patient Assessment

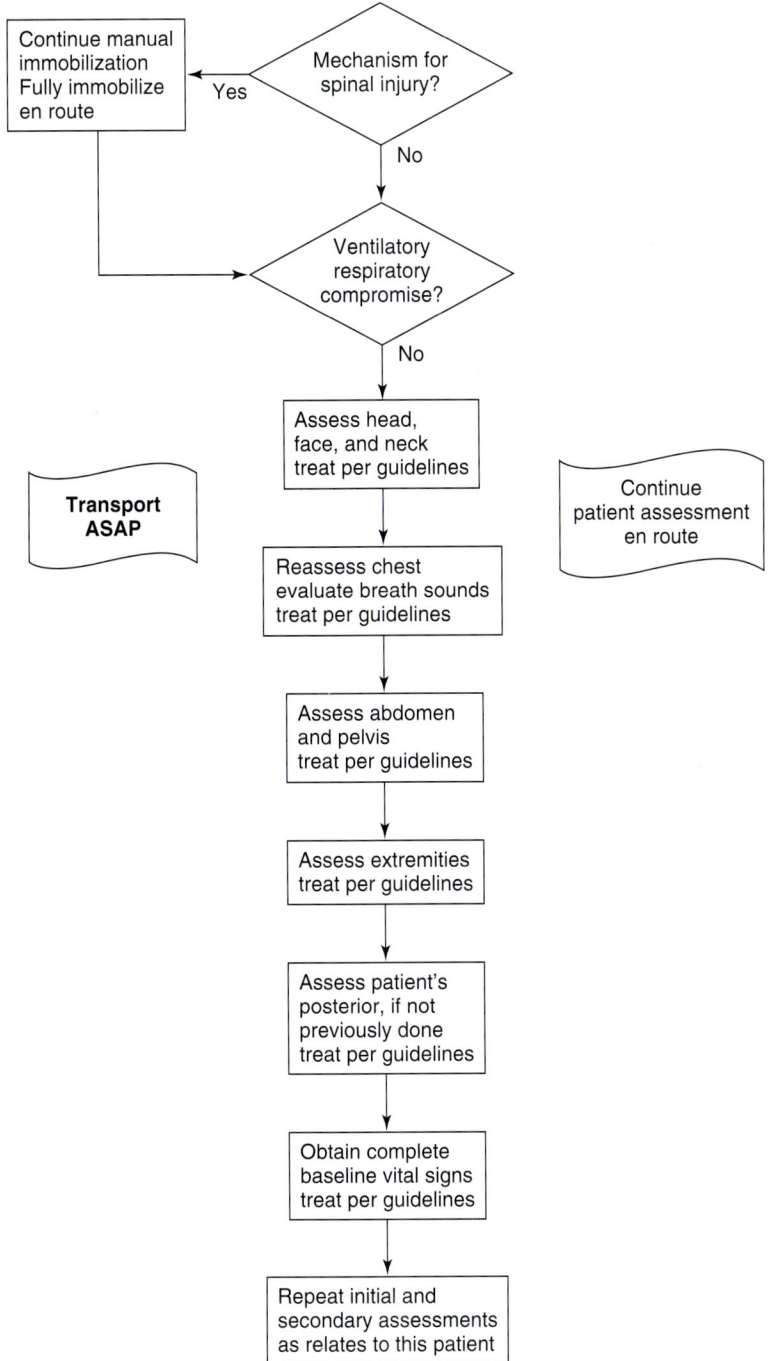

contains the alimentary canal, which is essentially a thick-walled hollow tube that consists of the mouth, esophagus, and GI tract (stomach, small intestine, and large intestine), rectum, and anus. The GI tract runs throughout the abdominal cavity; therefore a penetrating injury from any direction can damage the GI tract. A penetration to the intestines can introduce bacteria into the body in the same way that a penetration to the skin can introduce bacteria. This allows intestinal contents and bacteria to leak into the peritoneal cavity and produce an infection.

The solid organs in the abdominal cavity (e.g., liver, kidneys, and pancreas) do not move around much. This allows the EMT to predict what organs may be injured by examining the external location of the trauma. These organs are usually protected from injury by bony structures. However, the underlying organs can become vulnerable to injury if these bony structures are damaged.

Most of the **liver** lies in the right upper quadrant and is protected by the rib cage. The spleen is situated under the rib cage on the left side. The kidneys are located in the **retroperitoneal space** (behind the **peritoneum**) on either side of the body at the **costovertebral angle** (where the rib cage and spine meet). The **pancreas** is also located in the retroperitoneal space and is particularly vulnerable to anterior blunt trauma because it overlies the twelfth vertebra and there is no solid protection anteriorly. When a force, such as the steering column, stops the forward motion of the anterior abdominal wall and the motion of the posterior abdominal wall continues, the pancreas is trapped between the spine and the steering column. Compression across the vertebrae fractures the pancreas, causing the destructive pancreatic juices to leak into the retroperitoneal space (see Chapter 22).

The GI tract is vulnerable to most forms of penetrating trauma. For example, a moving bullet does not allow the GI tract or the solid organs to move out of the way. Penetrating objects will most likely injure the organs in the vicinity of its trajectory (see Chapter 22 for identification of the pathway of a bullet and entrance and exit wounds).

The mobility and location of the GI tract allow it to move out of the way of most forms of blunt trauma. However, compression of the abdomen by improperly worn seat belts does not allow the GI tract to escape. A bruise from the seat belt across the abdomen above the pelvis (seat belt sign) alerts the EMT to a condition with approximately 60% abdominal compartment injuries.

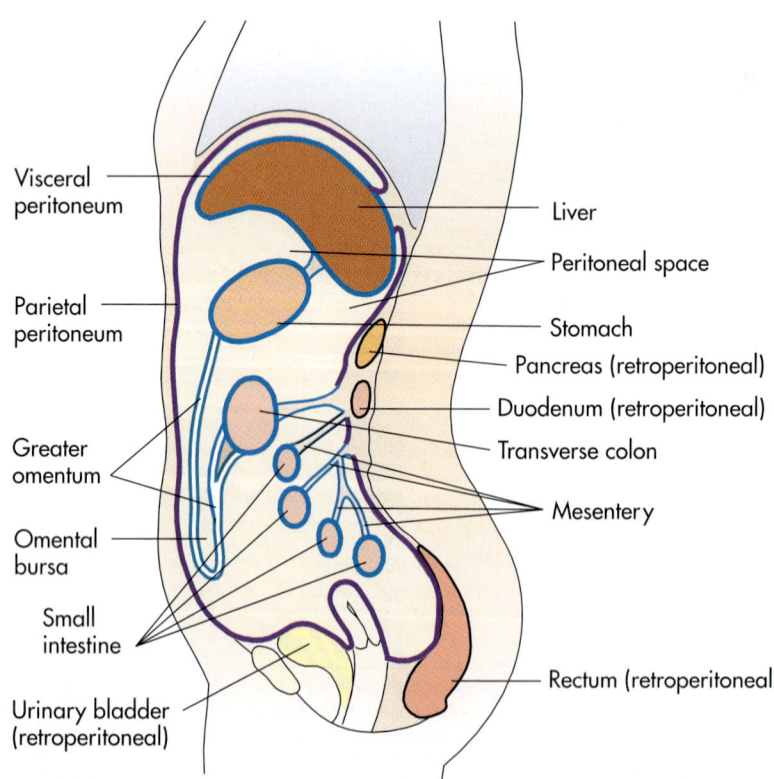

FIGURE 26.1 The abdomen is divided into two spaces: the peritoneal space and the retroperitoneal space. The retroperitoneal space includes the portion of the abdomen behind the peritoneum. The organs are not in contact with the peritoneal cavity. Injury to organs in this area does not necessarily produce peritonitis.

It is not necessary for the EMT to be an accomplished anatomist; however, the EMT must understand the general location of the various organs so that he or she can recognize trauma, pain, muscle guarding, or tenderness in a particular area as an important factor in assessing the patient and making decisions as to whether rapid movement to the hospital is critical.

Physiology and Pathophysiology

Although the EMT is not required to diagnose abdominal cavity problems in the field, the identification of patients who have serious or potentially serious complications of trauma and illness is the EMT's responsibility. The EMT can enhance his or her decision about what assessment findings may be important by understanding what is happening with the abdominal organs. The editors of this text believe that correct judgment decisions are based on a strong fund of knowledge. Knowledge of physiology and pathophysiology details is not required on any certification examination; however, the EMT can do the job better if he or she knows this information and can provide better care for patients. Therefore this text presents physiology and pathophysiology information for the reader's enlightenment and for the reader to use as he or she grows in the area of patient care and becomes a strong part of the health care team.

The EMT can evaluate conditions that affect the abdomen more easily by dividing them into medical and trauma conditions. Although both types can exist in the same patient and overlap may exist in the problems that the condition produces (e.g., acid leakage from the stomach caused by a perforated ulcer or a gun shot wound [GSW] to the stomach can produce the same problems), rapid assessment is much easier.

Hemorrhage

A large volume of blood from abdominal organs can be lost into the abdominal cavity, and there will be few if any early signs of bleeding. The EMT must evaluate the patient based on the kinematics of the event, the potential for hemorrhage, changes in the abdominal findings that indicate hemorrhage, and changes in the patient's hemodynamic state that indicate blood loss (see Chapter 9 for a more detailed discussion of hemodynamic changes). Blood in the abdominal organs can bleed into the free peritoneal cavity without the restriction that occurs in the compartments of the legs and arms. The abdominal cavity can easily hide 3 to 5 liters of blood in a short period of time, especially with injury to vascular organs such as spleen and liver. The liver is the most frequently injured organ in the abdominal cavity primarily because of its large size, and the spleen is the second most frequently injured organ; however, because of its vascularity the spleen loses blood more quickly.

Blood loss into the GI tract from a bleeding ulcer can produce the same signs of shock as blood loss from an injured intraabdominal organ but without the helpful history of trauma preceding the event.

Gastrointestinal Tract

Six general GI complications can occur: (1) **ulcers**, (2) perforation, (3) hemorrhage, (4) **abscess**, (5) **inflammation**, and (6) **fistula**. Whether these complications are secondary to trauma or to medical conditions, prehospital management consists of the EMT addressing hemodynamic accessibility and transporting the patient to a medical facility. Prehospital management of any of these conditions is otherwise limited.

Leakage of GI tract contents into the abdominal cavity produces either chemical inflammation of the peritoneal lining (hydrochloric acid from the **stomach**) or bacterial inflammation (bacteria from the **small intestine** or **colon**). The only difference between the two is that hydrochloric acid from the stomach usually produces sudden onset of abdominal pain and signs of an acute surgical abdomen, whereas bacterial **peritonitis** usually develops over a period of 24 to 48 hours after the insult (Figures 26.2 and 26.3).

The brain recognizes the peritoneal inflammation as pain. Movement of the peritoneal lining, which can result from physical examination (pushing on the abdominal), walking, jostling movement in an ambulance, or tight straps across the abdomen, increases this pain. The patient tries to prevent such sensation in any way possible (e.g., lying calmly in bed prevents jostling, lying in a rolled up in the fetal position prevents tightening of the abdominal musculature, or walking with the body listing to one side). During examination the patient will resist abdominal pain by tightening the overlying abdominal muscles, which is appropriately known as *guarding*. Guarding is described as minimal, moderate, severe, or rigid abdomen. A rigid abdomen is boardlike and is classically found in a patient with chemical peritonitis such as a perforated duodenal ulcer.

Other conditions that produce abdominal findings of peritoneal inflammation are discussed in the following sections, although they are not as severe as perforations into the cavity. These involve infection or inflammation of the organs and are often found in the section of the abdomen in which the affected organs lie. Gallbladder pain

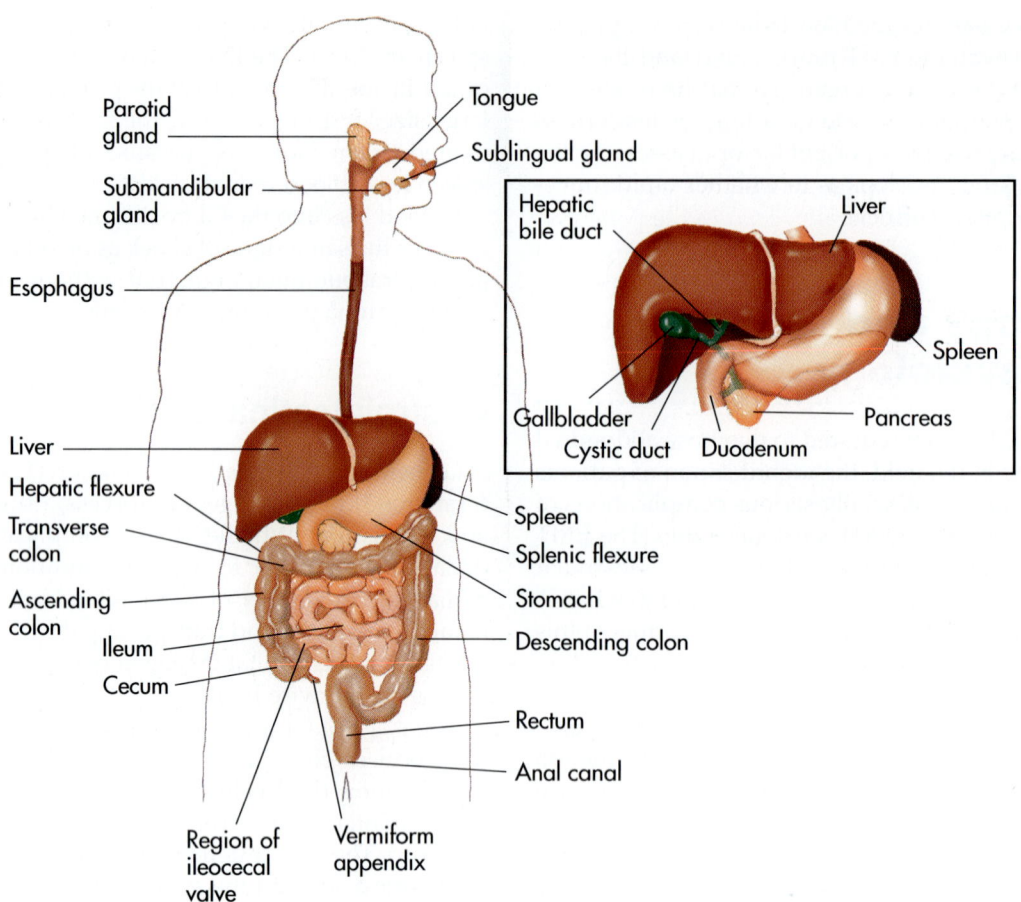

FIGURE 26.2 The organs inside the peritoneal cavity frequently produce peritonitis when injured. Organs in the peritoneal cavity include solid organs (spleen and liver), hollow organs of the gastrointestinal tract (stomach, small intestine, and colon), and the reproductive organs.

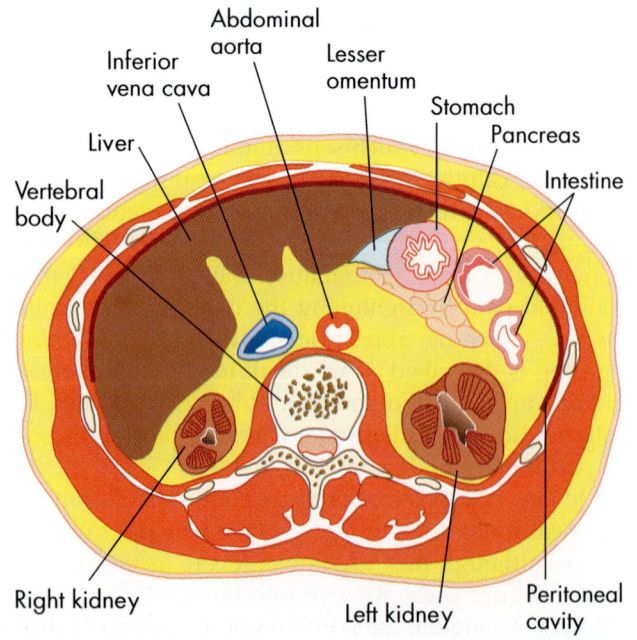

FIGURE 26.3 This transverse section of the abdominal cavity gives an appreciation of the organs' positions in the anteroposterior direction.

occurs in the right upper quadrant, pancreatic pain occurs in the midabdomen and back, renal pain is at the costovertebral angle, and pain of acute appendicitis occurs in the lower abdomen, particularly the right lower quadrant. Pain associated with the female organs of reproduction occurs in the lower abdomen and can be in the midline or either lower quadrant (Figure 26.4).

Gallbladder

Gallbladder disease is the result of chronic inflammation in the walls of the gallbladder, which allows stones to develop. The presence of fatty foods in the intestines causes the gallbladder to contract to empty the bile through the cystic duct, through the **common duct**, and into the **duodenum** to digest these fats. The smooth muscles that line the gallbladder are squeezed down. If a stone is present, it lodges in the cystic duct and prevents the outflow of bile. The continued force by the muscles increases pressure in the gallbladder, which stretches the wall of the organ and causes pain. When the contraction of these smooth muscles relaxes, the stone frequently falls free, allowing the bile to run out and preventing infection.

This condition is called *acute **cholecystitis** without infection*. Such a condition is most likely recurrent, is associated with fatty foods, and produces excessive flatulence; belching; and left upper quadrant, or epigastric, pain. Although this condition is painful to the patient, it is not an acute situation that requires hospitalization and operative management. However, if the stone does not fall free, the bile does not empty from the gallbladder and the gallbladder becomes stagnant and infected. This condition is called *acute cholecystitis with infection*. If not treated within 24 or 48 hours, this condition can deteriorate into severe inflammation leading to abscess formation in an extremely ill patient. It is difficult to distinguish between these two conditions, and it is impossible to do so outside of the hospital. Emergency department evaluation of these patients is usually necessary, although a physician who knows the history of the specific patient may be able determine whether infection is present.

Pancreas

The pancreas is divided into two parts that have separate functions:

1. *Endocrine part*. The pancreas produces insulin, which metabolizes glucose and carries it into the blood cells (see the diabetes section in Chapter 17 for a more detailed description of insulin production).
2. *Exocrine part*. The pancreas takes part in the digestion of food.

The exocrine part of the pancreas provides enzymes (e.g., **amylase** and **lipase**) to assist in the digestion of food, especially fats. The presence of food in the GI tract stimulates the pancreas to produce these enzymes. Some of the functions of this digestion are similar to those of the salivary glands, particularly the parotid gland. In is difficult for chemical analysis of the blood to determine whether the amylase is produced by the parotid gland or the pancreas.

Blockage of the ducts leading from the pancreas to the duodenum or inflammation of the pancreatic cells produces pain and sometimes leakage of the pancreatic enzymes into the tissue surrounding the pancreas. This inflammation can produce additional pain and can progress to hemorrhage or necrosis of the pancreas. Hemorrhagic pancreatitis and necrotic pancreatitis are critical illnesses that require intensive care unit (ICU) evaluation and management of the patient.

The presence of pancreatitis with back pain and epigastric pain associated with nausea and vomiting may indicate alcohol abuse. Such patients have frequent GI hemorrhage (cirrhosis of the liver), frequently vomit and aspirate, have a very distended abdomen, and are jaundiced.

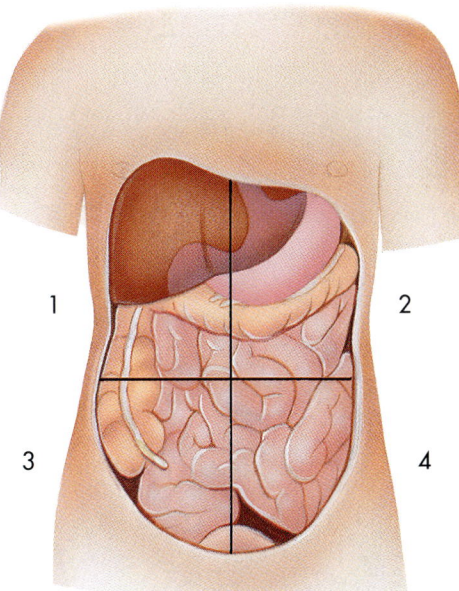

FIGURE 26.4 As with any part of the body, the better the description of pain, tenderness, and guarding, etc., the more accurate the diagnosis. The most common system of identification divides the abdomen into four quadrants: left and right upper, and left and right lower.

Appendix

Another cause of abdominal pain secondary to inflammation of the peritoneal lining is inflammation of the appendix, which is called **appendicitis**. If the opening in the appendix becomes obstructed, inflammation occurs within the lumen and the tissues become edematous, which leads to compression of the capillaries, ischemia, and perforation of the appendix. Such perforation can be into either the free peritoneal cavity or the fat surrounding the appendix, producing an abscess. The pain usually begins in the area around the umbilicus and is associated with nausea or other GI symptoms. The pain migrates over a period of 6 to 8 hours into the right lower quadrant. The localized inflammation in the right lower quadrant produces abdominal guarding and other signs of inflammation.

Kidneys

A kidney stone either in the pelvis of the kidney or along the length of the ureter can produce some of the most severe acute pain. Most often the patient is found pacing

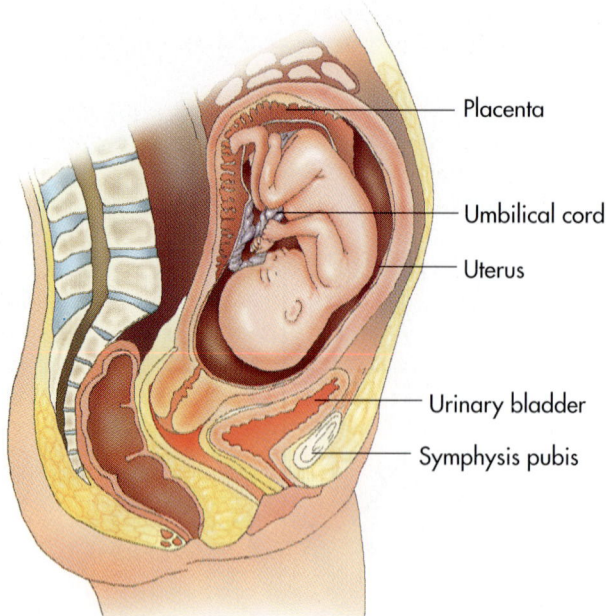

FIGURE 26.5 In a pregnant patient, as the uterus and fetus enlarge above the symphysis pubis, the fetus becomes more susceptible to both blunt and penetrating trauma.

the floor or "writhing" in pain. Pain associated with peritoneal inflammation is made worse by movement; however, since **renal (kidney) stones** do not cause inflammation of the peritoneum, pain in the ureter is not made worse by movement. The patient tends to move around a lot to try to get in a comfortable position as a distraction from the pain. Abdominal examination of a patient with kidney stones is frequently benign despite the fact that the patient is complaining of severe pain.

Female Reproductive Organs

Inflammation of the **gynecologic** organs can produce either chronic or acute pain. Because these organs are covered by peritoneum, the inflammation leads to pain. Inflammation of the gynecologic organs occurs in the lower abdomen or just to the right or left of the midline, depending on which parts of the organs are involved.

Assessment

The assessment of intraabdominal and retroperitoneal pain is frequently difficult in the hospital and even more difficult in the field. The only diagnosis that the surgeon caring for the patient usually makes is whether the patient needs exploration. Frequently the patient's condition is such that the diagnosis is too difficult to make effectively. It can be best diagnosed and handled by visualization of the organs, so the patient must go directly to the operating room. Exploration of the abdominal cavity identifies the pathologic process that is present, and steps are taken to fix or remove the affected organ.

If the surgeon makes the decision not to operate on the patient, then prolonged follow-up is often necessary. This can be extensive over the next 2 or 3 days with multiple x-ray, laboratory, and other evaluations, or it can be carried out on an outpatient basis with the patient reporting frequently to the physician from home.

Neither of these situations lends itself to prehospital evaluation. Therefore just as the surgeon must decide whether to operate on the patient, the EMT must decide whether to transport the patient to the hospital for evaluation and workup that is not available in the field. The EMT must decide whether the patient has an inflammatory or other acute intraabdominal problem that requires transportation to the hospital. Complex abdominal examinations in an attempt to make a specific diagnosis in the field are difficult in the hands of an older experienced physician and even more difficult in the hands of a younger EMT. Therefore the EMT should not waste time in the field with complex evaluations. The EMT should transport the patient to the emergency department where this evaluation can be done in a more controlled environment.

History

The EMT should take a careful history in the field or on the way to the hospital from the patient, family members, or friends who know about the condition or the circumstances that led up to the onset of the illness. Although it may not influence the decision to transport (the EMT may already have made that decision), this information may help the physicians in the emergency department make decisions regarding patient treatment. The patient may be unable or unwilling to provide this information. Those on the scene may not accompany the patient to the hospital; therefore if the EMT does not obtain this important information and provide it to the physicians, it may be lost and the outcome or management may be changed adversely for the patient.

Information should include the following:

- Duration of the patient's illness
- Time of onset
- Factors that may have influenced the onset (e.g., where, when, and types of food the patient ate; whether others ate the same food; whether they became sick)

- Recent trauma to the abdomen (falls or fights)
- Associated conditions such as pregnancy (Figure 26.5), sexual trauma, or assault
- Drug use (both legal and illegal)
- Medications that the patients is taking
- Recent hospitalizations

Physical Examination

The assessment of the abdomen of a trauma patient in the field is relatively simple. In a trauma situation the EMT first looks for penetrations, lacerations, exposed bowel, or bruising that indicate significant intraabdominal injury. Evidence of this nature indicates intraabdominal injury or pathology, and the EMT should transport the patient.

If there are no significant signs of trauma or severe medical illness, the second step is the physiologic evaluation. The EMT should consider the following questions:

- Is the patient hypotensive secondary to hypovolemia?
- Is the patient tachycardic?
- Does the patient have tachypnea or other symptoms of hypovolemia?
- Does the patient have a distended abdomen?
- Does the patient have a fractured pelvis?
- Does the patient have lower rib fractures?
- Is the patient's abdomen tender?
- Is the patient showing signs of guarding?

If the answer to any of these questions is yes, the EMT should transport the patient immediately for a more adequate evaluation.

Hemorrhage is the most critical of all these factors. If hemorrhage is allowed to progress unchecked, blood loss and complications of blood loss will continue, requiring more blood loss replacement. This can result in complications of blood replacement, in which case the patient's condition will become critical. Rapid transportation to the highest level of trauma care in the community is mandatory. The EMT should not take the patient to the closest hospital if it is not committed to the immediate management of major injuries.

Management

Management of intraabdominal trauma or suspected intraabdominal trauma is rapid transportation to a medical facility as is management of major medical conditions. En route to the medical facility, the EMT should protect these patients with supplemental oxygen. For the trauma patient, delivered oxygen (FiO_2) should be 0.85 or greater. For the medical patient, FiO_2 should be at least 0.40 during transportation.

Summary

- This chapter defines the difficulty in determining the severity of abdominal injuries based on the information that can be identified in the field. The possibility of injury must be determined, and if appropriate, the patient must be rapidly transported to the hospital.

Scenario Solution

This problem requires the EMT to use tact and his or her physiologic, pathophysiologic, and psychologic knowledge.

A. Kinematics
  1. Baseball bat to the rib cage
  2. Cavitation of the rib cage and underlying structures
  3. Compression of the solid organs
  4. Overpressure to the associated anatomic cavities

B. Anatomy
  1. Spleen
  2. Lungs
  3. Thoracic cavity
  4. Abdominal cavity
  5. Rib cage
  6. Diaphragm

Scenario Solution (cont'd)

C. Pathophysiology
1. Overpressure to the lungs
   a. Pneumothorax
      (1) Decreased lung expansion
      (2) Decreased ventilation
      (3) Decreased oxygenation
   b. Contusion of lung parenchyma
      (1) Decreased ventilation capacity
         (a) Hemorrhage into alveoli
         (b) Reduced circulation through contused area
2. Fracture of the ribs
   a. Hemorrhage from intercostal arteries and veins
   b. Reduction of ventilation
      (1) Pain from the fracture
      (2) Flail chest
3. Fracture of the spleen
   a. Severe hemorrhage
   b. Hypovolemia

D. Assessment
1. Open airway
2. Ventilation
   a. Tachypnea (30 breaths/min)
   b. Painful
3. Circulation
   a. Tachycardia (110 beats/min)
   b. Decreased blood pressure
   c. Decreased pulse pressure
   d. Normal blood flow

E. Impression
1. Compromised ventilation?
   a. Tachypnea
   b. Pain with ventilation
   c. Tachycardia
2. Hypovolemia (hemorrhage)?
   a. Tachypnea
   b. Tachycardia
   c. Decreased blood pressure
   d. Decreased pulse pressure
3. Anaerobic metabolism?
   a. Tachycardia

F. Analysis
1. Decreased ventilation
   a. Possible causes
      (1) Pneumothorax
      (2) Pain from multiple rib fractures
   b. Management
      (1) Transportation to hospital
      (2) FiO_2 of 0.85 en route
      (3) Detailed assessment by physician
      (4) Chest x-ray examination
      (5) Chest tube if indicated
      (6) Pain medication to improve ventilation if no other etiology
2. Hypovolemia
   a. Possible causes
      (1) Hemorrhage from fractured spleen
   b. Management
      (1) Transportation to hospital
      (2) FiO_2 of 0.85
      (3) Detailed assessment by physician
      (4) IV fluids as necessary
3. Other causes
   a. Excitement and stress of the event
      (1) Tachycardia certainly could result for this, but hypotension and reduced pulse pressure would not. Tachypnea could be a result of either.

G. Field treatment
1. Transport the patient to the hospital with above en route treatment.
2. Explain to the patient and coach that although the patient may have only fractured ribs, the chances of an injured spleen and a pneumothorax are great enough that the patient should have more evaluation than the EMT can provide in the field. His long-term chances of playing college baseball and professional baseball would be much better if he did not go into shock, which can lead to death.

Key Terms

Abscess Walled off infection that contains pus.
Amylase Enzymes measured in the blood from the pancreas.
Appendicitis Infection of the appendix.
Cholecystitis Infection of the gall bladder.
Colon Large bowel.
Common duct Connection from the liver to the duodenum.

Key Terms (cont'd)

Costovertebral angle Angle of the ribs and the spine.
Duodenum First part of the small bowel.
Endocrine Secretion of glands.
Fistula Abnormal connection between two organs or one organ and the outside of the body.
Gallbladder Sack that stores bile.
Gastrointestinal (GI) tract Food tract from the mouth to the anus.
Gynecologic Pertaining to the study of the diseases of the female reproductive organs.
Inflammation Infection.
Liver Large organ in the upper abdomen.
Lipase Secretion from the pancreas and salivary gland.
Pancreas Gland located in the abdomen that makes both digestive enzymes and insulin.

Paraspinal muscles Supporting muscles of the spine.
Peritoneum Serous membrane covering the organs and lining the abdominal cavity.
Peritonitis Infection of the peritoneum.
Rectus abdominis Large muscle in the center of the anterior abdominal wall.
Renal (kidney) stones Stones formed in the kidney.
Retroperitoneal space Space or potential space behind the abdomen.
Small intestine Duodenum, ileum, and jejunum.
Stomach Collection organ for food where digestion begins with hydrochloric acid.
Ulcers Chronic wounds in skin or muscle lining of the GI tract.

Review Questions

1. Signs of shock do not necessarily occur early with abdominal hemorrhage because:
   a. There are no organs in the abdomen that hemorrhage easily.
   b. The abdominal compartment and the capsules of the organs can contain hemorrhage for a short period of time.
   c. The liver and spleen do not have a large blood supply.
   d. The organs that bleed most easily are retroperitoneal organs.
2. All of the following contribute to the lack of early signs of an acute surgical abdomen except:
   a. Bacterial contamination from a hole in the intestine requires up to 24 hours to produce enough infection for significant abdominal pain.
   b. Free blood in the peritoneal cavity does not by itself produce enough irritation of the peritoneum to produce pain.
   c. Chemical irritation (such as hydrochloric acid from a perforated ulcer) is not an irritant of the peritoenum and therefore produces pain over a period of 12 to 24 hours.
   d. Bile alone in the peritoneal cavity does not produce pain.
3. Appendicitis is more common in the young adult or child and diverticulitis more often produces symptoms in the older adult because after 50 years of age the appendix closes off and cannot become infected. The two parts of the statement are:
   a. True, true and related
   b. True, false
   c. False, true
   d. False, false
4. All of the following are complications of GI tract disease except:
   a. Perforation
   b. Abscess
   c. Fistula
   d. Obstruction
   e. All of the above are correct.
5. Kidney stones produce all of the following except:
   a. Hemorrhage into the urine
   b. Pain without abdominal signs such as guarding and tenderness is rare
   c. Sharp and stabbing pain
   d. Some of the most severe pain associated with abdominal conditions
6. The bowel movements associated with upper gastrointestinal hemorrhage have all of the following characteristics except:
   a. Black color and tarry consistency
   b. Dark red port wine color with diarrhea
   c. White color and foamy appearance
   d. Foul smell
7. Sudden onset of severe abdominal pain is most often associated with which of the following conditions?
   a. Appendicitis
   b. Ovarian cyst
   c. Diverticulitis
   d. Perforated ulcer

Answers to these Review Questions can be found at the end of the book on page 866.

27

Spinal Trauma

Lesson Goal

Of all the injuries that can produce a lifelong debilitation, spinal cord trauma is the most severe. No young patient wishes to be a paraplegic or quadraplegic for the remainder of his or her life. If the patient has a spinal injury but without a cord injury, the EMT can protect the patient from further injury by providing proper immobilization. The use of the long or short back board to provide such stabilization is not difficult and does not prolong prehospital time more than a minute or two when properly applied. Patients who have spinal fractures but do not yet have cord injuries frequently do not have signs of symptoms that indicate this condition. Only with appropriate radiographs in the hospital can such injuries be ruled out. On occasion it is difficult to rule out such injuries even in the emergency department. Some patients may be in the hospital for several days before definitive studies can completely eliminate the possibility. Therefore the EMT-B spend excessive time in the field performing multiple neurologic examinations on the patient when it is easier and quicker to transport the patient to the emergency department where a more complete examination can be done is incorrect use of prehospital time and can delay life-saving care for other injuries.

Scenario

Hunter Scott fancies himself a pretty good rodeo clown. One day he was clowning around with his clown friends in a pasture, and unbeknownst to them there was a bull in the pasture. Unfortunately, Hunter Scott did not have his barrel with him to hide in and the bull came at Hunter at a full run. Luckily the bull did not have horns. Hunter's clown friends said he was thrown about "20 feet" into the air. Hunter is walking around "in a daze" state his friends, saying "all kinds of crazy things."

> **?** When you arrive on the scene, your partner gets the history from the bystanders while you go to Hunter Scott and manage his potential injuries. What do you do? Discuss the mechanism of injury. What does your mind's eye see when imagining the mechanism of injury? What complications and injuries will you be looking for? How would you treat this patient?

Spinal Trauma | Chapter 27   505

Key Terms to Know

Autonomic nervous system
Central nervous system
Cervical collar
Compression fracture
Diagonal slide
Distraction injuries

In-line stabilization
Intervertebral disk
Lateral bending
Long spine board (LSB)
Mandible
Motor nerves

Newton's first law of motion
Paraplegia
Peripheral nervous system
Quadriplegia
Sensory nerves
Short spine board

Somatic nervous system
Spinal column
Vertebrae

Learning Objectives

As an EMT-Basic, you should be able to do the following:

DOT

- Describe the central nervous system.
- Describe the peripheral nervous system.
- Define the structure of the skeletal system as it relates to the nervous system.
- Relate mechanism of injury to potential injuries of the head and spine.
- Describe the implications of not properly caring for potential spinal injuries.
- State the signs and symptoms of a potential spinal injury.
- Describe the method of determining if a responsive patient may have a spinal injury.
- Relate the airway emergency medical care techniques to the patient with a suspected spinal injury.
- Describe how to stabilize the cervical spine.
- Discuss indications for sizing and using a cervical spine immobilization device.
- Establish the relationship between airway management and the patient with head and spinal injuries.
- Describe a method for sizing a cervical spine immobilization device.
- Describe how to logroll a patient with a suspected spinal injury.
- Describe how to secure a patient to a long spine board.
- List instances when a short spine board should be used.
- Describe how to immobilize a patient using a short spine board.
- Describe indications for the use of rapid extrication.
- List steps in performing rapid extrication.
- State the circumstances when a helmet should be left on a patient.
- Discuss the circumstances when a helmet should be removed.
- Identify different types of helmets.
- Describe the unique characteristics of sports helmets.
- Explain the preferred methods for removal of a helmet.
- Discuss alternative methods for removal of a helmet.
- Describe how the patient's head is stabilized to remove the helmet.
- Differentiate how the head is stabilized with a helmet compared to without a helmet.
- Demonstrate opening of the airway in a patient with suspected spinal cord injury.
- Demonstrate evaluation of a responsive patient with a suspected spinal cord injury.
- Demonstrate stabilization of the cervical spine.
- Demonstrate the four-person logroll for a patient with a suspected spinal cord injury.
- Demonstrate how to logroll a patient with a suspected spinal cord injury using two people.
- Demonstrate securing of a patient to a long spine board.
- Demonstrate use of the short board immobilization technique.
- Demonstrate the procedure for rapid extrication.
- Demonstrate preferred methods for stabilization of a helmet.
- Demonstrate helmet removal techniques.
- Demonstrate alternative methods for stabilization of a helmet.
- Demonstrate completion of a prehospital care report for patients with head and spinal injuries.

Supplemental

- Name the five sections of the spinal column.
- Define Newton's law of motion.
- Describe the importance of determining mechanism of injury.
- Define *lateral bending*.
- Describe the importance of in-line stabilization.
- Describe the steps of nervous system assessment.
- Describe the methods of assessing the nervous system.
- Describe the difference between in-line immobilization and cervical traction.

Patient Care Algorithm

Trauma Patient Assessment

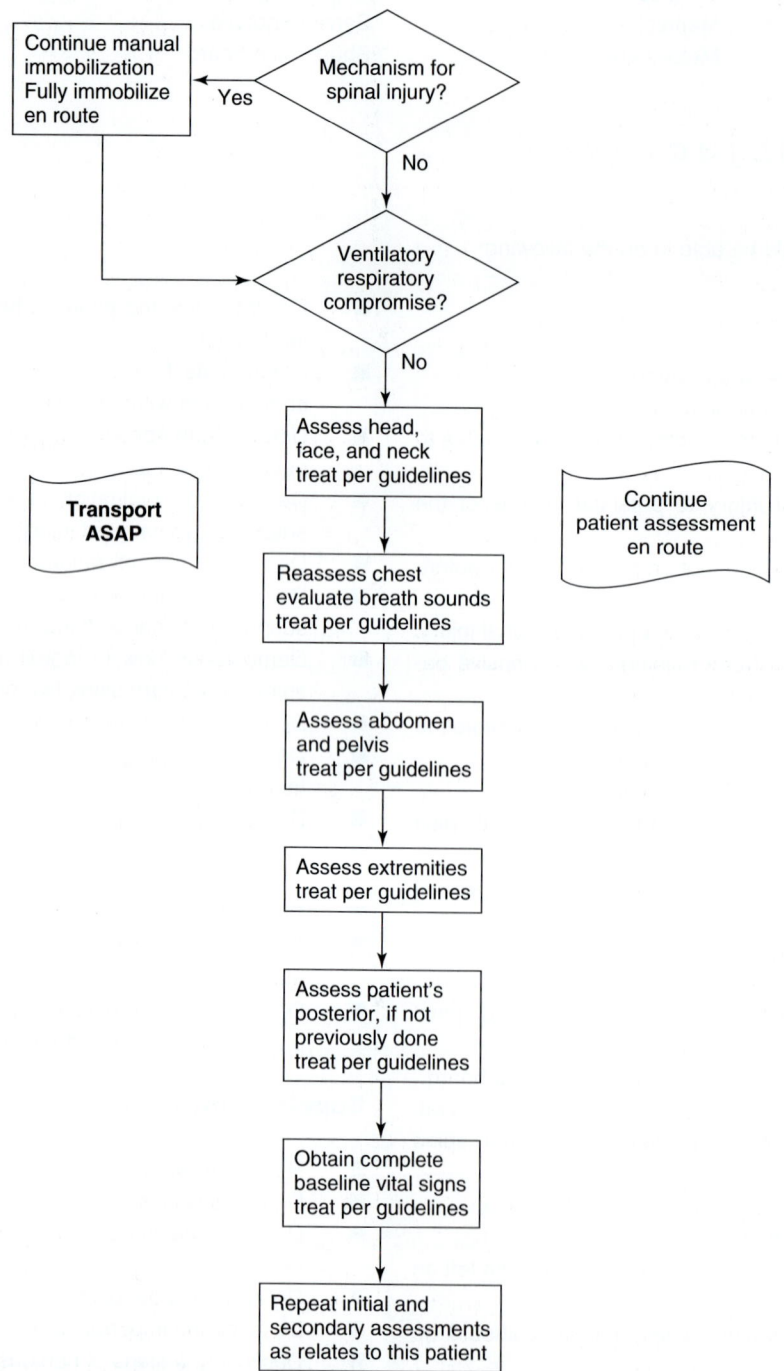

Throughout this text, *mechanism of injury* has been defined, explained, emphasized, and seen in each of the chapters in some way. Spinal precautions are one area where mechanism of injury is of utmost importance. Mechanism of injury will determine the use of spinal precautions and to some degree the definitive care the patient will receive in the hospital.

Spinal precautions are taken based on mechanism of injury. In most motor vehicle collisions, falls, trauma, and so on, spinal precautions are taken because of the mechanism of injury, and the care the patient receives in the hospital revolves around the information the emergency medical technician (EMT) relays to the hospital staff. Therefore the nervous system, level of consciousness, spinal anatomy, and spinal physiology are discussed in this chapter. All of this is tied into the building of knowledge received in other chapters, especially understanding the EMT's role in establishing the mechanism of injury.

The nervous system is an extremely complicated system that is not fully understood. Research continues into this vastly complex system. It is not the EMT-Basic's responsibility to understand the nervous system completely, only to understand enough to recognize a problem or something abnormal and correctly manage the potential condition. Is the patient's speech slurred because he or she has a head injury, or because of the amount of alcohol consumed? Is the patient combative because of hypoxia, head injury, hypoglycemia, or substance use? The EMT must make good use of bystanders and family to determine the normal activity of the patient and whether the patient is acting appropriately to the circumstances. A spouse or other family member or friend may say "he is just not acting right." Is that enough reason to take the patient to the emergency department (ED) and tell the ED staff that "the spouse states the patient isn't acting right"? Will the ED staff look at you like you are nuts, or will they gain a higher respect for you?

Although the nervous system is complicated, the basics are the most important for the EMT. This chapter discusses the different aspects of the nervous system, the divisions of the nervous system, the spinal cord and spinal column, and the difference between the two. Skills for the EMT-Basic and spinal precautions are discussed in detail. Immobilizing a patient on various spine boards and in various positions is also discussed. The EMT must know how and when to use the equipment that is available. Determining mechanism of injury and how to immobilize the patient is important to prevent further injury. One of the most important aspects of the Hippocratic oath is to do no harm. This chapter will help the EMT achieve that goal.

Nervous System

The nervous system is divided into two parts: the **central nervous system** and the **peripheral nervous system.** The central nervous system comprises the brain and the spinal cord. Its function is to decipher incoming messages and respond accordingly. A good way to remember its structure is to realize that it is the part of the nervous system that is enclosed within a bony cavity. The brain, of course, is encased in the cranial cavity, and the spinal cord is enclosed within the spinal column.

The peripheral nervous system comprises all the nerves that extend from the brain and spinal cord, which include the spinal and peripheral nerves. These nerves are the "phone lines" that carry nerve impulses to and from the central nervous system (Figure 27.1). These nerves, or *neurons,* the name of the particular type of cell, are not protected by a bony cavity, only by muscles and membranes.

The peripheral nervous system has two functional divisions: **sensory nerves** and **motor nerves.** The sensory nerves carry impulses from sensory receptors in the skin, muscles, or organs to the central nervous system—that is, to the spinal cord and then to the brain. They are the nerves that tell the brain something is wrong (or right). Sensory neurons provide the information, and the brain should respond accordingly. The sensory nerves provide all the information the brain receives. The motor nerves carry the response from the central nervous system to the organ or muscle. The part of the brain that received the message sends a response, which travels down the spinal cord and is sent to the area of the body needed to respond to the sensation.

The nervous system can also be broken down according to whether the action of the body is voluntary or involuntary. Activities that cannot be controlled by a person, such as the beating of the heart or the digestion of food, are controlled by the **autonomic nervous system.** This control is in contrast to that exerted by the **somatic nervous system,** which is the part of the nervous system that is voluntary. The somatic nervous system governs the kicking of a ball, the control of a pen, and the reading of this chapter.

The autonomic nervous system can further be divided into the parasympathetic and the sympathetic nervous system. The *parasympathetic nervous system* is that area of the system that concerns itself with the daily activities of the body—for example, the normal regulation of the heartbeat, motility of the gastrointestinal (GI) system, and the hormones the body must make and send to other areas to control everyday life of the body. The *sympathetic nervous system* is the part of the nervous system that the EMT usually sees the most of on calls. This is the

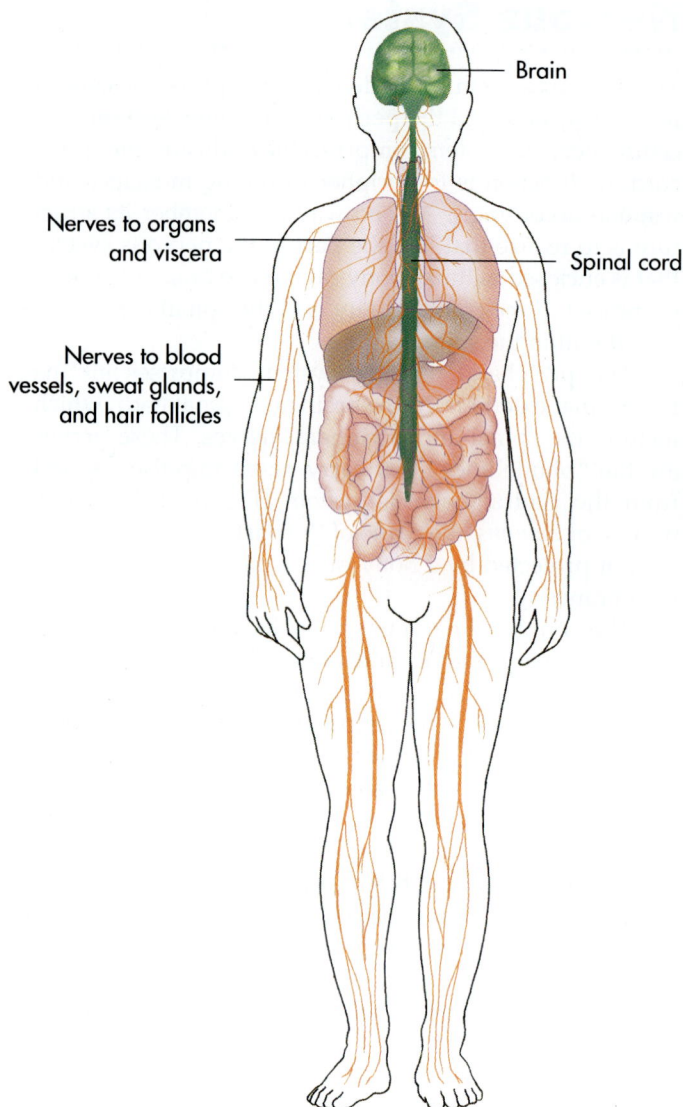

FIGURE 27.1 The central nervous system consists of the brain and spinal cord. The nerves make up the peripheral nervous system.

part of the system that responds during what is termed the *fight or flight syndrome.* A widely used analogy to describe the fight or flight syndrome is what happens physiologically to the body when one is faced with a bear. Because the brain is most concerned with running from the bear, the brain tells the heart rate to increase, delivering more oxygen to the cells so the body can run faster. The body also needs to see the bear, or to see how to run away from the bear, so the pupils dilate. The body is not concerned with the GI system, so the gastric motility, or the movement of the small intestine, slows down. Urine output decreases because the brain wants to save all of its energy to run. The blood vessels constrict so that the blood goes only to the parts of the body that need it most. The respiratory rate increases to ensure that the body has enough oxygen to be able to run away from the bear.

The EMT will often see the effects of the fight or flight syndrome in times of patient distress, for obvious reasons. Most or all of the signs and symptoms will be seen: increased heart rate, increased respiratory rate, vasoconstriction, pupil dilation, decreased urine output, and gastric motility. The EMT need not understand all aspects of the syndrome, but must be able to recognize and treat the effects. This syndrome is seen in patients with shock from any reason, shortness of breath, heart attack, anaphylactic reaction, hemorrhage, severe trauma, diabetic emergency, or delivery of an infant; it may also be seen in the EMT's own excitement en route to a call.

There are many divisions of the nervous system, and each serves an important function. It is a great network of vastly different and complex parts and responsibilities. As stated, it is not necessary for the EMT-Basic to understand all aspects of the nervous system, only to know they exist and how they respond to different stimuli.

Anatomy of the Spine

The skeletal system encloses and protects organs of the nervous system. The spinal cord is enclosed by the **spinal column.** This column is composed of 33 bones called **vertebrae.** The vertebrae function to protect the spinal column. Thus, because the spinal cord is enclosed by the bony structure of the spinal cord, the spinal column is part of the central nervous system.

There are 7 cervical, 12 thoracic, 5 lumbar, 5 sacral, and 4 coccygeal vertebrae (Figure 27.2). Vertebrae are identified by the first letter of the region in which they are found and their sequence from the top of that region. The first cervical vertebra is called C1, the third thoracic vertebra is T3, and so on. Each of the cervical, thoracic, and lumbar vertebrae is cushioned by an **intervertebral disk,** which provides for the elasticity and compressibility of the vertebral column. The disks allow the spine to flex and also act as shock absorbers (Figure 27.3). The intervertebral disks are disks of tough cartilage that is filled with fluid. This cartilage and fluid can absorb energy so that the spinal cord is not damaged (e.g., when someone is jumping on a hard surface, the intervertebral disks absorb some of the shock that would be sustained by the spinal cord or vertebrae). The disks also provide for compressibility, such as when the body sustains the up-and-over injury during a motor vehicle collision. The intervertebral disks also allow the spinal column to be able to roll the neck around in circles; enable a person to bend over to pick up a penny; and enable a person to twist around to call out someone's name. If the intervertebral disks were not in place, the vertebrae would grind into

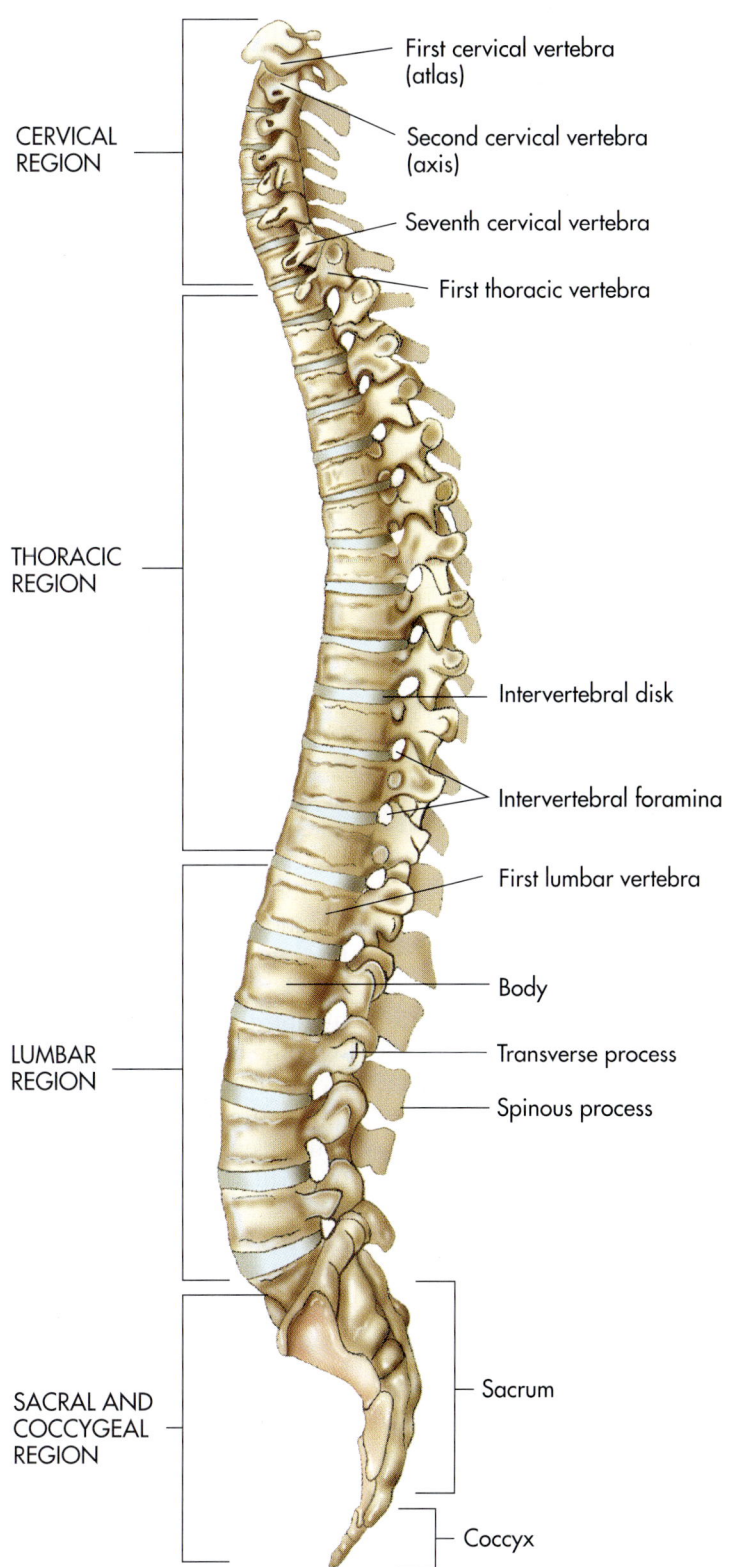

FIGURE 27.2 The spinal column is composed of 33 bones called vertebrae.

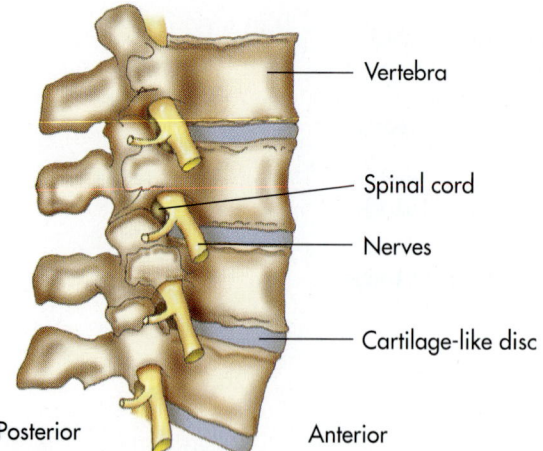

FIGURE 27.3 Each of the cervical, thoracic, and lumbar vertebrae is cushioned by an intervertebral disk that provides the elasticity and compressibility of the vertebral column. The disks allow the spine to flex and also act as shock absorbers.

each other and not protect the spinal cord as well, which is the function of the spinal column, the vertebrae, and the intervertebral disks.

Pathophysiology of the Spine

Mechanism of Injury

Determining the mechanism of injury is one of the crucial responsibilities of an EMT. The determination can begin while en route to the scene. The dispatcher will inform the crew of the type of call to be encountered, and from this information the EMTs can begin preparing for a possible spinal injury. Spinal injuries are seen in many situations. However, an EMT must always maintain a high index of suspicion, particularly when any of the following has occurred:

- Motor vehicle collision
- Pedestrian versus vehicle collision
- Fall
- Blunt trauma
- Motorcycle or bicycle collision
- Hanging
- Diving accident
- Unresponsive trauma victim

Newton's First Law of Motion

Newton's first law of motion states that an object in motion stays in motion until acted on by an outside force. As in all trauma, this law holds true in spinal injuries. In a motor vehicle collision, the torso continues moving until stopped by the seat restraint. If the torso is not stopped by the restraint, it continues its course until stopped by the steering wheel. The head, however, continues on its course until the torso is stopped, then proceeds further until the neck jerks it back. This force on the neck can cause many problems. This scenario is also true of pedestrian versus vehicle collisions; blunt trauma; penetrating trauma to the head, neck, or torso; and motorcycle or bicycle collisions. All of these situations can cause excessive flexion, extension, or rotation of the spine, specifically the cervical spine (Figure 27.4).

Flexion, Extension, Lateral Bending, and Rotation Injuries

As with all joints, the spinal column can also be hyperflexed or extended. There can be many causes; for example, in an motor vehicle collision the spine can be flexed or extended out of its normal range of motion by the impact of another car or object. The spine could be extended too far when the face is struck by a fist, baseball bat, or other object of force. This is why it is important to take spinal precautions in all patients with trauma above the clavicles. The force could be great enough to cause a flexion injury and damage the spinal cord or vertebrae. Rotation of the head and spine can also cause injury to the spinal column. Striking a head that is already turned could further rotate the spine past its normal range of motion. Physically forceful turning of the head simply with the hands can cause a rotation injury. A motor vehicle collision in which the car is left in a rotational spin may cause the spine and head to do the same. Spinal precautions must be taken in these instances to ensure that no further damage is done to the spine.

Lateral Bending

When evaluating the mechanism of injury, also consider **lateral bending** (bending of the spine from side to side). Lateral bending is seen most commonly in motor vehicle collisions involving a side impact. The impact to the side of the vehicle causes the spine to move in a lateral direction. Because of the center of gravity of the head, rotation provides a complicating factor of injury.

Compression Fracture

A compression injury is quite different from the previously mentioned kinds of trauma; however, results are the same injury to the spine. A **compression fracture** results in damage to the bones, specifically the vertebrae, produced by a force from above and below. This injury is seen in motor vehicle collisions in which the occupants are not restrained. Their heads strike the windshield and the skull stops, but the continued force of the forward motion of the torso provides pressure from below. Compression fractures also are seen in falls, diving into shallow water, and ejection from a motorcycle or automobile.

Distraction Injuries

Distraction injuries are those in which the spine is pulled apart. In this type of injury, ligaments and muscles are overstretched or torn. It is difficult to keep the vertebrae in proper alignment if the patient moves. This injury is seen in hangings or in certain collisions, such as a motor vehicle collision in which a child is restrained by a lap belt but no diagonal strap. The head acts as a distracting force, or a force that will allow separation of the vertebrae along the spine.

If you suspect or are not sure if the patient has spinal trauma, take spinal precautions. It is better to take a patient without a spinal injury to the hospital with full spinal precautions than to transport a patient with a spinal injury without spinal precautions. Overtreatment may result in using extra time and equipment, but undertreatment may result in **paraplegia** (paralysis from the waist down) or **quadriplegia** (paralysis from the neck down).

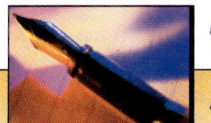

Tips from the Pros

A rule of thumb for spinal injuries is that for any trauma above the clavicle, the EMT should take spinal precautions.

✓ Determining the mechanism of injury is especially important in spinal management. Numerous types of injury can be determined from mechanism of injury, including compression, lateral bending, and distraction.

Assessment of Spinal Injuries

The signs and symptoms associated with spinal injuries range from quadriplegia and paraplegia to point tenderness and pain to no symptoms at all. Thus obtaining an accurate history of events and determining mechanism of injury are imperative. The patient's ability to walk should not determine whether the patient has a spinal injury. Approximately 15% to 20% of patients who required surgical repair of spinal injuries were found ambulatory on

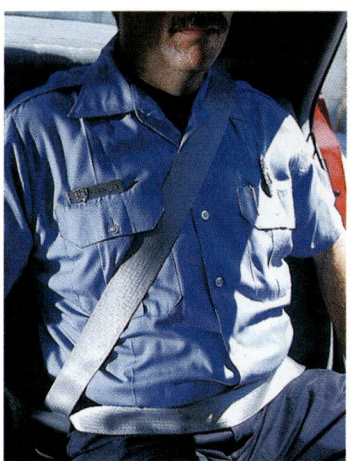

FIGURE 27.4 The restraint system absorbs impact energy.

the scene by the arriving EMTs, or the patients walked into the emergency department. In another incident, a man with a broken back walked 7 miles to a pay phone.

An unstable spine can be ruled out only by radiography. Thus the EMTs in the field should not guess if a patient has a spinal injury. When in doubt, take spinal precautions. In addition to the ability to walk, the ability to move extremities or feel sensation or the lack of pain to the spinal column also does not rule out the possibility of spinal column or cord damage.

As with all types of scenes the EMT will come into contact with, scene safety is the first assessment that must be made. Universal precautions must also be taken, and airway, breathing, and circulation (the ABCs) are the first things that are assessed. The only difference with the spinal patient may be assumption of spinal immobilization during the assessment of airway and breathing. The EMT should know before or immediately after arrival at the scene if spinal precautions are needed based on the mechanism of injury. If the decision has been made to take spinal precautions, the immobilization of the cervical spine (C-spine) is accomplished during airway and breathing. The EMT must always remember that scene safety, standard precautions, and assessment of ABCs are the first things to be accomplished and treated appropriately.

The best time to control the spine is before assessing the airway. The EMT is already at the patient's head and is in a perfect position to maintain the spine. Spinal immobilization should be maintained until spinal injury has been completely ruled out. See the Manual In-line Immobilization Skill Sheet at the end of this chapter.

Tenderness in the areas of injury is a symptom of possible cervical spine trauma. Pain provoked by movement is also an important finding. Do not ask the patient to move to try to elicit a pain response. If the patient experiences pain on palpation or movement, note this information and take special care to immobilize the patient's spine. Ask the patient not to move his or her head while answering questions but to give only verbal responses. If hypoxia is also suspected, causing the patient to be anxious and combative, assistance may be required to calm the patient and ensure his or her compliance. However, the patient must be kept still. In addition to spinal precautions, the patient should be given high-concentration oxygen.

Pain independent of movement or palpation is also an indication that the spine may be injured. This pain may be intermittent and is usually felt along the spinal column or in the lower legs. While palpating the spine, any obvious deformity of the spine should be noted. If deformity is found, do not aggravate it by palpating harder. Palpation may cause further damage. Any soft tissue injury noted to head or neck, shoulders or back, abdomen, or lower extremities is an indication of a possible spinal injury. These injuries may be indicative of injury to the cervical, lumbar, thoracic, or sacral spine, respectively. Any numbness, weakness, or tingling in the extremities can indicate loss of spinal integrity. Incontinence (inability to control bladder excretion) also can indicate spinal injury.

Of course, the single most obvious sign or symptom of spine injury is loss of sensation or paralysis below the suspected level of injury and loss of sensation or paralysis in the upper or lower extremities. It is important, if the patient's condition permits, to do a complete motor and sensory evaluation to provide a baseline identification of the level of injury. When approaching the scene, it can generally be determined if the patient is responsive. As mentioned earlier, the best time to gain control of the patient's spine is during the initial assessment. Be sure to inform the responsive patient about what is being done. Not only does the EMT have a legal obligation to inform the patient as to what is being performed, but it also reassures the patient, thus increasing the likelihood of compliance. A patient who is unresponsive may be able to hear. Talk to the patient in either situation.

After completing the initial assessment, and while still maintaining spinal immobilization, ask the patient what happened. This question is asked for several reasons. Not only is it necessary to ascertain the mechanism of injury, but it is also important to determine if the patient remembers what happened and if there was any loss of consciousness. If the patient answers coherently, or even incoherently, the EMT can determine a great deal concerning the severity of the patient's condition.

A number of questions can be asked of the patient with possible spinal injury. Where is the pain? What happened? Did the patient lose consciousness? Does his or her neck or back hurt? Can he or she move hands and feet? Can the patient feel the EMT touching the fingers or toes? Instruct the patient to answer verbally, not by moving the body or head.

While ensuring that a reliable person maintains the patient's spine, inspect for contusions, deformities, lacerations, punctures, penetrations, and swelling of the head, neck, shoulders, back, abdomen, and lower extremities. Palpate for areas of tenderness or deformity. Assess equality of strength of extremities by taking both of the patient's hands and asking the patient to grip and by asking the patient to gently push his or her feet against the EMT's hands. This test establishes if the patient has weakness on one side.

In the case of the unresponsive patient, the EMT must rely on bystanders to obtain an accurate history and to ascertain the mechanism of injury. Bystanders may have information about where the patient is found, damage to the vehicle, if the patient fell, if the patient was pulled from a pool, and so forth. The bystanders can also assist the EMT with assessing the patient's mental status before the arrival of emergency medical services (EMS). Any unresponsive patient who has evidence of trauma should be immediately suspected of spinal injury until proven otherwise by x-ray.

> ✓ Never ignore a patient. Treat the patient and explain carefully what is happening to the patient, even if the patient is not responsive and is unable to answer questions. The patient may still able to hear. Be careful what you say; it is not uncommon for a patient to recall everything you said, be it bad or good. Never talk about the patient as if he or she were not there.

> ✓ Signs and symptoms of spinal injuries range from quadriplegia to no symptoms whatsoever. An unstable spine can be ruled out only by x-ray. When in doubt, take spinal precautions. An unresponsive patient who has evidence of trauma is suspected to have spinal injury.

> ✓ Any patient who has trauma above the clavicles is suspected of also sustaining spinal injuries and must have spinal precautions taken immediately.

> ### McSwain-Paturas Spinal Assessment System (MPSAS)
>
> S—Suspicion of injury (kinematics)
> P—Pain in any part of the spine
> I—Immobilization of any part of the spine by the patient
> N—Neurologic examination of all extremities
> E—Examine the patient again after placing on the long board
>
> *Suspicion of injury.* On arrival at the scene, what happened? What motions did the patient go through at the time of impact? Would any of these potential motions stress the spine? If so, the spine must be protected.
>
> *Pain.* Is the patient complaining of pain in any part of the spine? Are there injuries in other parts of the body that would distract the patient's attention from pain in the spine?
>
> *Immobilization of the spine.* Is the spine held by the patient in an unusual position? Does the patient not move because of pain, or does the patient not move because some part of the body is paralyzed?
>
> *Neurologic examination.* A quick but complete neurologic examination should be preformed to detect any areas of the skin that are without feeling or if there are any muscles that are paralyzed.
>
> *Examination.* After the patient is secured to the backboard, the neurologic examination should be repeated to ensure that it did not change when the patient was moved to the board.

Management of Spinal Injuries

General Principles

Patients with a possible spinal injury can be found in almost any position, including horizontal position (supine, prone, or in a lateral recumbent position), sitting position, or in a vertical (standing) position. The position in which the patient is found does not minimize the possibility of spinal injury. In all cases, spinal in-line immobilization precautions must be taken immediately if the mechanism of injury so dictates. All three of these positions are discussed in this section.

It would be convenient if the patient was supine on the EMT's arrival at the scene; however, patients may be found in any number of positions. If the patient is found in a supine position, it is simple to maintain the spine and establish a patent airway. The EMT must put the patient's head in a neutral in-line position to open the airway, and this is an opportune time to establish control of the spine. Use a jaw-thrust lift without head tilt to establish a patent airway on an unresponsive patient with a suspected spinal injury (see Chapter 10).

Some patients are found in a prone or lateral recumbent position at the scene. Assuming the patient is in a horizontal position, maintain the spine in the position found and establish an open airway while another EMT performs a quick assessment for hemorrhage or possible fractures. The patient is then logrolled as a unit into the supine position, preferably onto a spine board. The EMT, in the span of approximately 10 to 15 seconds, has established an airway (either the patient has control of his or her own airway or the EMT performs a jaw-thrust maneuver), maintained in-line immobilization, performed a quick assessment to provide the crew with a general idea of the patient's injuries, and placed the patient in a position that is more desirable for the EMTs to perform a more thorough assessment and to extricate the patient. Once the patient is in a supine position, the EMT can more efficiently assess the patient's airway, as well as perform artificial ventilation or apply oxygen while maintaining in-line spinal immobilization.

The one drawback that exists in maintaining in-line immobilization is that one EMT must remain at the patient's head and must not move or relinquish this duty until the patient has been immobilized to the long backboard. The EMT is not free to assist his or her partner. However, if this duty is not performed or is performed incorrectly, the patient may sustain a lifelong or possibly fatal injury. Therefore maintaining in-line control of the spine may be the most important skill performed. Manual **in-line stabilization** must be constantly maintained until the patient is properly secured to a backboard with the head and body immobilized.

While one EMT maintains manual in-line immobilization, the other must continue the assessment while

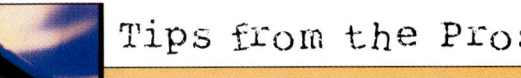

> **Tips from the Pros**
>
> The EMT at the head of the patient can use his or her knees to maintain in-line immobilization by sitting down on the ground with the lower legs tucked under the thighs and placing the patient's head between the EMT's knees. The EMT is then able to perform an initial assessment and focused assessment up to the patient's waist. The EMT at the patient's head who maintains in-line immobilization is in a perfect position to supervise all activities and should therefore be the "chief."

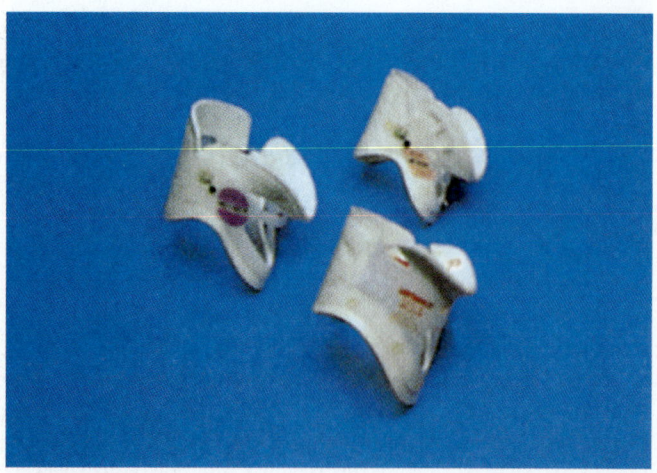

FIGURE 27.5 Types of rigid cervical spine immobilization devices.

paying close attention to assessing pulse, movement, and sensation in all extremities. Once the assessment is complete, assess the cervical region and neck and apply a rigid cervical spine immobilization device. Be sure to properly size the cervical spine immobilization device (if it does not fit, place rolled towels on each side of the head, tape head and towels to board, and have the other EMT hold the head manually). An improperly fitting immobilization device will do more harm than good.

Equipment

The basics of spinal immobilization equipment have sustained the test of time and have not changed much in the past 25 years. Newer models of backboards and cervical collars have become available that are more comfortable for the patient and more convenient and easier to use for the EMT.

Cervical Collar

The **cervical collar** is a valuable piece of equipment used for immobilization of the cervical spine and thus the entire spine. The cervical collar as a complete immobilizer, however, is a misnomer. The collar does not completely immobilize the spine but acts more as a reminder to the patient not to move his or her head. The cervical collar used to be made of a soft cushiony material, termed a *soft collar*, but the hard plastic collars are the preferred material prehospital. There are several manufacturers of cervical collars, and most EMTs have their own personal preference. Most EMS services also purchase a specific kind of cervical collar. The type of cervical collar used is usually the type the EMS uses.

Most cervical collars now are made of two pieces of hard plastic that Velcro together on the lateral aspects of the neck. They come in various sizes, usually pediatric, small, medium, large, and no-neck. It is extremely important to use the correct size of collar for the patient. If the collar is not sized correctly, the neck will either have too much area to move around in, or the neck will be hyperflexed, meaning the neck will not be in an in-line position. This may do more harm than good.

Long Spine Boards

The **long spine board (LSB)** is the device used to immobilize the body. LSBs can be made of wood, plastic, metal, or other substances. Wooden spine boards are no longer recommended by the Occupational Safety and Health Administration (OSHA) because wood absorbs body fluids, can become contaminated, and is harder to clean.

As with the cervical collar, use of specific types of spine boards is determined by the service that uses them. However, EMTs will develop their personal preference, usually by what they learn with or use most commonly. The type of LSB will depend on the situation and the equipment that will serve best to extricate the patient. For instance, for hip fractures it may be easier to use a scoop stretcher or an LSB. To anatomically immobilize a patient, in general, it is easier to use an LSB, or in the case of a sitting patient, a short spine board in conjunction with an LSB. With experience and instruction, the EMT will be able to use critical thinking skills to understand which of the devices should be used.

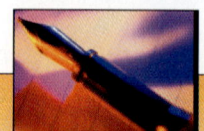

Tips from the Pros

Do not have a closed mind concerning the use of different types of equipment. Even though you may get used to using a certain kind of LSB, do not be afraid to try new kinds of LSBs, straps, and tape. You might find something else that you like better.

Skills

Spinal Immobilization

The rule of thumb for spinal immobilization is that it should be used for any trauma above the clavicles. This criterion, of course, includes most frontal or lateral motor vehicle collisions with major damage to the vehicle, rollover crashes, or any suspected injury to the spine based on mechanism of injury, history, or signs and symptoms.

Various types of rigid cervical spine immobilization devices are available today, and it is the responsibility of the EMT to be familiar with the device used by his or her service (Figure 27.5). An improperly sized cervical spine immobilization device may further injure the patient. It is

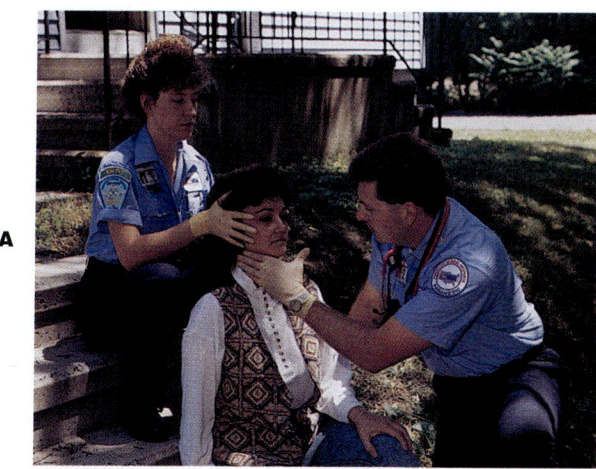 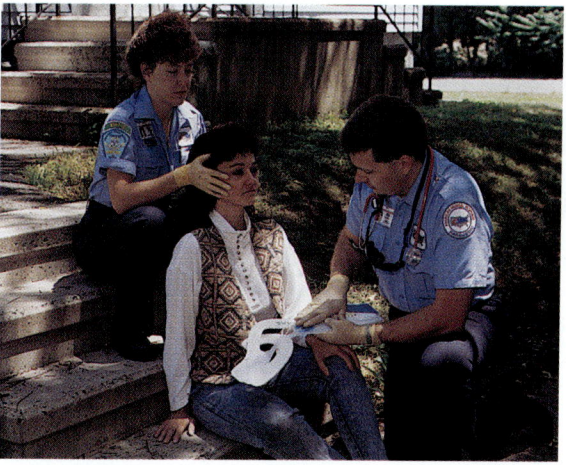

FIGURE 27.6 Sizing a cervical spine immobilization device. **A,** Measure the width of the patient's neck. **B,** Measure the device. Make sure the chin piece of the device will not hyperextend the patient's neck or lift the chin.

important to note that the rigid cervical spine immobilization device is more of a reminder to the patient not to move the head than it is an actual immobilization device. Instruct the patient not to move his or her head and to answer questions with a verbal response rather than shaking or nodding the head. Be sure not to obstruct the airway with a too-small collar. Always use cervical spine immobilization devices in conjunction with short and long backboards. Manual stabilization must always be used in conjunction with a cervical spine immobilization device until the head is secured to a spine board (Figure 27.6).

Some patients may feel that they cannot breathe with a cervical spine immobilization device in place, but in fact the device does not restrict breathing. If the patient can speak, the patient can breathe with the device in place. The patient might be more comfortable breathing through the mouth.

Long Spine Board

The long spine board, or backboard, provides full-body spinal immobilization. Several different types of long backboards are available. Among these are the traditional wooden backboards and the scoop stretcher. In recent years these devices have been improved, and they are now made of different materials. The use of the long backboard device should depend on familiarity and availability. As the EMT spends more time in the field, he or she will develop a preference for one type or the other; however, the EMT should be flexible and be able to use any type. Long backboards should be used on patients found in a supine, prone, lateral recumbent, standing, or sitting position. Sometimes these devices are used in conjunction with a **short spine board.**

When the patient is ready to be placed on the long spine board, one EMT maintains manual in-line immobilization. The other EMT positions the board next to the patient with the top of the board approximately 1 to 1.5 feet above the patient's head. The EMT at the patient's head directs the movement of the patient. It is this EMT's responsibility to ensure that the cervical spine stays in line with the rest of the body during the roll and to "count" the roll. One to three other EMTs control the movement of the rest of the body. On the "head" EMT's count, the patient's body should be rolled as a unit to a lateral position, maintaining the spine in line. Quickly assess the posterior body if not already done in the focused history and physical examination. Position the board under the patient. Roll the patient onto the board at the command of the EMT holding in-line immobilization (Figure 27.7).

Once the patient is on the board, a 1- to 1.5-foot space should be left at the top of the board. At this time, again on the head EMT's count, slide the patient up using a diagonal slide. A **diagonal slide** is a specific kind of movement in which the patient is moved from one side of the board and is slid up and diagonally until the patient is centered on the board. This procedure is accomplished with one EMT, positioned at the patient's hip level, sliding the patient onto the board. (If another EMT is available, additional help can be used at the patient's shoulders to move the patient more efficiently.) The EMT at the patient's head does not pull the patient, but simply maintains in-line stabilization. A lateral slide could compromise the spine, and using a diagonal slide helps eliminate

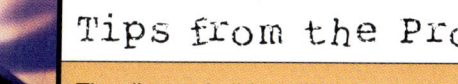

Tips from the Pros

The diagonal slide reduces the risk of compromising the patient's spine as compared with the traditional lateral movement of the patient onto the LSB.

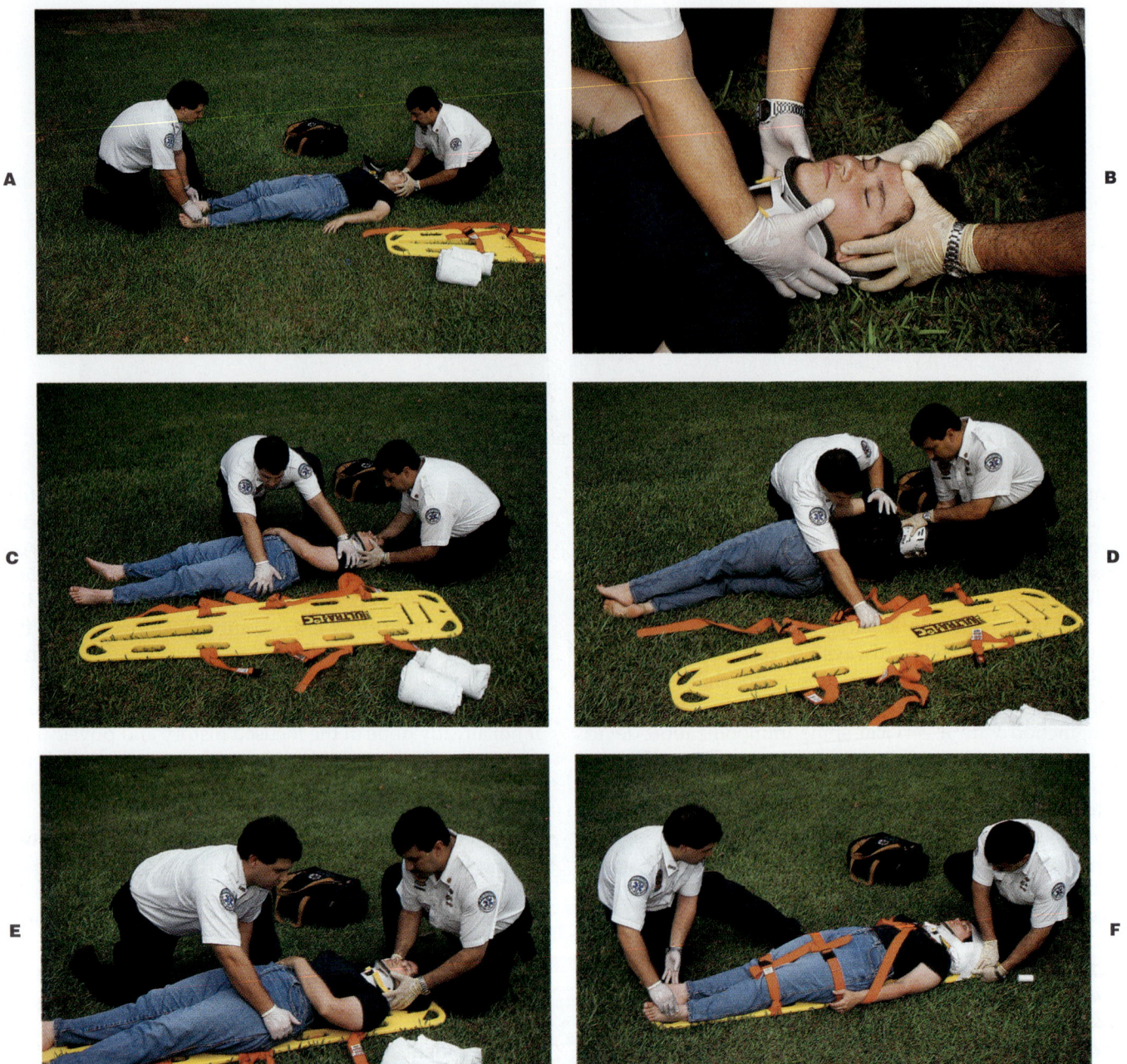

FIGURE 27.7 **A,** Patient is positioned flat on the ground while cervical inline positioning is maintained by the EMT at the head. **B,** Cervical collar is measured and placed. **C,** At the command of the EMT holding the patient's head, the EMT at the body rolls the patient from the shoulders and hips. The head inline position is maintained. **D,** While holding the patient steady, the EMT at the body positions the board next to the patient. **E,** Patient is rolled into position. Inline stabilization is maintained for the head through all motions. **F,** Padding is placed beneath the head and on each side (see Fig. 27.8) for proper neck positioning and taped into place.

this risk. The EMTs use either a slide, a proper lift, a logroll, or a scoop stretcher to keep movement to a minimum. The method chosen depends on the situation, scene, and available resources.

At this time, pad the voids (the spaces between the board and the patient). In the adult, the voids usually appear under the head and the small of the back (Figure 27.8, *A* and *B*). To demonstrate these voids, stand up against a wall with your heels flush against it. Now stand straight up. Note the void, usually a couple of inches wide, between the wall and your head. This area must be padded. If it is not padded, the void forces the head flush against the wall, or backboard, and causes hyperextension of the cervical spine, defeating the purpose of in-line

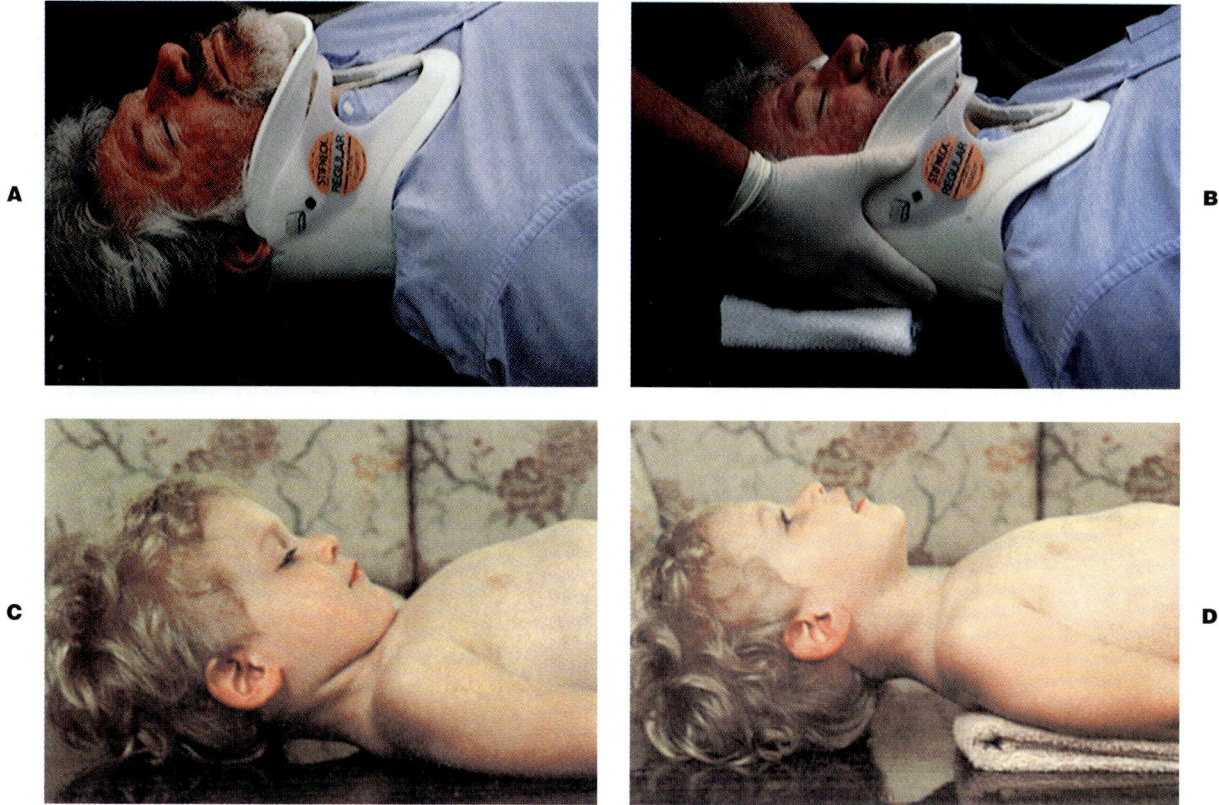

FIGURE 27.8 **A,** Head immobilization without padding. **B,** Adult on long board with padding behind the head. **C,** Child on backboard without padding. **D,** Child on backboard with padding.

immobilization. In children, padding is needed under the shoulders and the heels. When laying a child on a backboard and maintaining an in-line immobilized position, there is an excessive void under the shoulders. This void is due to the large circumference of the child's head (Figure 27.8, *C* and *D*).

Now that the patient has been placed on the backboard, the head EMT maintains in-line stabilization while the other EMTs immobilize the head and body. Immobilize the body first. If the patient needs to vomit, the EMT should lift one side of the backboard so as to make the board perpendicular to the floor. This action prevents the patient from aspirating the vomitus. If the board is lifted in this manner and only the head is secured, the patient's torso will slide off the backboard and will cause unnecessary movement of the spine. Straps must always be placed on the legs, hips, and chest. If extra straps are available, they may be used as shoulder straps to further support the body. The head is best immobilized by starting the tape on the board in the middle of the head, pulling the tape over the forehead, and securing it in the same area on the opposite side of the board (provided that the prevention of cervical spine movement will not be compromised, the tape that is placed over the forehead can be doubled over, or a gauze pad tucked under the tape can be used to promote comfort of the patient). The second piece of tape should start above the first, come down over the cervical spine immobilization device, and up above the end of the first tape. Thus the two pieces of tape cross each other. At this point, reassess pulse, movement, and sensation, and record. Now the patient is ready to be transferred to the ambulance (Figure 27.9).

> **Tips from the Pros**
>
> Be sure the backboard chosen is radiographically translucent. Make sure all equipment needed for backboarding is retrieved from the ambulance before you begin backboarding. Avoid running back and forth to the ambulance. Tape, Kerlix, triangular bandages, and sheets can be used in place of straps. Using straps is better, but if they are not available, improvise. Shoes, towel rolls, sheets, and blankets can be used for cervical spine immobilization devices. A sheet can be used for a cervical spine immobilization device. For a pediatric patient, a combination pad can be wrapped around the neck, like a scarf, and secured with tape. The head is stabilized on either side by sheets, shoes, or premade pads. Sandbags are thought to be too heavy for this purpose and may force the patient's head to the side in severe turning maneuvers.

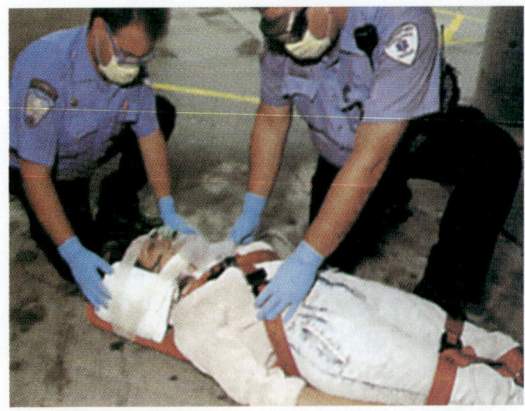

FIGURE 27.9 An adult being immobilized on a long board.

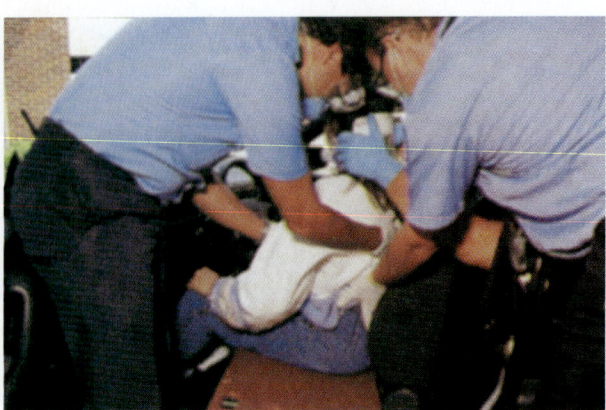

FIGURE 27.11 If the sitting patient must be moved urgently, he or she must be lowered directly onto a long board and removed with manual stabilization provided.

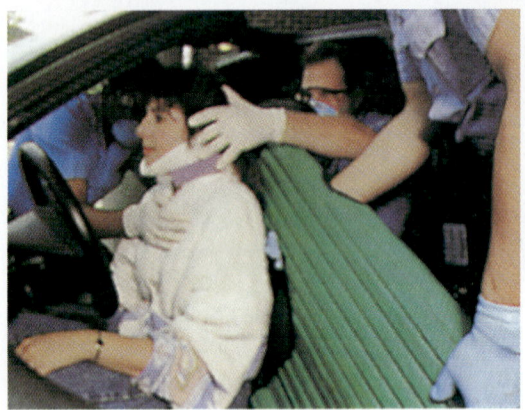

FIGURE 27.10 If a patient is found in a sitting position (and vital signs are stable), immobilize with a short spine immobilization device.

Short Spine Board

Several different types of short board immobilization devices exist. Among these are the vest type and the rigid short board (Figure 27.10). They all, however, have the same function, which is to provide immobilization of the head, neck, and torso. Which device to use depends on preference, familiarity, and the device provided by EMS. These devices are to be used to immobilize noncritical patients with suspected spinal injuries or as a long spine board for a pediatric patient. See the KED Skill Sheet at the end of this chapter.

If the patient is found in a sitting position in a chair, immobilize with a short spine immobilization device. However, if the patient must be removed urgently because of serious injuries, the need to gain access to others, or dangers at the scene, the patient must be lowered directly onto a long board and removed with manual stabilization provided (Figure 27.11).

The first EMT initiates manual spinal stabilization and performs the initial assessment. Stabilization can be accessed either from the front, the side, or behind the patient. The second EMT performs the focused assessment and prepares to apply the cervical spine immobilization device and the short spine board. The second EMT positions the device behind the patient. Be sure that the head end of the device is up. These areas are usually marked. As before, secure the torso to the board first. Evaluate torso fixation and adjust as necessary without excessive movement of the patient. Evaluate the void behind the patient's head, and pad as necessary to maintain neutral in-line immobilization. Secure the patient's head to the device. If the patient is sitting in a car, insert a long board under the patient's buttocks and rotate and lower the patient to the board. If the patient is sitting in a chair or on the ground, simply lift the patient and place him or her on the long spine board. Reassess pulse, movement, and sensation in all extremities, and record. Be sure to secure the short board to the long board. If the short board is not secured to the long board, the patient may slide off the long board while still attached to the short board. See the Extrication from Car with KED or KC Board Skill Sheet at the end of this chapter.

Standing Patient

If the patient is found in a standing position, one EMT stands behind the patient and maintains in-line stabilization. Another EMT should position the long board behind the patient. An EMT should stand on each side of the patient, and an additional EMT should stand at the foot, facing the patient. The EMTs at the sides of the patient reach under the arms to grasp the board and use the hand farthest from the patient to secure the head.

Once the position is ensured, the EMTs at the sides place their leg closest to the board behind the board and begin to tip the top backward. The EMT at the foot of the board secures the board and the patient to prevent slid-

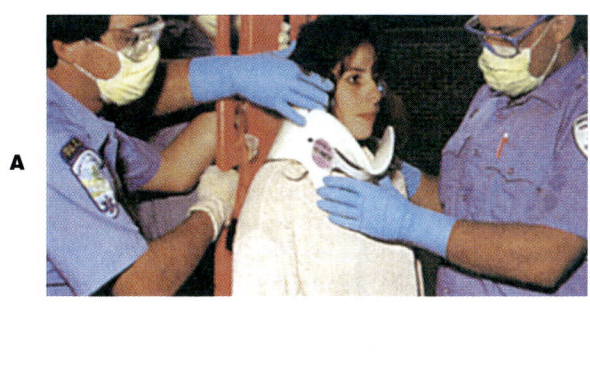
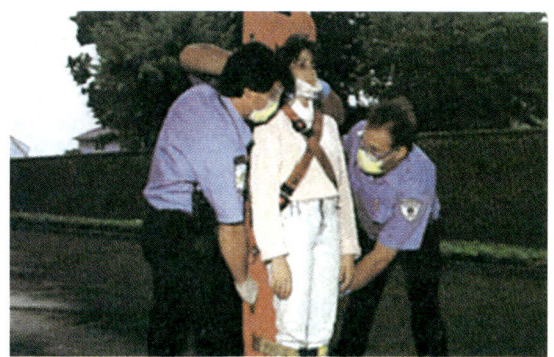
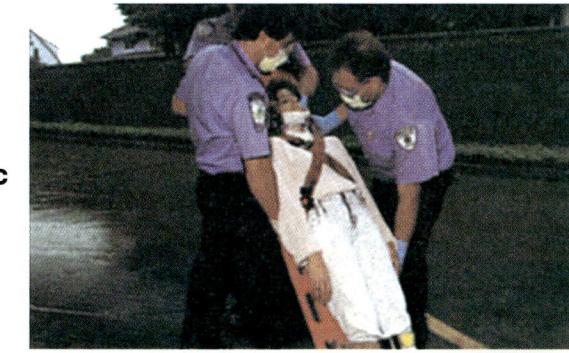
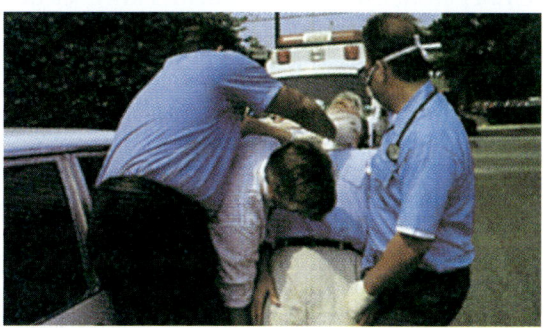
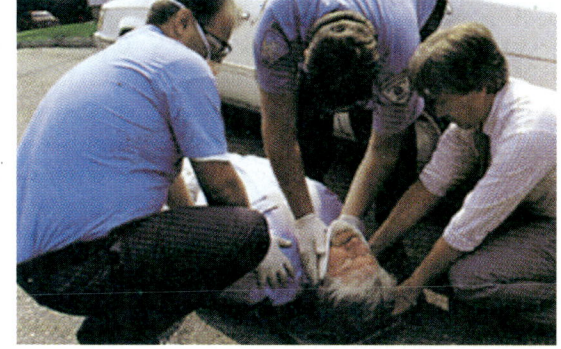

FIGURE 27.12 Standing patient. **A,** Apply manual in-line stabilization from behind the patient and apply a cervical spine immobilization device. **B,** Insert the long board behind the patient from the side. The EMT providing manual in-line stabilization keeps the board pressed against the patient with his or her hip and leg. One EMT at each side inserts his or her hand nearest the patient under the patient's armpit and grasps the nearest handhold on the board above the armpit. **C,** Another EMT or a bystander places a foot or hands at the bottom of the board to prevent movement. Each EMT grasps a handhold near the top of the board with his or her free hand. The EMTs lower the board partway to the ground, stopping about halfway down. **D,** The EMT holding the head rotates his or her hands as shown without losing stabilization. The EMTs at the sides may have to reposition their arms so they will clear those of the EMT at the head when the board is fully lowered. **E,** Lower the board to the ground. The EMT at the head must move from a standing to a kneeling position to avoid moving the head out of line. Immobilize the patient to the board.

ing, and the board is brought into a level horizontal position on the ground (Figure 27.12).

Rapid Extrication

The EMT occasionally will encounter a scenario that requires the rapid extrication of the patient. Few specific scenarios warrant a rapid extrication protocol. The first of these scenarios is the unsafe scene. The scene is too dangerous for the EMT and the patient to remain in for the time required to package the patient. The EMT's safety is the most important factor. If it appears that the scene is dangerous before the EMT enters, the EMT should not enter. In some situations, however, the scene progresses from safe to unsafe. In this situation, rapid extrication is called for.

A second consideration for rapid extrication occurs when a patient's life-threatening condition requires immediate transport to the appropriate facility. For these patients, the EMT will not progress beyond the initial assessment. The EMT concentrates on assessment of the ABCs and control of bleeding and not so much on the ongoing assessment unless correcting life-threatening conditions is warranted.

The most common scenario involving life-threatening conditions is a motor vehicle collision. On rare occasions, another patient, family member, friend, or stranger will prevent the EMT from caring for a patient. However unexpected this situation might be, it is the responsibility of the EMT to remove the patient from this type of unsecured environment. Police or fire department personnel are helpful in this type of situation to restrain the person who is inhibiting the care of the patient or to distract the person long enough to remove the patient. These kinds of scenarios, if not addressed properly, could endanger the life of the patient and the EMT and should be considered with scene safety.

As always, it is important to check ABCs before extrication.

> ✓ Patients are generally found in three positions: horizontal, vertical, or sitting. The EMT must be able to immobilize the patient in any position found. Once an EMT has taken control of spinal in-line immobilization, this duty may not be relinquished for any reason until the patient has been properly secured to a long spine board. The EMT must be familiar with all spinal immobilization equipment available to him or her.

Special Considerations

Patients with Helmets

The two basic types of helmets are sports helmets and motorcycle helmets. Sports helmets typically open in the front. This type of helmet makes for easier access to the patient's airway. Football helmets may require the removal of the pads beneath the ears before the helmet will easily come off. Caution during and after the removal of the football helmet is in order because the shoulders are lifted high off the ground or backboard, and this can result in severe hyperextension if the head is forced back to the board. The shoulder pads should be removed or the head must be padded off the board. Motorcycle helmets either are full face or have a shield over the face. A full-face helmet is much more difficult to remove because of the part of the helmet that covers the chin. While removing this part of the helmet, it is difficult to avoid snagging it on the nose; however, it can be done.

Helmets are an important piece of safety equipment; however, like seat belts, they must be worn properly. The helmet should fit well with little or no movement of the head inside the helmet. The helmet should protect against the impact of hard objects, especially ones traveling at high speed. If the helmet does not "fit like a glove," the head will bounce around inside the helmet and cause stress to the head and neck. According to Newton's first law of motion, the head does not stop moving until it hits the helmet. If the helmet fits properly, it absorbs the shock the head would have sustained without the helmet. If the helmet does not fit, it does no more good than an improperly fitted seat restraint or an air bag without the assistance of a seat restraint.

The appearance of the helmet itself should be considered with the mechanism of injury. Is the helmet damaged? Where is the damage? How much damage was done to the helmet? All of these things must be noted. It is a good idea to bring the helmet to the hospital with the patient. The helmet alone can give the EMT an overall view of the mechanism of injury. The EMT must consider whether or not the helmet should be removed. A helmet that allows little or no movement of the patient's head within it is reason enough to leave the helmet in place, provided that the patient has no impending airway or breathing problem. Removal of the helmet could further injure the patient. Proper spinal immobilization must be provided. This immobilization can be difficult because of the extra weight of the helmet, in addition to the added space at the back, which can prevent in-line immobilization. In addition to these considerations, as long as the EMT is able to assess and reassess airway and breathing and intervene if necessary, it is proper to leave the helmet in place and transport the patient.

> ✓ Helmets are an important piece of safety equipment. The EMT should include a helmet in his or her investigation of the mechanism of injury. The EMT must know how, when, and why to remove a helmet.

Helmet removal. The technique for removing a helmet depends on the type of helmet worn. This section gives the EMT general guidelines; however, every situation is different.

Be sure to remove the patient's eyeglasses before removing the helmet. One EMT stabilizes the helmet by placing his or her hands on each side of the helmet, with the fingers on the **mandible** (jawbone) to prevent movement. The second EMT loosens the strap under the chin. The second EMT then places one hand on the mandible at the angle of the jaw and the other hand posteriorly at the occipital region. The EMT holding the helmet pulls

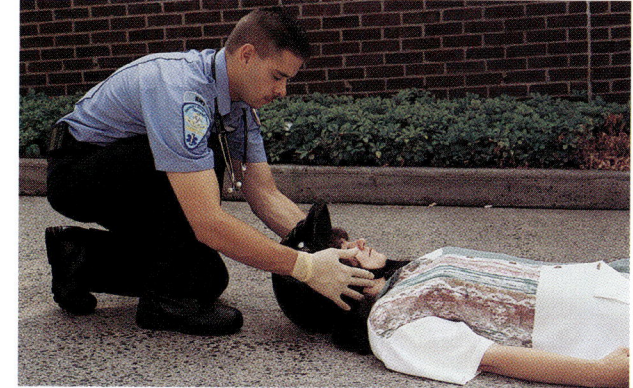
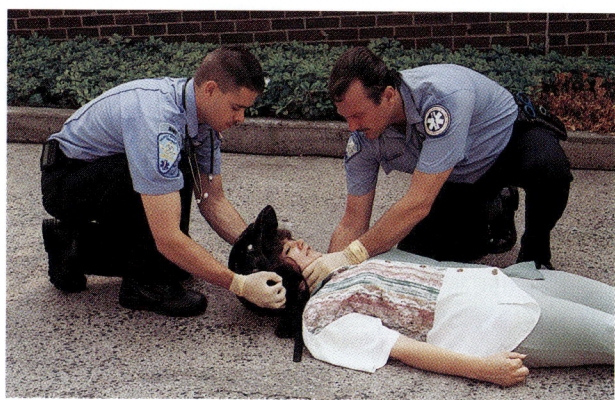
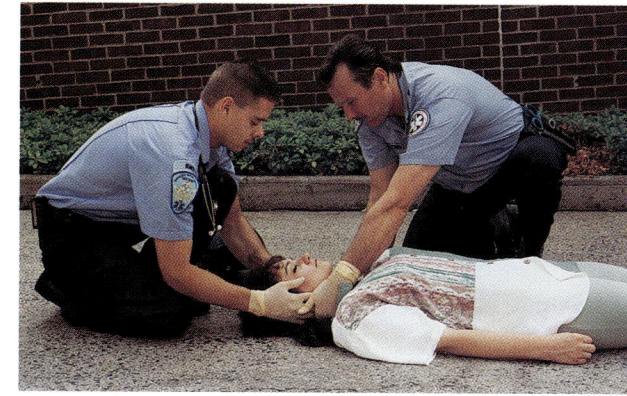

FIGURE 27.13 Helmet removal. **A,** One EMT stabilizes the helmet by placing his or her hands on each side of the helmet, with the fingers on the mandible to prevent movement. The second EMT loosens the strap under the chin. **B,** The second EMT places one hand on the mandible at the angle of the jaw and the other hand posteriorly at the occipital region. The EMT holding the helmet pulls the sides of the helmet apart and gently slips the helmet halfway off the patient's head, then stops. **C,** The EMT maintaining stabilization of the neck repositions and slides his or her posterior hand superiorly to prevent the head from falling back after complete helmet removal. After the helmet is completely removed, the EMT can proceed with spinal immobilization.

the sides of the helmet apart and gently slips the helmet halfway off the patient's head, then stops. The EMT maintaining stabilization of the neck repositions his or her hands by sliding the posterior hand superiorly to secure the head from falling back after complete helmet removal. Now, the helmet is completely removed. The EMT then can proceed with spinal immobilization as indicated in the spinal immobilization section (Figure 27.13).

> ✓ If the EMT is not able to assess or reassess airway and breathing, the helmet should be removed. Proper spinal immobilization must be maintained, and if immobilization cannot be maintained with the helmet in place, the helmet must be removed.

Infants and Children

If an infant is involved in a motor vehicle collision and was in a child seat, the infant can be immobilized in the child seat. Apply a cervical spine immobilization device (provided you can find one small enough), and then use tape to secure the infant in the seat.

Small children and infants not found in a car seat can be immobilized on a short spine board, provided the legs do not hang over the edge. This immobilization is accomplished by using the short spine board in the same way a long spine board is used for an adult. Children should be padded from the shoulders to the heels to maintain neutral immobilization.

Step-by-Step Procedure

Manual In-line Immobilization

Behind

1. From behind the patient's head, or sitting in the back seat of the car, place hands over the patient's ears without moving the head.

2. Place thumbs against the posterior aspect of the skull.

3. Place the little fingers just under the angle of the mandible (see Step 3).

4. Spread the remaining fingers on the flat lateral planes of the head and increase the strength of the grasp.

5. If head is not in a neutral in-line position, slowly move the head until it is.

6. Bring the arms in and rest them against the seat, the headrest, or your torso for support.

Side

1. Stand at the side of the patient.

2. Pass your arm over the patient's shoulder and cup the back of his or her head with your hand.

3. Place the thumb and first finger of your other hand, with one on each side of the face, on the cheeks in the notch where the upper teeth join the maxilla.

4. Tighten the anterior and posterior pressure of the hands (see Step 4).

5. If the head is not in a neutral in-line position, move the head slowly until it is.

6. Brace elbows on torso for support.

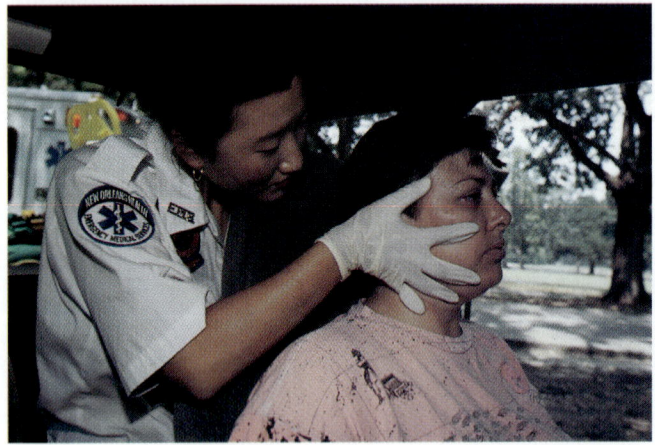

Step 3

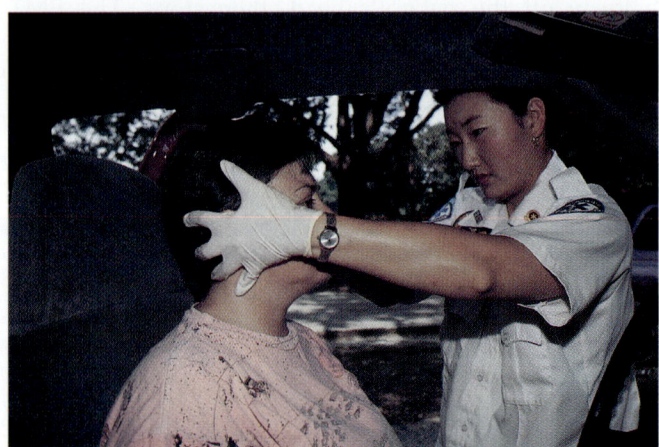

Step 4

Manual In-line Immobilization (cont'd)

Front

1. Stand directly in front of the patient.

2. Place the hands on the sides of the patient's head.

3. Place the little fingers at the posterior aspect of the skull.

4. Place one thumb in the notch between the upper teeth and the maxilla on each cheek.

5. Spread remaining fingers on the flat lateral places of the head and increase the strength of grasp.

6. If the head is not in a neutral in-line position, slowly move the head until it is.

7. Bring arms in and brace elbows against torso for support.

Supine

1. The little fingers are placed at the posterior aspect of the skull.

2. A thumb is placed in the notch between the upper teeth and the maxilla at each cheek.

3. The other fingers are spread across the flat lateral places of the head.

Step-by-Step Procedure

KED

1. Ensure scene safety.

2. Initiate body substance precautions.

3. EMT no. 1 initiates in-line immobilization from behind patient (see Step 3).

4. EMT no. 2 assesses pulse, movement, and sensation of upper and lower extremities (see Step 4).

5. EMT no. 2 applies cervical collar (see Step 5).

6. EMT no. 2 inserts KED between the patient's back and the seat. The head of the device should be inserted beside EMT no. 1's arms and then slid down the patient's back (see Step 6).

7. EMT no. 2 releases and prepares the straps. Unfasten the two long straps (groin straps) and the chest straps. Open the side flaps and place them around the patient's torso, under the arms.

8. EMT no. 2 holds the vest so that the top of the vest is level with the top of the patient's head.

9. EMT no. 2 correctly positions and fastens the middle strap first around the patient's chest. Connect the buckle, pull the strap snugly, and adjust the buckle.

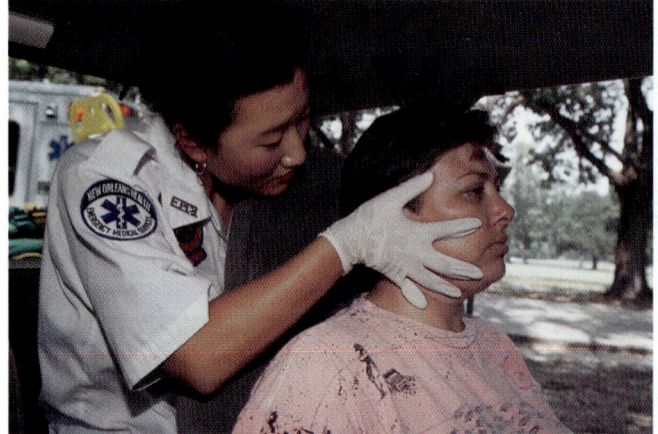

Step 3

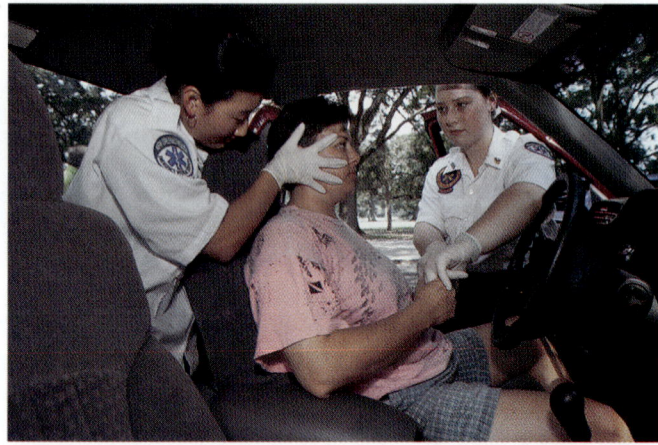

Step 4

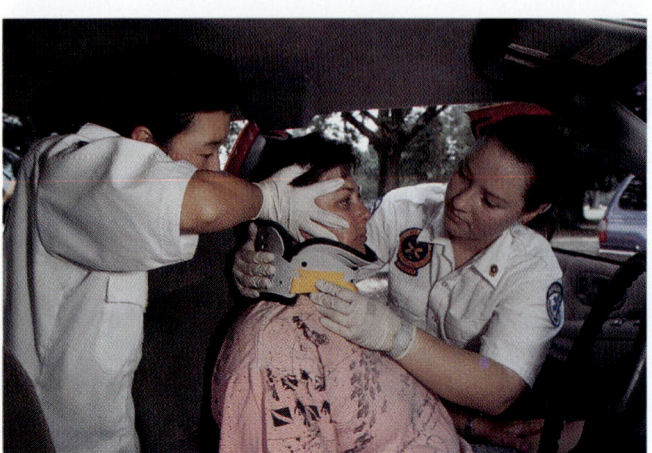

Step 5

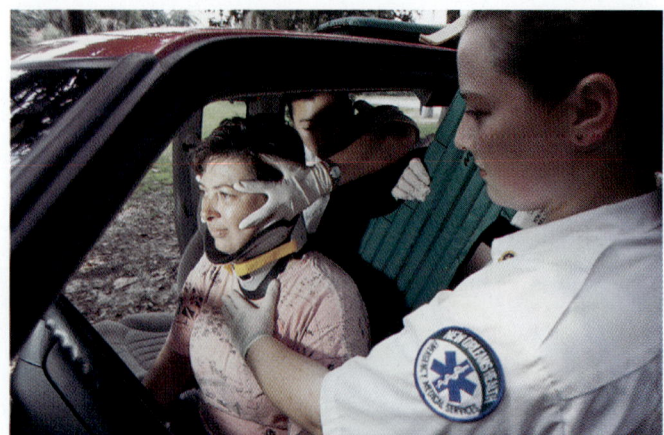

Step 6

KED (cont'd)

10. EMT no. 2 fastens the lower strap next, followed by the upper strap in the same manner. Do not fit the upper strap so tightly that it restricts breathing. Do not use force to secure the straps because it may cause movement of the spine and head (see Step 10).

11. EMT no. 2 now secures groin straps by grasping the top of the strap (near the vest) and the lower portion of the strap, and using a seesaw movement maneuvers the strap under the patient's leg so that it may be secured in the vest. The strap should form a straight line in the intergluteal fold from the back to the front.

12. Position it in the crotch on one side of the genitalia.

13. Bring the strap up the inner thigh and over the pelvis, and fasten it to the buckle on the same side of the vest so that the strap has formed a loop over one side of the pelvis.

14. EMT no. 2 repeats this procedure on the other side. Fastening and adjusting only one side at a time prevents unwanted movement of the patient's spine.

15. EMT no. 2 pads behind the head any voids.

16. EMT no. 2 positions the head flaps, coordinating this procedure with EMT no. 1 to maintain in-line immobilization (see Step 16).

17. EMT no. 1 maintains in-line immobilization with hands on top of the head flaps, and EMT no. 2 secures the head straps around EMT no. 1's hands.

18. EMT no. 2 applies the frontal strap first. This strap is brought from the back side of the head flap, over the frontal region, and secured to the opposite side behind the head flap.

19. EMT no. 2 secures the neck strap in the same manner, but the strap is brought around over the cervical collar.

20. EMT no. 1 releases in-line immobilization, because it is now being accomplished mechanically by the KED.

21. Both EMTs grasp the straps on the side of the KED, and on count move the patient onto the long spine board.

22. If the patient is inside a vehicle, the long spine board should be placed with the head end of the long spine board under the patient's buttocks, with the patient rotated and slid onto the long spine board (see Extrication Step-by-Step Procedure, step 5).

23. The KED must be secured to the long spine board using straps, tape, or Kerlix.

24. The patient is now secured to the long spine board using straps, tape, or Kerlix.

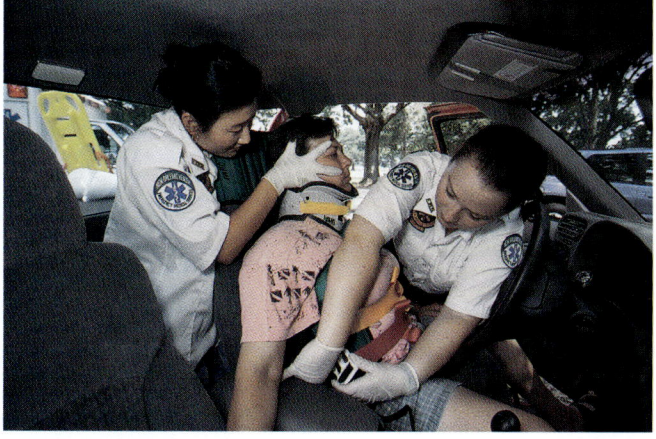

Step 10

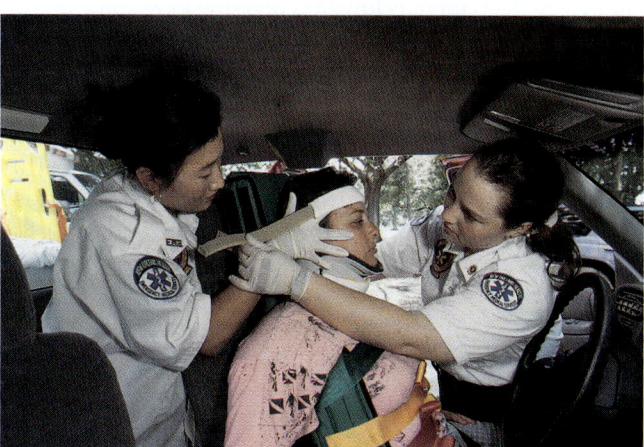

Step 16

Step-by-Step Procedure

Extrication from Car with KED or KC Board

1. If possible, the stretcher with a long spine board on it should be brought to the opening of the car door, next to the patient.

2. The foot end of the long spine board should be placed under or at least next to the patient's buttocks, so that one end is securely supported on the car seat and the head end is on the stretcher.

3. If the stretcher is not available, the head end of the long spine board can be held level by other EMTs or bystanders.

4. EMT no. 2 takes over in-line immobilization as EMT no. 1 positions himself or herself to regain immobilization so the patient can be extricated from the car.

5. EMT no. 1 maintains in-line immobilization while EMT no. 2 rotates the patient on EMT no. 1's count so that the patient's back is facing the outside of the car.

6. EMT no. 2 turns the patient onto the long spine board on EMT no. 1's count while maintaining in-line immobilization. EMT no. 1 watches spine to ensure that it remains in line.

7. Both EMTs lower the patient onto the board on EMT no. 1's count.

8. Once the patient is lowered onto the long spine board, the legs are straightened and the body is supine.

9. On EMT no. 1's count, the patient is slid out of the car on the long spine board until the patient is out of the car and on the long spine board completely. This step may take two or three counts based on the ease of extricating the patient from the car and onto the spine board (see Step 9).

10. EMT no. 2 lowers the legs onto the spine board. The groin straps may have to be loosened so as to extend the legs.

11. Position the long spine board on the stretcher.

12. Secure short spine board to the long spine board.

13. Secure patient to the long spine board.

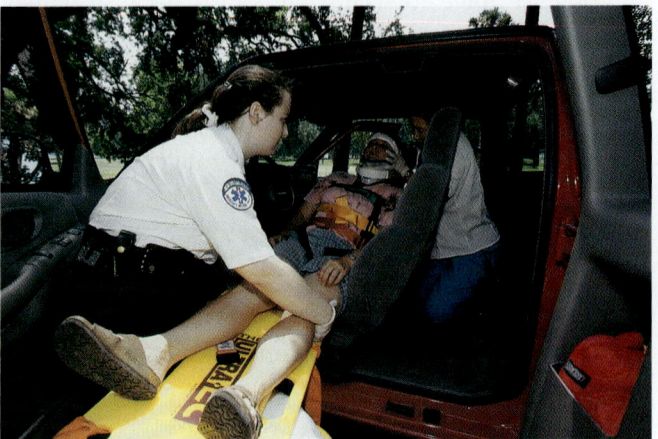

Step 9

Summary

- The central nervous system comprises the brain and spinal cord. Its function is to decipher incoming messages and respond accordingly. The peripheral nervous system comprises all nerves that extend from the brain and spinal cord. Its function is to send and receive all messages coming to and from the spinal cord.
- The spinal column is composed of 33 bones called the vertebrae. It is divided into five sections: cervical, thoracic, lumbar, sacral, and coccyx. Each of the first three sections is cushioned by an intervertebral disk that provides for the elasticity and compressibility of the vertebral column.
- Newton's first law of motion states that an object in motion will stay in motion until acted on by an outside force. This law is important in the pathophysiology of the spine.
- A compression fracture occurs when a bone has pressure from above and below it. Lateral bending is the bending of the spine in a side-to-side motion. A distraction fracture occurs when the vertebrae are pulled apart.
- Signs and symptoms of a spinal injury vary from no pain at all to quadriplegia. The mechanism of injury must be established.
- Any patient with trauma above the clavicle is suspected of spinal injury until ruled out by x-ray.
- Once in-line immobilization has been initiated, it must not be released until the patient is secured onto the long spine board.
- The patient's helmet must be inspected for evidence of damage and will help determine the mechanism of injury. Helmets are an important piece of safety equipment and must be worn properly.
- The EMT is responsible for understanding when, why, and how to properly immobilize any patient in any position.

Scenario Solution

The patient should be considered to have a spine injury because of the mechanism of injury. The patient should be immobilized using the standing technique. A complete but brief neurologic examination should be done after the patient is placed on the backboard.

Hunter Scott's initial contact with the bull rapidly moved Hunter's body from under his head, causing potential severe angulation at the neck. When Hunter fell back to the ground, there was potential to land on his head, absorbing the momentum of the torso on the cervical spine and producing hyperextension, hyperflexion, or compression injuries.

Key Terms

Autonomic nervous system Part of the nervous system that regulates involuntary vital functions, including the activity of the cardiac muscle, smooth muscles, and glands; divided into the sympathetic nervous system and parasympathetic nervous system.

Central nervous system Part of the nervous system comprising the brain and spinal cord.

Cervical collar Collar that provides partial spinal immobilization (about 50% range of motion in the three major motions of anterior/posterior, lateral bending, and rotation).

Cervical immobilization Reduction of motion of the spine by immobilization of the bones above and below the cervical spine (head and thoracic spine).

Compression fracture Bone fracture caused by forces from both above and below the bone.

Diagonal slide Movement used to place a patient on a long spine board.

Distraction injuries Injuries in which the spine is pulled apart.

In-line stabilization Immobilization of a bone or bones in the axis of the bones.

Intervertebral disk Padding between the vertebrae.

Lateral bending Injury caused by the head bending too far in one direction.

Long spine board (LSB) Device used to immobilize the entire body as a single unit.

Mandible Bone of the lower jaw.

Key Terms

Motor nerves Nerves that carry responses from the central nervous system to an organ or muscle.

Newton's first law of motion Physical law that states that an object in motion will stay in motion until acted on by an outside force.

Paraplegia Paralysis of the lower limbs and trunk.

Peripheral nervous system Part of the nervous system consisting of all the nerves that extend from the brain and spinal cord.

Quadriplegia Paralysis affecting all four extremities.

Sensory nerves Nerves that carry impulses from the sensory receptors to the central nervous system.

Short spine board Device used to immobilize the entire spine using the pelvis and the head as the bones above and below.

Somatic nervous system Part of the nervous system that is voluntary; used in activities such as kicking a ball or reading this text.

Spinal column Column of bones that encloses the spinal cord.

Vertebrae Circular bones that make up the vertebral column.

Review Questions

1. When removing a helmet in the field, the most important part of the process is:
   a. Removing the helmet quickly
   b. Ventilating the patient throughout the process
   c. Maintaining the stability and position of the spine
   d. Removing all of the padding inside the helmet before taking the helmet off

2. Stabilization of any fracture requires immobilization of the joint above and below the fracture. To achieve this goal with the spine, what two bones must be included in the splint?
   a. Skull and pelvis
   b. Skull and femur
   c. C1 and pelvis
   d. C1 and the thoracic cage

3. Management of the airway in a trauma patient includes:
   a. Placing the head in the partially extended and partially flexed position (sniffing position)
   b. Hyperextending the spine to open the airway
   c. Keeping the neck inline while moving the mandible forward
   d. Performing a spinal assessment first so that airway management can be done without harm to the patient.

4. An effective and safe way to immobilize the cervical spine is:
   a. With the patient in the supine position, apply traction to the head as the patient is logrolled onto the backboard
   b. Place the hands over the ears and the forearms on the clavicles
   c. Instruct two bystanders to lift the patient while you and your partner slide the long backboard under the patient
   d. After placing the patient is a good cervical collar, the spine is adequately immobilized for most rescue maneuvers

5. Which of the following describe proper padding for immobilization of the c-spine?
   a. Padding under the occiput of a child
   b. Padding under the occiput of an older adult
   c. Padding under the thoracic spine of an adult
   d. All of the above

Answers to these Review Questions can be found at the end of the book on page 866.

Musculoskeletal Trauma

Lesson Goal

Musculoskeletal system injuries are possibly the most common prehospital problem. This chapter addresses the simplicity and the complexity of those injuries. Although it is not the emergency medical technician's (EMT's) responsibility to make an ICD-9 (*International Classification of Diseases*, 9th Revision) diagnosis, it is the EMT's responsibility to diagnose and immobilize fractures.

Scenario

You are called to the scene of Gidge, a 5-year-old complaining of pain to her right shoulder. Her father is on scene and states that she and her older brother were "roughhousing" and jumping on the bed. The father states that that is all he knows and that neither of the children will say what happened. Gidge is crying and holding her left arm against her body.

After a lot of coaxing, she allows you to touch her. You notice that her left shoulder is deformed and that her left arm is longer than her right arm. During the assessment, she starts crying hysterically and will not let you touch her again. The older brother is standing at the edge of the room and is staring at the scene.

You and your partner notice that the bed is leaning to one corner. Your partner investigates and tells you that the bed is broken at that corner. At this point the mother comes into the house, says "What is going on?", and goes immediately to Gidge. Gidge is still upset, but she seems to be calming down with her mother at her side.

 How are you going to manage the scene and the patient's injuries?

Key Terms to Know

Anatomic positioning
Cardiac muscle
Closed fracture
Compartment syndrome
Crepitus
Dislocation
Internal fixation
Loss of skeletal integrity
Multisystem trauma patient
Open fracture
Open reduction
Smooth muscle
Sprain
Strain
Striations

529

Learning Objectives

As an EMT-Basic, you should be able to do the following:

DOT

- Describe the function of the muscular system.
- Describe the function of the skeletal system.
- List the major bones and bone groupings of the spinal column, thorax, upper extremities, and lower extremities.
- Differentiate between and open and a closed painful, swollen, deformed extremity.
- State the reasons for splinting.
- List the general rules of splinting.
- List the emergency medical care for a patient with a painful, swollen, deformed extremity.
- Demonstrate the emergency medical care for a patient with a painful, swollen, deformed extremity.
- Demonstrate completing a prehospital care report for patients with musculoskeletal injuries.
- List the complications of splint use.

Supplemental

- Describe the treatment of a fracture, a dislocation, and a sprain.
- Identify the signs and symptoms of a fracture, a dislocation, and a sprain.
- Describe the various types of muscles in the human body.
- Describe the importance of mechanisms of injury.
- Describe the principles of immobilization.

Musculoskeletal injuries are common in emergency medical services (EMS) situations. It is the emergency medical technician's (EMT's) responsibility to manage airway and patient oxygenation, to initiate shock management, and to immobilize possible fractures, dislocations, and sprains so that they produce minimal pain and do no further harm to the patient while en route to the hospital.

As in all calls the EMT will respond to, the most important aspects are scene safety, body substance isolation precautions, primary assessment, vital signs, and secondary assessment. These priorities do not change, even if there is a grossly deformed femur fracture evident on initial assessment of the scene. It does not matter if a patient has a fractured femur when he or she is not breathing—airway takes priority. Any complications found during the primary assessment must be addressed before continuing the assessment. Airway, breathing, and circulation (the ABCs) must come first.

Each trauma patient should be secured to a long spine board in a supine position. There may be rare occasions and unusual patient conditions when this is not possible. When such occurs, the critical thinking of the EMT must come into play. Supine position is the preferred method of transport, because it facilitates continued evaluation and resuscitation as required. This places the patient *almost* in the anatomic position. **Anatomic positioning** is defined as a supine position with the hands rotated out so that the palms are facing up. This position provides consistent meaning to the descriptive terms such as medial, lateral, anterior, and posterior. Understanding the position provides the EMT with the information to accurately describe the injuries in medical terms for clarity when discussing the patient with emergency department (ED) personnel.

The basic rule of fracture management is to splint the joints above and below the site of injury. This is easily accomplished in life-threatening conditions by strapping the entire body to the long backboard. This will effectively immobilize all of the bones in the body.

It is not the responsibility of the EMT to differentiate between the types of the various musculoskeletal injuries. However, it is the EMT's responsibility to identify the potential injuries and to treat the patient as if the most severe injury, the most unstable injury, or the injury that would cause the most harm is present. Even with the benefit of x-ray and computed tomography, it is not possible to identify every fracture or to distinguish between a fracture, sprain, dislocation, or hematoma producing swelling and pain. In the field, all these injuries can be managed using proper immobilization techniques, with the final diagnosis left to the ED personnel. The field diagnosis is "possible fracture—requires immobilization."

Frequently, final stabilization (definitive hospital care) requires **open reduction** (use of surgery to place bones in proper position) and **internal fixation** (use of wires, pins, and screws to place bones in proper position) of the fracture.

In each phase of patient care (prehospital, ED, operating room [OR], or intensive care unit [ICU]), as the continuum of care progresses, more sophisticated assessment and techniques are required. In the field, the EMT does not have x-ray and other diagnostic techniques to distinguish among the various types of injuries that may exist (fractures, dislocations, and sprains). However, the EMT can see, feel, and hear signs that indicate the possibility of **loss of skeletal integrity.** Loss of skeletal integrity may involve the shaft of the bone, the joint, or the supporting structures of the bone or joint.

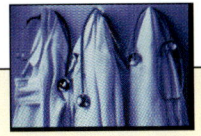

Physician Notes

There are four phases of patient care. In each situation that the patient is in, these phases become more complex. Musculoskeletal injuries demonstrate how assessment and management change from the field to the ED or OR and then to the ICU. Unfortunately for the EMT, the meaning of the terminology used by physicians and nurses can vary from that used in the field. This note will try to shed some light on that problem using musculoskeletal injuries as an example of the flow of care:

1. Identification and management of life-threatening injuries
2. Management of shock
3. Total body assessment
4. Definitive care

Example: Definitive care of the fracture or potential fracture in the field is to immobilize the potential injury so no further damage is done. It is not necessary to identify in the field whether the injury is a fracture or something else, hence the use of the term *deformed, painful, swollen extremity.* Treatment is to immobilize the patient and transport to the hospital.

Definitive ED care is to identify the presence or absence of a fracture, place the patient in a strong permanent splint, and transport the patient to the OR.

Definitive OR care would be to place an external fixator on the fracture or to perform open reduction with internal fixation (ORIF).

The descriptive term *definitive care* is correct for each situation, within the limitations of that situation.

Patient care is a team effort from the time the patient is injured until the patient returns to normal activity. The EMT is an important part of this team. EMTs must understand what will happen to the patient after he or she is admitted to the ED and understand the terminology that physicians and nurses use.

In practice, field management of fractures, sprains, and dislocations is the same: immobilization of the joints above and below the injury. The injured part is immobilized or stabilized so that the patient's pain is reduced and the two loose segments do not further injure structures in the vicinity. The EMT need only identify those signs and symptoms (pain, swelling, deformity) that indicate that one of the three types of injuries may be present and then take appropriate steps to provide immobilization.

Although it is only necessary for the EMT to recognize the possibility that such injuries exist, to provide the initial immobilization it is important that the EMT understand the mechanisms of injury, the pathophysiology, and the potential complications. Knowing and understanding these concepts will help EMTs use their judgment in overall patient care. In some instances, immobilization of the fracture is all that is required. In other cases, a decision must be made as to how the injury site should be immobilized based on other conditions that exist in the patient. For instance, the management of a potential fractured femur is very different in an elderly woman who has fallen in the bathroom as compared with a 20-year-old with a potential fractured femur who has been ejected from a motorcycle over a retaining rail and fallen 50 feet down a ravine. In this chapter, a more in-depth discussion of musculoskeletal injuries is presented so that the EMT can gain a general perspective of musculoskeletal injuries and their care.

Anatomy and Physiology

Skeletal System

The human body is composed of 206 bones of various size and shape to perform a variety of functions. The shape of the human body is primarily a result of the skeletal system. Because of these various shapes, the skeletal system forms many protective areas for the soft tissue organs found within them. The skull protects the brain. The rib cage protects the heart, lungs, and great vessels. The pelvic girdle protects the bladder, female reproductive organs, and major blood vessels. The spinal column protects the spinal cord. A joint is formed where two or more bones come together and is held in place by ligaments. Special tissues (ligaments) within the joint and between the bone ends allow for movement without pain. Bone joints give the human body its ability to move by contracting muscles that cross or whose tendons cross these joints.

Bone Structure

Bones of the skeletal system, like all other structures of the human body, are composed of tissues, which are composed of living matter called cells. Because of their compact, dense structure they are able to withstand significant amounts of stress without injury. A good example is the bone of the upper leg, the thigh bone. It is long and thick, which allows it to support the weight of the upper body and to absorb great amounts of stress when the foot strikes the ground, such as while running or jumping.

However, all bones have a breaking point and are not immune to injury. As bones become less dense and begin to lose calcium with age, they become more fragile.

Bones have a rich supply of blood vessels to support maintenance of structure and repair when necessary. Because of this rich supply of vessels, injuries to bones can bleed freely and can become life threatening if the bleeding is not properly managed.

Nerve supply to the periosteum (lining of the bones) indicates when the bones are broken or the supporting structures are injured. Because of this nerve tissue, fractures in bones are often extremely painful. This becomes beneficial to the patient as the surrounding muscles go into spasm to prevent the pain produced by movement and thereby aid in splinting the fracture.

The bone structure of young children is very flexible, and injuries to bones tend to be of a twisting nature rather than a clean break, such as found in adults. A good example is trying to break a green sapling from a tree. When twisted it does not break, rather it tends to split down the long shaft, or the branch breaks on one side but not the other. Bones in young children respond in a similar manner, and their injuries tend to be less severe.

Calcium is one of the essential components to healthy bone. As one grows older the amount of calcium needed for healthy bone diminishes. In an adult, the bones are hard and strong, and tend to break sharply. In the geriatric population, the loss of calcium results in bones that are more fragile. These brittle bones are weaker and are much more likely to break with minimal amounts of stress. An example is the elderly patient who is shopping at the grocery store and turns to pick something up from a shelf. All of the person's weight becomes centralized at the juncture of the joint, which is the femur, hip area, and its joint at the pelvis. Because of the weight concentration and stress, the hip fractures, causing the patient to fall to the floor. The fracture actually produces the fall, rather than the fall producing the fracture.

Bone Classification

Bones are classified according to their shape. Long bones, as the name implies, are longer than they are wide. An example is the long bone of the upper arm (humerus), or the long thigh bone (femur) of the upper leg. Short bones tend to be about equal in their length and width and include bones such as those found in the fingers and toes and the bones of the wrist (carpals) and feet (tarsals). Flat bones, as the name implies, tend to be flat by design, but not necessarily straight. Examples of flat bones include the breastbone (sternum), ribs, skull, and shoulder blade (scapula). All bones that do not fit into one of the first three categories are called irregular bones. Facial bones and the individual bones of the spinal column (vertebrae) are examples.

The EMT-Basic (EMT-B) is not required to learn all the names of the individual bones and muscles of the body. However, to aid in understanding of these two systems and the management of injuries, it is important to at least be able to identify the major bones and groupings of bones (Figure 28.1).

Muscular System

The human body has more than 600 muscles, which serve to support movement of the skeletal system, as well as other critical body functions. The majority of muscles in the body are those of the skeletal system and are attached to bone (Figure 28.2).

Composed of tissues, which are composed of individual cells, muscles are able to contract and relax as identified earlier. Muscles serve the body in many different ways. The development of muscle groups and their relationship to fat provides the body with its shape. Another important function of muscle is in providing protection. The large muscles of the abdomen serve to protect the internal organs. Because the skeletal muscle is attached to the outside of bone, it serves to protect the blood vessels and nerves found near the bone. All movement provided by the skeletal system is a result of muscle contraction.

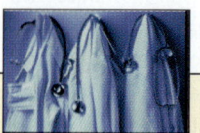

Physician Notes

Correct use of names of muscles and bones when describing the injuries and their prehospital management to ED personnel will tell them that you are a studious and conscientious EMT who is interested in the care of patients. This adds to the respect that physicians and nurses will have for you. In turn, they will be interested in teaching you how to be a better EMT and provide better for your patients.

Muscles are attached to bone by special tissues called *tendons*. These tough fibrous bands serve to attach a muscle to its *point of origin* (the bone that does not move during contraction) and to its *point of insertion* (the bone that moves during a muscle contraction). Tendons can be damaged from overextension or overuse. Tendon injuries are considered to be soft tissue injuries and are discussed later in this chapter.

Muscle and Bone Interaction to Produce Motion

As discussed earlier, it is the actions of muscles through their tendon attachments to the bone, along with the support of ligaments to stabilize the joints, that allows for

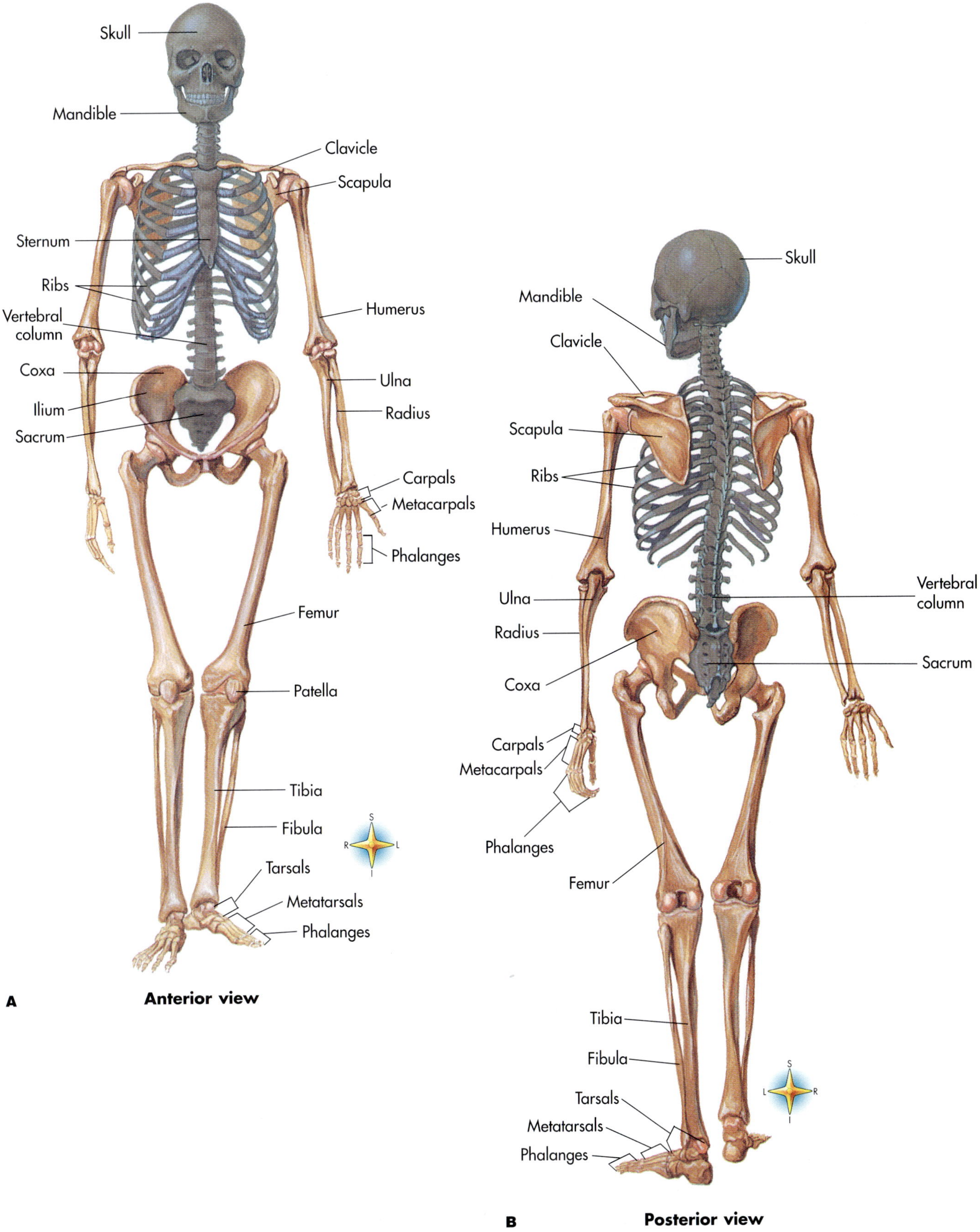

FIGURE 28.1 The skeleton. **A,** Anterior view. **B,** Posterior view.

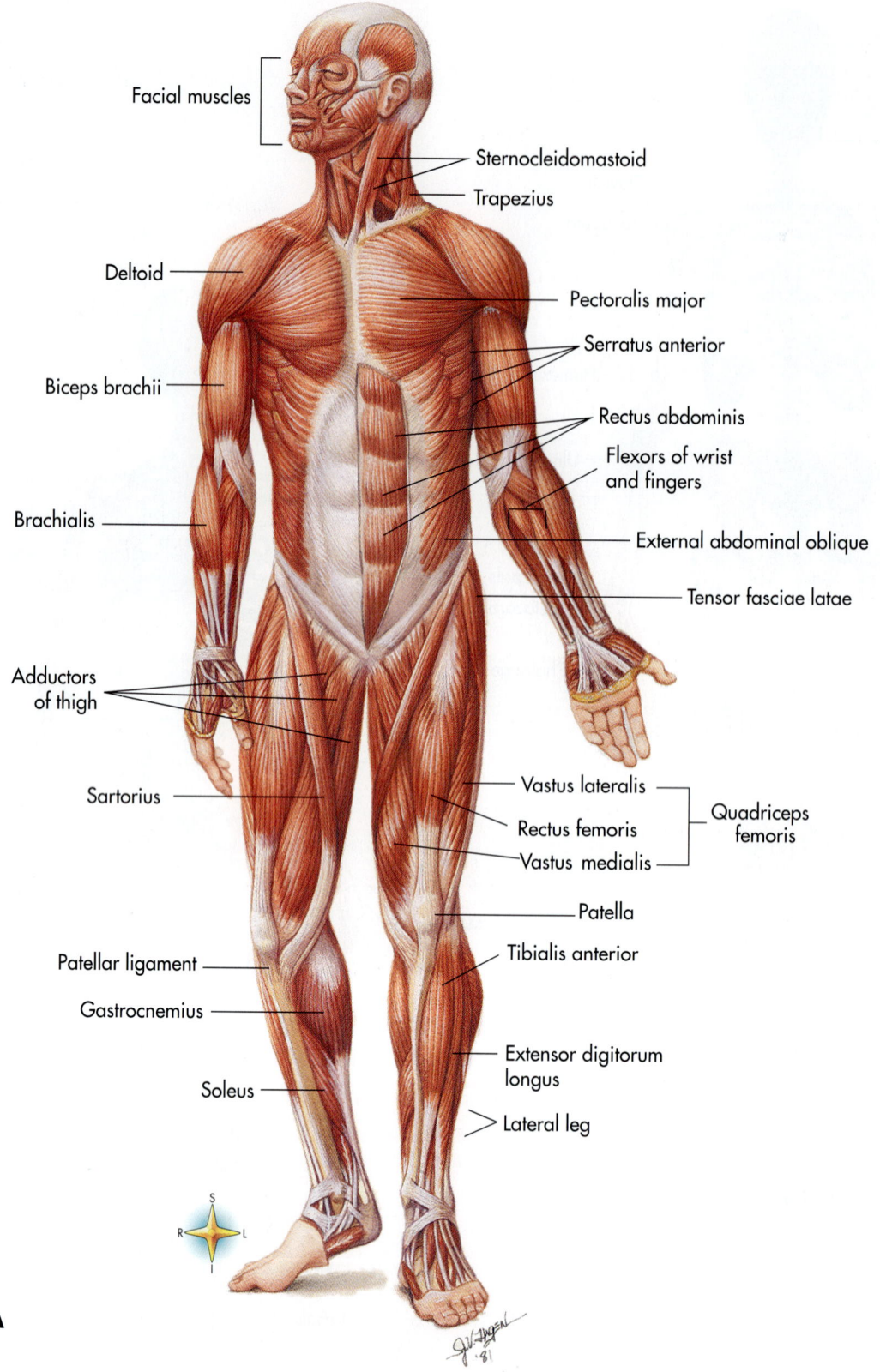

FIGURE 28.2 The muscular system. **A,** Anterior view.

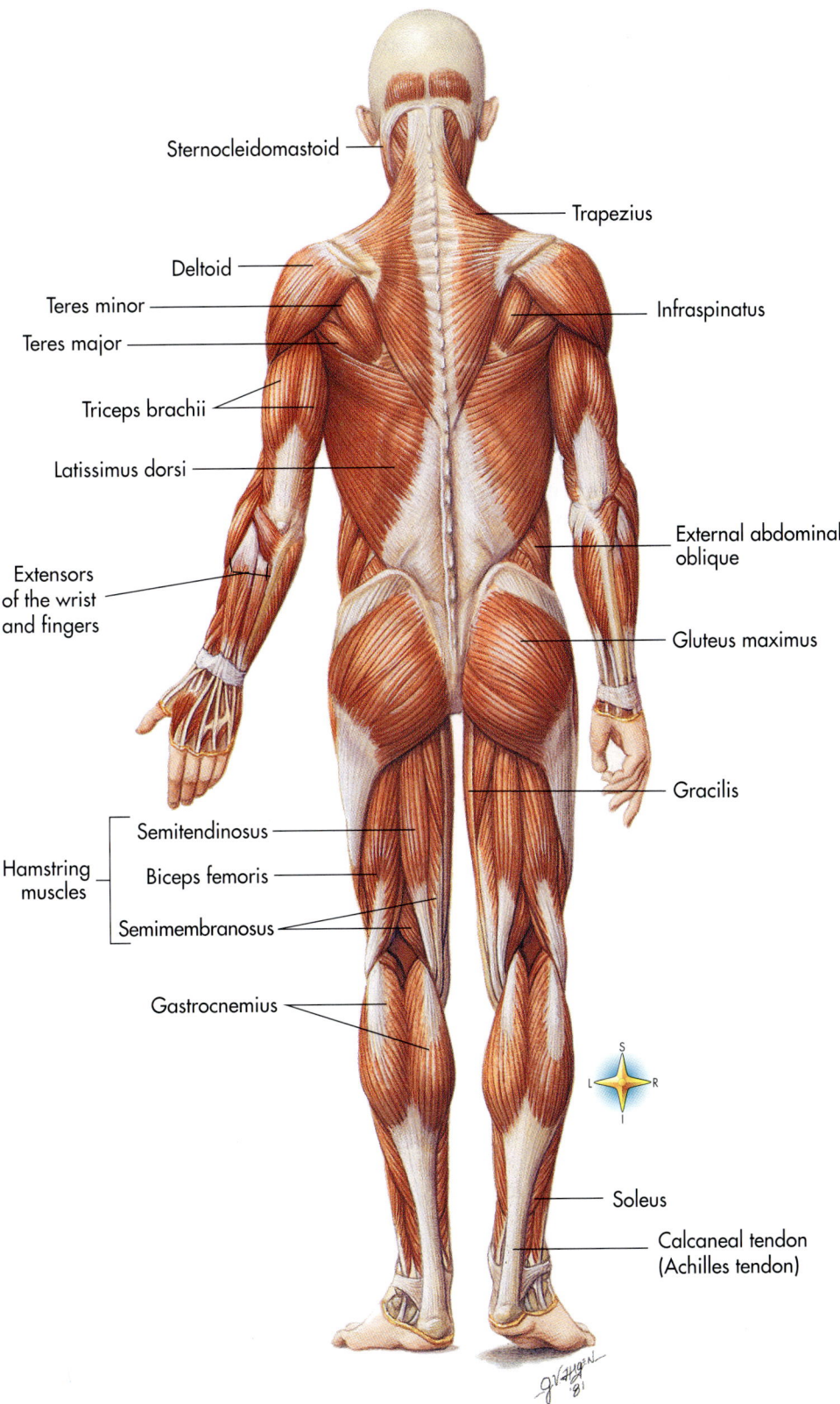

FIGURE 28.2, cont'd **B,** Posterior view.

movement of the skeletal system. An example is motion that occurs when the muscles of the arm contract or relax. The motion of flexing the elbow, moving the forearm up to the upper arm, is produced by contraction of the biceps muscle and relaxation of the triceps muscle. Extension of the forearm occurs by relaxation of the biceps and contraction of the triceps. Simplifying somewhat, all muscles of the skeletal system are arranged in pairs—the *agonist,* which moves a bone at its joint in one direction, and the *antagonist,* which slows and stabilizes the bone as this motion occurs. As the bones move in the opposite direction, the agonist-antagonist relationship changes. Not all movement is this simple to define, however. Even the movement of the elbow is not simply two muscles; others come into action as well. This complex action is illustrated by picking up an object with the hand, specifically between the thumb and forefinger. In accomplishing this seemingly simple task, numerous groups of muscles, starting in the shoulder, chest, and back and moving all the way down the arm to the hand, must work together in synergy.

Classification of Muscle

Muscles are classified into three groups based on their unique traits. Muscles found in the skeletal system are called skeletal muscles. Because of the design of skeletal muscle and the presence of **striations,** which serve to give it greater strength, it is referred to as striated muscle. Skeletal muscles are under voluntary control and respond to conscious thoughts; hence they are also called voluntary muscles.

Involuntary muscles are those found in the function and control of body organs, such as in the digestive system and respiratory system. They are also found in the blood vessels and help control blood pressure. This group of muscles is under involuntary control through the nervous system and controls functions vital to maintaining life. Involuntary muscle does not possess the strength of skeletal, striated muscle, but it has significantly greater endurance. Involuntary muscles do not possess the striations of skeletal muscle and are often referred to as **smooth muscle.**

The heart is made up of **cardiac muscle.** Possessing the strength of skeletal muscle and the endurance of smooth muscle, this unique muscle provides for movement of blood through the body on a continuous basis and responds to stimulation from the nervous system. Cardiac muscle is highly sensitive to lack of oxygen and will respond with pain in that area (angina pain). Skeletal and smooth muscle can tolerate much longer periods of anoxia (lack of oxygen) than can the heart. This is one reason why we say that injuries to the musculoskeletal system generally are not life threatening and should not take precedence over care of more serious, life-threatening situations, such as airway or circulation compromise.

> ✓ Tendons are the tough, fibrous structures that connect muscles to bone. Ligaments are similar fibrous structures that connect bone to bone across a joint.

> ✓ The EMT should be able to recognize the bones involved in a possible fractured extremity and understand the differences in muscle types.

Mechanism of Injury

The mechanism of injury is one of the most important facts that the EMT-B should determine when doing the survey of both the scene and the patient. The mechanism of injury provides valuable clues to what parts of the body may be injured and how serious the injury may be. Three forces cause bone and joint injuries:

- *Direct force,* such as would be found when a person is hit in the upper arm directly on the humerus, fracturing that bone at the point of impact
- *Indirect force,* such as would be found when a football player uses his outstretched hand to break a fall and the energy travels up the arm and results in a fracture near the elbow, the shoulder, or the clavicle
- *Twisting force,* such as would be found when a snow skier falls and the foot becomes planted in one spot, the rest of the body twists, and the energy is transmitted to the lower leg bone, resulting in a fracture (spiral)

Pathophysiology

Injuries to the Musculoskeletal System

If a bone is suspected of being fractured, the bone should be immobilized so that it does not continue to produce injury and pain to the patient. Movement of the sharp ends of bone inside the soft tissue of muscle and in the vicinity of arteries and nerves can produce additional damage. For example, if one took a tree branch and broke it in half, the ends of the branch would splinter. Picture these branch ends inside the body and imagine what the complications would be. The body tissues surrounding the injury could sustain lacerations to the arteries and veins, producing hemorrhage and compartment syndrome, or severed nerves, resulting in loss of feeling or motor function. These varied signs are why the term *swollen, painful,*

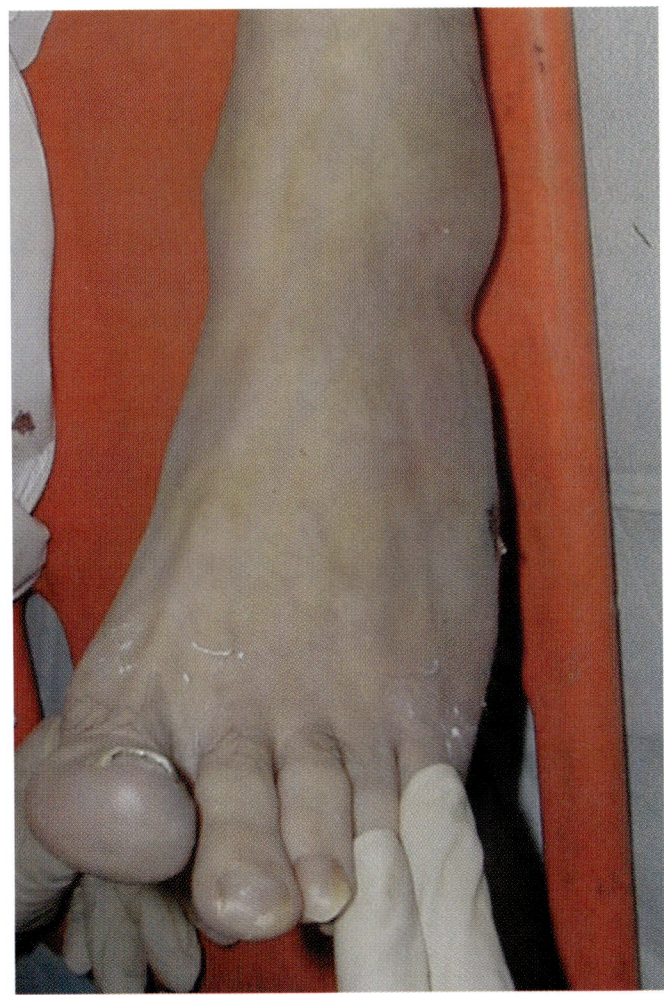
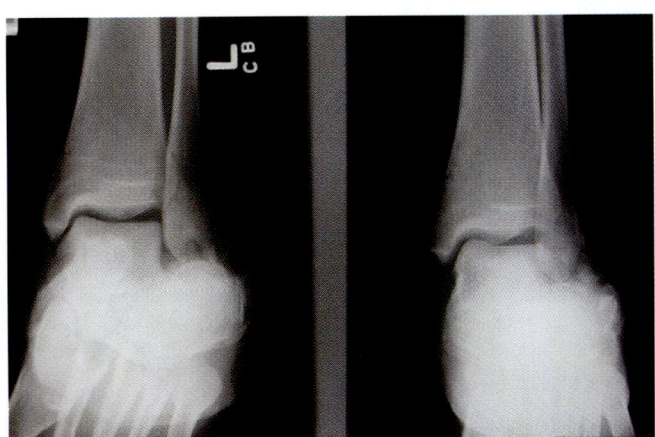

FIGURE 28.3 **A,** Sprained ankle with swelling. **B,** Radiograph of ankle showing no fracture.

deformed extremity has been introduced into the curriculum of the EMT-B training program. These are the signs that the injured extremity will cause in the field. Because the EMT cannot distinguish between a fracture, sprain, dislocation, or strain in the field, they all must be treated as if the worst type of fracture or dislocation exists. The extremity can be deformed on examination, painful when moved, swollen from blood or edema fluid, or all of these (Figure 28.3).

Fractures

Fractures can be described by the extent of the fracture, the possibility of contamination and infection (open or closed), the complexity of the fracture, or the relationship of one part of the bone to the other. Common fracture descriptions that are useful in prehospital management include the following:

Unstable—proximal and distal parts of the bone move freely in relationship to each other, as if a new joint has been created (Figure 28.4).
Impacted—jammed together so there is no motion between the proximal and distal bones (Figure 28.5).
Open versus closed—skin is open, allowing introduction of bacteria, dirt, and other foreign bodies, or skin is closed (Figure 28.6).
Fracture with dislocation—Fracture at the joint with injury to the supporting structures of the joint (Figure 28.7).

The muscle attachments that are usually proximal and distal to fractures involving the shaft of a bone tend to contract and shorten the extremity, producing overlapping of the bony ends. This overlapping can impinge on nerves, arteries, and veins that run in close proximity to the bones.

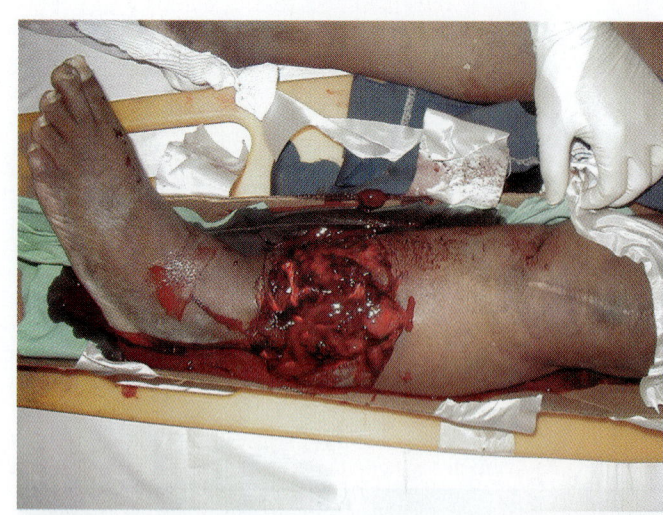
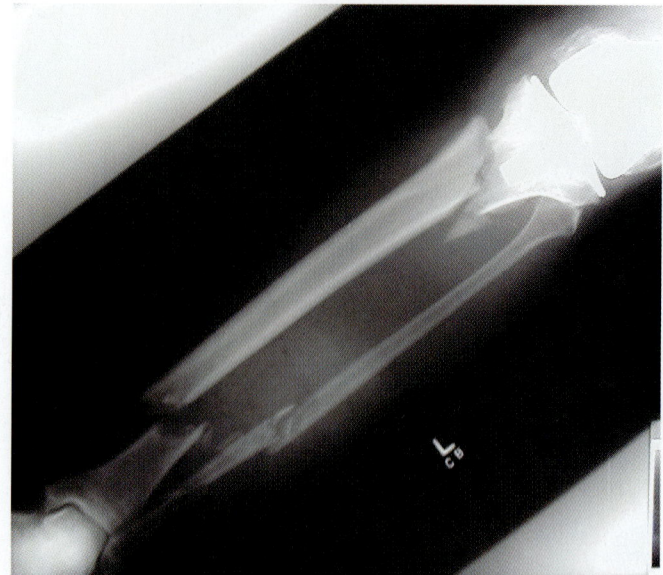

FIGURE 28.4 Unstable fracture.

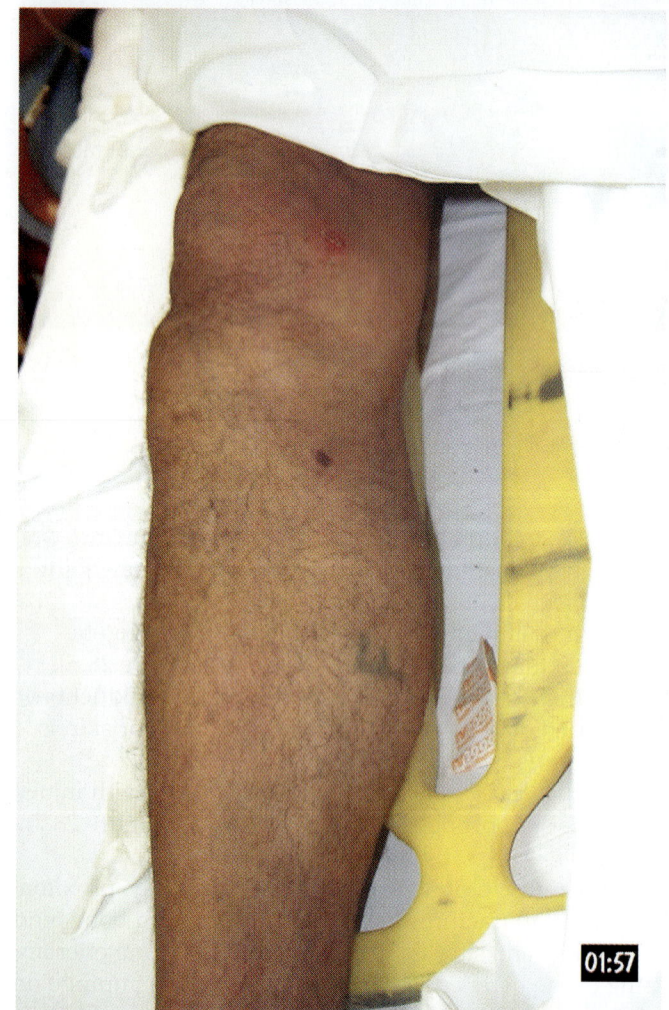
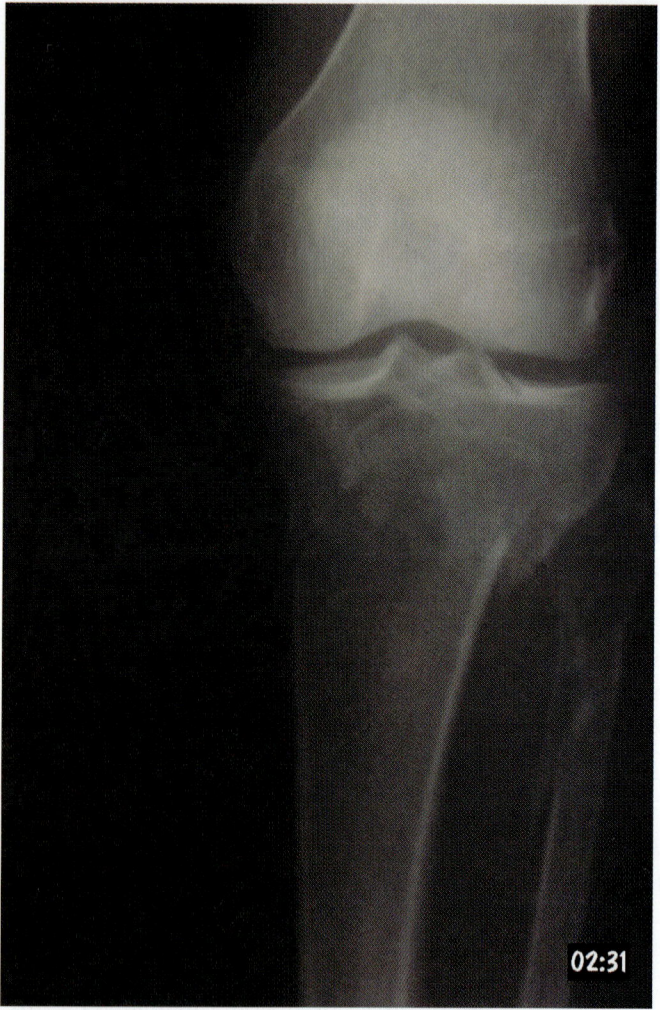

FIGURE 28.5 Impacted fracture.

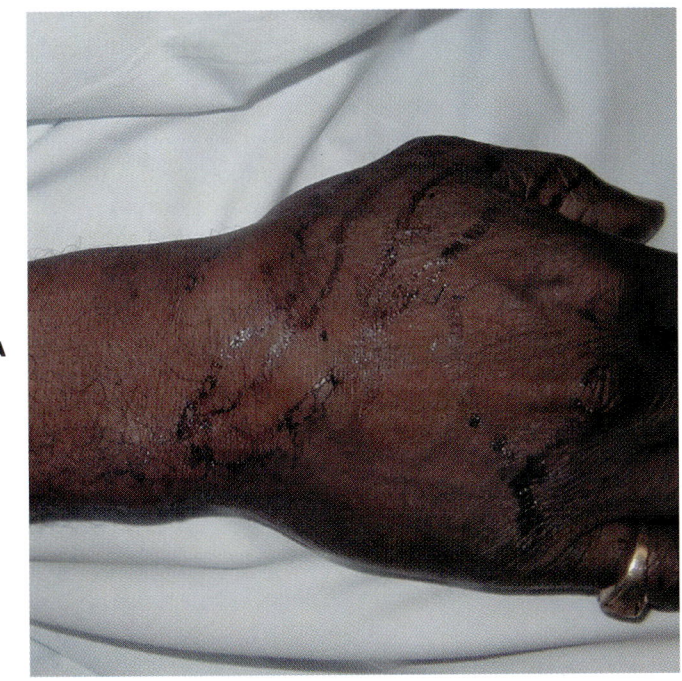 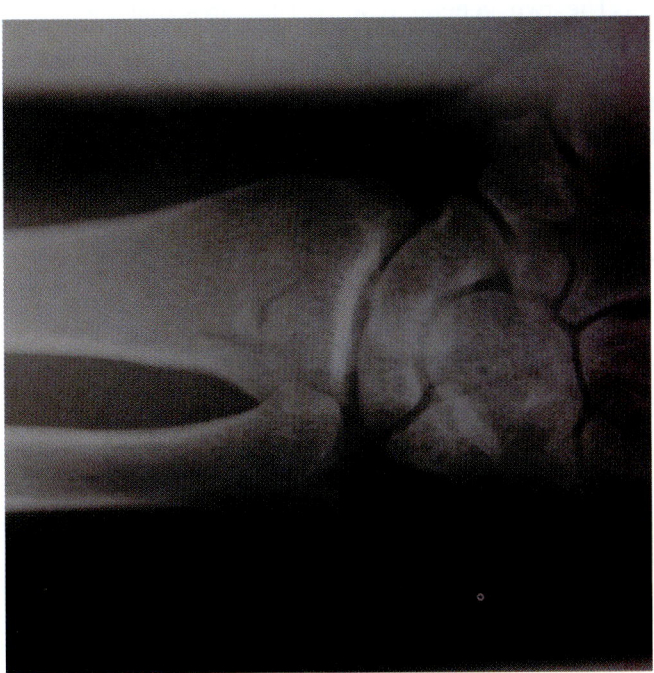

FIGURE 28.6 Open fracture.

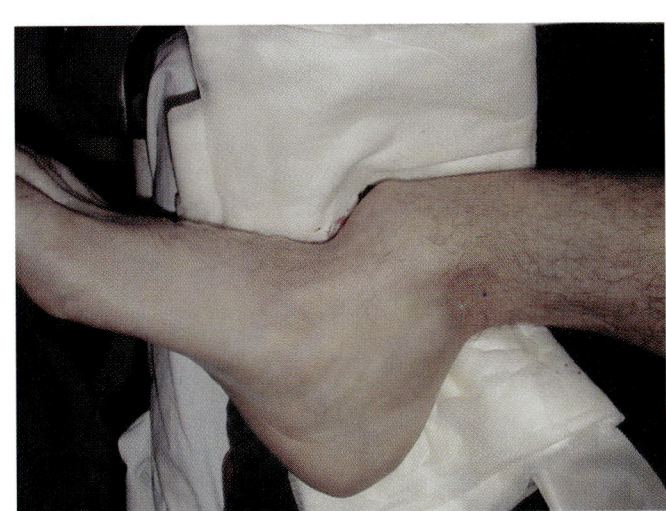 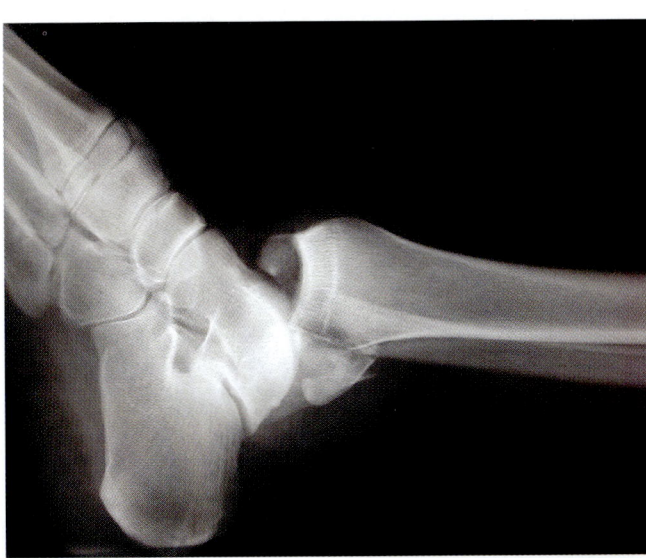

FIGURE 28.7 Fracture with dislocation.

The two general types of fractures that the EMT should recognize are open fractures and closed fractures.

Open fractures. An **open fracture** is one in which the integrity of the skin has been interrupted, which is usually caused by the bone ends breaking the skin from the inside (Figure 28.8). Usually the bone ends are still protruding through the skin, but it is possible for the bone to break the skin and then be pulled back inside the body due to the contraction of the muscles as they go into spasm.

Additional complications associated with open fractures include external hemorrhage, further damage to the muscles and nerves, and contamination. Do not try to push the bones back through the skin. However, the EMT should not worry if the ends of the bone "go back in" while the fracture is being stabilized.

> **Physician Notes**
>
> Reduction of the fracture ends back inside the skin will not cause an increase in the complication rate that already exists because of the initial contamination. The fact that the bone was out when first examined by the EMT should be reported to the ED physician at the time of the EMS report. The wound should be dressed with clean dressings.

Closed fractures. A **closed fracture** is one in which the skin integrity has not been compromised (Figure 28.9). The bone is broken; however, the skin is not lacerated.

Hemorrhage into the soft tissue surrounding the fracture site is a different but important complication of closed fractures for two reasons: compartment syndrome and blood volume loss. **Compartment syndrome** is any condition in which capillaries are compromised due to increased fluid into a closed space. This can be the result of hemorrhage, interstitial fluid, or swelling of the cells due to anoxia or direct injury. It can occur in the fascia compartments of the extremity, the abdomen, the pericardium, the chest, or the skull. This condition causes an increased pressure inside the compartment and can lead to death of the muscle tissue (ischemia) and may neces-

> ✓ Proper management of the extremity in the field can reduce the incidence of compartment syndrome. It is unusual for compartment syndrome to develop in the first few minutes after a fracture; therefore it is not something that the EMT should be overly concerned with, except as a condition that can result from poor field fracture management. However, compartment syndrome in the skull is of great concern to the EMT. This condition is discussed in Chapter 24.

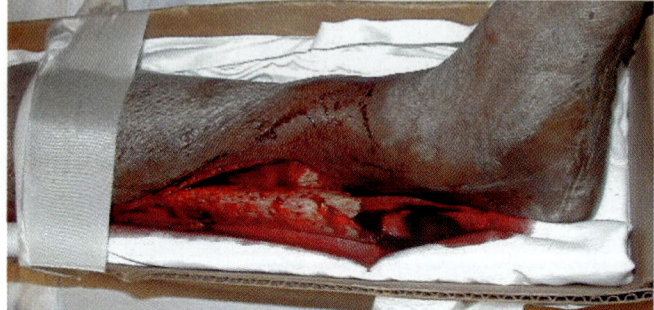
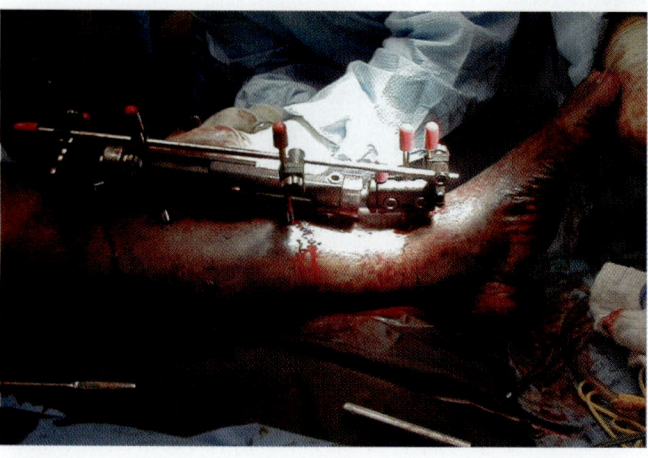
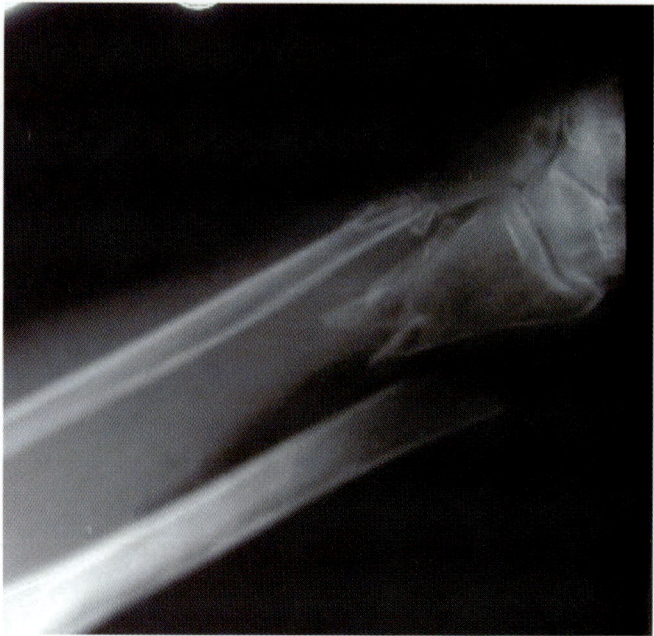

FIGURE 28.8 **A**, Open fracture. **B**, Radiograph of open fracture. **C**, Repair of open fracture with external fixator.

sitate amputation of the extremity involved. The condition is known by various names, such as pericardial tamponade, tension pneumothorax, closed head injury, or abdominal compartment syndrome, depending on the area of the body that is involved. In the extremity, the condition is simply called compartment syndrome. All result from the same pathologic process in which the pressure in the closed space increases to the point that the capillaries are compressed and blood flow to the cells is impaired.

In a closed fracture, in which the skin is not broken, the blood and fluid causing edema cannot escape. Blood loss into the tissue of a femur fracture can be as much as 500 to 1500 ml. This is a large amount of extra fluid in a closed space or compartment. As the hemorrhage continues and the pressure inside the compartment increases, capillaries, arteries, and veins that course through this compartment can become compressed. When this occurs, the blood flow to the cells in the compartment and to those cells distal to the compressed area is reduced. Ischemia develops, and the cells die. If edema is extensive, it can also produce the same result.

Dislocations

For the extremities to work properly, muscles attach to bones on either side of a joint. As the agonist muscles shorten and the antagonist muscles lengthen, they pull the two bones together and increase or decrease the angle of the joint. As long as the joint surfaces are in contact, such motion occurs in a smooth fashion. If an injury has pulled the joint surfaces out of contact, the joint can no longer move through its full range of motion or may not move at all. It may also impinge on nerves, arteries, and veins that are close to the involved joint. This dislodging of a bone from its normal position in a joint is called a **dislocation**. Frequently a dislocation is associated with a fracture (see Figure 28.7).

The bones that are in contact at a joint are held in place by ligaments that extend to the bones on either side of the joint, by muscles that attach on either side of the joint, or by a muscle-tendon complex in which the muscle is on one side of the joint but extends its influence to a bone on the other side of the joint by way of a tendon. The joint capsule itself keeps the joint surfaces in contact. Fluid inside the joint capsule lubricates the joint surfaces as they rub against each other.

Injury to any of these supporting structures, tendons, muscles, ligaments, or joint capsule, may not be severe enough to cause complete dislocation but can be severe enough to cause pain and swelling. It is also possible for the dislocation to occur at the time of the trauma and then to spontaneously reduce (or become "relocated") before the EMT arrives. Understanding this possibility allows the EMT to consider that such an event has occurred and to treat the patient accordingly.

Injuries to Muscle, Ligaments, and Tendons

Injuries to muscles are more common than injuries to bones. Most people will not call an ambulance for "twisting an ankle" or "pulling a back," unless the injury renders them nonambulatory (unable to walk). As has been noted, it is not the function of an EMT to differentiate between a muscle injury and a bone injury, because the field management of each is the same. However, it is important to recognize the difference between the two injuries and the pathophysiology of each.

Injuries to muscle, ligaments, and tendons occur when a joint or muscle is either torn or stretched beyond its normal limits. Two types of such injuries are strains and sprains.

Strains

A **strain** is a soft tissue injury or muscle spasm that occurs around a joint anywhere in the musculature (Figure 28.10). A strain is also known as a muscle pull. Strains do not involve injury to the surrounding ligaments, tendons, or joints, only to the muscle. Strains are characterized by pain with movement of the joint and little or no swelling.

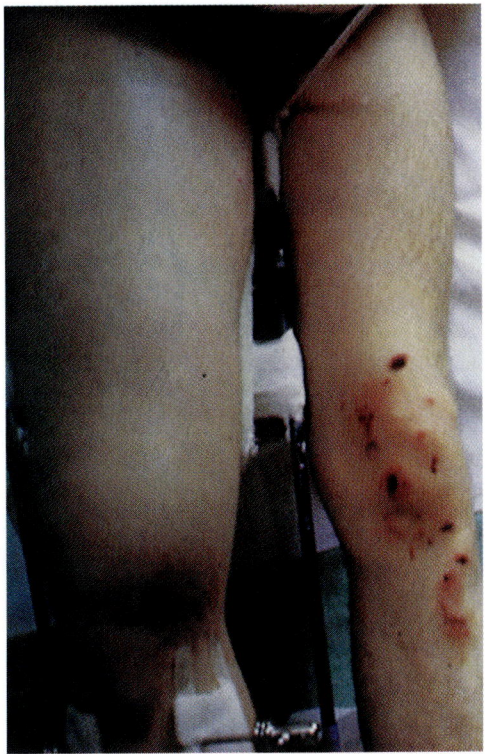

FIGURE 28.9 Example of a closed fracture. Note the massive swelling of the right thigh. The femoral artery had been partly torn, and the foot became ischemic. The patient subsequently lost his limb.

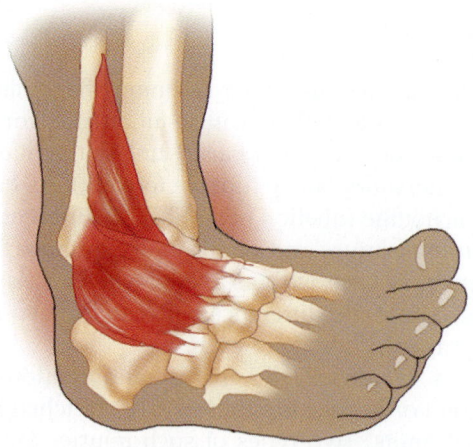

FIGURE 28.10 A strain is a soft tissue injury or muscle spasm that occurs around a joint anywhere in the musculature.

Sprains

A **sprain** is an injury in which ligaments are stretched or partially torn (Figure 28.11, A). Sprains are usually caused by a sudden twisting of the joint beyond its normal range of motion. A sprain can vary from mild to severe depending on the amount of damage the supporting ligaments sustain (Figure 28.11, B). Sprains are very painful, with swelling of the soft tissue surrounding the joint and possible discoloration. Sprains are sometimes confused with fractures; on scene they can appear the same. However, an x-ray of a sprain reveals no loss of integrity to the bones of the joint. Even though a sprain does not involve an actual fracture, it can and does produce significant pain for the patient that can last for several weeks (see Figure 28.3, A).

> ✓ It is important for the EMT to know that there are differences between a dislocation, a fracture, a strain, and a sprain. However, these injuries should all be treated as fractures (the most significant injury) because it is difficult, if not impossible, to diagnose a fracture in the field without an x-ray machine or other imaging equipment.

Assessment

The signs and symptoms that should lead the EMT to suspect a musculoskeletal injury are listed in Box 28.1.

Look

Mound or Swelling

Acute swelling of an extremity indicates hemorrhage and inflammation in the area. Hemorrhage can result from a fracture from the open ends of the bone and surrounding

---

Box 28.1 McSwain-Paturas Musculoskeletal Assessment System (MPMAS)

Look
- **M**—Mound of swelling around injury
- **U**—Unusual color—bruise or ecchymosis
  - Unusual position—deformity or angulations

Listen
- **S**—Sound progression down long bones

Feel
- **C**—Crepitus
- **U**—Unusual motion in the midshaft of the bone
- **L**—Loss
  - Nerve supply
    - Paralysis
    - Paresthesia
  - Blood supply
    - Pulse
    - Capillary refill
- **O**—*Ouch!* Pain and tenderness with palpation or movement

---

damaged tissue or a sprain in which torn structures bleed internally. Compartment syndrome should also be noted as a potential problem (Figure 28.12).

Unusual Discoloration

Hemorrhage into the subcutaneous tissue (fatty tissue just beneath the skin) gradually seeps into the interstitial space, producing purplish discolorations. This discoloration changes over a period of a few days to a week from purple to blue to green to yellow. The color then fades. This coloration can also travel distally as the blood runs "downhill." This change occurs over several days to weeks. The initial ecchymosis, or bruise, indicates subcutaneous hemorrhage associated with bone or soft tissue injury.

Unusual Position

Breaks in the bone or dislocations of the joint produce an extra bending point or extra angulation. Any deformity that does not show in-line positioning (normal linear position of the bone) of the extremity should raise the EMT's suspicions (Figure 28.13).

Listen

Sound progression along a long bone is diminished by a fracture or break in the continuity of the bone. By placing the stethoscope on the symphysis pubis, the sound of

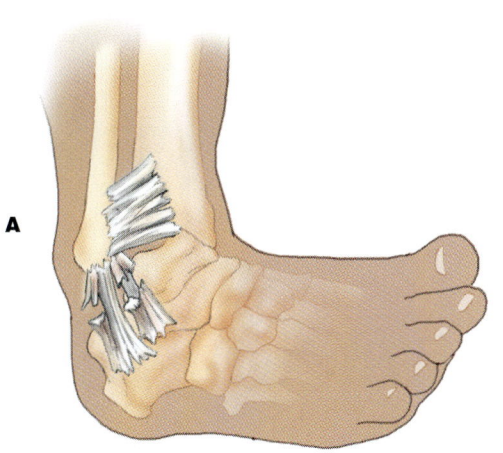 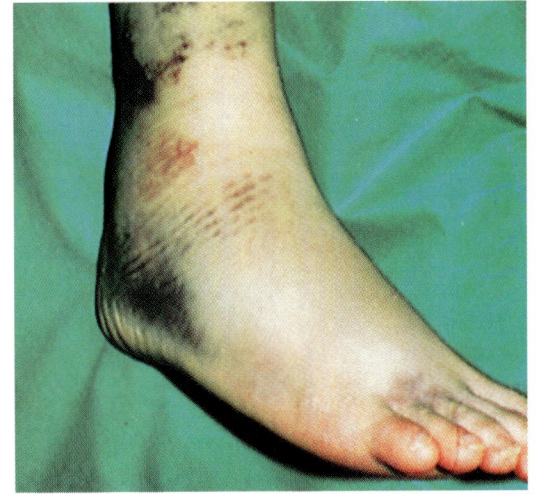

FIGURE 28.11 **A,** A sprain is an injury in which ligaments are stretched or partially torn. **B,** Example of a bad sprain, after 1 day.

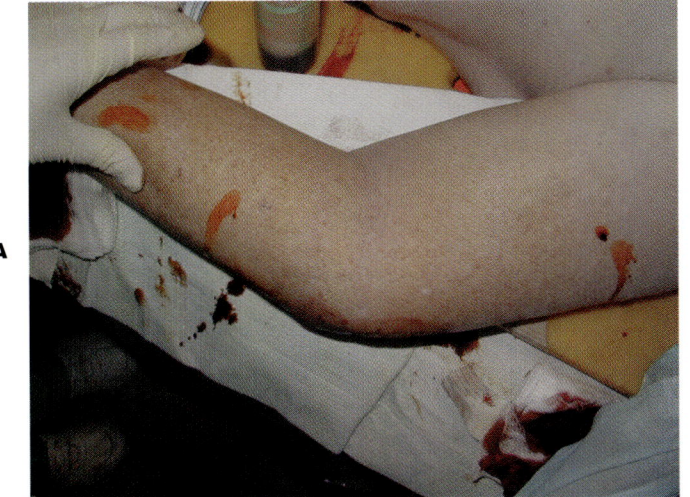 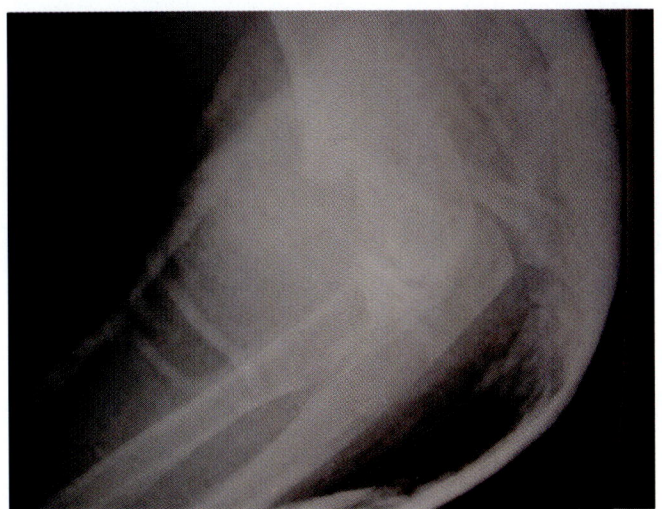

FIGURE 28.12 Mound or swelling.

percussion on the patella is easily heard if the femur is intact. If there is a fracture, the sound will be diminished when the patella is percussed on the side of the fracture.

Feel

Crepitus is both a sound and the feeling bones can make when they are fractured. It is caused by the grating of the bone ends against each other. An EMT can precipitate crepitus by palpating the site of injury. Crepitus sounds like a snap, crackle, and pop. Another analogy is the popping of bubble packing. Although the feeling of bones grating together is often felt during the assessment of the patient, it can produce further injury. Therefore the EMT should not try to produce it. Crepitus has a distinct sound and feeling; once recognized, it is not easily forgotten.

Loss of Nerve Supply (Paresthesia or Paralysis)

Loss of sensation of the part of the extremity distal to the injury indicates compression or laceration of the nerves in proximity to the fracture. This is more often associated with fractures than with sprains or strains. Inability to voluntarily move the extremity indicates nerve damage proximal to the muscle group in question.

Loss of Blood Supply (Pulselessness)

Blood supply to the region of the body that is distal to the injury can be interrupted by laceration of an artery,

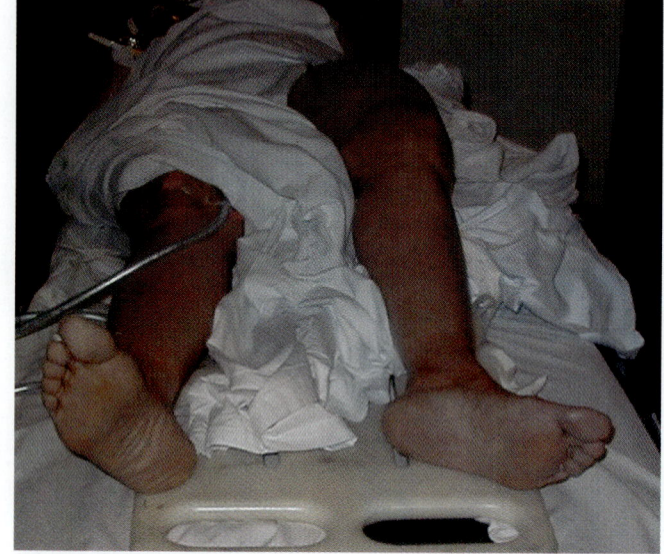
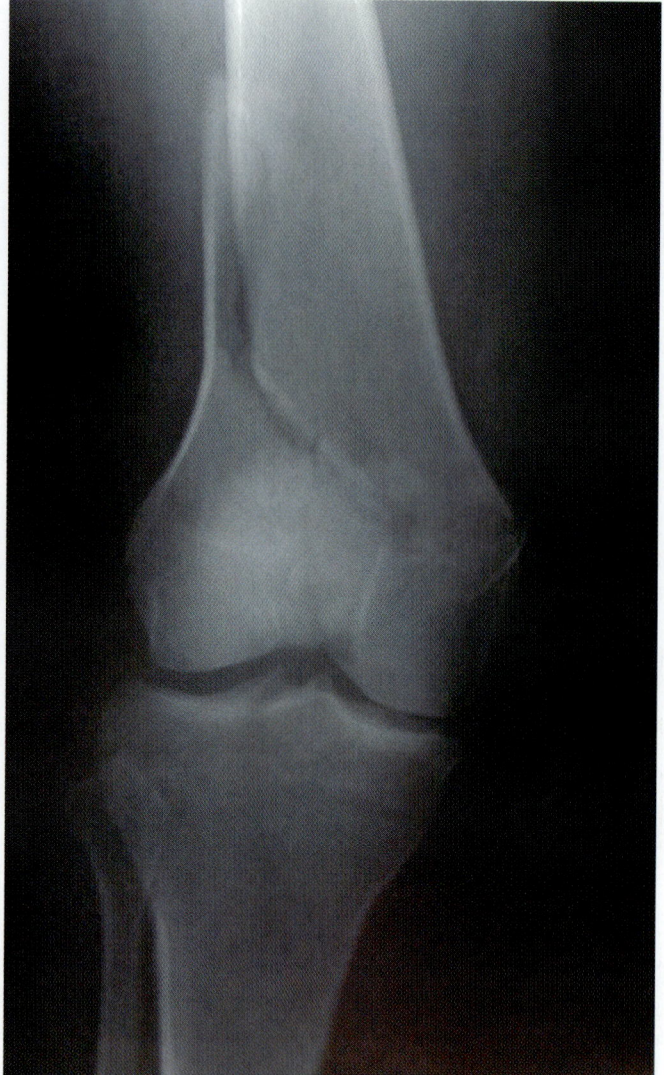

FIGURE 28.13 Unusual position.

compression of a vessel by an expanding hematoma, or a bone fragment encroaching on a blood vessel. If the blood flow is not returned to the extremity or the EMT does not recognize the significance of the injury, the result could be loss of the extremity.

Capillary Refill Time

Although other conditions, such as cold, may cause increased capillary refill time, if there is delay of capillary refill time one must be concerned that the blood supply has been interrupted or slowed to the extremity. The cause must be determined and treated.

Pain

The stretching or tearing of the periosteum (the external layer of tissue that surrounds the bone) produces an extremely painful area that is made worse by movement. Such signs and symptoms can be associated with dislocations, fractures, or sprains.

> ✓ Passive motion of the extremity by the EMT or active movement by the patient produces pain at the site of the fracture, dislocation, or strain. The EMT should not move the extremity unless necessary because movement could cause further injury to the patient.

The EMT must be able to identify the signs and symptoms of an extremity injury: pain; swelling; crepitus; discoloration; and an interruption of pulse, movement, or sensation (Box 28.2).

Management

General Principles

When arriving at a scene, it is easy for an EMT to be sidetracked by a gross deformity of an extremity or bleeding around a fracture site. As in any field situation, the initial assessment—looking for life-threatening conditions—is the most important lifesaving duty of the EMT. Assessment of the ABCs comes first, then control of gross hemorrhage, and then stabilization of fractures.

The joints above and below a fracture must be immobilized. Rotation and movement of the bone above and below the joint can be transmitted through the joint to the site of the fracture. Therefore the joint must be stable. To accomplish this goal, at least half of the bone above and below the joints that are above and below the fracture must also be immobilized; in critical situations, anatomic positioning must be done.

> ✓ A gross angulation or hemorrhage of a femur fracture, as dramatic as it may be, is not as important as the patient's airway. If the patient is not breathing, there is no sense in stabilizing a fracture or controlling a hemorrhage.

General Guidelines of Splinting

The following guidelines for splinting fractures are good general principles to follow. Each field situation is different, and each fracture is handled slightly differently. However, the following steps are helpful to memorize as a pattern to follow:

1. Assess pulse, motor, and sensation distal to the injury before and after splint application, and record findings.
2. Support the area of injury.
3. Remove or cut away clothing.
4. Cover open wounds with a sterile dressing, and control external hemorrhage.
5. If a severe deformity exists or the distal extremity is cyanotic or lacks pulses, align with gentle traction before splinting.
6. Do not intentionally replace the protruding bones, but it is acceptable if they return within the skin while the EMT is aligning and immobilizing the fracture.
7. Pad each splint to prevent pressure and discomfort to the patient.
8. When feasible, splint the patient's injury before moving the patient if no life-threatening conditions are evident.

Box 28.2

The National Standard Curriculum uses the mnemonic DCAP-BTLS as a teaching aid for injuries:
D = Deformities
C = Contusions
A = Abrasions
P = Punctures/penetrations
B = Burns
T = Tenderness
L = Lacerations
S = Swelling

9. If the patient shows signs and symptoms of shock, align the patient in supine position on the long backboard, treat for shock, and transport immediately.
10. If the extremity is deformed, gentle attempts at restoring alignment should be done. This realignment is frequently easier with traction.
11. When the patient has multiple injuries or is in shock, immobilizing the patient to the long backboard will immobilize all of the fractures at the same time.

Complications of Splinting

Any procedure has complications. Astute EMTs detect complications early by observing the following:

1. Constriction of blood supply
2. Compression on nerves

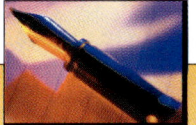

> **Tips from the Pros**
>
> Mark the site of a pulse once it is found, so that it can be relocated quickly and easily. Use a ballpoint pen to mark an X over the most prominent area of the pulse.
>
> It is possible to support the fracture site using the forearm to cradle the extremity, as one would an infant.

Special Considerations

Hemorrhage

After completing the ABCs, the next step is to control bleeding. Control of bleeding that is caused by an open fracture is much the same as controlling bleeding of any other part of the body: place a sterile dressing on the laceration and apply pressure to the site. An Ace bandage or roller gauze can be helpful in this situation because this frees the EMT's hands to further treat the patient. Once the

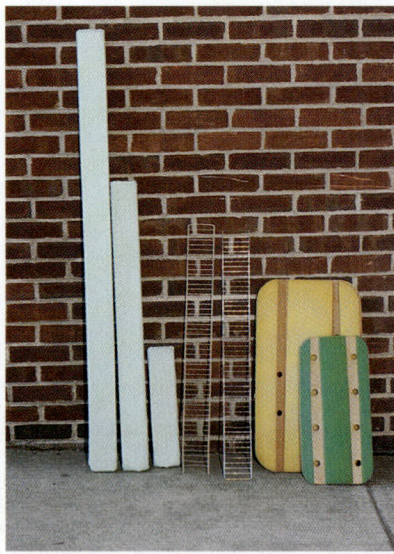

FIGURE 28.14 Examples of splints.

bandage becomes soaked with blood, do not remove the bandage but place more dressings over the original one.

Life-Threatening Injuries

If the initial assessment reveals that the patient has life-threatening injuries, precise stabilization of individual fractures is not a priority. In a **multisystem trauma patient** (a patient who has more than one body system injured) with non–life-threatening injuries to the extremities, the EMT must prioritize injuries and treat those that are life threatening. However, this prioritization should not minimize the need to stabilize fractures. Immobilization of fractures is done by complete immobilization of the body. Total immobilization of the body is accomplished by supporting all fractures and placing the patient on a long backboard and securing the patient to the board.

Interruption of Blood Supply, Movement, or Sensation

When assessing a possible fracture, the EMT may discover that the patient does not have a pulse distal to the injury or cannot move or feel sensation distal to the injury. In these situations, the priority level of the fracture increases. Attempts at restoring blood flow by using the standard splinting techniques should be done. However, these findings do not outweigh life-threatening injuries. This patient should be immediately transported to the hospital after the fracture is stabilized.

Practical Skills: Splinting

The following skills demonstrations describe only skills—they are not scenarios. In real life, the EMTs would have evaluated the scene and situation and ensured their safety and that of the patient. They would have also completed any higher-priority care and dressed all wounds before performing the demonstrated skill. The EMT should reassess the ABCs at any time during the procedure if the situation warrants. As always, use body substance isolation precautions.

> 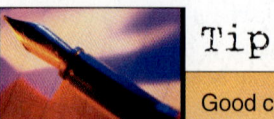 **Tips from the Pros**
>
> Good communication between partners and with the patient is always a must, especially when applying a splint. Communication ensures that each partner knows what the other is doing, and also informs the patient step by step what is being performed.

Long Bone Splint

Examples

Padded long board splint, gutter splint, and ladder splint (Figure 28.14).

Uses

Humerus, radius, ulna, tibia, and fibula.

Procedure

1. The first EMT supports the fractured extremity using one hand above the injury and one hand below the injury to prevent further movement of the extremity. For an upper extremity, hold the extremity under the site of injury, as opposed to a lower extremity, where it works better to hold the extremity above the injuries (Figure 28.15, A).
2. The second EMT assesses pulses, movement, and sensation and removes clothing. Movement is best assessed by asking the patient to wiggle his or her fingers or toes. Sensation is assessed by touching one of the patient's fingers or toes and asking, "Which finger/toe am I touching?" (Figure 28.15, B)

> ✓ The following general guidelines should be followed when splinting an extremity. Check pulses, movement, and sensation before, during, and after splinting an extremity. The extremity should be supported while being splinted, thus splinting requires two people. Interruption of pulse, movement, and sensation should be recognized as a serious problem. Immediate life-threatening injuries must be addressed first, and thus some fractured extremities may be splinted only with an anatomic splint (e.g., a long backboard).

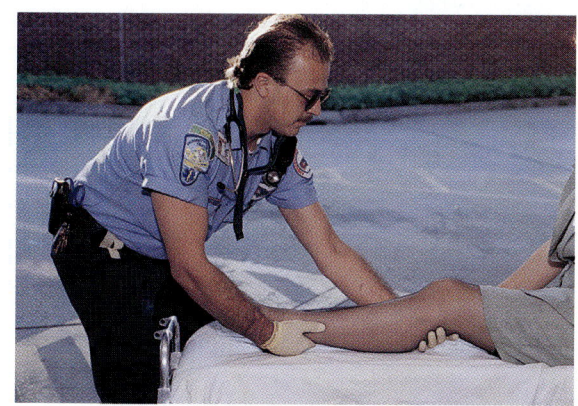
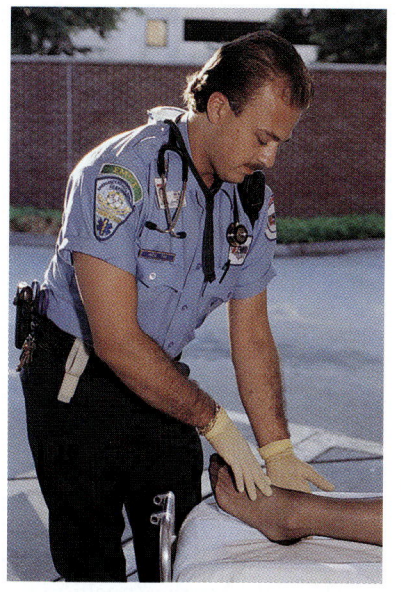
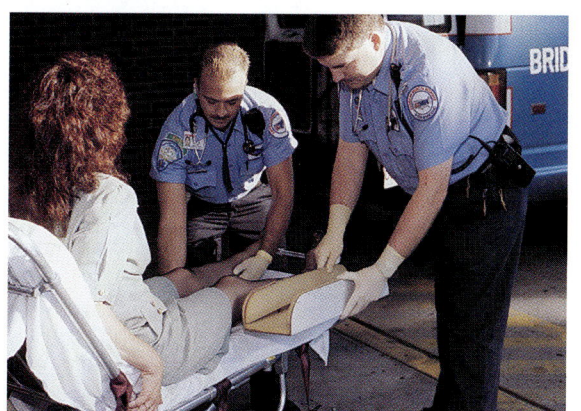
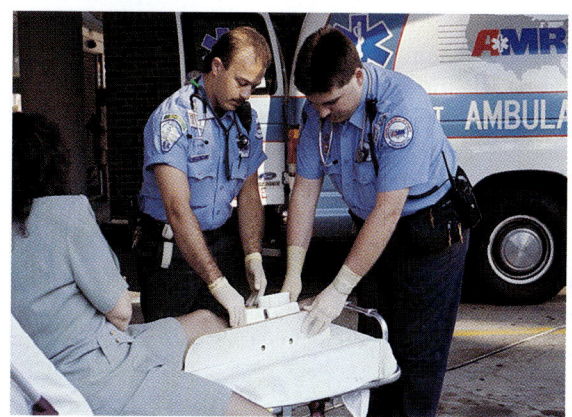
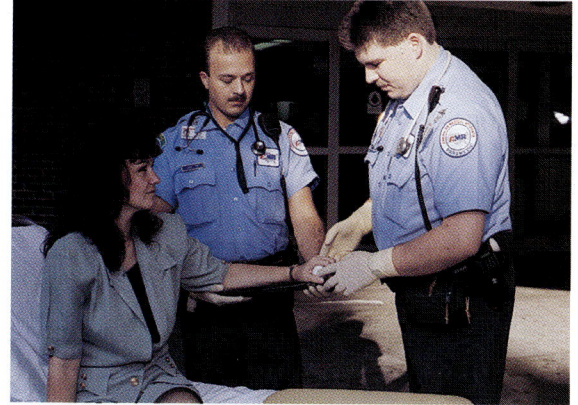
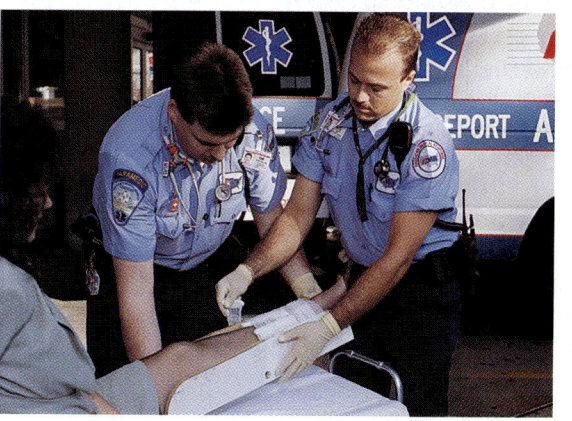
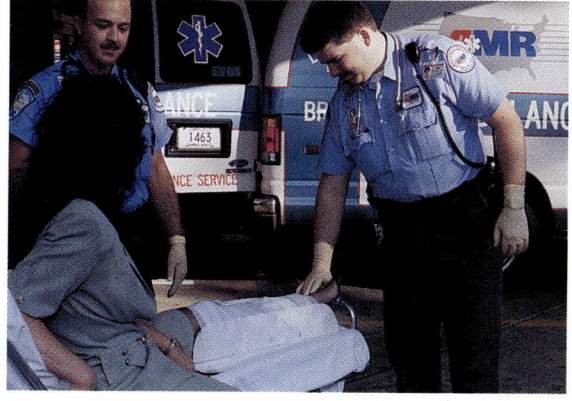

FIGURE 28.15 Long bone splinting. **A,** EMT #1 supports the fractured extremity using one hand above the injury and one hand below the injury. **B,** EMT #2 assesses pulses, movement, and sensation and removes clothing. **C,** While EMT #1 maintains stabilization of the injured extremity, EMT #2 measures the splint against the unaffected extremity. **D,** Pad voids between the splint and extremity. **E,** When immobilizing a radius/ulna or wrist fracture, the patient's hand must be placed in the position of function. **F,** Secure the splint to the extremity by wrapping the splint with roller gauze or tape. **G,** Reassess pulse, movement, and sensation of the extremity, and record.

3. While the first EMT maintains stabilization of the extremity, the second EMT chooses the best splint to apply and measures it against the unaffected extremity. Measurement is to ensure that the joints above and below the injured site will be immobilized (Figure 28.15, C).
4. When using a gutter splint, the first EMT supports the fracture site and lifts the extremity just enough so that the second EMT can slip the splint under the extremity.
5. Make sure that the joints above and below the injured site are included within the splint.
6. Pad voids between the splint and the extremity. Voids can be padded with combination pads, roller gauze, sheets, and so on (Figure 28.15, D).
7. When immobilizing a radius/ulna or wrist fracture, the patient's hand must be placed in the "position of function" for comfort. Position of function is accomplished by placing a roller gauze in the patient's hand and having the patient gently grasp the gauze. This procedure is done for the comfort of the patient and long-term management (Figure 28.15, E).
8. Secure the splint to the extremity by wrapping the splint with roller gauze or tape. The first EMT holds the splint, and the second EMT wraps tape or roller gauze around the splint. Leave fingers or toes uncovered to allow assessment of movement and sensation. Also, do not cover the site of the pulse for the same reason (Figure 28.15, F).
9. Assess pulse, movement, and sensation of extremity, and record (Figure 28.15, G).

Improvisation

If a commercial device is not available, pieces of wood that are long enough to reach above and below the injury site can be used, as well as rolled-up newspaper, cardboard, and so on.

Other

If possible, elevate the extremity and place an ice pack on the site of injury. This reduces both swelling and pain.

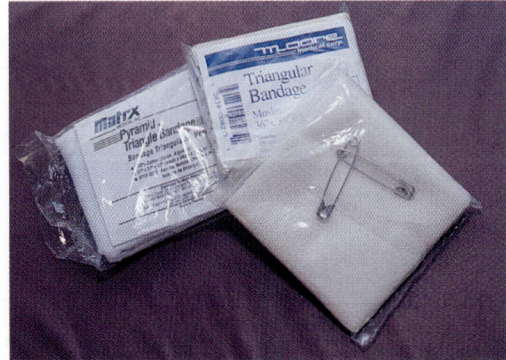

FIGURE 28.16 Triangular bandages, also called cravats.

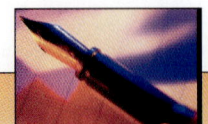

Tips from the Pros

Fractured extremities shorten due to the contraction and spasm of the muscles. Because of this shortening, always measure splints on the unaffected extremity.

Sling and Swathe

Examples
Triangular bandages, also called cravats (Figure 28.16).

Uses
Humerus, clavicle, scapula, radius, and ulna.

Procedure

1. The first EMT supports the fractured extremity using one hand above the injury site and one hand below the site (Figure 28.17, A).
2. The second EMT assesses pulse, movement, and sensation of the injured extremity and removes the patient's clothing (Figure 28.17, B).
3. When splinting the humerus, it is best to use a board splint to provide additional support. Secure the board splint on the lateral aspect of the arm, above and below the humerus (Figure 28.17, C).
4. While the first EMT supports the fractured extremity, the second EMT unwraps the triangular bandage and pulls one of the long ends up under the forearm and up around the neck (Figure 28.17, D).
5. The second EMT takes the other end of the triangular bandage and brings it up over the forearm and around to the other side of the neck (Figure 28.17, E). The sling should support the wrist and the hand, not just the radius and ulna alone.
6. The second EMT ties the two ends of the triangular bandage around the patient's neck, and the first EMT reassesses pulse, movement, and sensation (Figure 28.17, F).
7. A swathe is made by folding the triangular bandage in such a way that it is approximately 1 to 2 inches wide. Start by unwrapping the bandage and place the full length of it on a flat surface. Fold a square bandage into a triangle shape. Take the longer ends and fold them toward the shorter end, like a bandanna (Figure 28.17, G).
8. Ask the patient to hold the uninjured arm out to his or her side, and wrap the triangular bandage around the patient's body and the injured arm. Secure the bandage with a knot (Figure 28.17, H).
9. Assess pulse, movement, and sensation, and record.

Improvisation

Roller gauze can be used for a swathe if a triangular bandage is unavailable.

Other

When a humoral fracture is severely angulated or no pulse distal to the injury can be detected, the EMT should apply gentle traction to the injury site. This traction attempts to realign the arteries and nerves so blood supply can be regained. To apply gentle traction, grasp one hand distal to the injury, preferably at the elbow, and the other hand proximal to the injury, close to the axillary region. Pull gently in line to maintain position, and then check the pulse. If a pulse is present, splint the injury. If possible, elevate the extremity and apply an ice pack. This procedure also applies to radius and ulna fractures in much the same way.

Joints

Joints are more difficult to splint because joint injuries are more painful for the patient. Joint injuries must be handled more carefully so as not to damage the joint, muscles, tendons, or ligaments or cause more swelling. Splint joint injuries as found, however difficult this may be. This rule should not be hard to remember because patients are usually in so much pain that they will not allow the injured joint to be moved.

Example

Board splints are the most common kind of splint used for joint injuries (Figure 28.18).

Uses

Knee and elbow.

Procedure

See Joint Immobilization Step-by-Step Procedure at the end of this chapter.

1. Assess pulse, movement, and sensation distal to the injury, and remove the patient's clothing.
2. The first EMT supports the extremity as found.
3. While the first EMT supports the fracture site, the second EMT places one board splint on the medial

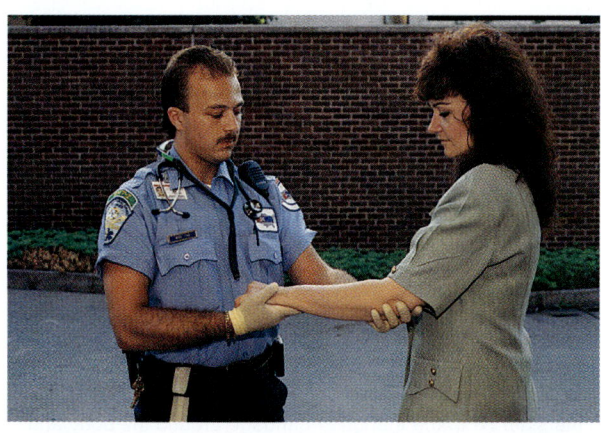
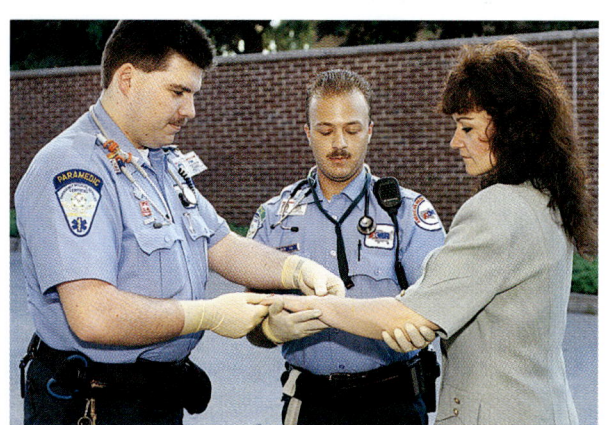
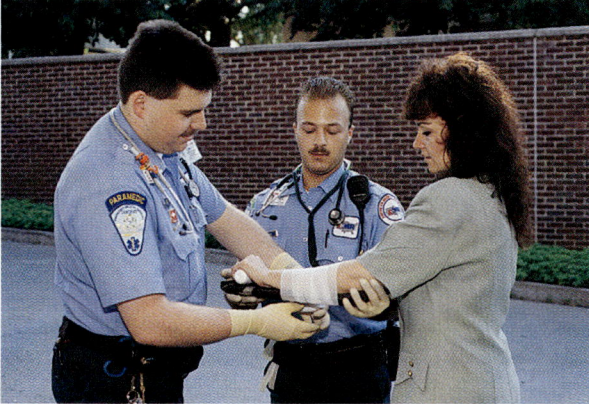
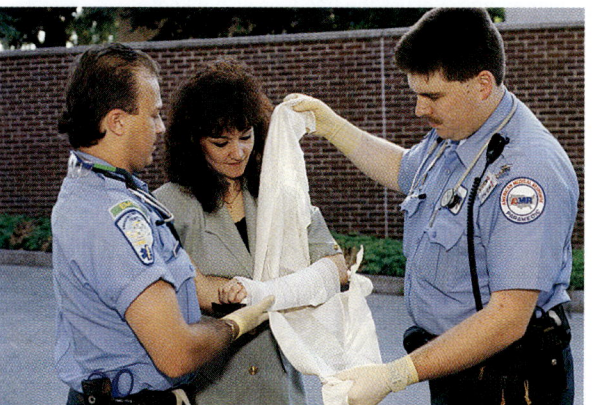

FIGURE 28.17 Sling and swathe. **A,** EMT #1 supports the fractured extremity using one hand above and one hand below the injury. **B,** EMT #2 assesses pulses, movement, and sensation and removes clothing. **C,** Secure the board splint above and below the humerus. **D,** While EMT #1 supports the fractured extremity, EMT #2 unwraps the triangular bandage and pulls one of the long ends up under the forearm and up around the neck.

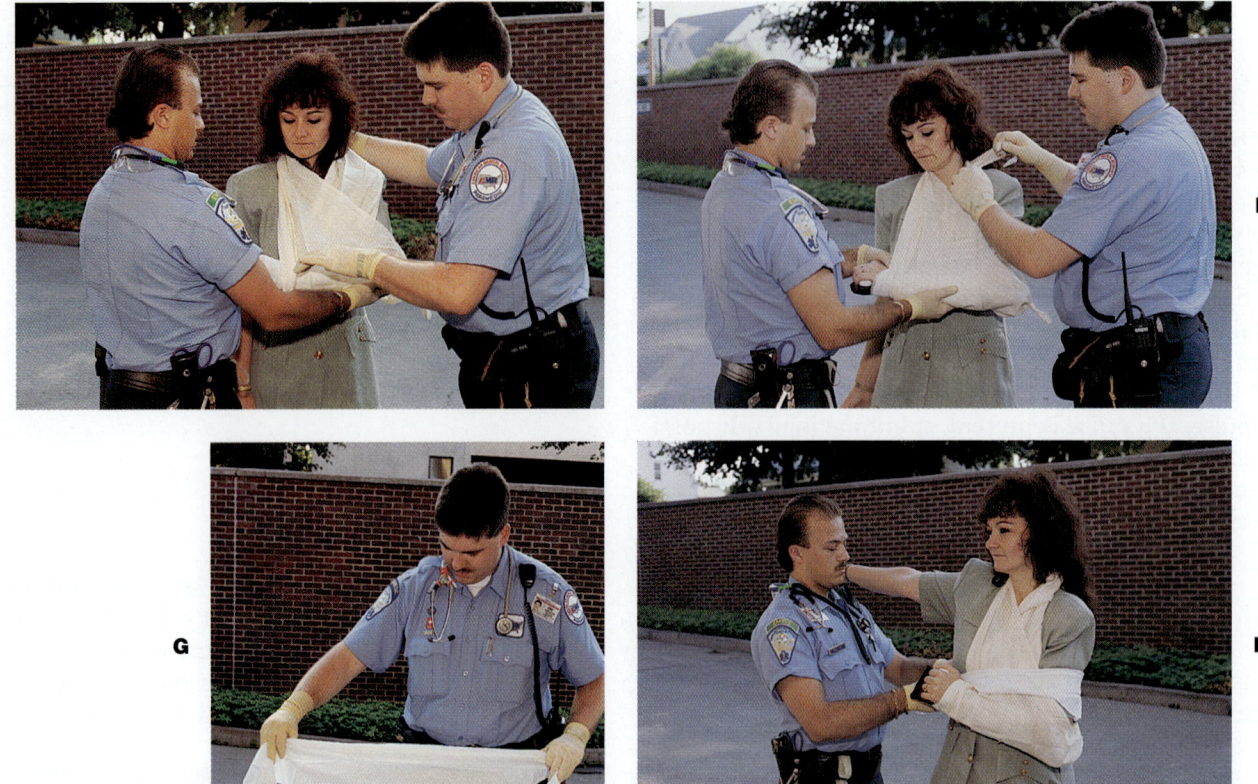

FIGURE 28.17, cont'd **E,** EMT #2 takes the other end of the triangular bandage and brings it up over the forearm and around the other side of the neck. **F,** EMT #2 ties the two ends of the triangular bandage around the patient's neck. EMT #1 reassesses pulses, movement, and sensation. **G,** A swathe is made by folding the triangular bandage so that it is approximately 2 inches wide. **H,** Ask the patient to hold the uninjured arm out to the side. Wrap the triangular bandage around the body and injured arm. Secure the bandage with a knot.

aspect of the extremity and another board on the lateral aspect of the extremity.
4. The two boards should now be secured to the extremity, and then to each other.
5. Assess pulse, movement, and sensation, and record.

Other

If no pulse is detected at the distal end of a fractured or dislocated extremity, transport to the hospital should not be delayed. A pillow can be placed under the knee for added support. If possible, elevate the extremity and apply an ice pack.

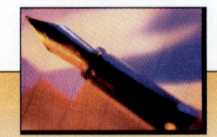

Tips from the Pros

When splinting joint injuries, be sure the board splint is not so long that it will be bumped en route.

Traction Splint

Examples

Thomas, Hare, and Sager splints (Figure 28.19).

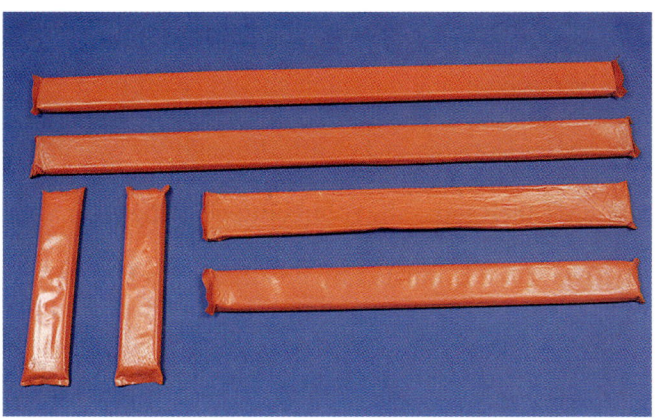

FIGURE 28.18 Board splints are the most common kind of splint used for joint injuries.

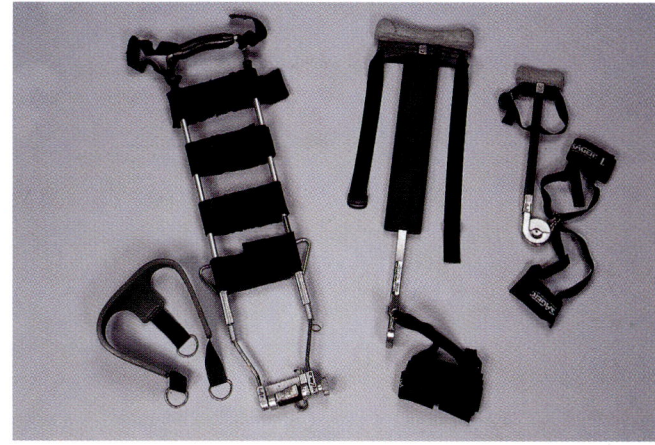

FIGURE 28.19 The Thomas, Hare, and Sager traction splints are used to immobilize femur fractures.

Uses
Femur fracture only.

Procedure
See Traction Splinting Step-by-Step Procedure at the end of this chapter.

1. The first EMT supports the femur. The second EMT removes the patient's clothing and assesses pulse, movement, and sensation.
2. The second EMT measures the appropriate length of the splint by measuring the splint against the uninjured leg. Because of the strength of the muscles of the femur, they tend to spasm more, and the leg shortens. The splint should be measured from the ischial tuberosity, approximately 10 to 12 inches beyond the foot. An ankle hitch (a device that wraps around the ankle and has a strap with a D-ring on the end so that the ankle hitch can be attached to the traction splint) is applied. A cravat can be used for an ankle hitch as well.
3. The first EMT applies manual traction to the leg. Traction is applied by placing one hand on the anterior aspect of the ankle and the other hand on the posterior aspect. The first EMT now leans back, pulling the leg toward him or her.
4. The second EMT places the splint and straps next to the injured leg and prepares the straps. Usually, four straps are used on a traction splint. One is placed above the fracture site, one above the knee, one below the knee, and one above the ankle. These straps should be prepared before placement, so that once the splint is applied to the patient the straps will not have to be manipulated into place and cause undue movement to the injured femur.
5. The first EMT, while still maintaining manual traction, lifts the leg slightly so that the second EMT can slip the splint under the injured leg. The padded part of the splint is placed under the patient's ischial tuberosity. The ischial strap is then applied. Padding along the femoral artery may be used to protect this vessel from compromise and reduce blood flow to the leg.
6. The second EMT hooks the loops of the ankle strap or cravat to the hook on the traction splint. The second EMT turns the wheel (or crank) on the splint to apply mechanical traction. Mechanical traction should be applied until the extremity is realigned. Frequently the pain is relieved by placing the bone back into its correct alignment. Now the first EMT can discontinue manual traction.
7. The first EMT assesses pulse, movement, and sensation, while the second EMT applies Velcro straps.

Other
The preceding steps describe the application of a Hare traction splint. Other traction splints may have different directions. If possible, elevate the extremity and apply an ice pack.

Pillow Splint

Pillow splints can be used for fractures to the wrist and ankle. Remember to leave a space to check pulse, movement, and sensation. See Pillow Splint Step-by-Step Procedure at the end of this chapter.

Air Splint

Uses
Arm, lower leg, and ankle.

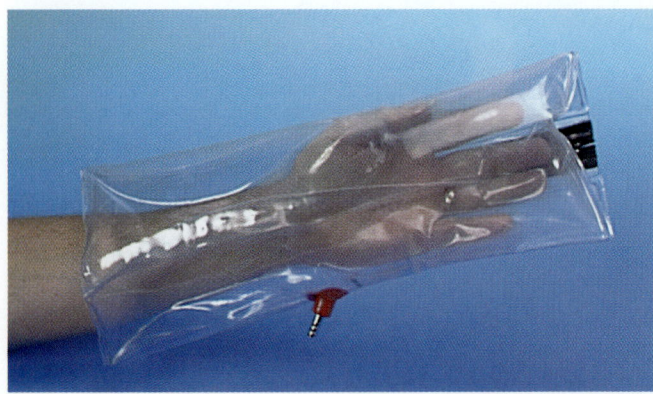

FIGURE 28.20 Air splints can be used to immobilize the arm, lower leg, and ankle.

Procedure

1. The first EMT assesses pulse, movement, and sensation and removes the patient's clothing. All skin to be placed inside the splint should be exposed.
2. The second EMT supports the extremity. The second EMT places his or her arm through the splint and grasps the patient's injured extremity. The second EMT then slides the splint onto the patient's injured extremity.
3. The splint is inflated by breathing into the hose attached to the splint. With proper inflation, the EMT should be able to make a small indentation in the splint by pushing gently on the inflated splint (Figure 28.20).
4. The first EMT assesses pulse, movement, and sensation, and records. Be sure these can be assessed with the splint in place. If not, the extremity must be re-splinted.

Step-by-Step Procedure

Joint Immobilization

1. Ensure scene safety.

2. Initiate body substance precautions.

3. Gather equipment: board splints; tape, Kerlix, or triangular bandage; ice pack.

4. EMT #1 assesses pulse, movement, and sensation. Mark pulse if possible (see Step 4).

5. EMT #2 removes clothing and supports extremity as found.

6. EMT #2 places one board splint on the medial and lateral aspects of extremity (see Step 6).

7. EMT #2 secures this board to the patient using tape, Kerlix, or triangular bandages.

8. EMT #1 reassesses pulse, movement, and sensation (see Steps 7 and 8).

9. A pillow may be placed for support of the extremity.

10. Elevate the injury and place an ice pack if possible.

11. Ensure joints above and below the injury are stabilized.

12. Document findings and treatment.

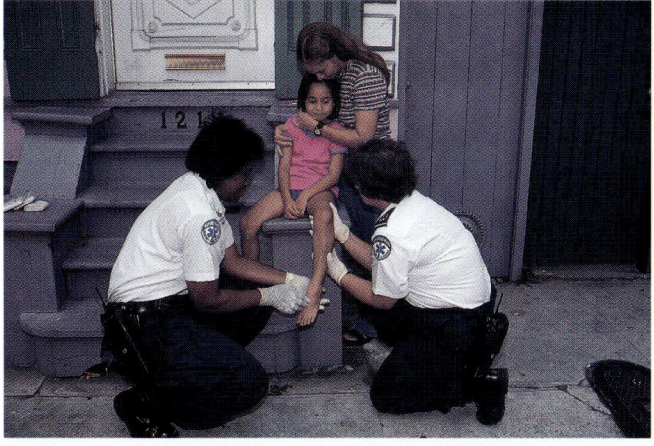

Step 4

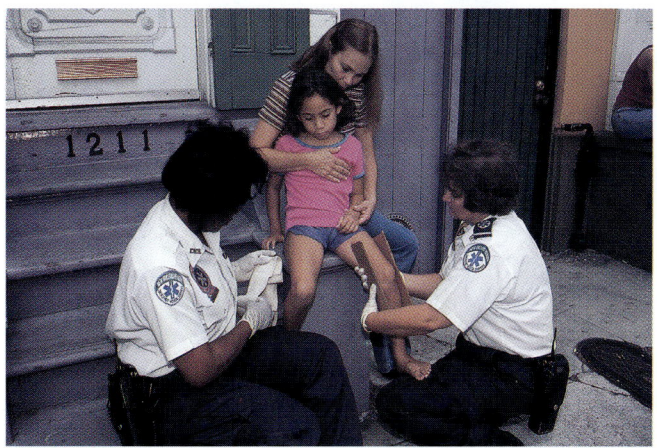

Step 6

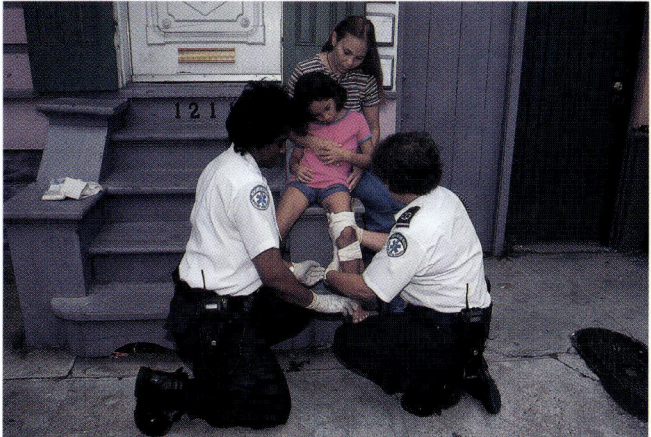

Steps 7 and 8

Step-by-Step Procedure

Traction Splinting

1. Ensure scene safety.

2. Initiate body substance precautions.

3. Gather equipment: traction splint, ankle hitch or triangular bandage, ice pack.

4. EMT #1 initiates manual stabilization of injured extremity.

5. EMT #2 assesses pulse, movement, and sensation. Mark pulse if possible (see Steps 4 and 5).

6. EMT #2 removes clothing from injured extremity (see Step 6).

7. EMT #2 measure traction splint against uninjured leg. Measurement should be from ischial tuberosity approximately 10 to 12 inches beyond the foot (see Step 7).

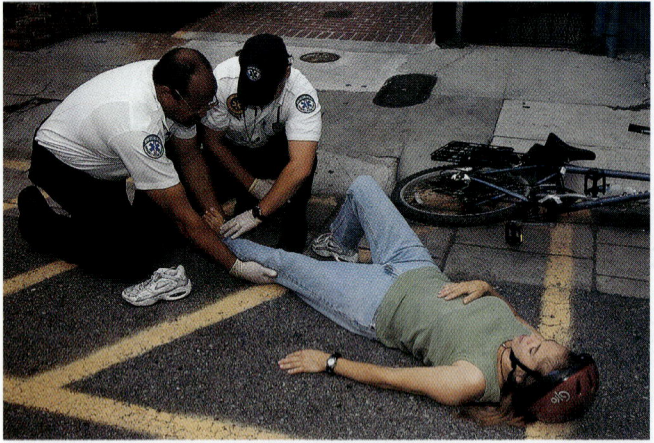

Steps 4 and 5

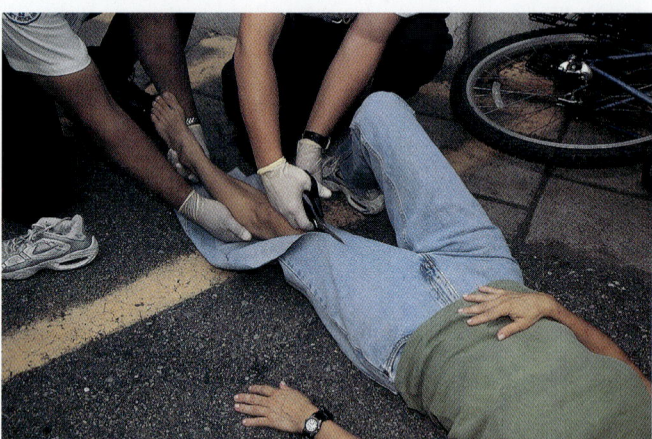

Step 6

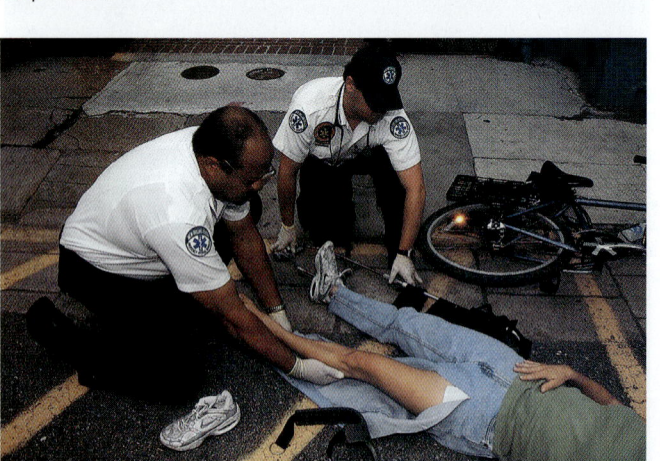

Step 7

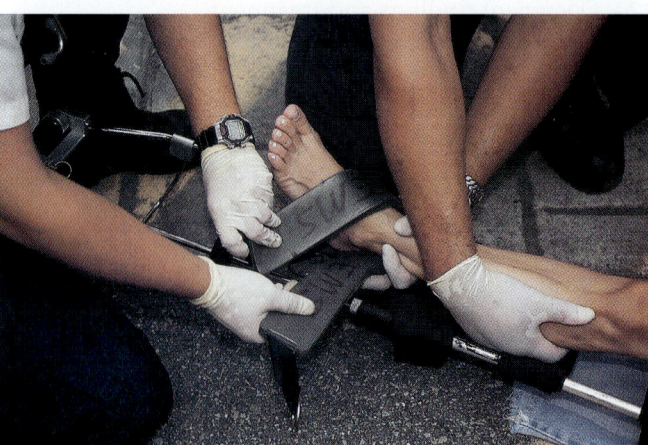

Step 7

Traction Splinting (cont'd)

8. EMT #2 applies ankle hitch to ankle, and EMT #1 initiates manual traction to the injured leg. Traction is applied by grasping ankle hitch and leaning back, pulling the leg. If no ankle strap is available, one can be made from a triangular bandage:
   a. While EMT #1 holds traction on the leg above the ankle, EMT #2 passes the folded triangular bandage around the ankle and crosses the end (see Step 8a).
   b. The ends are passed around and under the foot and then beneath the ankle portion (see Step 8b).
   c. The ends are tied together and attached to the hook (see Step 8c).

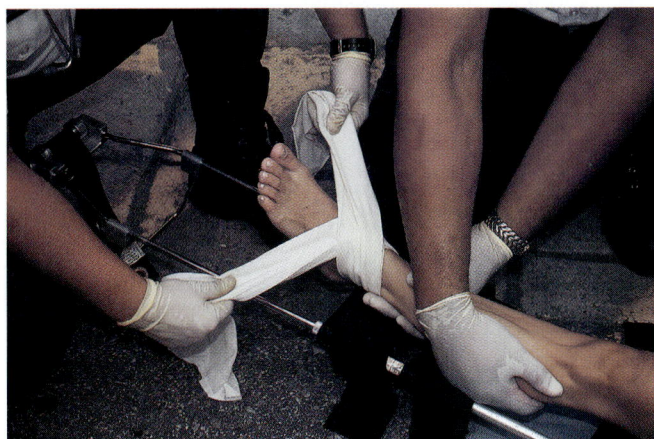

Step 8a

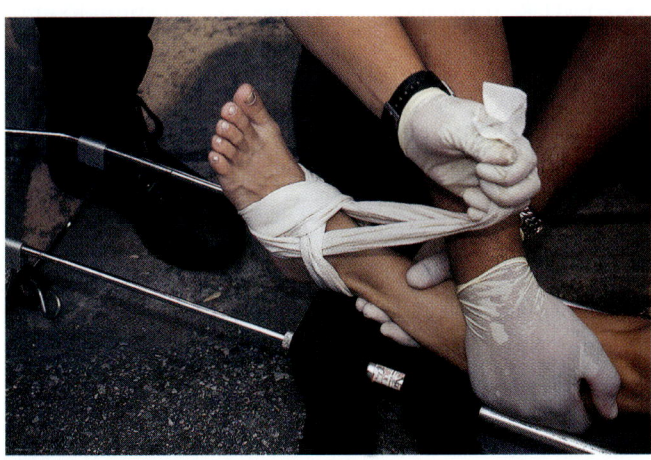

Step 8b

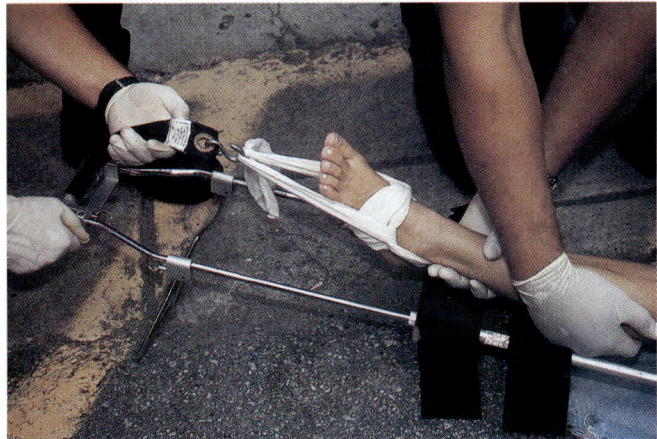

Step 8c

Traction Splinting (cont'd)

9. EMT #2 prepares straps on splint: one strap placed above the injury, one strap placed below the injury for support, one strap below the knee, and one strap above the ankle. Do not place straps on top of the injury or over the knee.

10. EMT #1, while maintaining manual traction, lifts leg slightly so EMT #2 can place traction splint under the ischial tuberosity (see Step 10).

11. Apply ischial strap. Pad the femoral artery region if necessary.

12. EMT #2 now hooks the D-rings of the ankle hitch to the hook on the traction splint.

13. EMT #2 turns the wheel of the traction splint to initiate mechanical traction from the splint (see Step 13).

14. Mechanical traction should be applied until the patient feels relief or the extremity is realigned. EMT #1 can now release manual traction.

15. EMT #1 assesses pulse, movement, and sensation (see Steps 14 and 15).

16. EMT #2 applies straps.

17. EMT #1 elevates the extremity by extending the stand on the posterior area of the traction splint (see Steps 16 and 17).

18. Ensure joints above and below injured site are stabilized.

19. Apply ice pack if possible.

20. Document findings and treatment.

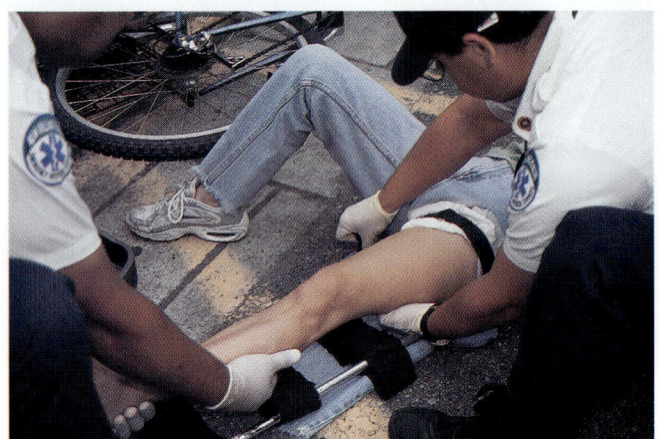

Step 10

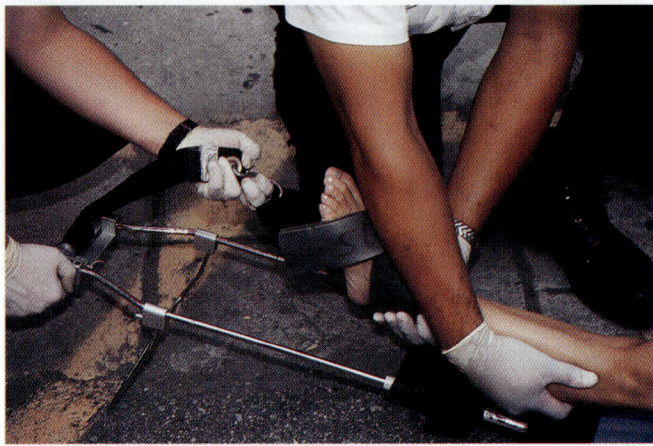

Step 13

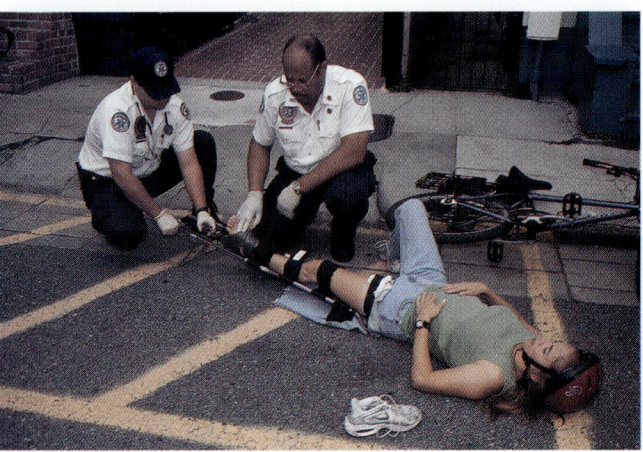

Steps 14 and 15

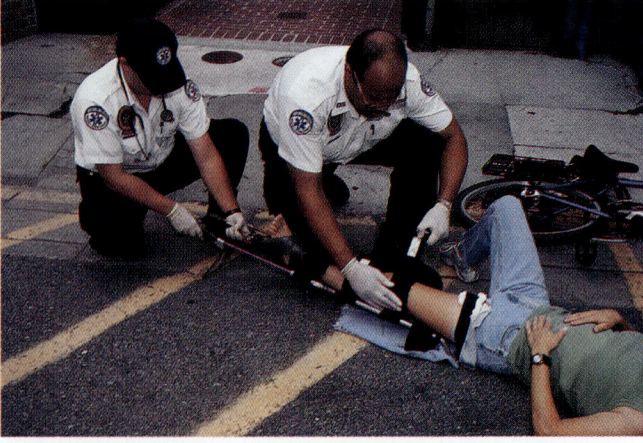

Steps 16 and 17

Step-by-Step Procedure

Pillow Splint

1. Ensure scene safety.

2. Initiate body substance precautions.

3. Gather equipment: pillow, triangular bandage or tape, ice pack.

4. This splint can be used for wrist or ankle strains, sprains, or fractures.

5. Remove clothing, socks, and shoes so injury can be observed.

6. Assess for pulse, movement, and sensation. Mark pulse if possible.

7. Place an ice pack over injury if possible.

8. EMT #1 supports and lifts injured extremity.

9. EMT #2 places pillow under injury.

10. Secure pillow around injury with triangular bandages, tape, or other. Be sure to leave an area open to reassess pulse, movement, and sensation (see Step 10).

11. Reassess pulse, movement, and sensation.

12. Ensure joints above and below injured site are stabilized.

13. Document findings and treatment.

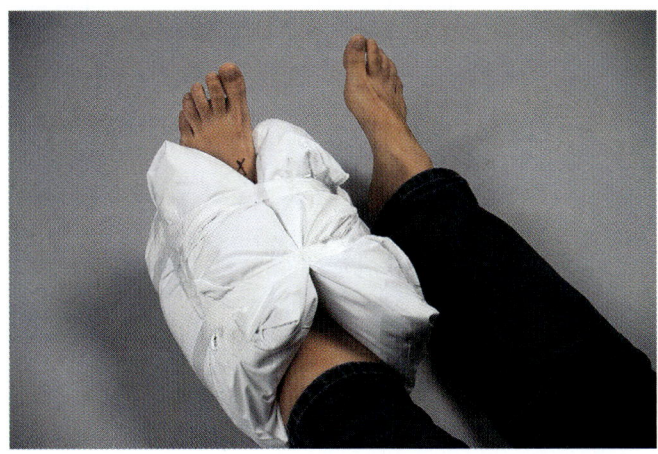

Step 10

Summary

- The important bones of the upper extremities that the EMT must recognize are the scapula, clavicle, humerus, radius, ulna, bones of the hand, and bones of the fingers. In the lower extremities, these bones are the pelvis, femur, tibia, bones of the foot, and bones of the toes.
- If a fracture exists, it is the responsibility of the EMT to immobilize these bones so that they do not continue to produce injury to the patient. Movement of sharp bone ends inside the soft tissue of muscle and in the vicinity of arteries and nerves can produce significant damage.
- Open fractures are those in which the integrity of the skin has been compromised. Closed fractures are those in which the integrity of the skin has not been compromised.
- Edema and hemorrhage are the most common complications of fractures. Edema can be so extensive it closes off surrounding arteries and veins. From a femur fracture alone, the patient can lose as much as 500 to 1500 ml of blood, either into the tissue space or out of the body.
- Dislocation of a joint is the dislodging of a bone from its normal position in a joint.
- A strain is a soft tissue injury or muscle spasm that occurs around a joint anywhere in the musculature. Strains are also known as muscle pulls. A sprain is an injury in which ligaments are stretched or partially torn.
- Signs and symptoms for which to look when assessing for a possible fracture are deformity, crepitus, swelling, discoloration, pain, loss of sensation or movement (paresthesia or paralysis), and interruption of blood supply.
- When splinting a fracture, immobilize the joint above and below the site of injury.
- It is not the responsibility of the EMT to differentiate between a dislocation, strain, sprain, or fracture. The EMT need only assess and determine the potential for one of these injuries and immobilize.
- Life-threatening injuries outweigh the importance of splinting each and every fracture separately. If the determination has been made that the patient has a life-threatening injury, fractures can be splinted using an anatomic splint, such as a long backboard.
- Remember to always expose the injury site. An EMT cannot assess what he or she cannot see. The price of clothing is not an issue.
- Always check pulse, movement, and sensation before and after splinting.
- The EMT must be familiar with the different types of splints that are accessible to him or her. The EMT must be able to choose the appropriate splint for the fractured extremity and be able to use it properly.

Scenario Solution

Let a few minutes pass so that Gidge can be reassured by her mother; if Gidge feels safer, she will be more compliant with your directions. During this time, you and your partner could split up and speak with the father and the brother. The brother probably does not want to tell what happened for fear of punishment. This is where your pediatric skills come into play. Try to convince the brother that you simply what to know what happened so you can help his sister. As you are speaking with him, you look over and notice that Gidge is still holding her arm against her body very tightly, which is immobilizing the dislocation for now and is acceptable as long as she continues to guard her arm. The father has no idea what happened, because he was in the kitchen making lunch. He heard a great crash and went immediately into the bedroom, saw the bed, saw Gidge crying, and called 911.

After you obtain this information, Gidge is more calm and states that she will let you put a sling and swathe on her arm as long as her mother can help. Because this is the only way to get compliance from Gidge, it is the best idea, and you and your partner instruct the mother how she can best help. This promotes trust from Gidge and her mother, which must be accomplished when working with pediatric patients. Gidge states that she did not hit her head, only landed on her shoulder after falling about 2 feet. You decide that cervical spine precautions are not indicated and call medical control for confirmation from the medical director. Gidge is placed on her "throne," as you call the stretcher, and is escorted by her mother into the unit. Gidge is happier, and her mother is satisfied with the service she and her daughter have received. You transport them to the hospital without further incident.

En route to the hospital, check the distal pulses again, and assess the potential fracture to ensure that the sling and swathe is doing a complete job of immobilizing the injury site.

Key Terms

Anatomic positioning Splinting the body by completely immobilizing on a long spine board and fully securing the patient to the long spine board.

Cardiac muscle Specialized muscle cell that is present only in the heart. Its internal makeup and function are different from other muscle cells in the body.

Closed fracture Fracture in which the skin integrity is not compromised.

Compartment syndrome Any condition in which nerves, arteries, or veins are compromised due to increased swelling in the interstitial space.

Crepitus A sound or feeling made by bones grating against each other.

Dislocation Separation of two pieces of bone at the joint.

Internal fixation Use of wires, pins, and screws to place bones in proper position.

Loss of skeletal integrity Condition in which bones are in a state of impairment, usually due to trauma.

Multisystem trauma patient Patient in whom trauma has either directly or indirectly caused more than one body system to fail.

Open fracture Fracture in which skin integrity has been broken.

Open reduction Use of surgery to place bones in proper alignment.

Smooth muscle Cells that can function without stimuli from the brain to contract and control the flow of food or digestive juices within the gastrointestinal tract.

Sprain An injury in which ligaments are stretched or partially torn.

Strain A soft tissue injury or muscle spasm that occurs around a joint anywhere in the musculature.

Striations Microscopic lines that differentiate voluntary muscle and give it its name of striated muscle.

Review Questions

1. Which of the following is *not* a function of the muscular system?
   a. Move bones
   b. Move skin
   c. Contract bowel
   d. Taste
2. All of the following are major bones in the upper extremities except:
   a. Humerus
   b. Ulna
   c. Metatarsal
   d. Radius
3. All of the following are major bones in the lower extremities except:
   a. Femur
   b. Humerus
   c. Tibia
   d. Fibula
4. Abnormal movement or position of a joint is best described as:
   a. Fracture
   b. Dislocation
   c. Sprain
   d. Strain
5. The ultimate goal of splinting is to:
   a. Hold the injury in the position as found
   b. Prevent as much movement of the injured part as possible
   c. Control hemorrhage
   d. Transport the patient
6. The purpose of a sling and swathe is to:
   a. Tie both feet together to prevent movement of the pelvis
   b. Immobilize the legs to the backboard
   c. Immobilize a fractured rib for pain control
   d. Immobilize the humerus to the chest wall
7. The importance of determining mechanism of injury is to:
   a. Report your finding to law enforcement personnel so that they can better describe the collision in court
   b. Predict the injuries that the patients may have
   c. Provide a report to the hospital for better patient billing
   d. Testify in court as to the nature of the injury and the potential pain suffered by the patient

Answers to these Review Questions can be found at the end of the book on page 867.

29

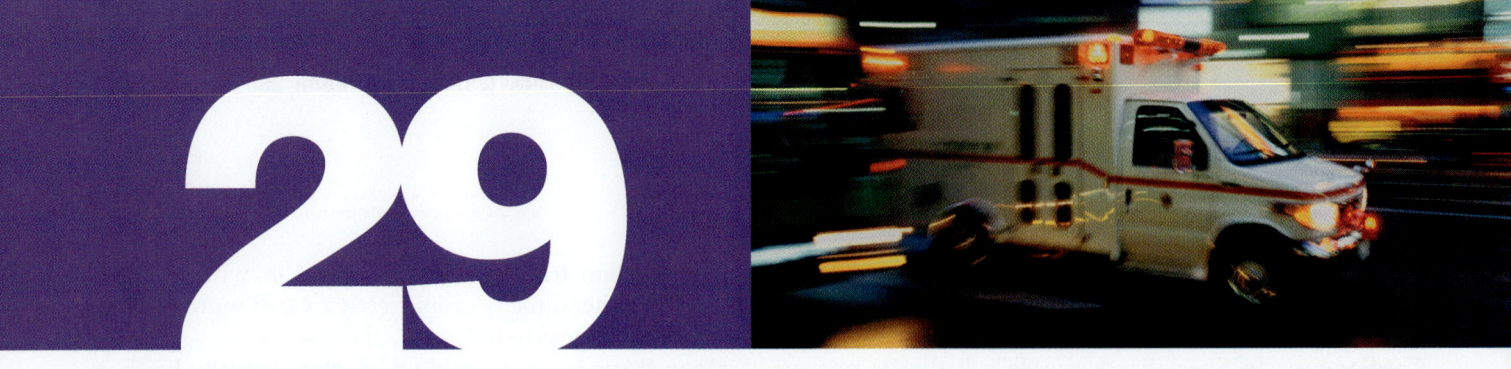

Environmental Emergencies

Lesson Goal

The goal of this chapter is to describe how the body regulates and maintains its internal or core temperature and the various ways that heat is lost by the body.

Scenario

"What a great day for a road race," you say to your partner as you pull into the first-aid tent area. You and your partner are assigned to the first-aid tent today to provide medical care for the annual "Run for History." This annual road race attracts between 200 and 300 runners each year who participate in a half-marathon. The proceeds from the race go toward the preservation of the historic district in town. Today has turned out to be a great day, with the temperature at race time expected to be in the mid-80s and the humidity at 72%, not bad for a day in late July.

After parking the vehicle, you and your partner go into the open-sided tent and set up your equipment. Shortly after completing your setup you start to see patients with a variety of minor complaints before the beginning of the race. After the race starts your area is empty of patients, so you and your partner step outside to watch the runners. The first-aid tent is set up in a grassy area along the racecourse at about the halfway point. From your vantage point you watch the runners as they race toward the finish line. As one of the last groups of runners passes your area, one of the runners leaves the group and heads toward the tent.

The runner, a woman in her midtwenties, comes into the tent and lies down on one of the cots. She lies on her left side and pulls her knees up to a fetal position, wrapping her arms around her knees. The patient is crying and states that she is dizzy with numbness and tingling in her fingers and has severe stomach cramps that began about 5 minutes ago.

On assessment you find that the patient's skin is warm to touch and pale in color, and her entire body is drenched in sweat. Further assessment reveals vital signs of respirations 30 and shallow, pulse 128 and bounding, and blood pressure 136/84. Your physical examination of the patient's abdomen confirms a rigid abdomen without any point tenderness and generalized pain. Additional questioning supplies you with a negative past medical history, taking no medications, no known allergies, and nothing to eat or drink yet today in preparation for the race. The patient states that this is her first race of the year and that she has lost 18 pounds since April by following a strict diet.

 What do you think is wrong with this patient? How would you treat her?

Key Terms to Know

- Ambient temperature
- Anaphylactic reaction
- Blanch
- Breathing
- Conduction
- Convection
- Core temperature
- Drowning
- Evaporation
- Frostbite
- Frostnip
- Full-thickness burns
- Heat cramps
- Heat exhaustion
- Heat index
- Heatstroke
- Humidity
- Hyperthermia
- Hypothermia
- Immersion
- Metabolism
- Near-drowning
- Partial-thickness burns
- Radiation
- Rule of nines
- Secondary drowning
- Submersion
- Superficial burns
- Toxin
- Windchill

Learning Objectives

As an EMT-Basic, you should be able to do the following:

DOT

- Describe the ways that the body maintains and/or loses heat.
- List the signs and symptoms of general and local exposure to cold.
- List the signs and symptoms of general and local exposure to heat.
- Detail the steps of emergency care for the patient exposed to cold or heat.
- Identify the signs and symptoms of water-related emergencies.
- Describe the complications of near drowning.
- Describe the emergency medical treatment of bites and stings.
- List the classifications of burns.
- Define *superficial burn*.
- List the characteristics of a superficial burn.
- Define *partial-thickness burn*.
- List the characteristics of a partial-thickness burn.
- Define *full-thickness burn*.
- List the characteristics of a full-thickness burn.
- Describe the emergency medical care of the patient with a superficial burn.
- Describe the emergency medical care of the patient with a partial-thickness burn.
- Describe the emergency care for a chemical burn.
- Describe the emergency care for an electrical burn.

Supplemental

- Describe the difference between an allergic reaction and anaphylaxis.

Any person with a prolonged exposure to a hot or cold environment can develop a medical or trauma emergency. Recognizing the signs and symptoms of exposure and knowing how to properly treat and transport exposed patients to an appropriate medical facility are essential goals in the care of environmental emergencies.

This chapter describes how the body regulates and maintains its internal or core temperature, and the various ways heat is lost by the body through such processes as convection, conduction, evaporation, and radiation. The external and internal effects on patients from prolonged exposure to either a hot or cold environment are discussed. Detailed signs and symptoms of several environmental emergencies, including thermal injuries, cold injuries, drowning, near-drowning, and bites and stings, also are discussed. The management of patients affected by environmental emergencies follows each major topic.

Anatomy and Physiology of Temperature Regulation

The human body strives to maintain a constant body temperature. Body heat is generated from the conversion of food (sugar) to energy, a process called **metabolism.** Heat is also produced by the body through such processes as muscle contractions during activity, exercise, and shivering.

The body controls its temperature though a complex system. A regular body temperature (oral) for healthy people is 98.6° F (37° C). Most of the time, the body is warmer than the surrounding air. Because heat always moves from warmer areas to cooler areas, body heat is constantly lost to the outside environment. The body counteracts this normal heat loss by producing still more heat. Everyday activities will usually replace the heat that is lost.

Patient Care Algorithm

Expose and Environment

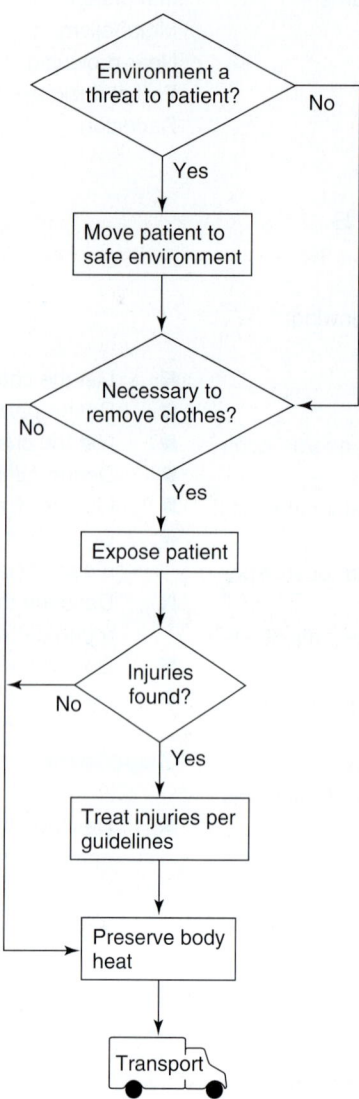

By monitoring both the environmental temperature and the internal temperature, or **core temperature**, the body balances the amount of heat lost with the amount of heat gained from the environment or manufactured within the body. When the amount of heat gained is greater than the amount of heat given off, **hyperthermia**, or higher than normal core temperature, exists. When the amount of heat gained is less than the amount of heat given off, **hypothermia**, or lower than normal core temperature, exists.

Cooling the Body

As the body's internal (core) temperature increases (becomes hyperthermic), the body tries to remove heat through the skin surface. Blood vessels closer to the skin surface widen (dilate) to bring more warm blood to the surface. Heat can then escape, and the body starts to cool. When the air temperature is very warm, dilation of blood vessels is less effective at removing internal body heat, and sweating increases. The body is also cooled by the

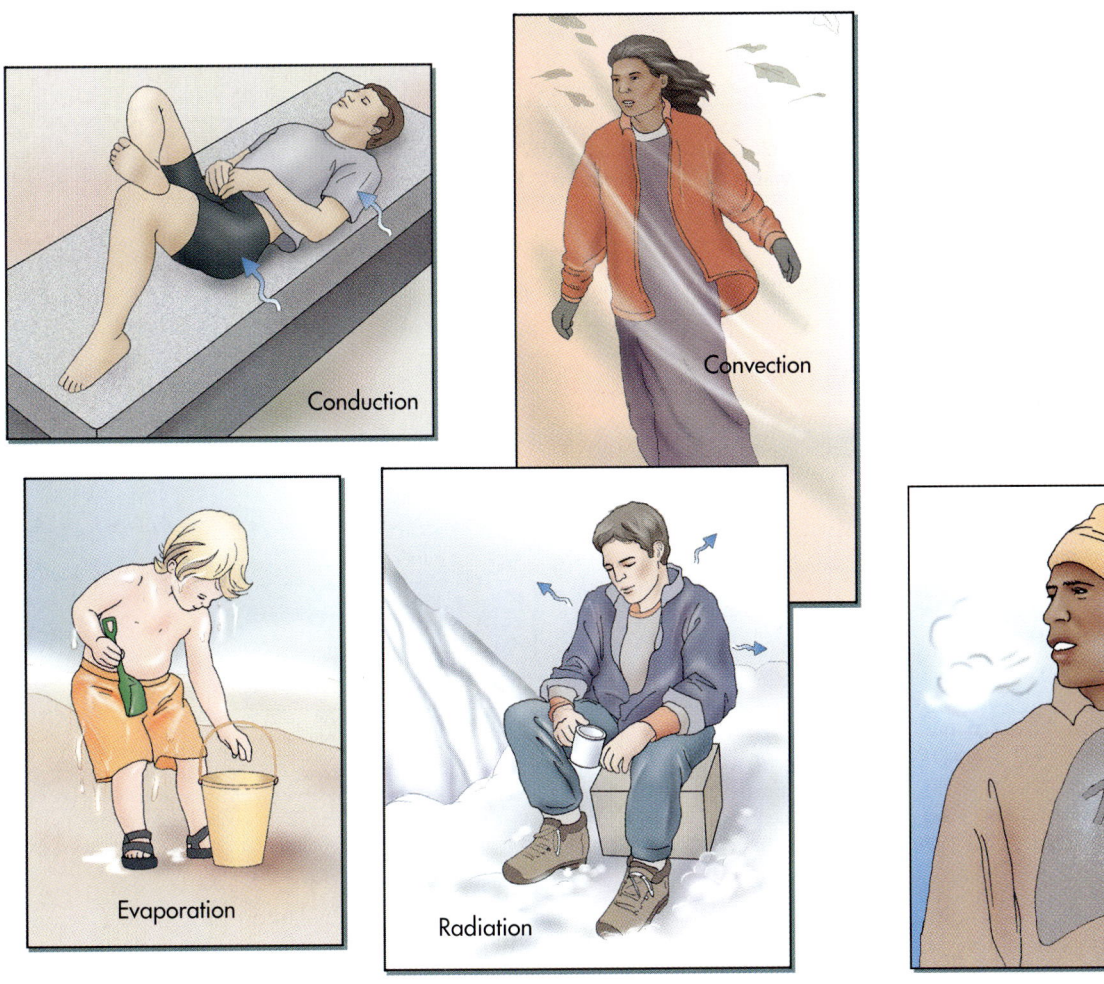

FIGURE 29.1 Mechanisms of heat loss.

evaporation of this sweat. When the humidity is high, generally greater then 70%, sweat does not evaporate as quickly. Instead, the sweat stays on the skin, acting as a barrier and actually causing the body's core temperature to increase.

The body can give off heat in five different ways: breathing, conduction, convection, evaporation, and radiation (Figure 29.1):

Breathing warms the air that is gathered within the lungs. Exhaling removes the heated air, and inhalation replaces it with cooler air from the external environment. The external environmental air is usually cooler than the body's internal temperature.

Conduction is the direct heat exchange that occurs when two or more surfaces of different temperature come into direct contact. The second surface can be either a solid, a liquid, or a gas that directly touches a patient's body. The transfer of heat will be from the surface with the greater temperature to the surface of lesser temperature. This transfer will continue if allowed until the surfaces involved are equal in temperature. For example, a patient's body will melt surrounding snow by the process of conduction.

Convection creates heat loss by air currents moving across an exposed surface area. Fanning or "blowing" on an exposed body surface creates heat loss by convection. This is especially true when surface areas of the body such as the head, neck, or torso are exposed.

Evaporation is the changing of a liquid into a gas, which requires heat. The evaporation of water or sweat from the patient's skin removes heat from the body.

Radiation is heat loss in the form of heat waves through the air or water. The heat moves from the patient to other objects without direct contact. An example of radiation is an oven. An oven heat element gets hot, warms the air, and then warms the food through radiation.

TABLE 29.1 Windchill

Estimated Wind Speed (in mph)	Actual Thermometer Reading (° F)											
	50	40	30	20	10	0	−10	−20	−30	−40	−50	−60
	Equivalent Chill Temperature (° F)											
Calm	50	40	30	20	10	0	−10	−20	−30	−40	−50	−60
5	48	37	27	16	6	−5	−15	−26	−36	−47	−57	−68
10	40	28	16	4	−9	−24	−33	−46	−58	−70	−83	−95
15	36	22	9	−5	−18	−32	−45	−58	−72	−85	−99	−112
20	32	18	4	−10	−25	−39	−53	−67	−82	−96	−110	−124
25	30	16	0	−15	−29	−44	−59	−74	−88	−104	−118	−133
30	28	13	−2	−18	−33	−48	−63	−79	−94	−109	−125	−140
35	27	11	−4	−21	−35	−51	−62	−82	−98	−113	−129	−145
40	26	10	−6	−21	−37	−53	−69	−85	−100	−116	−132	−148
(Wind speeds greater than 40 mph have little additional effect.)	Little danger. In <5 hr with dry skin. Maximum danger of false sense of security.				Increasing danger. Danger from freezing of exposed flesh within 1 minute.				Great danger. Flesh may freeze within 30 seconds.			
	Trenchfoot and immersion foot may occur at any point on this chart.											

From Sanders MA: *Mosby's paramedic textbook*, St Louis, 1994, Mosby.

Instructions: *Measure* local temperature and wind speed if possible. If not, *estimate*. Enter table at closest 10° F interval along the top with appropriate wind speed along left side. Intersection gives approximate equivalent chill temperature (that is, the temperature that would cause the same rate of cooling under calm conditions). Note that regardless of cooling rate, you do not cool below the actual air temperature unless wet.

Each individual process can remove heat from the body by itself, but in most situations, the body will remove heat by a combination of two or more of the processes.

Warming the Body

The body will also react when exposed to a cold external environment (hypothermic) to help maintain its normal core temperature. This reaction primarily will be opposite of the response that occurs when the body reacts to increased core temperature. After exposure to the cold, blood vessels closer to the skin surface will narrow (constrict). This narrowing results in less warm core blood being circulated near the skin surface and external environment. The result is that body heat is retained in the core. This process allows less heat to escape from the body through the skin surface, causing the body's core to maintain as much heat as possible. This preservation of core temperature is accomplished at the expense of the extremities, which often suffer damage (discussed later in this chapter) as a result of reduced blood flow. When blood vessel constriction fails to maintain adequate body heat, involuntary activities such as muscle shivering will begin and increase as needed to generate additional core heat. As stated previously, the body generates heat through the metabolic process. As we begin to feel cold, we increase muscular activities (stomping of feet, waving of arms, shivering, etc.) to increase the metabolic action, causing an increase in heat production.

> ✓ The body strives to maintain a normal internal, or core, temperature by employing different mechanisms. When exposed to an increase in core temperature, the blood vessels close to the surface can expand in size, allowing more blood to be carried to the surface and heat to escape. Excessive heat can also be eliminated by breathing and by sweating. When exposed to cold external temperatures, blood vessels close to the surface will constrict in size, retaining core heat. Involuntary activities such as shivering also generate heat. A low body core temperature is called hypothermia. An excessive body core temperature is referred to as hyperthermia.

Pathophysiology: Environmental Factors Affecting Body Temperature

Different environmental factors can affect how well the body maintains its core temperature: ambient temperature, wind, humidity, and heat index.

TABLE 29.2 Heat Index

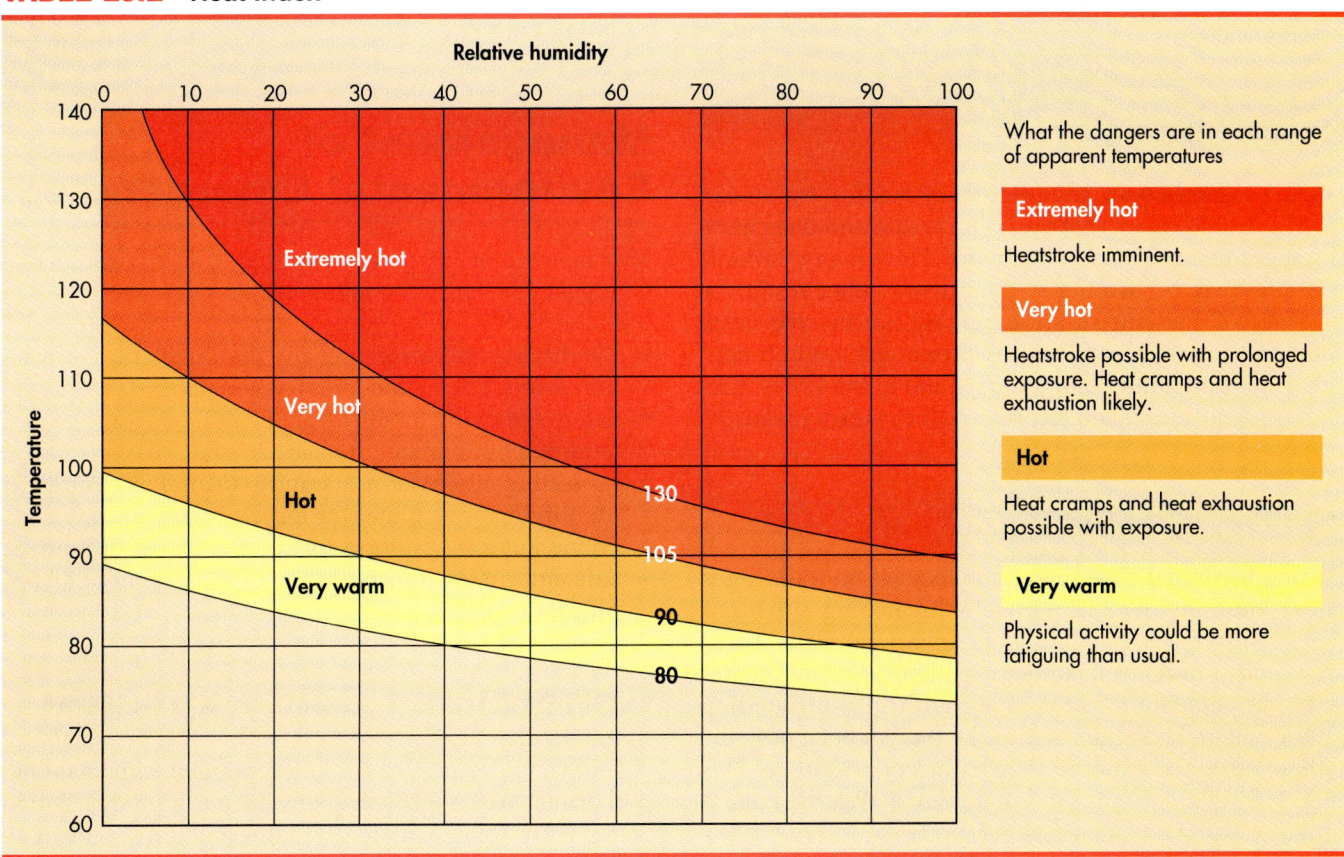

Ambient Temperature

A high or low temperature accompanied by high humidity or strong wind can increase **ambient temperature** (external temperature) effects. Different environmental conditions, such as humidity, may affect the ambient air temperature.

Wind

Ambient temperatures, combined with wind, create a **windchill** (Table 29.1). The windchill can quickly reduce body heat to dangerous levels if a person is not dressed appropriately. Like the heat index, the windchill suggests what the environment actually feels like. In certain conditions, it takes very little time for exposed flesh to be severely damaged.

Humidity

Humidity is a term used to refer to the amount of moisture in the air. High humidity levels hinder the evaporation of sweat from the skin surface. As the body continues to sweat without the benefit of evaporation, the sweat now acts as a shield, causing the internal body temperature to rise rapidly.

The **heat index** is a combination of the actual (ambient) air temperature and the relative humidity (Table 29.2). The resulting heat index suggests what the ambient air temperature will actually feel like and what effects it will have.

> ✓ External factors that can also affect the body's temperature include ambient temperature, wind, humidity, and heat index.

Assessment of Environmental Emergencies

Environmental emergencies can affect patients either locally (involving portions of the body, such as fingers, toes, or ears) or generally (involving the major systems of the body). Early recognition, intervention, and transportation to an appropriate medical facility will help in the survival and recovery of patients exposed to environmental emergencies.

Scene Size-up

During scene size-up, the emergency medical technician (EMT) should check that the scene is safe and determine the mechanism of illness or injury. How many patients will the EMT be dealing with and will other resources be needed? Patients in an extremely hot or cold environment or who are still exposed to a wet environment present a potentially dangerous scene to the EMTs. Precautions must be taken to protect all those involved.

Initial Assessment

During the initial assessment, the focus is on those signs and symptoms dealing with life-threatening situations and identifying the patient's immediate problem. These signs and symptoms include the patient's airway, breathing, and circulation status along with the surrounding environmental conditions. Has the patient been or is the patient currently exposed to extremes of heat or cold? Is there any evidence of a thermal injury? Was the patient bitten or stung by an animal or insect?

Focused Assessment

During the focused physical examination and history, the patient or bystanders can be questioned about the source of the exposure, as well as the environment. Some questions that should be asked and answered include the following:

- Was the patient in water or exposed to a wet environment?
- If exposed to water, what was the approximate temperature of the water?
- Was the patient working in a nonheated or air-conditioned workspace?
- How long was the patient exposed to the environment?
- Is the patient dressed inappropriately for the environment, either too many layers of clothing or not enough layers?
- Has the patient experienced a loss of responsiveness or a change in level of consciousness?
- Has the patient been bitten or stung by an insect or animal?

Bystanders or witnesses may provide better insight into the patient's recent history if the patient's level of consciousness is altered. The assessment of the signs and symptoms should reveal if the environmental effects are general or local in nature.

Management of Environmental Emergencies

Management of any patient exposed to an environmental emergency includes the following:

- Identifying and correcting any life-threatening condition found during the initial assessment.
- Safely removing or shielding the patient from the offending environment, if needed.
- Protecting all EMTs from environmental exposure.
- Identifying any animals or insects involved.
- Following local protocol for specific illness or injuries.
- Safe and timely transportation of the patient to an appropriate facility.

Generalized Cold Exposure

A general exposure to a cold environment can create hypothermia. Although less likely in parts of the United States with warm climates, hypothermia can occur in all climates of the United States and should be considered when assessing a patient who is found outside or who has been exposed to a cool or wet environment.

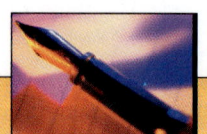

Tips from the Pros

Emergency medical services (EMS) personnel should be prepared for a variety of environmental conditions and should dress appropriately, especially in colder climates. You may respond from a 70° F emergency department to an extrication lasting an hour in 10° F weather. Many experienced EMS personnel dress with layers of clothing and can match their dress to the changing climate. Some sporting outfitters may be able to provide special protective weather gear for the climate. Exposed flesh (face, ears, nose) can develop frostbite as the wind speed increases over 15 miles per hour.

To keep their hands warm but still have use, some EMS providers use thermal liner gloves and wear protective rubber gloves over the liners to keep their hands warm during outside cold weather rescues. Others use rubber gloves under fingerless or fold-back mittens designed for shooting or skiing. Most important, protect the head and face from heat loss.

Exposure to cold environments can also predispose a patient to hypothermia. These environments can include such places as unheated rooms, warehouses, grain bins, the outdoors, and dwellings with the heat turned low or off. Often, the elderly or poor may live in buildings or apartments with the heat turned low or off for prolonged periods. Any of these types of exposures may lead to or add to hypothermia.

Factors That Predispose a Patient to Hypothermia

Factors that can predispose a patient to hypothermia are the patient's age, medical conditions, immersion or submersion, and the use of alcohol or drugs.

Age
Age contributes to a person's ability to regulate body heat. The elderly and the very young are less able to regulate their core temperatures. Infants and young children are small in total body mass but have large, exposed surface areas of skin. This ratio contributes to the rapid reduction of body heat (conduction, convection, evaporation, and radiation). Smaller muscle mass also means that children cannot shiver as much to generate internal heat. Young children may also have less fat to help retain body heat. The young generally need help with direction in dressing for the weather. Young children and elderly dependent-care adults usually cannot take off or put on their own clothing to help self-regulate their body temperature without assistance. Elderly persons may not feel the effects of the environment due to decreased peripheral circulation. Likewise, the reduced effectiveness of the peripheral circulation in the elderly also reduces their body's ability to compensate for changes in ambient temperature. This decrease in peripheral feelings will let a person feel fine for a longer exposure period. By the time the patient feels cold or hot, he or she may already have had significant exposure. Another place body heat is lost rapidly is through an exposed head. Persons with thin or no hair on their head will lose heat more rapidly than people who have full heads of hair or wear a hat or head scarf. Mental impairment of any kind can also cause patients to fail to dress properly for the environment.

Medical Conditions
Certain medical conditions increase the likelihood of the patient experiencing a change in body temperature. Shock prevents the dilation and constriction of the blood vessels to help regulate the internal temperature. Head or spinal cord injury can affect the central nervous system and alter the body's ability to control internal temperature. Burns or thermal injuries start to destroy the layers of skin and underlying structures, thus prohibiting the body's ability to sweat, trapping heat inside the body. As the burning process continues, the layers of the skin are destroyed and the body starts to release heat rapidly. Generalized infection can create a fever (rise in the body core temperature) and alter the body's ability to self-regulate. Medical conditions such as diabetes, hypoglycemia, and central nervous system disorders may also contribute to the body's ability to regulate its internal temperature.

Immersion and Submersion
Any **immersion** (to be completely soaked, as in being caught in the rain) or **submersion** (to actually enter a body of water such as a lake or pool) in water or wet conditions may predispose to hypothermia or cause a drop in the patient's core body temperature (hypothermia). Water that is colder then 70° F can cause hypothermia. Even heated pools or hot tubs may cause a patient's body temperature to drop when exiting the water. Through evaporation, body heat loss may be rapid. Immersion can also include a patient who has been in rain, sleet, or snow or an athlete who has been in sweat-soaked clothing in a cool area. Heat loss in water can be up to 32 times greater than heat loss to air alone.

Alcohol and Drug Use
The use of drugs or alcohol or the ingestion of poisons may interfere with the body's ability to regulate its internal temperature. Even prescription medications a patient is taking for other medical conditions can contribute to body temperature regulation problems. Problems encountered can occur from either an increase or decrease in vasoconstriction or an increase or decrease in the metabolic rate.

Assessment of Generalized Cold Exposure

Initial assessment for cold exposure should be included in the initial scene size-up. A rapid assessment that includes taking in the patient's environmental surroundings, before, during, and after the incident, can help determine an obvious exposure. For example, an obvious exposure might be a person in running shorts found in a snowdrift, or a child in pajamas playing outside on a frosty morning. Less obvious signs of exposure may be found at any point in the assessment. These signs may include alcohol or drugs, an overdose or poisoning, underlying illness, or major trauma including burns. Other times to consider a general exposure include resuscitation attempts conducted outdoors, immersion in water less then 70° F, or any other environment with a decreased temperature.

Patients with a generalized cold emergency will have cool abdominal skin. Assessment of cool or cold skin temperature, done with the back of the hand against the patient's abdomen underneath clothing, may help indicate an exposure to the cold. Skin conditions may also help show the extent and phase of the cold exposure. Initially, when exposed to a cold environment, the skin becomes red in color. As the cold exposure progresses, the skin becomes increasingly pale from the constriction of the blood vessels as the body tries to maintain its core temperature. If the exposure continues, the skin will become cyanotic, due to the continued constriction of the blood vessels and the decreased circulation. The skin may also feel stiff or hard due to the fluids freezing within the tissue.

Changes in the patient's level of consciousness or mental status can also indicate a possible environmental emergency. Signs or symptoms to look for include poor coordination, memory disturbances, reduced sense of touch or sensation, mood changes, a decrease in normal level of communication abilities, dizziness, and speech difficulties. The patient exposed to cold may also show poor judgement and may actually remove articles of clothing (Figure 29.2).

Vital Sign Changes in the Patient Exposed to the Cold

Depending on the extent of the exposure, the patient's vital signs may vary. Breathing may become rapid during the early stages of cold exposure and then become shallow or nonexistent during a later stage. Likewise, the pulse initially may be rapid and then slow and become absent during later stages. Blood pressure will typically be low to absent.

The detailed physical examination may reveal a patient with or without muscle shivering, stiff or rigid posture, or muscular rigidity. If responsive, the patient may also complain of joint or muscle stiffness.

Management of Generalized Cold Exposure

Patients exposed to the cold should be removed from the cold environment as soon as possible to protect them from further heat loss. Moving the patient should be done with consideration for known injuries or suspected injuries. Consider the dress and environmental preparedness of all the EMTs involved and use personal protective clothing as needed.

Handle these patients gently. Avoid unnecessary rough handling. Do not let the patients exert themselves or walk. Once in a warmed environment all wet clothing should be removed, and the patient should be covered with a blanket or other suitable material to help retain body heat. If not done as part of the initial assessment, high-concentration oxygen should be administered as soon as possible. This oxygen should be warmed and humidified whenever possible. Using warmed oxygen may begin the internal rewarming process.

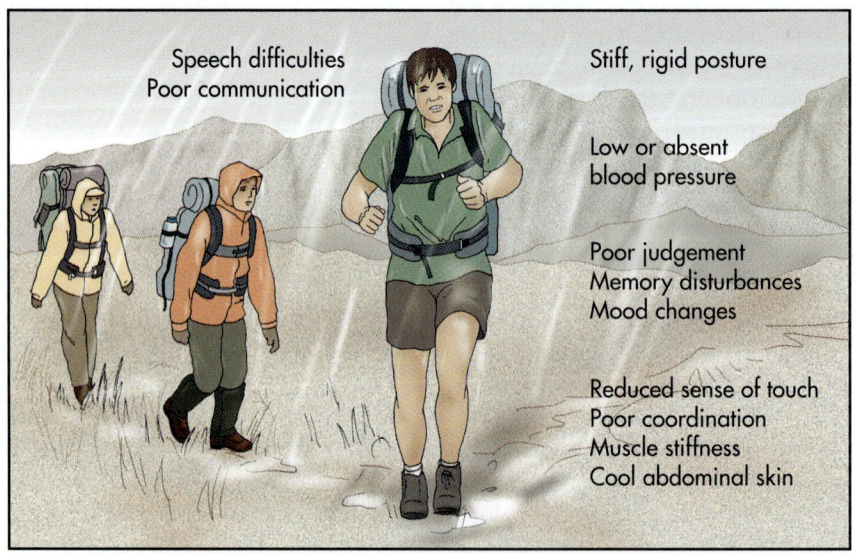

FIGURE 29.2 Signs and symptoms of generalized cold exposure.

Turn up the heat in the patient compartment of the ambulance. If the patient is alert and responding appropriately, actively rewarm the patient with warm blankets and heat packs or hot water bottles in the groin, axillary, and cervical regions. If actively rewarming the patient, care must be taken not to cause burns to the underlying tissues with the heat source. If the patient is unresponsive or not responding appropriately, passively rewarm the patient with warm blankets (Figure 29.3). Do not let the patient eat or drink anything, and do not massage the patient's extremities. Warming the patient's extremities without warming the core area may cause the cold blood from the extremities to circulate through the body core, causing a further decrease in the core temperature (rebound hypothermia).

If the patient is unresponsive, assess the pulse for a full 30 to 60 seconds before initiating cardiopulmonary resuscitation (CPR). In the profoundly hypothermic patient, pulses and respirations may be difficult to detect. A slow heart rate is common in hypothermic patients. If no pulse is detected, apply the automated external defibrillator immediately and follow protocol. Rough handling or even CPR may place the patient in a cardiac arrhythmia (e.g., ventricular fibrillation). Defibrillation may be ineffective until the patient's core temperature has been elevated to near normal. Normal cardiac care protocols may be ineffective during management of a patient exposed to the cold for an extended time.

> ✓ Four different conditions may predispose a person to hypothermia: age, preexisting medical conditions, immersion or submersion, and alcohol or drug use. The patient may initially shiver to help generate body heat, but as the body temperature decreases, the shivering stops. Patients may experience a decrease in level of consciousness, which may progress to unresponsiveness. Interventions include removing or protecting the patient from the environment as soon as safely possible. Actively rewarm the patient if he or she is alert and responsive. Passively rewarm those patients who are responding inappropriately or are nonresponsive.

Tips from the Pros

Prewarm oxygen from portable containers with a hot pack around the outlet where the tubing attaches.

Localized Cold Exposure

Injuries from exposures to the cold tend to be limited. Unprotected, poorly protected, or wet skin is the most likely area for a localized cold exposure. Localized cold injuries most often involve the skin surface of the ears, nose, face, and distal extremities (fingers and toes).

Assessment of Localized Cold Exposure

Much like burns, localized cold exposures are identified and classified according to the depth of injury to the involved area. **Frostbite** can be classified as either superficial frostbite (involving only the topmost layers of skin) or deep frostbite (involving the deeper layers of skin). Superficial frostbite injury, or **frostnip**, is best characterized by discoloration and loss of sensation. Often, the patient will not notice the condition until someone else points out the skin discoloration (grayish or yellow). Assessment of the affected area will reveal a local injury with clear demarcation (visible line of color change). Demarcation may not always be present during assessment at the scene. In superficial frostbite, the involved skin surface will still **blanch** (turn very pale or soft white when pressure is applied to it). Along with the blanching of the skin, the patient will complain of lost feeling or sensation in the involved areas. The tissue below the discolored area will be soft and malleable, much the same as normal tissue. Gently rewarming the involved skin surface, often with the patient blowing warm air on the affected part, corrects this condition. When rewarmed, the patient may

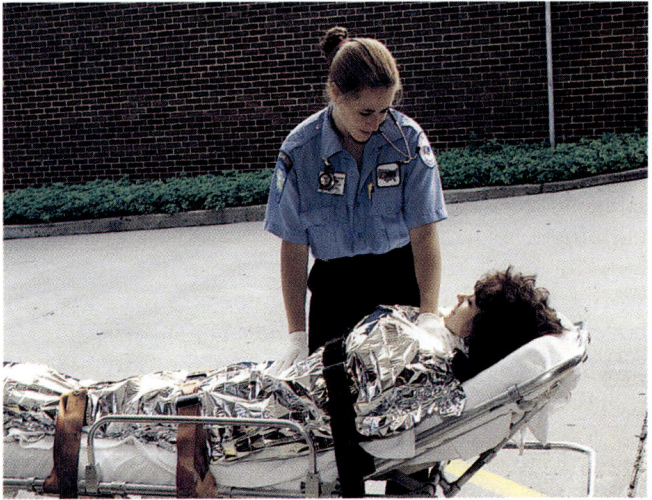

FIGURE 29.3 If the patient is alert and responding appropriately, actively rewarm the patient with warm blankets and heat packs or hot water bottles in the groin, axillary, and cervical regions.

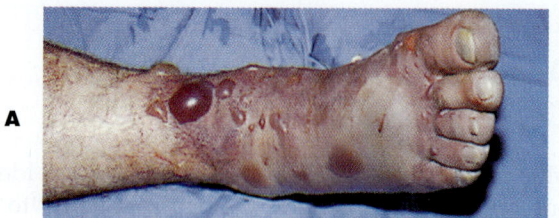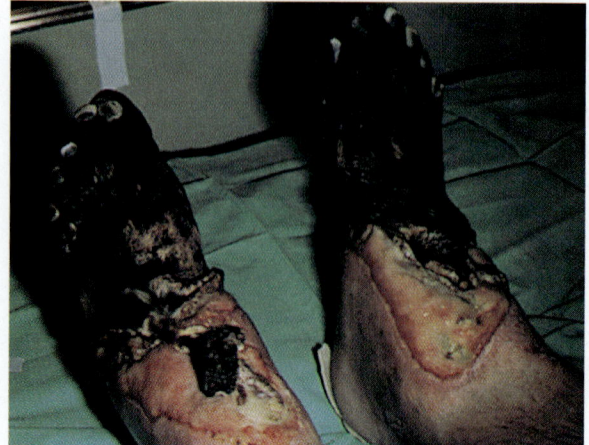

FIGURE 29.4 **A,** Edema and blister formation 24 hours after frostbite injury. **B,** Gangrenous necrosis 6 weeks after frostbite injury.

notice a tingling sensation, usually described as "pins and needles."

Frostbite is a more serious injury then frostnip. Frostbite usually occurs from a longer exposure to the cold and freezing of the involved body tissue. In deep frostbite, the skin becomes discolored, white, and waxy from lack of circulation. The skin feels firm to hard (frozen) on palpation. Gross swelling of the involved area or large, fluid-filled blisters may be present (Figure 29.4). If thawed or partially thawed, the skin may appear cyanotic or flushed, with blanched or mottled areas present.

Management of Localized Cold Exposure

Treatment of localized cold exposure follows the same guidelines as those used with the patient with general cold exposure. Remove the patient from the environment as safely and as rapidly as possible. Protect the cold-injured extremity or tissue from further injury. If not started during the initial assessment phase, administer oxygen. Remove any and all wet or restricting clothing.

The most superficial injury, frostnip, can be rewarmed by blowing warm air on the affected part or by covering the ears with warm hands. For superficial frostbite of an extremity, splint and cover the extremity. Do not rub or massage the injured part because this may cause damage to the underlying tissue by moving crystallized tissue over good tissue. Do not reexpose the injured areas to the cold. Bystanders may have folktales or myths about the care of frostbite, but it is not appropriate to rub frostbitten extremities, break the blisters, or pack the affected area in snow.

If the patient has deep frostbite, remove all jewelry from the affected area if possible and cover the injured area with dry clothing or dressings. Do *not* break any of the blisters; rub or massage the affected area; directly apply heat; rewarm the body part, unless following prescribed guidelines (see following paragraph); or allow the patient to walk on or use the affected extremity.

In circumstances in which transport is delayed or will be extremely lengthy, the affected body part should be actively rewarmed if possible (Figure 29.5). It is important to rewarm a frostbitten area correctly. Even when rewarming is done correctly, it can be painful for the patient. If possible, rewarming should be done in the emergency department. Immerse the affected body part in a warm water bath. The water temperature should be 100° to 105° F. If a thermometer is not available, make certain to test the water with your own hands. If it is uncomfortable to your touch, it is too hot for the patient to use. Monitor the water temperature throughout the bath. As the affected part is rewarmed, the water temperature will decrease, due to heat transfer. Keep stirring the water to aid in the heat transfer, and continue to do so until the affected part is soft to touch and the color and sensation have returned. After removing the affected extremity from the bath, pat the area dry (do not rub) and place dry sterile dressings over the area. Remember to place dry sterile dressings between the fingers and toes, if affected. Protect the body part against refreezing. Do not thaw the affected area if there is a chance of the part refreezing. If a body part is allowed to thaw and then is refrozen, a greater amount of permanent damage will occur. Expect the patient to complain of severe pain as the affected area regains sensations. Be prepared to provide psychologic support to the patient as needed.

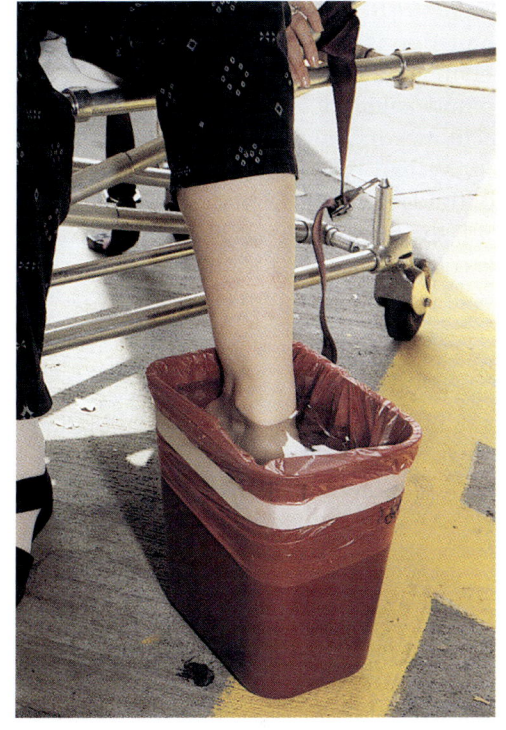 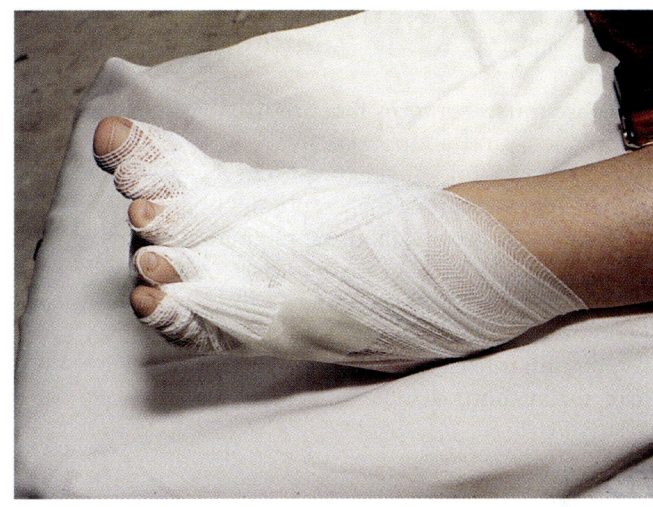

FIGURE 29.5 **A,** Immerse the affected part in a warm water bath (100° to 105° F). **B,** After removing the affected extremity from the bath, pat the area dry and place dry sterile dressing over the area. Place dry sterile dressings between fingers and toes if affected.

✓ Different categories of localized cold exposure include superficial frostbite or frostnip, frostbite, and deep frostbite. The most serious is deep frostbite. Frostnip is easily rewarmed with the use of warm air blowing on the affected body parts or pressure from warm hands. Frostbite injuries should be protected from the elements, and they should *not* be rubbed. Frostbitten areas should only be rewarmed if immediate transportation will be delayed and there is no chance of refreezing the injured part.

Heat Exposure

Environmental factors can also inhibit the body's natural ability to give off excess heat. A high ambient temperature will reduce the body's ability to lose heat by radiation (vessel dilation). High relative humidity will reduce the body's ability to lose heat through evaporation (sweating). High humidity or moist heat usually causes a person to tire quickly. This fact will prevent most people from harming themselves. Tiring rapidly will force most people to quit exerting themselves before any real harm is done. Some people will continue to push themselves, running the risk of a heat-related injury.

Activity in a warm environment with little or no moisture in the air, or dry heat, can be very deceiving. This environment can fool people into working and pushing their bodies beyond normal boundaries. Because of this reason, problems associated with dry heat exposure can be greater then those associated with exposure to a moist heat environment.

Exercise and activity can also challenge the body's ability to cool itself or eliminate excess heat. The body can lose more than 1 L of fluid (sweat) per hour. With this loss of fluid, there is also an accompanying loss of body electrolytes through the sweating process.

As with cold exposure, predisposing factors to a heat-related emergency include the patient's age, current and past medical conditions, medications, and reaction to any previous heat exposure.

The elderly may take medications that alter their body's heat-coping mechanisms such as vasoconstriction, vasodilation, and metabolic rates. Also, they are less mobile than their younger counterparts and less likely to be able to escape a hot environment as easily. Newborns and infants, too, have poor temperature regulation and cannot remove their own clothing. Preexisting illness and conditions such as dehydration, obesity, fever, fatigue, and diabetes can also make a person more likely to suffer the effects of a heat exposure.

Assessment of Heat Exposure

The initial scene size-up should reveal any obvious signs of heat exposure (Figure 29.6, Table 29.3). These signs might include a hot industrial site or a room with a greatly increased ambient temperature. Also, hot days with high humidity contribute to heat exposure and may be detected early in the assessment.

Heat Cramps

Heat cramps are muscle cramps that are usually limited to the patient's legs and abdominal area. These cramps are associated with a prolonged exposure to a warm environment. The temperature of this environment does not have to be that much greater than the temperature considered "normal." The patient sweats and often consumes large quantities of water or other fluids. As the sweating continues, water and salts are lost by the body, bringing on painful muscle cramps. The patient may also complain of exhaustion, dizziness, or even periods of faintness.

Heat Exhaustion

Heat exhaustion is a failure of the circulatory system to adequately maintain its normal functions due to the loss of fluids and salts. Heat exhaustion occurs after prolonged activities in a warm environment. The patient's circulatory system fails to maintain normal flow due to the loss of fluids and salts from the body. The patient may have rapid, shallow breathing; weak pulse; cold, clammy skin; pale color; heavy perspiration; total body weakness; dizziness; and sometimes unresponsiveness.

Heatstroke

Heatstroke is a true life-threatening emergency, resulting from the failure of the body's heat-regulating mechanisms. The body is unable to cool itself, and the core temperature is hyperthermic. When a patient is exposed to excessive heat and the body stops sweating, heatstroke will follow shortly. Most cases of heatstroke occur on hot, humid days; however, many cases occur from exposure to a dry heat. Heatstroke can occur in many locations, both indoors and outdoors.

Heatstroke patients may show the following signs and symptoms:

- Deep breathing followed by periods of shallow breathing
- Rapid, strong pulses, followed by rapid, weak pulses
- Dry, hot skin (may be red in color)
- Large (dilated) pupils
- Loss of consciousness
- Muscle twitching or seizures

Patients who have a heat-related exposure complain of muscle cramps, weakness or exhaustion, and dizziness or faintness. The patient's heart rate will be increased and an altered mental status or unresponsiveness may be noted. Skin will be pale in color, moist, and normal-to-cool to the touch. Hot, dry skin or overly moist skin suggests an emergency situation.

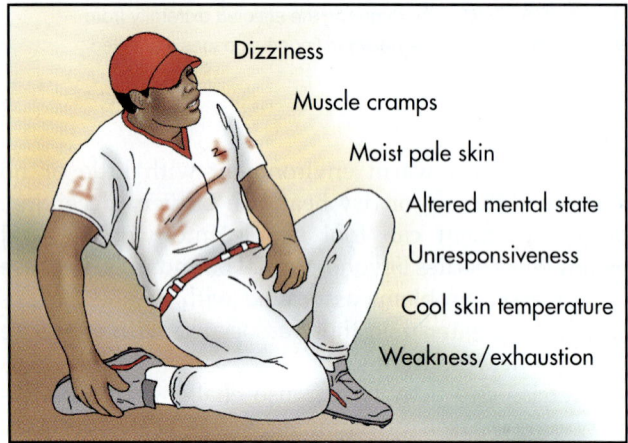

FIGURE 29.6 Signs and symptoms of heat exposure.

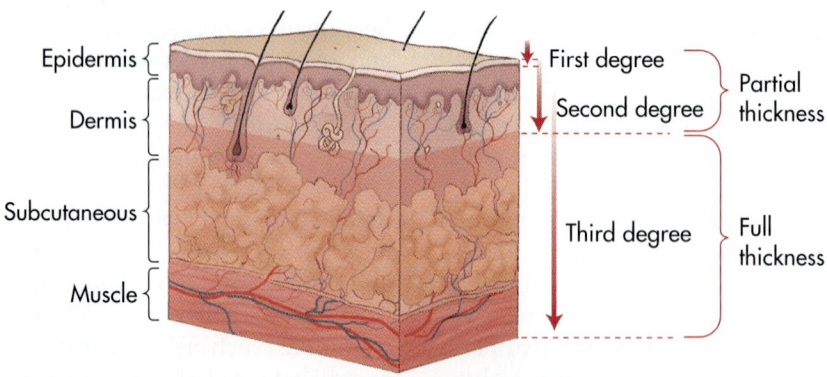

FIGURE 29.7 Parts of the skin damaged by different types of burns.

Management of Heat Exposure

The patient with skin that is moist and normal-to-cool in temperature should be removed from the hot environment as safely as possible and placed in a cooler environment, such as the patient compartment of the air-conditioned ambulance. Further cooling of the patient can be achieved by loosening or removing clothing and manually fanning the patient. The patient should be placed supine with legs elevated, if tolerated, to aid circulation. Supplemental oxygen should be started as soon as possible. If the patient is responsive and not nauseated and if it is not contraindicated, have the patient slowly drink water. If the patient is unresponsive or vomiting, place him or her in the recovery position (on his or her left side).

Some emergency medical services (EMS) agencies suggest and allow cold water submersion of patients suspected of having a heat-related exposure. If submersion is included in local protocols, be careful to fully protect the patient, especially if unresponsive. Remember that exposure to cold water will force the blood vessels to constrict, further reducing the body's ability to give off heat. This type of action may actually cause the core temperature to increase, the opposite effect of the desired action.

✓ Heat-related emergencies may manifest with muscular cramps, weakness, dizziness, and an altered level of consciousness. If the skin condition of the patient is moist and normal-to-cool in temperature to the touch, remove the patient from the hot environment as safely as possible. Cool the patient by loosening clothing and manually fanning. If the patient is responsive and not nauseated, have the patient slowly drink water. If the patient's skin is hot and dry or hot and overly moist to the touch, a serious medical emergency exists. Remove the patient from the hot environment. Remove the patient's clothing; apply ice packs to the groin, neck, and axillary areas; and sponge the patient with wet cloths. Medical direction may advise you to immerse the patient in cold water.

Burns (Thermal Injuries)

Most burns can be recognized during the initial assessment of the patient. Certain interventions may be started before arriving at the receiving facility. Burns are classified by their depth of involvement (Figure 29.7). The seriousness of a burn is evaluated based on both the depth of the burn and the percentage of body surface area (BSA) involved. As with any general environmental emergency, the elderly, the sick, and the young are less able to cope with burns than adults. Also, burns that are associated with other trauma such as head injury, spine injury, fractures, or patients having an underlying medical condition should be treated and managed aggressively.

Classification of Burns

Superficial burns, or first-degree burns, have the following general characteristics (Figure 29.8):

1. Reddened skin
2. No blisters (open or closed) present
3. Patient will complain of localized pain

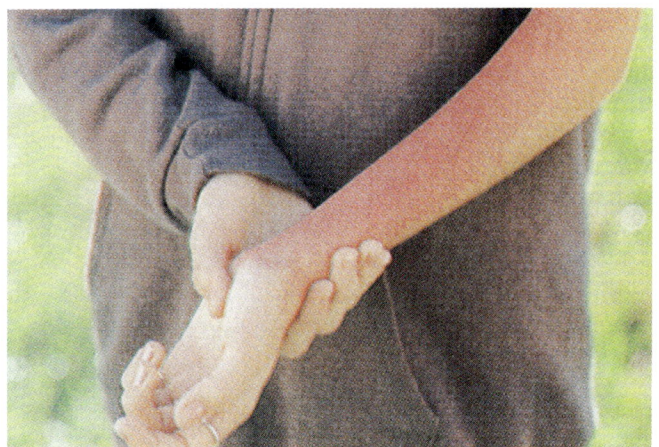

FIGURE 29.8 Superficial burn.

TABLE 29.3 Heat Related Emergencies

Heat-Related Condition	General Weakness	Muscle Cramps	Breathing Rates	Pulse Rates	Skin Condition	Sweat or Skin Moisture	Loss of Responsiveness
Heat cramps	Yes	Yes	Vary	Vary	Normal	Heavy	Seldom
Heat exhaustion	Yes	No	Rapid, shallow	Weak	Cold, clammy	Heavy	Sometimes
Heat stroke	Yes	No	Deep, then shallow	Full, rapid	Dry, hot	Little or none	Often

Partial-thickness burns, or second-degree burns, have the following general characteristics (Figure 29.9):

1. Reddened skin
2. Blisters (open, closed, or both) present
3. Patient will complain of localized pain

Patients with partial- and full-thickness burns usually have more than one type of burn and will probably experience localized pain from the lesser burn(s).

Full-thickness burns, or third-degree burns, have the following general characteristics (Figure 29.10):

1. Charring of the skin (black, white, or gray in color)
2. Tissue damage through the skin (epidermis and dermis layers) to underlying tissues
3. Patients with full-thickness burns alone may experience minimal to no pain as compared with patients with partial-thickness burns

Patients with partial- and full-thickness burns usually have more than one type of burn and will probably experience localized pain from the lesser burn(s).

Body Surface Area

The degree of BSA involved in burns is generally measured in the prehospital environment using the **rule of nines.** As Figure 29.11 shows, the human body can be subdivided into segments that account for approximately 9% of the total BSA. By combining these regions or portions of these regions, an effective estimation of the percent of body surface involved in the burn can be achieved. For smaller or less extensive burns, the hand can be used for a rapid measurement. An adult hand will cover approximately 1% BSA of an average adult body. For example, a burn area about the size of four adult hands would equal approximately 4% of the entire BSA.

Assessment of Critical Burns

Local protocols or treatment guidelines usually identify which burns are considered critical burns. For example, more than 20% BSA of partial- or full-thickness burns are typically considered to be critical, which requires special management. In addition, burns that involve the hands, feet, or genital region are usually considered critical burns also requiring special management. This assumption is based on the high use of these areas and their importance for everyday function. Any burn more than a superficial burn to these areas should be treated at a burn center. In fact, even superficial burns should be evaluated. Burns to the face are also considered critical because of the danger of involvement of the airway. The mucous membranes of the nose, mouth, and larynx are particularly sensitive to heat. The normal human reaction to suck in a breath when surprised often results in an inhalation injury. Once burned, the sensitive tissues of the airway can rapidly close and leave the patient with extreme difficulty breathing. Soot around the mouth or nose, singed or burned hair in the nostrils, or reddening or swelling of the oropharynx indicates the possibility of airway damage.

Chemical Burns

A chemical burn occurs when the skin comes in contact with various caustic agents. In most cases, dilution and washing away of the chemical with copious amounts of water is the first step because the chemical will continue to react until it is completely removed. The EMT must not waste time and begin flushing immediately. The EMT must not use neutralizing agents because they may cause further exothermic (heat) injuries from chemical reactions, producing sudden additional heat, burning, and tissue damage. The exact amount of time required for irrigation cannot be predicted. Therefore flushing should begin at the scene and continue until arrival at the hospital.

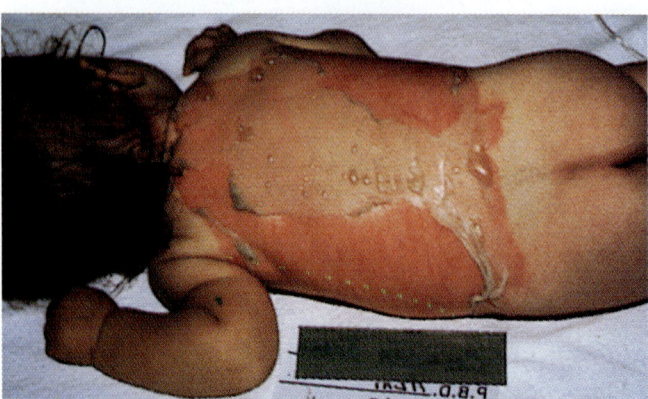

FIGURE 29.9 Partial-thickness burn.

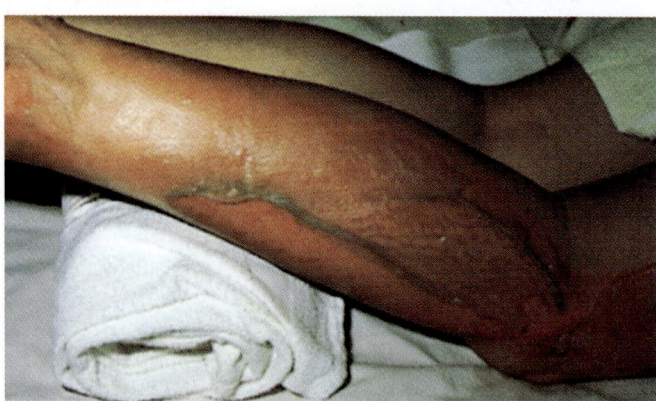

FIGURE 29.10 Full-thickness burn.

The EMT should notify receiving hospital in advance so that they can be ready to continue irrigation and to prepare a suitable area of the emergency department to contain the washed-off materials. If the EMT knows the identity of the chemical, he or she should relay this information so the receiving hospital can prepare special antidotes before the patient's arrival.

If the chemical is a dry powder, brushing off as much as possible before flushing will reduce the chemical concentration. While flushing is in progress, the EMT should remove patient's clothes. The EMT must remove the patient's shoes early to avoid pooling water that contains high chemical concentrations. The EMT must take care to avoid runoff or splattering on his or her clothing or skin. The EMT's own safety is paramount. Protective gloves and eye protection are necessary.

The EMT should irrigate chemical burns of the eye with large volumes of saline; topical anesthetic agents (such as tetracaine) may be applied if necessary to control eyelid movement. The EMT should continue irrigation en route to the hospital. He or she should take care to position the patient so that the runoff will not spill into the other eye.

The following chemicals require special treatment:

- Dry lime and soda ash, like any powder, should be brushed off because contact with water will form a corrosive substance. Contaminated areas should not be irrigated unless they are already wet. Large quantities of water should be used if the burning process has already begun.
- Phenol is widely used as a cleaning agent. Since it is not water soluble, alcohol should be used for flushing. When alcohol is not available, large amounts of water will suffice.
- Lithium and sodium metal are substances that react with water, releasing heat and toxic fumes. Therefore any large chunks remaining in or around the burn must be removed and placed in oil. After this has been done the burn should be washed with copious amounts of water. Irrigation should continue en route to the hospital.

For more exotic chemicals, the EMT should ask medical control to contact the nearest Poison Control Center or CHEMTREC at 1-800-424-9300.

Electrical Burns

The degree of tissue damage in an electrical burn is related to the amount of current involved and the duration of the exposure. The EMT's first priority is to determine if the patient is still in contact with the electrical source. If this cannot be determined with certainty, the EMT should not touch the patient. An electrocuted EMT only adds to the problems of scene management, adds to the number of patients that must be managed by the remaining EMS personnel, and takes up additional supplies that are needed. The EMT should not attempt to remove the patient from contact with an electrical source unless trained to do so. Electrical burns can cause cardiac arrest. CPR may be required with such patients.

Pathophysiology

Three types of electrical injuries occur:

1. *Direct contact burns,* with passage of current through tissue, cause extensive areas of necrosis along the current's pathway. Skin is often charred and in some

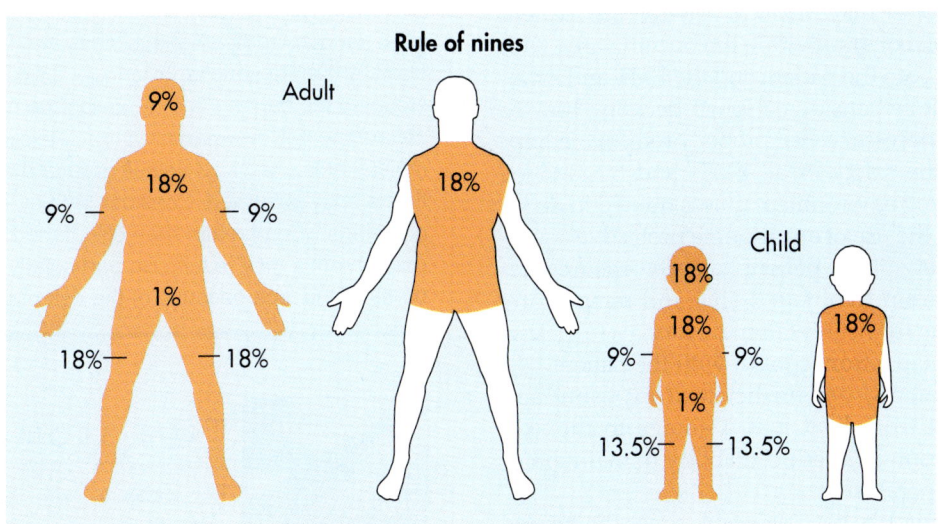

FIGURE 29.11 The rule of nines.

cases has exploded apart. Electrical contact burns may have entry and exit wounds that appear small on the surface. The EMT must assume that there are associated injuries to the nerves, bones, muscles, blood vessels, and other organs along the pathway between the entry and exit points.
2. *Arc injuries* occur by arcing of electricity between two contact points close together near the skin. With these injuries the skin can be exposed to temperatures of 4500° to 5400° F (2500° to 3000° C). This may produce significant cutaneous burns. Such injuries can be recognized by the loss or singeing of hair along the arc's pathway. The whole body may be involved.
3. *Flash burns* are seen when a victim is too close to an open electrical source. This results in thermal burns, usually to skin unprotected by clothing on the side next to the fire.

Management

Initial management for victims of electrical burns includes lactated Ringer's solution or normal saline intravenous runs wide open. This will aid in preventing kidney failure by gushing myoglobin, a by-product of muscle damage, through the kidneys. The following are key points to consider with electrical injuries:

- Do not become part of the circuit!
- Anticipate greater tissue damage than is visible externally.
- Examine for associated injuries to bones and internal organs.

Management of Burns

Remove the patient from the environment and stop the burning process. This may include having the patient "stop, drop, and roll" or smothering the burning area with a blanket. Safety of both the patient and the EMT and available materials must be considered when deciding how to put out the fire. If necessary, use proper protective equipment and ensure the safety of all EMTs and bystanders. Never enter a burning environment unless trained to do so, and then only with the use of appropriate protective equipment. After the safety of the patient has been ensured, remove all clothing from the injured area and remove any burning, smoldering, or heat-retaining materials (e.g., jewelry, belt buckles, snaps) from contact with the patient.

Protect the patient from further heat exposure and protect the patient from heat loss. Damage to the skin from a burn will result in a reduced ability to maintain or regulate body temperature.

Once the burning has been stopped, cover the injured areas to protect from further contamination and to help limit body fluid loss. Local protocols may once again dictate the type of dressings to use. Generally, if the involved areas equal less than 10% of the total BSA, cover with clean, dry, or moist dressings. The advantage of using moist dressings is that they will not stick to the burned tissue as much as dry dressings. Also, a cool, moist dressing may help reduce some of the localized pain associated with burns. If moist dressings are to be used, moisten them with sterile water whenever possible. If the total BSA burned is greater than 9%, clean, dry dressings should be used. A patient with more than 9% BSA burned will likely experience problems with excess body temperature loss through the burned tissue. Moist dressings, in this case, may increase the loss of body heat. The resulting hypothermia can further complicate the care and treatment of the patient.

High-concentration oxygen should be started as soon as it is safe to do so. Whenever possible, the oxygen should be humidified. Burns in the airway or the inhalation of the hot gas or steam during a fire can cause the airway to rapidly swell and reduce respiratory or ventilatory efficiency.

Definitive care for burn patients is a highly specialized field, and not every hospital is able to effectively provide for the care of these patients beyond initial stabilization. The medical community has long recognized hospitals that have the special knowledge, experience, and equipment to deal with the patient who has experienced critical burns. These hospitals are known as burn centers. Depending on local system resources and configuration, EMTs may be involved in transporting patients directly to a burn center from the scene, or the patient may need to be transported to the closest facility for initial stabilization. Local medical protocols or guidelines identify the appropriate course of action.

> ✔ Burns are classified by thickness and by the body surface area they cover. Superficial burns are the least serious, and partial-thickness and full-thickness burns are more serious. Treatment for all burns includes stopping the burning and removing the patient from the environment. Cover partial- and full-thickness burns with moist sterile dressings unless greater than 9% of the patient's body is burned. Consider the use of dry sterile dressings when greater than 9% of the BSA is burned (hypothermia may result). Be particularly cautious about burns to the face because of the risk of airway damage.

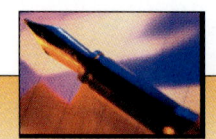

Tips from the Pros

For patients with facial burns, use clean dressings (4 × 4) to pad the oxygen mask against the burned skin.

Water-Related Emergencies

Statistics suggest that over 80,000 people are involved in water-related emergencies that claim 4600 lives annually. **Drowning** is defined as death by asphyxia after submersion. A water emergency can occur in almost any water, including home bathtubs, small streams, rivers, large lakes, and oceans. **Near-drowning** is submersion with at least temporary survival.

Management

During the scene size-up, safety must be a primary factor. Ensure the safety of all EMTs and bystanders involved. Specialized training in water rescue should be obtained by EMTs before attempting a water rescue. Ascertain the number of patients to be rescued. Make sure all people are accounted for at the beginning and end of the rescue effort.

Emotions can run high during water rescue, because the patients tend to be young. Television dramatizes impressive water rescues; however, would-be rescuers can quickly become additional patients if they are not properly trained water rescuers.

The temperature of the water plays a major role in the success of patient resuscitation. Any pulseless, nonbreathing patient who has been submerged in cold water (70° F or less) for a limited amount of time should be resuscitated. A crude but accurate saying among medical personnel is, "They're not dead until they're warm and dead." The longest documented survival without neurologic deficit is 66 minutes underwater. This instance involved a child who had been submerged in frigid water (37° F) and was resuscitated.

If the patient is known to have had a diving accident, or if it is uncertain, always suspect an injury and protect the spine. Application of spinal immobilization equipment on a patient in the water is very difficult and different than application on the usual trauma patient. If possible, practice applying spinal precautions and immobilization equipment to simulated "patients" in water rescue drills in the local swimming pool under controlled conditions.

If the patient is responsive and still in the water, and a spinal injury is suspected, use manual, in-line spinal stabilization techniques first and then employ a cervical collar and other devices as needed for complete immobilization. Secure the patient to a long backboard before removing him or her from the water.

If no spine injury is suspected, place the unresponsive patient on his or her left side after removal from the water. This position allows water, vomitus, and other secretions to drain from the upper airway. Use suction to clear the airway as needed, and administer high-flow oxygen as soon as possible. If the patient is not breathing, artificially ventilate the patient (see Chapter 10). If gastric distention interferes with the ability to adequately ventilate the patient, place the patient on his or her left side. After placing the patient on the left side, have suction readily available, place a hand over the epigastric region of the abdomen, and apply gentle pressure to help relieve the distention. This maneuver should only be done if the gastric distention interferes with the ability to ventilate the patient effectively.

If there is an absence of respirations or pulse, CPR and other resuscitative measures should be started. These may include use of the automated external defibrillator or the use of advanced life support.

Near-drowning patients who survive the initial submersion are faced with many complications following resuscitation. Eighty-five percent of patients involved in a near-drowning incident suffer a "wet" drowning, meaning that they have aspirated water into their lungs. Although this aspiration of cold water reduces body temperature and may help preserve the brain, the negative effect is that the water brought into the lungs destroys the protective substance that lines the alveoli. The loss of this protective lining causes the alveoli to collapse and additional fluids to accumulate in the lungs; this accumulation is called a **secondary drowning.** During this phase, which may be delayed for up to 24 hours after the initial immersion, the patient may experience increasing respiratory difficulty and may actually "drown" in his or her own body fluids.

The overall treatment of any near-drowning patient remains the same for EMT-Basics: protect the spine if injury is suspected or uncertain, protect and maintain the airway, ventilate the patient if necessary, retain body heat, and transport to the appropriate medical facility. Patients who have been submerged and who are now alert and responsive should be evaluated by a doctor. The following 24 hours can be just as lethal as the initial submersion.

> ✓ In water immersion, ensure the safety of all EMTs and bystanders as you begin the rescue. Do not attempt a rescue unless properly trained. Use spinal precautions as necessary when removing the patient from the water. If the patient is pulseless and apneic, begin CPR. If gastric distention interferes with ability to ventilate the patient, position the patient on the side and then place a hand on the epigastric region and press gently, have suction ready, and use as needed. Maintain the patient's body heat throughout the resuscitation and transport.

Cold Water Submersion

Studies by wilderness experts and the United States Coast Guard have shown remarkable results in resuscitating cold

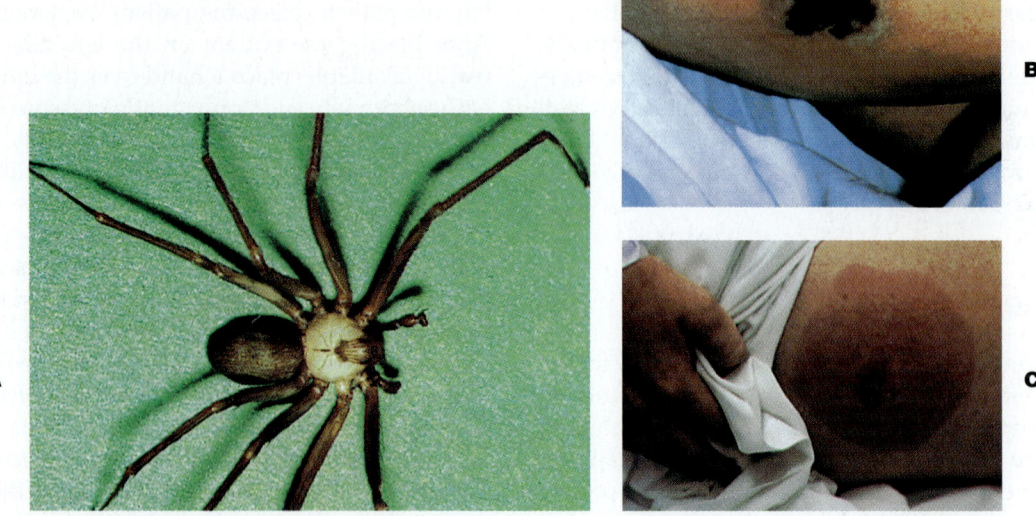

FIGURE 29.12 **A,** Brown recluse spider. **B,** Twenty-four hours after a brown recluse spider bite. **C,** Forty-eight hours after a brown recluse spider bite.

water drowning patients. Successful resuscitation without lasting neurologic impairment has been documented in cases of cold water submersion of up to 66 minutes. The physiologic mechanism behind these miraculous recoveries is not clearly understood. One theory is that the body has a natural ability, when exposed to a cold environment for an extended time, to slow down its normal functions such as respirations and circulation. This response also causes the blood to be shunted from the peripheral areas to the core area. This response is called the mammalian diving reflex. Although the existence and role of this reflex has not been clearly established scientifically, it has been identified as a possible mechanism that enables these patients to survive. Cold water is also thought to protect the central nervous system from the otherwise damaging effects of oxygen loss to the brain (cerebral hypoxia).

Several other factors may influence the patient's outcome from cold water submersion. These include the patient's age, other associated injuries or illness, length of time of submersion, water temperature, amount of struggle by the patient, water purity, quality of CPR performed, and other resuscitative measures. These factors appear to contribute to a patient's chance of successful recovery, based on ongoing research. Every submersion patient should have full resuscitation efforts made, regardless of the presence or absence of any of the factors.

Bites and Stings

Along with outdoor activities each year comes an increase in bites and stings. Many insect or animal bites are harmless, although the bites may contain a **toxin,** or a substance harmful to us. Some bites, however, can produce serious or life-threatening complications because some patients are more reactive (sensitive) to the venom or toxin than others. This can also be referred to as an **anaphylactic reaction,** a hypersensitivity or allergic reaction by the body to a foreign substance. An allergic reaction will usually involve a single, minor system of the body such as a rash produced by exposure to poison ivy. An anaphylactic reaction is a true life-threatening emergency. During an anaphylactic reaction the body's immune system rapidly responds to the invasion of a foreign substance in an attempt to rid the body of the invader. This response to the foreign substance by the immune system affects multiple systems of the body, the most severe involving the respiratory and cardiovascular systems. If an anaphylactic reaction is not recognized and treated promptly, it can cause respiratory or cardiac arrest.

Assessment

Many patients who seek care for an allergic reaction will relate a specific history of being bitten by a spider or snake

> ✓ Resuscitation of cold water submersion patients may be possible. Factors that influence the patient's outcome from cold water submersion include the patient's age, other associated injuries or illness, length of time of submersion, water temperature, amount of struggle by the patient, water purity, quality of CPR performed, and other resuscitative measures.

or having been stung by an insect, scorpion, or marine animal. Not all patients remember being bitten or stung and may not recognize that they have been bitten or stung.

During assessment the patient generally will complain of one or more of the following symptoms: localized pain, fatigue, weakness, dizziness, chills, fever, nausea, vomiting, and difficulty breathing. The EMT may observe such signs as unresponsiveness, wheezing with respirations, localized redness or swelling, hives, bite marks, or a visible stinger (Figures 29.12 and 29.13).

Management

If the patient has absence of respirations or pulse during assessment, begin resuscitative procedures. High-concentration oxygen should be started as soon as possible on all patients who do not need ventilatory assistance.

Examine all patients who have been bitten or stung for signs of an acute allergic reaction (anaphylaxis). Examine all injection sites for the presence of a stinger. If a stinger is still visible at the injection site, remove it by scraping along the skin with the edge of a stiff card. Do not use tweezers or forceps because the squeezing may push venom out of the venom sac and further inject the toxin into the patient.

Gently wash the area with soap and water and remove jewelry from the injured extremity before swelling begins. With some bites, extremities can swell two to three times their normal size. If possible, place the bite or sting site below the patient's heart level. Do not apply cold to snakebites, and consult medical direction regarding the use of a constricting band. Observe the patient for signs and symptoms of allergic reactions and dyspnea,

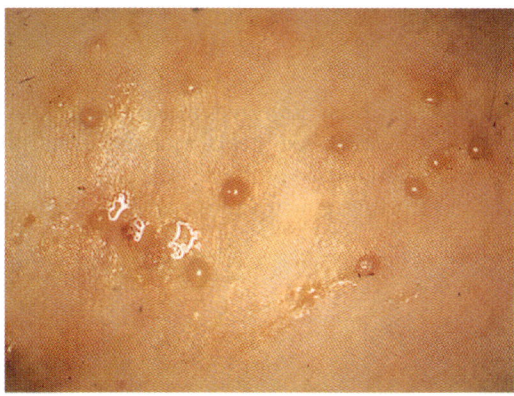

FIGURE 29.13 The result of fire ant stings, approximately 2 hours after injury.

and be prepared to manage the airway and ventilate the patient should the need arise.

Many patients who are allergic to bee stings carry a bee sting kit or an epinephrine self-injection pen. If they have not already done so, be prepared to assist the patient with the self-injection. For more on this procedure, see Chapters 13 and 18.

> ✓ For a bite or sting, remove all clothing and jewelry from the affected area. Thoroughly wash the area with soap and water. If a stinger is visible, remove it with the edge of a card; do not use tweezers. Monitor and treat the patient for any signs of respiratory difficulty or allergic reaction. If the patient has a prescription epinephrine self-injector, be prepared to assist the patient with this treatment.

Summary

- Cold- and heat-related injuries result from environmental conditions. An increase in the body's core temperature is called hyperthermia. A decrease in the body's core temperature is called hypothermia.
- Exposure to the cold can be a generalized condition. Signs and symptoms include a decrease in the level of consciousness to possible unresponsiveness, redness of the skin followed by paleness, and cool skin. Treatment includes removing and protecting the patient from the environment. Active rewarming (if patient is alert) and passive rewarming (if patient is not responding appropriately or is unresponsive) are also appropriate interventions.
- Localized cold exposure includes frostnip and frostbite. Frostnip is characterized by numbness and redness of the affected skin. Blowing on or rewarming the affected part with pressure is the appropriate intervention. Frostbite can be superficial or deep. In frostbite, tissues begin to freeze. Remove the patient from the cold environment. Do not rub the affected area. If directed by medical protocol, actively rewarm the body parts following careful guidelines.
- Heat exposure includes heat cramps, heat exhaustion, and heatstroke. Heat cramps can be treated with rest, fluids, and removal of the patient to a cool environment. Heat exhaustion and heatstroke

Summary (cont'd)

- are more serious. Remove the patient's clothing; apply ice packs to the groin, neck, and axillary areas; and sponge the patient with wet cloths. Medical direction may advise immersion of the patient in cold water.
- Burns may be superficial, partial thickness, or full thickness. Partial- and full-thickness burns should be evaluated by a burn center. Treatment for all burns includes stopping the burning and removing the patient from the environment. Cover partial- and full-thickness burns with moist sterile dressings. If the total BSA involved is greater than 9%, consider using dry sterile dressings to avoid causing hypothermia. Cover a superficial burn with a moist sterile dressing.
- Water emergencies may require a water rescue. Do not attempt a water rescue without adequate training. If you suspect spinal injury, use spinal precautions when removing the patient from the water. If the patient is pulseless and apneic, begin CPR. Maintain the patient's body heat throughout resuscitation and transport.
- Bites and stings from insects or land or marine animals may induce a severe anaphylactic reaction in some people. Maintain the patient's airway and transport to a medical facility. If the patient has an epinephrine injector, assist the patient with injecting the medication.

Scenario Solution

You feel confident with the patient's history and presentations that she is having heat cramps. You base this assumption on her vital signs, the ambient temperature, and her lack of fluid intake before and during the race.

Your partner starts the ambulance and turns on the air conditioner in the patient compartment to high cool. After moving the patient into the cooler patient compartment, you have her concentrate on slowing her breathing rate. You help her to remove her nylon running shirt down to her sports bra and place a cool, damp cloth on her forehead. After talking with medical control you have the patient start sipping cool water. After about 30 minutes of this treatment the patient's stomach cramping subsides.

Key Terms

Ambient temperature The outside or environmental air temperature that surrounds the body.
Anaphylactic reaction A hypersensitivity or allergic reaction by the body to a foreign substance.
Blanch The skin's ability to change from a lighter color to a normal color after slight pressure is applied to the area; indicates adequate circulation.
Breathing The act of inhaling and exhaling air, which involves taking in oxygen and giving off carbon dioxide.
Conduction Direct heat exchange that occurs when two or more surfaces come into contact; movement of heat will be from the surface of higher temperature to the surface of less temperature. A patient will lose body heat through conduction when lying on the cold ground.
Convection Heat exchange that occurs when air currents move across an exposed surface.
Core temperature Temperature in the center, or core, of the body.
Drowning Death resulting from asphyxiation following submersion in a liquid.
Evaporation Heat exchange that occurs when a liquid changes into a gas. When perspiration evaporates, it uses body heat as the energy source, resulting in a reduction of body heat.
Frostbite Injury to the skin caused by prolonged exposure to cold. The liquid content of the skin cells freezes and ruptures the cell membranes; may be superficial (frostnip) or deep.
Frostnip Frostbite that is superficial in nature; affects only the topmost layers of the skin.
Full-thickness burns Burns involving all skin layers and, in some cases, the underlying bone, muscle, and other tissues; characterized by charring of the skin and complete absence of feeling caused by destruction of nerve endings; also called *third-degree burn*.

Key Terms

Heat cramps First and mildest form of heat exposure; muscle cramping caused by excessive loss of body fluids and salts.

Heat exhaustion Heat exposure that occurs when the body's circulation system fails to maintain its normal functions because of excessive loss of body fluids and salts; patient has shocklike symptoms.

Heat index A measurement of the combined effect of temperature and humidity on the apparent temperature.

Heatstroke A life-threatening condition that results from the failure of the body's normal temperature regulatory processes; body temperature rises out of control, and critical body functions deteriorate.

Humidity Measurement, usually expressed in percent, of the amount of water or moisture in the air.

Hyperthermia A condition in which the core temperature of the body exceeds normal limits and begins to malfunction.

Hypothermia Abnormal and dangerous condition in which the core body temperature falls below 95° F (35° C) and the body's normal functions are impaired; usually caused by prolonged exposure to cold.

Immersion To be completely soaked by a wet substance (e.g., to be caught in the rain or to be drenched in sweat).

Metabolism Chemical reactions that take place within an organism to maintain life; the work of the cells.

Near-drowning Asphyxia following submersion with at least temporary survival.

Partial-thickness burns Burns involving the topmost and middle layers of the skin; often associated with blisters and intense pain; also called *second-degree burn.*

Radiation Form of heat exchange that occurs when heat is transmitted through air or water (e.g., the heat that can be felt when sitting in front of a fireplace).

Rule of nines A system of measuring the percent of body surface area (BSA) involved in a burn.

Secondary drowning The loss of the protective lining within the lungs caused by aspirated water, causing the alveoli to collapse and allowing additional fluids to accumulate in the lungs.

Submersion To enter a body of liquid (e.g., to dive or fall into a lake or pool).

Superficial burns The most minor of thermal injuries; involves the epidermis layer of skin and includes reddening of the skin without blistering.

Toxin Noxious or poisonous substance.

Windchill Measurement of the combined effect of ambient temperature plus wind velocity on exposed surfaces; in general, the higher the wind speed, the lower the temperature will seem.

Review Questions

1. List five different ways the body can give off heat.
2. List two factors that predispose a patient to hypothermia.
3. Water that is _____ degrees Fahrenheit (F) or less can cause hypothermia.
4. Using the rule of nines, estimate the percent of body surface area (BSA) involved when you have an adult patient who has sustained partial-thickness burns to the entire torso (front and back).
5. As a general rule of thumb, you should not cover burns with wet dressings unless they involve a total body surface area (BSA) of less then _____%.
6. A patient who exhibits a hypersensitivity or severe allergic reaction to an insect bite or sting is suffering from a(n) _____ reaction.

Answers to these Review Questions can be found at the end of the book on page 867.

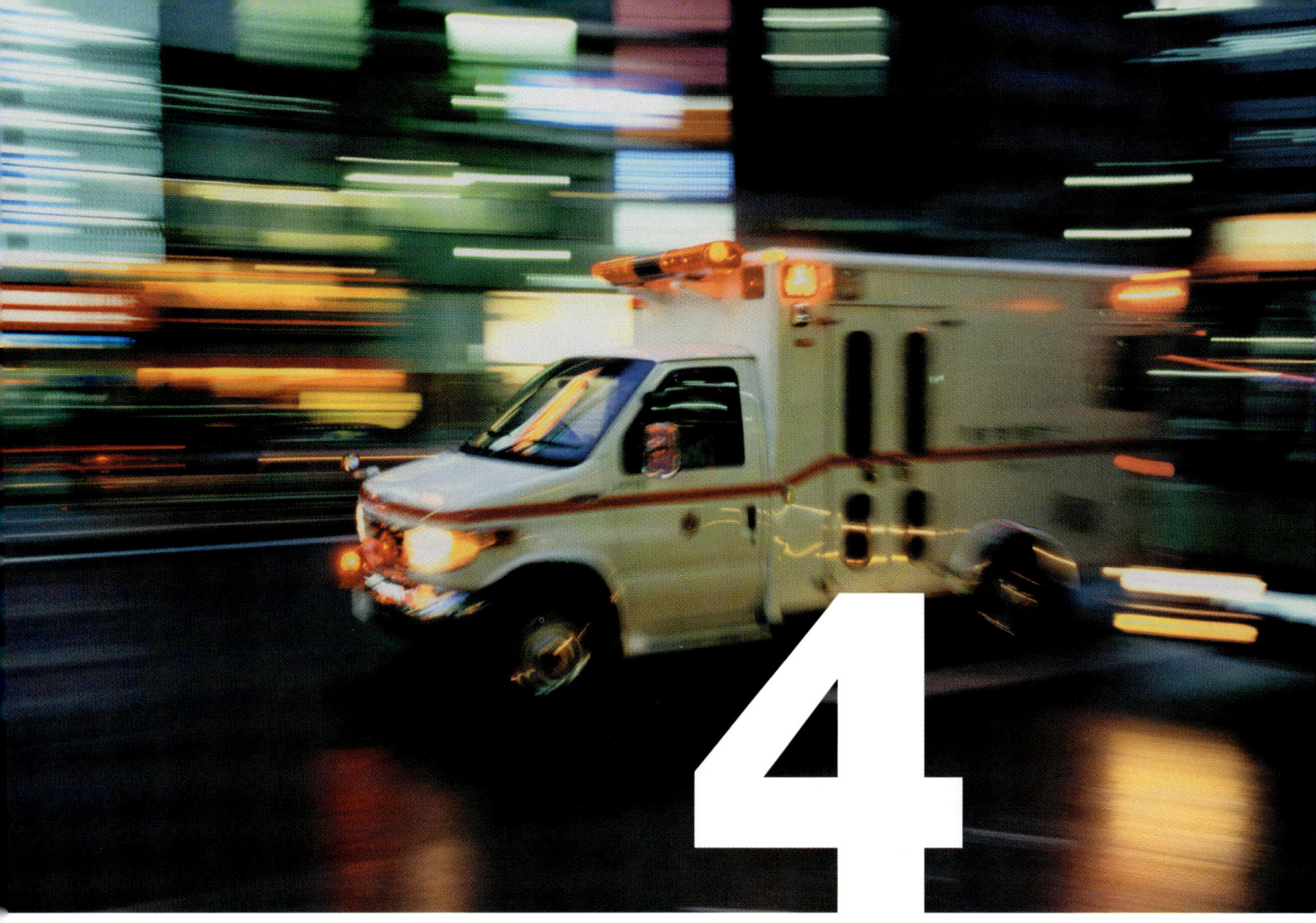

Section Four

Special Patient Populations

4

Special Patient Populations

30

Geriatric Patients

Lesson Goal

The goal of this chapter is to prepare the EMT-Basic for the challenges faced when dealing with the elderly. The EMT-Basic is presented with information on the management of illness and injury in the elderly that offers a different dimension than in the younger-age population.

Scenario

The dispatcher sends you to a reported "elderly fall." You recognize the address as one that you have previously responded to for a fall with a broken hip just 4 months ago. When you arrive at the house, you find an 85-year-old woman who lives alone who is alert and pleasant but confused and who has a deformity of her right wrist. In assessing the scene you note that she has a number of medication bottles on the kitchen table and that there are a number of loose throw rugs, poorly lighted areas, and appliance wires across the floor. Her vital signs are stable and you find no other injuries. You splint her wrist and transport her to the hospital.

 What is your assessment of this scenario? What may be contributing to this patient's repeated trauma?

Key Terms to Know

Activities of daily living
Aging
Dyspnea
Elder abuse
Elderly
Febrile
Gerontologists
Homeostasis
Hypercarbia
Kyphosis
Osteoporosis
Senescence
Syncope
Tinnitus

Learning Objectives

As an EMT-Basic, you should be able to do the following:

Supplemental

- Define the term *elderly*.
- State the leading causes of death of the elderly.
- Describe the process of gathering patient information for the elderly person.
- List the steps in assessing an elderly patient.
- Describe communication basics used with an elderly patient.
- Describe trauma assessment in the elderly.
- Describe acute illness assessment in the elderly.
- State the nature of the problem of elder abuse.
- List the categories and characteristics of elder abuse.

The term **elderly** traditionally refers to persons 65 years of age and older. The elderly represent the fastest-growing age group in the United States. The term *elderly* as defined by **gerontologists,** medical specialists who study and care for the elderly, is more specific. Middle age comprises persons 50 to 64 years of age; late age, 65 to 79; and older age, 80 and above. The elderly currently represent 11% of the population of the United States, or approximately 26 million persons. By the year 2030, the elderly will achieve a projected 18% of the U.S. population.

The elderly present EMTs with significant emergency medical care management challenges. The emergency medical management of sudden illness and trauma in the elderly has different emergency medical care dimensions than in younger patients.

Aging

Aging, or **senescence,** is a natural biologic process. Aging is sometimes referred to as a process of biologic reversal that begins during the years of early adulthood. Organ systems have reached maturation and a turning point in physiologic growth has been reached. The body gradually loses its ability to maintain **homeostasis** (state of relative constancy of the internal environment of the body), and viability declines over a period of years until death occurs.

The fundamental process of aging occurs at the cellular level and is reflected in both anatomic structure and physiologic function. The period of old age is characterized, in general, by frailty, slower mental processes, impairment of psychologic functions, diminished energy, the appearance of chronic and degenerative diseases, and decline in sensory acuity. Functional abilities are lessened, and the well-known superficial signs and symptoms of older age appear, such as skin wrinkling, changes in hair color and quantity, osteoarthritis, and slowed reaction time and reflexes.

Aging is a set of predictable, inevitable changes in biologic and psychologic function, some of which are detrimental, that occur in healthy persons with the passage of time. Changes caused by the aging process in physical structure, body composition, and organ function, in addition to physical changes, often affect emergency medical care. Varying patterns of mental health must also be considered because of the impact they have on the elderly's functioning and activities of daily living. **Activities of daily living** are activities usually accomplished during a normal day, such as washing, dressing, and eating. The mental status of the elderly may be a major factor in finding out what emergency medical problems exist. The elderly are also considered at high risk for many mental health problems.

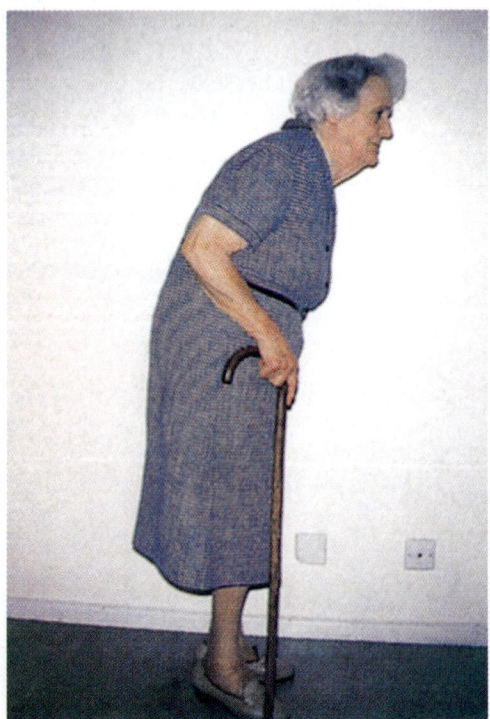

FIGURE 30.1 Kyphosis, commonly caused by osteoporosis.

Some elderly individuals have reached an advanced age with minimal medical problems. Another group, those with chronic illnesses controlled by modern medical means, also have attained advanced age. The latter group may deteriorate more rapidly in an emergency medical situation.

The leading cause of death in the elderly is cardiovascular disease. Risk factors affecting the death rate in the elderly are age over 75 years, living alone, recent hospitalization, recent death of a significant other, incontinence, immobility, and unsound mind.

People in the elderly years are estimated on average to have two or more chronic health conditions such as arthritis, stroke, lung disease, or heart disease. These conditions, when superimposed on other medical or traumatic emergencies, often complicate emergency medical care and often increase patient mortality and morbidity rates.

The elderly are more susceptible to disease and injury. Acute illness or trauma is more likely to be accompanied by a chronic disease. In addition, acute illness and trauma are more likely to alter organ systems beyond those initially involved. For example, an elderly patient who has fallen and fractured a hip may also be suffering from a lung disorder.

> ✓ The leading cause of death in the elderly is conditions resulting from cardiovascular disease. Risk factors affecting the mortality rate in the elderly are age over 75 years, living alone, recent hospitalization, recent death of a significant other, incontinence, immobility, and unsound mind.

Anatomy and Physiology

The aging process occurs in all the body systems; however, the discussion here is limited to the major systems.

Skeletal System

Bones lose minerals as they age. The loss of bone is unequal between the sexes. Bone mass in young adulthood is greater in women than in men. There is a decrease in the total weight of skeletal muscle. Bones widen and become weaker. There is degeneration of the joints. The emergency medical technician (EMT) must be alert to an increase in the probability of fractures even with minor injuries; there is a marked increase in the risk of fractures of the vertebrae, hips, and ribs. However, bone loss is more rapid in women, and after menopause it accelerates. The incidence of **osteoporosis** (increased porosity of bone) is greater in women as well. Older women have a greater probability of fractures, particularly of the neck of the femur (thigh).

Older persons are sometimes shorter than they were in young adulthood because of dehydration of the vertebral disks. As the disks flatten, a loss of approximately 2 inches in height occurs between ages 20 and 70 years. Contributing to this shortness is **kyphosis** (curvature of the spine) in the thoracic region. This condition commonly is caused by osteoporosis (Figure 30.1).

As the bones become more porous and fragile, erosion occurs anteriorly or compression fractures develop. As the thoracic spine becomes more curved, the head and shoulders appear to be pushed forward (see Figure 30.1). If chronic obstructive pulmonary disease (COPD), particularly emphysema, is present, the kyphosis may be more pronounced because of the increased development of the accessory muscles of breathing.

Osteoarthritis, a form of arthritis in which joints degenerate, is characterized by stiffness, deformity, swelling of the joints, and pain. Osteoarthritis usually involves changes in the hands and feet, particularly in the proximal and distal interphalangeal joints, and in the hips and spine (Figure 30.2).

Changes in the contours of the face result from resorption of the mandible, in part because of absence of teeth (edentulism). The characteristic look is an infolding and shrinking of the mouth. The nose and ears are more elongated than in earlier years because of the continuous growth of cartilage (Figure 30.3). The increased tendency to flex the legs makes the arms appear longer even though no change in their anatomic length has actually occurred (Figure 30.4).

> ✓ Changes in the skeletal system include loss of bone mass, which may lead to osteoporosis, kyphosis, and fractures. Osteoarthritis is another condition that may be linked to aging of the bones.

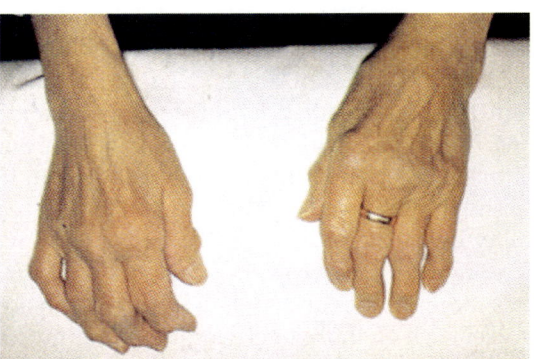

FIGURE 30.2 Osteoarthritis.

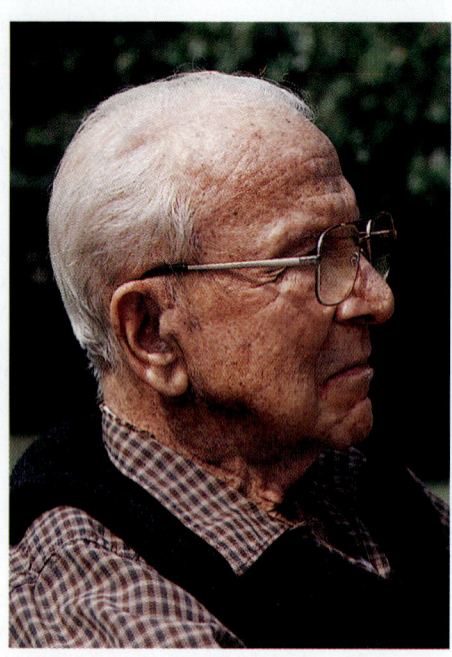

FIGURE 30.3 Changes in the contour of the face.

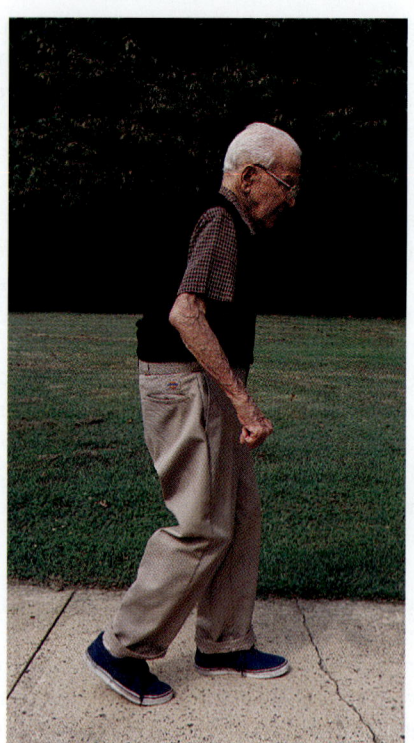

FIGURE 30.4 Because of the tendency to flex the legs, the arms appear longer.

Muscular System

As muscles age, loss of muscle mass occurs, estimated at 30% between ages 30 and 80 years. Deficits that relate to the musculoskeletal system, such as less ability to flex the hip or knee, predispose the elderly to falls. Muscle fatigue in the elderly can cause many problems affecting movement, falls being one of the most common.

Skin

As the skin ages, sweat and sebaceous glands are lost. Loss of sweat glands reduces the body's ability to regulate temperature. Loss of sebaceous glands, which produce oil, makes the skin dry and flaky. Production of melanin (the pigment that gives color to skin and hair) declines, causing an aging pallor. The skin thins and appears translucent, primarily due to changes in connective tissue. The thinning and drying of the skin also reduces the ability of the skin to protect the body from invasion by microorganisms. As elasticity is lost, the skin stretches and falls into wrinkles and folds, and more so in areas of heavy use, such as those overlying the facial muscles of expression. In addition, loss of fatty tissue predisposes the elderly to hypothermia and hyperthermia.

> ✓ As muscles age, loss of muscle mass occurs. The skin thins and sweat and sebaceous glands are lost. The elderly may have trouble regulating internal body temperature.

Respiratory System

Respiratory function declines in the elderly, partly as a result of the inability of the chest cage to expand and contract, as well as stiffening of the airway. Vital capacity decreases by as much as 50%. The increased stiffness in the chest wall is associated with a reduction in intercostal muscle (muscles that assist in expansion of the chest wall) power and stiffening of the connections of the ribs. As a result of these changes, the chest cage is less pliable. With the decline in the efficiency of the respiratory system, it takes more exertion for the elderly to carry out activities of daily living.

Changes also occur in the alveoli. The alveoli become smaller and shallower, reducing the alveolar surface. Reduction in the number of cilia (hairlike processes that propel foreign particles and mucus from the bronchi) predisposes the elderly to problems from inhaled particulate matter. Elderly people exposed over a long period of time

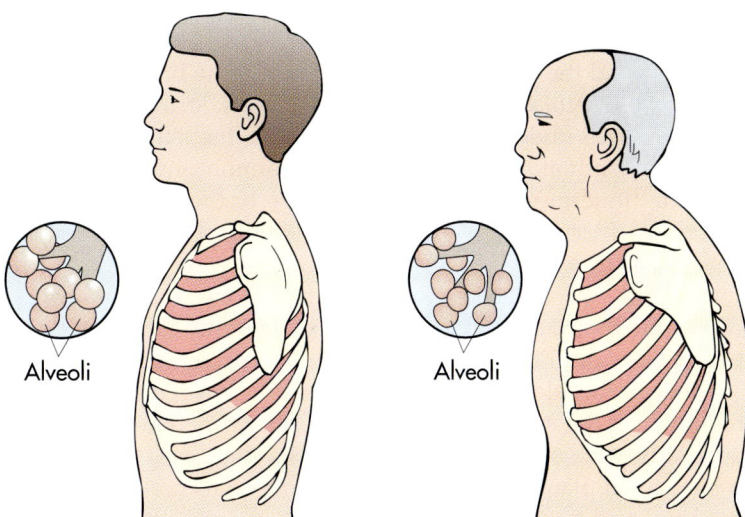

FIGURE 30.5 Spinal curvature can lead to an anteroposterior hump, which can cause respiratory difficulties. Reduction in the size of the alveoli can also reduce the amount of oxygen that is exchanged in the lungs.

to particle-laden air have difficulty removing material from the lungs. Oxygen uptake is decreased by the occlusion of the already reduced alveolar surface.

Another factor in decreased compliance of the chest wall is change in spinal curvature. Spinal curvature changes, accompanied by an anteroposterior hump, often lead to additional respiratory difficulty (Figure 30.5). Changes affecting the diaphragm also contribute to respiratory problems. Due in part to stiffening of the rib cage, older people rely more on diaphragmatic activity to breathe. This increased reliance on the diaphragm makes the older person especially sensitive to changes in intraabdominal pressure. Thus a supine position or an overly filled stomach from a large meal may provoke respiratory insufficiency. Obesity also plays a part in diaphragm restriction, especially when fat distribution tends to be central.

As the lung loses its elasticity, it empties less completely on expiration so that the elderly person breathes at higher lung volume levels. In addition, decreased responsiveness to hypoxia and high concentrations of carbon dioxide in the blood (**hypercarbia**) may occur, which often are aggravated by drugs (e.g., salicylates used in making aspirin) or sedatives. The ability to acquire and deliver oxygen to the cells is also decreased. Hypoxia is a much more likely consequence of hypovolemia than it is in the young.

Cardiovascular System

Diseases of the cardiovascular system are the major cause of death in the elderly. Cardiovascular disease accounts for more than 3000 deaths per 100,000 persons over 65 years of age. For persons over 65 years of age, it is well acknowledged that cardiovascular diseases are the most important group of diseases causing death. Moreover, with advancing age, cardiovascular diseases increase their role in death rates.

The following cardiac emergency situations are most consequential in the care of geriatric patients:

- Acute chest pain
- Arrhythmias
- Coronary artery disease
- Pericarditis
- Thoracic aortic dissection

Changes in the cardiovascular system structures may lead to decreased cardiovascular function. There is degeneration of heart muscle cells and fewer pacemaker cells, making the elderly prone to changes in electrical conductivity of the heart and leading to various arrhythmias. The

> ✔ In the respiratory system, the chest cage becomes less pliable. Alveoli become smaller, and the number of cilia in the lungs is reduced. Loss of lung elasticity predisposes the elderly to hypercarbia, whereas reduction in the size of alveoli reduces the amount of oxygen that is exchanged in the lungs. Loss of cilia may result in more infections and illnesses associated with inhaled particulate matter. Another factor is that bacteria are more likely to be present in the oropharynx, leading to the possibility of more respiratory infections.

heart and blood vessels rely greatly on their elastic, contractile, and distensible properties to function properly. With aging, these properties decline, and the efficiency of the cardiovascular system to move circulatory fluids around the body decreases. The arteries undergo structural changes due to an increase in smooth muscle and fibrous tissue (collagen). The intima (innermost coat of a blood vessel) thickens.

Arteriosclerosis is the name given to a group of diseases characterized by thickening and loss of elasticity of arterial walls. The cause may be due to accumulation of fibrous tissue, fatty substances (lipids), or minerals.

Atherosclerosis is a narrowing of the blood vessels. Atherosclerosis is a condition in which the inner layer of the artery wall thickens and fatty deposits build up within the artery. These deposits, called plaque, protrude above the surface of the inner layer and decrease the diameter of the internal channel of the vessel. One of the results of the narrowing of the diameter of the arteries is hypertension (high blood pressure), a condition that affects one out of six adults in the United States.

Another risk associated with narrowing and eventual obstruction of the coronary arteries is heart attack (myocardial infarction). Risk factors for heart attacks are smoking, hypertension, high blood-cholesterol levels, and a family history of premature coronary death or early death from myocardial infarction.

The heart itself shows an increase in fibrous tissue and size (myocardial hypertrophy). Calcification and sclerosis may adversely affect conduction pathways and valvular integrity. At rest, these changes in the heart's structure may not be a problem. Under stress, overall performance may be affected, which is demonstrated by a decrease in heart rate and cardiac output. A major result of the aging process as it affects the heart is reduced capability to respond to critical incidents. During incidents of acute illness or trauma, the ability of the heart to respond will affect resuscitation efforts. It is common following trauma for the elderly patient to have a low cardiac output without hypoxia and have no lung injury.

> ✓ Cardiovascular changes associated with aging include loss of the elastic properties of arteries, atherosclerosis, and arteriosclerosis. These changes may result in hypertension and may increase the risk of heart attack. Changes in the heart itself may reduce the ability of the heart to withstand acute illness or trauma.

Nervous System

As individuals age, brain weight and the number of neurons, or nerve cells, decrease. The weight of the brain reaches its peak at approximately age 20 years (1.4 kg [3 lb]). By age 80 years the brain loses about 100 g (about 3.5 oz). As the brain mass decreases, there is an effect on the venous structure. The dura mater adheres more closely to the skull, which makes epidural hemorrhage less common and subdural hemorrhage more common. Because of the atrophy of the brain there can be significant subdural hemorrhaging with minimal clinical findings. The speed with which nerve impulses are conducted along certain nerves decreases. Despite these decreases, only small effects on behavior and thinking result. There may be subtle changes in mental function. Reflexes are slower, but not to a significant degree, and compensatory function is usually adequate.

The elderly may learn more slowly than the young, but once materials are learned, retention is good. General information and vocabulary abilities rise or are maintained, whereas decline is observed in those functions requiring mental and muscular activity (psychomotor ability). The intellectual functions involving verbal comprehension, arithmetic ability, fluency of ideas, experiential evaluation, and general knowledge tend to increase after age 60 years in the elderly who continue learning activities. Exceptions are those who develop senile dementia and other disorders such as Alzheimer's disease.

The normal biologic aging of the brain is not a predictor for diseases of the brain. It is important, however, that emergency medical personnel consider that the decreases in the cortical structure of the brain may be involved in mental impairment. As changes occur in the brain, memory loss, personality changes, and other reductions in brain function often result in behavioral problems. These changes may involve the need for some form of mental health service; approximately 10% to 15% of the elderly require professional mental health services.

> ✓ As a person ages, brain weight and the number of neurons decrease. Although these changes may not result in any reduction in brain function, approximately 10% to 15% of the elderly require professional mental health services.

Sensory Changes

The National Center for Health Statistics reports that more than 1 in 4 elderly persons has hearing problems, and more than 1 in 10 suffers impaired vision. Men tend to be more likely to suffer hearing problems. Both sexes have similar shares of eye-related problems. Overall, approximately 28% have hearing problems and 13% have visual problems.

Vision

Loss of vision is considered a problem at any age, and for the elderly, it may be more so. Reliance on the sense of sight to carry on the activities of daily living is essential. For example, the inability to read directions on a prescription vial may lead to disastrous effects.

The elderly experience decreases in visual acuity, ability to differentiate, and night vision. The decreases are mainly the result of defects in the renewal of cells that occur in all body systems. As abnormal molecules are not degraded as rapidly as before, the effects of aging begin to appear. The lens of the eye is particularly affected.

The cells of the lens of the eye are mostly inert and are incapable of restoration to their original molecular structure. One of the destructive agents over the years is ultraviolet radiation. Eventually, the lens loses its capability to increase in thickness and curvature. The result is almost universal farsightedness (presbyopia) in persons over 40 years of age.

As a result of changes in the various structures of the eye, it is more difficult for the elderly to see in dimly lighted environments. Decreased tear production leads to dry eyes, as well as to itching, burning, scratchiness, and the inability to keep the eyes open for long periods of time.

Cataracts refer to any impenetrability of light rays (opacity) in the lens. In a cataract, the compression of the lens leads to gradual opacity, like a glass of water to which milk is added one drop at a time. The milky lens blocks or distorts light entering the eye and blurs vision.

Hearing

Hearing loss is a serious disability in the elderly and contributes to a lack of well-being and inability to carry on the activities of daily living. Almost all parts of the auditory system undergo changes with age.

Factors that affect hearing loss should be observed when taking the focused medical history. These factors may include hereditary, metabolic, vascular, and other systemic lesions affecting the ear and central nervous system. Factors that can produce or result in a hearing deficit include the following:

- Trauma
- Diabetes
- Vascular lesions
- Middle ear disease
- Barotrauma
- Hypertension
- Benign bony growths
- Arteriosclerosis
- Accumulation of earwax (cerumen)

The role of environmental noise is not altogether clear but is suspected, especially in men, to be a factor of considerable impact.

Ringing in the ears (**tinnitus**) is associated with a number of conditions and should not be dismissed casually. It should always be considered as symptomatic of a disease or syndrome.

 Loss of visual and hearing abilities is a common sign of aging.

Thermoregulation

The elderly are more susceptible to changes in the ambient environmental temperature. They have decreased ability to respond to hot and cold environments, have decreased heat production, and suffer from greater heat loss. This may be due in part to imbalance of electrolytes (e.g., potassium depletion), hypothyroidism, and diabetes mellitus. The basal metabolic rate is decreased; there is a decreased ability to shiver (which produces heat) and less ability to detect feelings of heat or cold. Some of the thermoregulatory problems may also be due to arteriosclerosis or the effects of drugs, alcohol, or other agents. Increases in body temperature may be related to stroke, diuretics, antihistamines, and antiparkinsonian agents. The elderly do not tolerate rapid rise in body temperature and are at grave risk when heatstroke is present. Hypothermia is often more of a problem because of decreased metabolism, less body fat, poor nutrition, and less efficient peripheral vasoconstriction. An elderly person living in a home or apartment with the internal ambient temperature at less than 68° F may suffer hypothermia.

Dehydration and Feeding

The elderly can rapidly dehydrate and have a decreased thirst response. The kidneys have a problem in meeting the challenge of injury, and as their ability to concentrate urine decreases, dehydration worsens. There is decreased body fat and total body water (15% to 30%). Nutrition often affects fluid balance in the body. Many elderly have increased dependence on others for feeding or do not eat or hydrate themselves adequately. Sometimes this is due to decreased mobility caused by osteoarthritis.

Dementia and Alzheimer's Disease

Altered comprehension resulting from neurologic disorders is a significant problem for many elderly persons. Impairments can range from confusion to dementia of the Alzheimer type. Not only may these patients have difficulty in communicating with the EMT, but they may also not be able to comprehend or assist in the assessment. They may be restless or combative. Firmness; reassurance; and clear, simple, and repeated questioning may be helpful. Often, a family member or friend can be of assistance in reassuring the patient.

Dementia is the loss of intellectual abilities, especially those higher-order functions measured by memory, judgment, abstract thinking, reasoning, and visual-spatial relations, in the context of preserved alertness. Approximately 15% of persons over 65 years of age have some degree of dementia, although most of these persons are not severely impaired. Dementia must be differentiated from delirium, which is a clouding of consciousness with decreased awareness of both external and internal environment and a decrease in the ability to maintain attention evident by disordered thinking and agitation. Memory impairment takes the form of absentmindedness, such as misplacing things. Another common difficulty is recalling names, particularly proper names. Dementia develops slowly, is progressive, and can be present for many months or years. The terms *senile dementia, chronic brain syndrome,* and *Alzheimer's disease* are commonly and mistakenly interchanged. The first sign of dementia may be a report that an elderly family member is staring out of the window more often, or not responding to questions as quickly, or beginning to make mistakes while balancing the checkbook, or perhaps just repeating sentences or having difficulty naming familiar objects. Psychiatric evaluation of the patient with dementia is vital and may be lifesaving because depressive illness in the elderly is important.

Given the increasing growth of the elderly population and the fact that 10% of Americans may have Alzheimer's disease, EMTs will see more patients with this problem. Alzheimer's disease results from an accumulation of plaque around nerves and unusual bundles of cells in the cerebral cortex, the part of the brain responsible for memory and reason. A person with Alzheimer's lives an average of 8 years after diagnosis, although many live longer. During this period the patient grows forgetful, suffers personality changes, and loses the ability to perform everyday tasks such as shopping, preparing meals, and driving a car. In the final stages, patients often become incontinent and mute and are unable to recognize friends and family.

> ✓ Memory loss, asking repeated questions, trouble using words, confusion, and disorientation are classic indications of Alzheimer's disease.

Patients with Alzheimer's often have behavioral problems that accompany the disease. Agitation, rage, paranoia, and hallucinations are common behavioral problems and are often the first sign of the disease. Some Alzheimer's patients become apathetic and do not speak unless spoken to. Others behave like unruly 2-year-olds, saying no to every request. Still others exhibit signs of depression, such as feelings of sadness or hopelessness, or disruptions of eating and sleeping patterns. Some patients become fixated on certain tasks such as turning off and on lights or washing dishes; some may hide and hoard food. Possibly because of becoming overtired, patients' behavioral problems may worsen in the evening in what is known as the "sundown syndrome." It seems to occur more frequently with patients who suffer from dementia. Many people with Alzheimer's disease have low sleep efficiency, spend a high percentage of sleep time in "early sleep time," and experience more arousals and awakening. Some of the reversible causes involve drug-related toxicity, infections, dehydration, and drug-drug interactions. Napping during the day may help consolidate the sleep schedule, but a long nap may interfere with nighttime sleep.

New screening tests have been developed for Alzheimer's disease. These include a short test that measures the following:

- *Orientation to time.* The patient is asked to identify the day of the week, month, and year.
- *Clock drawing.* The patient is asked to draw a clock showing a specific time.
- *Verbal fluency.* The patient is asked to name as many words in a specific category (e.g., meats) as he or she can in 1 minute.

Assessment: General Considerations

In the prehospital emergency setting, when the elderly are managed for acute illness or trauma, the EMT must be alert to advanced disease states that may cloud initial patient assessment. These include the following:

- Failure of the heart to provide adequate circulation
- Respiratory insufficiency
- Auditory and visual loss
- Reduced red blood cells (anemia)

Because older persons are more susceptible to critical illness and trauma than the general population, the EMT must consider a wider range of complications in patient assessment and intervention. In treating the elderly, EMTs must be able to render care that is different than that for younger patients.

The range of disabilities from which the elderly suffer is enormous, and field assessment may take longer than with younger patients. Difficulties in assessment can be expected due to sensory deficits (e.g., hearing, vision), senility, and physiologic changes.

> ✓ One of the most important considerations in the assessment of the elderly is mental health problems. The range and extent of mental health problems are considered serious factors in the elderly. The recognition of mental health problems in emergency medical situations will become more important because of the significant effect on the elderly person's health.

Basics

Assessment of the elderly in the prehospital environment must involve determining the presenting acute illness. Interviewing family members, friends, caretakers, senior citizen center workers, or significant others can be helpful and critical to the assessment. Remember that assessing the elderly often takes longer and may be more difficult to conduct due to communication problems such as the following:

- Visual impairment
- Hearing loss
- Fatigue
- Distractions in the immediate environment

Elderly patients appreciate factual information from health care personnel; they are more discerning in evaluating matters based on their life experiences. They desire more privacy, do not like quick decisions, and generally do not respond to messages or directions that force them to make quick decisions. Remember that the exact sequence of assessment of the elderly may have to be modified because of the presence of sensory deficits.

When assessing the elderly patient, the EMT should do the following (Figure 30.6):

- Pay attention to the possibility of impaired hearing, sight, comprehension, and mobility.
- Make eye contact.
- Grasp the hand and feel for temperature, grip, and skin condition.
- Address the patient by last name.
- Minimize noise, distractions, and interruptions.

- Observe for behavior, dress/grooming, ease of rising and sitting, fluency of speech, involuntary movement, cranial nerve dysfunction, and difficult respiration.
- Note whether movement is easy, unsteady, or unbalanced.
- Note whether the patient appears well nourished, thin, or emaciated.

Assessment of the elderly requires using different assessment skills. Ask for specific versus general information. The elderly tend to respond "yes" to all questions during the assessment process. Asking open-ended questions is a useful tool in evaluating most patients, but with the elderly it is sometimes necessary to help them by providing specific details from which to choose when dealing with a problem. For example, "Describe the pain in your hip" and "Describe your chest pain" are open ended and may lead to imprecise responses from the patient. The following questions are more specific and may help the patient give better information:

- "Is the pain in your hip sharp, stabbing, or dull?"
- "On a scale of one to five, with five being the most intense pain, what number describes your pain?"

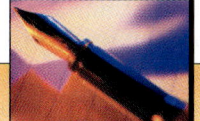

Tips from the Pros

When assessing an elderly patient, ask precise questions. Asking the patient "What is wrong?" may bring about more answers than needed.

Ask precise questions. If the patient has a history of difficulty breathing (dyspnea), you may need to investigate

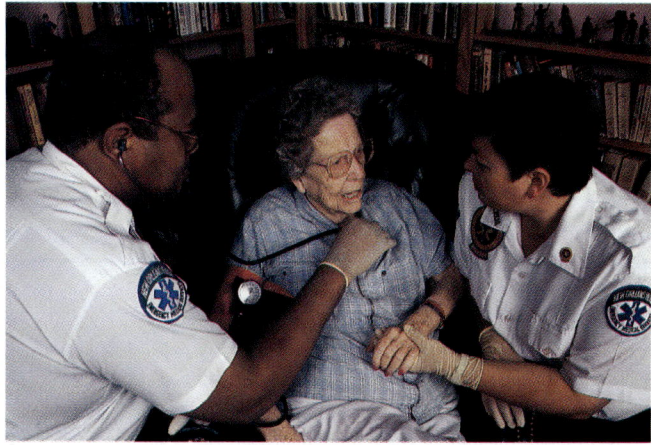

FIGURE 30.6 Proper assessment of a geriatric patient.

further and ask about the changes in the patient's difficulty in breathing, for example, "Do you have to rest several times when walking to the kitchen?"

Involve a significant other. With the patient's permission, involving the caregiver or spouse may be necessary to gather valid information. Some elderly patients may be reluctant to give information without assistance of a relative or supportive person.

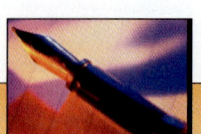

Tips from the Pros

The elderly patient may not want any other person present for a host of reasons, one of which may be an abuse problem. The elderly patient may fear punishment for telling the EMT why he or she has multiple bruises in the presence of the abuser.

There may be some problems about which the patient feels embarrassed and does not want the family member to know. Information from the family, however, may be important; for example, "Dad has not been acting normally for the past few days," or "Mom has been soiling her undergarments frequently."

Pay attention to sensory deficits (hearing, vision, smell, taste, touch, and position). Given the usual presence of these deficits, maintaining eye contact and speaking more slowly than usual and with suitable volume is important in gathering patient information.

Note altered comprehension. Neurologic disorders are a significant problem for many elderly patients. Impairments can range from confusion to senile dementia of the Alzheimer type. These patients have difficulty in communicating with the EMT and may not be able to comprehend or help in the assessment. They may be restless or combative.

Tips from the Pros

Firmness, reassurance, and clear, simple (and repeated) questioning may be helpful. Often, a family member or friend can be of assistance.

✓ Assessment of the elderly may require different communication skills than assessment of younger patients because of the possibility of hearing, vision, and neurologic deficits. Involving family members and asking precise questions may aid in assessing the elderly patient.

Communication

- Be respectful.
- Address the patient by his or her last name unless invited by the patient to use his or her first name: "Mrs. Doe, my name is Jack Smith. What would you like to be called?"
- Relieve anxiety. Say, "I am John Doe, and I am here to help you." Sit close to the patient and ask, "May I shake your hand?" This gesture helps communicate compassion and expresses friendliness and reassurance.
- Reassure appropriately. Do not say, "Everything will be all right." This will only increase anxiety.
- Talk more slowly than usual. Remember to consider a hearing deficit; talk to the "better" ear, if the patient has one, and face the patient.
- Slow down the interview pace. More information will be obtained.
- Be specific with your questions. When asking about medications, mention the organ system: "Are you taking anything for your heart?"

Medications and the Elderly

Many elderly persons take some form of prescribed medication, as well as over-the-counter drugs. Many elderly patients take multiple medications, and drug interactions are not uncommon. Many hospital admissions are the result of drug-induced illness. Underdosing is usually more of a problem than overdosing. Causes of underdosing include the following:

- Confusion
- Forgetfulness
- Arthritis of the hands, making it difficult for the patient to open bottles and take the proper amount of medication
- Trying to save money

Overdosing must be considered for a number of reasons:

- Confusion
- Vision impairment
- Arthritis of the hands; inability to take the proper amount of medication
- Taking the wrong medication
- Self-destruction (suicide)

One factor that may be responsible for both underdosing and overdosing is "brown bagging" the drugs (in plastic lunch sacs or brown lunch bags, hence "brown bagging"). In this activity elderly patients either "save up" the drugs and take them all at one time, or take a few at a time. Elderly persons often do this to save money or because they think more of the drug at one time will be better for them or because they are confused about the directions for taking the drug.

The absorption and use of medications (drug pharmacokinetics) are altered in the elderly. These changes depend on the particular drug and patient. Causes of these alterations include the following:

- Decline in kidney function (decreased excretion)
- Poor nutritional state
- Decline in liver metabolic activities
- Changes in body composition, such as increased fat and decreased lean body mass
- Decline in plasma volume and total body water

> ✓ In an elderly patient, be alert to the possibility of overdosing or underdosing of prescribed or over-the-counter medications, as well as drug interactions.

Initial Assessment

The initial assessment is no different in the elderly than in other age groups. The patient's airway, breathing, and circulation (ABCs) and level of consciousness require immediate assessment and intervention if deficits are determined (see Chapter 8).

Assessment and Emergency Medical Care of Acute Illness

In assessment of acute illness, the following factors are important, after managing urgent life support problems (ABCs):

- Plan for more than the average time in gathering information and taking a history.
- Patience is necessary, probably more than usual, due to the condition of the patient and probable sensory deficits, among other factors.
- Empathy and compassion are essential.
- Do not underestimate the patient's intelligence merely because communication may be difficult or absent.
- If the patient has close associates or relatives, ask them to participate in giving information or to be nearby to help validate information.
- Obtain a list of medicines and drugs taken or bring medicines and drugs to the hospital. Many elderly participate in the Vial of Life program, in which listings of drugs are kept in a vial stored conspicuously in the refrigerator.
- Make sure the patient can hear you; stand directly in front of the patient so he or she can see you speaking. Repeat questions if you are not sure that the patient has heard you.
- Observe the current health situation for specific abnormalities, specific illnesses, high-risk factors, nutritional status, mental status, activities of daily living, coping ability, and current environment (living space and arrangements).

> ✓ The initial assessment of the elderly patient should include general assessment of the ABCs and assessment of specific abnormalities and illness, risk factors, general nutritional and mental status, activities of daily living, coping ability, and current environment.

Acute Chest Pain

The number of conditions related to thoracic pain is substantial. Some conditions may not be life threatening, but, until ruled out, a high index of suspicion must be maintained for the possibility of myocardial infarction. Acute chest pain has a variety of causes, among them dementia and chronic medical illnesses. Chest pain must be assessed promptly, due to the high mortality rate of conditions such as myocardial infarction, aortic dissection, transection of the aorta, and tension pneumothorax. Less urgent conditions such as pneumothorax, pneumonia, pleurisy, pericarditis, and pulmonary embolism can be assessed following those conditions that are life threatening, with definitive diagnosis being made by the emergency department physician.

Myocardial Infarction

Myocardial infarction is responsible for over 550,000 deaths annually. Fifty percent of these deaths involve individuals over 65 years of age. The elderly tend to have larger infarctions, and their symptoms may be atypical and therefore unrecognized by emergency medical care providers. The typical presentation of chest pain, **dyspnea** (shortness of breath), **syncope** (fainting), weakness, vomiting, and confusion may not be seen. Myocardial infarction is often silent in elderly persons. The usual presentation of substernal pain, with referral to the jaw and left arm, may not be seen. Pain may be referred to different areas as a result of cervical arthritis, shoulder bursitis, or dental disease. The elderly may also delay activating prehospital emergency medical services. Because of the high mortality rate within the first hours of onset of symptoms, early assessment and emergency management are critical.

> ✓ The EMT must assess the patient rapidly, provide supportive care, and transport immediately to the emergency department. The presentation of myocardial infarction may be equivocal, and therefore rapid intervention by advanced life support personnel is important.

Aortic Dissection

Aortic dissection is usually the result of chronic hypertension and age. The wall of the aorta deteriorates, beginning with its inner lining. The deterioration eventually leads to bleeding into the medial lining. The patient commonly complains of severe tearing or ripping chest pain. The pain may be excruciating or, depending on the type of dissection, may be mild or even totally absent. The patient may have nausea, vomiting, and sweating and may experience a fainting (syncopal) episode. The pain may be anterior or in the upper back. There may also be pulse deficits of the upper extremities. If the carotid arteries are occluded by the dissection, there may be neurologic symptoms as well, such as paralysis of half of the body (hemiplegia) or inability to speak (aphasia). The carotid pulse may be diminished or absent on the affected side. Hoarseness and unilateral external jugular distention also may be seen.

Aortic dissection is a difficult assessment to make, and the medical diagnosis is often missed. The EMT should consider chest pain, hypertension, neurologic signs, left hemiplegia and hypotension in the right arm, chest pain radiating to the back, and unilateral jugular venous distention as signs and symptoms of possible aortic dissection. The onset can be acute, and the mortality rate is high. This patient requires supportive care and prompt transportation to the emergency department.

> ✓ Chest pain in the elderly may have numerous causes, including myocardial infraction (heart attack) and aortic dissection. Patients with chest pain should be transported immediately.

Syncope

Syncope is a brief loss of consciousness characterized by unresponsiveness and loss of postural tone. The most common cause is decreased cerebral blood flow (hypoperfusion). Decreased blood flow may be caused by hypovolemia, cardiac arrhythmias, orthostatic hypotension (occurs when a person assumes an erect position from a supine position), vasodilation, cerebrovascular diseases, and other cardiovascular pathologies (e.g., angina pectoris, anemia, and arterial insufficiency in the legs). Other coexisting diseases may be implicated as well, including COPD, chronic renal failure, and diabetes mellitus. A number of drugs are related to syncopal episodes, including diuretics, antiarrhythmics, antihypertensives, nitrates, calcium channel blockers, psychotropics, beta blockers, and digitalis.

In the elderly, syncopal episodes, particularly when they occur in patients with cardiac problems, have a high mortality rate. These patients require prompt transportation to the emergency department.

> ✓ Syncope is a brief loss of consciousness. In the elderly, this may indicate a life-threatening condition. These patients should be transported immediately.

Assessment and Emergency Medical Care of Trauma

Airway

Dentures

The existence of dentures, which is common in the elderly, may affect airway management. Ordinarily, dentures should be left in place because maintaining a seal around the mouth is more difficult without dentures in place. Partial dentures (plates) may become dislodged during the emergency and occlude or partially block the airway; remove the dentures in this event.

Preexisting Pathology

Previous disease in both upper and lower airway structures may affect airway management. Elderly patients who have had laryngectomies (partial or full removal of voice box structures) or chest surgery or who have a lateral curvature of the spine may have respiratory difficulty.

Breathing

Chronic Obstructive Pulmonary Disease

COPD is prevalent in the elderly population. In patients with COPD, respiratory drive does not depend on carbon dioxide levels but on diminished oxygen levels.

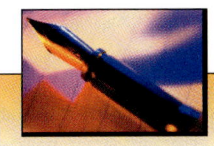

Tips from the Pros

Never withhold oxygen from a patient who needs it—even a COPD patient.

Lung Volumes

Stiffness of the chest wall increases in the elderly. In addition, reduced chest wall muscle power and stiffening of the cartilage make the chest cage less flexible. These and other changes lead to reductions in lung volumes. Respiratory support may be needed in such cases.

Cervical Spine

Protection of the cervical spine, particularly in trauma patients who have sustained multiple-system injury, is an expected standard of care. In the elderly, this standard of care must apply not only in trauma situations but also in acute medical situations, in which attempts to maintain airway patency are a priority. Degenerative arthritis of the cervical spine may subject the elderly patient to spinal cord injury while maneuvering the neck, even if there is no injury to the spine. Another consideration with improper or accidental movement is the possibility of carotid occlusion. A carotid occlusion (a blockage of the carotid arteries that supply the brain with blood) could produce symptoms ranging from an altered level of consciousness to a stroke.

Circulation

Bleeding (hemorrhage) in the elderly is managed no differently than in the young. However, a higher index of suspicion must be maintained for the potential of shock (hypovolemia) when an elderly patient's systolic blood pressure is less than 120 mm Hg.

Altered Level of Consciousness

Besides the usual mechanisms that lead to an altered level of consciousness, other factors in the elderly must be considered. Chief among these factors may be the use of medications to help with sleeping disorders, antidepressants, or medications prescribed for cardiovascular diseases such as hypertension.

Central Nervous System

Assessing neurologic deficit in the elderly may be difficult due to preexisting conditions or pathology. It may be difficult to decide whether the cause of the elderly patient's neurologic deficit is the result of a previous stroke or if the deficit is a result of the current trauma or illness. In addition, many medications may interfere with central nervous system function in times of trauma or acute medical illness. In any event, a rapid neurologic evaluation using the AVPU method is necessary (A, alert; V, responds to verbal stimuli; P, responds to painful stimuli; U, unresponsive). Any decrease in the level of consciousness usually means decreased flow of oxygen to the brain, inadequate circulation, or both.

> ✓ In trauma assessment of the elderly patient, special considerations must be kept in mind while assessing airway, breathing, and circulation, as well as the central nervous system. Cervical spine immobilization may be needed in both acute medical emergencies and trauma situations.

Environmental Problems

The ability of the elderly patient's body to adjust to variations in the temperature of the surrounding area or atmosphere depends on many factors, including the state of the patient's health, existence of pathologic conditions such as hypothyroidism and diabetes mellitus, diet, and the capability to alter environmental conditions. Altered thermoregulatory mechanisms due to altered cardiovascular, respiratory, and central nervous system functions affect the body's ability to adjust to climatic changes. Use of multiple medications, a common factor in the elderly, also may drastically alter neurologic control, circulation, electrolyte balance, or excretory function and thereby affect temperature regulation.

Heat Illness

Heat illness encompasses several entities, ranging from heat edema, the least severe, to heatstroke, the most severe. Heatstroke (hyperpyrexia) is a catastrophic illness, and mortality rate from heatstroke in the elderly reaches 80%. In the elderly, it is not likely that EMTs will see environmentally induced heatstroke resulting from exercise. The type of heatstroke likely to be seen is nonexertional and related to a disorder of the thermoregulatory center of the central nervous system. Heatstroke typically occurs during summer heat waves when the weather has been hot and humid for several days, the environmental temperature reaches 100° F (37° C), and the humidity is high (over 50%).

The elderly patient at risk of heatstroke is usually debilitated and taking drugs that alter fluid balance or temperature regulation. Risk of hyperpyrexia increases in patients with any of the following conditions:

- Preexisting **febrile** illness
- Infection
- Skin disease
- Heat cramps, heat exhaustion
- Chronic dehydration
- Reduced potassium in the body (hypokalemia)

Drugs may also increase the risk of heatstroke, including diuretics, antihistamines, and antiparkinsonian medications.

The classic presentation of hyperpyrexia includes hot, dry skin and no perspiration; high body temperature, 100° to 106° F (37.8° to 41.1° C); and altered mental status. Other signs and symptoms include headache, dizziness, muscle cramps, hyperventilation, vomiting, diarrhea, fatigue, and weakness.

Heatstroke is an acute medical emergency requiring rapid and aggressive intervention. The first goal, after airway management, is the rapid and immediate cooling of the body. Prompt transportation to the emergency department is needed. See Chapter 29 for more detailed information.

Hypothermia

Hypothermia is a serious and often fatal emergency in the elderly. Factors contributing to hypothermia include exposure to the cold, living in inadequately heated quarters, decreased ability to cope with the effects of changes in ambient temperature, decreased metabolism and fat, less efficient peripheral vasoconstriction, poor nutrition, and lower income. Emergency medical services (EMS) providers may not immediately recognize the problem as hypothermia because of associated problems such as trauma and pulmonary and cardiovascular failure. Factors other than exposure to a cold environment may contribute to hypothermia, such as alcohol use or abuse. Alcohol use may significantly alter central nervous system regulation of temperature and cause hypoglycemia, resulting in a reduction of metabolic energy sources.

Assessment of hypothermia includes the following:

- Body temperature below 95° F (34° C)
- Lack of coordination, lethargy, stiffness of muscle, and rigidity as temperature drops
- Shivering (ceases when hypothermia progresses)
- Altered mental status: level of consciousness impaired, progressing to coma

Emergency medical care depends on the degree of hypothermia. The first consideration after airway management has been ensured is raising the patient's temperature. Reduce heat loss by insulating the patient with blankets. If oxygen is administered, it should be heated and humidified. Prompt transportation to the emergency department in moderate and severe cases is required. See Chapter 29 for more detailed information.

> ✓ The elderly are at greater risk for both heatstroke, which is a serious medical emergency, and hypothermia. Both conditions require prompt transportation.

Geriatric Cases

Identify the medical problems involved in the following cases.

Case 1

A 75-year-old woman has a chief complaint of back pain, severe and very low; tenderness over the sacrum; and pain in the hips and legs, especially on movement of the lower extremities of the trunk. The patient states that any weight bearing, even trying to turn in bed, is painful and uncomfortable. There is no history of trauma.

Answer

This patient probably has suffered a fracture, perhaps pathologic, of the hip.

Case 2

A 65-year-old man has a cough with rusty sputum, is running a fever (temperature 102° F), has a pulse rate of 110, has chills, is dyspneic, has chest pain, and has a toxic appearance. The patient tells you that these symptoms came on abruptly. On examination of the chest, you find rales, rhonchi, bronchial breath sounds, and percussion dullness of some regions of the lung.

Answer

This patient likely has a lung infection, probably pneumonia.

Case 3

You have been called to a nursing home. The patient, a 73-year-old man, has been bedridden with several chronic illnesses and has a psychiatric history. The patient complains of a severe colicky pain, has a distended abdomen, complains of nausea, and has vomited; there is no muscle guarding. On palpating the right lower quadrant you find a soft rubbery mass. There is no marked tenderness.

Answer

This patient is probably suffering from a volvulus, a twisting of the bowel on itself, causing intestinal obstruction.

Case 4

An 82-year-old man suddenly experiences numbness and weakness in his left hand and arm. The episode resolves completely within the next 5 minutes, but over the next 2 months it recurs with increasing frequency until he is having five such episodes each day, lasting 10 minutes.

Answer

This patient is probably suffering from an epidural bleed.

Case 5

A 55-year-old woman has had poor appetite and has been losing weight over the past 2 weeks. She has not been sleeping well, exhibits psychomotor agitation, complains of loss of energy, and is quickly fatigued. Her daughter said she has not been able to concentrate or think clearly and has been self-reproachful and expressed feelings of guilt for her current condition.

Answer

This patient is probably suffering from a psychologic condition, possibly depression.

Case 6

It is December, and the temperature is 20° F. A 67-year-old man, living in a two-room home heated by wood stove, called his daughter and complained of headache, irritated eyes, and dyspnea. The daughter went to her father's home to check on him. When the EMS unit arrives, the patient and daughter are both exhibiting nausea, decreased vision, impaired judgment, fatigue, and loss of dexterity. The father also complains of angina-type pain.

Answer

This is a case of carbon monoxide poisoning.

Suicide

Suicide is a major problem among the elderly. Consider the following checklist to assess serious depression, which may lead to self-destructive acts:

- A persistent, sad, anxious, or "empty" mood
- Loss of interest or pleasure in ordinary activities
- Decreased energy, fatigue, or feeling "slowed down"
- Sleep problems (e.g., insomnia, oversleeping, early-morning awakening)
- Eating problems (e.g., loss of appetite, weight loss or gain)
- Difficulty concentrating, remembering, or making decisions
- Irritability
- Excessive crying
- Recurring aches and pains that do not respond to treatment
- Feelings of pessimism or hopelessness
- Feelings of guilt, worthlessness, or helplessness
- Thoughts of death or suicide or making a suicide attempt

Elder Abuse

Last Thursday, the city-financed cleaning service, along with a social worker, arrived at the home of Joseph, a 79-year-old man. They found him frozen to death in his second-floor apartment. For months, his neighbors tried to get help for Joe as he seemed less and less able to care for himself in his tiny studio apartment, which was cluttered with garbage. They gave him money for food, and ran an extension cord to his apartment when his electricity first stopped working. On the day of his death, the radiator in Joe's apartment was working, but much of the heat was lost through a jagged opening in a broken windowpane. It was so cold on that day that a half-empty beer can near the window in the apartment was frozen. The apartment was littered with filthy clothing and sheets, soiled mattresses, and paint chips. Near the window, someone, presumably Joe, had scrawled: "Life will never be the same."

Mary, 72 years of age, was confined to her home with Alzheimer's disease. Her daughter-in-law, Esther, with whom she lived, worked all day as a housekeeper and was Mary's primary support provider. Mary's spouse,

Phil, had been a maintenance man at a local factory and was a chronic alcohol abuser with a history of violence directed at his family. One evening, a neighbor heard a loud disturbance from within the house and then saw a chair crash through the kitchen window. The neighbor called the police. On arrival, the police found Esther unresponsive on the kitchen floor and, in the bedroom, found Mary gagged and tied to the bed with ropes. There were feces and urine all over her body. When the EMS unit arrived, the EMTs, while attempting to move Mary onto the gurney, found that the bedsprings of the mattress had physically invaded her skin. She was extremely malnourished and dehydrated.

Reports and complaints of abuse, neglect, and other related problems among the nation's elderly are believed to be on the rise. The exact extent of **elder abuse** is not known for several reasons. One reason is that elder abuse has been a problem largely hidden from society. Another is the varying definitions of abuse, neglect, and the elderly. Other obstacles involve the reticence of elders or others to report the problem to law enforcement agencies or human and social welfare personnel. In 1981 the House Select Committee on Aging concluded that 4% of the elderly nationwide were victims of some kind of abuse, representing more than 1.1 million persons. The typical victim of elder abuse may be a parent who feels ashamed or guilty because he or she raised the abuser. The abused person may also feel traumatized by the situation or fearful of reprisal by the abuser. Some jurisdictions also lack formal reporting mechanisms, and some states lack statutory provisions requiring the reporting of elder abuse.

The physical and emotional signs of abuse—those of rape, spouse beating, or nutritional deprivation—are often overlooked, or perhaps not accurately identified. Older women in particular are not likely to report incidents of sexual assault to law enforcement agencies. Sensory deficits, senility, and other forms of altered mental status (e.g., drug-induced depression) may make it impossible or extremely difficult for them to report the maltreatment.

Definition of Abuse

Abuse is defined as any action on the part of an elderly person's family (any relative); associated persons who have daily household contact (housekeeper, roommate); any person on whom the elder is reliant for daily needs of food, clothing, and shelter; or a professional caretaker who takes advantage of the elder's person, property, or emotional state.

Profile of the Abused

Elderly persons likely to be abused fall into the following profile:

- Over 65 years of age, and especially over 75 and female
- Frail
- Multiple chronic medical conditions
- Dementia
- Impaired sleep cycle, sleepwalking, shouting
- Incontinence of feces, urine, or both
- Dependent on others for their daily activities of living or incapable of independent living

Assessment of Elder Abuse

In the overall assessment of abuse, it is important to pursue an adequate explanation of the presenting incident. The astute emergency medical service provider looks for the indicators of concealment or avoidance to answers of questions that attempt to discover causation of the injury.

Answers that are implausible or doubtful, from anyone other than the patient who has sustained alleged abuse or reliable significant witnesses to the alleged injury, require aggressive investigation. Questions by the EMT that may provide valuable clues to the existence of maltreatment include the following:

"Exactly where did this happen?"
"What was he or she (the victim) doing, exactly?"
"What time did it happen?"

A sense of suspicion should develop when the medical history raises questions such as "Does this make sense?" and "Do I really believe this story?"

Burns, especially cigarette burns (a sign of abuse), or physical marks indicative that certain portions of the body have been systematically scalded are warning signs that abuse must be suspected. Emergency medical service providers may be the first health care providers to observe possible abuse. In gathering the elderly person's medical history, information should be sought that may be related to violent incidents. Information about the following medical incidents may be important factors in assessment of potential abuse:

- Repeated visits to emergency department or clinic
- A history of being "accident-prone"
- Soft tissue injuries
- Implausible explanation of injuries
- Simplistic, often vague explanation of injuries
- Psychosomatic complaints

- Pain, especially chronic pain
- Self-destructive behavior
- Eating and sleep disorders
- Lack of energy
- Depression
- Substance abuse
- Sexual abuse

It is important to remember that many patients suffering abuse are terrorized into making false statements for fear of retribution. In the case of elder abuse by family members, fear of removal from the home environment may be the cause of lying about the origin of the abuse. In other cases of elder abuse, sensory deprivation or dementia may preclude adequate explanation. The significance of these assessments is important in uncovering pathology, as well as identifying abuse that often is not reported by the patient for fear of reprisal, because of embarrassment, or because of incapability of reporting. Some of these assessments will involve definitive diagnostic procedures by the physician, such as x-rays or magnetic resonance imaging. Others, such as malnutrition, can be observed by visual examination. Still others can be determined by palpation, as with the swelling of an extremity.

In addition to the implicit lifesaving care that must be administered during the assessment, one of the significant concomitants of a thorough examination involves reducing further trauma from abuse through its very identification. It is well known that in child abuse the cycle of repeat abuse has a high mortality rate. It can be extrapolated from the data on child abuse that one of the preventive measures in reducing additional maltreatment of the elderly is the knowledge of its existence uncovered or identified by emergency medical providers. Uncovering abuse allows for referral to the protective services of human, social, and public safety agencies.

> ✔ EMTs who treat the elderly must be alert to the signs of elder abuse. Knowing the profiles of the typically abused and the abuser and questioning signs and responses that do not make sense may uncover the existence of elder abuse.

Categories of Abuse

Abuse may be categorized as follows:

- Physical: assault, neglect, dietary, poor maintenance of habitat, poor personal care
- Psychologic: benign neglect, verbal, infantilization, deprivation of sensory stimulation
- Financial: thefts of valuables, embezzlement, failure to notify

The signs of physical abuse or neglect may be obvious (e.g., the imprint left by an item such as fireplace poker) or subtle (e.g., undernutrition in the fragile elderly person). A comprehensive and thorough physical examination, in which findings are recorded and documented, is mandatory in the clinical setting. Indeed, the medicolegal implications for not doing so are enormous. In general, the physical factors to look for, particularly when there is inadequate explanation, are inflicted bruises, burns, head injuries, chest injuries, abdominal injuries, bone injuries, failure to thrive, sexual abuse injuries, and urogenital injuries.

> ✔ Elder abuse may be physical, psychologic, or financial. Signs of physical abuse include bruises, burns, head injuries, chest injuries, abdominal injuries, bone injuries, failure to thrive, sexual abuse injuries, and urogenital injuries.

Summary

Abuse of any person presents the emergency medical service provider with many challenges, including assessment and maintenance of basic life support functions. The clinical signs of abuse are often missed because the particular and usual mechanisms of trauma are not considered. It is abundantly and often distressingly clear, however, that the progress of the pathophysiologic insult is the same—high rates of mortality and morbidity.

In developing an assessment of possible abuse, the following key factors should be kept in mind:

- Eyewitnesses may be available who can relate what they saw. They may also identify the perpetrators. The perpetrator may also confess.
- Unexplained injuries are suspect first and ruled out only after careful analysis of all the evidence gathered, both personal and clinical.
- Implausible histories need thorough investigation before being accepted as valid.
- Alleged self-inflicted injuries must be carefully analyzed as to their origin; psychologic screening may be necessary to diagnose self-destructive behavior.

Summary (cont'd)

- Delay in seeking medical care in the adult, except when altered mental status exists, is always questionable.

  The management of abuse that results in physical violence is always fraught with many concerns. Detection of its existence by astute emergency medical service providers may be the single most important factor in its reduction by providing the proper medical care, referral, and protection afforded by social, human welfare, and public safety agencies. The high mortality rate involved when the vicious abuse circle closes is all too well known.

- Recognizing the special and urgent problems of the elderly faced by EMS providers is the key factor in rendering emergency medical care. Providing emergency medical care is fraught with unusual and challenging decisions that often demand extraordinary courses of intervention.
- The aging process affects the physical structure, body composition, and organs, including the skeletal system, muscular system, cardiovascular system, respiratory system, skin, and nervous system, including the sensory organs.
- Intervention in these instances also requires the EMT to consider a host of presenting problems and assessment strategies.
- The various medications an elderly person takes may contribute to medical problems. The elderly person may underdose or overdose on his or her medications.
- Two common presenting acute illnesses are acute chest pain and syncope.
- Trauma assessment in the elderly includes assessment and management of airway, breathing, and circulation. Special consideration must be given to the cervical spine and assessment of level of consciousness.
- The elderly are more susceptible to heat and cold illnesses, and EMTs must be alert to the presence of these conditions.
- Elder abuse is another consideration to which EMTs must be alert. Clues to the presence of elder abuse include eyewitnesses, confession by a perpetrator, unexplained injuries, implausible histories, alleged self-inflicted injuries, and delay in seeking medical care in the adult, except when altered mental status exists.

Scenario Solution

The repeated trauma may be exacerbated by medications that the patient is taking or by uncorrected factors in the home, such as loose carpets, poor lighting, and objects that can trip the patient. In addition to reporting the obvious injury to the emergency department physician, you also report your concerns about the risk factors that you have noted. Before the patient's discharge, after reduction and casting of her fractured wrist, a home visit is arranged with the local social services agency to correct the hazards that you identified in the home.

Key Terms

Activities of daily living The activities usually accomplished during a normal day (e.g., eating, dressing, washing).
Aging A set of expected, inevitable changes in biologic and psychologic function, some of which are detrimental, that occur with the passage of time.
Dyspnea Difficulty breathing or shortness of breath.
Elder abuse The physical, psychologic, or financial mistreatment of the elderly.
Elderly Traditional term given to those persons 65 years of age or older.
Febrile Pertaining to elevated body temperature; a body temperature of over 100° F is commonly considered febrile.
Gerontologists Specialists who treat the elderly.
Homeostasis State of relative constancy of the internal environment of the body.
Hypercarbia High concentration of carbon dioxide in the blood.
Kyphosis Curvature of the thoracic spine.

Key Terms (cont'd)

Osteoporosis Increased porosity of bone, occurring most frequently in postmenopausal women and sedentary or immobilized persons.

Senescence Aging; growing old.
Syncope Brief loss of consciousness.
Tinnitus Ringing in the ears.

Review Questions

1. When faced with an elderly patient with diminished hearing, what is the best way to communicate?
    a. Speak loudly and rapidly into the patient's ear.
    b. Talk slowly and face the patient unless the patient directs you to speak into one ear or the other.
    c. Do not bother to try to get additional history because you will only be wasting your time.
    d. There is no reason to change your usual pattern of interaction.
2. The findings in the elderly who are likely to be abused include:
    a. Dependent on others for their daily activities of living or incapable of independent living
    b. Presence of dementia
    c. Impaired sleep cycle, sleep walking, shouting
    d. Incontinence of feces, urine, or both
    e. All of the above
3. True or False: In the event of respiratory distress requiring bag-valve-mask assist, the patient's dentures should always be removed.
4. Medication may cause problems in the elderly by:
    a. Errors in dosing, either high or low
    b. Unexpected levels due to changes in kidney function
    c. Interactions with other medications prescribed for the patient
    d. All of the above
5. The leading cause of death in the elderly is:
    a. Cancer
    b. Cardiovascular disease
    c. Diabetes
    d. Trauma
6. Discuss why the elderly, when involved in a trauma situation, require different and more challenging emergency medical treatment. Include in your discussion physiologic and anatomic issues, comorbidity, and the age of the patient.
7. Many elderly people take some forms of prescribed and nonprescribed (over-the-counter) drugs and medications. Discuss why drug-induced illnesses are a problem for the elderly patient.
8. Elder abuse is a growing national problem with as many as 3 million cases per year. Describe important factors in assessing potential abuse. List the three categories of abuse with an example of each. How should the EMT-B manage a suspected case of elder abuse?
9. Describe how the EMT-B would asses and manage the following scenario:

    A 70-year-old male is found face down on a snowy sidewalk near his home. A neighbor has placed a coat around him and tells you that the man looked like he was having a seizure when he found him. On assessment, you find the patient responsive to your verbal commands and his pupils are dilated with the right pupil larger than the left. His pulse is 84 beats/min, and his blood pressure is 140/90 mm Hg. He is able to move his extremities in response to your commands. A medical identification bracelet notes that the patient is taking digoxin and coumadin. As you continue your assessment, the patient's condition deteriorates; he no longer can speak or follow commands and becomes nonresponsive.
10. What are the characteristics of demntia in the elderly? Describe what you may do to assess this condition. Consider orientation, recall, and attention questions to help in this assessment.

Answers to these Review Questions can be found at the end of the book on page 867.

31

Infants and Children

Lesson Goal

The goal of this chapter is to highlight the characteristics and developmental issues specific to infants and children when the EMT-Basic is presented with a medical emergency.

Scenario

You are called to an urban apartment for a reported "child with difficulty breathing." On arrival to the third floor walk-up you find a 9-month-old child who is seated in his mother's lap. When approaching the child, you hear a high-pitched inspiratory noise and intermittently "barking" cough. The child appears to have a mild degree of respiratory difficulty and slight cyanosis. You note a respiratory rate of 50, and when you auscultate the chest you hear a heart rate of 180. When you auscultate the chest, the child becomes more agitated and the respiratory noise and distress increases.

 How would you assess this patient? What interventions would you perform?

Key Terms to Know

Absence	Cyanosis	Hyperextension	Paresthesia
Acidosis	Dehydration	Hypersensitivity	Perfusion
Allergens	Diaphoresis	Hypothermia	Postictal
Anaphylaxis	Epiglottis	Hypovolemia	Renal failure
Asthma	Epiglottitis	Hypovolemic shock	Seizure
Aura	Epilepsy	Intracranial	Sepsis
Autonomic	Esophagus	Laryngotracheobronchitis	Septic shock
Autonomic nervous system	Flexion	Lethargy	Status asthmaticus
Brainstem herniation	Gastroenteritis	Malnutrition	Status epilepticus
Bronchioles	Gastrointestinal	Meninges	Stridor
Bronchiolitis	Glottis	Meningitis	Tachycardia
Cerebral edema	Hematoma	Needle cricothyrotomy	Trachea
Convulsive	Hemothorax	Paralysis	Tracheostomy

604

Learning Objectives

As an EMT-Basic, you should be able to do the following:

DOT

- Identify approach strategies for different pediatric developmental stages.
- Recognize the signs and symptoms of shock in the infant and child.
- Describe differences in anatomy and physiology of the infant, child, and adult patient.
- Differentiate the response of the ill or injured infant or child (age specific) from that of an adult.
- Indicate various causes of respiratory emergencies.
- Differentiate between respiratory distress and respiratory failure.
- List the steps in the management of foreign body airway obstruction (see Appendix A).
- Summarize emergency medical care strategies for respiratory distress and respiratory failure.
- Describe the methods of determining end-organ perfusion in the infant and child patient.
- State the usual cause of cardiac arrest in infants and children versus adults.
- List the common causes of seizures in the infant and child patient.
- Describe the management of seizures in the infant and child patient.
- Differentiate between the injury patterns in adults, infants, and children.
- Discuss the field management of the infant and child trauma patient.
- Summarize the indicators of possible child abuse and neglect.
- Describe the medicolegal responsibilities in suspected child abuse.
- Identify the developmental considerations for infants, toddlers, preschool-age children, school-age children, and adolescents.
- Recognize the need for emergency medical technician debriefing following a difficult infant or child transport.
- Demonstrate the techniques of foreign body airway obstruction removal in the infant and child (see Appendix A).
- Demonstrate the assessment of the infant and child.
- Demonstrate bag-valve-mask artificial ventilations for the infant and child.
- Demonstrate oxygen delivery for the infant and child.

Supplemental

- Recognize the signs and symptoms of increased respiratory effort in the infant and child.
- List three techniques to accomplish effective bag-valve-mask ventilation in the infant and child.
- List three characteristics of the following diseases: croup, epiglottitis, asthma (reactive airways disease), and bronchiolitis.
- Describe the treatment of an infant or child in status epilepticus.
- Identify the signs and symptoms of an infant or child with meningitis.
- Identify the signs and symptoms of an infant or child with dehydration.
- List the causes of pediatric injuries in the order of most common to least common.
- List three activities that may cause spinal trauma in the pediatric patient.
- List three of the most common types of poison in children.
- List five risk factors for child maltreatment.
- List five indicators of child abuse.

Pediatric patients represent a special challenge to the emergency medical technician—basic (EMT-B). This chapter highlights the characteristics and developmental issues specific to infants and children. Techniques for basic life support are reviewed, and selected advanced skills are outlined for those EMT-Bs approved to perform these skills. Several medical and trauma emergencies are discussed, including assessment and treatment modalities.

Pediatric Patients

Epidemiology

In rural and urban areas, approximately 10% of all emergency medical services (EMS) calls are for children under 14 years of age. Of those children, children between 5 and 14 years of age are most commonly seen because of trauma. Medical illness is the most frequent reason given for children below 5 years of age. In children under 2 years of age, serious illness, including cardiopulmonary arrest, is most common.

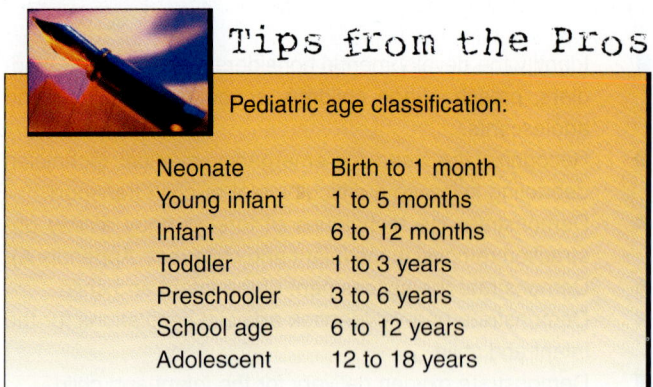

Tips from the Pros

Pediatric age classification:

Neonate	Birth to 1 month
Young infant	1 to 5 months
Infant	6 to 12 months
Toddler	1 to 3 years
Preschooler	3 to 6 years
School age	6 to 12 years
Adolescent	12 to 18 years

It is critical that EMTs are trained to deal with emergencies involving infants and young children. Once trained, the prehospital provider must maintain those skills, particularly in areas in which pediatric field experience is limited. Workshops, continuing education programs, and other clinical opportunities are available to EMTs to enhance and maintain the level of care rendered to pediatric patients.

Emergency Medical Services for Children

The management of critically ill and injured children has received a great deal of national attention. Congress authorized the Emergency Medical Services for Children (EMSC) program in 1985. Administrated by the Maternal and Child Health Bureau of the United States Department of Health and Human Services, EMSC has had a significant effect in the United States. Over the past 10 years many individuals and organizations across the country have worked to enhance and expand EMS for the pediatric sector through EMSC funding (Figure 31.1).

The seven basic components of an effective EMSC system are system description, education, prevention, research and data collection, medical direction and supervision, quality assurance and improvement, and ongoing funding. Many communities have incorporated these elements into their EMS systems, and their efforts have contributed significantly to improved prehospital care for children.

However, the work is not done. It is up to you as a primary provider of EMS to become educated and take full advantage of the data, information, and programs now available. Share this information with your colleagues. Help educate the public so that parents, school personnel, and other caretakers of our nation's children can recognize the ill or injured child; provide first aid, including cardiopulmonary resuscitation (CPR), when necessary; activate the EMS system; and know what type of emergency care is available in their communities.

> ✓ Children represent approximately 10% of all EMS calls. EMTs must take advantage of educational programs and information to provide the best level of emergency care to children and to educate communities about prevention.

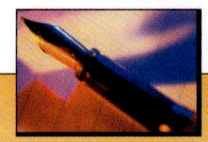

Tips from the Pros

EMSC informational materials and the Institute of Medicine report can be obtained from:

The National Maternal and Child Health Clearinghouse
8201 Greensboro Drive, Suite 600
McLean, VA 22102
Telephone: (703) 821-8955, extension 254 or 265

Emergency Medical Services for Children (EMSC)

- Focuses on the impact of pediatric emergencies on children and their families
- Develops and implements a body of knowledge concerning types, frequencies, and characteristics of pediatric emergencies and how existing emergency medical services systems address them
- Develops comprehensive EMSC systems ranging from prevention to identification, acute care, and rehabilitation related to severe illness and injury of children
- Trains and educates emergency medical services personnel to deal with pediatric emergencies
- Develops and maintains state and local support for EMSC

Source: Maternal and Child Health Bureau, 1994.

FIGURE 31.1 Emergency medical services for children (EMSC).

Approaching the Pediatric Patient

Children can present unique challenges simply because of their age and level of understanding. Figure 31.2 reviews the various stages that children go through as they grow and how you should handle each stage. Incorporate this information into your assessment and treatment of pediatric patients.

Before you begin to interact with a child, ask yourself several questions:

- What is the child's chronologic age?
- What is the child's level of understanding? (Note: It may not always match the child's *chronologic* age.)
- Is someone present whom the child knows or trusts (e.g., parents, older siblings, caregivers, teachers) who can offer reassurance and emotional support?
- Does anyone know the child's medical history or other information that may be helpful to the EMTs (e.g., details of the accident, type of seizure activity)?
- Are any special circumstances present (e.g., language barrier, physical or mental disabilities, special equipment)?

To adequately care for children, it is also essential to have equipment specific to the pediatric population. Table 31.1 includes the minimum pediatric equipment recommended by the American College of Emergency Physicians. Work with personnel in your area to ensure access to the appropriate pediatric equipment.

> ✓ When approaching the child, keep in mind specific developmental characteristics for each age group. Use these characteristics as guidelines. In addition, have equipment available to you that is appropriate for pediatric patients.

Vital Signs: Normal Pediatric Values

Pediatric patients include the spectrum from birth through adolescence and encompass a wide range of vital signs. In addition, "normal" vitals signs can vary from patient to patient. Table 31.2 gives examples of values common for pediatric patients. Height and weight are included as additional resources.

Text continued on p. 611

Developmental Stages and Approach Strategies for Pediatric Patients

INFANTS

Major Fear:
 Separation and strangers

Approach Strategies:
 Provide consistent caretakers.
 Decrease parent's anxiety (transmitted to infant).
 Minimize separation from parents/caregivers.

TODDLERS

Major Fear:
 Separation and loss of control

Characteristics of Thinking:
 Primitive
 Inability to recognize views of others
 Little concept of body integrity

Approach Strategies:
 Keep explanations simple.
 Choose words carefully.
 Let toddler play with equipment (stethoscope).
 Minimize separation from parents/caregivers.

PRESCHOOLERS

Major Fears:
 Bodily injury and mutilation
 Loss of control
 The unknown and the dark
 Being left alone

Approach Strategies:
 Keep explanations simple and concise.
 Choose words carefully.
 Emphasize that a procedure will help the child be more healthy.
 Be honest.

Continued on next page

FIGURE 31.2 Developmental stages and approach strategies for pediatric patients.

Developmental Stages and Approach Strategies for Pediatric Patients—(Continued)

PRESCHOOLERS—(continued)

Characteristics of Thinking:
- Highly literal interpretation of words
- Inability to abstract
- Primitive ideas about their bodies (fear all blood will "leak out" if bandage removed)

SCHOOL-AGE CHILDREN

Major Fears:
- Loss of control
- Bodily injury and mutilation
- Failure to live up to expectation of others
- Death

Approach Strategies:
- Ask child to explain what is understood.
- Provide as many choices as possible to increase the child's sense of control.
- Assure the child that he or she has not done anything wrong and that necessary procedures are not punishment.
- Anticipate and answer questions regarding long-term consequences (such as what the scar will look like, how long activities may be restricted, etc.)

Characteristics of Thinking:
- Vague or false ideas about physical illness, body structure, and function
- Ability to listen attentively without always comprehending
- Reluctance to ask questions about something they think they are expected to know
- Increased awareness of significant illness, potential hazards of treatment, lifelong consequences of injury, and the meaning of death

ADOLESCENTS

Major Fears:
- Loss of control
- Altered body image
- Separation from peer group

Approach Strategies:
- When appropriate, allow adolescents to be part of decision making about their care.
- Give information sensitively.
- Express how important their compliance and cooperation are to their treatment.
- Be honest about consequences.
- Use or teach coping mechanisms such as relaxation, deep breathing, and self-comforting talk.

Characteristics of Thinking:
- Ability to think abstractly
- Tendency toward hyperresponsiveness to pain (reactions not always in proportion to event)
- Minimal understanding of the structure and workings of the body

FIGURE 31.2, cont'd Developmental stages and approach strategies for pediatric patients.

TABLE 31.1 American College of Emergency Physicians and the National Association of Emergency Medical Technicians Guidelines for Ambulance Equipment

Category	Basic Life Support Equipment	Advanced Life Support Equipment (in addition to Basic Life Support Equipment)
Airway management and ventilation	Oxygen tank (fixed and portable) with tubing	Laryngoscope handle with extra batteries and bulbs; pediatric and adult
	Humidification source for long transports	Laryngoscopes blades
	Oxygen masks (transparent, nonrebreathing) in infant, child, and various adult sizes	Sizes 0, 1, and 2 straight Sizes 3 and 4 straight or curved
	Nasal cannulas; infant, child, and various adult sizes	Endotracheal tubes (minimum of 2 each size) Sizes 2.5 to 5.0 mm uncuffed
	Oral airways; infant, child, and various adult sizes	Stylettes for endotracheal tubes; pediatric and adult
	Nasopharyngeal airways with lubricant; infant, child, and various adult sizes	Magill forceps (pediatric and adult)
	Self-inflating resuscitation bags; 750 and 1000 ml with oxygen reservoir	Lubricating jelly (water soluble)

	Masks for use with resuscitation bags; neonate, infant, child, and various adult sizes	Nasogastric tubes
		   Pediatric sizes 5F and 8F
		   Adult sizes 14F, 16F, and 18F

	Portable suction unit with tonsillar and flexible suction catheters, 5F to 14F	
	Bite stick	
Patient assessment	Blood pressure cuff; infant, child and adult; standard and thigh cuff	
	Stethoscope	
	Flashlight (with extra bulb and batteries)	
	Thermometer with low temperature capability	
Monitor/defibrillator	Automated external defibrillator is strongly recommended for systems that lack immediate response from an advanced life support service.	Portable, battery-operated, cardiac monitoring defibrillator with recorder, quick-took paddles or hands-free patches, pediatric and adult electrodes and paddles, with capability to provide electrical discharge (below 25 watt-seconds)
Obstetrics	Sterile preassembled delivery kit (includes towels, bulb suction, gauze, sterile scissors or other cutting utensil, cord clamp or umbilical tape, sterile gloves)	
	Thermal absorbent blanket and head cover	
	Appropriate heat source for ambulance compartment	
Immobilization	Femur traction splint with padded ankle hitch, padded pelvic support, and traction strap; child and adult	
	Firm upper and lower extremity splints to include joint above and below injury, rigid with padding	
	Backboard; short and long appropriate securing straps, with padding for children	
	Rigid cervical collars; for children >2 years old; infant, child, small, medium, large adult	
	Neck immobilization device (firm padding or commercial product)	
	Triangular bandages	

Personal protection	Infectious disease prevention materials
	   Gloves
	   Goggles or face shield
	   Masks
	   Gowns
	   Appropriate disinfectants for hands and equipment	

	Protective helmet	

From American College of Emergency Physicians.

Continued

TABLE 31.1 American College of Emergency Physicians and the National Association of Emergency Medical Technicians Guidelines for Ambulance Equipment—cont'd

Category	Basic Life Support Equipment	Advanced Life Support Equipment (in addition to Basic Life Support (Equipment)
Personal protection—cont'd	Protective coat with reflective materials	
	Shoe covers	
	Sharp object disposal containers	
Communications	Two-way communications equipment between dispatcher, ambulance, and physician	
Bandaging	Burn pack; standard package, gel burn, sheet, or towels for children	
	Sterile gauze sponges, 4″ × 4″	
	Sterile trauma dressings of various sizes	
	Sterile gauze rolls of various sizes	
	Adhesive tape in various sizes	
	Elastic bandages in various sizes	
Vascular access		Intravenous catheters, 14g–22g
		Intraosseous needles of choice
		Tourniquet/rubber bands
		Syringes of various sizes including tuberculin
		Needles; sizes 14g–24g
		Blood sample tubes; adult and pediatric
		Intravenous administration sets; microdrip, macrodrip, pediatric burette infusion set, and in-line blood pump (as differentiated from intravenous tubing with an in-line blood filter)
		Intravenous arm boards; adult and pediatric
Medications		Activated charcoal
		Adenosine
		Albuterol or other inhaled bronchodilator of choice
		Atropine sulfate
		Bretylium tosylate
		Crystalloid solution (lactated Ringer's solution or normal saline)
Other	Length-based tape or chart for equipment sizing	Length-based tape or chart for equipment sizing and medication dosage
	Scissors capable of cutting heavy material	Povidine-iodine prep pads
	Sterile saline irrigation fluid	Alcohol prep pads
	Disposable bedpan	Finger-stick blood glucose reagent strips with analyzer
	Disposable urinal	
	Disposable emesis bags or basins	
	Cold packs	
	Blanket(s)	
	Wheeled cot	
	Folding stretcher(s)	
	Patient care flow chart	
	Disaster tags	
	Warning flares/signal devices	
	Fire extinguisher	

From American College of Emergency Physicians.

TABLE 31.1 American College of Emergency Physicians and the National Association of Emergency Medical Technicians Guidelines for Ambulance Equipment—cont'd

Category	Basic Life Support Equipment	Advanced Life Support Equipment (in addition to Basic Life Support (Equipment)
Investigational	Pneumatic antishock garment	Pulse oximetry
		End-tidal CO_2 detectors
		Transcutaneous cardiac pacemaker
		Portable automatic ventilators
		Magnesium sulfate

From American College of Emergency Physicians.

TABLE 31.2 Vital Signs—Normal Pediatric Values

Height and Weight Range for Pediatric Patients

		Range of Mean Norms	
Group	Age	Height (Average)	Weight (Average)
Newborn	Birth–6 weeks	51–63 cm	4–5 kg
Infant	7 weeks–1 year	56–80 cm	4–11 kg
Toddler	1–2 years	77–91 cm	11–14 kg
Preschool	2–6 years	91–122 cm	14–25 kg
School age	6–13 years	122–165 cm	25–63 kg
Adolescent	13–16 years	165–182 cm	62–80 kg

Pulse Rates for Pediatric Patients

Group	Age	Beats/Min	Assume a Serious Problem Exists (Bradycardia or Tachycardia)
Newborn	Birth–6 weeks	120–160	↓100 or ↑110
Infant	7 weeks–1 year	80–140	↓80 or ↑120
Toddler	1–2 years	80–130	↓60 or ↑110
Preschool	2–6 years	80–120	↓60 or ↑110
School age	6–13 years	(60–80)–100	↓60 or ↑100
Adolescent	13–16 years	60–100	↓60 or ↑100

Respiratory Rates for Pediatric Patients

Group	Age	Breaths/Min	Suspect Possible ↓ Minute Volume and Need for Ventilatory Assist with BVM
Newborn	Birth–6 weeks	30–50	↓30 or ↑50
Infant	7 weeks–1 year	20–30	↓20 or ↑30
Toddler	1–2 years	20–30	↓20 or ↑30
Preschool	2–6 years	20–30	↓20 or ↑30
School age	6–13 years	(12–20)–30	↓20 or ↑30
Adolescent	13–16 years	12–20	↓12 or ↑20

Blood Pressure in Pediatric Patients

Group	Age	Expected Mean for Blood Pressure	Lower Limit of Systolic BP
Newborn	Birth–6 weeks	74–100 mm Hg 50–68 mm Hg	↓70 mm Hg
Infant	7 weeks–1 year	84–106 mm Hg 56–70 mm Hg	↓70 mm Hg
Toddler	1–2 years	98–106 mm Hg 50–70 mm Hg	↓70 mm Hg
Preschool	2–6 years	98–112 mm Hg 64–70 mm Hg	↓70 mm Hg
School age	6–13 years	104–124 mm Hg 64–80 mm Hg	↓80–90 mm Hg
Adolescent	13–16 years	118–132 mm Hg 70–82 mm Hg	↓80–90 mm Hg

It is difficult to remember all of this information. A more practical method is to keep some type of reference in the ambulance. A "resuscitation tape" developed by Broselow and colleagues is an example of a tool that can be used (Figure 31.3).

✓ Be familiar with normal values regarding vital signs for infants and children. Use references whenever possible to help you remember the ranges.

Pathophysiology

Respiratory Status

Respiratory distress in a pediatric patient can be a life-threatening event. For this reason, prompt assessment of the child's respiratory status must be accomplished immediately. Approximately 90% of pediatric cardiopulmonary arrests start as respiratory problems. Early identification and intervention is the best way to prevent pediatric cardiac arrest and can significantly enhance the child's future quality of life.

The first sign of respiratory distress in an infant is usually a rapid rate of breathing. Other signs of respiratory distress that may be present in infants or children are increased respiratory effort, diminished breath sounds, decreased level of consciousness or response to parents or pain, poor skeletal muscle tone, and **cyanosis.**

As the child's respiratory effort increases, other signs and symptoms will be present:

- Nasal flaring
- Intercostal, subcostal, and suprasternal inspiratory retractions
- Head bobbing
- Grunting
- Stridor
- Prolonged expiration

If an infant or child is acutely ill, a slow or irregular respiratory rate is a serious sign. This sign usually indicates that the child's status is declining due to fatigue, central nervous system depression, or hypothermia. Many times the child will be breathing rapidly for a period of time, become fatigued from working so hard, and slow his or her rate of breathing. Do not be fooled into thinking the child is improving because the respiratory rate drops. In reality, the child may progress to respiratory arrest and possibly cardiac arrest if not treated appropriately.

The child should have equal breath sounds on both sides of the chest. Listen to the front of the chest, the back, and under the arms to do an adequate assessment. Breath sounds can be easily transmitted throughout the chest because the child's chest wall is so thin, and it may be difficult to identify areas of decreased function on one side because you can hear sounds from the lung on the other side. Do not rely solely on breath sounds. Look at the overall status of the child.

Circulatory Status

Normal heart rates for infants and children are shown in Table 31.2. A rapid heart rate at the high end of the range may be normal for some children. This increased rate can also occur as a result of stress due to **hypovolemia** (an abnormally low circulating blood volume), decreased oxygen, anxiety, fever, pain, increased carbon dioxide, or cardiac problems.

A slow heart rate usually occurs when the child can no longer maintain adequate tissue oxygenation. This decreased rate usually precedes cardiopulmonary arrest and should be treated quickly. Many times, proper oxygenation will cause the heart rate to rise, thus increasing the child's cardiac output.

Circulation Assessment

Infants have short, chubby necks, which makes it extremely difficult to palpate the carotid artery. Palpate the brachial artery on the inside of the upper arm between the infant's elbow and shoulder (Figure 31.4), or the femoral artery in the middle of the groin crease between the abdomen and thigh. The carotid artery can be used for children older than 1 year of age (Figure 31.5). Capillary refill can also be used to determine status of circulation.

Shock

The leading cause of shock in children across the world is **gastroenteritis** (inflammation of the stomach and intestines) with **dehydration** (excessive loss of water from the body tissues). Infection and diarrhea cause dehydration, and the severe loss of fluid can lead to hypovolemic shock (state of physical collapse caused by inadequate

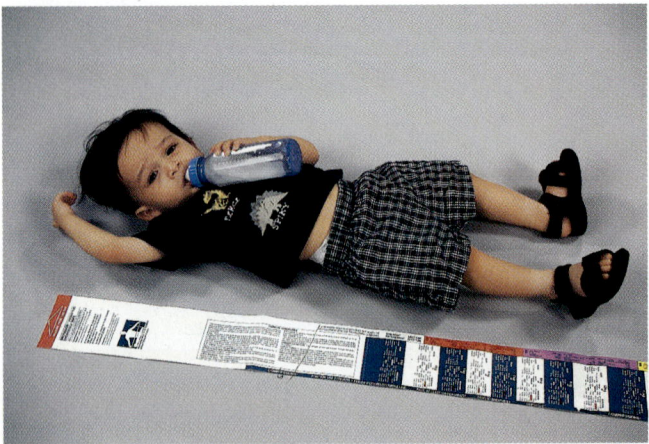

FIGURE 31.3 Broselow tape.

circulating volume leading to circulatory dysfunction, and inadequate tissue perfusion).

Blood loss such as that seen with trauma is another cause of **hypovolemic shock.** Massive bleeding is most common in the following situations:

- Injury to the liver or spleen
- **Hemothorax** (accumulation of blood and fluid in the chest cavity usually caused by trauma)
- Bleeding into the soft tissues of the thigh from a femur fracture
- Multiple extremity fractures or pelvic fractures
- Scalp lacerations

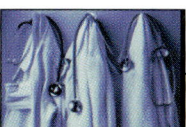

Physician Notes

In children with a primary head injury who also have a low blood pressure, always consider the possibility of some other source of bleeding. Only infants who have a soft spot on top of their heads have adequate space to allow for enough **intracranial** (within the cranium or skull) bleeding to cause hypotension.

Another cause of hypovolemic shock is burns. Partial-thickness burns (second-degree burns) and full-thickness burns (third-degree burns) damage the skin and allow fluid to escape through the burn surface. Sometimes fluid seeps into tissue outside of the blood vessels. In either case, it is not available to the circulating volume, and the child's blood pressure drops.

Other reasons for shock in the child are **sepsis** (systemic infection or contamination), **anaphylaxis** (life-threatening allergic reaction), and neurogenic (spinal) shock. In each of these types of shock there is decrease in the tone of the blood vessels without an increase in the total amount of blood volume to fill the larger space, resulting in *relative* hypovolemia. The child with meningitis or some other type of infection can develop sepsis, which can lead to **septic shock.** Anaphylaxis is most common due to insect stings, drug allergies, and food allergies. Neurogenic shock is seen with spinal cord injuries when the nervous system tone controlling the blood vessel size is lost.

Signs of shock include the following:

- Altered level of consciousness (confusion to irritability to **lethargy** [sluggishness] to coma)
- Increased respiratory rate leading to respiratory failure
- Rapid heart rate
- Normal blood pressure progressing to low blood pressure
- Cool or cold, clammy skin
- Decreased peripheral pulses
- Prolonged capillary refill
- Low urine output (ask if child has urinated recently or how many diapers the child has wet within the last 24 hours)
- **Acidosis** (abnormal increase in hydrogen ion concentration in the body)

✓ Approximately 90% of cardiopulmonary arrests in infants and children start as respiratory problems. Therefore it is crucial to recognize changes in the pediatric patient's respiratory status as early as possible. Be alert to changes in the circulatory status as well, including the causes, signs, and symptoms of shock.

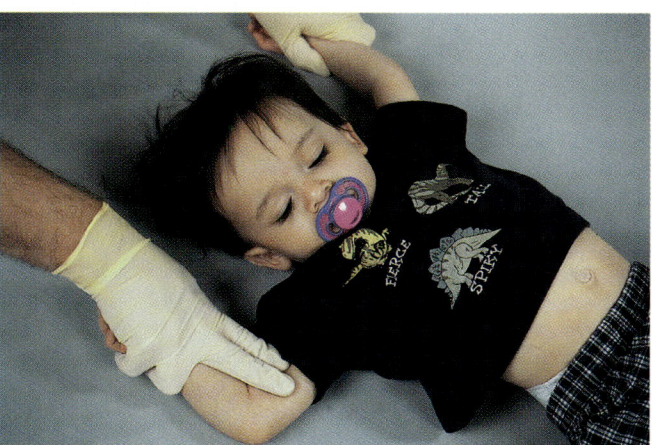

FIGURE 31.4 Palpation of the brachial artery.

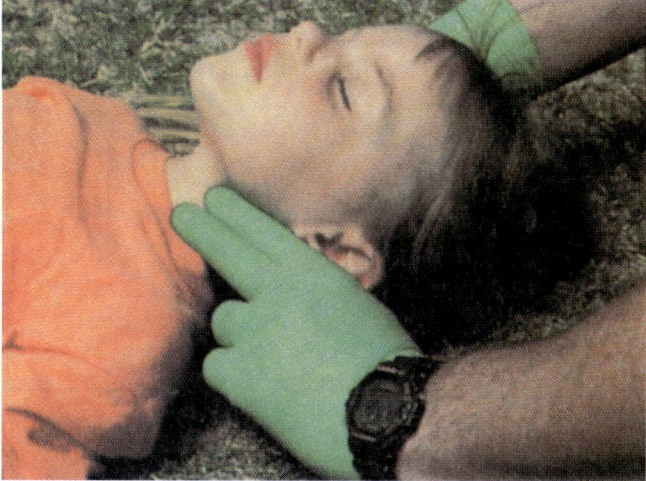

FIGURE 31.5 Palpation of the carotid artery.

Pediatric Basic Life Support

It is crucial that basic life support measures be started as soon as respiratory or circulatory problems are identified. Adequate artificial ventilation can buy critical minutes and also may be just enough to delay further respiratory or circulatory problems.

If an infant or child suddenly develops respiratory distress with coughing, gagging, **stridor** (high-pitched sound caused by an obstruction in the trachea), or wheezing, a foreign-body airway obstruction should be suspected. More than 90% of deaths from this cause occur in children younger than 5 years of age. Sixty-five percent of those victims are infants. Objects such as hot dogs, balloons, small toys, nuts, grapes, and round candies are common culprits.

Provide effective chest compressions when necessary by keeping the pediatric patient on a hard, flat surface. For infants and small children, the EMT's hand or forearm may be used to provide a hard surface under the back while carrying the patient.

Frequently reassess the infant or child. Many infants and children can compensate for a serious injury longer than an adult because they are usually healthy before the onset of illness. However, they rapidly get worse when they can no longer maintain that state.

> ✓ It is important for the EMT-B to maintain proficiency in CPR for infants and children. Include techniques for clearing an obstructed airway in these age groups. Remember that pediatric patients can compensate longer for serious injuries and then decompensate rapidly. Reassess them frequently.

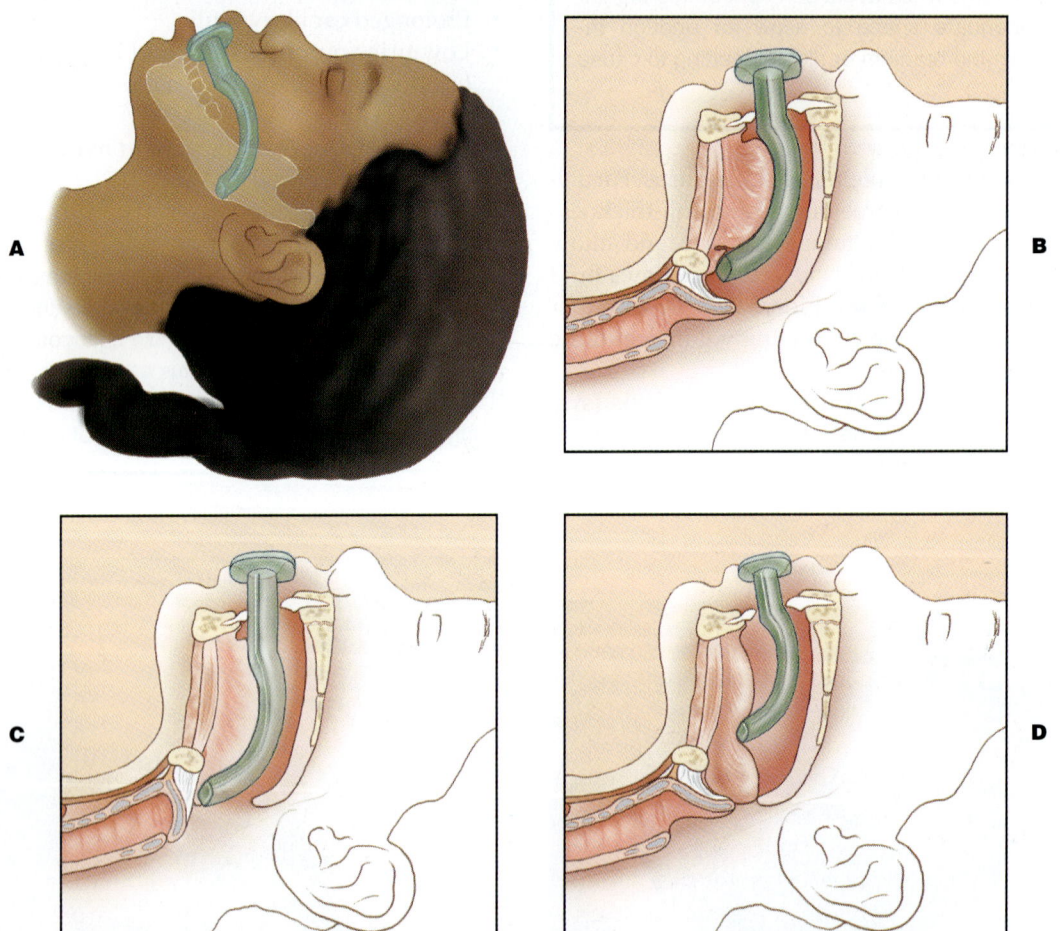

FIGURE 31.6 **A,** The airway should react from the corner of the mouth to the angle of the jaw. **B,** A properly sized and inserted airway keeps the tongue out of the way and opens an effective air passage. **C,** An airway that is far too large may block the airway, instead of opening it. **D,** An airway that is too small may not keep the tongue from blocking the airway.

Pediatric Basic Airway and Respiratory Adjuncts

Oropharyngeal Airway

An oropharyngeal airway can be used on an unresponsive infant or child to maintain a clear, unobstructed airway. *Be sure to select the proper size airway* so that no harm is done to the child. Measure the airway in the same way as for an adult. The airway should reach from the corner of the patient's mouth to the angle of the jaw (Figure 31.6).

In children, the oropharyngeal airway should be inserted using the tongue blade to depress the tongue. It is inserted straight back toward the back of the throat. This insertion technique minimizes the potential for soft tissue injury in the child's mouth. Remember to maintain correct positioning of the child's head to ensure a patent airway.

Nasopharyngeal Airway

Again, it is important that the nasopharyngeal airway is the proper size. Measure the length of the nasopharyngeal airway from the tip of the nose to the outside of the ear in front of the opening to the inner ear. Lubricate the airway and gently insert it into one of the child's nostrils (Figure 31.7). This device may need to be suctioned to keep it open.

Nasal Cannula

An example of low-flow oxygen is the nasal cannula. Use the pediatric size, and insert the two plastic prongs into the child's nares. Use a flow rate of 2 to 4 L/min. Higher rates irritate the nasal passages and do not substantially improve the child's oxygenation. If more oxygen is needed, switch to a face mask.

Nonrebreather Oxygen Mask

Children can use a nonrebreather face mask depending on the factors surrounding the illness or injury. This mask includes a reservoir bag, which should be inflated with oxygen with a flow of 10 to 12 L/min before application to the child's face. It also has two valves: one to prevent inhalation of room air, and another to prevent flow of exhaled gas into the bag. The patient inhales directly from the reservoir bag and receives an oxygen concentration of 95%. The mask must fit tightly against the child's face to obtain the concentration previously described.

The pediatric size should be used to provide a proper fit on the child's face and adequate oxygen concentration. Many children, however, do not tolerate the face mask because they feel restricted or suffocated. You may administer oxygen via the "blow-by" method by having the child or parent hold the mask in front of the child's face instead of directly on it, but remember that this is a much less effective means of delivery.

> **Tips from the Pros**
>
> Try using a paper cup for a child who will not tolerate a face mask. Punch a small hole in the bottom of the cup and insert the oxygen tubing. Have the child pretend to "drink" out of the cup. By doing this the child will be inhaling oxygen every time he or she takes a "drink."

Suction Equipment

If the child is crying, he or she will swallow air and be prone to vomiting. Frequent suctioning may be necessary because of the presence of vomit, saliva, mucus, blood, teeth, and so on. Be careful not to use a force greater than 120 mm Hg for an infant or child to avoid damaging the airway during the procedure.

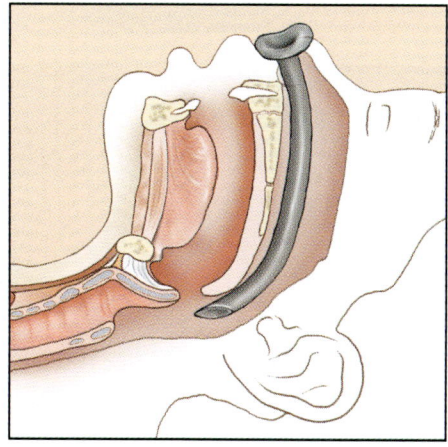

FIGURE 31.7 Nasopharyngeal airway.

Also, use a flexible plastic catheter whenever possible. A large-bore (tonsil-tip) catheter may be used for larger or thicker amounts of material, but be cautious that you are not too vigorous. Do not cause soft tissue damage to the mouth and increase the obstruction because of bleeding.

Frequently check the infant's or child's pulse during suctioning. Stimulation of the back of the throat, vocal cords, or **trachea** may produce stimulation that causes the heart rate to drop. If the heart rate drops, stop the procedure and rapidly ventilate the child with high-concentration oxygen.

Bag-Valve-Mask Ventilation

Bag-valve-mask (BVM) ventilation is best performed by two rescuers—one manages the mask and ensures an adequate seal, and one performs the bagging. In the event that two rescuers are not available, bagging must be done with two hands. One hand holds the mask on the face with the thumb and index finger forming a C around the ventilation port and maintains the head tilt–chin lift maneuver at the same time, and the other hand squeezes the bag to deliver the ventilations. When treating infants and toddlers, support the jaw with the middle or ring finger. For older children, place the fingertips of the third, fourth, and fifth fingers under the jaw to hold it forward and extend the head (which accomplishes the jaw-thrust maneuver) (Figure 31.8, *A*).

If one EMT is having difficulty ventilating the child, a two-person approach is mandatory. One EMT uses both hands to maintain the airway maneuver and mask seal on the face while the second EMT performs the ventilation (Figure 31.8, *B*).

Maintenance of the head in a neutral position without **hyperextension** is usually adequate for infants and toddlers. Hyperextension can actually close off the infant's soft airway. Children over 2 years of age do well with padding behind the occiput to move the cervical spine forward (Figure 31.8, *C*).

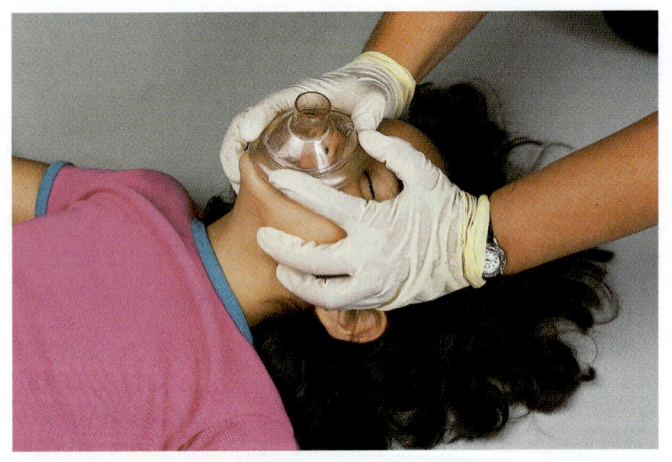
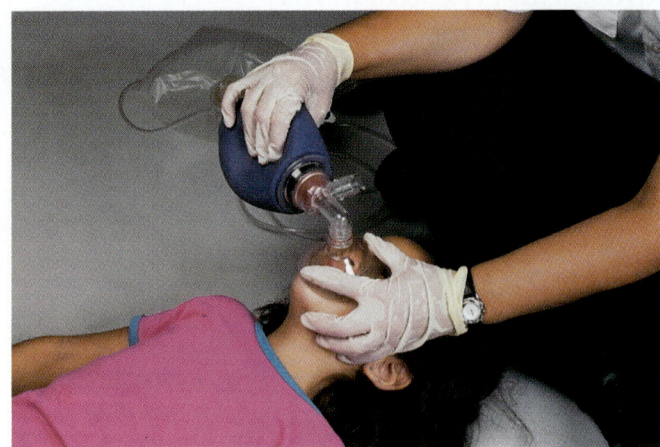
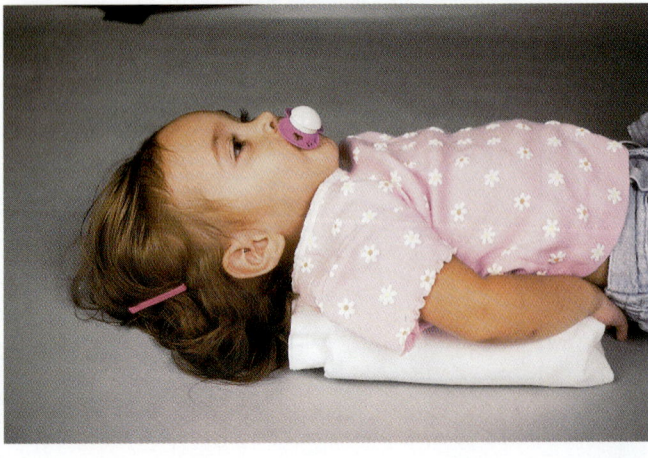
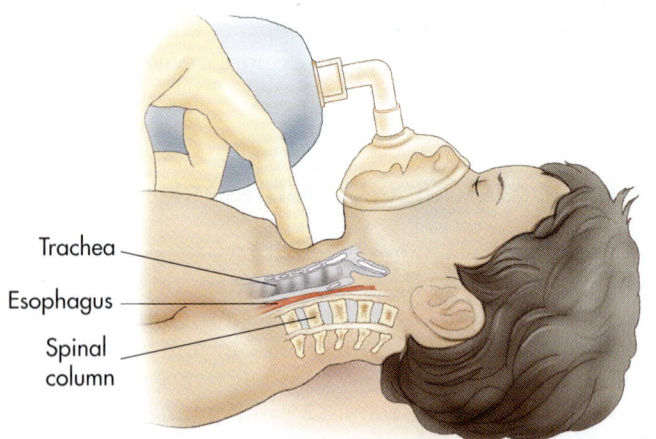

FIGURE 31.8 **A** and **B**, Oxygen devices and bag-valve-mask ventilation. **C**, Padding can help maintain position of the airway. **D**, The Sellick maneuver may prevent abdominal distention and vomiting.

Obviously, if a cervical spine injury is suspected, all airway maneuvers and ventilation should be done with the head in a neutral, in-line position. A trauma jaw-thrust or trauma chin-lift can be used to maintain airway patency.

The goal is to achieve effective ventilation. Consider the following if effective ventilation does not occur:

- Reposition the head.
- Make sure the mask is snug against the face.
- Lift the jaw.
- Suction the airway.
- Check the bag for damage.
- Verify an adequate source of oxygen.

Watch for swelling of the abdomen, which is common during BVM ventilation. Air gets into the stomach and causes the abdomen to swell. Have appropriate suction available. If the infant or child is unresponsive, apply pressure to the front of the throat (Sellick maneuver) to decrease swelling of the stomach and possible vomiting (Figure 31.8, *D*). This maneuver compresses the **esophagus** between the trachea and the cervical spine. The second EMT should apply this pressure with one fingertip in infants and the thumb and index finger in children. Do not use excessive pressure, which can cause tracheal obstruction in infants.

Last, it is critical to use a BVM system that delivers at least 450 ml of air for full-term infants and children. Neonatal BVMs only deliver about 250 ml and should not be used. However, do *not* use an adult BVM and attempt to give smaller puffs. The child who is not breathing presents a very stressful situation, and it may be difficult to give only small breaths. However, large volumes of air will cause the lungs to overinflate, leading to rupture.

It is crucial to the child's ongoing survival to provide adequate oxygenation and ventilation. If you need to request additional personnel to accomplish oxygenation and ventilation, do so early and without unnecessarily delaying transport of the pediatric patient.

> ✓ Select the appropriate oropharyngeal or nasopharyngeal airway depending on the size of the infant or child. Be careful not to use a device that is too large for the patient because this will cause harm. Use a nasal cannula or nonrebreather mask to provide oxygen as appropriate for the patient's condition. Remember to have suction equipment available because infants and children are prone to vomiting. Last, ventilate as necessary using the appropriate bag-valve-mask system.

Pediatric Resuscitation

Once basic life support (BLS) skills have been performed on the infant or child, consideration should be given to more advanced procedures. The EMT must continue to reassess the patient to determine if these skills should be attempted at the scene, en route to the hospital, or not at all. Efforts should be made to request advanced life support (ALS) assistance if deemed necessary. These ALS providers may come directly to the scene or meet the BLS unit at some point during transport.

Once the decision has been made to initiate an advanced airway procedure, intubation remains the skill of choice. Intubation provides the most effective airway control and allows direct ventilation of the lungs. In some states, EMT-Bs are permitted to perform this skill. See Chapter 11 for information on intubation of pediatric patients.

In infants and children, cardiac arrest usually results from decreased oxygen in the blood, as well as acidosis caused by respiratory insufficiency or shock. The utmost attention must be given to establishing and maintaining a patent airway, effective ventilation, adequate oxygenation, and circulatory stabilization.

EMT-Bs may assist ALS providers during resuscitation of an infant or child. This assistance may include intubation, preparing the child for monitoring, gathering equipment for intravenous (IV) line insertion, and medication administration. Only ALS providers, however, can give many of the drugs used. Work with your medical director to clarify what you are permitted to do and how you may assist the ALS members of your team.

Because most pediatric patients do not go into cardiac arrest as a result of ventricular fibrillation, defibrillation is not a primary skill in pediatric resuscitation. Currently, the American Heart Association (AHA) does not recommend using automatic external defibrillators (AEDs) during most pediatric cardiac arrests. Children should receive no more than 4 J/kg of energy during defibrillation, and most AEDs can only deliver a minimum energy level of 200 J. This level is simply too high for infants and some children. The AHA does recommend AED use for patients in cardiac arrest who are older than 8 years of age or who weigh more than 55 lb (25 kg).

> ✓ Determine the need for ALS assistance during pediatric resuscitations. If appropriate, request ALS providers to the scene or meet them en route. Assist with those procedures within your scope of practice that have been approved by your medical director.

Assessment and Management of Common Pediatric Medical Emergencies

Croup

Also known as **laryngotracheobronchitis,** croup is a respiratory illness that occurs in children between 3 months and 3 years of age. It is a viral infection that has an unusually abrupt onset, usually after the child has had an upper respiratory infection and low fever. Inflammation of the larynx or vocal cords and the surrounding tissues causes the primary symptoms.

Usually the child will be hoarse with a respiratory stridor and a characteristic "barking" cough. The stridor is due to edema below the **glottis,** the slitlike opening between the vocal cords, and the barking cough is from edema of the vocal cords. If the lower airways are involved, wheezing will be heard.

The emergency frequently occurs during the middle of the night. The child wakes up with a barking cough and may show signs of respiratory distress. The amount of swelling usually dictates the severity of the situation. Be aware, however, that the child is at risk of complete airway obstruction from the narrowed diameter of the trachea.

High-concentration oxygen should be administered (cool and humidified when possible), and the patient should be transported in a comfortable position. Monitor vital signs and the cardiac rhythm. Many times the outside environment (if air is cool and humid) during transfer from the home to the emergency department may cause an improvement in the child's condition. Be sure to reassess frequently to detect any changes or signs of airway obstruction.

Epiglottitis

Epiglottitis is an inflammation of the **epiglottis** that most often occurs in children 3 to 7 years of age. It is caused by bacteria and progresses rapidly. Fortunately, since the availability of the *Haemophilus influenzae* type B (HIB) vaccine, this has become a rare disease. It is a true emergency because the child can progress to complete airway obstruction and respiratory arrest if the epiglottis swells over the opening of the trachea.

This child will look critically ill, will be quiet, and will be doing everything possible just to keep breathing. The child will sit upright and lean slightly forward on his or her hands with the neck extended forward (tripod position). The mouth is usually open with the tongue protruding. Swallowing is difficult, so the child will be drooling. In addition, the child will usually show signs of respiratory distress and, in severe cases, hypoxia. A muffled voice and stridor may also be present.

Do *not* make any attempt to examine the airway. Manipulation of this child's airway can lead to complete obstruction and respiratory arrest. *All* efforts should be made to keep the child comfortable and as calm as possible. Allow the child to remain with parents or caregivers in a sitting position. Give high-concentration, humidified oxygen via either a mask or the blow-by method, depending on what the child will tolerate. Monitor the child's cardiac rhythm and vital signs if doing so does not further agitate the child.

Be prepared to ventilate using positive pressure through a BVM device. You should be able to force enough oxygen past the obstruction to buy some time until you get to the hospital. ALS personnel may attempt intubation or **needle cricothyrotomy** in some cases after consultation with the medical director, but this procedure is difficult to perform on small children. Intubation should be done only by those highly experienced in the skill and in an environment where an emergency cricothyrotomy or **tracheostomy** can be performed if the intubation is not successful.

Communicate with medical direction so that everyone at the receiving facility is prepared. Optimal treatment includes intubation and IV antibiotics once the child reaches the hospital.

Table 31.3 shows the differences between epiglottitis and croup.

TABLE 31.3 Differences Between Epiglottitis and Croup

Epiglottitis	Croup
Usually caused by bacterial infection	Usually caused by viral infection
No seasonal preference	Usually occurs during late fall and early winter
Occurs in ages 3 to 7 years	Occurs in ages 3 months to 3 years
Rapid onset	Slow onset
Patient will sit upright in a "tripod" position	Patient will either lie down or sit up
No "barking" cough	"Barking" cough present
Pain on swallowing causing drooling	No drooling
Temperature >104° F	Temperature <104° F

Asthma (Reactive Airways Disease)

More commonly known as **asthma,** reactive airways disease is considered the most common chronic illness among children and the leading cause of school absences. It is a respiratory illness in which the **bronchioles**, the small airways of the respiratory system in the lungs, become temporarily narrowed. Spasm of the muscles around the bronchioles and edema of the airways cause difficulty breathing and wheezing. The patient may also cough up mucus as it accumulates in the air passages.

Asthma is usually caused by an **autonomic** (related to the **autonomic nervous system,** which regulates involuntary vital functions of the body) problem or sensitizing agents. Factors such as **allergens** (substances that can produce a **hypersensitivity** reaction in the body such as food, environmental agents, or medications), viral infection, emotional stress, weather changes, exercise, and other irritants may precipitate an asthmatic episode.

EMS may be requested because the child is having an episode of difficulty breathing and increased wheezing. Treatment is focused on opening the air passages to make breathing easier. Provide humidified oxygen, and monitor the child's cardiac rhythm and vital signs. Communicate with medical direction, and follow local protocols concerning the administration of drugs. In some locales, EMT-Bs may be permitted to assist patients in administration of their asthma inhalers. In the event that a patient requires assistance, you should contact medical direction after ensuring that the medication is the patient's and has not passed the printed expiration date on the canister.

In severe cases, respiratory failure can occur. If the child has been struggling for a while, he or she may finally tire and stop breathing altogether. Have equipment available to assist the child's ventilation if necessary. Circulatory support may also be necessary if the ventilatory support is not adequate.

When treating a child with asthma, do not be fooled by a cooperative, lethargic child who is not wheezing. This child's bronchioles may be so tight that he or she cannot move *any* air.

Status asthmaticus is a life-threatening situation in which an asthma attack is severe, prolonged, and cannot be broken with traditional bronchodilators. The child should be transported rapidly in a position that is most comfortable for him or her. Monitor the airway and cardiac rhythm, and be prepared to provide ventilation.

Bronchiolitis

Bronchiolitis is an infection of the lower respiratory tract that is most often caused by a virus. It usually affects children between ages 6 and 18 months.

Usually the child has a mild fever, cough, and runny nose, which progress to respiratory distress. Edema and increased mucous secretions block the bronchioles. This condition is different from asthma because a virus causes it, and bronchospasm may not always respond to medications.

Provide high-concentration, humidified oxygen, and transport the child to the hospital for further evaluation. Monitor the respiratory and cardiac status, as well as the vital signs. Keep the child as calm as possible to maximize respiratory effort.

If the respiratory distress increases, provide ventilatory support to include intubation if necessary. Medical direction should be contacted with an update. Sometimes epinephrine or an albuterol treatment through a nebulizer may decrease the respiratory symptoms.

See Table 31.4 for the differences between asthma and bronchiolitis.

Seizures and Epilepsy

Seizures account for approximately 8% of pediatric prehospital transports. In many children, seizures are a complication of a fever. In fact, approximately 1 out of every 20 children at some time between birth and age 7 years will have a seizure resulting from a fever. Seizures are thought to occur because of the rapid rise of temperature and not the absolute temperature.

However, seizure disorders or epilepsy may also be a primary problem in some patients. It is estimated that approximately 12 million people in the United States have seizures each year.

Some children with epilepsy continue to have seizures on a regular basis despite aggressive medical therapy. The seizures interfere with the daily life of the child and his or her family and therefore are a chronic problem. Also, the growth and development of the child may be affected. Injuries often result, at which time EMS may become involved.

By definition, a **seizure** is associated with sudden, abnormal electrical activity in the brain. This activity results in an involuntary change in sensation, behavior, muscle

TABLE 31.4	Differences Between Asthma and Bronchiolitis
Asthma	Bronchiolitis
Occurs at any age	Occurs between 6 and 18 months of age
More common in winter and spring	Can occur at any time
Response to allergy, exercise, or infection	Caused by a virus
Family history of asthma	Usually no history of asthma
Drugs reverse bronchospasm	Drugs may not always be effective

activity, or level of consciousness. Seizures usually result from irritated, overactive brain cells. Therefore any condition that affects the structure of the cells of the brain or alters the brain's chemical metabolic balance may trigger seizures. Causes include hypoxia, head trauma, low blood sugar, tumors, drug toxicity, meningitis, epilepsy of an unknown origin, poison ingestion or exposure, or failure to take anticonvulsant medication as prescribed.

Other terms commonly associated with seizures include the following:

- **Epilepsy** is defined as two or more unprovoked seizures.
- **Aura** is the period of time immediately preceding the seizure. The patient experiences a certain feeling or sensation that warns of an impending seizure.
- **Postictal** refers to the period of time immediately following the seizure. During this time the child may be sleepy, or lethargic, agitated or confused, or have some short-term **paralysis,** depending on the etiology of the seizure disorder.

Seizures are usually defined as either partial or generalized. Partial seizures occur in one particular part of the brain and have specific symptoms. They are considered simple if the child's level of consciousness does not change and complex if the child experiences some loss of consciousness. Generalized seizures, on the other hand, involve the entire brain and produce a variety of symptoms. They are divided into those seizures producing motor activity (**convulsive**) or those producing some loss of consciousness (**absence** [pronounced *ab-saunce*]).

Symptoms vary depending on the type of seizure. Some patients may have a sudden jerking of a specific body part or a feeling of pins and needles in that extremity. Others may exhibit repetitive activity such as lip smacking, picking at their clothes, or fumbling. The child may stare or fall to the ground with rigidity or jerking of the extremities. During a generalized seizure, the patient may be cyanotic for the length of the seizure or become incontinent.

If there is no change in the level of consciousness, the child may be aware of the seizure activity, such as an arm or leg shaking. If the level of consciousness does change, the child may not be arousable during the seizure activity. In addition, some infants and children will be postictal and have symptoms ranging from mild confusion to a deep sleep.

Assessment of patients experiencing seizures includes thorough primary and secondary surveys. If no major life-threatening conditions are discovered, attention is then directed toward the seizure itself. Make note of the following:

- Duration of the seizure
- Presence of any aura
- Level of consciousness
- Part(s) of body involved
- Eye deviation and direction (if present)
- Postictal period (if present)

Find out if the child has a history of seizures and under what circumstances they usually occur. Determine what happened before this recent event, if more than one seizure occurred, what medications may have been taken, and so on.

If a seizure is witnessed, the child should be gently assisted to a side-lying position with the head turned to the side. In addition, the area should be cleared of hazardous items that might cause injury during the seizure activity.

Do not insert anything into the mouth if the teeth are clenched. A nasal airway is an appropriate alternative adjunct for this situation. The airway should be maintained and suctioned as necessary.

Ventilations should be assisted with a BVM device if hypoventilation or apnea occurs for a prolonged period. Remember that short periods of apnea occur with most tonic-clonic seizures. Respirations then return at the completion of the seizure. Only ventilate if the apnea is prolonged.

When the seizure has subsided, reassure the patient and the family. If a postictal period occurs, continue to maintain the airway as appropriate. If a fever is present, attempts to reduce the child's body temperature may be appropriate (e.g., sponging the child with a moist washcloth or 4×4 dressing or removing the child's clothing).

For some seizures an IV line and administration of diazepam (Valium®) or lorazepam (Ativan®) may be required to stop the seizure activity. ALS personnel per local protocols may give these medications. Recently, rectal diazapam (Diastat®) has become available, as well as a new formulation of fosphenytoin (Cerebyx®), which may also be used in some EMS systems.

Status epilepticus is a continuous seizure or a series of seizures in which the patient does not regain responsiveness. If this condition occurs, immediate intervention is necessary. Complications include aspiration of blood or vomitus, hypoxia resulting in brain damage, long bone and spinal fractures, and hypoglycemia and hypothermia from prolonged muscle activity. Maintain the child's airway and monitor cardiac activity. For those EMT-Bs permitted to initiate IV therapy, IV glucose (25% to 50% depending on the size of the child) may be ordered to correct hypoglycemia from the prolonged seizure activity. Specific drugs may be necessary to attempt to break the seizures. Request assistance from ALS personnel so that these drugs can be given. If ALS assistance is delayed, transport the child immediately to the hospital while oxygenating the child as best as possible.

Meningitis

Meningitis involves an inflammation within the **meninges**, the covering that surrounds the brain and spinal cord. It is caused by viruses, bacteria, or other microorganisms and may follow infections such as tonsillitis or an ear infection.

In younger patients, signs and symptoms of meningitis may include the following:

- Fever
- Rash, particularly one that does not fade when pressed with a finger (petechiae)
- Dehydration
- Lethargy
- Bulging fontanelle or soft spot in an infant
- Irritability (infant or child does not want to be touched or held)
- Loss of appetite
- Poor feeding (may be a sign in young infants)
- Vomiting
- Seizures
- Respiratory distress
- Cyanosis

In the older child, in addition to the previously mentioned signs and symptoms, the following may be present:

- Stiffness of the neck
- Pain when extending the legs or moving the hip
- Pain when flexing the neck
- Headache

As the bacteria or virus spreads, the child will become increasingly more ill. Complications may include cerebral edema (accumulation of fluid in the brain tissues), which can lead to increased intracranial pressure with brainstem herniation.

Treatment focuses on maintaining the child's respiratory and circulatory efforts. Monitor vital signs and cardiac status. Provide high-concentration oxygen, and assist ventilations as necessary. If permitted to start an IV, infuse lactated Ringer's solution in boluses of 20 ml/kg as necessary to manage shock. Make the child as comfortable as possible, and transport immediately if meningitis is suspected. Notify medical direction and frequently reassess the child, watching closely for any seizure activity.

> ✓ Meningitis is considered a true emergency in infants and children.

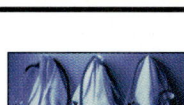

Physician Notes

For your own protection, talk with personnel at the receiving facility after the call is completed. Ask to be notified if the child is diagnosed with bacterial meningitis. In those cases, you may be given medication to prevent you from contracting the disease.

Bacterial meningitis is contagious by respiratory droplet transmission. When you first consider meningitis as a possible diagnosis, appropriate body substance isolation precautions with respiratory precaution (mask) should be used. The risk of transmission to EMTs who do not provide prolonged care in a closed environment or mouth-to-mouth resuscitation is low, but for your protection take precautions.

Dehydration

Vomiting, diarrhea, fever, burns, and poor fluid intake can contribute to a loss of body fluids. These symptoms can lead to dehydration, which poses a threat to the infant and child. The subsequent decrease in cardiac output from a smaller circulating volume can lead to **renal failure** (kidney failure), shock, and death if not treated properly.

Think about illness in a child. A fever can cause **diaphoresis** (secretion of sweat) and **tachycardia** (heart rate greater than 100 beats per minute). If a viral **gastrointestinal** disorder is present, the child may be nauseous or have vomiting or diarrhea. These last symptoms may cause the child to refuse food and fluids, which further jeopardizes the fluid balance. This cycle continues until the child is lethargic and in danger of circulatory collapse.

Infants are particularly susceptible to this loss of fluid because a greater proportion of their bodies is composed of water. In addition, their fluid needs are higher. For example, 65% of an infant's total weight is water. If an infant weighs 22 lb (10 kg), approximately 14 lb (7 kg) is water.

During the assessment, look for signs and symptoms of dehydration (Table 31.5). The dehydration can be mild, moderate, or severe depending on the clinical signs you find during the assessment. In fact, you may discover signs and symptoms of mild dehydration as you assess the child for another chief complaint (e.g., a febrile seizure).

Ask the parents or caregivers, or the child (if he or she is old enough and developmentally appropriate), specific questions about the history. Was there any fever, vomiting, or diarrhea? If so, how high was the fever? How much or how often has the child vomited or had diarrhea? When did the child last have something to drink (by cup or bottle)? How many bottles has the infant taken within the past 24 hours? Is the child urinating or wetting his or her diaper in the usual manner? How many diapers have been wet with urine or diarrhea within the past 24 hours?

No special treatment is necessary if mild dehydration exists. It is important, however, to reassess the child in case the dehydration progresses.

TABLE 31.5 Signs and Symptoms of Dehydration

Clinical Findings	Mild	Moderate	Severe
Vital signs			
Heart rate	Normal	Increased	>130 beats per min
Respiratory rate	Normal	Increased	Tachypneic
Blood pressure	Normal	Normal	Systolic <80
Peripheral pulses	Normal	Diminished	Absent
Capillary refill	Normal	2 to 3 seconds	>2 seconds
Mental status	Alert	Irritable	Lethargic
Fontanelle	Flat	Depressed	Sunken
Skin			
Turgor	Normal to slightly decreased	Decreased	Markedly decreased
Mucous membranes	Dry	Very dry; may see some tears	Parched; no tears
Temperature	Warm	Cool	Cool; clammy
Eyes	Normal	Darkened; sunken	Sunken; soft
Thirst	Increased	Intense	Intense if responsive

From Eichelberger M: *Pediatric emergencies: a manual for prehospital care providers,* Englewood Cliffs, NJ, 1992, Prentice-Hall.

In moderate to severe cases, provide high-concentration oxygen. Monitor the child's vital signs. Assist ventilations if necessary. If the patient is hypovolemic and you are permitted to start an IV line, give a 20 ml/kg bolus of normal saline or lactated Ringer's solution. Repeat this procedure in 5 minutes if the child's vital signs do not improve. Further boluses may be necessary to restore an adequate blood pressure and subsequent tissue perfusion. Prepare for immediate transport, and maintain contact with medical direction. CPR may be required.

> ✓ Pediatric medical emergencies include croup, epiglottitis, asthma, bronchiolitis, seizures, meningitis, and dehydration. Be familiar with the signs and symptoms of each entity. Assess the infant or child and provide the appropriate management.

Pediatric Trauma

Children have a particular injury pattern and physiologic response to trauma. These responses depend on the child's size, level of maturation, and overall development. However, basic life support and the assessment of airway, breathing, and circulation (ABCs) are still critical to the child's survival.

Prevention

The most frightening fact about pediatric trauma is that 20% to 40% of the deaths that occur are preventable. Many EMS and trauma systems are now focusing more of their efforts on trauma prevention. Educational activities, for example, are directed toward children and their families and may include such things as helmet safety, bike rodeos, seat belt use, proper use of car seats, swimming pool safety, spinal injury prevention programs, and antiviolence campaigns.

Unique Pediatric Characteristics

Blunt trauma continues to be the most common pediatric mechanism of injury. However, penetrating injuries have increased to almost 15%. Causes of pediatric injuries are categorized from the most to least common as follows:

1. Falls (most frequent in children less than 5 years of age)
2. Vehicular-related trauma
3. Sports-related injury
4. Assaults

Children may not show many external signs of injury. Therefore it is important to expect multiple-system injuries as opposed to single-system injuries until other-

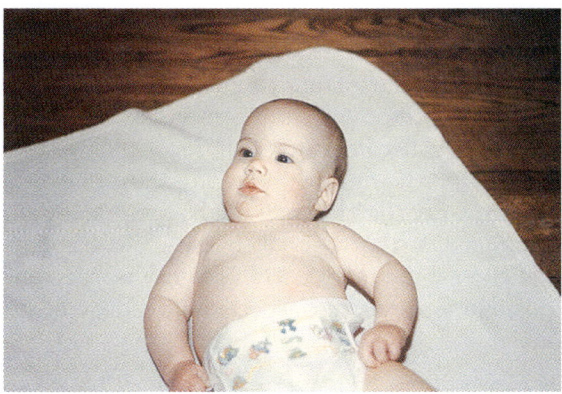 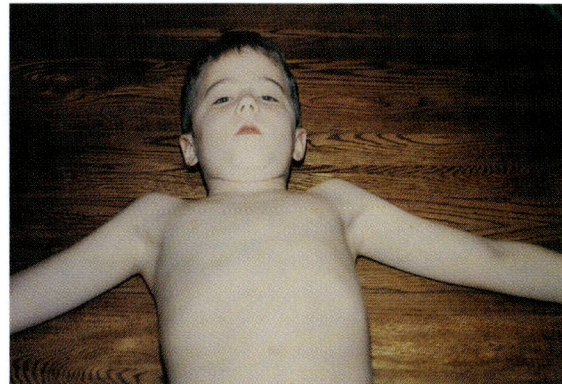

FIGURE 31.9 A comparison of the torsos of an infant and a school-age child.

wise confirmed (which usually takes place once the child reaches the hospital).

Several factors contribute to the differences in injury patterns between children and adults:

- In infants and younger children, the head is larger in proportion to the rest of the body.
- A child has a lower amount of body fat.
- The child's connective tissue is more elastic.
- The child's organs are much closer together. Therefore more organs can be injured when energy is released during a traumatic situation (Figure 31.9).
- The child's skeleton is not completely calcified and has many active growth centers. This difference makes the skeleton more resistant to injury so that a severe injury may exist to the underlying organs without any broken bones. Children can withstand a higher level of energy without signs of external injury.
- The child has a larger surface area in relation to body weight and can lose heat more quickly.

Remember that the child's future growth and development may be adversely affected by trauma and subsequent injuries. The injuries may heal, but the child may be left with lifelong physical, mental, or psychologic disabilities that can affect his or her future productivity and contribution to society. In addition, the costs for rehabilitation and subsequent care can be staggering. You directly influence not only the immediate survival of the child but also the long-term functioning of that child.

> ✓ The most common causes of pediatric trauma include falls, vehicular-related trauma, accidental injury, sports-related injury, and assaults (in that order). More important, many deaths from pediatric trauma are preventable. Keep in mind the specific differences between children and adults when treating injured pediatric patients.

Assessment

Thorough initial and ongoing assessments are performed on the pediatric patient just as on the adult. It is even more critical to recognize the potential for life-threatening injuries during the primary assessment. Even if the child appears stable during the ABC assessment phase, go with your instincts if you think the child has sustained a substantial force that may cause serious injury. Initiate rapid transport to a pediatric trauma center if you believe the child's condition may continue to worsen.

If a life-threatening situation does not exist, continue with the ongoing assessment. Pay close attention to anything that could possibly cause permanent damage, such as injuries resulting in paralysis or **paresthesia** (sensations such as numbness, tingling, or a feeling of "pins and needles"). In addition, any isolated extremity injury may require hospital evaluation to determine if the growth plate has been damaged.

Keep in mind that the three most common reasons infants and children die from trauma are the same as in the adult: hypoxia, overwhelming central nervous system trauma, and massive hemorrhage. If you are not quick to recognize these situations or the possibility of life-threatening conditions, you will contribute to the child's death or long-term disability.

> ✓ Proper initial and ongoing assessments are crucial in infants and children. Treat life-threatening injuries as they are found, and pay special attention to the child's respiratory status. Rapidly transport the patient to a pediatric trauma center when necessary.

Head Trauma

In the pediatric patient, head injury is the most common cause of death. Children have large heads relative to the

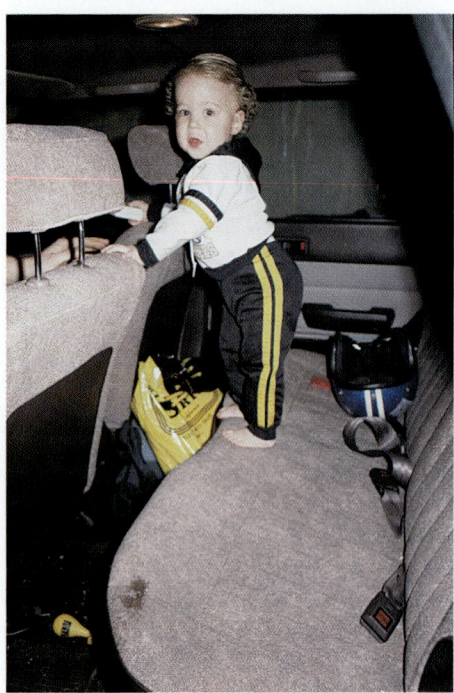

FIGURE 31.10 Laws require children to be restrained while riding in an automobile.

rest of their bodies and tend to land on their heads when they fall. Closed head injuries often result and range from a momentary loss of responsiveness to coma to death. Adequate assessment, resuscitation, and transport to a suitable facility designed to manage pediatric trauma are critical.

It is crucial to initially manage the airway and provide ventilation and supplemental oxygenation in an attempt to prevent further damage and to sustain neurologic function. Prevention of hypotension and hypoxia is vital to prevent further brain injury. Hyperventilation, which was previously recommended, is now believed to be more dangerous than helpful, because it can reduce the flow of blood and oxygen to the brain tissue, resulting in further injury. Hyperventilation should be done only in a controlled setting where oxygen and carbon dioxide levels can be monitored.

Even if the child has lost consciousness only briefly, it is important for the child to be evaluated. Cerebral edema, **hematoma** formation, and decreased **perfusion** can still occur, and serious secondary injury must be ruled out.

> ✓ Head injury is the most common cause of death in pediatric patients. Any change in level of consciousness is reason for evaluation. Managing blood pressure and ensuring adequate ventilation are the most effective ways to minimize secondary brain injury.

Spinal Trauma

The spine in the infant or child has not calcified, has more active growth centers, and is more flexible. Serious injury to the spinal cord can occur (e.g., pinching, stretching, bruising, or tearing) without any signs of external injury. In fact, x-ray changes may not be present once the child is evaluated at the hospital. If the child has any signs of deficit or if the mechanism of injury was significant, serious injury should be suspected and adequate precautions taken.

Causes of Spinal Trauma

Despite an increase in the use of car safety seats, the potential for injury to infants and young children still exists. Many parents buckle their infants into the seats and forget to secure the seats in the vehicles. If an accident occurs, the seat bounces around the inside compartment. The result can be injury to the child or injury to other occupants in the vehicle.

Motor vehicle collisions are also an origin of spinal trauma for older children. Many children, especially those between ages 4 and 10 years, ride completely unfastened despite laws requiring them to be secured in the car (Figure 31.10). Too many parents simply do not adhere to the law and do not serve as good role models themselves. For example, many parents who own a minivan, station wagon, or pickup truck allow their children to ride unrestrained in the cargo area. During an accident, these unrestrained children become missiles and are susceptible to serious spinal and other traumatic injury.

Those children who do wear seat belts or ride in secured car safety seats may also suffer spinal injury, but their susceptibility to injury is not nearly so great as those who are not restrained. Use of a lap belt may cause injury to the abdomen or lumbar spine, so it is important to examine the placement of the belt on the child. Is it high on the abdomen, or is it secured across the pelvis (Figure 31.11)? Also, with more vehicles now having a shoulder harness as standard equipment in the front and back seats, the shoulder strap at times falls across the smaller child's neck or face, thus contributing to a possible cervical spine injury.

Children riding on dirt bikes, on all-terrain vehicles, or as passengers on a motorcycle can also suffer spinal trauma. Observe the mechanism of injury, the vehicle involved, and what type of safety equipment may or may not have been used.

Last, warm weather tends to mean more children will be outside and therefore will be prone to more injuries. Riding bicycles, skateboarding, playing kickball in the street, swimming, and so forth are recreations in which serious injury may occur.

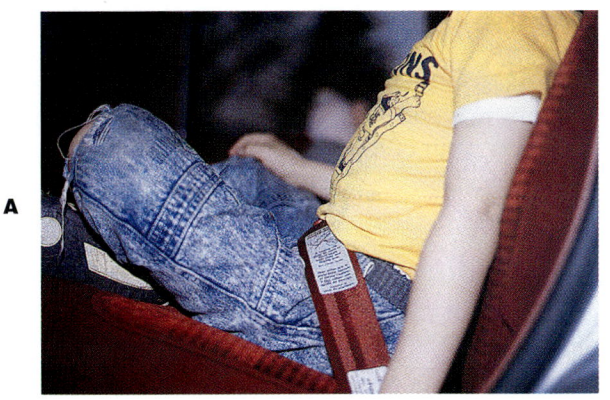 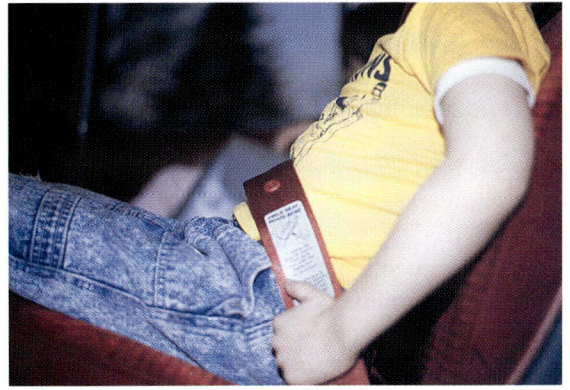

FIGURE 31.11 Correct (**A**) and incorrect (**B**) positions for lap belts on children.

Initial Assessment

Initial evaluation of the scene and mechanism of injury is crucial to performing a good assessment on any patient. When called to an incident involving possible pediatric spinal trauma, it is especially important to notice what type of equipment, if any, was being used at the time of the incident. Has the equipment, such as a bicycle, sustained any damage? Was the surface on which the child landed cement, grass, padded material, or dirt? If it was a bicycle accident, was the child wearing a helmet? If so, is it still in place or was it knocked off the head on impact? Was the helmet damaged? This information, if available, can tell you a great deal about the injuries that may have occurred.

Pay particular attention to playgrounds and the different types of equipment available to children. Many playgrounds now have cedar chips or some similar material on the ground under the equipment. This material provides a softer surface on which the child may land if he or she falls while playing. It is important to make note of this surface when evaluating the mechanism of injury and to relay this information to the personnel at the emergency department (Figure 31.12).

A thorough initial assessment with frequent reassessment is important in the pediatric patient. Evaluation of the airway with special attention to the cervical spine, in addition to assessment of breathing and circulation, should be done first. Then perform a quick neurologic examination and expose the patient to complete the initial assessment. Once you rule out any life-threatening injuries, you can then begin the ongoing assessment, which involves an entire "toe-to-head" approach.

Remember, children between ages 12 and 17 years have bodies with the same anatomic ratios as adults. Children 7 years of age and younger, however, are significantly different in their anatomic configurations. The most notable difference is the size of the head.

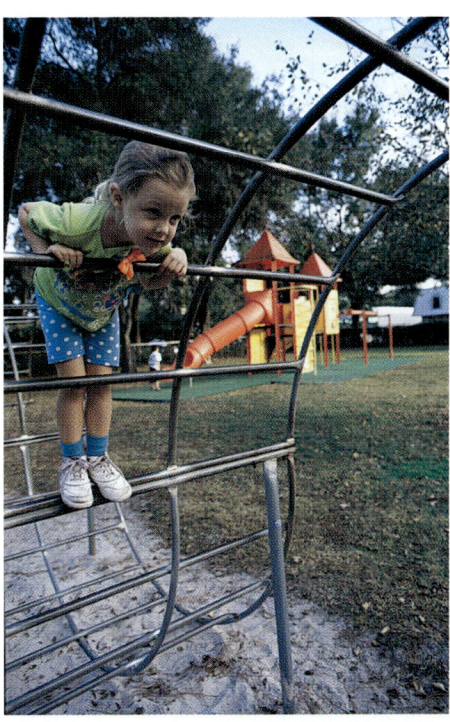

FIGURE 31.12 It is important to pay attention to playgrounds and the types of equipment available to children.

✓ Evaluate the mechanism of injury before ruling out spinal trauma. Serious internal injury can occur without any external injury. Perform a thorough initial assessment and reassess pediatric patients frequently because of their ability to compensate longer than adults.

Management

The indications for pediatric immobilization are based on the same criteria used for adults: evaluation of the mechanism of injury, one or more injuries suggesting some type of violent interaction, or specific signs and symptoms indicating spinal trauma such as numbness, tingling, and so forth. However, the mechanism of injury should be a key determination for immobilization even if the patient has no symptoms. If you believe the child may have been exposed to a force great enough to cause violent or sudden movement of the spine, the child must be properly immobilized.

Once you have identified the possible existence of cervical or other spinal trauma, you should begin management. The goal is to secure the child in a neutral, in-line position to a rigid board (Figure 31.13). Although this procedure may sound the same as that for an adult, the process is different for children. Box 31.1 outlines a step-by-step approach for infants and children up to 10 years of age.

Special Considerations

When faced with a potential spinal injury in a child, remember to rule out life-threatening injuries before turning your attention to full-body immobilization. Initial manual stabilization of the head and cervical spine should begin immediately as you assess the airway. Further immobilization should not occur until adequate assessment and treatment have been completed. When immobilization can be performed, select the best equipment you have available.

Immobilization Devices

Regardless of the immobilization equipment used, some padding may still be necessary depending on the size of the child. Use your best judgment in padding the open areas.

Child Safety Seats

If the child is small and is found in an infant safety seat, chances are that the thoracic and lumbar spine may have been protected. However, the cervical spine is susceptible to maximum **flexion**, especially if the seat is not in the backward position as recommended for infants.

Other seats accommodate a child until approximately 4 years of age or 40 lb. In these seats, the child actually extends beyond the margin of the seat and may be susceptible to all types of trauma. Also, if the child's head is above the back of the seat (more common in older models), the neck may be hyperextended during a rear-end collision.

If the child is critically injured or the child's condition has the potential to worsen, the car seat should not be used for immobilization. Instead, the child should be gently extricated from the seat onto a rigid board. Short backboards work well for this. Maintain manual stabilization of the head, and move the child as a unit onto the board (Figure 31.14). The child can then be secured to a backboard.

Box 31.1 Immobilization of Infants Through Children 10 Years of Age

1. Ensure scene safety, and quickly evaluate the mechanism of injury.
2. Approach the child, and manually hold the head.
3. Bring the head into a neutral, in-line position. If any resistance is met or pain is elicited, stop any movement and stabilize the head in that position.
4. Perform an initial assessment to rule out any life-threatening injuries. If any are found, immediately begin treatment.
5. Apply a rigid cervical spine immobilization device to the neck *only if it fits properly.* If a properly fitting device is not available, use towels, washcloths, or other material to immobilize the head as best as possible.
6. If no life threats are found, continue with the ongoing assessment.
7. Perform any other management necessary (administer oxygen, immobilize fractures, etc.).
8. Logroll the child onto a rigid board, and fasten the torso to the board.
9. Secure the torso as appropriate. Pad as appropriate.
10. Fasten the head securely to the board. Manual stabilization can be discontinued at this time.
11. Secure the board to the stretcher, and reassess the patient.
12. Prepare to transport, and manage the patient as necessary.

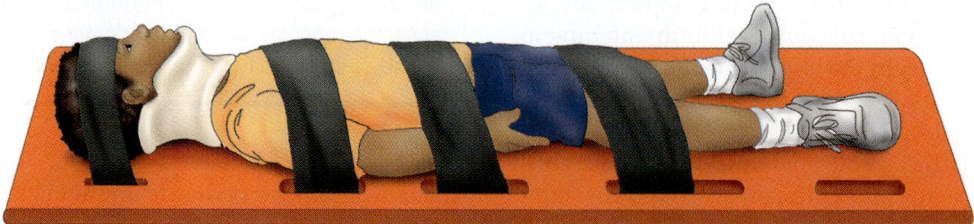

FIGURE 31.13 The goal of spinal immobilization is a neutral and in-line position.

No one can be an expert with every device, so the following guidelines should be used:

- When an infant or child is found in a safety seat, it can be used for immobilization only after a brief inspection. Has the car seat sustained any major structural damage as a result of the accident? In other words, can it still effectively support immobilization? Can it be secured appropriately in the ambulance? If the answer to either of these questions is no, the seat should not be used.
- If the seat includes a protection plate over the baby's chest, it should be removed so the patient's thoracic area can be easily accessed, permitting adequate lung assessment and manual chest compressions if necessary. Usually the plate can be lifted and taped to the back of the seat. If that is not possible, the straps should be cut and the plate completely removed from the seat. The child's torso can then be secured using cravats and padding.
- If a chest plate is not present, use the straps to secure the infant in place whenever possible. You may need to put additional padding or cravats between the straps and the child or tighten the straps.
- padding for all open areas around the child's body so that the child does not move. Padding should also be placed around the head and neck if a properly sized rigid cervical spine immobilization device is not available.
- Once adequately immobilized, the patient and seat should be transferred to the ambulance. The seat should then be carefully secured to the stretcher or captain's seat so that it is not mobile during transport to the hospital.

Cervical Spine Immobilization Devices

A rigid cervical spine immobilization device is recommended for any patient who may have sustained a cervical spine injury. In pediatric patients, however, make sure the device does not hyperextend the child's neck because of improper sizing. If the device is too large, do not use it. If a cervical spine immobilization device cannot be used, improvise with padding to attempt to keep the neck immobile. Also, remember that a cervical spine immobilization device alone is not adequate immobilization. Manual stabilization must continue until the child is completely secured to a long backboard or equivalent device.

Backboards

A short or long backboard can be used depending on the height of the child. If the short backboard is used to secure an infant, for example, it should be turned around so the head can be immobilized to the larger end, and some type of immobilizing device can be applied to both sides of the head (e.g., commercial pads, towels).

Keep in mind that children have proportionally larger heads than adults and have less-developed back muscles, which causes a natural flexion when the child is supine. The torso may need as much as 2 inches of padding to bring the spine into a neutral, in-line position. A flat blanket should be placed under the back from the upper margin of the pelvis and extended out to the left and right edges of the board. All open areas should then be additionally padded.

When the child has been strapped to the backboard, you may notice open areas between the straps and the edge of the board. Additional padding is also necessary along the outside of the torso and around both sides of the legs so that the board can be tilted without any movement of the child from side to side (Figure 31.15).

For a smaller child, use cravats instead of straps. This is important when securing the pelvis. Young children have abdomens that extend past the iliac crest of the pelvis. Abdominal movement is a necessary part of ventilation until approximately age 7 years, and a strap could restrict that process. Cravats are also recommended, instead of straps,

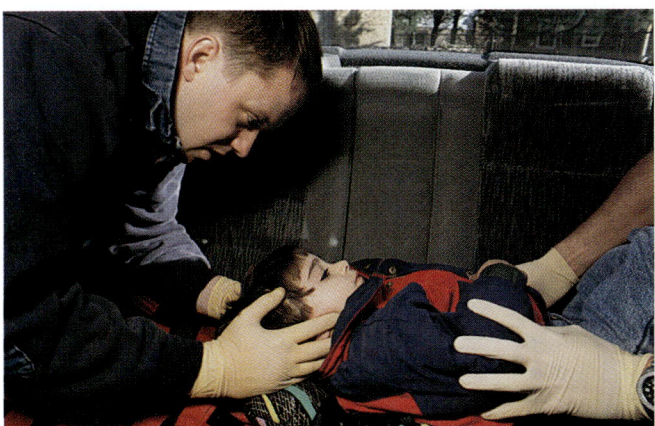

FIGURE 31.14 Maintain manual stabilization while moving the patient to the board.

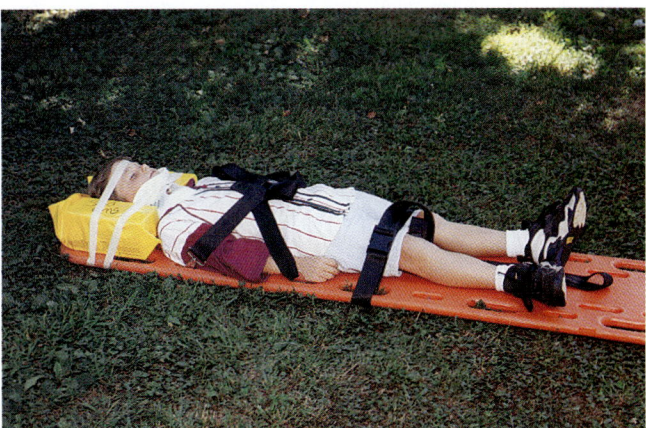

FIGURE 31.15 Pad any voids so that the board can be carried without patient movement.

for under the armpits. Large, wide straps can inhibit brachial circulation and actually cause more damage. If cravats are not available, tape may be used.

Vest Devices

Although in many parts of the United States an adult vest device such as the Kendrick extrication device is used to immobilize children, this method is not recommended. Using this device in a manner other than that for which it was intended has not been proven to be beneficial. For example, wrapping an adult vest device around the child like a papoose raises several concerns. One problem is that respiratory distress can occur if the thorax and abdomen are not permitted to expand adequately. Another concern is that in-line spinal immobilization is not achieved in many instances. More studies are needed before this method can be recommended.

Helmets

With so much attention being given today to encourage children to wear helmets during biking, skateboarding, and so on, an injured child may be wearing a helmet. What should be done? Should immobilization occur around the helmet, or should it be taken off as recommended for adults?

According to the American College of Surgeons Committee on Trauma, helmet removal is recommended so that other vital functions can be assessed and immobilization can be maintained. No distinction is made between adults and children. In fact, it may be even more critical to remove a child's helmet so that flexion of the child's head is not increased from the helmet when in the supine position (Figure 31.16). Also, because cartilage in children may not be calcified, airway compromise can occur easily during hyperflexion.

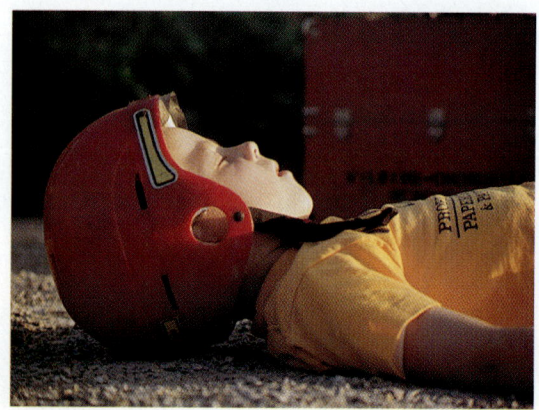

FIGURE 31.16 Neck flexion caused by a helmet on child.

> ✓ Make the decision to immobilize based on obvious injury or mechanism of injury. Use equipment properly sized for the child—do not use equipment that is too large or that inhibits respiratory or abdominal movement. For a child on a long backboard, pad all open areas, including the area beside the legs, so that the child can be turned onto his or her side if vomiting occurs.

Chest and Abdominal Trauma

The child's rib cage is extremely resilient, and the chest can suffer major internal injury without any bony fractures. If rib fractures do occur, they are associated with a high mortality rate.

Carefully observe for respiratory distress and the signs and symptoms of shock when treating a child with trauma to the chest and torso. Evaluate the mechanism of injury, and suspect injury even if the child appears to be fine.

Assess for any signs of blunt trauma to the abdomen, such as bruising (e.g., from a lap belt in a motor vehicle); an unstable pelvis; abdominal swelling, rigidity, or tenderness; or signs and symptoms of unexplained levels of shock. Children under 8 years of age also tend to be "belly breathers," and respiratory distress may also be a sign of abdominal trauma.

If the child is crying, it may be difficult to do an abdominal examination. Guarding and swelling can be missed if the child is upset. Remember, however, that a crying child is one whose brain function and blood pressure are reasonably intact. Become concerned if the child suddenly quiets down and allows an assessment of the abdomen.

The ideal treatment is the same as for an adult: definitive care at the hospital. Provide high-concentration oxygen, and prepare for rapid transport to an appropriate facility. Monitor vital signs, and make the child as comfortable as possible. Do *not* waste time in the field if you suspect chest or abdominal trauma in the pediatric patient, even if the child appears to be stable. This patient can deteriorate rapidly.

> ✓ Major internal thoracic injuries can occur without any bony fractures because the child's rib cage is so resilient. Bruising, an unstable pelvis, or signs and symptoms of unexplained levels of shock, as well as abdominal swelling, rigidity, or tenderness, may indicate blunt trauma to the abdomen. Prepare for rapid transport if you suspect chest or abdominal trauma even if the child appears to be stable.

Hypothermia

Children are susceptible to hypothermia due to their large body surface area in comparison with their weight. In addition, their compensatory mechanisms such as shivering are not well developed. Newborns in particular can quickly become hypothermic because they have little subcutaneous fat.

Hypothermia is defined as a core body temperature below 95° F (35° C). It often occurs in children as a result of prolonged exposure to cold temperatures. Leaving the child uncovered in a cool environment during examination and treatment can also lead to hypothermia. Other causes include metabolic disorders (e.g., low blood sugar), infection, and trauma or other brain disorders that interfere with the body's temperature regulating system. If alcohol or drugs have been ingested, the peripheral blood vessels dilate, and the body cannot conserve heat. Hypothermia often develops.

> **Tips from the Pros**
>
> Be sure to protect yourself if exposed to a cold environment. Do not become a victim of hypothermia while trying to resuscitate a child. Dress warm and in layers when the temperature is below 50° F.

During the assessment, obtain information about the incident. How long was the child exposed to the cold, rain, or snow? Was the child in any type of water? What was the approximate temperature of the water? Is it known if the child ingested any alcohol or drugs? Does the child have a history of diabetes or an ongoing infection?

Look for specific signs and symptoms of hypothermia (Table 31.6). Types of hypothermia include mild, moderate, and severe depending on the core body temperature.

In addition, look for areas of frostbite on the hands, fingers, feet, toes, ears, or nose. If the child complains of pain and a burning feeling, superficial frostbite has probably occurred. If the child reports no pain or feeling and the body part is blistered, a deeper injury may be present.

When treating this patient, move him or her to a warmer environment as quickly as possible. If trauma is suspected, briefly immobilize the child before moving. Remove all wet clothing, and wrap the child in blankets. Once the blankets become wet, apply new, dry blankets. If the child is responsive, give warm liquids by mouth. Under no circumstances should anyone give the child any form of alcohol to increase warmth (some people think a "hot toddy" will help the rewarming process).

If the hypothermia is moderate to severe, the first priority is maintenance of the airway. Provide high-concentration oxygen by face mask or ventilate with a BVM device if necessary. If there is no pulse, begin chest compressions. Transport the child rapidly, and continue CPR until you reach the hospital. Do *not* discontinue the resuscitation until the child's temperature has returned to normal. At that time a decision can be made to stop or continue the resuscitation.

If a pulse is present, do not provide any stimulation, beyond what is needed to maintain adequate oxygenation and ventilation such as endotracheal intubation, CPR, or suctioning. The goal is to prevent the onset of ventricular fibrillation. In addition, do not waste time attempting to start an IV. Continue with BLS and rapidly transport to the hospital.

Use heat packs as long as they do not directly touch the skin. Place them under the armpits and in the groin area over the blanket (Figure 31.17). If frostbite has occurred, wrap the affected extremities in a blanket. Do *not*

TABLE 31.6 Signs and Symptoms of Hypothermia

Mild (32–35°C)	Moderate (28–32°C)	Severe (<28°C)
Slurred speech	Progressively lowered consciousness	Coma; unresponsive
Mild incoordination	Decreased respiratory rate; bradycardia	Dilated and fixed pupils
Shivering	Cyanosis	Ventricular dysrhythmias
Poor judgment	Edema	Respiratory arrest
	Muscle rigidity; no shivering	

From Eichelberger MR: *Pediatric emergencies: a manual for prehospital care providers*, Englewood Cliffs, NJ, 1992, Prentice-Hall.

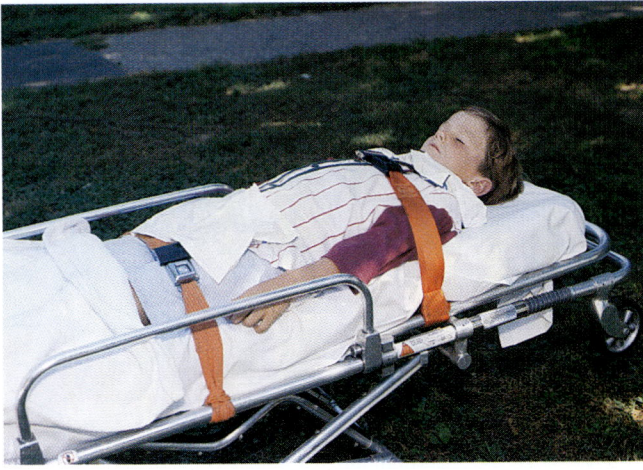

FIGURE 31.17 A child with heat packs in place, under the armpits and in the groin area.

agressively rub the part or expose it to dry heat, which may cause tissue damage.

> ✓ Children have a large body surface in comparison with their weight and can easily become hypothermic. Newborns have little subcutaneous fat and also are susceptible to hypothermia. Know the signs of hypothermia, and warm the pediatric patient as quickly as possible. Maintain ABCs for the child who is severely hypothermic. Last, protect yourself so that you, too, do not become hypothermic.

Other Pediatric Problems

Poisoning

Poisoning is a preventable emergency. Young children are at high risk for accidental poisonings because of their inquisitive nature and tendency to explore the environment by tasting and placing things in their mouths. As the child grows older, poisoning may occur from drugs or alcohol as the child experiments with mind-altering substances or intentionally overdoses when angry or depressed.

Poison is defined as any substance that produces harmful physiologic or psychologic effects. Children ages 18 months to 3 years account for approximately 30% of all accidental ingestions of poisons. The most common types of poisons are as follows:

- Household products (e.g., petroleum-based agents, cleaning agents, and cosmetics [Figure 31.18]).
- Medications (prescription and nonprescription)
- Toxic plants (e.g., poinsettia plants during the Christmas season)

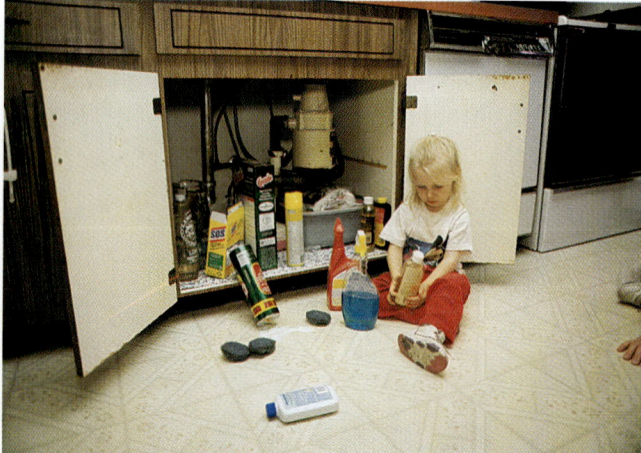

FIGURE 31.18 Children are at a great risk for accidental poisoning because they are very curious and want to explore everything.

- Contaminated foods (e.g., potato salad left out all day at a summer picnic)

Between school age and adolescence, the most common poisons are as follows:

- Alcohol
- Organic solvents (hydrocarbons and fluorocarbons, which are present in gasoline, typewriter correction fluid, and airplane glue)
- Mind-altering drugs (marijuana, hashish, LSD, PCP, mescaline)
- Narcotics (heroin, morphine)
- Central nervous system depressants (barbiturates)
- Central nervous system stimulants (amphetamines, cocaine, crack)

For more information and specific treatment of poisons, see Chapter 19.

> ✓ Poisoning is a preventable emergency. Young children run a high risk of being poisoned because they are so inquisitive. Older children may be poisoned as they experiment with mind-altering drugs or intentionally overdose.

Child Abuse and Maltreatment

Child abuse happens to more than 1 million children annually. It involves the maltreatment of children by their

TABLE 31.7 Risk Factors for Child Maltreatment

Child	Family
Prematurity	Alcohol dependency
Prenatal drug exposure	Drug dependency
Developmental disability	Childhood history of maltreatment
Physical disability	Belief in use of corporal punishment
Chronic illness	Rigid expectations regarding child's behavior
Product of multiple birth	Negative parental perceptions of child
	Unrealistic expectations of child
	Single parent
	Social isolation
	Psychologic distress
	Low self-esteem
	Extreme poverty
	Acute and chronic stressors

From *Emergency nursing pediatric course*, 1993, Emergency Nurses Association.

parents, guardians, or other individuals responsible for their care. Although reporting of child abuse increased 31% from 1985 to 1990, it is still difficult to know how many cases actually occur each year, despite the fact that reporting is mandatory by law in all 50 states.

Certain factors can place families and children at a greater risk to abuse or be abused. Table 31.7 shows some risk factors for child maltreatment.

Child abuse can be divided into the following four major types:

- **Physical abuse:** Any physical injury intentionally delivered to the child by a caregiver
- **Sexual abuse:** Any sexual activity between a child and an older child or adult
- **Emotional or psychologic abuse:** Behaviors inflicted on the child that are degrading, terrorizing, isolating, or rejecting
- **Neglect:** Failure to meet the child's basic needs (e.g., food, clothing, shelter, medical care, safety)

Figure 31.19 and Box 31.2 list some indicators of possible child abuse.

As difficult as it may be, the most important role for the EMT-B is to be nonjudgmental. Do not accuse anyone of child abuse even if abuse appears obvious to you. That type of approach may make the potential abuser angry and may even place the EMT-B in danger. Instead, carefully document in objective terms exactly what you see or have assessed on the child. Some states mandate that EMTs report suspected abuse. This means you may be required by law to report your concerns to the state's child protection agency. Unless the report was made in a malicious or knowingly false manner, you are generally shielded from civil action by the individual being reported. State laws vary; know what they are in your jurisdiction.

Whether your state requires mandatory reports or not, you should make a direct report of your concerns to the triage nurse or attending physician in the emergency department on arrival. Your run form documentation should include your observations. In writing the report,

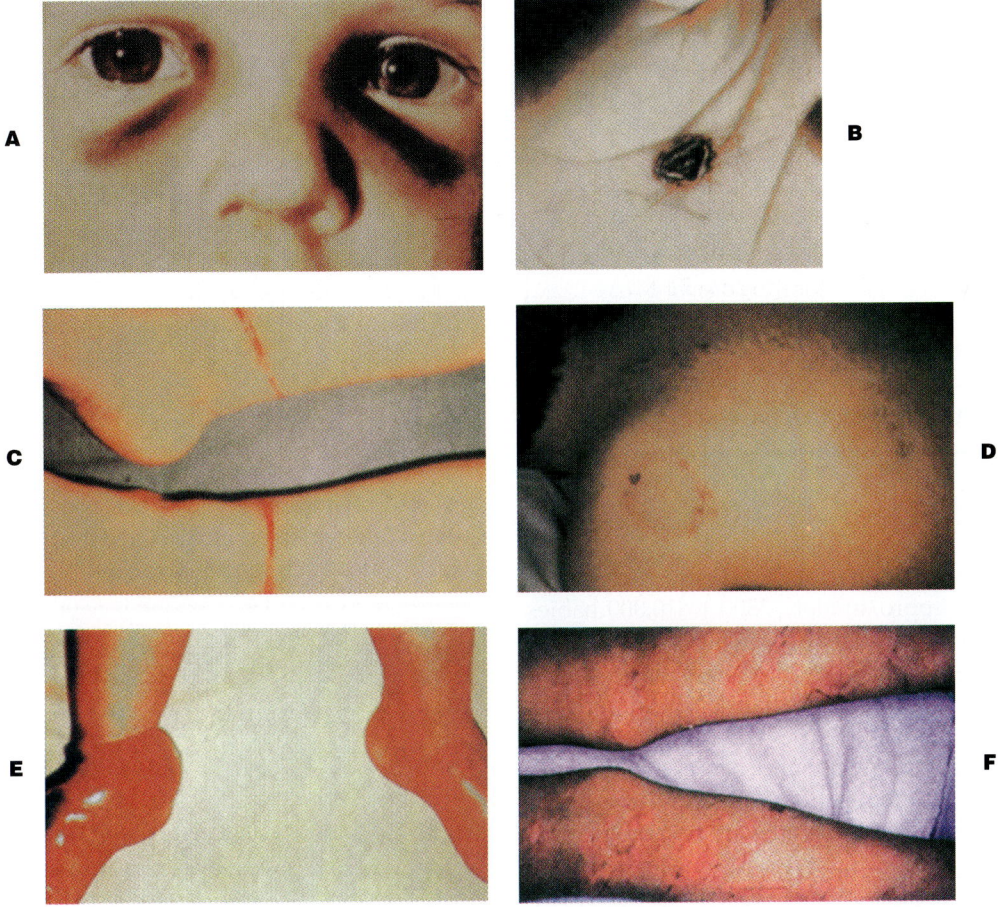

FIGURE 31.19 Indicators of possible abuse. **A,** "Raccoon eye," or periorbital bruising, possible indication of anterior fossa skull fracture. **B,** Fresh cigarette burn to palm. **C,** Fresh abrasions of restraint injury. **D,** Human bites. **E,** "Dunking" burns to the feet. **F,** Welts and abrasions to legs as a result of an electrical cord.

> **Box 31.2 Indicators of Possible Abuse**
>
> 1. Any obvious or suspected fractures in a child under 2 years of age
> 2. Injuries in various stages of healing, especially burns and bruises
> 3. More injuries than are usually seen in other children of the same age
> 4. Injuries scattered on many areas of the body
> 5. Bruises or burns in patterns that suggest intentional infliction
> 6. Suspected increased intracranial pressure in an infant
> 7. Suspected intraabdominal trauma in a young child
> 8. Any injury that does not fit the description of the cause given
> 9. An accusation that the child injured himself or herself intentionally
> 10. Long-standing skin infections
> 11. Extreme **malnutrition**
> 12. Extreme lack of cleanliness
> 13. Inappropriate clothing for the situation
> 14. Child who withdraws from parent
> 15. Child who responds inappropriately to the situation (e.g., quiet, distant, withdrawn)

avoid the use of terminology such as "suspected child abuse" or similar comments.

> ✓ Physical abuse, sexual abuse, emotional or psychologic abuse, and neglect are four major types of child abuse or maltreatment. Learn to recognize potential situations in which child abuse may occur. Be nonjudgmental, and simply document what you see.

Sudden Infant Death Syndrome

Sudden infant death syndrome (SIDS) is a disease that claims the lives of approximately 7500 to 10,000 babies every year. SIDS is one of the most difficult and challenging emergency medical calls an EMT faces. The deaths are sudden and unexpected and happen to apparently healthy babies.

In spite of the years of experience and recent research efforts, little is known about this disease and the actual cause of death in these infants. There are several theories about the cause of SIDS, ranging from some type of viral infection to the possibility that a congenital defect impairs the infant's ability to breathe while sleeping. Medical researchers have yet to identify a specific pathophysiology. In fact, the diagnosis of SIDS can be made only at autopsy after ruling out all other possible causes of death.

The SIDS case is a challenge to the EMT for several reasons. First, the EMT is faced with an apparently healthy infant who is in full cardiac and respiratory arrest. Most likely, the patient will be dead. This type of call creates strong emotions within the EMT; it is often a great challenge to remain focused on providing basic emergency care. The second challenge for the EMT is dealing with the family. For them, this is an unbelievably heartbreaking experience. The parents had a perfectly healthy baby when they strapped the child into their car seat for the long ride or put the child to bed that night. Now, suddenly and unexplainably, their loved one is extremely ill or dead. The family is completely distraught with anxiety and grief.

Emergency care in the case of SIDS is aimed toward the infant and the parents. The EMT should implement complete BLS procedures for the infant, including CPR and rapid transport to the closest medical facility. The rapid initiation of ventilation, chest compression, and transportation will give the child the best possible chance of survival. The EMT should make sure that the parents of the infant also receive attention in this situation. The parents are in a highly emotional state and may require emergency care for the extreme emotions that they are experiencing. The EMT should tell the parents about what is being done for their child and where their child will be taken. Rapid initiation of BLS and rapid transport will give the parents some measure of reassurance that everything possible is being done for their child.

On arrival at the medical facility, the EMTs should give the hospital staff a complete report of their assessment and findings on the scene. The EMTs should also make sure that the parents have arrived safely and that their presence is known to the hospital staff.

> ✓ SIDS is an extremely challenging situation for the EMT. Emotions are high, and there are many patients who require the EMT's attention. The infant requires rapid BLS and transportation, and the parents require strong emotional support.

Children with Special Needs (Disabilities and Special Health Care Needs)

Children with special needs may include pediatric patients with disabilities, chronic illnesses, acquired injuries, or special equipment needed to sustain or maintain that child's level of function (Figure 31.20). The EMSC program, sponsored by the Maternal and Child

Health Bureau and the National Highway Traffic Safety Administration, provides these definitions of children with special health care needs:

> A child with a preexisting condition is one who experiences an acute illness or injury that results in a change in status or extra education for care required at home. Examples include children who are technology dependent, require 24-hour-a-day care, or have a structural or functional anomaly.
>
> A child with an acquired special health care need is one who experiences an injury or medical condition (disease) that interrupts his or her established developmental pathway necessitating adjustments in the child's life and the lives of the child's family. These adjustments may require special resources.

Assessment and management modalities may need to be adjusted for the child with a special need. See Chapter 32 for more information.

Pain Control in Infants and Children

A common myth regarding children is that they do not experience pain in the same way as an adult, and for this reason do not require pain management. Thankfully, this erroneous belief is fading and pediatric patients may benefit from some form of pain control during painful emergency procedures. Many air medical services use various drugs to control pain for pediatric patients during transport. The use of pain-killing drugs during ground transports is not as widespread but is expected to increase as more emphasis is placed on providing EMS for children. At the basic level in lieu of drug therapy, several techniques can be performed that directly improve the care given to ill and injured children.

Providing emotional support to the pediatric patient and the family can make an emergency scenario more tolerable for everyone. Making the child more physically comfortable may also decrease the anxiety experienced by the child and family during various procedures.

Children view things differently than adults and experience more pain and anxiety. During a traumatic or medical emergency, even the most routine procedures can be frightening to a child. Measures such as verbal reassurance and distraction techniques may have some value.

> ✓ Children experience increased pain and anxiety during a medical or trauma emergency. Provide emotional and physical support whenever possible.

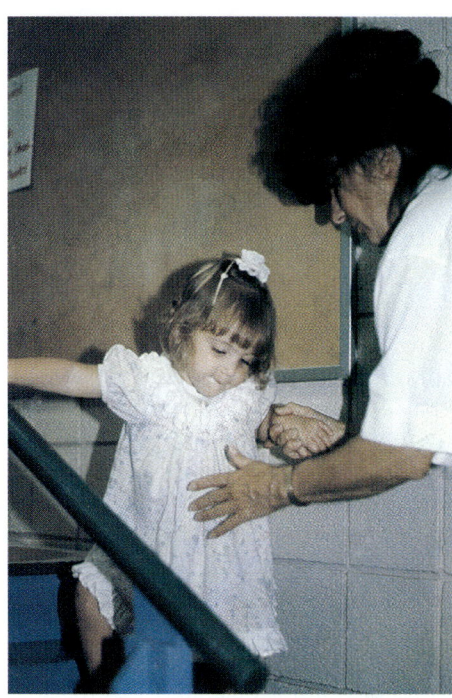

FIGURE 31.20 Children with special needs require a unique approach to assessment and treatment.

General Considerations

Remember to involve the parents, caregivers, or teachers throughout the call, because it is often emotionally as well as physically traumatizing to the child and the family. In addition, if the accident occurs in a crowded area such as a school or playground, other children or the patient's brothers or sisters may be in the area. They also may be frightened by the entire experience and need some extra emotional support.

Try to speak to the child as much as possible to explain what is happening. For a young child, simple distraction from the activities at hand may be better than trying to logically detail all of your actions. Diversionary tactics such as playing with a toy or teddy bear can be helpful.

When faced with a potential spinal injury in a child, remember to rule out life-threatening injuries before turning your attention to full-body immobilization. Initial manual stabilization of the head and cervical spine should begin immediately as you assess the airway. Further immobilization should not occur until adequate assessment and treatment have been completed. When immobilization can be performed, select the best equipment you have available.

Pediatric trauma can be frightening to even the most experienced EMS provider. On those days when you are not too busy, take the opportunity to review the equipment you would use to immobilize the pediatric patient. Practice with your own children or children of other EMS or fire department members. This role-playing is great experience for the EMT-B, as well as for the children. As they say, "Practice makes perfect." Become more confident with the equipment so that efforts can be directed toward patient care.

Summary

- Assessing and treating infants and children can be rewarding, as well as frightening at times. Use the same basic principles of care that apply to all patients. However, concentrate on the differences in the pediatric patient when providing that care. Remember to appreciate the developmental needs of this population, as well as the needs of the child's family.
- Assess the infant or child depending on the appropriate level of development. Include the family or other caregivers during this process. Be familiar with pediatric vital sign ranges and use these as a reference during the assessment.
- The first sign of respiratory distress in an infant is usually a rapid rate of breathing. Other signs include an increase in breathing effort, diminished breath sounds, a decrease in level of consciousness or response to parents or pain, poor skeletal muscle tone, and cyanosis. Further signs and symptoms may include nasal flaring, retractions, head bobbing, grunting, stridor, and prolonged expiration. A slow or irregular respiratory rate in an acutely ill infant or child is a serious sign.
- A decreased heart rate usually occurs when the infant or child can no longer maintain adequate tissue oxygenation. Provide oxygen quickly to decrease the possibility of cardiopulmonary arrest.
- Shock in infants and children can be caused by gastroenteritis, dehydration, blood loss, burns, sepsis, and anaphylaxis. In a child with a head injury and low blood pressure, always look for another source of bleeding. Signs and symptoms of shock include a change in the level of consciousness, increased respiratory rate, increased heart rate, a normal blood pressure that progresses to low blood pressure, cool and clammy skin, decreased peripheral pulses, increased capillary refill, and decreased urine output.
- Maintain proficiency in infant and child CPR and techniques for clearing an obstructed airway. Select airway and respiratory adjuncts based on the size of the patient and the ventilatory support needed (e.g., insert an oropharyngeal airway and ventilate with a bag-valve-mask and oxygen at 15 L/min for a pediatric patient with a respiratory rate of 4). Only use a bag-valve-mask that delivers at least 450 ml of air to provide the full-term infant or child with an adequate tidal volume. Remember to have suction equipment available because pediatric patients are prone to vomiting.
- If ALS will be needed, request assistance as early as possible. Meet the ALS personnel at the scene or en route to minimize delays in transport.
- Infants and children are susceptible to a host of medical emergencies that may include croup, epiglottitis, asthma, bronchiolitis, seizures, meningitis, and dehydration. Review each situation and become familiar with the signs and symptoms of each. Provide management specific to the emergency, and prepare for immediate transport when necessary.
- Falls, vehicular-related trauma, sports-related injury, and assaults are the most common causes of pediatric injury in order of most common to least common. Review the differences between children and adults, and incorporate this information into your assessment process.
- For head trauma, ensure adequate ventilation and circulation to provide good cerebral perfusion and avoid secondary brain injury. For spinal trauma, concentrate on the mechanism of injury and immobilize as needed. Pad under the head or upper back and along the sides of the child when on a long backboard, depending on the child's age and size. Use immobilization equipment that properly fits the infant or child.
- For chest or abdominal trauma, pay special attention to the infant's or child's respiratory status. Manage respiratory distress or shock if present. Remember that children under 8 years of age tend to be "belly breathers," and therefore respiratory distress may be a sign of abdominal trauma.
- Children are susceptible to hypothermia because of their large body surface area in relation to body weight. Watch for signs and symptoms of hypothermia, and make a special effort to keep the pediatric patient warm.
- Because young children are very inquisitive, they are at a high risk for accidental poisonings. Older children may experiment with mind-altering substances.

Summary (cont'd)

- Child abuse or maltreatment includes physical abuse, sexual abuse, emotional or psychologic abuse, and neglect. Child abuse or maltreatment should be considered when the child or family has risk factors for this behavior or your physical examination reveals indicators of possible abuse.

- Remember to consider physical and psychologic measures that may relieve pain and anxiety in the pediatric patient. Also, work with the family or significant others when providing care to the infant or child.

Scenario Solution

You assess that the child appears to have croup and to be in mild respiratory distress. Because you are familiar with developmental stages, you recognize that this child has a normal degree of stranger anxiety that exacerbates her respiratory distress; therefore you choose to allow the child to be transported properly restrained in an infant car seat with the mother holding "blow-by" oxygen at the child's face. You note that the child becomes less agitated, her respiratory distress decreases, and her color improves. You complete the transport to the hospital.

Key Terms

Absence A seizure characterized by a sudden, momentary loss of consciousness; also called *petit mal seizure*.

Acidosis An abnormal increase in hydrogen ions in the body; blood pH below 7.40 (normal: 7.5).

Allergens Substances that can produce a hypersensitive reaction in the body; not always harmful (e.g., pollen, dust, animal dander, feathers, various foods).

Anaphylaxis An exaggerated, life-threatening hypersensitivity reaction to a previously encountered antigen.

Asthma A respiratory disorder characterized by recurring episodes of sudden onset of breathing difficulty, wheezing on expiration/inspiration due to constriction of the bronchi, coughing, and thick mucous bronchial secretions; also termed *reactive airways disease*.

Aura Period of time immediately preceding a seizure.

Autonomic Having the ability to perform independently without outside influence; pertaining to the autonomic nervous system.

Autonomic nervous system Part of the nervous system that regulates involuntary vital functions, including the activity of the cardiac muscle, smooth muscles, and glands; divided into the sympathetic nervous system and the parasympathetic nervous system.

Brainstem herniation Portion of the brain containing the medulla oblongata, pons, and mesencephalon that is forced down through the foramen magnum when pressure inside the cranium is increased.

Bronchioles Small airways of the respiratory system extending from the bronchi into the lobes of the lung.

Bronchiolitis Acute viral infection of the lower respiratory tract that occurs primarily in infants under 18 months of age; characterized by expiratory wheezing, respiratory distress, inflammation, and obstruction at the level of the bronchioles.

Cerebral edema Accumulation of fluid in the brain tissues. Because the skull cannot expand to accommodate the increase in pressure, the brain is compressed; early symptoms are changes in level of consciousness, sluggish or dilated pupils, and gradual loss of consciousness; can be fatal.

Convulsive Producing motor activity, as in a seizure.

Cyanosis Slightly bluish, grayish, slatelike, or dark purple discoloration of the skin caused by a deficiency of oxygen and excess carbon dioxide in the blood.

Dehydration Excessive loss of water from the body tissues; signs include poor skin turgor, flushed and dry skin, coated tongue, low urine output, irritability, and confusion.

Diaphoresis Secretion of sweat.

Epiglottis The leaf-shaped structure just above the larynx that prevents food and liquid from entering the trachea during swallowing.

Epiglottitis Inflammation of the epiglottis; a bacterial infection seen most often in children. The epiglottis becomes swollen and may cause airway obstruction; patients often have excessive drooling.

Key Terms (cont'd)

Epilepsy A group of neurologic disorders characterized by recurrent episodes of convulsive seizures, sensory disturbances, unusual behavior, loss of consciousness, or all of these; uncontrolled electrical discharge from the nerve cells of the cerebral cortex.

Esophagus Muscular canal extending from the back of the mouth to the stomach.

Flexion Movement allowed by certain joints of the skeleton that decreases the angle between two adjoining bones, such as bending the elbow.

Gastroenteritis Inflammation of the stomach and intestines that accompanies numerous gastrointestinal disorders; symptoms are lack of appetite, nausea, vomiting, abdominal discomfort, and diarrhea.

Gastrointestinal Of or pertaining to the organs of the gastrointestinal tract, from mouth to anus.

Glottis Slitlike opening between the vocal cords.

Hematoma Damage similar to a contusion but more extensive with larger blood vessels torn and more blood collected in deep tissues.

Hemothorax Accumulation of blood and fluid in the pleural cavity usually caused by trauma.

Hyperextension Portion of a joint in maximum extension.

Hypersensitivity Abnormal condition characterized by an excessive reaction to a stimulus.

Hypothermia Abnormal and dangerous condition in which the core temperature of the body falls below 35° C (95° F) and the body's normal functions are impaired.

Hypovolemia Abnormally low circulating blood volume.

Hypovolemic shock State of physical collapse caused by massive blood loss, circulatory dysfunction, and inadequate tissue perfusion.

Intracranial Within the cranium (skull).

Laryngotracheobronchitis Inflammation of the major respiratory passages usually causing hoarseness, nonproductive cough, and difficulty breathing; also called *croup*.

Lethargy State or quality of being indifferent, apathetic, or sluggish; stupor or coma resulting from disease or hypnosis.

Malnutrition Any disorder of nutrition; may result from an unbalanced, insufficient, or excessive diet or from the impaired absorption or metabolism of foods.

Meninges One of three highly vascular membranes that separate the cranium from the brain; includes the dura mater, pia mater, and arachnoid.

Meningitis Any infection or inflammation of the meninges.

Needle cricothyrotomy Insertion of a needle into the cricothyroid membrane to create a temporary airway opening.

Paralysis Loss of muscle function, loss of sensation, or both.

Paresthesia Any subjective sensation experienced as numbness, tingling, or a "pins and needles" feeling; may be a symptom of hyperventilation or spinal cord injury.

Perfusion A state of inadequate supply of oxygen and nutrients to the tissues; ability of the circulatory system to distribute blood containing nutrients and oxygen to the tissues.

Postictal Period of time immediately after a seizure.

Renal failure Inability of the kidneys to excrete wastes, concentrate urine, and conserve electrolytes.

Seizure Sudden, abnormal electrical activity in the brain.

Sepsis Infection; contamination.

Septic shock Form of shock that occurs from an infection when toxic products are released from pathogenic bacteria into the bloodstream.

Status asthmaticus An acute, severe, and prolonged asthma attack; hypoxia, cyanosis, and unconsciousness may follow.

Status epilepticus Continuous seizure lasting more than 30 minutes or a seizure in which the patient does not regain consciousness.

Stridor An abnormal, high-pitched, musical sound caused by an obstruction in the trachea or larynx; usually heard during inspiration.

Tachycardia Condition in which the heart contracts at a rate greater than 100 beats per minute.

Trachea Cylinder-shaped tube in the neck composed of cartilage and membrane that extends from the vocal cords to approximately the level of the fifth thoracic vertebra where it divides into two bronchi; also called the windpipe.

Tracheostomy A surgical opening through the neck into the trachea through which an indwelling tube may be inserted.

Review Questions

1. The following are signs and symptoms of increased respiratory effort in the infant or child:
   a. Grunting
   b. Nasal flaring
   c. Intercostal and substernal retractions
   d. All of the above

2. Sizing of an oropharyngeal airway may be estimated by measuring:
   a. The length of the child's pinky finger
   b. The distance from corner of the patient's mouth to the angle of the jaw
   c. The distance from the tip of the nose to the ear
   d. The distance from the chin to the sternal notch

3. A disease characterized by occurrences during the middle of the night in children 3 months to 3 years with a barky cough is known as:
   a. Epiglottitis
   b. Bronchiolitis
   c. Asthma
   d. Croup

4. All of the following are signs and symptoms of severe dehydration except:
   a. Sunken fontanel
   b. Cool, clammy skin
   c. Alert mental status
   d. Blood pressure less than 80

5. A 7-year-old boy has been struck by a car while riding his bike. He was not wearing a helmet. Initial assessment shows him to be unresponsive with a large abrasion on his forehead from where he hit the road. He is breathing 6 times per minute and has a pulse rate of 60. Your initial action after maintaining cervical spine precautions is to:
   a. Cleanse the abrasion and place a bandage on his forehead
   b. Ventilate the child using bag-valve-mask and 15 L/min of oxygen
   c. Attempt to find the boy's parents to get permission for treatment
   d. Complete the assessment to discover any other injuries

6. All of the following are useful when approaching adolescents except:
   a. When appropriate, allow the adolescent to be part of the decision-making about his or her care.
   b. Be honest about consequences.
   c. Direct all communication to the child's parent or caregiver.
   d. Recognize and acknowledge the adolescent's concern about altered body image.

7. The EMT would document the level of consciousness, presence of an aura, body part(s) involved, and the presence of a postictal period for which emergency?
   a. Meningitis
   b. Seizure
   c. Head trauma
   d. Dehydration

8. A 12-year-old girl was playing softball as the pitcher and was struck in the abdomen by a line drive. Signs of blunt trauma include:
   a. Numbness and tingling in the legs
   b. Distant bowel sounds and a pulsating mass
   c. Swelling and tenderness of the abdomen
   d. Vomiting and diarrhea

Answers to these Review Questions can be found at the end of the book on page 868.

32

The Patient with Special Needs

Lesson Goal

The goal of this chapter is to give the EMT-Basic information about how to interact with and treat patients with special needs.

Scenario

You are called to the local child care center for a 4-year-old girl having trouble breathing. When you arrive at the scene, a teacher meets you at the door and takes you to the preschooler room. She tells you that the girl has mental retardation, does not speak, and does not always understand what is explained. You see a crowd of children around another teacher and a little girl. You hear stridor as you approach the crowd.

 What would you do at this point?

Key Terms to Know

Advocate	Colostomy	Ileostomy	Paraplegia
Apnea monitor	Developmental disabilities	Immunosuppressive	Physical disabilities
Arnold-Chiari malformation	Down syndrome	Ketogenic diet	Quadriplegia
Asthma	Epilepsy	Mental retardation	Special needs
Cerebral palsy	Gastrostomy tube	Myelomeningocele	
Chronic	Hydrocephalus	Ostomy	

The Patient with Special Needs | Chapter 32   639

Learning Objectives

As an EMT-Basic, you should be able to do the following:

Supplemental

- Discuss methods of providing care to patients with special needs.
- Identify developmental considerations for patients with special needs.
- Describe examples of physical and developmental disabilities.
- Identify feelings of the family and caregivers in relation to an ill or injured patient with special needs.
- Explain the need for knowledge and skills in treating patients with special needs.
- Discuss the provider's own emotional response to caring for a patient with special needs.
- Develop methods of providing emergency care while appreciating the unique needs of each patient and family.

The purpose of this chapter is to give the emergency medical technician—basic (EMT-B) information about how to interact with and treat patients with special needs. With the increased usage of specialized technology, infants survive life-threatening illnesses and birth anomalies to become productive adult citizens. Children and adults are successfully resuscitated from critical illness or injury only to require rehabilitation or special adaptive devices to function. This population is at a higher risk for emergencies, and it is important to be proactive and learn about this unique group before being called to treat them (Figure 32.1).

Patient Care Algorithm

Disability Assessment

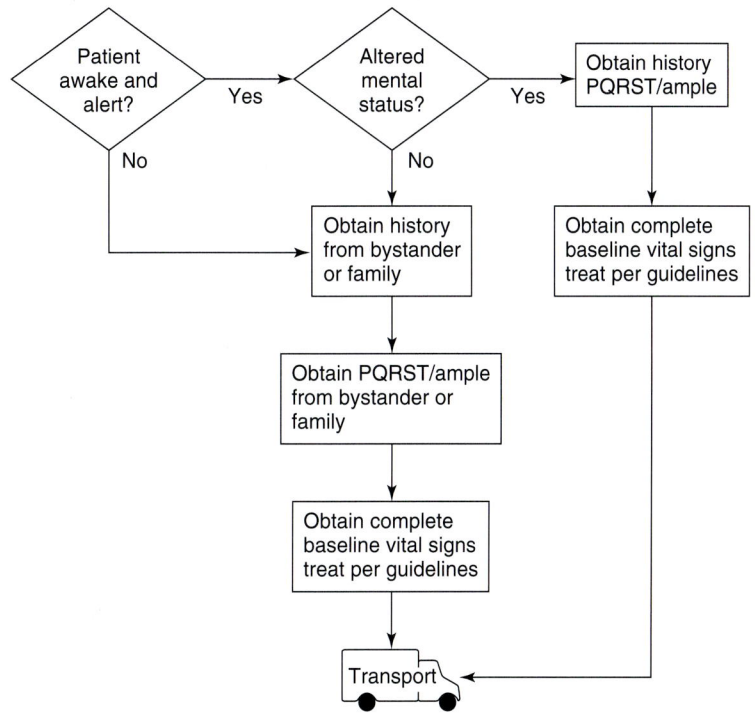

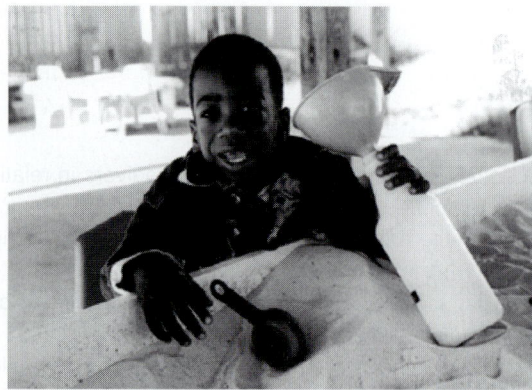

FIGURE 32.1 Many myths and prejudices surround individuals with disabilities.

Many myths and prejudices surround individuals with disabilities. Many people erroneously believe that if something is different about a "part" of a person, the "whole" person is affected. For example, health care professionals tend to talk about a child with mental retardation instead of talking to that child (Figure 32.2). In this chapter, the EMT-B will learn the importance of treating illness or injury first and the disability second.

Pathophysiology

Special needs are conditions with the potential to interfere with usual growth and development. These conditions may involve physical disabilities, developmental disabilities, chronic illnesses, and forms of technologic support.

Developmental Disabilities

Developmental disabilities involve some degree of impaired adaptation in learning, social adjustment, or maturation. A developmental disability results in a substantial functional limitation in three or more areas of major life activity, such as self-care, receptive and expressive language, learning, mobility, self-direction, capacity for independent living, and economic self-sufficiency. Causes include the following:

- Metabolic disorders
- Infections
- Intracranial hemorrhage
- Anoxia
- Inherited disorders (e.g., Down syndrome)
- Trauma
- Any other entity that damages the brain

Some of these disorders can occur at any age. The patient is usually said to have a learning disability, mental

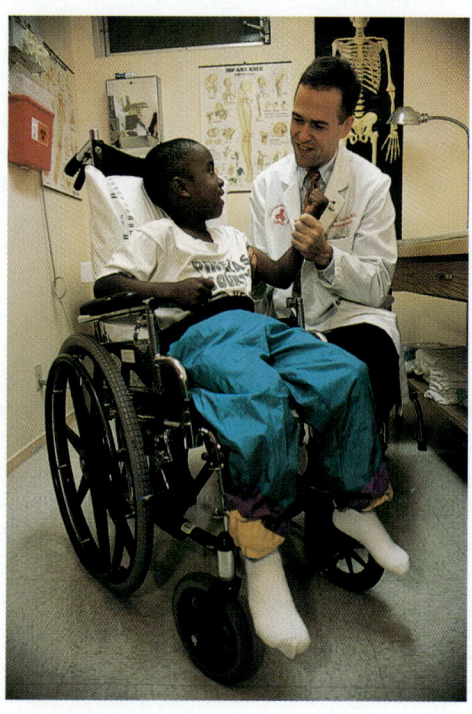

FIGURE 32.2 In the initial assessment, "disability" refers to the patient's neurologic status, *not* the disabling condition. Perform assessments on individuals with special needs in the same way you would for patients without these needs.

retardation, or some form of developmental delay. **Mental retardation** is an example of a developmental disability. Approximately 1 of every 10 Americans is directly involved with a person with mental retardation as a member of his or her family. In addition, approximately 2.4 million children and adolescents under age 21 years have mental retardation.

Down syndrome is an example of a congenital anomaly that causes mental retardation. Children and adults with Down syndrome range from severely retarded to having average intelligence. Most people, however, have a mild to moderate range of retardation.

The diagnosis of mental retardation or developmental delay is no longer an automatic sentence for seclusion in a long-term care facility. Children and adults with mental retardation may be involved in the community, hold jobs, vote, and so on, depending on their level of ability (Figure 32.3).

Physical Disabilities

Physical disabilities involve some type of limitation of mobility. Causes include the following:

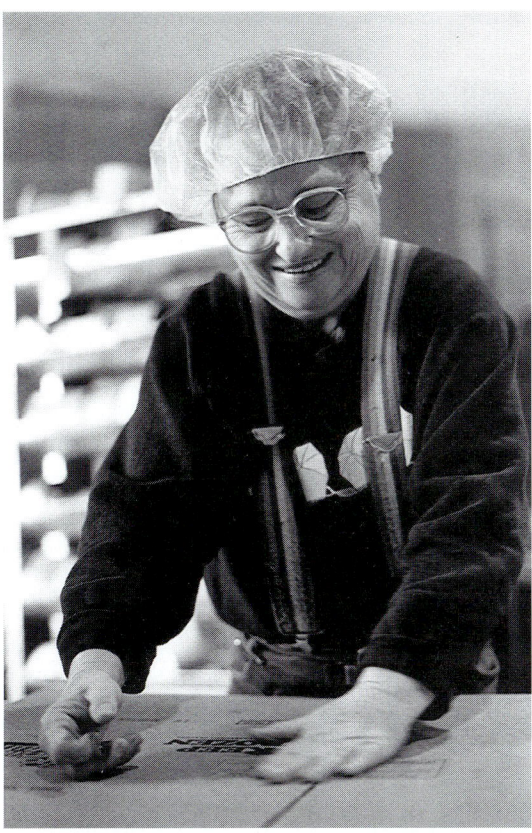

FIGURE 32.3 Children and adults with mental retardation may be involved in the community, hold jobs, vote, and so on, depending on their level of ability.

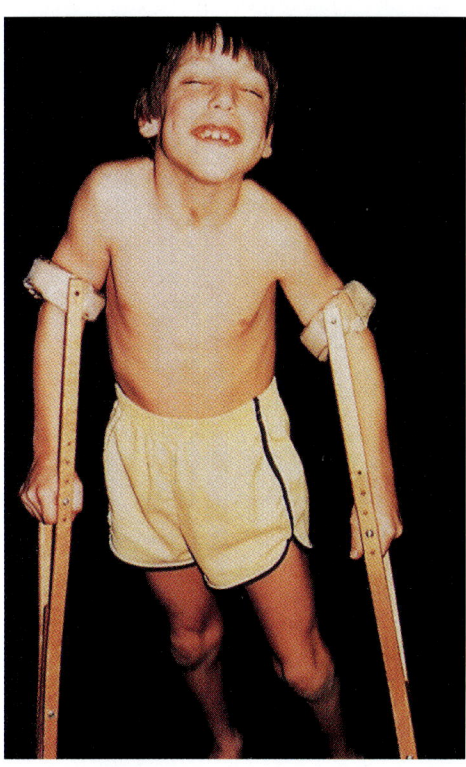

FIGURE 32.4 Cerebral palsy is a neuromuscular disability consisting of difficulty in controlling the voluntary muscles as a result of damage to a portion of the brain.

- Birth anomalies (e.g., spina bifida)
- Head and spinal cord injuries
- Infections resulting in paralysis (e.g., meningitis)
- Disease processes

Cerebral Palsy

Cerebral palsy (CP) is a neuromuscular disability. A person with CP has difficulty controlling the voluntary muscles due to damage to a portion of the brain. The disability can range from mild to severe and is fixed, meaning that it does not become progressively worse as the patient ages (Figure 32.4).

Most people with CP have a normal level of intelligence. They are not mentally retarded and may in fact be highly intelligent. Many children with CP develop keen thinking skills because their physical activities are usually limited.

In individuals with severe CP, swallowing may be compromised, which puts them at a higher risk for respiratory difficulties. Airway obstruction can occur from increased secretions or food.

The spastic type of CP presents the most common evidence of motor disability. Certain muscle groups have an unusually strong tone that can keep portions of the body, particularly the extremities, in characteristic positions. For example, the legs may be crossed with the toes pointed. In addition, the patient's fists may be clenched with the upper arm pressed against the wall of the chest. Also, the head may be extended with the back arched. It is important not to forcefully manipulate the patient when performing the physical examination. Gently attempt to move the extremity to the position you desire. If this movement is not possible, document the posturing and continue your assessment. For instance, if the patient's right arm is flexed across the chest, extending the arm to check a blood pressure may not be possible. Use the other arm or document why a blood pressure was not taken if both arms are involved. If possible, wrap a cuff around the patient's thigh and use the popliteal artery behind the knee.

> ✓ In patients with cerebral palsy, pay special attention to the respiratory status. Be prepared for airway obstructions caused by increased secretions or food. In addition, be gentle when moving the patient during the physical examination so as not to cause any further harm.

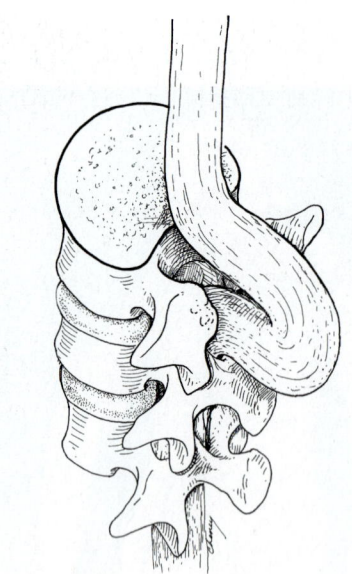

FIGURE 32.5 Myelomeningocele.

Spina Bifida

Spina bifida is the number one disabling birth anomaly in the United States. The back portion of the vertebrae fails to close, usually in the area of the baby's lower back. Meninges, the spinal cord, or both may protrude through this opening. **Myelomeningocele,** in which the defect involves protrusion of the meninges and the spinal cord, is the most serious form of spina bifida.

In most cases, a sac forms on the back of the fetus before birth and is detected when the baby is born (Figure 32.5). It is usually repaired as soon as the infant is able to undergo surgery, which helps prevent infection and preserve whatever neurologic function remains.

A common occurrence in spina bifida is the presence of **hydrocephalus,** in which cerebrospinal fluid accumulates in the brain (Figure 32.6). Depending on the type of spina bifida, the child may be at high risk for developing mental retardation and other neurologic complications such as seizures if this fluid buildup is not treated properly.

Hydrocephalus may require lifelong treatment. A shunt or tube is inserted from the brain to another place in the body, such as the peritoneum in the abdomen, to drain the excess fluid. As the child grows, the shunt must be revised or replaced. The shunt can become infected at any time, with the first 2 months after insertion being the time of greatest risk. The patient with an infected shunt will have the usual signs of infection (fever, irritability, etc.) in addition to malfunction of the shunt and abdominal pain (if the shunt ends in the peritoneum). Sepsis, meningitis, bacterial endocarditis, wound infection, and ventriculitis (infection in the ventricles of the brain) are some of the complications that can develop.

These shunts can also become blocked. Blockage produces signs of increased intracranial pressure such as a bulging soft spot on the head of an infant, changes in mentation in an older child or adult, headaches, vomiting, lethargy, seizures, or irritability. Immediate evaluation by a physician (i.e., neurologist) is needed. Document the patient's initial neurologic status and any changes that occur during treatment and transport.

Another potential complication is the presence of an **Arnold-Chiari malformation,** which occurs in approximately 90% of patients with spina bifida. The brainstem and cerebellum extend down through the foramen magnum into the cervical portion of the vertebrae. If the patient's head is hyperextended, pressure is put on the brainstem and cerebellum. Apnea may occur as a result of this pressure. Therefore avoid hyperextension of the head and use in-line stabilization when performing airway maneuvers. If the patient needs ongoing airway control, immobilize the cervical spine just as you would for a trauma patient.

Box 32.1 Items That May Contain Latex

Adhesive bandage strips
Airways
Blood pressure cuff and tubing
Bulb syringe
Catheters
Dressings
Elastic bandages
Electrode pads
Endotracheal tubes
Gloves
Intravenous tubing and bags
Medication vials
Nasogastric tubes
Oxygen masks and cannulas
Pulse oximeter
Spacer (from metered-dose inhaler)
Stethoscope tubing
Suction tubing
Syringes (disposable)
Tape
Tourniquet

Fom Wertz E: *Providing out-of-hospital care to infants and children,* Albany, NY, 2000, Delmar.

TABLE 32.1 Classifications of Hearing Loss

Conductive	Related to problems of the outer or middle ear
	Most common
	Interference with loudness of sound
Sensorineural	Result of problems with inner ear or auditory nerve
	Also called *perceptive* or *nerve deafness*
	Distortion of sound and problems with discrimination of sound (identifying one sound from another)
Mixed	Combination of conductive and sensorineural
	Interference with transmission of sound in the middle ear and along the neural pathways

From Wertz E: *Providing out-of-hospital care to infants and children,* Albany, NY, 2000, Delmar.

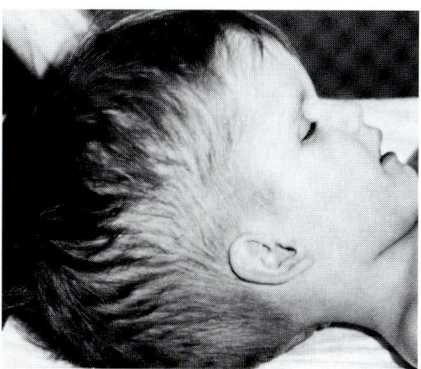

FIGURE 32.6 A child with hydrocephalus.

> ✓ In patients with spina bifida, observe for signs and symptoms of increased intracranial pressure (change in the patient's usual mentation, seizures, etc.) related to the presence of a malfunctioning shunt. When performing airway maneuvers on a patient with spina bifida, keep the head and neck in an in-line, neutral position even if trauma is not involved. Note preexisting paralysis, areas of decreased sensation, and so on.

In 1989 latex allergy was found to be a serious problem in children with spina bifida. As a result of repeated exposure to products containing latex (e.g., catheters, gloves), children become sensitive to the latex and develop life-threatening allergic reactions. These allergies continue into adulthood.

It is important to know immediately if the patient is sensitive to latex. If a sensitivity or allergy is present, the patient must not come into contact with any latex products or even be near equipment with latex (Box 32.1). Assemble a latex-free kit that can be stored in the ambulance for use when needed.

Spinal Cord Injuries

Spinal cord injuries also result in varying degrees of ability after the injury. Most instances result in some degree of paralysis or weakness. For instance, if the patient has been in a motor vehicle collision, he or she may have **paraplegia,** or paralysis from the waist down. If the accident involves diving, damage to the spinal cord in the cervical area may result in **quadriplegia,** or paralysis from the neck down. These individuals usually have a normal level of intelligence unless some other type of brain damage has also occurred.

> ✓ Note preexisting paraplegia or quadriplegia in patients who have had a previous spinal cord injury. Also look for areas of weakness.

Visual Impairment

Some patients have preexisting visual impairment that varies from complete loss of sight (i.e., blindness) to blurred vision. Causes may include genetic, prenatal, medical, and traumatic conditions. One example is the older patient with cataracts. The patient's decreased sight may have caused the injury for which the ambulance has been requested (e.g., fall from tripping over an object that was not seen).

These patients may be very frightened during an emergency because they cannot see what is happening. Orient the patient to whatever care or treatment is being provided, and explain any movements in position (moving the stretcher from the home to the back of the ambulance). Remember that people with any type of visual impairment may have heightened hearing or smell to compensate for their visual loss.

Some individuals with visual impairments use a seeing-eye dog for assistance. This animal is not a pet and has been highly trained. The patient may be very concerned about the dog to the point where he or she will not agree to treatment until plans are made for the dog. Enlist the assistance of a caregiver, friend, or spouse. If no one is available and willing to care for the dog, request assistance from the local police to make sure someone assumes responsibility for care of the dog.

Hearing Impairment

Some patients may have preexisting hearing loss. This impairment ranges from complete hearing loss (i.e., deafness) to a patient who is simply hard of hearing (Table 32.1).

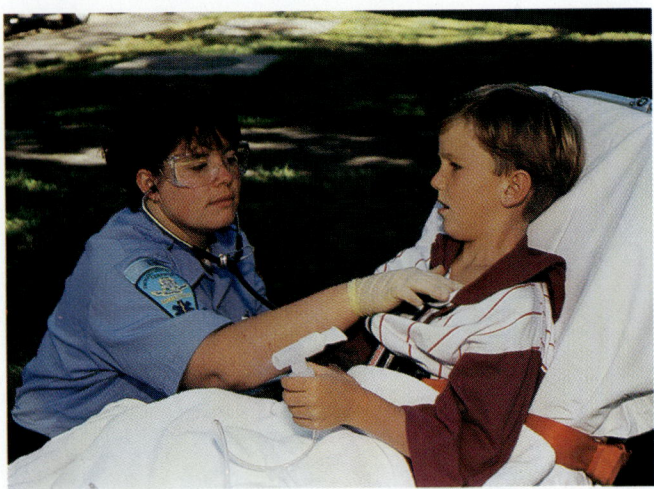

FIGURE 32.7 Asthma is considered the most common chronic illness among children and the leading cause of school absences.

The patient may have been born with a hearing loss or acquired one after an infection, head trauma, reaction to a medication (e.g., aspirin, furosemide), or through the usual aging process.

A hearing aid may amplify sound, enabling the person to hear. These devices may be attached to the person's glasses or be worn in or behind the ear. A whistling noise may be present if the device is not secured into the ear.

Communication is usually the greatest challenge. Determine the child's or adult's usual method of communication by talking to the family, school personnel, or long-term care personnel. If the patient reads lips, face the person whenever speaking. Try not to use complicated language or large words. Talk at a slow and even pace. If the patient uses sign language, ask for assistance from anyone present. Remember that an injury to the hands or upper extremities may greatly inhibit the patient's ability to communicate through sign language.

This patient will notice nonverbal communication much more readily. Remain calm, use a gentle touch when treating the patient, and establish eye contact whenever possible. Actively demonstrate your intent to understand what the patient is trying to communicate.

Chronic Illnesses

Many conditions fall under the category of chronic illnesses. Any disease, condition, or situation that extends for a prolonged period of time is considered **chronic.** Examples of chronic illnesses include the following:

- Reactive airways disease (e.g., asthma, bronchospasm)
- Diabetes
- Epilepsy
- Cancer
- Heart disease
- Cystic fibrosis

A few of these chronic illnesses are discussed in this chapter.

Reactive Airways Disease

More commonly known as **asthma,** reactive airways disease is considered the most common chronic illness among children and the leading cause of school absences. It also occurs in adults and accounts for multiple missed days at work. Asthma is a respiratory illness in which the bronchioles in the lungs become temporarily narrowed. The muscles around the bronchioles spasm, causing dyspnea and wheezing. The patient may also cough up mucus as it accumulates in the air passages.

Children and adults with asthma usually are seen frequently in the emergency department for episodes of wheezing. Treatment is focused on opening the passages to make breathing easier. The EMT-B must recognize this emergency and provide specific interventions (Figure 32.7). See Chapters 13 and 14 for more information.

Do not be fooled by the patient with asthma who is lethargic, cooperative, and without wheezing. This person may have bronchioles so tight that he or she cannot move any air. *This situation is life threatening and will be fatal if appropriate intervention is not started.*

Seizures and Epilepsy

One of the more common complications in children and adults with disabilities, especially those with a neurologic focus, is the occurrence of seizures. However, seizure disorders, or **epilepsy,** may also be a primary problem in some patients. Approximately 2.3 million Americans have seizures and epilepsy. In addition, approximately 8% of pediatric prehospital transports are for children having seizures.

It may be difficult to think of seizures alone as a disability. However, approximately 25% of all children and adults have multiple seizures that resist control despite aggressive medical and surgical therapy (Table 32.2). The seizures interfere with the daily lives of these patients and their families and subsequently constitute a chronic problem. In children, growth and development are often affected by the number of seizures, as well as the side effects of multiple medications.

Some children with uncontrolled seizures may be on a special diet called the **ketogenic diet.** This diet is high in fat, low in carbohydrates, and low in protein. It is thought to achieve some seizure control through the ketosis that results from the metabolism of fat instead of

TABLE 32.2 Seizure Chart

Type	Duration	Seizure Symptoms	Postictal Symptoms
Simple partial	30 seconds	Vary: Sudden jerking of a specific body part; Sensory phenomena such as a pins and needles sensation; Flushing, sweating; Feeling of fear or deja vu	No loss of consciousness
Complex partial (also called psychomotor or temporal lobe)	1–2 minutes	May have aura; Staring; Automatisms such as lip-smacking, picking at clothes, fumbling, etc.; Unaware of environment; May wander	Amnesia for seizure events; Mild to moderate confusion
Absence (formerly called petit mal)	2–15 seconds	Staring; Eyes fluttering	Amnesia for seizure events; No confusion; Able to resume activity
Generalized tonic-clonic (formerly called grand mal)	1–2 minutes	A cry; Fall; Tonicity (rigidity); Clonicity (jerking); May have cyanosis	Amnesia for seizure events; Confusion; Deep sleep
Atonic (also called drop attacks)	10–60 seconds	Sudden collapse and fall	Amnesia for seizure events
Myoclonic	Varies	Brief, massive muscle jerks	No loss of consciousness
Infantile spasms	Varies	Clusters of quick, sudden movements	No loss of consciousness

From Epilepsy Foundation of America, 1989.

glucose. These children should not be given any glucose solutions either orally or intravenously.

Transplant Recipients

Many patients who have had organ transplantations must take antirejection drugs and are continually monitored by their physicians. This situation constitutes a chronic illness even though the transplanted organ(s) may be functioning well. These individuals are usually at a higher risk for infection due to the **immunosuppressive** effects of their medications. Signs and symptoms of an infectious process may be the reason for a request for assistance.

> ✓ In the patient with a chronic illness, make note of any medications, side effects, or other disabling circumstances. For example, in the child with uncontrolled epilepsy, two to three seizures per day may be the routine and not a result of the present emergency.

Technologic Aids

As previously discussed, technology has made a tremendous difference in the lives of many people. This technology includes an array of medical equipment such as apnea monitors, tracheostomies, gastrostomy tubes and buttons, and so on. Patients, families, and caregivers usually receive education about caring for the specific equipment or device while in the hospital before discharge. However, they may experience a great deal of anxiety once the patient returns home.

Once at home, it can be very frightening if a malfunction occurs or the device does not operate as it did in the hospital. Emergency medical services (EMS) may be called at the first sign of trouble, especially in the first few weeks during the adjustment phase. The EMT-B may be expected to "save the day" without having actual experience with the equipment in use.

It may be helpful to meet with personnel from the social services departments in the hospitals in your area. Encourage them to notify the ambulance service with

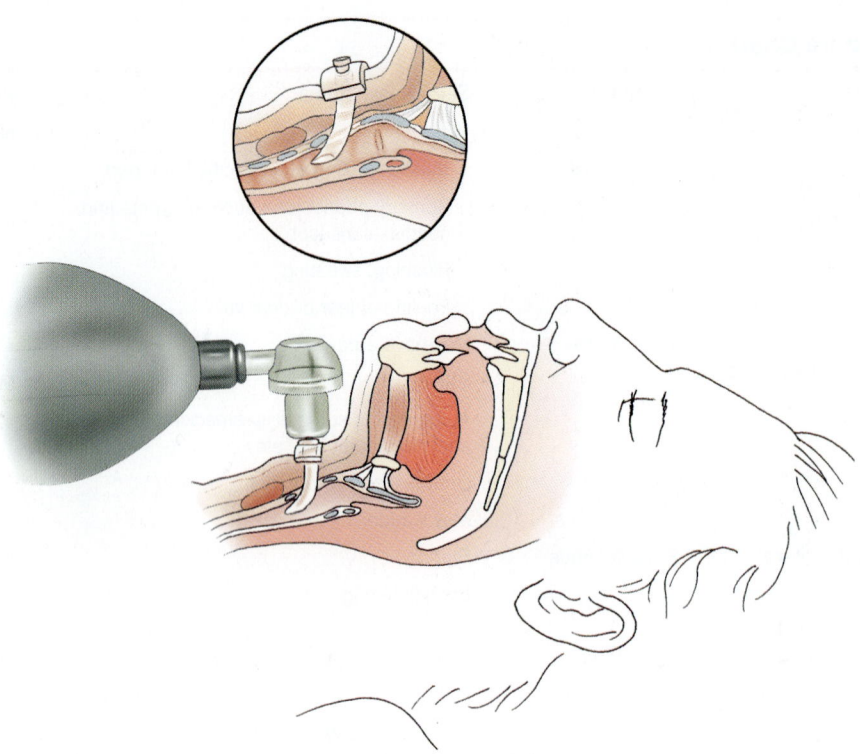

FIGURE 32.8 A tracheostomy is an opening through the neck into the trachea through which a tube may be inserted.

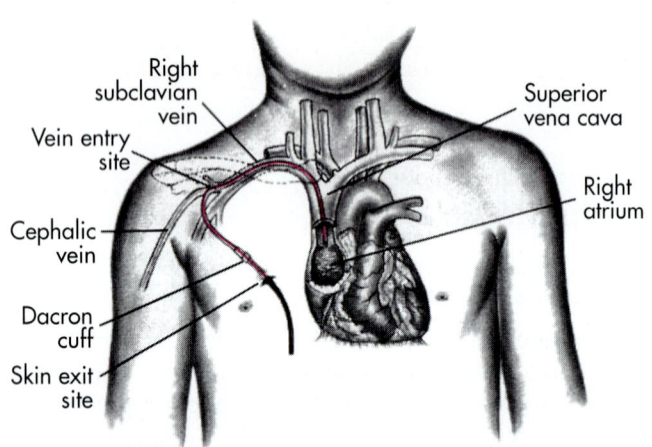

FIGURE 32.9 Central venous catheter insertion and exit site.

whom the patient may be in contact regarding the presence of specialized equipment in the home. These details can precipitate a visit to the residence in which more information is gathered from all parties involved. It may also be helpful to review what procedures should take place if a disaster (e.g., earthquake, tornado, flooding) or other event occurs that can cause a loss of power.

Tracheostomy

A tracheostomy may be used as a temporary or permanent device. In some patients it provides protection against secretions that could be aspirated. In other patients, it may be necessary because of direct trauma to the airway, weakened respiratory muscles, or prolonged mechanical ventilation (Figure 32.8).

Obstruction of the tracheostomy requires immediate action. Difficulty clearing secretions, improper positioning, or incorrect insertion of the tube during replacement may lead to obstruction. Place the patient in a sitting position as long as trauma is not suspected. Removal of the tube and direct suctioning of the stoma may be necessary to relieve the blockage.

Central Venous Access Devices

Some patients who require frequent intravenous medications, repeated blood testing, administration of blood products, or administration of large quantities or concentrations of fluids may have a central venous access device inserted. This device provides extended access to a vein without the need for repeated venipunctures or infusions.

There are several types of devices (Table 32.3). All catheters end at the superior vena cava or the right atrium (Figure 32.9). Some of them may be used for fluid resuscitation or medication administration in an emergency. Follow local protocols or consult with the medical command physician. Medication and fluid may be given directly through the tubing for a peripherally inserted central catheter and through the injection cap for Hickman® and Broviac® catheters (Figure 32.10). The im-

TABLE 32.3 Central Venous Access Devices

Type of Catheter	Benefits	Maintenance Considerations
Peripherally inserted central catheter (PICC)	Used for therapy of short to moderate duration Less costly	Antecubital vein most common site (may limit movement of arm) Risk of infection May become dislodged easily (most are not sutured into place)
Tunneled catheter Hickman® Broviac®	Used for long-term therapy Easy to use for self-administered infusions	Daily heparin flushes required Must be clamped or have clamp ready at all times Site must be kept dry Risk of infection Protrudes from body Susceptible to damage May be pulled out May alter body image of child
Implanted ports Port-A-Cath® Infus-A-Port® Mediport®	Used for long-term therapy Reduced risk of infection Only slight bulge on chest; completely under skin Increased safety (under skin and no maintenance care) Reduced cost for family Regular physical activity (including swimming) not restricted Heparinized monthly and after each infusion	Must pierce skin to access port Pain associated with needle insertion (may use local anesthetic, e.g., EMLA cream) Special needle (Huber) required to access port Must prepare skin before injection Catheter may dislodge from port, especially if child "plays" with site Generally not allowed to engage in vigorous contact sports Difficult for self-administered infusions

Adapted from Wong D: *Whaley and Wong's nursing care of infants and children,* St Louis, 1999, Mosby.

planted devices can only be accessed using a special needle called a Huber needle (Figure 32.11).

Vagus Nerve Stimulator

Some patients with seizures that have not responded to medication may have a vagus nerve stimulator in place. These devices are used in patients over 12 years of age and provide a pattern of stimulation to the vagus nerve to stop the progression of seizure activity. The generator is implanted under the skin and can also be activated by the patient if necessary. If the patient's heart rate is slow, consider a problem with this stimulator. Relay its presence to the medical command physician, and treat the patient for bradycardia.

Apnea Monitor

Many infants born prematurely may need an **apnea monitor** at home to warn caregivers of any cessation of breathing (Figure 32.12). Some monitors also warn of bradycardia and tachycardia. Patches are applied to the baby's chest and connected to the monitor. If the device does not detect a breath within a specific time frame or if

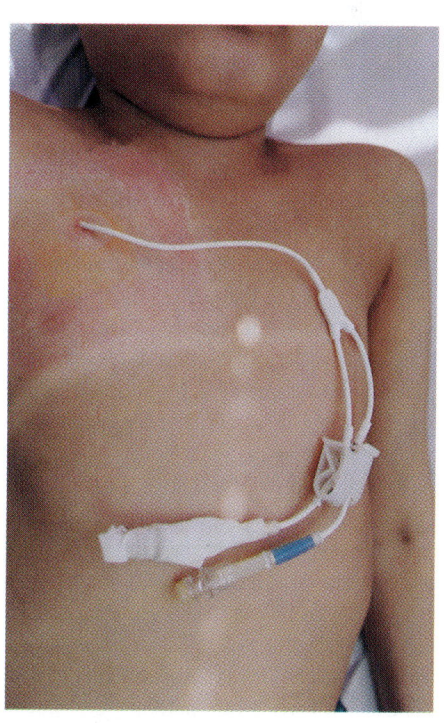

FIGURE 32.10 External venous catheter.

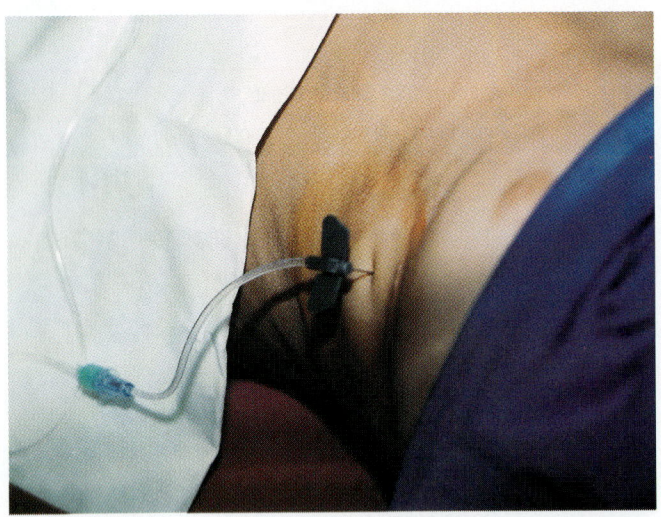

FIGURE 32.11 Implanted venous access device with Huber needle placement.

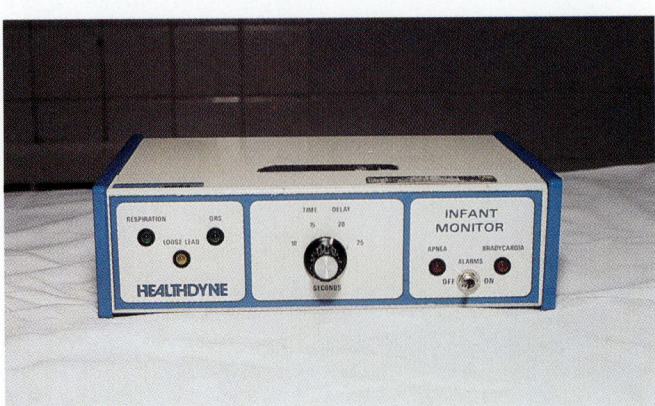

FIGURE 32.12 Apnea monitor.

the infant's heart rate is too slow or too fast, an alarm sounds.

Many different models are available. Newer apnea monitors are computerized and can store information. A printout can be given to EMS providers or hospital personnel that includes an electrocardiogram tracing, heart rate, respiratory rate, and time. It is best to visit the family before an emergency occurs so that they can show you the features of their particular monitor. This visit may also help boost the family's confidence by letting them know that trained members of the health care team are available to assist them.

Gastrostomy Tube or Button

People who cannot take food by mouth for an extended period of time may require a **gastrostomy tube** or button for feeding. This device is common in some chronic diseases, central nervous system disorders, disorders of the digestive system, or situations in which the developmental ability of the person hinders feeding.

There are multiple types of gastrostomy tubes and buttons with different methods for inserting and securing them (Figure 32.13). No unusual measures are necessary from an emergency standpoint. Be aware that if the tube was surgically sutured in place and is now dislodged, additional bleeding will occur inside the stomach. In this situation, further evaluation is necessary by a physician in a hospital setting.

Assessment

Perform initial and ongoing assessments on individuals with special needs using the same method as indicated for patients without these needs. Evaluate the ABCs (airway, breathing, and circulation). In the initial assessment, which includes the ABCs, is the *D* for "disability," which still refers to the patient's neurologic status and not the disabling condition. The patient should still receive a complete initial assessment.

If any life-threatening situations are discovered during the initial assessment, it is necessary to begin intervention immediately as you would do for someone without a disability. The adult's or child's disability is usually an ongoing process; therefore focus on treating the acute problem.

During the ongoing assessment, spend more time gathering information about the patient's overall condition, as well as the disability. Ask pertinent questions of the patient, parent, or caregiver such as the following:

- "Does your child take medications for his or her seizures?"
- "Are you able to remove the brace on your leg so that I can examine your foot?"
- "Is your child able to take anything by mouth?"
- "Can you feel me touching your leg?"
- "What is different today that prompted you to call for an ambulance?"

> ✓ If special aids are used, make every effort to gather this information before an emergency occurs. Meet with the family and become familiar with the device. Share that information with other members of the service who may respond when help is requested.

If the patient is a child, ask the parent, caregiver, or school nurse if an *Emergency Information Form* is available. In October 1999 the American Academy of Pediatrics and the American College of Emergency Physicians finalized a document that provides standard information that would be helpful to emergency personnel (Figure 32.14). They authored a joint policy statement advocating the use of this form for children with special health care needs (Figure 32.15). Medic Alert® also participates in the project and stores the information if the child has a Medic Alert® bracelet or necklace.

The document is completed and updated by the child's primary care physician. It is then given to the parents, day care provider, school nurse, or anyone with whom the child spends a part of his or her day. During an emergency, this form relays pertinent information that may affect treatment.

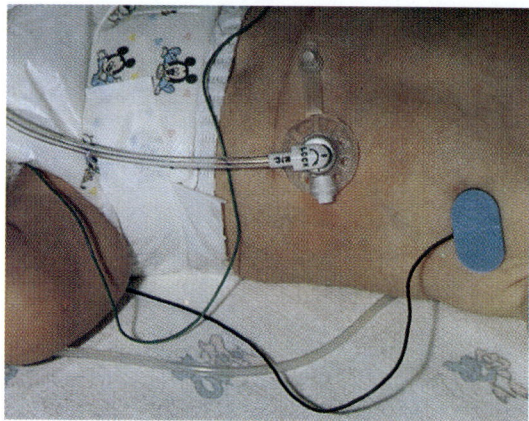

FIGURE 32.13 A gastrostomy is the surgical creation of an artificial opening in the stomach through the abdominal wall, performed to provide a means of feeding the patient. In this child, a feeding tube is connected to a gastrostomy button.

Developmental Disabilities

In most circumstances, the actual physical examination is essentially unchanged. The most prominent differences will be in the patient's level of understanding and ability to communicate. It is important to explain everything that is done even if it seems that the patient does not understand.

Approach the patient in a manner consistent with his or her developmental level. Talk with the patient, parent, or caregiver to determine the patient's level of ability. Direct your questions in a positive light. For example, ask, "Mrs. Binder, can you tell me what Sean is able to do?" In this manner, the focus is on the patient's abilities instead of his or her disabilities.

Physical Disabilities

During the assessment, it is important to know whenever possible what type of deficit existed before the present emergency. Was the patient already paralyzed, or is the numbness and tingling the patient reports a result of the present injury?

The amount of sensation in the body is usually different from person to person. Some people with physical disabilities may be able to feel parts of their lower extremities, whereas others have no sensation from the waist down. Individuals with no sensation are particularly susceptible to hazards such as burns or other injuries because they cannot feel dangerous things (e.g., scalding water or hot grease). They also may not feel an ankle being caught in the spokes of a wheelchair. Remember to determine the mechanism of injury and maintain a high level of suspicion for hidden trauma.

The level of bladder and bowel function may also vary. Some people accomplish elimination of waste products through a surgically created opening on the abdomen called a *stoma*, or **ostomy** (Figure 32.16, *A*). More common terms are **ileostomy** and **colostomy** for feces (Figure 32.16, *B*). Urine and feces are collected in special appliances or clear plastic containers that attach directly over the opening (Figure 32.16, *C*). These appliances, or pouches as they are also known, are emptied and changed periodically.

Many people with physical disabilities use some type of adaptive device, including a wheelchair, braces, crutches, or a combination of devices. Some people also may use corrective splints at different times during the day or night. Ask the patient, parents, or caregivers to explain the particular device. Use their knowledge to examine underlying tissue when it is necessary to perform an adequate physical examination. Remember that splints or braces can serve as tools for immobilization if trauma is suspected, as long as there is no damage to the equipment. However, if circulation or breathing is impaired or major bleeding is present, these devices should be removed. If a wheelchair is used, make sure someone assumes responsibility for getting it back to the patient's room, home, or personal care facility.

Technologic Aids

When a patient uses a technologic aid, incorporate information about the device into your assessment. Do not, however, be distracted by the equipment, because it is

650 Section Four | Special Patient Populations

Emergency Information Form for Children With Special Needs

American College of Emergency Physicians®   American Academy of Pediatrics

| Date form completed By Whom | Revised | Initials |
| | Revised | Initials |

Name: | Birth date: | Nickname:
Home Address: | Home/Work Phone:
Parent/Guardian: | Emergency Contact Names & Relationship:
Signature/Consent*: |
Primary Language: | Phone Number(s):

Physicians:

Primary care physician: | Emergency Phone:
 | Fax:

Current Specialty physician: Specialty: | Emergency Phone:
 | Fax:

Current Specialty physician: Specialty: | Emergency Phone:
 | Fax:

Anticipated Primary ED: | Pharmacy:
Anticipated Tertiary Care Center:

Diagnoses/Past Procedures/Physical Exam:

1.

2.

3.

4.

Synopsis:

Baseline physical findings:

Baseline vital signs:

Baseline neurological status:

*Consent for release of this form to health care providers

Last name:

FIGURE 32.14 Emergency Information Form for Children with Special Health Care Needs.

Diagnoses/Past Procedures/Physical Exam continued:

Medications: _____ Significant baseline ancillary findings (lab, x-ray, ECG): _____

1. _____ _____
2. _____ _____
3. _____ _____
4. _____ Prostheses/Appliances/Advanced Technology Devices: _____
5. _____ _____
6. _____

Management Data:

Allergies: Medications/Foods to be avoided _____ and why: _____

1.
2.
3.

Procedures to be avoided _____ and why: _____

1.
2.
3.

Immunizations

Dates					Dates				
DPT					Hep B				
OPV					Varicella				
MMR					TB status				
HIB					Other				

Antibiotic prophylaxis: _____ Indication: _____ Medication and dose: _____

Common Presenting Problems/Findings With Specific Suggested Managements

Problem	Suggested Diagnostic Studies	Treatment Considerations

Comments on child, family, or other specific medical issues:

Physician/Provider Signature: _____ Print Name: _____

© American College of Emergency Physicians and American Academy of Pediatrics. Permission to reprint granted with acknowledgement.

FIGURE 32.14, cont'd Emergency Information Form for Children with Special Health Care Needs.

> Emergency physicians and pediatricians provide medical care to many children with special needs because of chronic, complex medical illnesses. Care of these children may be complicated by the lack of patient history information and unusual and uncommon disease processes.
>
> To optimize emergency care of children with special needs, the American College of Emergency Physicians supports these principles:
>
> - A mechanism should be available to quickly identify the child with special health care needs when that child presents for emergency care.
> - Records of each child's special needs should be maintained in an accessible and usable format.
> - The exact form in which relevant information is stored may vary depending on individual physician and patient preference.
> - A universally accepted form should be disseminated for use by prehospital providers, parents, physicians, and other child advocates.
>
> Approved by the American College of Emergency Physicians Board of Directors and the American Academy of Pediatrics, December, 1998

FIGURE 32.15 American College of Emergency Physicians Policy Statement Emergency Information Form for Children with Special Health Care Needs.

still necessary to complete adequate initial and ongoing examinations. For example, if the patient has a tracheostomy, include an inspection of this device as part of your assessment. Is it patent? Are secretions present, and if so, what color are they? Is bleeding present around the tracheostomy site? Request suction equipment to clear away any secretions to maintain patency.

> ✓ Focus the assessment on the present chief complaint. Incorporate information about a particular disability or device as appropriate.

Management

Keep several considerations in mind when caring for patients with special needs. A summary of conditions and management issues is provided in Table 32.4.

1. *Focus on the patient's abilities, not disabilities.* Focusing on what this person is able to do promotes self-esteem and a positive self-image. Be sensitive to the particular situation. Saying to a parent, "What is wrong with your child?" or "Your child isn't normal, is he?" may create parental anger and resentment. Asking the parent what is special about his or her child promotes trust and understanding.

    Avoid using the "N" word—*normal*. Normalcy is relative and is not always reflected in growth charts and developmental screening tests. Asking the parent, "Is this your child's usual behavior (or posture, color, etc.)?" implies acceptance of the child's health condition and avoids the normal/abnormal merry-go-round.

2. *Develop creative means for communication.* Never assume that the patient cannot understand what you are saying. Communicate in a manner appropriate to the disability. Allow the person to use a specialized communication board or device if he or she is used to doing so. If the patient can read and write, provide pencil and paper so the patient can write down key words during your examination. Use sign language only if you are skilled in that technique. Speak loudly only if you know that the person is able to hear you at a louder tone. Resist the temptation to simply shout at someone with a hearing impairment. Shouting usually does not improve the communication and may increase the level of frustration for you and your team members. These techniques open patterns of communication between the patient, family, and emergency care personnel.

    Another crucial level of communication is notification of the receiving facility. Make sure the receiving hospital is aware of the patient's special needs. In some cases, diversion to a more appropriate facility designed to handle these special circumstances, such as a hospital with a spina bifida program, may be suggested.

3. *Treat this patient with the same respect afforded other patients.* It is easy to forget the patient's modesty during emergency treatment, especially when an "unusual" physical finding is present or the EMT-B assumes that the patient is not aware of what is happening. Keep exposure to a minimum by using sheets or blankets as appropriate. Also, do not be tempted to "show" the patient's disability to the remainder of the crew or other people at the scene.

    Some patients may not realize that they can refuse repeated examinations and can ask for specific

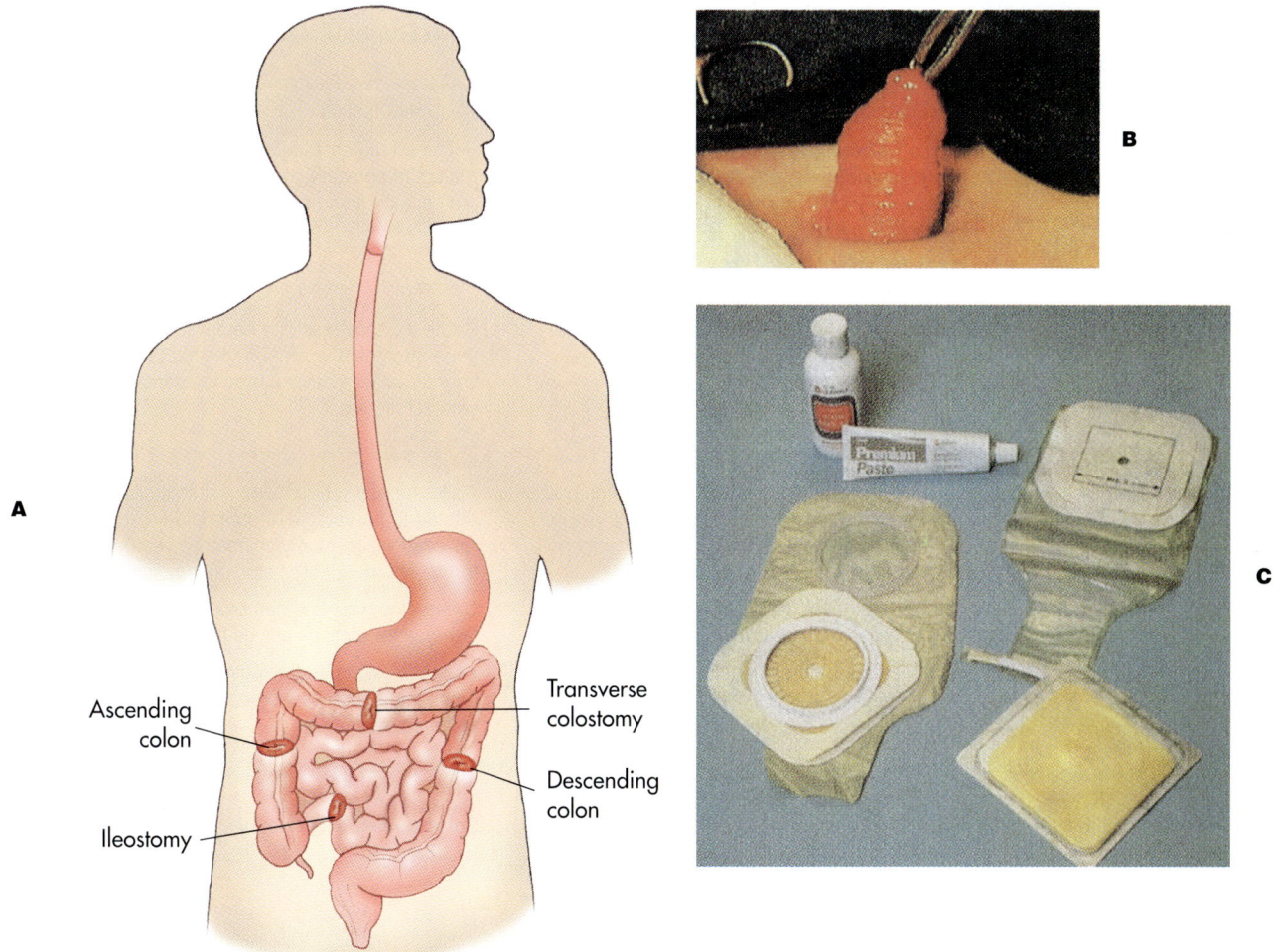

FIGURE 32.16 A, Ostomy sites. **B,** An ileostomy is a surgical formation of an opening of the ileum onto the surface of the abdomen, through which fecal matter is emptied. **C,** Ostomy pouches.

information about their health condition. Serving as the patient's **advocate** assists in the maintenance of dignity. Do not perform needless examinations, and provide as much information as possible.

> ✓ Concentrate on the patient's abilities rather than disabilities. Show respect for the patient. Involve other members of the health care team in providing additional support if necessary.

4. Other factors include the following:

   - When treating the patient with a physical disability, special features of the disability may come into play. For example, a patient with cerebral palsy may routinely have a large amount of secretions that may interfere with airway procedures. Be prepared to suction the airway or provide high-concentration oxygen as necessary. In patients with rigid body parts, do not forcefully manipulate that part to make the patient conform to your equipment (e.g., forcing someone with an arched back to lie flat on a long backboard).
   - When assessing the patient with special needs, look for a medical identification bracelet or necklace. Although its absence does not rule out a chronic condition, its presence can be helpful during assessment and treatment.
   - Obtain from the parent, caregiver, or other family member a list of the patient's current medications and their schedules. Ask the time of the last dose. Vomiting and diarrhea can alter the medication's absorption. Ask about the presence of side effects.
   - Other health care professionals may be able to help when caring for the patient with special needs. Once at the hospital, people such as social services personnel, medical specialists, child life specialists,

TABLE 32.4 A Sampling of Health Conditions Related to Patients with Special Needs—Implications for Providers of Emergency Care

Special Need	General Characteristics	Treatment Issues
Mental retardation	May see physical signs such as unusual formation of teeth or low set ears; soft neurologic signs such as microcephaly and poor fine or gross motor coordination	Focus on patient's abilities, not disabilities; include patient in conversation whenever possible; ask patient's opinions and concerns
	Cognitive function variable, ranging from educable to needing complete care	
Permanent disabilities	Physical: obvious deformities of limbs, craniofacial malformations, paralysis, etc.	Same as above; ask for help if special equipment is used such as a ventilator, gastrostomy tube, central venous access device, braces, artificial limbs, a wheelchair, etc.
	Sensory: difficulty in hearing, vision, tactile perceptabilities	
	Cognitive: alterations in thinking abilities	
Neurologic conditions	Congenital malformations such as spina bifida and Arnold-Chiari malformation; chromosomal anomalies; Dandy-Walker malformation; hydrocephalus	As for mental retardation; assess for further findings related to paraplegia or quadriplegia, mental retardation, ileostomy/colostomy, ventriculoperitoneal shunt, spasticity, posturing, seizure activity
	Perinatal causes such as infections, anoxic encephalopathy, birth trauma, cerebral palsy	Conduct a complete neurologic assessment; ask the family what findings are usual or unusual
	Postnatal causes such as head and spinal cord trauma, neoplasms, demyelinating diseases (multiple sclerosis)	Watch for signs and symptoms of altered neurologic functioning such as increased intracranial pressure, seizures, etc.
	Seizure disorders such as infantile spasms, Lennox-Gastaut syndrome, epilepsy	
Neuromuscular conditions	Anterior horn cell diseases such as Werdnig-Hoffmann's disease	Same as neurologic conditions
	Neuromuscular function diseases such as myasthenia gravis	
	Muscular dystrophies	
Cardiovascular conditions	Congenital cyanotic heart diseases such as tetralogy of Fallot, transposition of the great vessels	Ask if the cardiac anomaly has been repaired and if more surgery is needed
	Congenital acyanotic heart diseases such as atrial or ventricular septal defects, coarctation of the aorta	Ask about the medication schedule; ask about the use of oxygen at home
	Other anomalies such as dextrocardia	Ask about the person's usual status (i.e., Is the patient more cyanotic or dyspneic than usual?)
Respiratory conditions	Congenital such as softening of the larynx of trachea, underdeveloped or improperly developed lungs; cystic fibrosis	Perform a complete respiratory assessment; place the patient in a position of comfort
	Acquired such as pulmonary neoplasms	Assess the presence and patency of an artificial airway (tracheostomy)
	Others such as asthma, chronic bronchitis, or bronchopulmonary dysplasia	Maintain airway patency through suctioning and oxygenation; have replacement trach tubes available (same size and one size smaller)
		Ask if respiratory status is usual or unusual (i.e., Is stridor or are the retractions more severe than usual?)
Immunologic conditions	Acquired such as HIV, hepatitis leukemia, carcinomas	Isolate patient from other people as much as possible; gather information about the patient's medication schedule
	Induced such as immunosuppression for organ transplants (heart, heart-lung, lung, liver, kidneys, visceral) or bone marrow transplant	Relay information about a central venous access device if present
		Recognize the signs and symptoms of organ rejection and chemotherapy rejection

physical and occupational therapists, and nutritionists can provide the necessary care to help the patient reach his or her potential. Some patients or family members may feel too proud to ask for assistance or may not be able to afford such services. Social service personnel can visit the family in the emergency department and develop a plan for future home care as necessary (Figure 32.17).

Family Considerations

Families of adults and children with special needs are forced to become experts in the care and treatment of their loved one. Use these resources as much as possible to gather information, assist with treatment, or communicate with the patient. Because they spend a great deal of their time with this person, recognize their knowledge and encourage their participation.

People with special needs may require frequent prehospital interventions, visits to the emergency department, and hospitalizations. Some patients and families may be familiar with the emergency routine and may seem nonchalant or unconcerned. Others may be overly defensive as a result of frustration about repeated medical treatments that do not appear to be working. This roller coaster of emotions is typical of families of people with special needs. Acknowledging their frustration and helping to make the emergency situation more tolerable strengthens everyone's coping abilities.

If the patient is a child, the siblings of this child may also require attention. Their lives are also disrupted by their brother's or sister's emergency treatments and hospitalizations. They may have anger or resentment that their parents' time is taken up with the child with special needs. When they grow older, they may be ashamed of their "different" brother or sister. Allow the sibling to assist whenever possible, such as retrieving a favorite blanket or stuffed animal, and to ask questions. Praise the brother or sister for helping and being good. These measures help the sibling to develop a positive self-image, as well as receive some much-needed attention.

> ✓ Pay special attention to the patient's family, and include them in the care whenever possible. Rely on these resources to assist with communication, explanation of special equipment, and so on. Interact with the patient's sibling(s) when present to promote self-esteem.

EMT-B Considerations

Caring for a patient with special needs can be intimidating. The equipment may be unfamiliar, or the lack of communication ability on the patient's part may be frustrating. Develop a relationship with the discharge planners at the local hospitals in your service area. Make sure they contact someone at the ambulance service when a person with complex medical needs is being discharged into the community. Whenever possible, make a visit to the person's home, the child's school, or the long-term care facility before an emergency occurs to become somewhat familiar with the situation, the patient, and the associated equipment or devices used to sustain that person outside of the hospital setting.

Box 32.2 Guidelines for Disability Awareness

Use the word "disability" instead of handicapped.

Refer to the person first and the disability second.

Never refer to someone as "wheelchair bound" or "confined to a wheelchair" because a wheelchair actually makes the person more mobile.

Avoid negative descriptions whenever possible. Do not use "invalid," "afflicted with," or "suffers from." Do not refer to persons with Down syndrome as "mongoloids" or to persons with epilepsy as "epileptics." Do not call seizures "fits."

Do not use "normal" to describe people who do not have disabilities. Use "typical" or "people without disabilities."

Do not refer to a person's disability unless it is relevant.

Adapted from *Talking about disability: a guide to using appropriate language,* Nashville, TN, 1993, Coalition for Tennesseans with Disabilities.

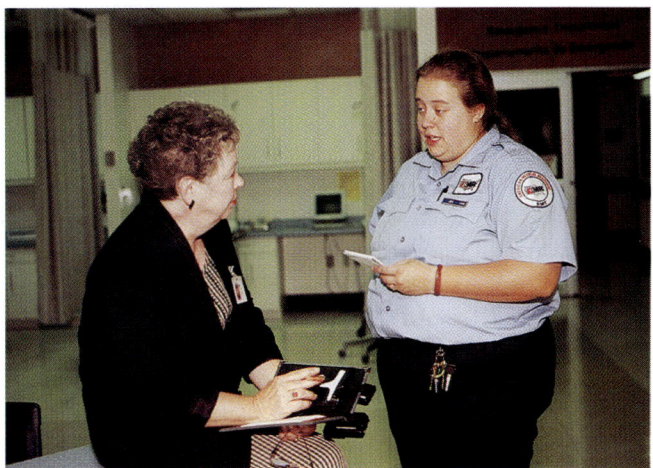

FIGURE 32.17 It may be helpful to meet with social services personnel in the hospitals in your area.

Guidelines for Disability Awareness

With the passage of the Americans with Disabilities Act in July 1992, people with disabilities have finally received the attention they deserve. These individuals now have legislative support to function in the community alongside their peers without disabilities. However, it will take much longer to educate the public and decrease the discrimination and poor attitudes that still exist. Box 32.2 lists suggestions to help increase awareness and promote equal treatment for everyone.

> ✓ Think "person first, disability second." Whenever you interact with someone with a disablity, think of him or her as a person who just happens to have something unique or different about him or her.

Summary

- Many people now survive life-threatening illness and injury. Therefore individuals with special needs are present in the community and require additional attention when an emergency occurs.
- If the patient has a developmental disability, take extra time to explain what is being done even if it seems that the person does not understand you. Use terminology that is appropriate to the patient's level of ability.
- If the patient has a physical disability, gather informaton about the circumstances or special equipment involved. Minimize exposure when assessing and treating the patient.
- If a chronic illness is present, ask about preexisting medical conditions (e.g., wheezing, seizures). Relay this information to other members of the health care team.
- If the patient uses specialized equipment, provide reassurance to the patient and family. Make every effort to visit this person before an emergency to get a better understanding of the equipment and why it is being used.
- Perform initial and ongoing assessments as you would routinely do on individuals without disabilities. However, you may need to modify your actions based on the particular disability present (e.g., take a blood pressure using the arm that is not flexed and rigid or using the patient's thigh and popliteal artery).
- Pay special attention to family members, and provide support as necessary. Rely on them as a resource, and trust what they tell you. Allow siblings to assist whenever possible.
- In general, be aware of people with disabilities in the community. Use the appropriate guidelines when interacting with these individuals.

Scenario Solution

Initial Assessment and Treatment

Your partner goes to talk with the director of the center to get more information. Find out the child's name, and use it. The child begins to cry when you approach her. You suggest to the teacher that she hold Nicole (the patient) in her lap. Nicole calms down a bit when sitting in her teacher's lap. Your examination reveals the following:

Airway. Stridor is audible. You ask her to stick her tongue out at you after you demonstrate it to her. You repeat your action twice, and Nicole then sticks her tongue out at you. When you visually inspect her mouth, no foreign bodies are seen.
Breathing. Rapid and shallow in between crying; expiratory wheezes are heard in both lung fields.
Circulation. Carotid and radial pulses palpable (tachycardic); skin pale, cool, and diaphoretic.
Disability. Awake; responds to simple verbal commands; pupils equal and reactive.
Expose. No obvious bleeding or trauma noted.

Ongoing Assessment and Treatment

The potential airway compromise is your first priority. You try not to agitate Nicole in any way. Blood pressure is 108/68, and pulse is 128, strong, and regular. Respirations are 36. Apply high-concentration oxygen via a pediatric nonrebreather face mask. If Nicole does not tolerate the face mask, consider having her pretend to drink from a plastic cup with oxygen tubing placed in the bottom of it.

The director is attempting to reach the girl's parents. Ask another teacher to distract the other children as much as possible. Talk in a soothing voice to the child as you are treating her.

Scenario Solution (cont'd)

Use the Broselow tape you have in your pediatric kit. Once you determine her length, identify the equipment and drugs you would use for her. Administer epinephrine according to your protocols and the information from the tape.

Move the child to the ambulance and begin transport. In the ambulance, connect Nicole to the ECG monitor so that you can monitor her cardiac status. Repeat vitals every 5 minutes after the epinephrine.

If family members arrive at the scene before you transport, briefly explain your actions. Allow them to stay with the child as much as possible as long as they are emotionally capable of doing so. *Do not delay transport.* Attempt to gain more information about the child's history and any current health concerns.

Continue to reassess the child, and make contact with the receiving facility. Remember to document all assessment findings and interventions (see Chapter 35).

Throughout the call, talk softly to the child. Hold her hand, and stroke her hair or face. Provide as much support as possible to help calm her. Try to limit the number of providers touching her.

Once at the hospital, provide a verbal report to the nurses and physicians in attendance. Leave a copy of your documentation, and replace your supplies. If the family has arrived, spend a few minutes giving them an update of what happened while you were with their child.

Key Terms

Advocate A person who assists another person in carrying out desired wishes; an EMT should function as a patient's advocate in all aspects of prehospital care.

Apnea monitor A technologic aid used to warn of cessation of breathing in a premature infant; also may warn of bradycardia and tachycardia.

Arnold-Chiari malformation A complication of spinal bifida in which the brainstem and cerebellum extend down through the foramen magnum into the cervical portion of the vertebrae.

Asthma Respiratory disorder characterized by recurring episodes of sudden onset of breathing difficulty, wheezing on expiration/inspiration due to constriction of bronchi, coughing, and thick mucous bronchial secretions; also termed *reactive airways disease.*

Cerebral palsy Neuromuscular condition in which the patient has difficulty controlling the voluntary muscles due to damage to a portion of the brain.

Chronic Long, drawn out; applied to a disease that is not acute.

Colostomy Incision in the colon for the purpose of making a temporary or permanent opening between the bowel and the abdominal wall.

Developmental disabilities Disabilities that involve some degree of impaired adaptation in learning, social adjustment, or maturation.

Down syndrome A genetic syndrome characterized by varying degrees of mental retardation and multiple physcial defects.

Epilepsy A group of neurologic disorders characterized by recurrent episodes of convulsive seizures, sensory disturbances, unusual behavior, loss of consciousness, or all of these; uncontrolled electrical discharge from the nerve cells of the cerebral cortex.

Gastrostomy tube A tube placed in a person's stomach that allows continuous feeding for an extended period of time.

Hydrocephalus "Water on the brain"; can cause increased intracranial pressure if allowed to accumulate.

Ileostomy Surgical creation of a passage through the abdominal wall into the ileum.

Immunosuppressive Prevention of formation of immune responses.

Ketogenic diet Special diet high in fats and low in carbohydrates and protein; produces a state of ketosis in which fat is used for energy instead of glucose; used for children with ongoing seizures that do not respond to customary medication and other therapies.

Mental retardation Developmental disability characterized by a lower than normal IQ.

Myelomeningocele Developmental anomaly of the central nervous system in which a hernial sac containing a portion of the spinal cord, the meninges, and cerebrospinal fluid protrudes through a congenital cleft in the vertebral column; occurs in approximately 2 of every 1000 live births, is readily apparent, and is easily diagnosed at birth.

Ostomy Surgical opening that allows the passage of urine or feces through an incision, or stoma, in the wall of the abdomen.

Paraplegia Paralysis of the lower limbs and trunk.

Physical disabilities Disabilities that involve limitation of mobility.

Quadriplegia Paralysis affecting all four extremities.

Special needs Conditions with the potential to interfere with usual growth and development; may involve physical disabilities, developmental disabilities, chronic illnesses, and forms of technologic support.

Review Questions

1. True or False: When assessing a patient with special needs, *D* in ABCD refers to the person's developmental or physical disability.
2. Which of the following are examples of chronic illnesses?
   a. Diabetes
   b. Down syndrome
   c. Epilepsy
   d. Answers a and c only
3. How should the family of a person with special needs be treated?
4. True or False: The presence of a medical identification bracelet or necklace may indicate a chronic condition.
5. The head is placed in a neutral position when performing airway maneuvers on a patient with spina bifida because:
   a. It makes it easier to use a bag-valve-mask without a partner.
   b. An Arnold-Chiari malformation may be present.
   c. It reduces intracranial pressure.
   d. None of the above.
6. *Mental retardation* is an example of a _____.
7. True or False: The EMT-B should know how to use all specialized medical equipment that may be found in the home of a person with special needs.
8. True or False: It is not necessary to explain procedures to a person with a developmental disability.
9. A shunt can become infected and lead to:
   a. Meningitis
   b. Sepsis
   c. Ventriculitis
   d. All of the above
10. Children with spina bifida are prone to what type of allergy?
11. The _____ diet is used for children with uncontrolled seizures.
12. A _____ may be present in a patient requiring repeated blood testing, frequent intravenous medications, or large quantitites or concentrations of fluids.
13. Patients who cannot eat by mouth for whatever reason may be fed through a/an:
    a. Ileostomy
    b. Colostomy
    c. Gastrostomy
    d. None of the above
14. Two organizations collaborated to produce the *Emergency Information Form for Children with Special Health Care Needs.* Name those organizations.
15. True or False: The patient's wheelchair should be transported with the patient.

Answers to these Review Questions can be found at the end of the book on page 868.

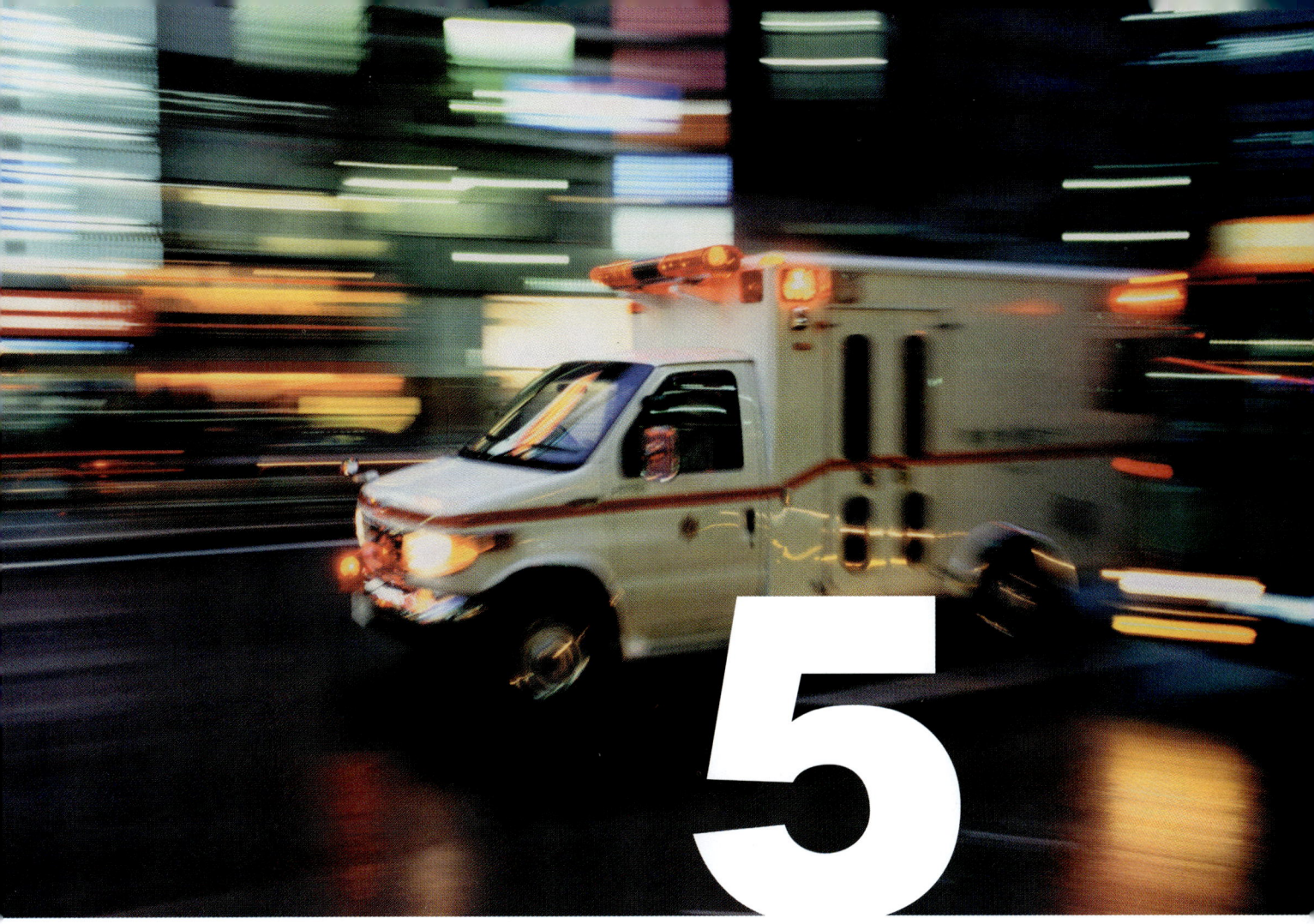

Section Five

EMS Operations

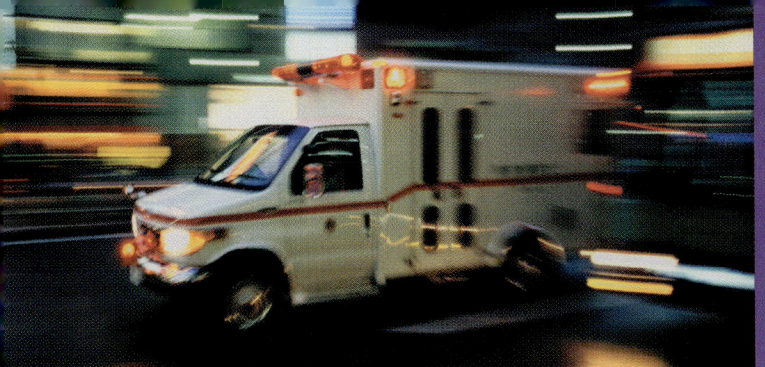

33

Lifting and Moving Patients

Lesson Goal

This chapter provides the basis of the EMT-Basic student's classroom practice and real-life applications. Reviewing and practicing the procedures described in this chapter will minimize the possibility of sustaining a personal injury when lifting and moving patients.

Scenario

It is 18:00 on a cold and rainy evening. You are called to the home of a 77-year-old woman who has fallen in her upstairs bathroom. You find an alert and oriented female with the only complaint being pain in the right hip. The only abnormal findings on examination is rotation and shortening of the right leg and pain in the right hip. Your assessment of the house reveals that the only exit is down the steep and narrow front stairs.

? What devices can you use to move this patient safely and efficiently without causing undue movement? How are you going to package this patient for the move outdoors into the cold and rainy environment? Could advanced life support (ALS) (paramedic) intervention be of use for this patient?

Key Terms to Know

Bent-arm drag
Blanket drag
Clothing drag
Direct ground lift

Emergency move
Extremity lift
Flexible stretcher
Inline drag

Nonurgent moves
One-person stretcher
Portable stretchers
Recovery position

Sheet drag
Time dependent
Two-person stretcher
Urgent move

Learning Objectives

As an EMT-Basic, you should be able to do the following:

DOT

- Define *body mechanics.*
- Discuss guidelines and safety precautions that must be followed when lifting a patient.
- Describe guidelines and safety precautions for carrying patients and equipment.
- Describe the safe lifting of cots and stretchers.
- Describe correct and safe carrying procedures on stairs.
- State the guidelines for reaching, pushing, and pulling.
- Identify seven standard patient carrying devices and their applications.
- State three situations that require the use of an emergency move.
- Discuss one-handed carrying techniques.
- Describe correct reaching for logrolls.
- Discuss the general considerations of moving patients.
- Working with a partner, prepare each of the following devices for use, transfer a patient to the device, properly position the patient on the device, move the device to the ambulance, and load the patient into the ambulance:
  - Wheeled ambulance stretcher
  - Portable ambulance stretcher
  - Stair chair
  - Scoop stretcher
  - Long spine board
  - Basket stretcher
  - Flexible stretcher
- Working with a partner, demonstrate techniques for the transfer of a patient from an ambulance stretcher to a hospital stretcher.

Supplemental

- Describe time-dependent problems as they relate to trauma patients and medical patients.
- Explain why transportation is often the most important intervention in prehospital care.
- List the factors to be considered when assessing the trauma patient for prompt transportation.

Although emergency medical technicians (EMTs) are taught various skills for the treatment of patients in the prehospital setting, including proper lifting and moving techniques, prompt transportation remains one of the most important therapeutic interventions. Most definitive care of emergency patients takes place within the confines of the hospital. Therefore it should be the EMT's goal in most patient encounters to efficiently evaluate, stabilize, and package the patient for transportation. However, the decision making involved in preparing for transportation is one of the most complex issues facing prehospital providers.

Because each patient presents unique and challenging problems, decisions regarding when to transport a patient, how quickly to transport, what lifting or moving technique is safest and most efficacious, and what procedures to perform before transportation can be difficult. Transportation decisions are influenced by various factors that often are not under the control of EMTs. Such factors include access to the patient, scene safety, availability of personnel or other resources, the type of medical problem, and so forth. Although some medical problems are more time-dependent than others, the EMT should make every effort to minimize the total prehospital time without harming the patient or the crew.

Every day thousands of patients are prepared for transportation to a hospital emergency department. During this preparation patients are lifted and moved in the prehospital setting. Unfortunately, many EMTs use improper lifting techniques that can result in a career-ending, lifetime injury. The fact that most of these injuries could have been prevented is distressing.

Various patient conditions and circumstances, such as stairs, elevators, and tight hallways, factor into the decision for patient "packaging." Environmental factors also come into play. In cold climates, ice and snow cause problems with footing. Darkness and rain soaked roads and sidewalks also pose potential for slips and falls. The EMT should select a specific piece of equipment and appropriate lift and carry procedure after considering all of the factors. EMTs have many pieces of equipment available to them for lifting and moving patients. EMTs should select the piece of equipment that will allow him or her to do the job effectively and safely.

Time-Dependent Medical Problems

The treatment of most medical conditions is **time dependent**. To maximize the effectiveness of any treatment, it should be delivered within a certain time frame.

During the initial patient assessment, the EMT must determine what interventions are going to be required for the patient within the on-scene time frames. In the case of a patient who presents in cardiac arrest from an acute myocardial infarction (AMI), it is relatively easy for the EMT to decide to initiate immediate on-scene treatment of cardiopulmonary resuscitation (CPR) and rapid defibrillation. However, the EMT must take extra care when moving the patient to the ambulance and subsequently the emergency department. Because of the patient's condition, the EMT may need to move additional equipment at the same time as the patient. In addition, in the EMT's haste to get the critical patient to more definitive care, he or she may inadvertently skip proper lifting techniques and potentially injure himself or herself or his or her partner.

If an EMT is called to evaluate a patient with an isolated lower-extremity injury that may be either an ankle sprain or a fracture, the need for immediate intervention is not as critical to the long-term survival of the patient at it is for the patient with an AMI. Assuming that the patient has no significant neurovascular damage in the extremities, definitive treatment for this patient will be administered at the hospital and may even be delayed for a few days. Treatment in the field in this case is not time dependent and should be directed toward splinting the extremity for comfort, stabilizing the patient, initiating proper lifting and movement, and safely transporting the patient.

Many other clinical presentations fall between these two extreme examples. No matter what type of patient encounter the EMT is presented with, he or she must make a host of difficult decisions regarding how quickly a patient is transported and what resources will be required to accomplish the movement and transportation effectively. Such a case may involve a patient in a motor vehicle crash (MVC) who has sustained blunt traumatic injuries to a variety of body systems. If the patient is awake and oriented, he or she may complain of neck, chest, and abdominal pain in addition to extremity injuries. Although any of these complaints may be life threatening, it is often difficult in the prehospital setting to determine whether a serious condition exists. If the initial assessment of a patient raises suspicion of a life-threatening scene, the EMT should not spend too much time on the scene and package the patient as quickly and efficiently as possible.

> ✓ Time-dependent medical problems require treatment interventions that must occur within certain time frames. In prehospital care, initiation of care and preparation for transportation must occur within minutes.

Minimization of Risk

The concept of minimizing risk in medicine is not new. Virtually every treatment or intervention that is administered to a patient has an associated risk-benefit ratio. Unfortunately, many of the interventions in prehospital care have not been studied thoroughly. It is unknown whether a basic procedure such as spinal immobilization is clearly beneficial for patients with cervical spine fractures. Although this procedure seems to make sense based on the mechanism of injury, the EMT must also consider the possibility that in some cases it may offer no substantial benefit to patients. This procedure may also increase the patient's chances for further injury to the spine. For example, how much damage to the spinal cord is sustained while logrolling a patient onto a rigid backboard? Are there occasions when a patient is so hemodynamically unstable that the time required to carefully immobilize him or her actually presents a risk to the patient's life?

No easy answers exist to these kinds of questions, and a full discussion of all of the risks and benefits of prehospital treatment procedures is beyond the scope of this chapter. Assuming that no immediate life threats are present on the scene, a good rule of thumb is to perform most treatment while en route to the hospital. The EMT should refer questions regarding when and where to start treatment to local medical direction.

Because on-scene treatment may delay transportation, EMTs must understand potential risks before transportation begins. This same logic can be applied to patient assessment (Figure 33.1). When estimating the risk-benefit ratio of prehospital interventions, it is helpful to know whether the risk of delaying transportation is outweighed by the benefit of performing the intervention on the scene.

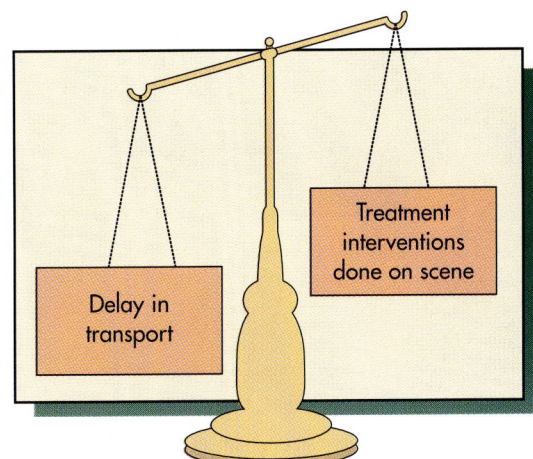

FIGURE 33.1 Weighing the risks of a delay in transportation versus the benefit of treatment interventions performed on the scene.

No matter what decision the EMT reaches when preparing the patient for transportation, he or she must initiate proper lifting and moving techniques and consider the best methods of transportation.

Mechanics of Lifting

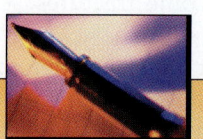

Tips from the Pros

Experienced EMTs agree that the back is the most vulnerable part of the body to the demands of EMS. Youth and strength alone do not prevent back injuries. Lift smart.

The human body is capable of lifting a tremendous amount of weight. EMTs may never be called on to lift several hundred pounds, but they regularly lift patients weighing up to 300 lb (136 kg) as part of their job.

Training and practice are the keys to mastering lifting skills. As the EMT trains, he or she should practice these techniques, keeping the following points in mind:

- Always get as close as possible to the person or piece of equipment that you are going to lift.
- Keep your arms and the weight you are lifting close to your body to create leverage and help maintain your balance.
- Stand with your feet shoulder's width apart, and place one foot slightly in front of the other. This stance provides the best support for lifting.
- Bend at the knees while keeping your back as straight as possible. Practice this simple movement until it begins to feel natural.
- Lift only the stretcher with a partner.
- Place weights or a person on the stretcher in increasing weight increments.
- Be realistic about your progress, and do not expect overnight success. Training takes time.

The EMT should recognize his or her physical abilities and limitations. The EMT should call for backup when it is needed and not attempt to lift a patient who is beyond his or her ability. To do so puts at least three people at risk: the patient, the EMT, and the EMT's partner.

General Guidelines for Safe Lifting

The following are general guidelines for the safe lifting of patients. These guidelines are based on body mechanics and are tried and found to be true by experienced EMS personnel.

1. Consider the weight of the patient together with the weight of the stretcher or other equipment and determine if additional help is needed. Note that some kinds of stretchers weigh up to 50 lb (23 kg) when they are empty.
2. Know your physical ability and limitations. Lifting is easiest when partners are evenly matched in height and ability. However, matching partners of-

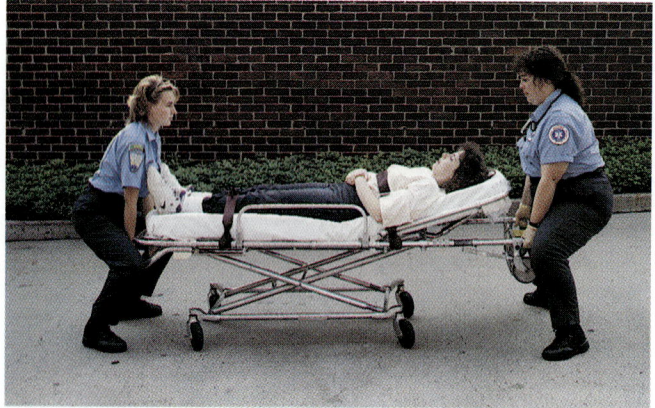

FIGURE 33.2 The power lift or squat lift position. Keep the feet flat and shoulders width apart.

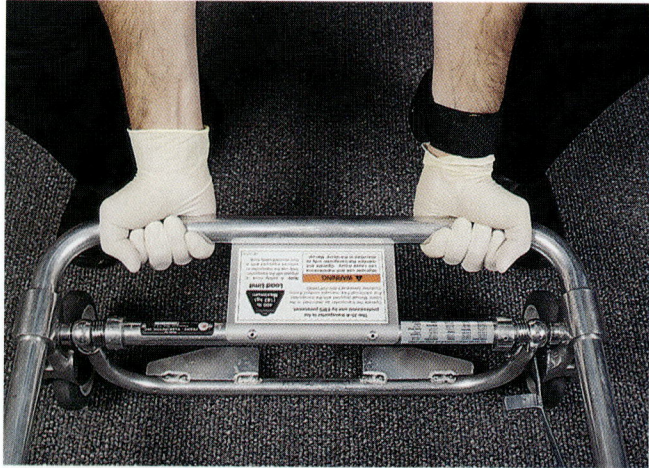

FIGURE 33.3 Hands should be a minimum of 10 inches apart, and palms face up with palm and fingers in complete contact with the stretcher bar.

ten is not possible because schedules and partnerships are based on many other factors. Know your ability and the combined ability with your partner and be realistic. If necessary ask other emergency personnel on the scene, such as firefighters and police officers, for assistance. If absolutely necessary, ask bystanders to help. One team member should always give clear, concise direction. This way all members of the team will act as one unit.

3. Lift without twisting. Avoid any kind of twisting or swinging motions when lifting. Muscles must be used within the range of motion for which they are intended. Twisting is an invitation for injury.

4. Position your feet shoulder's width apart with one foot slightly in front of the other. Wear proper boots that go above the ankle to protect your feet and that help keep a firm footing. Boots should have nonskid soles, good traction, and reinforced toes. As an EMT you will be walking over broken glass, climbing steep terrain, and working in all kinds of weather conditions. Do not minimize the importance of proper footwear.

5. Communicate clearly and frequently with your partner. Communication is the key to efficient moves and transfers of patients. Plan the sequence of a lift or move with your partner. Decide ahead of time the verbal indicators (e.g., "lift on the count of three"), and then use them routinely. Planning communication and sequences in advance is particularly important for new EMTs and when changing partners. As always, remember to communicate with the patient. Tell the patient what you are going to do before you do it. A startled patient may reach out or grab onto something and cause a loss of balance.

> ✓ When lifting, use the legs, not the back. Training and practicing will help in the mastering of lifting skills.

Guidelines for Safe Lifting of Cots and Stretchers

Back injuries caused by improper lifting techniques are among the most common causes of injury and disability for prehospital personnel. Some of these injuries are unavoidable because of the environmental conditions in which the lifting is done. However, the EMT can avoid most of these injuries by keeping the following guidelines in mind:

- If possible, know or find out the weight to be lifted.
- Use a minimum of two people to lift, even if a one-person stretcher is being used.
- Ensure that enough help is available. Use an even number of people to maintain balance during the lift.
- Know the weight limitations of the equipment you use. Know what to do with patients who exceed the weight limitations of the equipment. Be familiar with local protocols.
- Use the power lift or squat lift position. The feet are kept flat and shoulder's width apart. The back is tight, and the abdominal muscles lock the lower back in a slight inward curve. Distribute the weight to the balls of the feet or just behind, keeping both feet fully in contact with the floor. While standing, keep the back locked in because the upper body comes up before the hips (Figure 33.2).
- Use a power grip to get maximum force from the hands. The hands should be positioned a minimum of 10 inches apart. The palms should face up with palms and fingers in complete contact with the stretcher bar (Figure 33.3).
- Lift while keeping your back in the locked-in position (Figure 33.4).
- When lowering the cot or stretcher, reverse the steps.
- Avoid bending at the waist.
- Avoid twisting. "Feed" the stretcher into the ambulance while facing across the patient.

> ✓ When lifting a patient, consider the weight of the patient together with that of the stretcher. Lifting is easiest when lifting partners are equally matched in size and strength. Lift without twisting and with feet positioned properly, and communicate clearly with your partner.

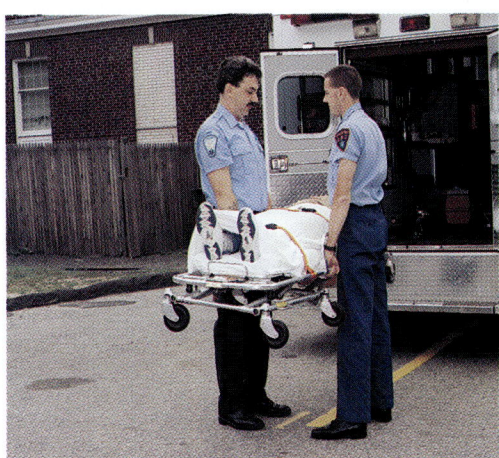

FIGURE 33.4 Lift while keeping the back in a locked-in position.

Guidelines for Carrying Patients and Equipment

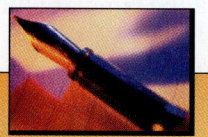

Tips from the Pros

Many EMTs use aids to support their backs. Commercial braces are designed to support the backs of people who do a significant amount of standing or lifting during their work. EMTs use lightweight, yet strong, reinforced fabrics with Velcro closures to supplement their back muscles.

Whenever possible, the EMT should move patients on devices that can be rolled. They should minimize the distance needed to carry patients by planning ahead and remembering the following points:

- Know or find out the weight to be carried.
- Know the limitations of the crew's abilities.
- Work in a coordinated manner and communicate with partners (Figure 33.5).
- Keep the weight as close to your body as possible.
- Keep your back in a locked-in position and refrain from twisting.
- Flex at the hips, not the waist, and bend at the knees.
- Do not hyperextend your back (do not lean back from the waist).
- Whenever possible, partners should have similar height and strength (Figure 33.6).

When carrying equipment by hand, the EMT should try to balance the weight and bulk evenly from side to side. When carrying only one piece of equipment, the EMT should resist the tendency to lean to the side to compensate for the imbalance. The EMT should always try to keep his or her body evenly centered (Figure 33.7).

 Follow the same guidelines for carrying patients and equipment as those provided for lifting patients.

Guidelines for Safe Carrying Procedures on Stairs

Stairs provide a special challenge for EMTs. As always, the EMT should begin to develop a plan with the initial scene survey. Stairs can be steep, have overhangs or narrow footings, and be covered with material that is not secured well. Stairs may have sharp corners or be circular with narrow, triangular treads. If the EMT finds potential problems with the stairs while approaching the patient, he or she should ask if there is another way out. Often the EMT may find that an elevator or an easier way of egress is available. If no other means is available, the EMT should remove all items from a stairway and check it carefully before carrying a patient up or down. The EMT

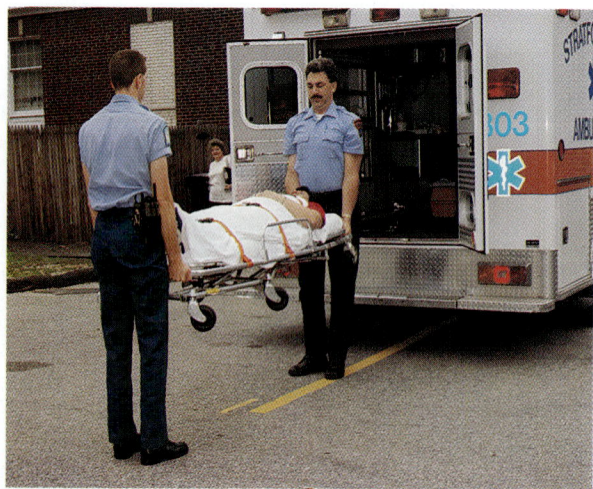

FIGURE 33.5 A patient carried from the end-to-end position.

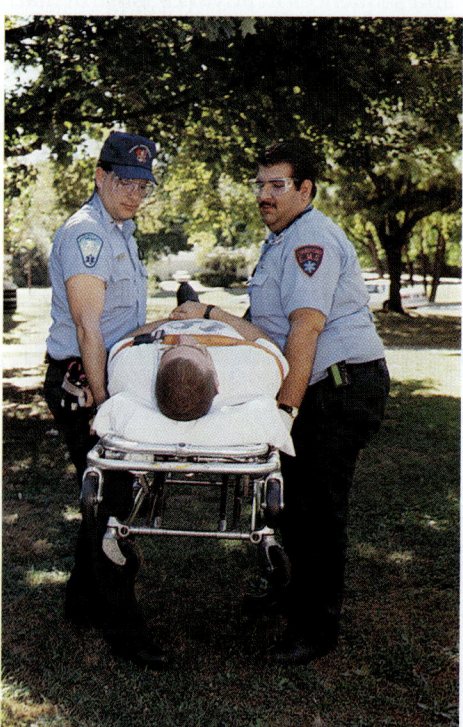

FIGURE 33.6 A patient carried from the side-to-side position.

should try to have other emergency personnel stand behind him or her while backing up, especially if going down stairs. This extra person acts as a guide so that the EMT does not have to twist to look where he or she is going. The guide lets the EMT know how many steps remain and may provide stabilization in the event of a slight loss of balance (Figure 33.8).

One of the most difficult carries that an EMT must perform is to carry a patient backward up a stairway. This carry requires strong quadriceps muscles in the thighs because the legs are doing all of the lifting. If the EMT is required to carry a heavy patient up a stairway, he or she should have two people at the top if the stairway is wide enough to fit both people shoulder to shoulder (Figure 33.9). The EMT should observe the following guidelines when carrying a patient on stairs:

- Always carry patients head first up the stairs and feet first down the stairs. The slant created is most comfortable and least frightening for the patient when using this method. Most equipment is designed for use in this direction.
- When possible, use a stair chair if the patient's condition allows it. If the patient is unable to sit upright or is unconscious, the EMT can use devices such as the scoop stretcher, canvas stretcher, or long backboard (Figure 33.10).
- Keep your back in a locked-in position.
- Flex at the hips, not the waist, and bend at the knees.

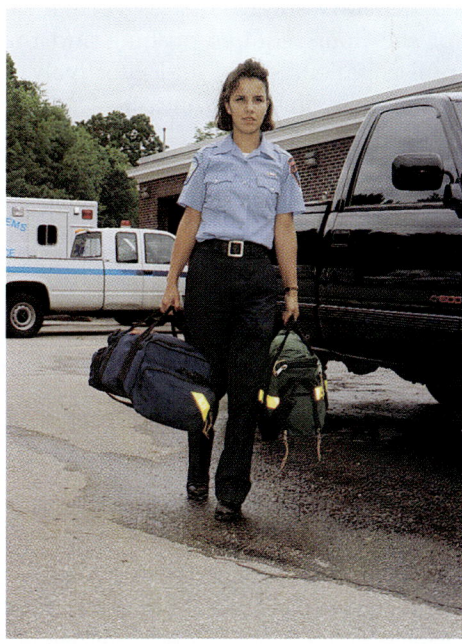

FIGURE 33.7 When carrying equipment by hand, try to balance the weight and bulk evenly from side to side.

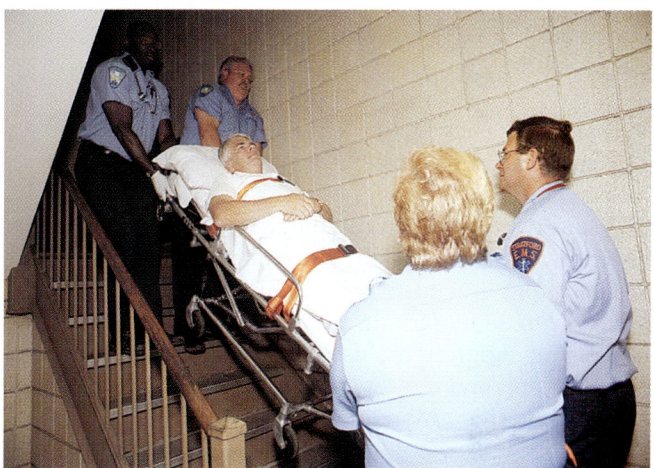

FIGURE 33.9 If you are required to carry a heavy patient up a stairway, it is preferable to have two people at the patient's head.

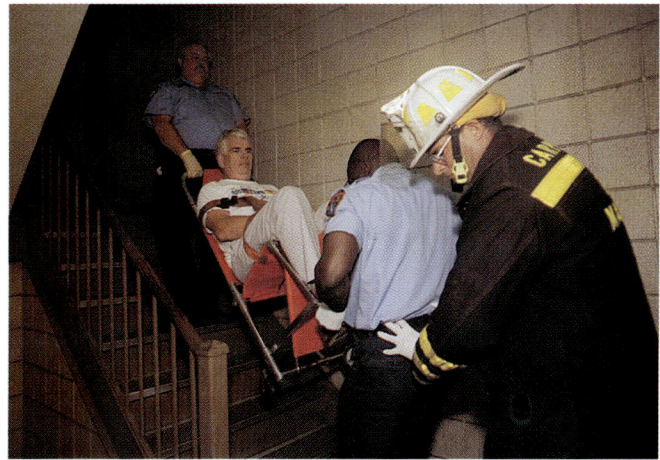

FIGURE 33.8 When moving a patient down stairs, have another EMT or emergency personnel available to act as a guide.

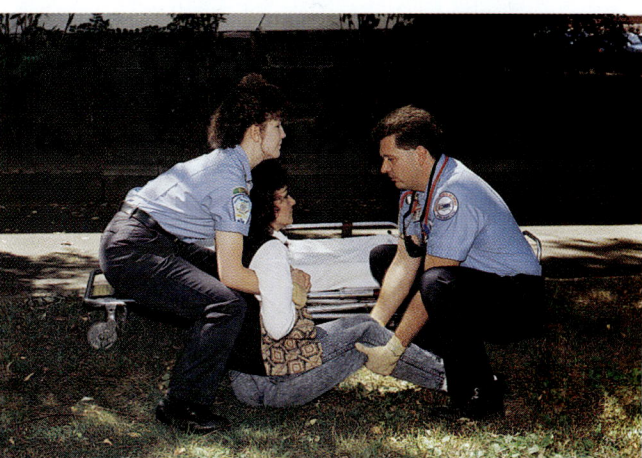

FIGURE 33.10 Extremity lift.

- Keep the weight and your arms as close to your body as possible.
- Instruct the patient not to reach out. This may cause injury to the patient and loss of balance for the EMT.

> ✓ When carrying patients on stairs, the EMT should try to use a stair chair if possible. If one is not available, the EMT should use the extremity lift. Also, if possible, an extra EMT should be available to "spot" the EMT who moves backward on the stairs. Communication between partners is crucial in this carry.

Guidelines for Reaching

Reaching is a common activity; however, reaching for patients is a different matter. The following guidelines will maximize the EMT's reaching ability while minimizing the possibility of injury:

- Keep your back in a locked-in position.
- When reaching overhead, avoid stretching or overreaching.
- Avoid twisting when reaching.
- Keep your back straight when leaning over patients.
- Lean from the hips when reaching.
- Use your shoulder muscles to help with logrolls while reaching. Logrolls are used to turn the patient as a whole unit and are covered in detail in Chapter 24.
- Avoid reaching more than 15 to 20 inches in front of your body.
- Avoid situations requiring reaching and strenuous effort for more than 1 minute to avoid injury.

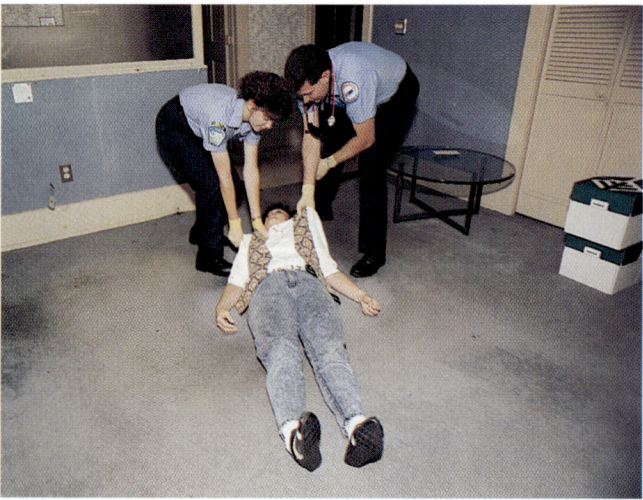

FIGURE 33.11 Clothing drag.

> ✓ Guidelines for reaching include avoiding stretching, overreaching, and twisting; keeping the back straight; leaning from the hips; using shoulder muscles when logrolling; avoiding reaching more than 15 to 20 inches in front of the body; and avoiding prolonged reaches.

Guidelines for Pushing and Pulling

Moving a patient on a surface such as a bed, the front seat of a car, or the floor requires pushing and pulling. To push or pull a patient safely and effectively, the EMT should use the following guidelines:

- Keep your back in a locked-in position.
- Keep your elbows bent with your arms close to your sides.
- Keep the line of pull through the center of your body by bending your knees.
- Keep the weight close to your body.
- Push at a level between your waist and shoulders.
- If the weight is below your waist level, use a kneeling position when practical.
- Avoid pushing and pulling from an overhead position.

> ✓ Guidelines for pushing and pulling include keeping the back locked-in and elbows bent, keeping the line of pull through the center of the body, keeping the weight close to the body, pushing at a level between the waist and shoulders, using a kneeling position when the weight is below the waist level, and avoiding pushing and pulling from an overhead position.

Principles for Moving Patients

All patients need to be moved to transport them to the hospital. Moves are categorized emergency, urgent, or nonurgent.

Emergency Moves

Criteria: The EMT should move the patient immediately with an **emergency move** only when an immediate danger is present to the patient or the EMTs, including the following:

- Fire or danger of fire
- Danger of explosives or other hazardous materials
- Inability to protect the patient from other hazards at the scene
- Further violence erupting on the scene
- Inability to gain access to other patients, in a vehicle or other location, who need lifesaving care
- Inability to provide care because of location or position (e.g., the patient in cardiac arrest who is sitting in a chair or is found between the toilet and bathtub)

When a situation requires an emergency move, the greatest danger to the patient is the possibility of aggravating a spine injury. In an emergency, the EMT should make every effort to pull the patient in the direction of the long axis of the body to provide as much protection to the spine as possible. If the situation is an MVC, this ideal cannot be met. It is impossible to remove a patient from a vehicle rapidly while providing as much protection to the spine as possible using spinal precautions and immobilization devices. The EMT should only move a patient in this manner when immediate danger exists. To move a patient needlessly may cause the patient a lifetime of paralysis.

If the patient is on the floor or ground, the EMT can use an **inline drag** to pull the person to safety. The most common inline drags include the **clothing drag**, **sheet drag**, **blanket drag**, and **bent-arm drag**.

Clothing Drag

If the patient is wearing a shirt, jacket, or other article of clothing on his or her upper body, the EMT can use it to support the patient's neck and head while pulling the body (Figure 33.11). The EMT should take the following steps to perform a clothing drag:

1. Tie the patient's wrists together if you have something readily available, such as a triangular bandage, gauze wrap, or strips of cloth. If no such material is handy, tuck the patient's hands into his or her waistband to prevent the arms from being pulled upward.
2. Clutch the patient's clothing on both sides of the neck to form a support for the head.
3. Pull the patient toward you as you back up, watching the patient at all times. Be careful not to strangle the patient. Concentrate the pulling force under the armpits, not the neck.

Sheet Drag

A sheet, large towel, or some articles of clothing can be used to create a harness for pulling the patient. The EMT should take the following steps to perform a sheet drag:

1. Fold or twist a sheet or large towel lengthwise.
2. Place the narrowed sheet across the patient's chest at the level of the armpits.
3. Tuck the sheet ends under the armpits and behind the patient's head.
4. Grasp the two ends behind the patient's head to form a support and a means for pulling.
5. Pull the patient toward you while observing the patient at all times.

Blanket Drag

The blanket drag is an easy way for one person to move a patient to safety. It is the most effective drag for moving the patient more than just a few feet (Figure 33.12). The EMT should take the following steps to perform a blanket drag:

1. Lay a blanket lengthwise beside the patient.
2. Kneel on the opposite side of the patient and roll him or her toward you.
3. As the patient lies on his or her side while resting against you, reach across and grasp the blanket.
4. Tightly tuck half of the blanket lengthwise under the patient and leave the other half lying flat.
5. Gently roll the patient onto his or her back.
6. Pull the tucked portion of the blanket out from under the patient and wrap it around his or her body.

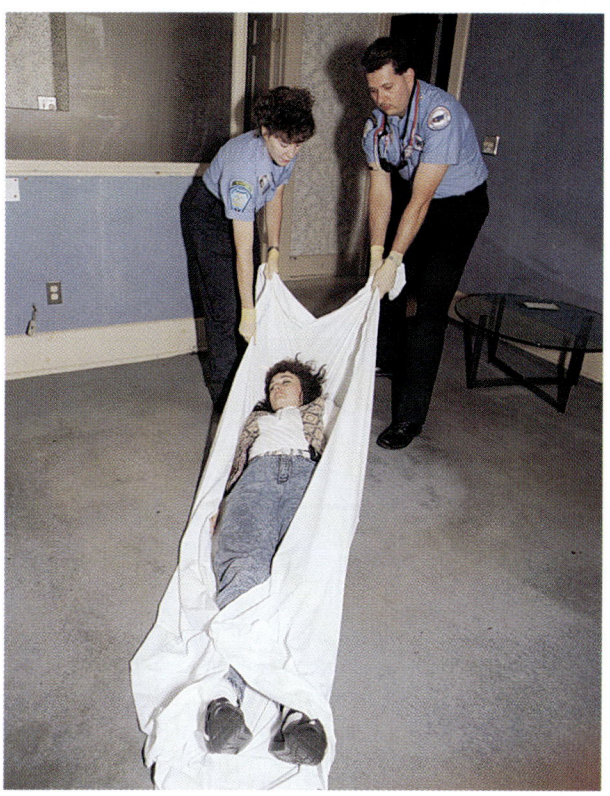

FIGURE 33.12 Blanket drag.

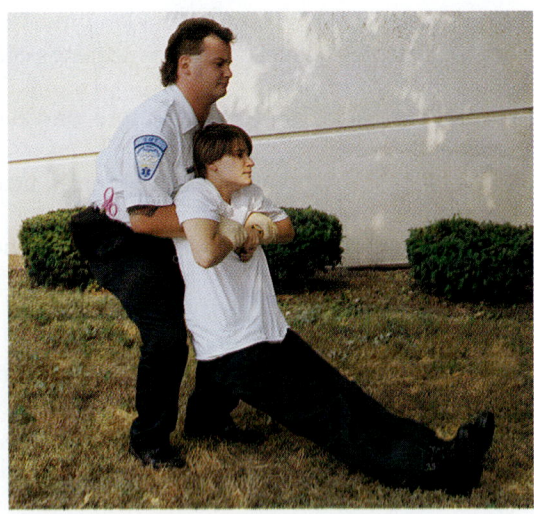

FIGURE 33.13 Bent-arm drag.

7. Grasp the blanket under the patient's head to form a support and a means for pulling.
8. Pull while backing up and while observing the patient at all times.

Bent-Arm Drag

The bent-arm drag is the most rapidly executed drag because it does not require additional supplies. The EMT should take the following steps to perform a bent-arm drag:

1. Reach under the patient's armpits from behind and grasp his or her forearms or wrists, depending on your hand size.
2. Use your arms as a cradle for the patient's head and keep the arms locked in a bent position by your grasp.
3. Drag the patient toward you as you walk backward, observing the patient at all times (Figure 33.13).

> ✔ Emergency moves are those that move a patient out of immediate danger. These moves include in-line drags such as the clothing drag, sheet drag, blanket drag, and bent-arm drag.

Urgent Moves

Criteria: Sometimes the EMT must move a patient more quickly than usual for reasons of an urgent nature. Examples include extreme weather conditions, hostile or interfering bystanders, or environmental conditions such as rapidly rising water. Factors at the scene that the EMT determines to be contributing or may contribute to a decline in the patient's status or risk to the EMTs justify the use of an **urgent move**.

> ✔ Urgent moves are those that move a patient more quickly than usual for reasons of an urgent nature, such as extreme weather conditions or hostile bystanders. Rapid extrication is considered an urgent move.

Nonurgent Moves

Criteria: Most moves required for patients are **nonurgent moves**. After ensuring scene safety, assessing the patient, completing necessary intervention, and deciding to transport, the EMT needs to determine the best way to make the move. The EMT bases his or her decision on the patient's illness or injury, factors at the scene, and resources available, including equipment and personnel.

Extremity Lift

The EMT should only use the **extremity lift** when he or she does not suspect a spinal injury. The EMT bears more weight at the head of the patient during this move. The extremity lift is best used for short distances (Figure 33.14). The EMT should take the following steps to perform an extremity lift:

1. One EMT kneels at the patient's head, and the other EMT kneels at the patient's side by the knees.
2. The EMT at the head reaches under the patient's arms at the shoulders and grasps the patient's wrists. If the patient is unresponsive or uncooperative, the other EMT may assist by lifting the patient's wrists to within the reach of the partner. You may achieve additional stability by grasping the patient's left wrist with your right hand and the patient's right wrist with your left hand. In other words, the patient's arms become crossed over the chest, creating a more secure hold with less give.
3. The second EMT reaches under both knees with one arm and under the buttocks with the other arm.
4. The EMTs rise to a crouching position, then simultaneously stand and move with the patient to the stretcher.

Direct Ground Lift

The **direct ground lift** is only used for the patient who does not have a suspected spine injury. However, it is helpful to use a backboard for this patient without the associated spinal precautions. The EMT should take the following steps to perform a direct ground lift (see the Direct Ground Lift Step-by-Step Procedure at the end of this chapter):

1. Two or three EMTs line up on the same side of a supine patient.
2. The EMTs all kneel on one knee (preferably all right or all left).

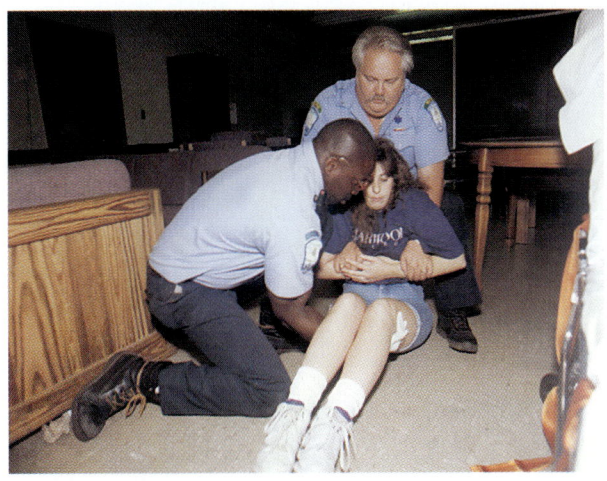 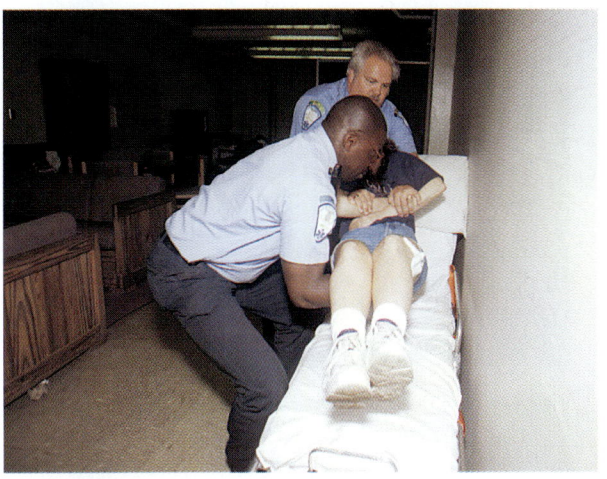

FIGURE 33.14 Extremity lift. **A,** One EMT kneels at the patient's head, and the second EMT kneels at the patient's side by the knees. The EMT at the head reaches under the patient's arms at the shoulders and grasps the patient's wrists. The second EMT reaches under both the patient's knees with one arm and under the patient's buttocks with the other arm. **B,** The EMTs rise to a crouching position, then simultaneously stand and move with the patient to the stretcher.

3. The patient's arms are crossed on the chest if injuries do not prevent it.
4. The EMT at the head places one arm under the patient's head and shoulders, cradling the head. The EMT places the other arm under the patient's lower back.
5. The second EMT places one arm directly below the first EMT's arm in the small of the patient's back. The second EMT places the second arm under the patient's knees.
6. If a third EMT is available, this EMT slides both arms under the patient's waist. The other EMTs adjust their arms slightly higher and lower accordingly.
7. On signal, the EMTs lift the patient to their knees and roll the patient in toward their chests.
8. On signal, the EMTs stand and move the patient to the stretcher.
9. On signal, the EMTs lower the patient onto the stretcher, which has been positioned at waist level.

Transfer of Supine Patient from Bed to Stretcher

The most common ways of moving a patient from a bed to a stretcher are the direct carry and the draw sheet methods.

Direct carry

The EMT should take the following steps to perform a direct carry:

1. Position the stretcher at a right angle to the patient's bed with the head end of the stretcher at the foot of the bed.
2. Prepare the stretcher by unbuckling the straps, removing other items, and lowering the closest railing.
3. Both EMTs stand between the stretcher and the bed, facing the patient.
4. The EMT at the head of the stretcher slides one arm under the patient's neck and shoulders, cupping the far shoulder with his or her hand and cradling the head.
5. The second EMT slides one arm under the small (lumbar) portion of the patient's back, slides the arm under the buttocks (toward the hips), and lifts slightly to allow the first EMT to slide an arm under the waist.
6. The second EMT reaches under the patient's lower legs.
7. The EMTs pull the patient to the edge of the bed, then lift and curl the patient toward their chests.
8. The EMTs rotate to be inline with the stretcher, then place the patient onto it gently (Figure 33.15).

Draw sheet method

The EMT should take the following steps to perform the draw sheet method:

1. Loosen the bottom sheet, or draw sheet, on the patient's bed.
2. Prepare the stretcher, adjusting it to a height equal to the bed, lowering both rails, unbuckling the straps, and removing all items on it.
3. Position the stretcher directly beside and touching the bed.
4. The EMTs position themselves on each side of the patient.

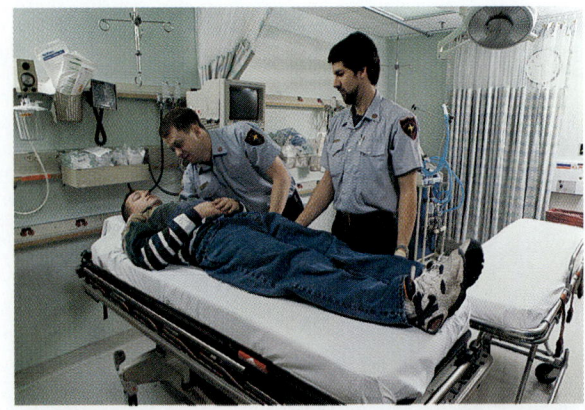 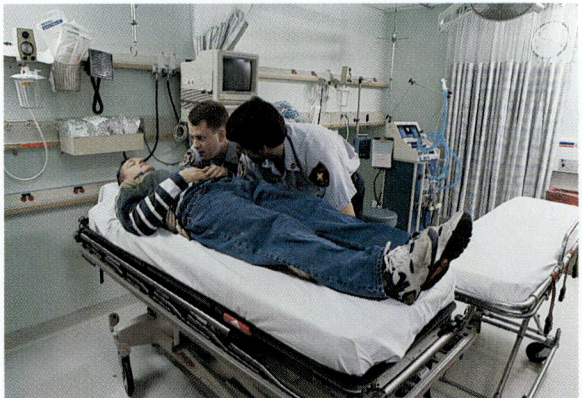
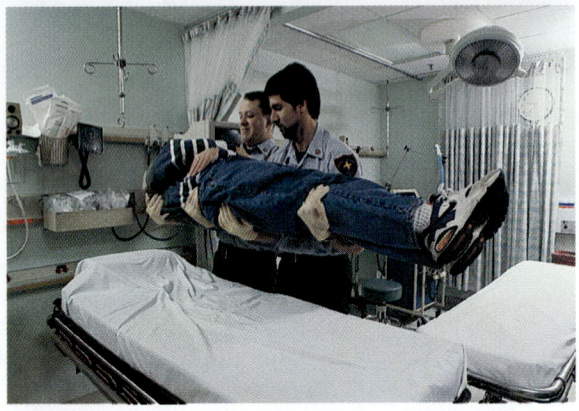 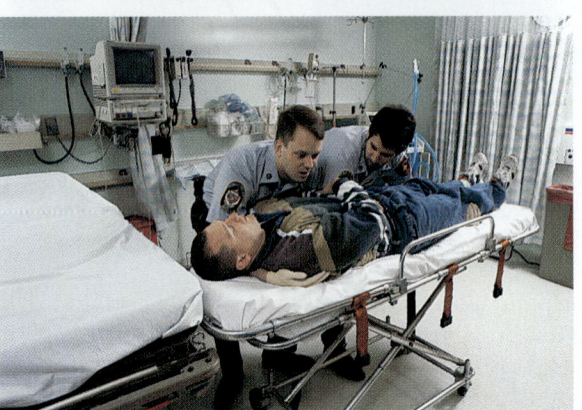

FIGURE 33.15 Direct carry. **A,** The stretcher is positioned perpendicular to the patient's bed with the head of stretcher at the foot of the bed. The EMT at the patient's head slides one arm under the patient's neck and shoulders, cupping the far shoulder with his or her hand and cradling the patient's head. **B,** The second EMT slides one arm under the lumbar portion of the patient's back, slides toward the patient's hips, and lifts slightly to allow the first EMT to slide an arm under the patient's waist. The second EMT reaches under the patient's lower legs. **C,** The patient is pulled to the edge of the bed, then lifted and curled toward the EMT's chest. **D,** The EMTs rotate perpendicularly to be in line with the stretcher, then place the patient gently onto it.

5. Slide the patient gently across and onto the stretcher. If additional emergency personnel are available, they may give assistance by lifting the patient's lower extremities.

✓ Nonurgent moves include the extremity lift, direct ground lift, and transfer of supine patients from a bed to a stretcher (direct carry and draw sheet methods).

Equipment for Moving Patients

Wheeled Stretcher

The piece of equipment that EMTs use most often for moving patients is the wheeled stretcher. Most ambulance stretchers weigh 60 to 80 lb (27 to 36 kg) and are made to hold patients weighing up to 400 lb (182 kg) (Figure 33.16).

The two basic types of ambulance stretchers used in North America are the **two-person stretcher**, which requires two EMTs to lift the stretcher from each side when loading and unloading from the ambulance, and the **one-person stretcher**, which has special loading wheels at the head to allow it to be rolled in and out of the ambulance by one person if needed. The advantage of the one-person stretcher is that the EMT can roll it instead of lifting it into the ambulance. Most stretchers allow for height adjustment to facilitate patient transfers to and from beds. The head can be adjusted to several angles, from completely flat to 90 degrees for the upright patient. Some stretchers allow for elevation of the legs or knees or for the shock (Trendelenburg) position. Additional pieces of equipment can be attached to the stretcher for carrying oxygen, intravenous lines, and cardiac monitors or defibrillators. The EMT must be familiar with the manufacturer's specifications for the stretchers that he or she is using. Before an EMT starts working with a new type of stretcher, he or she must practice loading and unloading the stretcher to become efficient in its operation. The EMT should look for the location of the operating levers on the stretcher and be comfortable using the stretcher. The scene of the emergency is no time to learn its operation.

Guidelines for Moving the Wheeled Stretcher

The EMT can accomplish patient safety and smooth movement of the stretcher by practicing the following guidelines:

- Always handle the stretcher with a minimum of two team members who preferably have both hands on the stretcher. Ask other emergency personnel or bystanders for assistance in carrying equipment to enable you and your partner to focus on moving the stretcher and observing the patient.
- Never leave the patient alone on the stretcher. An unattended patient may roll to one side of the stretcher, causing it to overturn.
- The foot of the stretcher should go first, except when loading the patient into the ambulance or going up stairs.
- When rolling the stretcher along the floor or ground, position one EMT at each end of the stretcher. The EMT at the foot pulls while the EMT at the head pushes and guides.
- While rolling the stretcher, always maintain a firm grip to prevent it from tipping if a wheel catches a crack or bump.
- On rough ground it may be necessary to carry the stretcher end to end while facing one another. In this situation, the stretcher should be lowered before beginning the carry.
- On extremely rough terrain, it is safer and more stable to use four EMTs with one at each corner of the stretcher.
- Roll the stretcher at a safe and smooth pace.
- Turn corners slowly and squarely, avoiding sideways movement of the stretcher that might cause the patient to become dizzy. If you encounter tight corners, it may be necessary to elevate the head of the stretcher and push in the grab bar. This will shorten the length of the stretcher and allow a tighter turning radius.
- Lift the stretcher over rugs, grates, door jambs, and other such articles on the floor or ground.
- Secure the patient with the stretcher belts at all times whether the stretcher is moving or stationary.
- Recognize that not all stretchers are interchangeable. A stretcher from one ambulance may not fit into another.

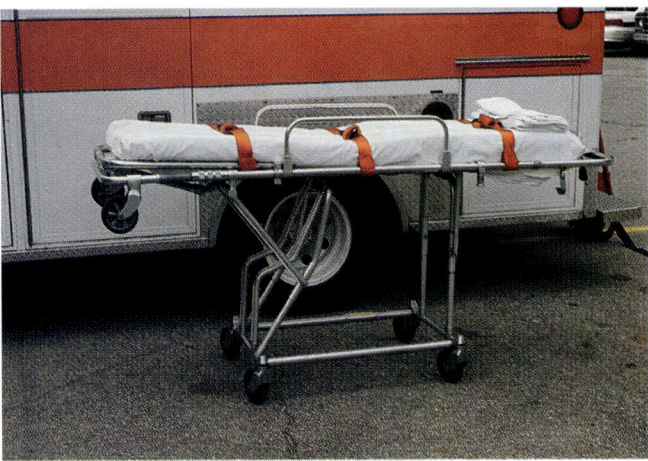

FIGURE 33.16 Wheeled stretcher.

- Load portable stretchers before the wheeled stretcher. This can easily be done by placing the portable stretcher on the wheeled stretcher. Then load the wheeled stretcher into the ambulance. Once inside the ambulance, move the portable stretcher onto the squad bench and secure it. Then remove the wheeled stretcher so that another patient can be placed on the main stretcher. As a general rule, the more stable patient is placed on the squad bench and the more critical on the main stretcher.
- Ensure that all patients and stretchers are secure before moving the ambulance.

Loading the Two-Person Stretcher into an Ambulance

Loading and unloading the stretcher into the ambulance is a prime time for injury to occur to the EMT. By working together and following the steps as outlined, EMTs are able to avoid preventable strain to themselves:

1. Place the head of stretcher close to the bumper of the ambulance, and make certain that it is locked at the lowest level.
2. The EMTs should stand on opposite sides of the stretcher, bend at the knees while keeping their backs straight, and grasp the lowest bar of the stretcher.
3. Hands are positioned at each end of the lowest bar with both palms facing up.
4. On signal, both EMTs stand and move toward the rear of the ambulance until the front wheels rest on the floor at the back of the ambulance.
5. Roll the stretcher forward and guide it into the front of the stretcher catch. Lock the foot of the stretcher into place.

Loading the One-Person Stretcher into an Ambulance

See the One-Person Stretcher Step-by-Step Procedure at the end of this chapter.

1. With the stretcher in the highest position, place the head into the rear of the ambulance.
2. One EMT lifts the head of the stretcher, causing the wheels on the head of the stretcher to contact the floor of the ambulance.
3. The second EMT ensures that the safety catch on the head of the stretcher engages with the hook on the floor of the ambulance.
4. The second EMT instructs the EMT at the foot of the stretcher to pull the wheel adjustment lever on the left foot of the stretcher.
5. The second EMT lifts the wheels of the stretcher, and the EMT at the foot rolls it forward into the ambulance. Secure the stretcher to the ambulance.

Unloading the Two-Person Stretcher from an Ambulance

1. Unlock the latch at the foot of the stretcher catch and pull the stretcher until the rear wheels are at the end of the floor.
2. Grasp the lowest bar on each side of the stretcher with your palms facing upward as it is rolled out.
3a. Once the head of the stretcher is clear of the ambulance, keep the stretcher level and lower it to the ground by bending at the knees while keeping the back straight. The stretcher then can be raised from the same side-to-side position or from end to end by triggering the appropriate release handle and lifting on the main stretcher bar (Figure 33.17).
3b. *Alternative.* Once the head of the stretcher is level and clear of the ambulance, the driver's side EMT triggers the handle release and the base of the stretcher is allowed to "slide" down the legs of

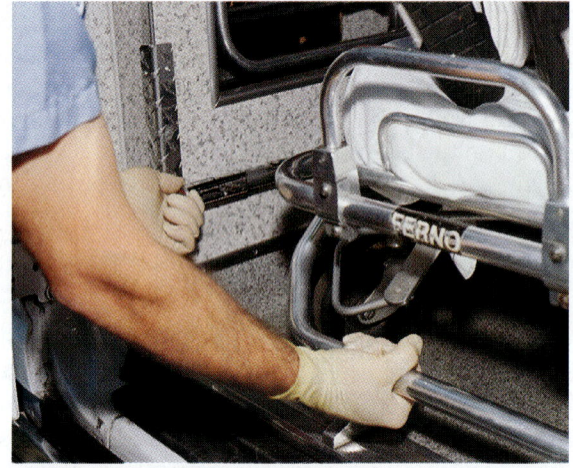
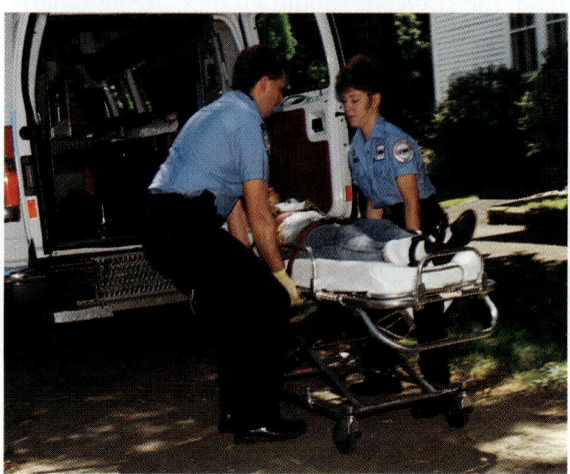
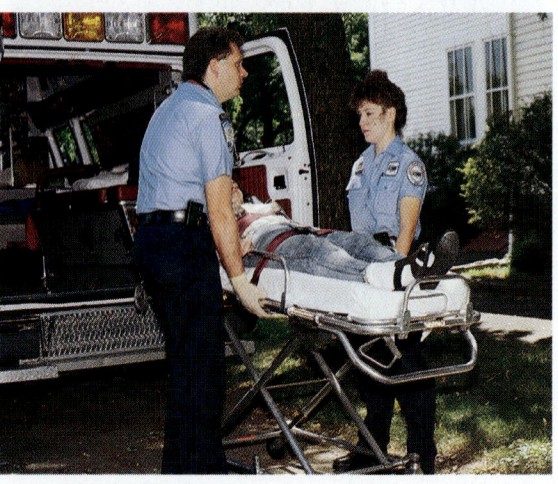

FIGURE 33.17 Two-person stretcher. **A,** Unlock the latch at the foot of the stretcher catch and pull the stretcher until the rear wheels are at the end of the floor. **B,** Grasp the lowest bar on each side of the stretcher with the palms facing upward as it is rolled out. Once the head of the stretcher is clear, keep the stretcher level and lower it to the ground by bending at the knees (keeping the back straight). The stretcher may then be raised from the side-to-side position or from end to end by activating the appropriate release handle and lifting on the main stretcher bar. **C,** *Alternative*: Once the head of the stretcher is level and clear of the ambulance, the EMT on the driver's side triggers the handle release and the base of the stretcher is allowed to "slide" down the legs of the EMTs. This alternative method avoids the extra lift from the ground but requires the use of the main stretcher bar for lifting and simultaneous release of the handle.

the EMTs. This alternative avoids the extra lift from the ground but requires the use of the main stretcher bar for lifting and simultaneous release of the handle.

Unloading the One-Person Stretcher from an Ambulance

1. Position yourself at the foot of the stretcher. Disengage the floor mount, freeing the stretcher from the ambulance.
2. Pull out on the stretcher while lifting up slightly on the foot of the stretcher. This will engage the wheels on the head of the stretcher.
3. Pull the stretcher out until the safety catch is engaged. Pull the wheel lever and lower the wheels.
4. The second EMT then disengages the safety catch once the wheels are securely down.

> ✓ The wheeled stretcher can either be a one- or two-person stretcher. EMTs should learn and practice guidelines for moving, loading, and unloading these stretchers.

Portable Stretcher

Portable stretchers are sometimes referred to as "folding stretchers." These stretchers weigh 8 to 15 lb (3.5 to 7 kg) and have a load capacity of 350 lb (159 kg). The portable stretcher is usually folded for storage. They are less bulky than the wheeled stretchers and are more easily used for carrying patients down stairs, downhill, or over rough terrain (Figure 33.18).

The portable stretcher is also used in multiple casualty situations. Once the EMTs load the patient onto it, they can suspend the portable stretcher from the ceiling of the ambulance by using special brackets, but more commonly it is secured to the squad bench. The EMTs carry the portable stretcher end to end and can load it into the ambulance this way or from side to side.

> ✓ Portable, or folding, stretchers are used most often in multiple casualty incidents. They are carried end to end and loaded in this manner or from side to side.

Stair Chair

Stair chairs are designed for patients who can assume a sitting position while being carried from a residence or scene to the ambulance. The EMT must not use stair chairs for patients who are unresponsive, who have possible spine injuries, or who can not sit upright. Stair chairs are most useful for taking patients up or down stairs, through narrow halls or doorways, or into small elevators. The EMT may also use them to move patients in narrow aisles in airplanes or buses. This piece of equipment is not meant for transporting the patient, so the EMT must transfer the patient to the main stretcher after arriving at the ambulance (Figure 33.19).

The EMT uses the extremity lift to place the patient onto the stair chair. The EMT secures all belts and straps and instructs the patient to cross the arms over the chest and not reach out. If the patient is disoriented, the EMT can loosely tie the wrists to prevent the patient from grabbing onto fixtures and causing the EMT to lose balance. The EMT then tilts the stair chair slightly backward to allow movement along the floor by the weight of the chair and the patient resting on the wheels. An additional EMT or other emergency personnel should guide the EMTs when going down stairs as described previously in this chapter.

> ✓ EMTs use the stair chair to carry patients on stairs. EMTs use the extremity lift to place the patient into the chair. EMTs should use stair chairs only for patients who can safely assume a sitting position.

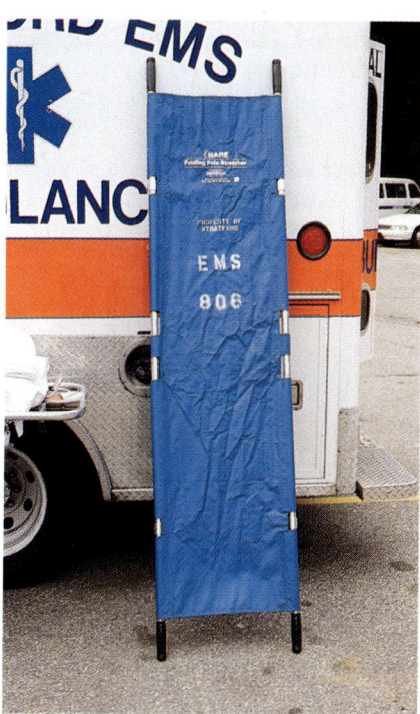

FIGURE 33.18 Portable stretcher.

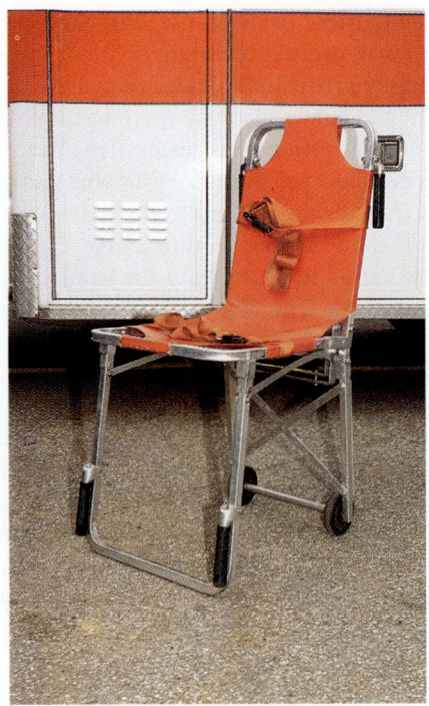

FIGURE 33.19 Stair chair.

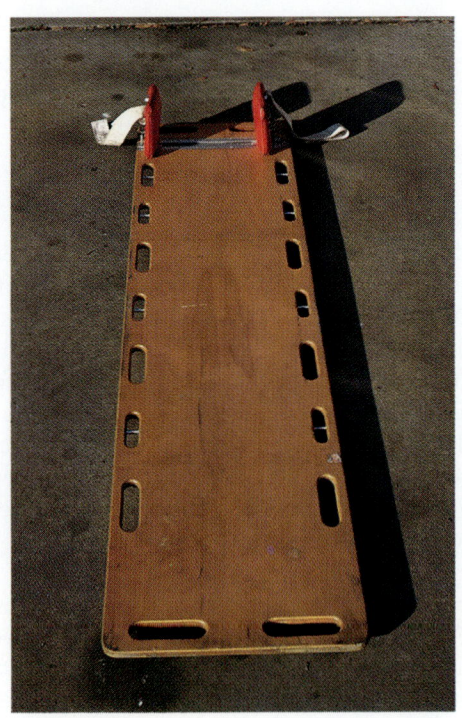

FIGURE 33.21 Miller backboard.

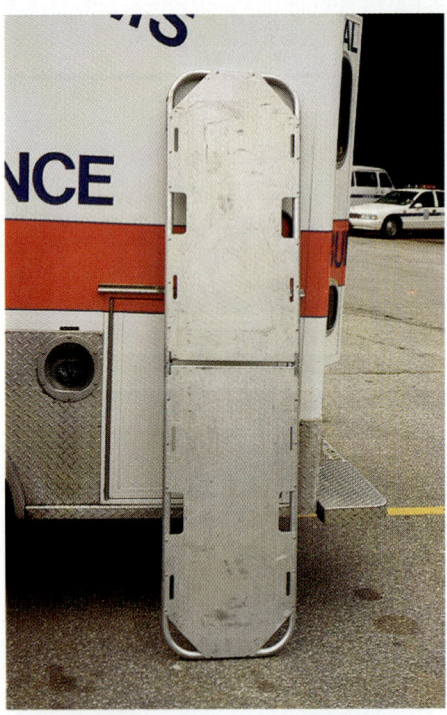

FIGURE 33.20 Aluminum backboard.

Long Backboard

Many styles of backboards are available (Figures 33.20 to 33.22). The Ohio style is coffin-shaped to easily fit into a basket stretcher or helicopter. The Farrington style is rectangular with rounded corners. Some services use aluminum backboards because of their ability to fold in half and store easily. Disadvantages of an aluminum backboard are that it conducts cold to the patient in cold climates and it makes x-ray examination difficult. Many manufacturers make backboards from molded plastic for durability and easier decontamination of body fluids. The vacuum backboard or mattress molds to the patient once the patient is positioned on it.

Whichever style of backboard is used, it is a invaluable tool for moving patients. The backboard's uses include the following:

- Immobilizing the spine of a patient suspected of having a spinal injury
- Moving patients
- Removing the patient from a vehicle during rapid extrication
- Providing secondary support when a short spineboard is used

The procedures for positioning and securing a patient on the long backboard are covered in Chapter 24.

✓ The long backboard is used for immobilizing the spine, moving patients, and providing secondary support when a short backboard is used.

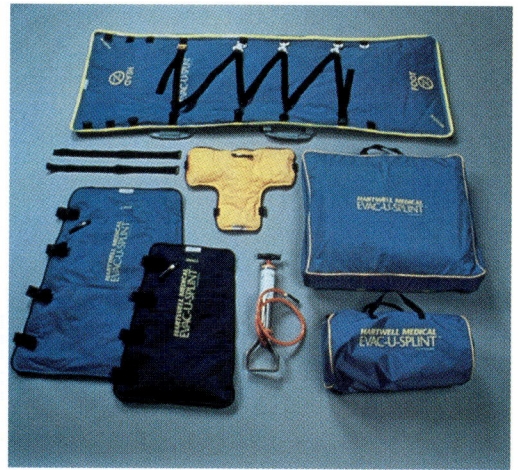
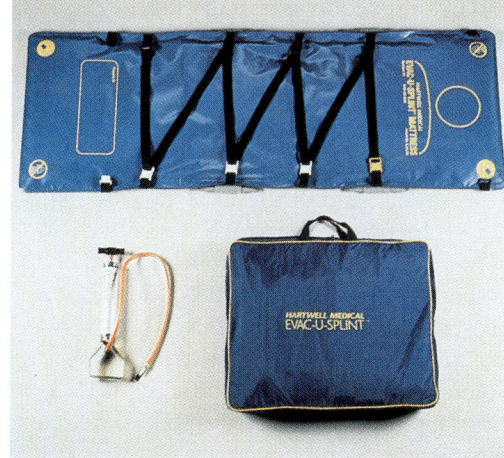

FIGURE 33.22 Vacuum backboard.

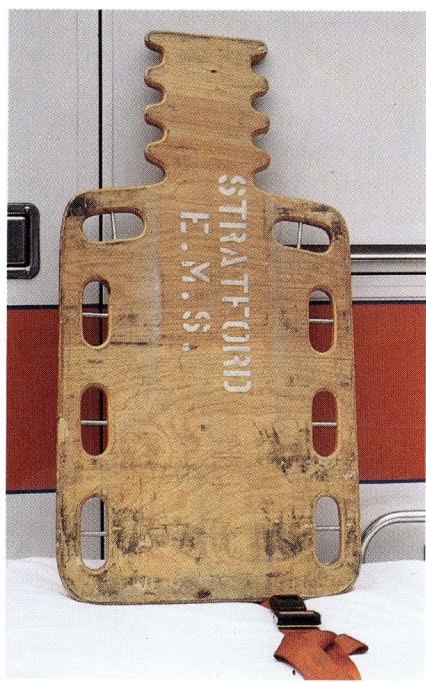

FIGURE 33.23 Wooden short backboard.

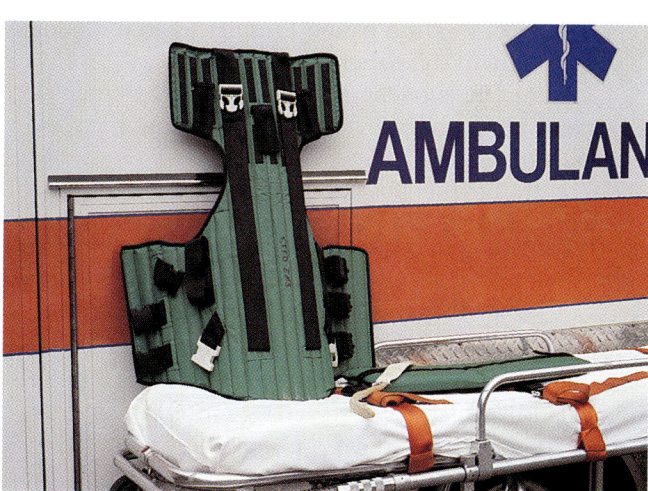

FIGURE 33.24 Vest style short backboard.

 Short backboards are used for immobilizing the spine of a patient found in a sitting position.

Short Backboard

A short backboard is used to immobilize a patient with a suspected spinal injury who is found in a sitting position. Short backboards may be made from wood, aluminum, or plastic (Figure 33.23). Another common type of short backboard is the vest style (Figure 33.24). This style wraps around the patient and has all of the straps attached or enclosed. The vest style is especially useful when a patient is found in a compact or sports car.

The procedures for positioning and securing a patient on a short backboard are covered in Chapter 24.

Scoop (Orthopedic) Stretcher

The scoop stretcher is specially designed to easily lift supine patients. The stretcher is made of aluminum tubing with V-shaped lifts to "scoop" patients from the floor or ground without changing their position. The greatest advantage of the scoop is that it can be used in confined spaces where other stretchers cannot fit. Another use of the scoop stretcher is for isolated hip and pelvic injuries. By design the EMT applies the scoop stretcher with minimal patient movement, limiting pain to the patient. Unlike the long backboard, the scoop stretcher provides lateral support to the hip and pelvic area.

The EMT can use the scoop to initially lift the patient with a suspected spinal injury from the ground or floor; however, it cannot provide full spinal immobilization. For this reason the EMT should place the patient on a long backboard for full immobilization. Experienced EMTs often prefer to logroll the patient directly onto the long backboard to save a step. If the EMT does not suspect a spinal injury, he or she can place the patient and scoop onto the stretcher for transportation, and the scoop can be used at the hospital to move the patient onto a bed. Both the logroll and the scoop allow some movement of the spine, so the EMT should use them with great caution in any patient with suspected spinal injury.

The following steps describe the use a scoop stretcher (see the Scoop Stretcher Step-by-Step Procedure at the end of this chapter):

1. Adjust the length of the scoop stretcher on the ground beside the patient. Adjust to accommodate the height of the patient.
2. Separate the stretcher halves and place one half on each side of the patient. Do not lift equipment over the patient.
3. Slightly lift the clothing on one side of the patient while another EMT slides one half of the scoop under the patient's side. Repeat on the other side. If a spinal injury is suspected, another EMT must maintain cervical spine control at all times.
4. Lock the head of the scoop in place, then bring the foot together until the assembly is locked. If any resistance is met, have an EMT gently lift one side of the patient. This move prevents the patient's clothing from being caught or his or her skin from being pinched. Scoop stretchers are especially useful in patients with suspected hip and pelvic injuries.
5. Attach the padded head support strap if so equipped.
6. Use at least three straps to secure the patient to the scoop stretcher before lifting.

 Scoop stretchers are used to easily lift supine patients.

Flexible Stretcher

The **flexible stretcher**, or pole stretcher (Figure 33.25), is designed for the following situations:

- When space is limited to access the patient
- On stairs or around cramped corners
- When there is a shortage of other available equipment

The EMT should not use the flexible stretcher for patients with suspected spinal injury because they do not provide the support necessary to immobilize the spine. As their name indicates, these stretchers are flexible and lightweight and are able to be stored in a small space.

Equipment Maintenance

All of the equipment presented in this chapter for patient lifting and moving comes with manufacturer's instructions. The EMT should review the instructions carefully for

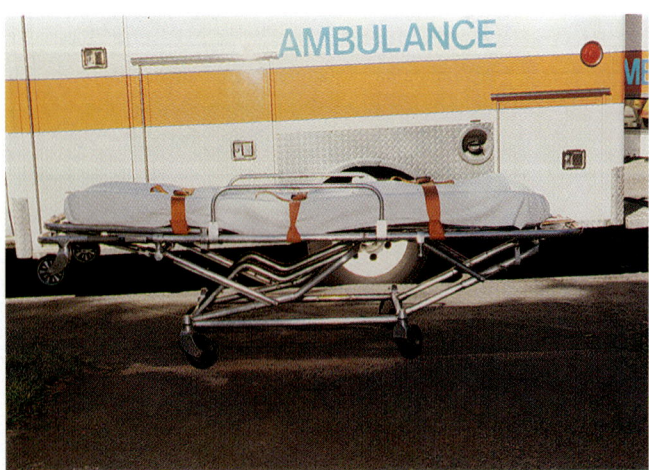

FIGURE 33.25 Flexible style stretcher.

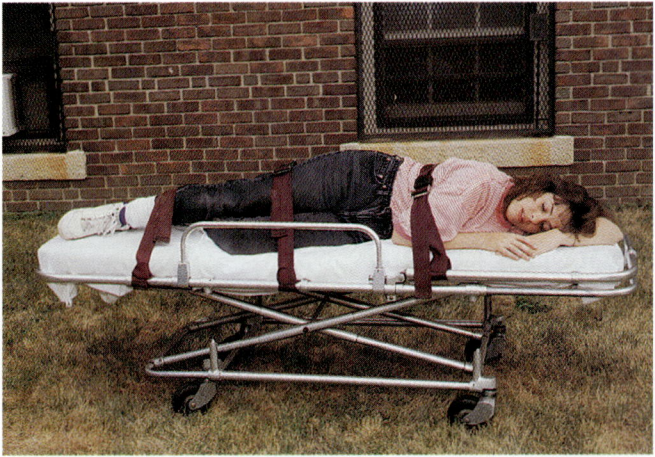

FIGURE 33.26 An unresponsive patient without suspected spinal injury should be placed in the recovery position on his or her left side.

operation, cleaning, inspection, repair, and maintenance. Many services have dedicated personnel responsible for equipment preventive maintenance, but the EMT must check the equipment at the beginning of every shift. If the EMT finds a piece of equipment to be in need of repair, he or she must bring it to the supervisor's attention. There is nothing more unprofessional or potentially life threatening to the patient than to arrive on scene with missing or broken equipment. The EMT should take time to ensure that the equipment is clean and functioning correctly.

Patient Positioning

This chapters has introduced several devices and pieces of equipment for lifting and moving patients. The EMT must consider which piece of equipment to select and how to position the patient based on his or her condition. Subsequent chapters in this text cover specific positioning techniques as part of the care for patients with various conditions. The following general rules apply:

1. The EMT should place unresponsive patients without suspected spinal injury in the **recovery position** on their left side (Figure 33.26). The left side is preferred when transporting by ambulance because the patient then faces the EMT who is caring for him or her. The recovery position keeps the patient on his or her side by positioning the arms and legs for support and balance.
2. The EMT should never walk the patient with chest pain, chest discomfort, or difficulty breathing to the ambulance. The EMT should always move a patient with these signs and symptoms on a stretcher. Once in the ambulance, the EMT should elevate the head of the stretcher to a comfortable position.
3. The EMT must fully immobilize a patient with a suspected spinal injury on a long backboard and transport the patient flat on the stretcher.
4. The EMT may elevate the legs of a patient with the signs and symptoms of shock 8 to12 inches.
5. An early intervention for the pregnant patient with hypotension (low blood pressure) is to place the patient on her left side.
6. Infants and small children should be transported in an approved child restraint device appropriate to their weight and age. When possible, the EMT should use an infant's or child's own car seat. The EMT can secure the car seat to the main stretcher using the restraint straps on the stretcher. He or she may use additional straps if necessary. If the child is a second patient, the EMT can secure the car seat to the jump seat located at the head of the stretcher. Using the child's own seat reduces the child's fear and minimizes unnecessary movement. With padding and tape it can also serve as an immobilization device for a noncritical child (Figure 33.27). Commercially available car seats for EMS use are available. Some models are inflatable for situations in which storage space on the ambulance is an issue.
7. The EMT should transport trauma patients with multiple injuries on the long backboard. This provides full body immobilization and allows easy movement of the patient.
8. The EMT should use discretion when moving and positioning physically disabled patients. The nature of their disability dictates how the EMT should compensate. Visually- and hearing-challenged patients may require extra communication to ease their anxiety. The EMT should place patients with twisted limbs or other obvious deformities in the position of greatest comfort. The EMT should take extra care when securing them with straps and use pillows or rolled towels and blankets to pad, support, and create a comfortable position.
9. Older adult patients should be placed in as comfortable position as allowed by their condition. Osteoporosis (bone degeneration), preexisting injuries, or conditions such as arthritis require extra time and care with the older adults patient.

> ✓ Many situations that you will encounter in your EMS career will require you to modify the way that you lift and move patients. Your ability to "think on your feet" while following the basic concepts of lifting and moving will lead to a successful outcome for you and your patients.

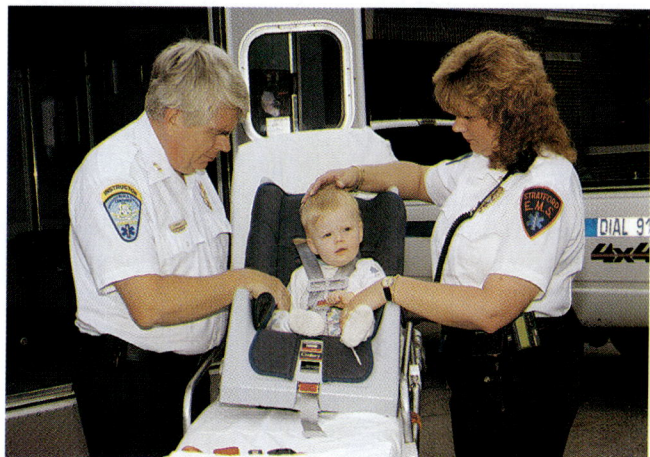

FIGURE 33.27 When possible, and infant's or child's own car seat should be used for immobilization. The car seat then can be secured to the main stretcher with the straps and the head of the stretcher used to regulate the position.

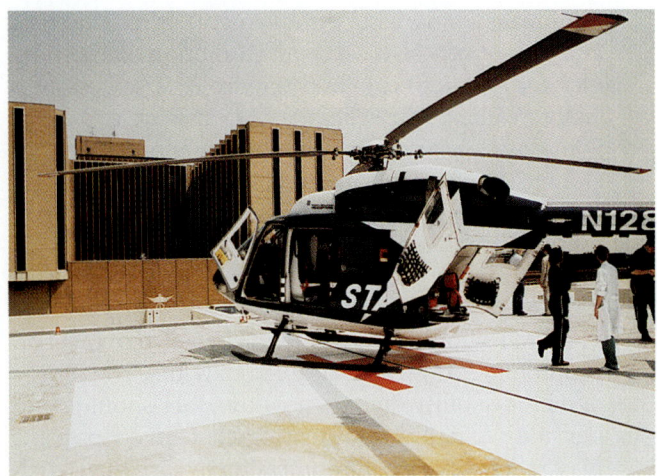

FIGURE 33.28 When considering aeromedical transport, the risk-benefit ratio must be weighed.

Transportation Considerations

Now that the patient has been properly packaged and moved to the air, sea, or ground ambulance, it is time for transportation to the emergency department. The EMT should consider the method of transportation as soon as enough information is gathered and life-threatening conditions are managed. The EMT should consider transportation time to a medical facility that can best meet the patient's needs when preparing a patient for transportation.

Helicopter transportation minimizes transportation time and thereby makes up for a longer on-scene time. In some situations, it may be more reasonable to initiate ground transportation and rendezvous with a helicopter at a more convenient landing zone or at a point closer to the medical center. A good working knowledge of the capabilities of the local EMS system will dictate whether the patient is immediately transported to a hospital or an advanced life support (ALS) intercept is made. This process involves arranging to meet a paramedic-level crew at a predetermined place before arrival at the hospital. When ALS intercept is used, the EMTs at the scene must decide whether it is more appropriate to remain at the scene until arrival of an ALS unit or a rendezvous with that unit en route to the hospital would be more efficient. The EMT can understand the importance of each of these factors by considering how they may come into play in various emergencies.

Transportation is an intervention that the EMT must prioritize and accomplish in a safe manner. The EMT often decides the most appropriate mode of transportation and the destination hospital long before assessing, treating, and packaging the patient. Choosing one hospital over another depends on patient request, proximity, specialized care, emergency department patient diversion status, and local protocols. Local (city, county, state) laws and rules may vary regarding hospital bypass. Some legislation forbids it, some permit it, and some require bypass of one hospital and transportation to a trauma center.

When considering aeromedical transportation, the EMT must weigh the risk-benefit ratio (Figure 33.28). Usually a helicopter is warranted if rapid access to a higher level of care is required (hospital to hospital) or for scene response when hospital access time to the correct hospital can be shortened. Another consideration is access to an appropriate landing zone (see Chapter 38). For most patients, the best and most commonly used method of transportation is the ground ambulance.

Mastering and maintaining safe driving techniques are as important for any EMT as understanding clinical care. All of the prehospital care and transportation decisions are worthless if the patient never arrives at the hospital or the crew is injured in the process. Furthermore, rough transportation of a patient may aggravate their injuries or conditions (e.g., in a patient with orthopedic injuries). The rough or violent movement of the ambulance can cause these patients increased pain. In the case of a medical patient, nausea and vomiting may ensue on an uneasy ride to the hospital. In a noncritical patient, the 2 to 3 minutes saved is not worth the poor ride to the hospital. The EMT must use his or her judgment to determine the speed and route of transportation for the patients that they are treating.

The EMT will make the decision to transport the patient in relationship to the patient's best interest, which may or may not be the closest medical facility to the incident. Patient transportation is an important treatment intervention of the EMT.

Step-by-Step Procedure

Direct Ground Lift

1. Ensure scene safety, or at least enough to be able to retrieve patient.

2. Initiate body substance precautions.

3. Keeping back straight, EMT #1 kneels by the patient's head.

4. Keeping back straight, EMT #2 kneels by the patient's waist on the same side as EMT #1 (see Step 4).

5. EMT #1 places one arm under the patient's head and shoulders, cradling the head.

6. EMT #1 raises the patient's upper body to be able to place the other arm under the patient's lower back.

7. EMT #2 places one arm directly below EMT #1's arm in the small of the patient's back and the other arm under the patient's knees.

8. Keeping back straight, knees bent, on EMT #1's count, lift the patient to their knees and roll the patient toward their chests.

9. On EMT #1's count, keeping back straight, both EMTs stand straight up with the patient curled against their chests.

10. On EMT #1's count, keeping back straight and knees bent, both EMTs lower their bodies onto one knee in front of the stretcher and gently lower and roll patient onto it (see Step 10).

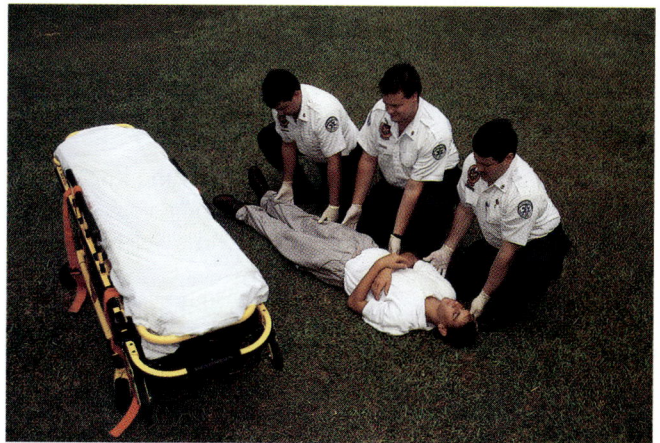

Step 4

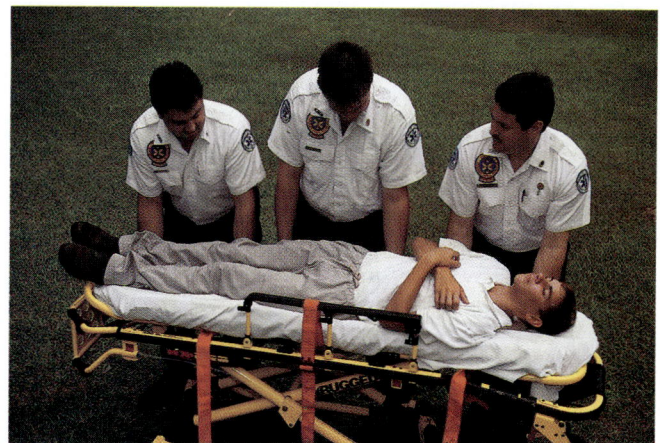

Step 10

Step-by-Step Procedure

One-Person Stretcher

1. *Unloading the stretcher:* Unlock the latch at the foot end of the stretcher catch by pushing inward on the bar and pulling the stretcher out of the catch by moving the stretcher away from the lock.

2. Stand at the foot of the stretcher, keeping knees bent and back straight, grasp and pull the lever, and gently guide the stretcher out of the unit (see Step 2).

3. Pulling the lever unlocks the legs of the stretcher and allows the legs to "fall" as the stretcher comes out of the unit.

4. *Loading the stretcher:* EMT #1 stands at the foot of the stretcher and guides the front wheels into the unit.

5. EMT #2 stands to the right of the stetcher and, with knees bent and back straight, kneels to the feet of the stretcher.

6. EMT #1 pulls the lever at the foot of the stretcher and lifts up slightly on the stretcher.

7. EMT #2 gently lifts the feet of the stretcher and helps guide it into the unit (see Step 7).

8. EMT #1 "walks" the stretcher into the unit and locks it into place.

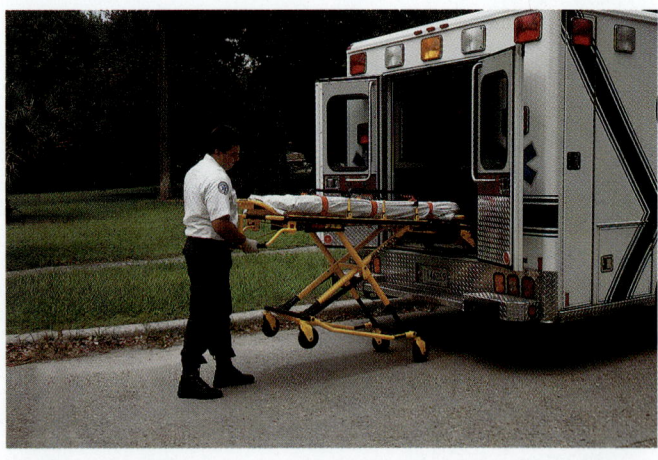
Step 2

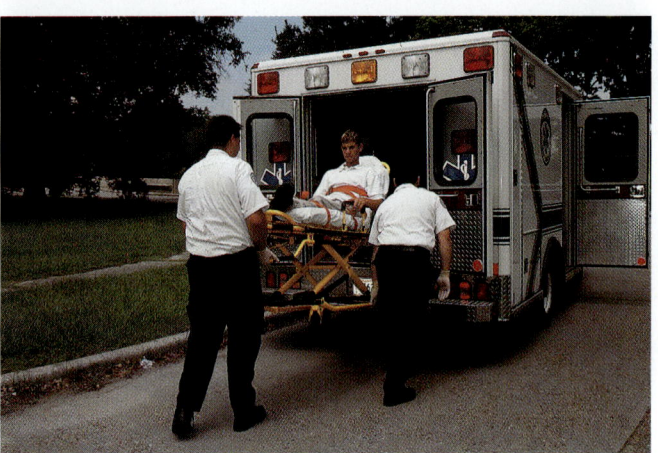
Step 7

Lifting and Moving Patients | Chapter 33

Step-by-Step Procedure

Scoop Stretcher

1. Lay the scoop stretcher beside the patient.

2. Adjust the scoop stretcher height according to the patient's height.

3. The scoop stretcher height can be adjusted by turning the lever at each side of the stretcher. The levers are located at about the knee level and need to be turned and pulled out. Then pull the lower end of the stretcher down to meet the height of the patient.

4. To separate the scoop stretcher, EMT #1 kneels at the head of the scoop stretcher and EMT #2 kneels at the foot. Push the button at the end of each side and pull the two halves apart.

5. Place one half on either side of the patient. Do not lift equipment over the patient.

6. Slightly lift the clothing on one side of the patient while another EMT slides one half of the scoop stretcher under the patient's side (see Step 6).

7. Repeat on the other side of the patient.

8. The patient may need to be rolled from side to side to get the scoop stretcher under the patient.

9. Lock the head end of the scoop stretcher in place by rejoining the top ends. The ends should lock into place using a slight bit of force and putting the two ends together. If any resistance is met, have an EMT gently lift one side of the patient with a small logroll (see Step 9).

10. Lock the feet together in the same manner.

11. Secure the patient to the scoop stretcher using straps, tape, or Kerlix.

12. The patient can now be moved onto the stretcher (see Step 12).

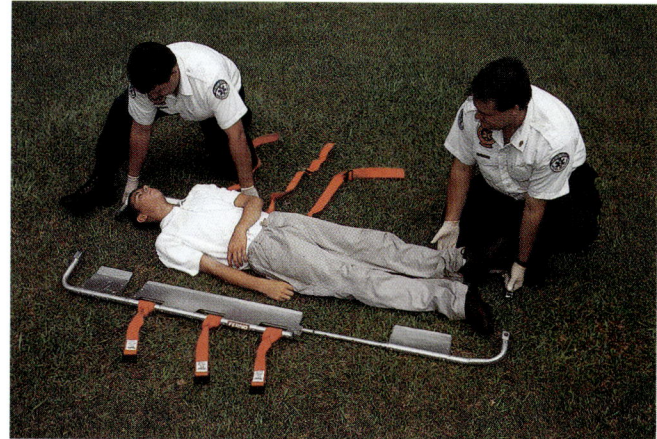
Step 6

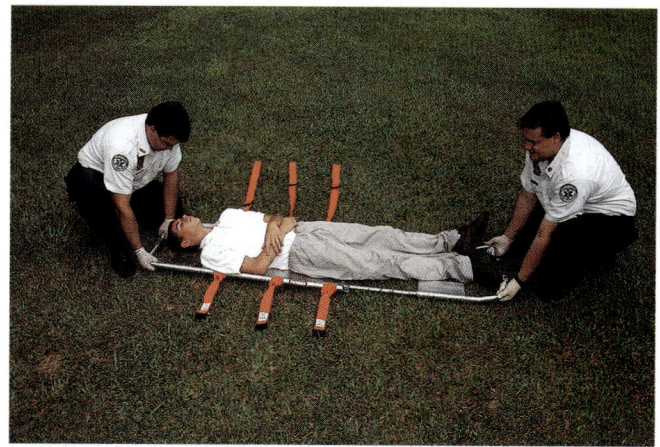
Step 9

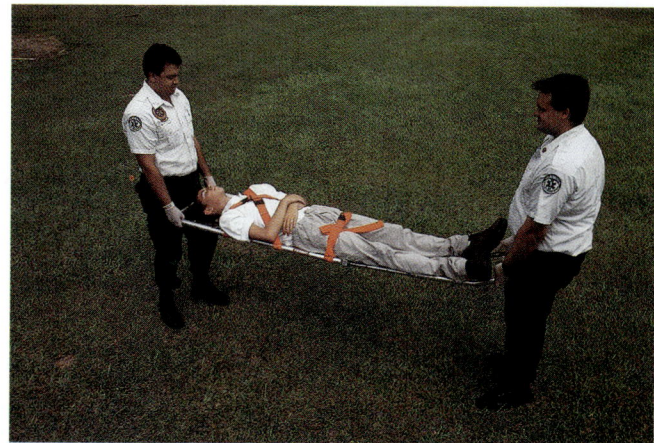
Step 12

Summary

- EMTs need to understand body mechanics and be aware of their own physical abilities and limitations. To avoid injury when lifting and carrying patients, EMTs must communicate in advance with one another, lift without twisting, wear appropriate footwear, position their bodies correctly, and know their equipment.
- Stairs demand additional help, if available. A spotter or guide allows the EMTs to concentrate on lifting without twisting to see where they are going. Other body movements such as reaching, pushing, and pulling require extra care when the weight of a patient is involved.
- EMTs may need to initiate an emergency move if the patient or EMTs are in immediate danger. EMTs can use inline drags, such as the clothing, sheet, blanket, or bent-arm drag. An urgent move may be required if a factor at the scene may contribute to the patient's decline, such as an unstable vehicle or environmental conditions. A nonurgent move allows the best care possible for a patient and is dependent on patient status and the presence of a safe, stable setting. Types of nonurgent moves include the direct ground lift, extremity lift, direct lift, and draw sheet lift.
- Specially designed ambulance equipment takes space and functionality into consideration. The most common devices for carrying and moving patients include the one- or two-person wheeled stretcher, portable stretcher, stair chair, long backboard, short backboard, scoop stretcher, and flexible stretcher. EMTs must check equipment regularly to ensure that it is functioning properly before it is needed. General rules apply to the positioning of patients on the equipment. By using all of the equipment available and using it as it is intended, EMTs can avoid unnecessary strain on their bodies during their years in EMS.

Scenario Solution

This patient scenario is commonly seen in the day-to-day work of EMTs. Assessment of the patient revealed only right hip pain with shortening and rotation of the affected leg. In this situation you must carefully select the device for transferring the patient. It must provide support and immobilization for the hip and leg and have the ability to be easily carried down the stairs. You can rule out the stair chair because this patient must remain supine (on her back). Acceptable devices include a scoop (orthopedic) stretcher, Reeves, or canvass stretcher. You may also use a long backboard, but you should place additional padding on the backboard before application.

You should carry the patient down the stairs feet first, with an effort to keep the head and feet as level as possible. Once on the ground floor, you should take the environmental factors into consideration. The ambulance should be parked as close to the door a reasonable. You should place the patient on the main stretcher and cover her appropriately for the cold and rain. You should use blankets to cover her body and place a towel around her head like a bandana. The move to the ambulance should be as quick as possible, but use caution. The use of ALS in this patient may be warranted for pain control. Paramedics carry medication that can ease the pain. This can be very beneficial to patients with orthopedic injuries.

Key Terms

Bent-arm drag A type of inline drag using the patient's arms in a bent position to provide leverage for dragging the patient away from immediate danger.

Blanket drag A type of inline drag using a blanket placed under the patient to pull him or her away from immediate danger.

Clothing drag A type of inline drag using the patient's clothing to pull him or her away from immediate danger.

Direct ground lift A lift used for patients who are not suspected of having a spinal injury; allows the movement of the patient from the ground to a piece of equipment.

Emergency move Any move that is initiated because of immediate danger to the patient and rescuer.

Extremity lift A lift used for patients who are not suspected of having a spinal injury; uses the patient's arms and legs to move him or her a short distance.

Key Terms (cont'd)

Flexible stretcher A piece of equipment, also known as a *pole stretcher,* designed for use when space is limited.

Inline drag A move used to drag a patient to safety when immediate danger is present.

Nonurgent move A type of move designed to provide the best care based on the patient's status in a safe, controlled environment.

One-person stretcher Piece of equipment designed to allow one person to load the stretcher into the ambulance, if necessary.

Portable stretcher A piece of equipment designed to easily carry patients down stairs or over rough terrain; sometimes referred to as *shippers* or *folding stretchers.*

Recovery position Position in which an unconscious patient is placed on his or her side and balanced by the positioning of the arms and legs.

Sheet drag A type of inline drag using a sheet placed under the patient to pull him or her away from immediate danger.

Time dependent The relationship of the effectiveness of many medical interventions to the time at which they are implemented.

Two-person stretcher A piece of equipment designed for two people to carry, move, and load the patient.

Urgent move A move performed when any factor at the rescue scene may contribute to the patient's decline or the rescuer's safety; requires that the patient be moved more quickly than usual.

Review Questions

1. List the seven guidelines for carrying patients and equipment.
2. List the devices that can be used to move a patient down a flight of stairs. List the advantages and disadvantages of each.
3. Describe the two most common types of wheeled stretchers used in EMS today. Describe the loading and unloading procedures of each.
4. List medical emergencies that would require immediate transportation.
5. What factors should the EMT consider when making transportation decisions in multisystem trauma patients?

Answers to these Review Questions can be found at the end of the book on page 868.

34

Communication

Lesson Goal

This chapter characterizes the basic components of an EMS communication system and describes the principles of each component.

Scenario

A lazy afternoon in a mountain resort soon tests the emergency medical services (EMS) system. Nick and Beth are grandparents who are watching their grandchildren ride their bicycles while the childrens' parents are waterskiing on the lake. As the grandchildren start to get brave on their bikes, a few try a big jump. One grandchild, Alex, is known to be fearless. He attempts a big jump and injures his leg and arm.

Nick yells to Beth, "Call 911. Alex has been hurt!" She dials 911 and starts to worry about what to say. She does not know the address or what town she is in, and the rental cabin has no information or address listed. Beth questions whether an EMS is in the area. The 911 call is answered.

While Beth is making the call, Nick uses his cellular phone to call Alex's parents and tell them that their son has been hurt. The parents misunderstand the conversation and call 911 immediately from their cellular phone. Nick stays with Alex while all the other kids try to help. Alex's brother rides his bike to the fire station in an attempt to activate the EMS system in a different way. The other kids, grandparents, and parents are all scared, nervous, and worried. They are in a strange place in a tough situation. They all need the best EMS system to help save life and limb. They wait for help to arrive, but they were the first to activate the EMS system and start the communication loop.

 What happens when someone calls 911? How are resources sent? What are the basic communications needed to access the EMS system? How are the people, equipment, and facilities orchestrated to make the EMS system work?

Key Terms to Know

Base station
Digital radio equipment
Emergency medical dispatch (EMD)
Mobile radios
Repeaters
Six-way communications model
Systems status management (SSM)
Telemetry
UHF band
VHF high band
VHF low band

Learning Objectives

As an EMT-Basic, you should be able to do the following:

DOT

- List the proper methods for initiation and termination of a radio call.
- State the proper sequence for delivery of patient information.
- Identify the essential components of the verbal reports.
- Describe the attributes for increasing the effectiveness and efficiency of verbal communication.
- State the legal aspects to consider in verbal communication.
- Discuss the communication skills that should be used to interact with the patient.
- Discuss the communication skills that should be used to interact with the family members, bystanders, and individuals from other agencies while providing patient care.
- Discuss the difference between skills used to interact with the patient and those used to interact with others.
- List the correct radio procedures in the following phases of a typical call:
  - To the scene
  - At the scene
  - To the medical facility
  - At the medical facility
  - To the station
  - At the station
- Perform a simulated, organized, concise radio transmission.
- Perform an organized, concise patient report that would be given to the staff at a receiving facility.
- Perform a brief, organized report that would be given to an advanced life support (ALS) provider arriving at an incident scene at which the EMT-Basic was already providing care.

Supplemental

- Demonstrate appropriate use of radio communication with the dispatch center in various phases of an ambulance call.
- Describe the importance of communication in an EMS system.
- Identify the components of an EMS communication system.
- Describe the various methods that are available to the public to access the EMS system.
- Explain the basic principles of emergency medical dispatch.
- Describe the process for dispatching EMS agencies, including the use of computer-aided dispatch.
- Describe the role of radio communication between the EMT and medical direction.
- Identify the six elements of the "six way" communications model

---

In emergency medical services (EMS), communication is essential. The ability to communicate clearly and efficiently is required in almost every component of the system. Patients must be able to access the system, and the system must have a method for dispatching individual units. Emergency medical technicians (EMTs) must have a method for communication with medical direction and with the receiving facility, and EMTs must be able to accurately communicate vital information about their patients to other medical personnel, both by radio and in person. Perhaps most importantly, the EMT must be able to communicate with the patient and his or her family members (Figure 34.1).

> ✓ A picture is worth a thousand words. Unfortunately, the EMT must paint a picture in few words. The goal of good communication is to paint the best possible picture of the patient with as few words as possible.

This chapter describes the basic components of an EMS communication system. Each system component is characterized, and important principles of use described. Medical communication and communication principles between the EMT and hospital are reviewed.

The need for effective communication is a theme that is woven throughout this book. In any EMS system, EMTs are required to communicate with the patient; his or her partner; and the physician, nurse, or paramedic. The most skillful EMT who has poor communication abilities is not effective. This chapter provides the basic information necessary to successfully master communication.

Components of an EMS Communication System

The EMS communication system is a complex network composed of people, equipment, and facilities. The system is designed and constructed to meet the specific communication needs of the individual geographic service area of the EMS system. The communication system includes the equipment and people necessary to receive

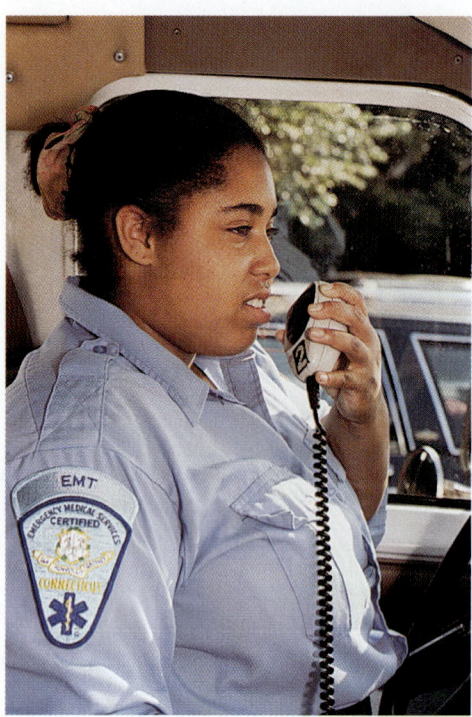

FIGURE 34.1 Communication is an essential piece of any EMS system and a skill that the EMT must master.

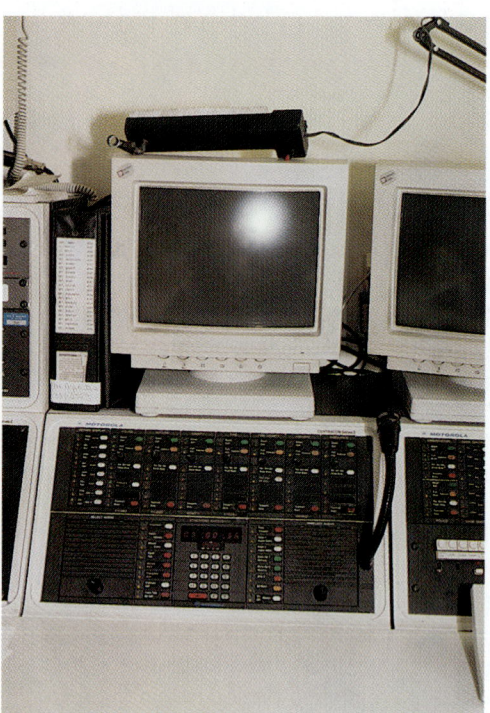

FIGURE 34.2 A base station radio is located at a fixed site such as a hospital or dispatch center.

calls for assistance from the public, dispatch and coordinate the response of EMS agencies, and provide for communication between the scene and the medical facility.

Equipment

One of the crucial elements of an EMS communication system is the actual equipment or hardware that operates in the system.

Base Station

A **base station** is a radio operated from a fixed site, such as a dispatch center or a hospital. It usually runs with community electrical power as opposed to battery power and transmits at a much higher power than do smaller, portable radios. In addition to the normal electrical power source, a base station often has an alternative power source, such as a generator or a set of batteries, for power outages (Figure 34.2).

Mobile Two-Way Radios

Mobile radios are mounted in vehicles such as ambulances or fire engines. Mobile radios are much more powerful than portable radios, but they broadcast with significantly less power than base stations. Under normal circumstances, a mobile radio's range is less than 20 miles at a broadcast strength of less than 50 watts (Figure 34.3).

Portable Handheld Radios

Portable radios are handheld units that are often referred to as *walkie-talkies* or *handi-talkies*. They are designed to be carried or worn by individuals and operate with a small internal battery pack. The transmission power of portable radios is generally under 5 watts, and the range is limited. Portable radios typically are used for short-range communication (e.g., between the scene and a mobile radio or a repeater). Portable radios allow communication to take place directly from the patient's side (Figure 34.4). Portable radios also may provide for a safer workforce as a result of the EMTs constant link to the dispatch center.

Often portable radios have coverage deficiencies in different areas of the radio system. These may include large buildings and areas blocked by terrain. The EMT should learn these areas in his or her local system and understand that communications may be compromised in certain areas. The drawbacks of the portable radio do not outweigh its benefits, as this small radio is used regularly by most EMT's everyday.

Repeaters

In many EMS systems, units operate at such great distances from the base stations that **repeaters** are required. A repeater is a radio unit that receives a signal from another radio unit and rebroadcasts it, boosting the signal strength in the process. Several different types of repeaters are available, depending on the needs of a particular system.

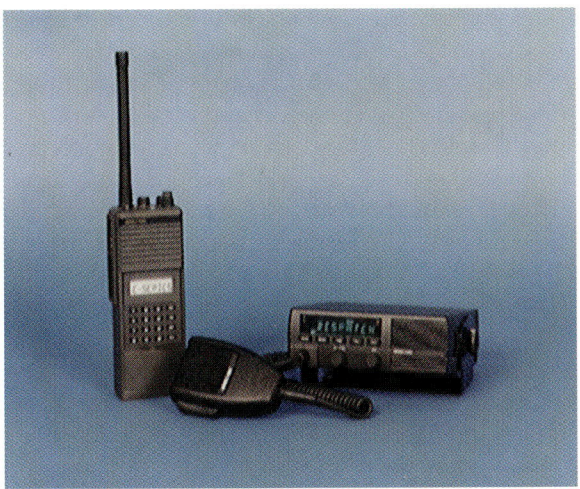

FIGURE 34.3 A mobile radio is mounted in a vehicle and operates with the vehicle's battery.

For example, mobile repeaters receive a signal from portable radios and rebroadcast to the base station. In mountainous regions, mountaintop repeaters enable radio signals to be picked up and rebroadcast over or around significant obstacles (Figure 34.5). Some repeaters rebroadcast the signal by radio, and others convert the signal to a microwave signal. The repeater may also convert the signal to a telephone signal and send the communication through public or dedicated telephone lines.

Radio Frequencies

Radio communication is conducted using radio frequencies or channels. The radio channels are divided into groups called *bands*. EMS radio communication takes place in the VHF low band, VHF high band, and UHF band. The radio waves in each band have unique properties that give each band advantages and disadvantages.

VHF low band. The **VHF low band** is the set of radio frequencies between 32 and 50 megahertz (MHz). Radio waves in this band are able to curve and follow the shape of the earth or other obstacles, thus allowing communication over long distances. However, frequencies in this band are also most susceptible to interference from buildings, electrical equipment, or weather. Many of these low-band systems are being replaced with VHF high band or UHF band.

VHF high band. The **VHF high band** is the set of radio frequencies between 150 and 174 MHz. These radio waves travel in a straight line and do not bend to follow the curve of the earth or around obstacles. They are limited to line of sight (i.e., the straight line between the transmitter and the receiver needs to be clear and free

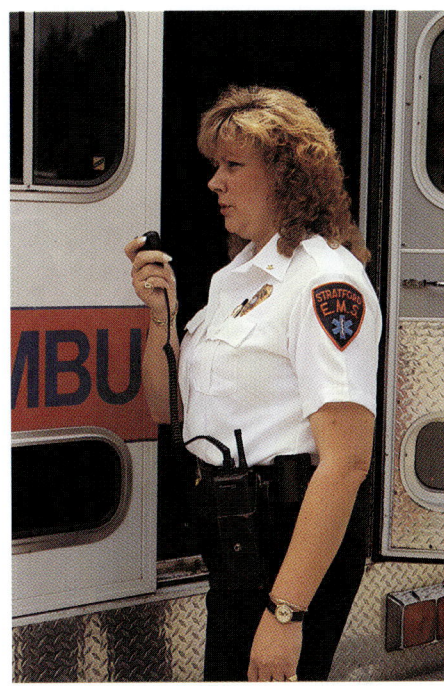

FIGURE 34.4 Portable radios give the EMT the freedom to communicate without being confined to the vehicle.

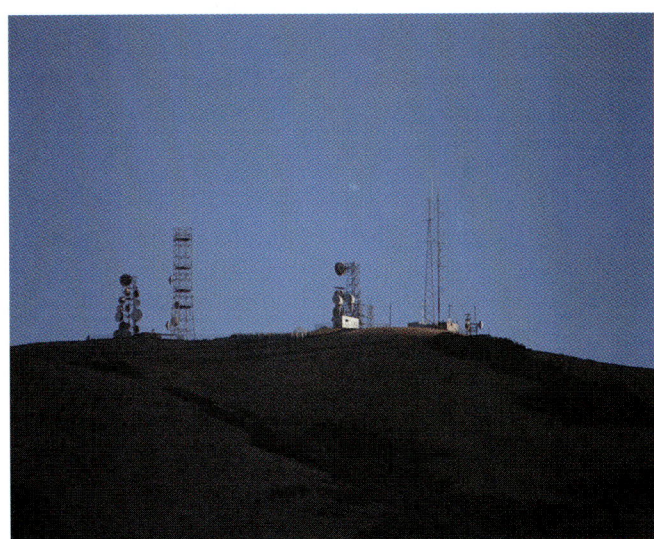

FIGURE 34.5 Repeaters allow radio broadcasts to cover larger distances and avoid significant obstacles.

from substantial obstructions like mountains, buildings, or the earth itself). VHF high-band frequencies are less susceptible to the interference that bothers low-band communication, but interference is still possibile.

UHF band. The **UHF band** is the set of radio frequencies between 450 and 470 MHz. These frequencies are almost interference free, offering some of the cleanest

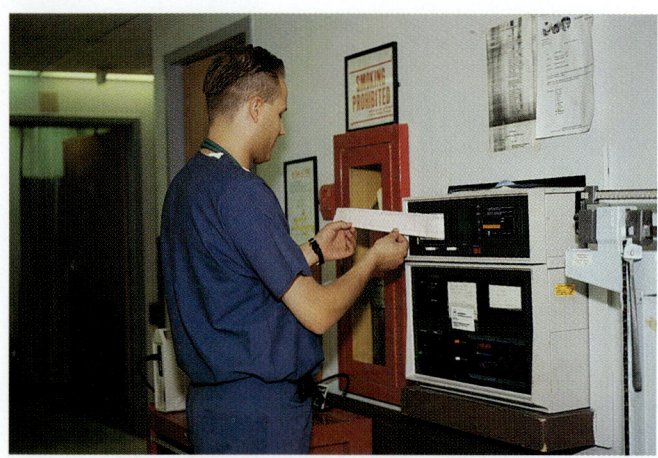

FIGURE 34.6 Telemetry allows the transmission of electrical signals such as electrocardiograms between the scene and the hospital.

communication frequencies available. The disadvantage is that they only travel short distances and are limited to line of sight. Because of the lack of interference, UHF frequencies are used most often for telemetry. **Telemetry** is the transmission of electronic signals over the radio. In EMS, the most frequent telemetry transmission is the electrocardiogram (Figure 34.6).

Digital Radio Equipment

The need for more frequencies for EMS providers became evident in the mid-1970s when it became difficult to obtain more radio channels. Many EMS agencies saw increases of 100% of their service requests from the 1970s until the late 1990s, with radio systems installed in the 1970s. This has created new communications needs that were unforeseen at the time. Currently, many EMS systems have critical weaknesses in their current radio systems. Another problem was the need for different agencies to talk on the same frequency during large EMS incidents. With these two needs and the advances of computer and radio technology, the 800-Megahertz (MHz) range of frequencies was put in service.

Radio waves in this frequency range are clean and interference free. Sophisticated radio equipment allows the identification of many more discrete channels than are available in the other bands. Using computer technology known as *trunking*, simultaneous communication can take place between different agencies or to the same units because the radio selects the available channels as needed. This **digital radio equipment** is computer controlled, highly reliable, and error free. However, the 800-MHz frequencies have some concerns. Currently, the equipment is costly and has the shortest range. Any system based on 800 MHz requires numerous repeaters. It is common for many EMS agencies to combine with one another to form joint power agencies to combine the needed money to operate these systems more cost-effectively.

New advances in personal pagers have put them in use for some EMS systems. In some cases, these small one-way devices are used as a primary or secondary communications tool. Pagers have alphanumeric, voice, or simple numeric readouts for the EMT to read. Many portable radios have this function available as an option.

Cellular Telephones

Cellular telephones are becoming more common in urban, suburban, and rural locations. The cellular technology combines radio frequencies above the 800-MHz range with telephone lines to accomplish a cost-effective and readily available form of mobile communication. For EMS and other emergency services, the chief advantages of cellular communication are low cost and high efficiency. The disadvantage is that there are no protected channels or frequencies for EMS as there are in the VHF, UHF, and 800-MHz bands. The EMT should not expect to use a cellular phone during many moderate to large-scale emergencies. Many EMTs report that during emergencies cellular phones are almost useless because of high cellular usage by the public, other responders, and the news media. The EMT should always anticipate that every radio or television station that responds to an emergency scene will be using the same cellular communication system, and all available channels will be used up quickly.

In many systems, selected phones have priority and are allowed to access the cellular site when the general public is not. The EMS system must arrange this in advance with the cellular provider. Furthermore, during extended EMS operations, the cellular company may set up a temporary cellular site to provide cellular phone communications specifically for an emergency.

Automatic Vehicle Location

The location of ambulances for dispatching is always a concern for EMS managers. The dispatcher must determine which ambulance is closest to the medical emergency. Most early dispatchers used the dispatcher's brain and a rough status board to locate units. Automatic vehicle location (AVL) devices, which forward ambulance and emergency response vehicle locations to the communications center to ensure fast response to medical emergencies, have replaced the status boards. An on-board positioning system calculates the location of an ambulance using a combination of a global positioning system (GPS) and dead reckoning technology. This information is sent to the communications center by an 800-MHz trunking radio system. The communications system adds this information to the computer-aided dispatch (CAD) system, which selects the closest resource.

Automatic Crash Notification

Currently, research is being conducted for a communicating crash recorder that sends data via wireless telecommunications. This system is known as *automatic crash notification* (ACN). This new system will contact EMS providers and notify responders, in less than 1 minute, of a calculation of serious injuries in a vehicular crash. This system can direct EMS providers to the exact location of a vehicular crash. ACN technologies using crash sensors, global positioning systems, and wireless telephones have been installed in production vehicles. These vehicles, upon impact, have crash sensor measurement, which instantly are translated into a rating of injury probability. The EMT can use these data to determine the need for other resources (air ambulance) before arrival on the scene, therefore saving precious time. Medical records of occupants of the vehicle can be sent to the emergency department or the EMT. Information like medications, drug reactions, or blood type can assist in emergency treatment and save time. Future software for ACN will notify EMS providers with information about absence or presence of fire, air bag deployment, and the total number of occupants in the vehicle and their seat location.

> ✓ EMS radio communications occur over a broad range of radio frequencies and use a variety of equipment. Each frequency band and piece of equipment offers a distinct set of advantages and disadvantages. EMTs must be familiar with the frequencies and equipment used in the system in which they will be functioning.

Personnel

In addition to equipment, the people who operate the EMS communication system are also crucial to its success. In the hospital, nurses, physicians, and technicians may operate the communication system with specific radio communication responsibility. In the field, EMTs, paramedics, and other health care providers may be involved in communication. The center of the communication system, called the *dispatch facility*, employs dispatchers and public safety communications specialists to receive calls for assistance and dispatch emergency personnel and vehicles.

Emergency services' dispatching is a profession in its own right. It requires highly specialized education and experience to function in the modern dispatch center. Several states have legislation or regulations in place that establishes training and performance standards for dispatch personnel.

Public Access

For any emergency service system to function, the public must have a way to access the system. For EMS in particular, the access method must be simple and easy to remember because the caller is often in a highly emotional or stressful state. EMS system access has evolved over the years and is far from being completely effective or uniform throughout the United States. The public's access to an EMS system is influenced by several factors, including the following:

- Capability of local telephone company equipment
- Public service budgets of local and regional governments
- Formal politics between differing jurisdictions
- Competition within single political jurisdictions over control of public access

Behind the budgets, politics, and turf battles, EMS system access, from the public perspective, boils down to the simple question, "What number do I call to activate the EMS?"

Seven-Digit Access Number

The most common method for accessing the EMS system is the telephone. Although some systems and geographic locations may offer alternatives such as roadside call boxes, the telephone remains the most-used tool for contacting emergency assistance. Until the late 1970s and early 1980s, emergency services were contacted by dialing a seven-digit telephone number. Which number to dial was determined by which community the call was made from. Often, separate seven-digit emergency numbers existed for police, fire, and ambulance. If traveling or away from home, a caller had to use a phone book if one was available or contact the telephone operator to try to find help.

911

In the late 1970s and early 1980s, awareness grew throughout the United States that a simpler, more efficient, and more user-friendly method of public access was needed. Advances in telephone and computer technology soon made it possible to construct telephone systems in which a single access number could be used everywhere. Telephone company computers and switches would ensure that calls were routed to the appropriate dispatch center based on the origin of the call. A caller would not need to worry about which number to call; they would

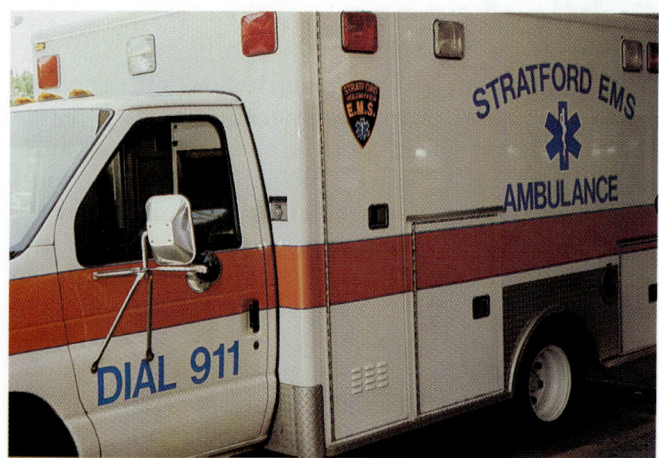

FIGURE 34.7 911 has become the standard number for public access to emergency services in the United States. Although not yet in place in every community, this number will eventually be in place everywhere.

simply dial 911, and the computers and switches would take care of the rest.

All 911 calls arrive in a single location, known as a public safety answering point (PSAP). The PSAP may be operated by one of the emergency services in a community or may be a separate operation. The PSAP may perform the actual dispatch functions or channel calls to the appropriate emergency response agency (Figure 34.7).

In theory, the system sounds simple. However, in practice it has proved to be challenging to implement for reasons previously mentioned. Currently, more than 10 years after the concept began to gain widespread acceptance, vast areas of the United States are still without access to 911 service. Nevertheless, in communities that have implemented 911, public access to EMS has been made much simpler.

Enhanced 911

Enhanced 911, or E911, is a new access technology that builds on the original principles of 911. In this type of system, additional computer technology enhances the simplified public access in regular 911 systems. The dispatcher can immediately see the street or billing address of the incoming call based on telephone company records. This display speeds up the transfer of location information between the caller and the dispatcher. It has also proved helpful in reducing the number of false alarms.

E911 is not foolproof; it also has difficulties. Calls from cellular phones are routed to the dispatch center closest to the cell tower site, not necessarily to the dispatch center for the responsible jurisdiction. Occasionally, the billing address for a telephone has nothing to do with the actual street location; they may be separated by long distances. The telephone systems in large buildings with switchboards, such as large factories, hotels, and high-rise apartment buildings, do not allow the E911 system to distinguish any location more detailed than the street address for the building. In addition, E911 requires even more sophisticated telephone equipment and involves even greater cost than simple 911 systems.

✓ Public access to emergency services is changing. It is becoming easier and more user-friendly through the phase-out of seven-digit access numbers and the increasing availability of 911 and E911 systems.

Emergency Medical Dispatch

As mentioned previously, in recent years the position of emergency services dispatcher has evolved into a specialized field of its own. People make careers in emergency dispatch or communication, and specialized training is essential. In the EMS field, recent advances have led to the development of a concept known as **emergency medical dispatch (EMD)**.

General Principles

EMD involves the dispatcher in the delivery of emergency medical care. Using carefully designed sequences of questions and directions, dispatchers provide emergency medical instructions to callers to assist the victim until EMS units arrive on the scene. The simple instructions focus on life-saving techniques such as cardiopulmonary resuscitation (CPR) and control of bleeding. Although the value of giving prearrival instructions is clear, this dispatch service is not yet universally available.

An additional facet of the EMD concept is having the dispatcher get information about what is going on at the scene. The dispatcher uses this information to make decisions about the priority or type of EMS response that is required and to relay important information to responding units. EMD training encompasses the basic EMS skills and provides prearrival" instructions for childbirth, altered mental states, shock, and allergic reactions.

Dispatch Methods

After the dispatch center receives a request for emergency medical assistance and decides which EMS units to send, the dispatch takes place. Notification of the responsible units occurs in a variety of ways, depending on the technologic capabilities of the EMS system. In systems in which EMS units are housed in fixed locations, such as fire stations, dispatch may occur via dedicated telephone lines or teletype transmission. When EMS units are moving either out of the station or in a constantly changing pattern in an attempt to anticipate call location, dispatch will be accomplished by radio (voice or pager).

A term that the EMT confronts in many EMS systems in the United States is **systems status management (SSM)**. SSM is a method of deploying EMS resources (people and vehicles) in a dynamic pattern that is based on anticipated call volume and location. Using sophisticated computer equipment and software, EMS vehicles are kept constantly moving in an attempt to provide maximum coverage with the least amount of resources expended. The goal is maximum efficiency with minimal sacrifice in quality of care.

In modern dispatch systems that include EMD programs, the dispatch information usually includes information about the relative priority of the call and the actual nature of the call.

En Route Communication

As the alerted EMS unit responds, EMS personnel should notify the dispatch center that the unit is en route. Methods for performing this notification vary from system to system. Some response notification methods are simple, involving repetition of the address or other relevant information. EMTs should become familiar with the practices in the system in which they will function.

While en route to the scene, the dispatch center may be able to provide additional specific information about the incident. This dispatcher obtains this information from the caller or other responding units that are already on the scene. The goal is to give the responding EMS personnel the opportunity to prepare, medically and mentally, for the situation they will face on the scene.

EMS personnel should also advise the dispatch center when the unit arrives on the scene. In the past, practice was to perform this notification when the vehicle arrived at the street address of the incident. However, in recent years, on-scene notification has changed to reflect the actual time that providers arrive at the patient's side. Time of arrival at the patient may be dramatically different from the time that the unit pulls to a stop in the street, particularly in large factories or buildings.

✔ Modern EMS communication systems actively involve the dispatch personnel in the chain of emergency medical care. Dispatchers provide life-saving instructions to callers and gather detailed information to help responding units mentally prepare for what they will find on the scene.

General Guidelines For Radio Communication

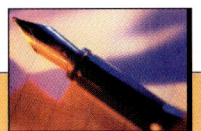

Tips from the Pros

The scene of an EMS call is full of noise and distraction. In addition, the stress of an emergency call often "gets the adrenaline going" in EMTs, and emotions are often high. This combination of background noise and emotion often creates a chaotic atmosphere that impedes the delivery of a good patient report to the hospital. Unless the situation absolutely dictates otherwise, it is often best for the EMT to search out a relatively quiet place, away from all of the noise and distractions, to pick up the radio and talk to the hospital. If the EMT cannot go somewhere to find this quiet spot, he or she should ask for quiet for a few minutes while this important conversation takes place. Before picking up the radio, the EMT should organize his or her thoughts. Some EMS systems provide notepads with space for notes in the proper order. The EMT should take a deep breath and calm down. He or she should close his or her eyes, if necessary, to shut out distractions. The objective is to make a full and complete report all at one time in a volume and tone of voice that is easily understood. A lot of background noise, speech that is too rapid, or shouting will not help the EMT convey information. Say it once and say it right.

Six-Way Communications Model

An EMS system must have a communications program. Equipment designators, a standard set of words and phrases, lines of communications, and frequencies to use should all be in a written format. If special codes are used, they should be listed in *this written format*. Training on these procedures is paramount for a successful communications system. This chapter deals primarily with radio communication; however, the EMT must remember that face-to-face communication is the most effective form of communication. When using radios and other electronic devices, the EMT must follow certain steps to ensure the effectiveness of communication. In review of accidents and injuries, improper communication has played a major role. By diminishing the problems associated with poor communication, the safety and effectiveness of the EMT needs to be increased.

The six-way communications model consist of the following:

Step One—Think. The sender **thinks** the idea (thinking, "I need help."). Before the sender sends a message, he or she needs to think about exactly what it is that he or she needs to say. If this is not clear, the receiver will not be clear. The message should be concise; long messages increase the chance of a misunderstanding.

Step Two—Transmit. The sender **transmits** about the message (dialing telephone, squeezing microphone, verbalizing). The first part of this step is to get the attention of the receiver. Without this step, the communication effort may fall on "deaf ears" and could be ineffective.

Step Three—Transfer. The sender **transfers** the message through a medium (over telephone lines, over radio transmitter). The sender should keep in mind the medium being used (e.g., telephone, radio, fax machine, or face to face). All of these media require standard language and terminology to be effective. Nicknames are not appropriate for quality communication.

Step Four—Obtain. The receiver **obtains** the message (through telephone receiver, radio receiver). The receiver has the responsibility to listen, read, or watch. The receiver must keep background noise to a minimum and not allow himself or herself to become distracted.

Step Five—Interpret. The receiver **interprets** the message (use of brain, logic, or education). Most people take a few seconds to read or decipher the received information. The sender must avoid pushing the receiver to understand more quickly. Interpretation is in the eyes, ears, and brain of the receiver.

Step Six—Confirm. The receiver **confirms** the message (provides feedback and closes the communication loop). Without this step all of the previous steps may be lost. Confirmation "closes" the communication loop, letting the sender and receiver know that the intended communication has been completed.

Specific procedures for use of a radio to communicate with the dispatch center or hospital are often explained in standard operating procedures or instructions provided by individual EMS agencies or dispatch centers. However, a few general principles of radio use apply to almost any system:

1. Ensure that the radio is turned on and properly adjusted.
2. Listen to the frequency to ensure that there is no other traffic before transmitting.
3. Think through the message *before* pushing the transmit button. Assemble notes if it is a patient report.
4. Press the push-to-talk switch on the microphone and wait 1 second before speaking.
5. Speak clearly and distinctly.
6. Use plain English. Systems used to rely heavily on the use of codes, but codes cause problems with miscommunication. Most modern EMS systems use plain English.
7. Keep transmissions brief, and avoid the use of unnecessary phrases such as "thank you" or "please."
8. Remember that every word is being transmitted over radio waves, which can be picked up by anyone with a scanner (including the general public and the news media). Protect the patient's privacy. Many systems do not allow transmission of the patient's name for this reason.

Example of the Six-Way Communications Model

Sender (thought): "I need another ambulance here!" **(Step One—Think)**

Sender (get the attention of the receiver): "Dispatch, Ambulance 12." **(Step Two—Transmit)**

The sender sends though the medium **(Step Three—Transfer)**

Receiver: "Ambulance 12, this is dispatch. Go ahead."

Sender: "Dispatch a second ambulance to this incident." **(Step Four—Obtain)**

Receiver (thought): "The CAD shows that ambulance 11 is the next available. I'll send it." **(Step Five—Interpret)**

Receiver: "Ambulance 12. Sending ambulance 11 to your incident." **(Step Six—Confirm)**

Communication with Medical Direction or Destination Facility

Most modern EMS systems provide the capability for EMTs to talk from the scene or from the ambulance to the hospital and/or a physician. This communication to the physician or hospital may be required in some systems and optional in others, but it occurs with two objectives in mind:

1. It provides the opportunity for EMTs to receive instructions or advice from a physician. This is known as direct or on-line medical direction. Chapter 4 discusses this topic in more detail.

2. Notify the receiving hospital and personnel so that they can make preparations to receive the patient in an efficient manner. Pre-notification of the receiving hospital can dramatically reduce the time between arrival at the emergency department and initiation of definitive treatment or interpretive services (for non–English-speaking patients) (Figure 34.8).

Essential Elements and Proper Sequence of Patient Report

Keeping in mind the two goals of medical communication described previously, the EMT needs to address normal or essential elements of the verbal report in each communication with the hospital. A generally preferred sequence or order exists for delivering this information. General guidelines are discussed in this section, but the EMT also needs to be familiar with local protocols or standard operating procedures. The essential elements of a radio report to the receiving facility, in the order they should be given, are as follows:

1. *Identify unit and level of provider.* This information serves as an introduction and allows those at the receiving facility or the physician to know to whom they are talking and what level of care they are capable of providing.
2. *Estimated time of arrival (ETA).* The EMT must deliver this information early in the patient report because it has a direct influence on the treatment instructions that the physician may select. It also has a direct influence on the speed with which the hospital must prepare itself to receive the patient. An ETA of 2 minutes with a cardiac arrest creates a different sense of urgency in the emergency department than would a 30-minute ETA with the same cardiac arrest.
3. *Age and sex of the patient.* This information begins the verbal process of "painting a picture of the patient." This picture enables the medical personnel on the other end of the radio to develop a clinical picture of what is wrong with the patient. In some systems, the estimated weight of the patient may also be included at this stage because it may effect drug dosage recommendation.
4. *Chief complaint.* As discussed in Chapter 8, the chief complaint is a brief description of the symptoms of which the patient is complaining. If the patient is unresponsive, the chief complaint is a description of what appears to be wrong or the mechanism of injury.
5. *Brief, pertinent history of the present illness.* This information involves a brief review of the details behind the chief complaint, including what happened, when, for how long, and other types of historical questions about the current illness.
6. *Major past illnesses.* The EMT should review significant previous illnesses or injuries that may influence diagnosis or treatment of the current illness.
7. *Mental status.* The EMT should describe the patient's state of responsiveness and alertness.
8. *Baseline vital signs.* The EMT should review the patient's temperature, blood pressure reading, pulse rate, respiratory rate.
9. *Pertinent findings of the physical examination.* The EMT should report significant findings detected during the initial or follow-up assessments.
10. *Emergency medical care given.* The EMT should summarize what has been done for the patient so far.
11. *Response to emergency medical care.* The EMT should describe how the patient responded to the medical care.

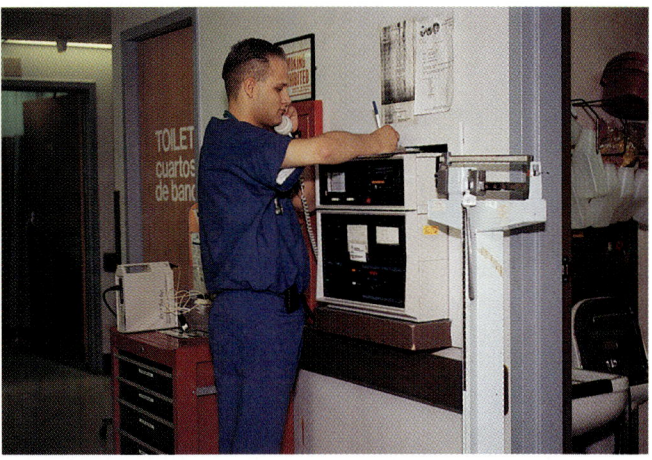

FIGURE 34.8 Radio provides the connection between the EMT and medical direction. It also provides the emergency department with advanced warning about an impending patient arrival.

This medical communication may occur at the scene or it while en route to the receiving facility (Figure 34.9).

> ✓ The medical report, provided over the radio by the EMT, is the bridge between the prehospital environment and the emergency department. It is the first contact between the physician and the patient, and it begins the process of definitive medical care.

Communication en Route to the Hospital

Once the EMS unit has left the scene and is en route to the hospital, communication is still important.

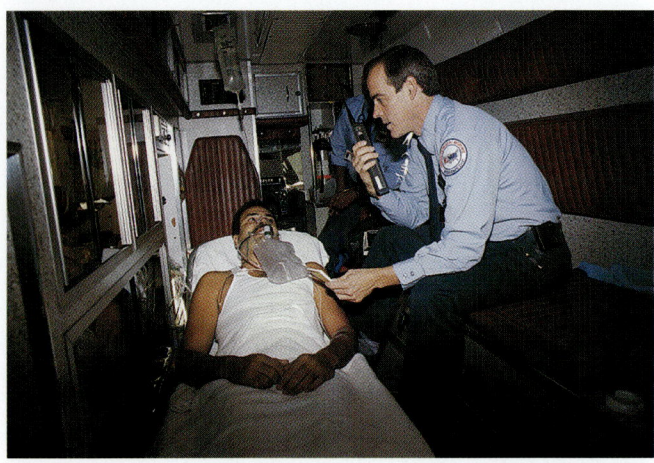

FIGURE 34.9 The EMT is responsible for presenting all important patient information to the hospital in a standard order.

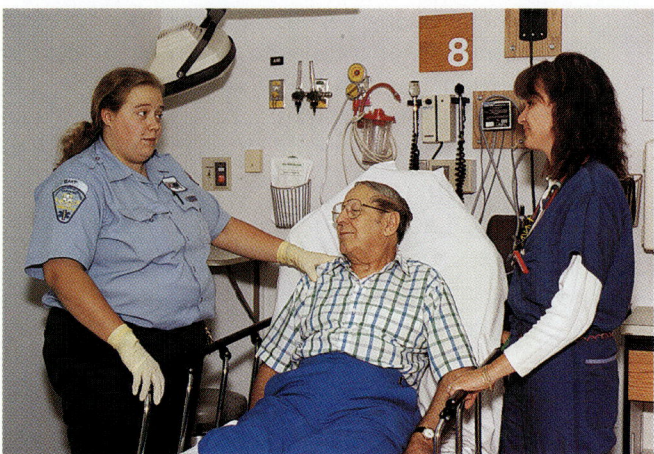

FIGURE 34.10 The EMT's verbal report to hospital personnel is an essential component of transferring responsibility for the patient to the emergency department.

Departure from the Scene and En Route

EMS personnel should notify the dispatcher as soon as the unit leaves the scene with the patient. This notification informs the dispatcher that work on the scene is concluded and the transportation phase has begun. Many systems include prompts or alarms in the dispatch center if a unit is out of contact on the scene for too long a period of time.

While en route, the EMT continues to assess and provide care for the patient. The EMT should report significant changes in the patient's condition or response to treatment to the receiving facility.

Arrival at the Hospital

The EMS unit should also notify the dispatch center on arrival at the hospital. This notification informs the dispatcher that the unit has safely completed the transportation phase and that personnel can be reached at the hospital if necessary.

> ✓ The dispatch center must be kept constantly informed about the location and status of EMS vehicles. This information is important for both operational and safety reasons.

In-Person Communication with Facility Staff

As the patient is delivered to the receiving hospital (probably the emergency department), the EMT must report verbally to hospital personnel. This report is a critical phase in patient care. At the hospital, the EMT hands over responsibility for the patient to appropriately qualified staff in the emergency department. *Appropriately qualified staff* means someone who is at least as capable as the EMT of providing care for the patient. For example, the EMT should turn responsibility for a patient over to a physician, nurse, or other trained medical staff member. However, the EMT should not turn medical responsibility for a patient over to a nonmedical member of the emergency department staff (e.g., an admissions clerk). This transfer of medical responsibility requires the complete and orderly transfer of information from the EMT to the hospital staff (Figure 34.10).

Essential Elements

The verbal report to the hospital staff is similar to the radio report, but some of the elements are different:

1. Identify the EMT and unit.
2. Introduce the patient to the hospital personnel.
3. Summarize the information that was provided over the radio:
   Chief complaint
   Other pertinent history not previously relayed

4. Describe additional interventions made en route.
5. Describe significant changes in vital signs or response to interventions noted en route.

Essential Principles of Interpersonal Communication

As has been described in this chapter, communication is an essential element of a successful EMS system. Communication involves the transfer of information between people. A real danger of miscommunication exists any time that people interact (i.e., the message does not get through at all or as intended). EMTs need to be students of interpersonal communication. Communication with others requires a set of skills that must be learned and constantly refined for the EMT to be successful in the field. The following are general principles of interpersonal communication (Figure 34.11):

1. Act and speak in a calm and confident manner.
2. Make and maintain eye contact with the patient.
3. Speak clearly, slowly, and distinctly.
4. Treat the patient with respect. Ask the patient how he or she would prefer to be addressed.
5. Use words that the patient can understand. Avoid complex medical terminology or abbreviations.
6. Be honest and direct with the patient.
7. Be constantly aware of both the patient's and your body language.

> ✓ Success as an EMT requires the study of much more than medical knowledge and skills. The EMT must learn and practice interpersonal communication skills, which are perhaps just as important as medical knowledge.

Communication with Special Patients

Emergency medical work places the EMT in various situations that involve communication challenges. For example, the noise and confusion at almost any EMS scene sometimes makes communication impossible. Other special situations may also cause communication challenges.

Hearing- or Speech-Impaired Patients

The hearing-impaired patient presents a unique set of challenges for the EMT. Because many hearing-impaired

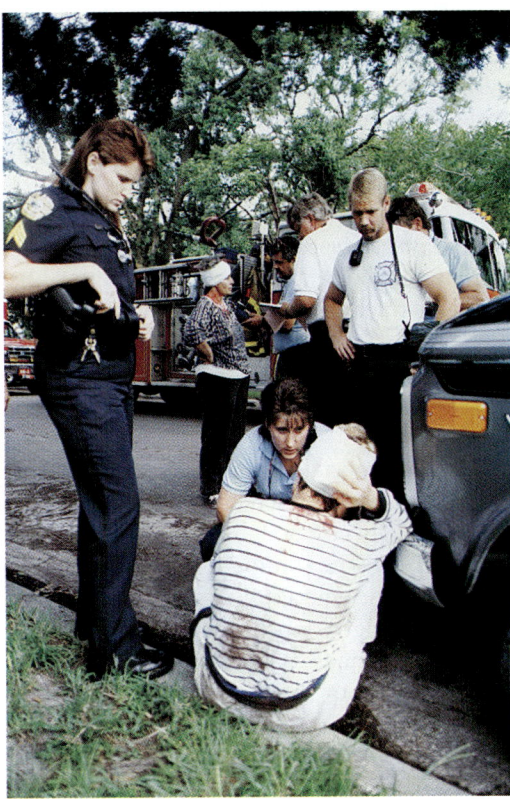

FIGURE 34.11 Successfully communicating with patients requires that the EMT keep general principles of communication in mind at all times.

patients are capable of reading lips, the EMT should always speak clearly with lips clearly visible to the patient. The speech-impaired patient may or may not be able to hear the EMT. Many EMTs learn basic sign language to communicate with these patients. If all else fails and if the patient is capable, the EMT can exchange written notes with the patient as a means of communication.

Non–English-Speaking Patients

Non–English-speaking patients are found in almost every EMS system in the United States. Many EMS systems encourage or require that personnel learn a second language if a prominent non–English-speaking population lives in the area (e.g., Spanish is a valuable language for EMT providers in communities near the southern border). If the EMT cannot communicate in the patient's language, the first step is to try to speak with a family member or friend who is capable of communicating with the patient. If no one on the scene is capable of communicating with the patient, the EMT should attempt to find out what language the patient speaks and notify the hospital. Many hospitals have call rosters of interpreters available, and they may be able to have an interpreter waiting by the time the patient arrives at the hospital.

If verbal communication is not possible, the EMT will need to be innovative and imaginative to communicate with the patient. The EMT will still need to do all that can be done to assess the patient and begin the process of stabilization. The EMT should proceed slowly and cautiously and demonstrate or gesture to indicate what will be done. The should remember that many foreign cultures have different attitudes toward the human body and illness.

Children

Children present special communication challenges. Although they can often understand the words that adults use, they are usually emotionally overwhelmed by what is happening to them. The stimulation of the illness or injury, the excitement of the emergency response vehicles, and the fear caused by strangers touching them and, in some cases, hurting them combine to make communication difficult.

Although many of the principles of communication described previously apply, the EMT must remember that children are not little adults, either physically or emotionally. The EMT must win the trust and confidence of the child before meaningful communication can take place. Parents or siblings may be of help, although they may also aggravate the emotional situation.

Chapter 31 discusses the unique aspects of communicating with children in more detail.

Older Adults

Older adults are another patient population that often presents unique communication challenges. Older patients occasionally have difficulty hearing. In most cases, effective communication can be achieved simply by speaking louder or more clearly. Older patients also often have poor vision. Many common disease processes in older patients also contribute to disorientation or confusion. In addition to speaking clearly and distinctly, the EMT should speak slowly and take time to make sure that the patient understands what is being said and what is taking place.

> ✓ EMTs will often face communication challenges with special patients. EMTs should prepare themselves with alternatives for dealing with these patients and should be familiar with the other resources available in their system, such as interpreters.

Legal Concerns

The EMT should be concerned about legal issues in communications because this is a litigation-prone society. Many things that are done in EMS require information for future reference. All EMTs must realize that what they say and do during EMS situations needs to be recorded. The best way to manage this concern is to keep good records of what was said to whom. Often litigation may become an issue many years later and the EMT should strongly consider keeping a record of all pertinent communications. This record may be in the run report, as a separate log, or maintained by the EMS system in radio tapes.

Summary

- Communication is required throughout all phases of EMS. Telephone and radio communication is essential to EMS system access and operation. Interpersonal communication in a face-to-face setting is essential to dealing with patients and medical personnel at the receiving facility.
- EMS communication systems are complex arrangements of equipment and people that are organized in such a manner as to provide the connection between people who require emergency medical care and those who provide it. Equipment includes various types of radio and computer equipment. Personnel include specially trained dispatchers in many systems.
- Communication between the scene and the hospital occurs with two goals in mind: (1) the communication provides the opportunity for the EMT to receive on-line or direct medical direction from a physician, and (2) it serves to warn the facility of the impending patient arrival so that advance preparations can begin. The radio communication with the receiving facility has essential components that should be delivered in a specific order.
- The EMT should keep the dispatch center informed of the EMS unit's location and status throughout the EMS call. This notification is essential for record-keeping purposes, but it also serves a valuable safety

Summary (cont'd)

function in that it allows the dispatcher to maintain ongoing contact with the EMTs.
- EMTs often will be exposed to situations that present special communication challenges. Advanced preparation and careful attention to the general principles of interpersonal communication and the six-way communications model will help in many of these situations.

Scenario Solution

The public safety answering point answers the phone, "Mountain Dispatch. Do you need sheriff, fire, or ambulance?" Beth explains the situation quickly but tells the dispatcher, "I don't know where we are." The dispatcher takes a few seconds and advises her of her location using the E911 screen and assures her of a quick response to her location. The brother on the bike who rode to the fire station is frantically relating the story to the firefighters: "He is hurt badly. Please hurry." Even though Andrew does not know the address, he gives good directions. The fire captain contacts dispatch, which confirms the address with the same dispatch center and responds. At the same time a cellular phone is being routed from another dispatch center 30 miles away to the Mountain Dispatch Center. The cellular phone "found" the closest cell site at another dispatch center; therefore, the PSAP center at the state highway patrol took a few seconds to define the area served by mountain dispatch and forward it. Now the Mountain Dispatch Center has received three phone calls for this response and used all three calls to confirm the address and get more information.

Sandy, the dispatcher, keeps Beth on the phone and gets more information. "What is the injury?" Beth answers, "His leg is badly broken and bleeding." The second dispatcher is sending out the emergency response as requested in the CAD within 1 minute over an in-house paging system and VHF radio system. The automatic vehicle locator (AVI) shows fire and ambulance personnel on scene, and both units confirm by radio. Sandy, who has been giving prearrival information to Beth, assures her that her grandson is in the best possible care. Beth hangs up the phone and is introduced by the fire captain and paramedic on the scene. Alex is being splinted and pain management measures are helping him through this injury. The EMT contacts the hospital, the Mountain Dispatch Center keeps in communication with all units, the emergency crew keeps in communication with the entire family, and all members keep in communication with one another. Emergency care and transportation are just starting, but the communication loop is always in motion.

Key Terms

Base station A radio that is operated at a fixed site such as a dispatch center, a hospital, or another location that does not move; usually runs with community electrical power (as opposed to battery power) and transmits at a much higher power than do smaller, portable radios.

Digital radio equipment Computer-controlled radio equipment that is used in a sophisticated communication system, usually in the 800-MHz range.

Emergency medical dispatch (EMD) An approach to the dispatch function of an EMS system that involves the dispatcher in making decisions about the type and priority of EMS response that is necessary, providing critical information to responding units while they are en route, and providing prearrival instructions to callers until the EMS units are on the scene.

Mobile radios A vehicular mounted radio that operates with the vehicle's electrical supply; has a range of approximately 20 miles and a broadcast strength less than that of a base station.

Repeaters A radio unit that receives a signal from another radio unit and rebroadcasts it, boosting the signal strength in the process; used to overcome distance or geographic obstacles, such as mountains.

Six-way communications model Consists of the following steps: (1) the sender *thinks* of the idea that he or she wishes to convey to another member, (2) the sender *transmits* the message, (3) the sender *transfers* the message through a medium, (4) the receiver *obtains* the message, (5) the receiver *interprets* the message, and (6) the receiver *confirms* the message.

Key Terms (cont'd)

Systems status management (SSM) An approach to deployment of EMS resources (personnel and vehicles) that seeks to achieve maximum efficiency with minimal sacrifice in quality of care. SSM uses computer modeling techniques to predict EMS call volume and location, thereby allowing systems to preposition vehicles in the most efficient locations.

Telemetry The transmission of electronic signals over the radio. In EMS, the most frequent telemetry transmission is the electrocardiogram. To be useful, telemetry requires a "quiet," or interference-free, frequency.

UHF band Set of radio frequencies between 450 and 470 MHz; almost interference-free but are limited to line of sight and travel only short distances.

VHF high band Set of radio frequencies between 150 and 174 MHz; less prone to interference than VHF low band but are limited to line of sight communication because they cannot bend around obstacles or the curve of the earth.

VHF low band Set of radio frequencies between 32 and 50 MHz; can travel great distances but are subject to interference.

Review Questions

1. The type of radio installed in the ambulance is called:
   a. A base station
   b. Mobile
   c. Portable
   d. Manual
2. The cellular telephone is:
   a. A great tool in EMS communications because it allows for constant communications.
   b. A great tool in EMS communications because it always has special EMS channels.
   c. Considered as a communications tool, but it has limitations during peak times or emergencies.
   d. Considered as a communications tool for personal use only.
3. The following "codes" must be used over the radio:
   a. 10-4
   b. Code sixty
   c. 10-200
   d. Most modern EMS systems have diminished or eliminated 10 codes
4. Some EMS systems require communications to the hospital. List the two reasons why prehospital personnel need to communicate with the hospital.
   a. Provides the EMT instructions or advice from the physician, and allows the hospital to prepare to receive the patient
   b. Allows for hospital billing to start, and provides for the administrators to prepare
   c. Allows for the hospital to prepare for the patient and to notify the next of kin
   d. Provides the EMT instructions on travel to the hospital
5. The primary purpose to have a communications system use EMD is:
   a. To provide postincident review information.
   b. To provide prearrival instructions to callers.
   c. To provide prearrival instructions to EMTs.
   d. To allow for dispatchers to oversee EMTs.
6. The six-way communications model ends with which step?
   a. Transfer
   b. Obtain
   c. Confirm
   d. Think

Answers to these Review Questions can be found at the end of the book on page 869.

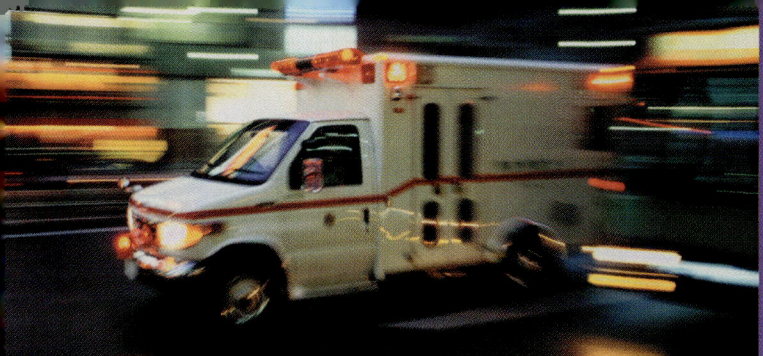

35

Documentation

Lesson Goal

This chapter presents guidelines on the rules for documentation of the patient care report. It also reviews the legal implications of proper documentation and its importance in the transmission of information.

Scenario

"Would you please read to the court your written account of the events that led to the reason for these proceedings?"

You scan the photocopy of a photocopy of a call that occurred over 3 years ago, and try to remember this specific call. Your mind draws a blank as you begin to read your report out loud:

"Male, obviously drunk with slurring speech involved in fight. Injury noted: laceration to forehead. Patient refusing care."

"Did you ask my client what caused the laceration?"

"I don't remember."

"Did you ask my client if he lost consciousness?"

"I don't remember."

"Did you perform an examination on my client prior to allowing him to refuse care?"

"I don't remember."

"Did you inform my client as to the possible ramifications of refusing care after sustaining a cut to the head from an unknown source?"

"I don't remember."

"One last question. When did you find out my client suffered permanent brain damage that was a result of an intracranial bleed caused by a blow to the head on the night of this call? An intracranial bleed that was not diagnosed by a doctor until my client passed out at home the next evening and his wife brought him to the emergency room?"

"I found out when I received a summons for deposition and immediately contacted my employer."

"It's too bad for my client you weren't as quick to take care of him as you were yourself. No further questions."

 If you have been in a court of law and placed under oath to review a case that may have likely happened years before, this is what it can be like. Would you be prepared to answer the questions accurately? Would your documentation support your verbal responses? Would your run report have documented that you rendered proper care and treatment to this patient?

Key Terms to Know

Computer-based report
Field assessment card
Glasgow Coma Scale
History of the present illness or injury
Injury location chart
Intervention
Multiple casualty incident (MCI)
Patient care report (PCR)
Patient data
Pediatric trauma score
Pertinent negative
Pertinent past medical history
Pertinent positive
Physical assessment
Reportable incident
Revised trauma score (RTS)
Run data
SOAP method
Written report

Learning Objectives

As an EMT-Basic, you should be able to do the following:

DOT

- List, explain, and apply the components of essential patient information in a written report.
- Identify the various divisions of the written report.
- Describe the information required in each section of the patient care report and how it should be entered.
- Discuss the legal implications associated with the written report.
- Define the special considerations concerning patient refusal.
- Discuss all state and local record-keeping and reporting requirements.
- Complete a prehospital care report.

Supplemental

- Explain the reasons for appropriate documentation and reporting of patient care information.
- Explain the purpose of gathering and reporting information.
- State the proper sequence of delivery of patient information.

Documentation is often seen as a necessary evil in emergency medical services (EMS). However, it is one of the most important nonclinical skills an emergency medical technician (EMT) possesses. Proper prehospital documentation provides a source of information about patient care:

- Provides a record of scene information that may not be available from any other source
- Provides information for the continuity of patient care from one health care professional to another
- Provides a record of specific prehospital interventions performed or attempted
- Provides medicolegal evidence
- Reveals any significant changes in the patient's condition
- Provides an internal tool for statistics, budgeting, quality assessment or improvement, and education
- Reveals problems with record-keeping procedures

Like any other EMT skill, the ability to document patient and emergency care information develops with practice. The **patient care report (PCR)** documents the **intervention** provided by the EMS crew in the prehospital setting based on the presentation of the patient or the mechanism of injury. It is a confidential legal document in many states and often becomes part of the patient's hospital record. An accurate and complete PCR is just as important as the nurses' notes or physician's report because it documents the reason for the call, pertinent medical history, the assessment and care of the patient, and other relevant data. Should the care of the patient ever be called into question, the PCR will be the EMT's first line of defense. PCRs are also used in quality improvement review, service reimbursement, and statistical review.

Although rules for documentation are not carved in stone and can vary from service to service, several universal guidelines can be applied to any PCR and can serve as a foundation for documentation of prehospital care. This chapter presents those guidelines, as well as the different parts of the PCR.

Patient Care Report

The PCR is the official documentation of an EMS call. Its importance cannot be overstated. It is considered a legal document that serves as an official record of care given by

EMS. It also provides valuable information regarding service crew information, run times, and mechanism of injury. As the only record of the prehospital care provided, the PCR could be the first line of defense if questions are raised about the incident, either now or at some time in the future (months or years later). Therefore the PCR must be thorough and complete.

> ✓ The patient care report is a legal document that should provide all the necessary information regarding that particular patient.

Use of the Patient Care Report

Two different types of PCRs are used in EMS systems. The first is the traditional **written report**, which typically provides check boxes and a narrative section for the EMT to complete in writing (Figure 35.1). The second is the **computer-based report**, which is generated on an electronic clipboard or mobile data terminal (Figure 35.2). The EMT enters the information by a special instrument or keyboard and then either downloads the information or prints a hard copy at the hospital or ambulance base.

A PCR typically has three divisions: (1) run data, (2) patient data, and (3) narrative. The **run data** typically consists of the service name and unit number, crew license numbers and names, location of the ambulance call, response times, and mileage. The **patient data** consists of the patient's name, address, date of birth, age, and sex; the nature of the call; the mechanism of injury; the location of the patient; the patient's level of consciousness, sensation, pupillary response, skin color, moisture and temperature, vital signs, pertinent medical history, and trauma or medical assessment (as appropriate); care administered to the patient; and any medical care provided before the arrival of the EMT, as well as who performed that care.

The narrative section is provided for the EMT to document observations at the scene, **physical assessment** findings, care delivered by the EMS crew, and changes in the patient's condition. Here, important observations about the scene should be noted. For example, was a weapon involved? What kind of weapon was it? If it was a handgun, what caliber? If it was a knife, how long was it? If it appears the patient was attempting to commit suicide, was a note left? Are empty pill bottles nearby? If the patient was involved in a motor vehicle accident, what kind of damage was there to the car? Is the windshield broken? Was the headrest in the raised or lowered position? Was the patient restrained at the time of the accident? Where did the impact occur—front, rear, or side?

> ✓ The PCR may be in a written or computer-based format. In either format, the PCR contains three sections: (1) run data, (2) patient data, and (3) narrative.

Completing the Patient Care Report

The PCR should document the care delivered to the patient at the scene and en route to the hospital, as well as any medical care delivered before the arrival of the EMS crew. It must be detailed and legible, and it must provide a clear and accurate picture of the patient, the chief complaint, and any special scene situations that may have affected care of the patient (e.g., extended extrication time, difficulty in reaching the patient due to severe weather). Proper spelling and general neatness are imperative to convey professionalism. To assist in obtaining complete patient information, a **field assessment card** may be used for taking notes during the assessment process. Information from the field assessment card is then transferred to the PCR at the appropriate time.

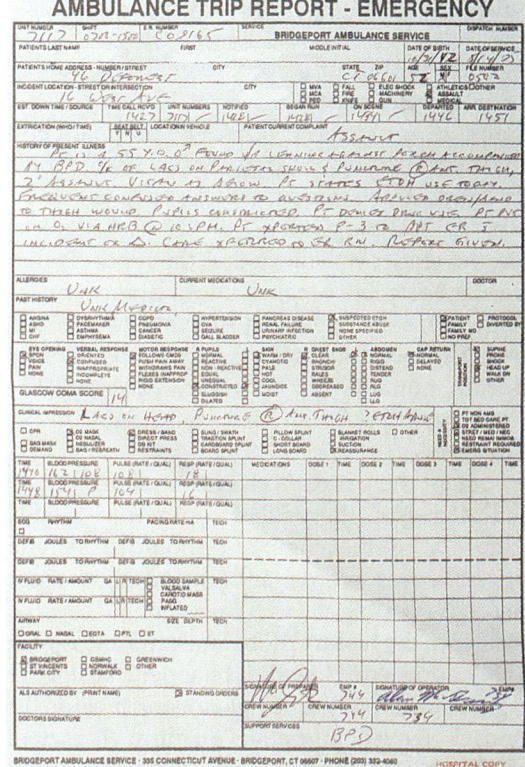

FIGURE 35.1 A written patient care report (PCR).

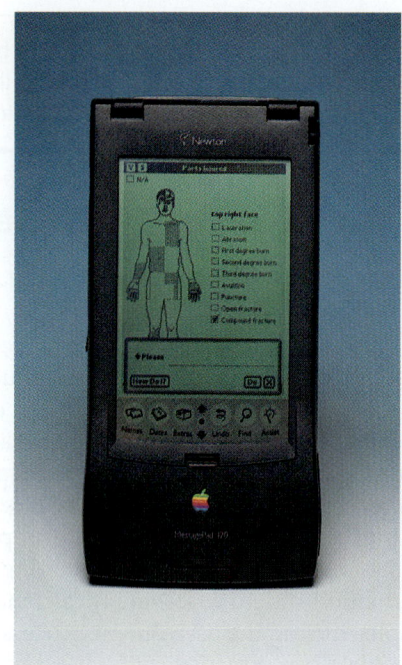

FIGURE 35.2 A computer-based report system.

General Guidelines

General guidelines for completing the PCR are as follows:

1. Collect all patient information (e.g., name, date of birth, age, sex, address). Depending on the service and the report form, insurance or billing information may also be required.
2. Complete *all* blanks and check *all* pertinent boxes on the call report form. Do not leave spaces intentionally blank. If the item does not apply to this patient, mark it "Not Applicable" or "N/A." Blank spaces lead the reader to believe that the report is not thorough or complete because information is missing.
3. Begin the narrative by documenting the patient's level of consciousness (LOC), age, and how he or she appears initially. For example, "20-year-old male found supine on the living room floor, responsive and alert."
4. Document the patient's chief complaint. What is the medical reason the patient summoned medical assistance? The chief complaint should be stated in the patient's own words and included in quotation marks, if possible.
5. Document the **history of the present illness or injury**. What happened? How did it happen? History should be given in chronologic sequence and include the time of onset, frequency, location, quantity, character of the problem, setting, and anything that aggravates or relieves the problem. Use the OPQRST format:

   O—Onset. What time did the problem start?
   P—Provokes. What was the patient doing when the pain or problem started? What makes the pain worse?
   Q—Quality. Is the pain sharp or dull? How does the patient describe the pain?
   R—Radiates. Does the pain radiate anywhere?
   S—Severity. On a scale of 1 to 10, with 10 being the worst pain, how does the pain rate?
   T—Time. How long has the problem or pain lasted?

6. Document physical assessment findings, including any pertinent positives or pertinent negatives. For example, in a patient complaining of abdominal pain, finding that "the abdomen is soft and nontender to palpation" is a **pertinent negative**. In a patient with difficulty breathing, finding that the lung sounds are diminished on one side is a **pertinent positive**. When information of a sensitive nature (e.g., communicable disease) is documented, the source of that information (e.g., the patient, patient's family, a bystander) should also be documented: "Patient states . . ."
7. Document any significant **pertinent past medical history**, including surgeries, hospitalizations, illnesses, or injuries. *Significant* is the key word here. The broken toe Grandma suffered 12 years ago probably has little bearing on the heart attack she's having now.
8. Document allergies and current medications. Accurately list each drug the patient is taking and the dosage.
9. Document interventions, who performed them, and the patient's response or lack of response to the intervention. Include the time of each intervention and either the name or license (certification) number of the EMT performing the skill.
10. Document vital signs and any orders received from the medical direction physician. Record the time a set of vital signs is taken. Any orders received from medical control should be documented along with the name of the physician providing the orders. In some systems, it may be required that a physician sign for his or her orders on the PCR.
11. Attach electrocardiogram documentation (where applicable) with date, time, and patient's name on it. When an automated external defibrillator is used, a copy of the electrocardiogram tracing or summary printed by the machine should be attached to both the hospital copy and the original PCR. The documentation should be plainly marked with the date, time, patient's name, and PCR number (if applicable).
12. Complete the **Glasgow Coma Scale** with times when indicated. Many PCRs provide the Glasgow Coma Scale on the report. If not, consider carrying an appropriate pocket card or other reference (Figure 35.3).

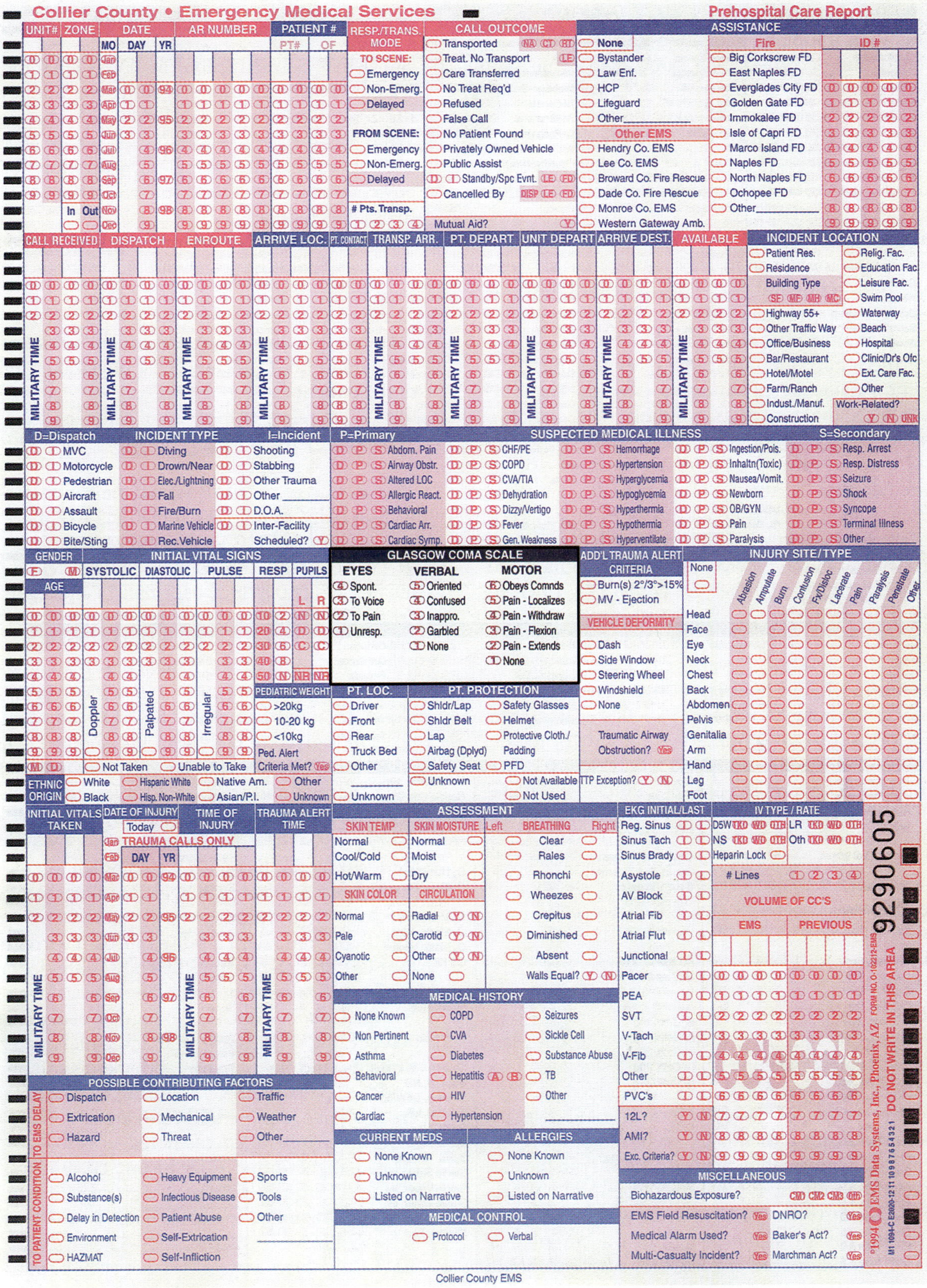

FIGURE 35.3 The Glasgow Coma Scale can usually be found on the PCR.

13. Complete the **revised trauma score (RTS)**, or rule of nines, if required, with times, when indicated. In patients with traumatic injury, the RTS should be calculated and recorded. The same holds true with burn victims and the rule of nines. As with the Glasgow Coma Scale, the RTS may be printed on the form, thus allowing the EMT to simply fill in the appropriate numbers to calculate the score. In pediatric patients, a **pediatric trauma score** should be calculated and recorded.
14. Complete the **injury location chart**, if indicated. Some PCRs contain an injury location chart showing both the anterior and posterior surfaces of the body. The EMT may indicate the area of injury by placing a mark on the chart (Figure 35.4).
15. Sign the report and obtain the receiving nurse's or doctor's name or signature as needed. The EMT must sign the report as required. The signature should be legible or should be followed by the EMT's name printed in a legible manner. The requirement for a nurse's or physician's signature varies from state to state and even from service to service. In states in which it is required, the nurse or physician attending the patient usually signs the report after receiving either the verbal or written report from the EMT.
16. Leave a copy of the report with the patient's chart. Again, this requirement varies from state to state. In systems in which a multipart form is used, one copy is left at the hospital with the patient's chart. Multipart forms provide continuity in the care of the patient as other health care providers review the PCR to better understand the patient's initial condition.

> ✓ A professional and organized approach is vital to successful documentation. Incomplete or inaccurate reports cast doubt on the care delivered and on the EMT who delivered it.

Writing the Narrative

When writing the narrative, it is important to use plain language and correct spelling and to avoid slang terms or abbreviations that are not widely recognized and accepted. If the spelling of a word or term is not known, the EMT should consult a dictionary or use another word. Specific types of information may be necessary in the narrative depending on the type of call. Examples are provided in Box 35.1. The narrative may be written based on either the assessment of the patient or the chronologic progress of the call. In either case, the narrative should begin with the patient's age, sex, and chief complaint, and how the patient was found initially.

SOAP method. One method for documenting based on patient assessment is the **SOAP method**:

S—Subjective. Subjective information is what the patient tells the EMT regarding his or her condition: What's hurting? Where is the pain? How did it happen? What was the patient doing when it happened? Does the patient have any allergies (medication, food, or environment)? Are there any medications that the patient takes regularly?

O—Objective. Objective information is what the EMT observes about the scene and any obvious patient injuries.

A—Assessment. Assessment is the EMT's evaluation of the situation, the patient, the patient's chief complaint, and findings based on a physical examination of the patient.

P—Plan. Plan refers to the plan of action and the care delivered by the EMT.

For example, a SOAP-format narrative for a man with chest pains might look something like this:

S—47-year-old male complaining that his "chest began hurting while playing basketball." Pain described as "sharp, stabbing" and radiates down left arm and into left jaw. Pain began suddenly at approximately 0900 hours today while patient was playing game of basketball. On a scale of 1 to 10, with 10 being the worst, pt. states pain is an "8.5." Pt. states that he takes nitroglycerin tablets for his angina. He has taken three already with no relief. Pt. denies any drug allergies and states that his last meal was breakfast today and that he feels slightly nauseous.

O—EMS arrives to find male patient, responsive and alert, sitting on the bench. Pt. complaining of stabbing-type chest pain, which radiates down his left. At 0910 hr the patient is noted to be pale, cool, and diaphoretic with a pulse rate of 106 irregular, BP 144/100, and respirations 28 and slightly labored. Pt. denies difficulty breathing other than being "winded" from exercise. No jugular vein distention noted. Lung sounds are clear and equal bilaterally in all fields, and the patient's abdomen is soft and nontender to palpation. No pulsating masses noted in the abdomen, and pedal pulses are felt bilaterally. No signs of peripheral edema noted.

A—Male patient with cardiac history currently experiencing substernal chest pain with radiation to his left arm and jaw following basketball game. Pt. appears to be in moderate distress.

P—EMT Gage placed pt. on oxygen at 15 L/min via nonrebreather mask at 0915. Pt. moved on stretcher to the ambulance. Vital signs rechecked at 0915,

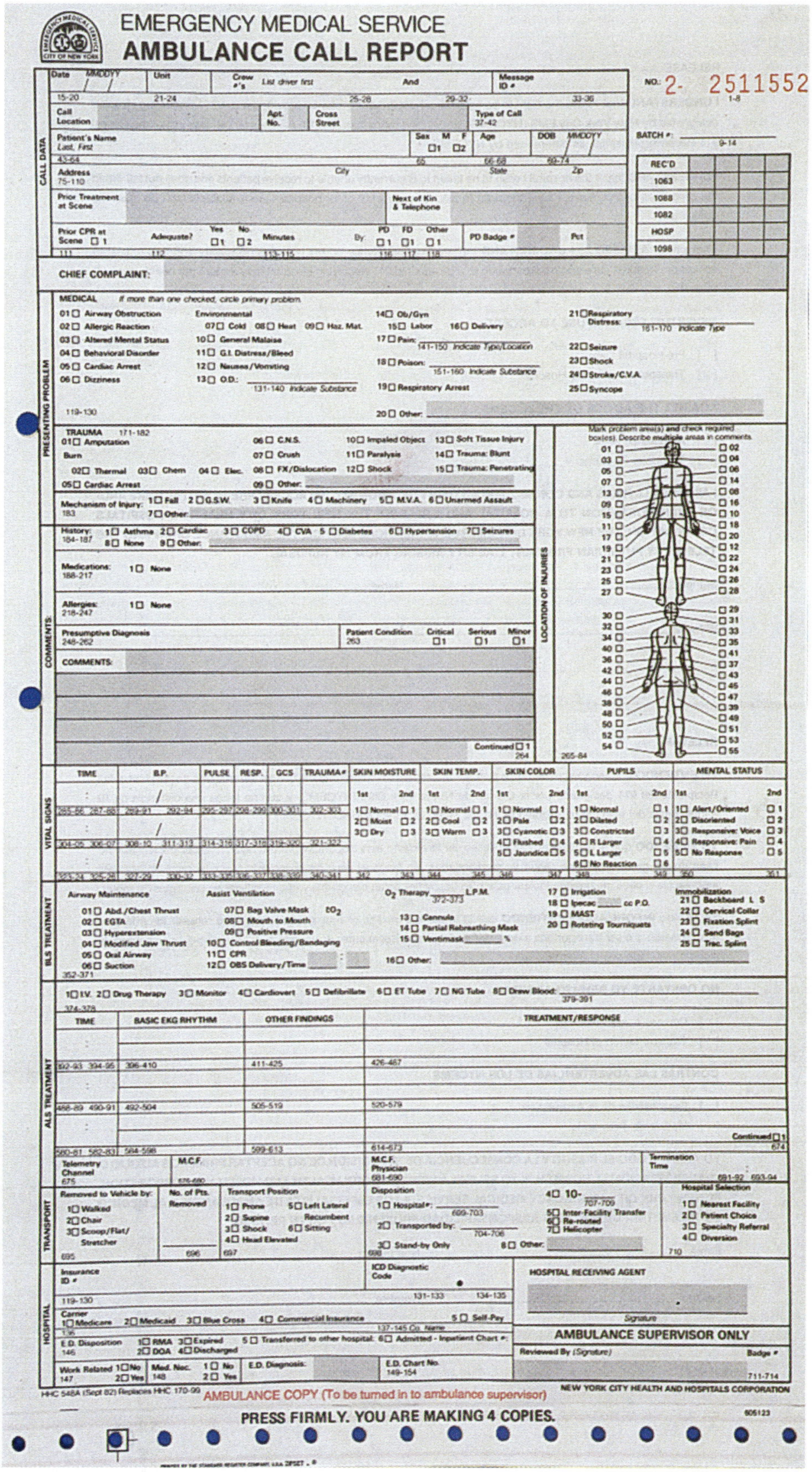
EMERGENCY MEDICAL SERVICE
AMBULANCE CALL REPORT

NO. 2- 2511552

CALL DATA: Date MMDDYY / Unit / Crew #'s List driver first And / Message ID #
Call Location / Apt. No. / Cross Street / Type of Call
Patient's Name Last, First / Sex M F / Age / DOB MMDDYY
Address / City / State / Zip
Prior Treatment at Scene / Next of Kin & Telephone
Prior CPR at Scene / Adequate? Yes No / Minutes / By: PD FD Other / PD Badge # / Pct

BATCH #: / REC'D 1063 1088 1082 HOSP 1098

CHIEF COMPLAINT:

PRESENTING PROBLEM
MEDICAL If more than one checked, circle primary problem.
01 Airway Obstruction; 02 Allergic Reaction; 03 Altered Mental Status; 04 Behavioral Disorder; 05 Cardiac Arrest; 06 Dizziness
Environmental: 07 Cold; 08 Heat; 09 Haz. Mat.; 10 General Malaise; 11 G.I. Distress/Bleed; 12 Nausea/Vomiting; 13 O.D.: indicate Substance
14 Ob/Gyn: 15 Labor; 16 Delivery; 17 Pain: indicate Type/Location; 18 Poison: indicate Substance; 19 Respiratory Arrest; 20 Other:
21 Respiratory Distress: indicate Type; 22 Seizure; 23 Shock; 24 Stroke/C.V.A.; 25 Syncope

TRAUMA
01 Amputation; Burn: 02 Thermal 03 Chem 04 Elec.; 05 Cardiac Arrest
06 C.N.S.; 07 Crush; 08 FX/Dislocation; 09 Other:
10 Impaled Object; 11 Paralysis; 12 Shock; 13 Soft Tissue Injury; 14 Trauma: Blunt; 15 Trauma: Penetrating
Mechanism of Injury: 1 Fall 2 G.S.W. 3 Knife 4 Machinery 5 M.V.A. 6 Unarmed Assault 7 Other:

History: 1 Asthma 2 Cardiac 3 COPD 4 CVA 5 Diabetes 6 Hypertension 7 Seizures 8 None 9 Other:
Medications: 1 None
Allergies: 1 None
Presumptive Diagnosis / Patient Condition: Critical, Serious, Minor
COMMENTS: / Continued

LOCATION OF INJURIES: Mark problem area(s) and check required box(es). Describe multiple areas in comments.

VITAL SIGNS: TIME / B.P. / PULSE / RESP. / GCS / TRAUMA# / SKIN MOISTURE (1 Normal, 2 Moist, 3 Dry) / SKIN TEMP. (1 Normal, 2 Cool, 3 Warm) / SKIN COLOR (1 Normal, 2 Pale, 3 Cyanotic, 4 Flushed, 5 Jaundice) / PUPILS (1 Normal, 2 Dilated, 3 Constricted, 4 R Larger, 5 L Larger, 6 No Reaction) / MENTAL STATUS (1 Alert/Oriented, 2 Disoriented, 3 Responsive: Voice, 4 Responsive: Pain, 5 No Response)

BLS TREATMENT
Airway Maintenance: 01 Abd./Chest Thrust; 02 EGTA; 03 Hyperextension; 04 Modified Jaw Thrust; 05 Oral Airway; 06 Suction
Assist Ventilation: 07 Bag Valve Mask; 08 Mouth to Mouth; 09 Positive Pressure; 10 Control Bleeding/Bandaging; 11 CPR; 12 OBS Delivery/Time
O_2 Therapy L.P.M.: 13 Cannula; 14 Partial Rebreathing Mask; 15 Ventimask %; 16 Other:
17 Irrigation; 18 Ipecac cc P.O.; 19 MAST; 20 Rotating Tourniquets
Immobilization: 21 Backboard L S; 22 Cervical Collar; 23 Fixation Splint; 24 Sand Bags; 25 Trac. Splint

ALS TREATMENT
1 I.V. 2 Drug Therapy 3 Monitor 4 Cardiovert 5 Defibrillate 6 ET Tube 7 NG Tube 8 Draw Blood
TIME / BASIC EKG RHYTHM / OTHER FINDINGS / TREATMENT/RESPONSE
Telemetry Channel / M.C.F. / M.C.F. Physician / Termination Time

TRANSPORT
Removed to Vehicle by: 1 Walked 2 Chair 3 Scoop/Flat/Stretcher
No. of Pts. Removed
Transport Position: 1 Prone 2 Supine 3 Shock 4 Head Elevated 5 Left Lateral Recumbent 6 Sitting
Disposition: 1 Hospital #: 2 Transported by: 3 Stand-by Only 4 10- 5 Inter-Facility Transfer 6 Re-routed 7 Helicopter 8 Other:
Hospital Selection: 1 Nearest Facility 2 Patient Choice 3 Specialty Referral 4 Diversion

HOSPITAL
Insurance ID # / ICD Diagnostic Code
Carrier: 1 Medicare 2 Medicaid 3 Blue Cross 4 Commercial Insurance 5 Self-Pay
E.D. Disposition: 1 RMA 2 DOA 3 Expired 4 Discharged 5 Transferred to other hospital 6 Admitted - Inpatient Chart #:
Work Related 1 No 2 Yes / Med. Nec. 1 No 2 Yes / E.D. Diagnosis: / E.D. Chart No.
HOSPITAL RECEIVING AGENT / Signature
AMBULANCE SUPERVISOR ONLY / Reviewed By (Signature) / Badge #

HHC 548A (Sept 82) Replaces HHC 170-99 AMBULANCE COPY (To be turned in to ambulance supervisor) NEW YORK CITY HEALTH AND HOSPITALS CORPORATION
PRESS FIRMLY. YOU ARE MAKING 4 COPIES.

FIGURE 35.4 Injury location chart. The EMT notes sites of injury by marking the chart.

Box 35.1 Documentation by Call Type

The following lists are specific pieces of information that may be necessary for complete and accurate documentation. This information is not in prioritized order. These lists indicate suggested items that should be included in your documentation.

Car Crash
- Patient location in auto
- Seatbelt or shoulder harness usage
- Loss of consciousness
- Velocity of accident
- Type of accident (head-on, roll-over)
- Type of vehicle damage
- Patient trapped or pinned
- Delay in extrication
- Patient ejected from vehicle
- Patient ambulatory at scene

Chest Pain
- Activity at time of pain onset
- Radiation
- Pain on movement
- Onset (gradual or sudden)
- Breath sounds (presence, quality, and quantity)
- Dyspnea
- Nausea or vomiting
- Diaphoresis
- Jugular venous distention
- Peripheral edema
- Pain character (sharp, dull)

For any type of pain, the OPQRST format can be used: O—Onset, P—Provokes, Q—Quality, R—Radiates, S—Severity, and T—Time.

Coma
- Sign or history of trauma
- History of diabetes or seizure
- Drug or alcohol ingestion
- Last seen conscious by whom and when
- Position found
- Scene survey
- Pupils
- Response to painful or verbal stimulus

Diabetes
- Level of consciousness
- Insulin-dependent or oral hypoglycemics
- Last meal
- Amount of exercise
- Last insulin injection and how much
- Any recent illnesses
- Gradual or rapid onset of symptoms
- Kussmaul breathing
- Alcohol or other drug use

Gunshot Wound
- Number of wounds
- Location of wounds
- Type of weapon (handgun, rifle, or shotgun)
- Patient's position at time of shooting
- Perpetrator's position at time of shooting
- How many shots heard
- Head-to-toe assessment
- Note caliber of weapon, if it can be confirmed
- Amount of external hemorrhage noted
- Police notification

No Transport Call
- Clear documentation
- Patient demographic information
- Patient informed of consequences of not being transported
- Methods used to encourage patient to accept treatment/transportation
- Alcohol or other drug usage
- Level of consciousness
- Patient's reason for contacting EMS
- Individual responsible for contacting EMS, if not the patient
- Vital signs
- Physical examination
- Cancellations en route noted (e.g., police, fire, dispatch)
- Patient's cooperation with your attempt to deliver care and transport
- Signature of patient
- Signature of witnesses

Overdose
- Level of consciousness
- Whether overdose was witnessed or not
- Medication or substance ingested
- Amount ingested
- Time of overdose or best approximation
- Any associated alcohol or drug consumption
- Prior overdose or suicide attempts
- Patient admission of intent to harm self
- Police notification

Pediatric
- Level of consciousness (crying, uninterested)
- Parent recognition
- Consolable
- Head bob
- Fontanelles (full, flat, or sunken)

> **Box 35.1 Documentation by Call Type—cont'd**
>
> **Pediatric—continued**
> - Child's weight
> - Skin condition
> - Sucking reflex
> - Finger grasp
> - Response to pain
> - Fever
> - Length of illness
> - Medications or treatments administered
>
> **Pregnancy**
> - Last menstrual period
> - Estimated due date (if known)
> - Number of pregnancies (gravida)
> - Number of pregnancies carried to term (para)
> - Prenatal care history (none, some, continuous)
> - Complications with this pregnancy
> - Complications with other pregnancies
> - Water broke
> - Back pain
> - Urge to push
> - Vaginal discharge
> - Multiple births
> - Type of pain
> - Duration of pain
> - Regularity of pain
> - Interval between pains
> - Progress during transport
>
> **Respiratory Distress**
> - Level of consciousness
> - Skin color and temperature
> - Amount of distress (mild, moderate, or severe)
> - Audible respiratory sounds (wheezes, rales)
> - Onset of distress (gradual or sudden)
> - Activity at time of onset
> - Cardiac history
> - Chronic obstructive pulmonary disease history
> - Breath sounds (present, absent, wheezes, rales)
>
> **Seizure**
> - Level of consciousness
> - History of seizures
> - History of alcohol or other drug usage
> - History of diabetes
> - Sign or history of injury
> - Number of seizures
> - Duration of seizures
> - Motor activity observed during seizure (e.g., where began and spread)
> - Medication history (i.e., takes seizure or diabetic medications regularly)
> - Pupils
> - Breath sounds
> - Head-to-toe assessment
> - Cardiac history
>
> **Stab Wounds**
> - Number of wounds
> - Location of wounds
> - Amount of external hemorrhage noted
> - Patient's position at time of stabbing
> - Perpetrator's position and knife angle at time of stabbing
> - Head-to-toe assessment
> - Scene survey
> - Police notification
>
> **Trauma**
> - Level of consciousness
> - Type of accident
> - Ambulatory after accident
> - Head-to-toe assessment
> - Special circumstances
> - Scene survey

pulse 114 irregular, BP 146/94, and respirations 30. Pt. remains pale, diaphoretic, and nauseated. Transport to the emergency department at Bay Harbor Medical Center. Contacted the ED en route with pt. report and 8-minute ETA; no orders requested. En route, pt. stated that breathing was somewhat easier but chest pain is still at 8–8.5 on a scale of 1 to 10. At 0920, pulse is 106 irregular, BP is 144/92, and respirations are 24. Arrived Bay Harbor ED at 0925 with pt. in stable condition. Care transferred to ED staff, report to E. Butcher, RN.

Head-to-toe method. Another method is to document the assessment the way you performed it—head-to-toe. Begin your report with the patient's age, sex, and level of consciousness, and how the patient was found initially. Then list the results of your initial assessment and focused history and examination, concluding with the interventions and care delivered to the patient. An easy way to write this kind of report is to imagine the patient lying on the stretcher with a sheet over him or her. As the sheet is rolled down, the various body regions are assessed, noting pertinent findings. Let's use the same patient but write a head-to-toe format report:

EMS arrives to find a 47-year-old male responsive and alert complaining of his "chest hurting," sitting on a bench at the basketball court. Pt. states pain began suddenly around 0900 hours today while he was playing basketball. Pain is described as substernal, "sharp, stabbing," and radiates down the left arm and up into the left jaw. Pt. states pain is an "8.5" on scale of 1 to 10, with 10 being the worst. Pt. states history of "heart problems" and says that he has already taken three nitroglycerin tablets with no relief. Pt. denies drug allergies, states that his last meal was lunch today and he now feels nauseous. INITIAL ASSESSMENT shows pt. to be pale, cool, and diaphoretic at 0910. Vital signs are BP 144/100, pulse 106 and irregular, respirations 28 and labored, and lung sounds clear and equal bilaterally in all fields. Pt. denies difficulty breathing other than being "winded" from exercise. FOCUSED HISTORY AND EXAMINATION shows no jugular vein distention, abdomen is soft and nontender with no pulsatile masses noted. Pedal pulses are palpable in both lower extremities. No signs of peripheral edema noted.

INTERVENTION: Placed pt. on oxygen at 15 L/min by nonrebreather face mask at 0915 and placed him on the stretcher with assistance from health club personnel. Pt. was moved to ambulance for emergency transport to Bay Harbor Medical Center. Pt. remains pale, diaphoretic, and nauseated. Vital signs rechecked at 0915: BP 146/94, pulse 114 irregular, and respirations 30. Transport begun. ED contacted and pt. report given with 8-minute ETA—no orders requested. En route, pt. states breathing is easier but chest pain is still at 8–8.5 on scale of 1 to 10. Vital signs at 0920: BP 144/92, pulse 106 and irregular, and respirations 24. Arrived at Bay Harbor's ED at 0925 with pt. in stable condition. Transferred care to ED staff, report to E. Butcher, RN.

Chronologic method. Documentation based on the chronologic progress of the call begins with the time of arrival on the scene. An exception would be if difficulties were encountered in reaching the scene, in which case that entry (with time) would precede the arrival time entry. Each entry begins with a time notation followed by the pertinent information for that time frame. Here is an example using the same patient:

0910—Arrived on scene to find 47-year-old male responsive and alert, complaining of his "chest hurting" while playing basketball, found sitting on a bench. Pt. states pain began suddenly at 0900 hours today and describes it as substernal, "sharp, stabbing" type pain, which radiates into his left arm and left jaw. On scale of 1 (least) to 10 (worst), pt. states pain is an "8.5." Pt. further states history of "heart problems" and says he has taken three nitroglycerin tablets today without relief.

0910—Initial assessment completed—shows pt. to be pale, cool, and diaphoretic. Vital signs: BP 144/100, pulse 106 and irregular, respirations 28 and labored. Lung sounds clear and equal bilaterally in all fields. Placed pt. on oxygen at 15 L/min per nonrebreather mask. Pt. denies difficulty breathing except for feeling "winded" after exercise.

0913—Focused examination and history completed and shows pt. to be in moderate distress. Pt. states his last meal was lunch today and he now feels nauseous. Pt. denies any drug allergies. No jugular vein distention noted. Abdomen is soft and nontender on palpation, and pedal pulses are palpable bilaterally in the lower extremities. No signs of peripheral edema noted.

0915—Pt. placed on stretcher with assistance from health club personnel and moved to ambulance for emergency transport to Bay Harbor Medical Center.

0915—Pt. remains pale, diaphoretic, and nauseated. Vital signs reassessed: BP 146/94, pulse 114 irregular, respirations 30 and labored. Transport begun. Bay Harbor ED contacted with pt. report and 8-minute ETA.

0918—Pt. states breathing is easier but chest pain remains at 8–8.5.

0920—Vital signs: BP 144/92, pulse 106 irregular, and respirations 24.

0925—Arrived Bay Harbor's ED with pt. in stable condition. Transferred care to ED staff, report to E. Butcher, RN.

No matter which format you use, the narrative may be longer than the space provided. Use a supplemental sheet to complete the narrative, making sure to include the patient's name, the date, and the report number (if used) at the top of the supplemental sheet. Make sure that a copy of the supplemental sheet is left with the copy of the PCR at the hospital.

> ✓ The narrative section of the PCR is used to describe the findings of the scene, physical assessment, and the interventions delivered by the EMT in a simple, straightforward format. By using a systematic approach in writing the narrative, a complete and accurate story can be told.

Considerations

If you make a mistake while writing the narrative or any part of the PCR, do not erase or mark out the mistake. Doing so only gives a later reader the impression that something was done wrong and is being covered up. Rather, the EMT should simply draw a single line through the error and then place his or her initials beside the line. Some EMS agencies require that the word "error" be written above the line. The correct information may then be written following the correction. When a mistake is discovered after the completion or submission of the report, the EMT should draw a single line through the error (preferably with a different color ink), initial and date it along with the time, and add a note with the correct information. In the event that information was omitted, adding a note with the information, the date, and the EMT's initials is appropriate.

When an error in patient care occurs, under no circumstances should the EMT try to cover up the mistake. Rather, the EMT should document what did or did not happen and what corrective action (if any) was taken. Falsifying information on the PCR is harmful to the patient, because it may lead other health care providers to a false impression of the patient's condition, assessment, and care provided. It may also lead to suspension or revocation of the EMT's certification or license and other legal action.

As mentioned earlier, the PCR is considered a confidential document. Laws regarding confidentiality vary from state to state, so it is important for the EMT to be familiar with the laws in the state of practice. Although a legal obligation may not exist for confidentiality, the EMT certainly has an ethical obligation to protect a patient's privacy, and this ethical obligation includes the patient's PCR. As a medical document, distribution of the document is also regulated by law. Local and state regulations determine how and where copies of the document should be distributed. Once again, familiarization with the appropriate regulations will assist the EMT in complying with them.

> ✓ The PCR is a legal document and must be treated as such. Any mistakes made, in either the care of the patient or documentation of care, should be carefully noted and corrected. Copies of the PCR are distributed in accordance with state and local regulations, and all EMS personnel should be aware of those regulations.

Special Situations

Patient Refusal of Care

In some instances, the patient may refuse care from the EMS crew. Laws regarding a patient's right to refuse medical attention vary from state to state. In general, adult patients who competent to make their own decisions may refuse care and transportation from an EMT. The EMT must ensure that the refusing patient is indeed able to make a rational, informed decision and is not under the influence of drugs, alcohol, or any effects of an illness or injury. Because the patient, family member, co-worker, or bystander believed that the situation required an EMS response, every attempt should be made to persuade the patient to go to a hospital. The patient should be informed of why he or she needs to go to the hospital and what may happen if he or she does not. For example, a patient involved in a motor vehicle crash who complains of neck pain but refuses care should know that a cervical spine injury is possible. The patient should also be informed that such an injury could result in paralysis if not diagnosed and treated appropriately.

If the patient continues to refuse care, the patient should then sign a refusal form provided by the EMT (Figure 35.5). A police officer, bystander, or family member should sign as a witness to the refusal. If the patient refuses to sign the refusal form, a witness should sign the form verifying that the patient refused to sign. Contact with medical control should be made as directed by local protocol for refusal situations.

When documenting the refusal situation, the EMT should include all of the following in the narrative:

1. Complete patient assessment, including vital signs, or the refusal of assessment.
2. Care that the EMS crew wished or offered to provide to the patient.
3. Statement that the EMT explained to the patient the possible consequences of refusing care, including adverse effects and potential death. In the case of a minor patient, the possible consequences would be explained to the parent or legal guardian and documented.
4. Offer of alternative methods for accessing care.
5. Statement of the EMS crew's willingness to return should the patient's condition change or the patient decide to seek medical attention.

More specific items for documentation of refusal of care are shown in Box 35.1.

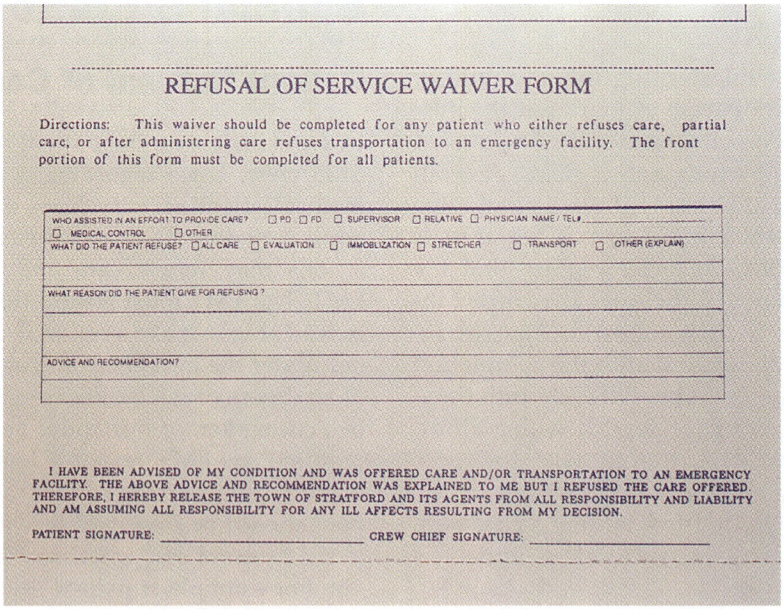

REFUSAL OF SERVICE WAIVER FORM

Directions: This waiver should be completed for any patient who either refuses care, partial care, or after administering care refuses transportation to an emergency facility. The front portion of this form must be completed for all patients.

WHO ASSISTED IN AN EFFORT TO PROVIDE CARE? ☐ PD ☐ FD ☐ SUPERVISOR ☐ RELATIVE ☐ PHYSICIAN NAME / TEL# ____ ☐ MEDICAL CONTROL ☐ OTHER

WHAT DID THE PATIENT REFUSE? ☐ ALL CARE ☐ EVALUATION ☐ IMMOBLIZATION ☐ STRETCHER ☐ TRANSPORT ☐ OTHER (EXPLAIN)

WHAT REASON DID THE PATIENT GIVE FOR REFUSING ?

ADVICE AND RECOMMENDATION?

I HAVE BEEN ADVISED OF MY CONDITION AND WAS OFFERED CARE AND/OR TRANSPORTATION TO AN EMERGENCY FACILITY. THE ABOVE ADVICE AND RECOMMENDATION WAS EXPLAINED TO ME BUT I REFUSED THE CARE OFFERED. THEREFORE, I HEREBY RELEASE THE TOWN OF STRATFORD AND ITS AGENTS FROM ALL RESPONSIBILITY AND LIABILITY AND AM ASSUMING ALL RESPONSIBILITY FOR ANY ILL AFFECTS RESULTING FROM MY DECISION.

PATIENT SIGNATURE: ____ CREW CHIEF SIGNATURE: ____

FIGURE 35.5 A patient refusal form.

Box 35.2 Cases Reportable Under Law in Most States

- Neglect or abuse of children
- Neglect or abuse of older adults
- Rape
- Gunshot wounds
- Stab wounds
- Animal bites
- Certain communicable diseases

Multiple Casualty Incidents

A **multiple casualty incident (MCI)** presents a number of challenges for EMS personnel, not the least of which is documentation of the patients involved. Depending on the situation, the PCR may not be completed right away and, in fact, may be completed some time later. Local MCI plans should include both a means for temporarily recording important patient information and guidelines for completion of the PCR in an MCI situation. Triage tags are ideal sources of information for completion of the report at the conclusion of the incident.

Special Situation Reports

In some instances, a special report or addendum is indicated. In situations in which the narrative exceeds the section provided, a supplemental or addendum report is needed and should be attached to the original PCR, with a copy attached to each copy of the PCR distributed. In other circumstances, a separate report may be required for an infectious disease or body fluid exposure, a line-of-duty injury, or a **reportable incident** (Box 35.2).

> ✔ Special situations require particularly close attention to documentation. Local protocols may dictate specific guidelines to follow in those instances, and the EMT should be familiar with those situations and protocols.

Summary

- Documentation is the most important nonclinical skill possessed by the EMT. The patient care report must be accurate and report both subjective and objective findings, physical assessment results, care and treatment rendered by the EMS crew, and any significant observations about the scene.
- The PCR is used for a number of different purposes, such as providing medicolegal documentation of

Summary (cont'd)

- patient care, ensuring continuity of care among health care providers, administrative functions (e.g., billing, statistics), research, and continuous quality improvement.
- The PCR is considered a legal document that serves as an official record of care given by EMS. As the only official record of the patient care provided by the EMT, the PCR could be the first line of defense if questions are later raised about the incident.
- The PCR contains three sections: run data, patient information, and narrative. Run data includes the service name and unit number, crew license numbers or names, location of the ambulance call, response times, and mileage. Patient data consists of the patient's name, address, date of birth, age, and sex; the nature of the call; the mechanism of injury; the location of the patient; the patient's level of consciousness, sensation, pupillary response, skin color, moisture and temperature, vital signs, history, and trauma or medical assessment (as appropriate); care administered to the patient; and any medical care provided before the arrival of the EMT. Narrative includes the EMT's observations at the scene, physical assessment findings, and care and treatment delivered by the EMS crew.
- The narrative can be written using the SOAP, head-to-toe, or chronologic method.
- In the event that a patient refuses care, the EMT must carefully document the following information in the narrative: complete patient assessment, including vital signs, or refusal of assessment; the care that the EMS crew wished or offered to provide to the patient; a statement that the EMT explained to the patient the possible consequences of refusing care, including adverse effects and potential death; an offer of alternative methods for accessing care; and a statement of the EMS crew's willingness to return should the patient's condition change or the patient decide to seek medical attention.
- Special situations, such as mass casualty incidents, require specific documentation.

Scenario Solution

In this scenario, the lack of accurate and appropriate documentation has dire consequences. The assessment and treatment were cursory at best, and the documentation was even worse. The EMT cannot remember, and the report is of no value.

Had the EMT performed a complete assessment and properly documented the findings, the patient's refusal of care, and the consequences of refusal of care, the EMT would have had no problem answering the attorney's questions. Instead, her incomplete narrative casts great doubt on the care she provided.

Key Terms

Computer-based report One format for a patient care report. A computer-based report is completed using an electronic clipboard or mobile data terminal in which the information is entered by a special instrument or keyboard. The information can then be downloaded or printed at the hospital or ambulance base.

Field assessment card A form used for making notes during the assessment and history-taking process; serves as a way for the EMT to organize information informally before entering it on the patient care report.

Glasgow Coma Scale Standardized rating system used to evaluate the degree of consciousness impairment based on eye opening, motor response, and verbal response. Points are scored for the patient's best response in each of the three categories.

History of the present illness or injury Events or complaints associated with the patient's current health problem; it should correspond to the reason the patient is now seeking medical attention.

Injury location chart Anterior and posterior anatomic figure diagram located on the prehospital care report; used to diagram the patient's injuries.

Intervention An action or skill performed by the EMT in response to finding the initial assessment or focused history and examination.

Multiple casualty incident (MCI) Commonly accepted definition is any incident involving one or more patients that cannot be handled by the first responding unit or units to a scene (e.g., the bombing of the Murrah Federal Building in Oklahoma City).

Key Terms (cont'd)

Patient care report (PCR) The official or formal documentation of the physical assessment and care provided to a particular patient; may either be in written or computer-based format.

Patient data Specific information about a patient that is documented on the patient care report. This information may include, but is not limited to, the patient's name, address, date of birth, age, and sex; the nature of the call; the mechanism of injury; the location of the patient; the patient's level of consciousness, sensation, pupillary response, skin color, moisture and temperature, vital signs, history, and trauma or medical assessment (as appropriate); care administered to the patient; and any medical care provided before the arrival of the EMT.

Pediatric trauma score Standardized injury severity index used in pediatric patients.

Pertinent negative Absense of a sign or symptom that helps substantiate or identify a patient's condition (e.g., in a patient complaining of abdominal pain, finding that the abdomen is soft and nontender is a pertinent negative and should be documented).

Pertinent past medical history Any prior or current medical conditions, surgeries, hospitalizations, illnesses, or injuries suffered by the patient; specific attention is focused on major problems that might be relevant to the patient's current medical condition.

Pertinent positive Presence of a sign or symptom that helps substantiate or identify a patient's condition (e.g., if a patient falls and complains of wrist pain, the positive sign is deformity of the wrist).

Physical assessement Head-to-toe, hands-on examination.

Reportable incident Any incident that is to be reported to the appropriate authority under local, state, or federal regulation or law (e.g., in some states, health care providers are required to report suspected child or elderly abuse).

Revised trauma score (RTS) Standardized injury severity index that incorporates the Glasgow Coma Scale and the measurements for the systolic blood pressure and respiratory rate.

Run data Specific information about the ambulance call that is documented on the patient care report. Run data may include, but is not limited to, ambulance service name and unit number, crew license numbers or names, location of the ambulance call, response times, and mileage.

SOAP method A specific format used in completing the narrative section of the patient care report. SOAP is an acronym for the components of the narrative: subjective findings, objective findings, assessment, and plan of action for caring for the patient.

Written report One format for a patient care report; typically consists of a specific form that includes check boxes and a section for writing a narrative of the patient scenario, assessement, and interventions provided or attempted.

Review Questions

1. All of the following are reasons for accurate documentation *except*:
   a. It provides a record of scene and patient information
   b. It reveals any significant changes in the patient's condition
   c. It provides medicolegal evidence
   d. It cannot be held against you if it is unknown how you treated a patient
2. Define "SAMPLE" and "OPQRST" and explain how they relate to documentation.
3. Information regarding response times, crew information, and ambulance service information could be found in which of the following?
   a. The patient information section of the PCR
   b. The narrative section of the PCR
   c. The run data section of the PCR
   d. None of the above
4. True or False: A patient should not be informed of the possible consequences of refusing treatment because it may unduly bias him or her into making a decision about seeking further medical attention.
5. When a mistake is made while documenting, which of the following should be done?
   a. Scratch out the mistake with multiple lines.
   b. Draw a single line through the mistake.
   c. Draw a single line through the mistake and initial after.
   d. Put parentheses around the mistake, then correctly finish writing the report.

Answers to these Review Questions can be found at the end of the book on page 869.

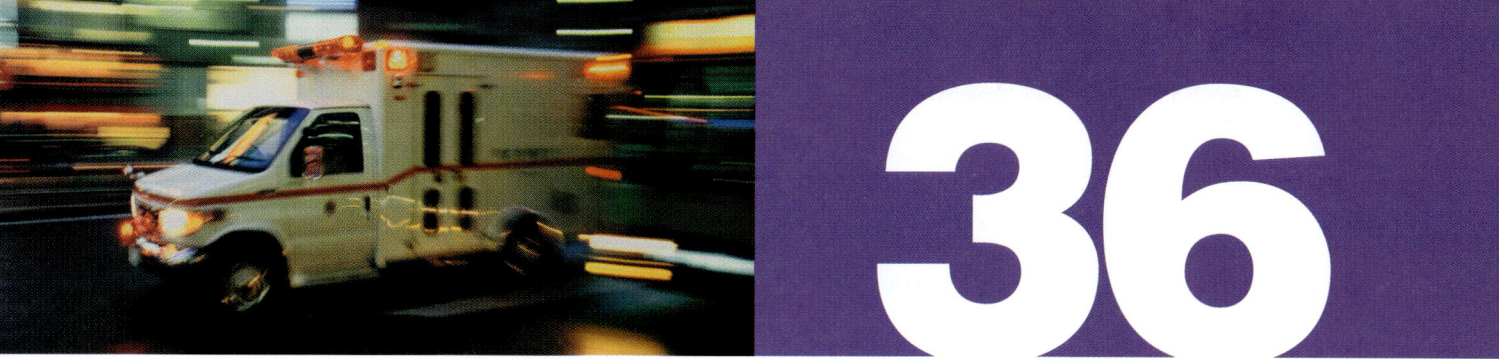

Quality Improvement

Lesson Goal

This chapter reviews the basic concepts of quality measurement and evaluation. It also reviews the basic components of a performance improvement program and the role that the EMT-Basic plays in improving the quality of care provided.

Scenario

Your new service medical director walks into the station about 15 minutes after your shift begins. Your supervisor tells you that Dr. Quentin is going to be riding with you and your partner for the shift. After grabbing a cup of coffee, you show Dr. Quentin to the ambulance bay and go over the ambulance and equipment with him. Just as you begin to show him the rest of the station, the tones sound and you are dispatched to a motor vehicle accident involving a motorcycle. As you arrive on the scene, you observe a car with damage to the driver's side, a motorcycle on its side next to the car, and a male patient lying prone on the side of the road. The driver of the car is trying to talk to the motorcyclist. The driver tells you, "I don't know if he's breathing or not." You determine that the patient is unconscious; is responsive to painful stimuli only; and has bilateral femur fractures, a closed head injury, and multiple abrasions. The patient is quickly immobilized and placed in the ambulance.

You and Dr. Quentin continue to treat and reassess the patient en route to the local trauma center. Once patient care has been turned over to the trauma team, you and your partner begin to replace equipment and clean the ambulance. Dr. Quentin assists in replacing linen on the stretcher and asks you how you felt the call was handled. You indicate that you wish the logroll and immobilization had gone smoother, but overall you are happy with the care provided. Dr. Quentin tells you that he thought the logroll and immobilization were done very quickly and appropriately. After further discussion and completion of the report, the three of you realize your on-scene time was only 6 minutes. Dr. Quentin congratulates you and your partner on a job well done as you return to quarters. You appreciate the immediate feedback on your patient care and notice that your nervousness about having the medical director ride with you has quickly disappeared.

? What type of quality evaluation methods are being used in this scenario? What benefits does Dr. Quentin receive from this type of activity? How is patient care improved by this type of activity?

Key Terms to Know

Case review
Concurrent evaluation
Continuing education
Continuous quality improvement
Data collection
Prospective evaluation
Quality assurance
Remediation
Retrospective evaluation

Learning Objectives

As an EMT-Basic, you should be able to do the following:

DOT

- Define *quality improvement* and discuss the EMT-Basic's role in the process.

Supplemental

- Define *quality assurance* and *continuous quality improvement*.

- Define the terms *prospective evaluation, concurrent evaluation,* and *retrospective evaluation* as they apply to quality assurance.
- Describe four methods used in a continuous quality control program in which an EMT is likely to become involved.

Quality is a vital issue in the health care system. The medical community and society have come to learn that simply providing any kind of health care is not good enough. Instead, the focus has shifted to taking the necessary steps to ensure that the best health care possible is being provided to all patients. Accomplishing this goal requires a concentrated effort to evaluate care provided and to make necessary changes to systems, equipment, and personnel.

The concepts of quality management have been growing since shortly after World War II, when Deming introduced his theories on quality management to the Japanese. Although many experts believe that his theories were the key to Japan's industrial success, others believe that his theories are significantly flawed. Instead, whole new theories on quality, how to identify it, and how to achieve it have evolved. Tremendous debates have raged for years over what is the best theory. Debates also continue over what percentage of "flaws" are due to systems, equipment, or people. As the theory has evolved, new terminology has developed. The theories are identified by a variety of names, including *quality assurance, quality management, quality control, total quality management,* and *continuous quality improvement.* Hundreds of books are available on these theories, and the ardent advocates of each theory can take hours to justify why their particular theory is best.

In emergency medical services (EMS), each of these theories has had its day. For the emergency medical technician (EMT), and particularly for the EMT student, it is less important to try to sort out the subtle theoretical differences than it is to understand the general principles of providing quality emergency medical care. These general principles include collecting data; evaluating the care that is provided (from the perspectives of both process and outcome); and taking what is learned and putting it back into the system, equipment, and people so that care is improved. It is imperative to understand that whatever the process is called, it should not be a punitive one. Instead, the goal of any quality process in EMS must be to provide for excellence in patient care. Although some cases may require punitive action, particularly after repeated problems, this should be the exception rather than the rule.

The EMT is a vital participant in any effort to enhance the care that is provided in an EMS system. This chapter introduces the basic concepts of quality measurement and evaluation. It reviews the basic components of a quality assurance program and how the EMT is likely to participate in improving the quality of care provided by the EMS system (Figure 36.1).

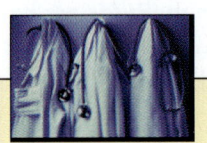

Physician Notes

EMS systems must realize that the quality assessment process consumes time and resources. A commitment to a quality evaluation program should also mean a commitment to spend the money and provide the necessary staff support to make the program successful.

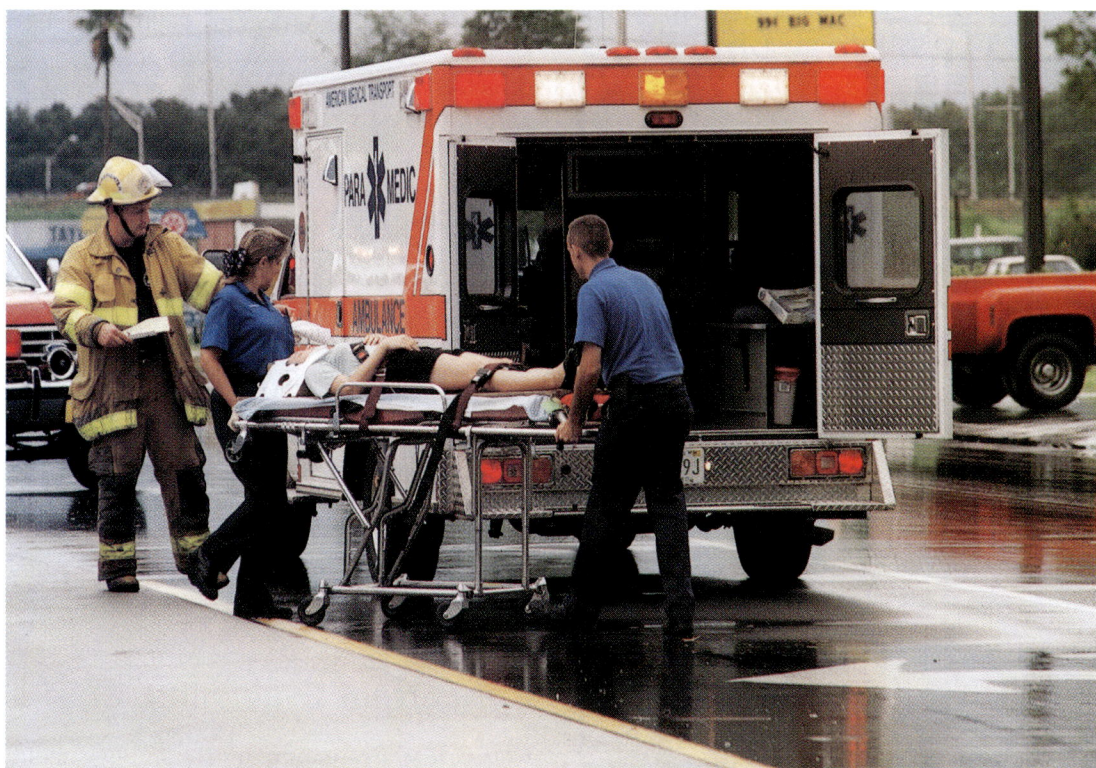

FIGURE 36.1 EMTs must play an active role in the quality assurance process to ensure that they provide the best patient care possible.

Quality Assurance

Quality assurance is defined as a mix of activities designed to evaluate how well the EMS system and EMTs take care of patients. System performance is measured in a variety of ways to determine if care is delivered in a timely, efficient, and medically sensible manner (Box 36.1). Certain predefined standards are used for comparison. For example, cardiac arrest survival rates are available for a number of EMS systems in the United States and Europe. In addition to looking at the system, an important aspect of quality assurance includes evaluating each EMT's training, performance, and patient care. For example, does a particular EMT have unusual difficulty with a specific skill, such as blood pressure measurement?

Continuous quality improvement differs from quality assurance in that it strives to continuously improve how the system takes care of patients. Many experts in health care have replaced the traditional methods of quality assurance with continuous quality improvement. Continuous quality improvement examines the performance of all aspects of the EMS system and makes changes to continuously improve the system. Improving the quality of continuing education and updating treatment protocols are examples of continuous quality improvement.

✓ Quality assurance measures performance of the system or an individual against a certain standard, whereas continuous quality improvement uses evaluation to continuously improve the EMS system.

Box 36.1 Examples of Items Trackable for Quality Improvement

Almost any aspect of health care delivery can be identified and tracked for quality improvement by the service manager, the medical director, or the quality committee in charge. These are some commonly tracked items in various EMS systems:

- Types of calls
- Response times
- On-scene times
- Patient survival rates
- Percentage of extrications done in less than 15 minutes

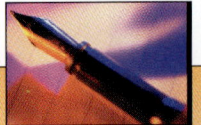

Tips from the Pros

The medical director should, at the very least, be involved in the following elements to improve quality of any EMS system:

- Chart review and audit and improving EMT performance with training when appropriate
- Use of skill training as a prospective evaluation tool
- Active participation in the hiring of personnel (volunteer or paid)

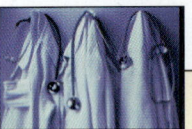

Physician Notes

EMS medical directors should complete formal training in medical direction. Although this type of training is not routinely provided in medical schools or residencies (even emergency medicine residencies do not consistently provide information on this subject), a number of continuing education courses are devoted to this topic.

Quality Assessment Methods

Both quality assurance and continuous quality improvement are important to an effective EMS system and the development of good patient care skills by the EMT. The medical director and EMS system staff must be able to evaluate how well care is delivered by EMTs. These tools assist in collecting information so that the medical director can assist the EMTs in providing the best possible patient care. Three basic methods are available to medical directors to evaluate quality: prospective, concurrent, and retrospective evaluation (Box 36.2).

Prospective Evaluation

Prospective evaluation tools are designed to improve the care delivered by the EMS system before responding to a call. This type of evaluation is the most valuable because it allows care to be improved before the emergency call takes place. Evaluating the quality of training, continuing education, and periodic skill check-offs are prospective evaluation tools that may be used by the medical director. Medical directors should have input in deciding continuing education topics, patient care equipment that should be carried, and hiring of personnel. These issues can all affect the quality of care (Figure 36.2).

Concurrent Evaluation

Concurrent evaluation in continuous quality improvement programs includes the direct observation of care delivered by the EMT. The medical director or a member of

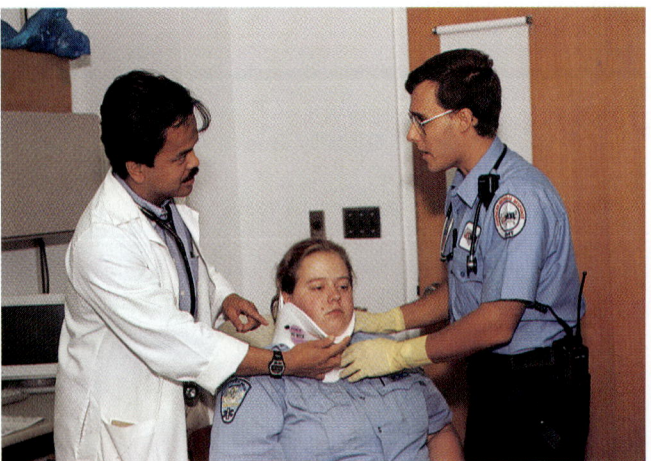

FIGURE 36.2 Skills check-off is one of the most valuable quality assessment methods.

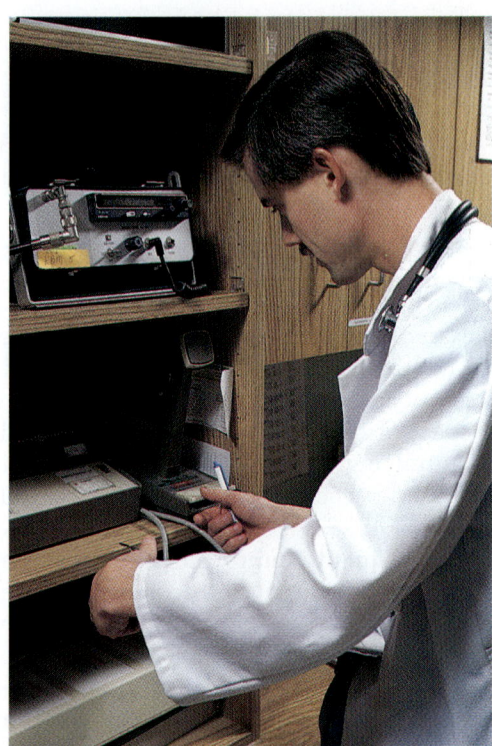

FIGURE 36.3 Concurrent evaluation methods include EMT–physician interaction with on-line medical direction.

the staff, such as an EMS coordinator or field instructor, "rides along" with the EMT to observe patient care delivered in the field. Concurrent evaluation may include observations in the hospital or clinic or occur briefly as the EMT and medical director interact in the emergency department. Concurrent evaluation also can be performed during the clinical and field training portion of a training program or when a physician provides on-line medical direction. Concurrent evaluation is the most useful kind of evaluation to the medical director. The physician can personally observe the EMT's skills and provide positive feedback about how patient care can be improved (Figure 36.3).

Retrospective Evaluation

Retrospective evaluation includes methods that are applied after an EMT has completed a call. Although these methods of evaluation take place "after the fact," they are the most commonly used because of ease and cost. Medical directors may use chart audits, case reviews, and debriefings to review what happened after an EMS call. Many methods include reviewing the quality of documentation and monitoring how closely the EMT followed established protocol (Figure 36.4).

> Quality assessment methods involve three categories of techniques: retrospective, concurrent, and prospective. Prospective is the most beneficial because it occurs before an EMS response takes place.

Quality Improvement Loop

Measurement of quality is useless if it is not acted on. Quality improvement is a constant cycle of evaluation and improvement (Figure 36.5). The loop concept is useful in that it emphasizes that each step of the quality evaluation process feeds another. Data collection feeds analysis or evaluation. The results of analysis cause changes in the system, people, or equipment. Once changes are made, data must be collected, the effect of the change evaluated, and so on. Quality improvement loops are used to ensure that quality is measured and improved—continuously. EMTs become involved in this loop as data collectors, valuable participants in the analysis phase, and the subjects of change (either in training or individual performance). Ultimately, continuous quality improvement assists all personnel in improving the care they deliver to patients.

> The quality improvement loop is used to continuously improve the care an EMT delivers to the patient.

Box 36.2 Three Basic Quality Methods

- *Prospective evaluation:* the quality evaluation method used before an EMS response. Skills check-off is an example of prospective evaluation.
- *Concurrent evaluation:* evaluating the quality of care as it is being given. Physician ride-along is an example of concurrent evaluation.
- *Retrospective evaluation:* the quality evaluation tool used after an EMS response has occurred. Run sheet review is an example of retrospective evaluation.

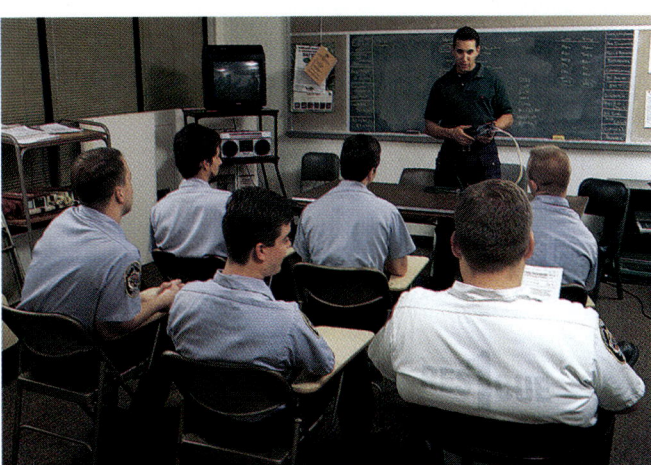

FIGURE 36.4 Retrospective evaluation often includes reviewing of actual calls with EMT case reviews.

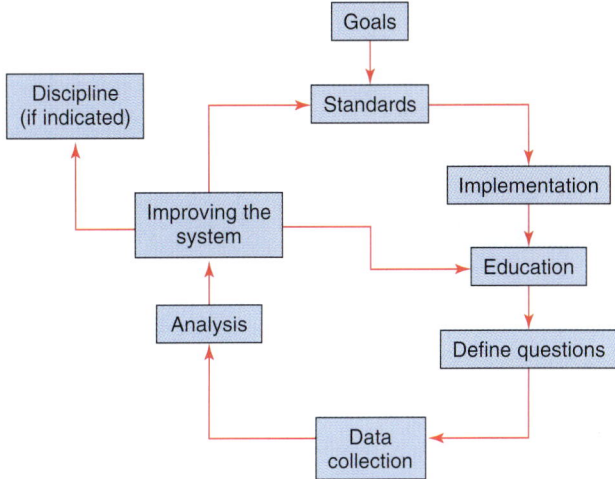

FIGURE 36.5 The continuous quality improvement loop in which quality is continuously evaluated and improved.

Run Report

Date of Run: Mo Day Century Year

Ambulance Service #

Vehicle ID #

MARYLAND HEIGHTS FIRE PROTECTION DISTRICT

Ambulance Service Name

Patient Information

Last Name First Name M.I.

Street, Route, etc. City

County State Zip

Date of Birth: Mo Day Century Year

Race: 1 Black 2 White 3 Hispanic 4 Other

Sex: 1 Male 2 Female

Location of Pickup

Name of Hospital, Nursing Home, Clinic, or Street, Route, Highway #

City County State Zip

Patient Destination

Name of Hospital, Nursing Home, Clinic, Ambulance Service, Home, Etc.

City State

Type of Run

TO SCENE

- 1 Emergency response requested
- 2 Non-emergency response (routine)

FROM SCENE

- 01 Life threatening, transported
- 02 Urgent, transported
- 03 Routine, transported
- 04 Dry run, no transport

Times

- Call Received
- Unit Dispatched
- Unit En Route
- Arrive Location
- Depart Location
- Arrive Destination

Place of Incident

- 0 Home
- 1 Farm
- 2 Mine/Quarry
- 3 Industrial Place
- 4 Recreation/Sport
- 5 Street or Highway
- 6 Public Building
- 7 Residential Institution (hospital)
- 8 Other
- 9 Unspecified

Call Detail

Units On Scene: ☐ 4417 ☐ 4410 ☐ 4422 ☐ 4426 ☐ Other: ____________

Call Received From: ☐ 911 ☐ MHPD ☐ Other: ____________ Subdistrict: ________

Medical Control (MD/RN name/Hospital): ____________

Care Transferred to (X):

Driver: ____________ Attendant #1: ____________

Mileage to Hospital: ____________ Attendant #2: ____________

In Service Time: ____________

License No.

- Driver
- Att. #1
- Att. #2

Vital Signs

- Systolic Blood Pressure
- Respiratory Rate
- Glasglow Coma Score

Protective Equipment

- 1 None
- 2 Unknown
- 3 Seat Belt
- 4 Child Seat
- 5 Air Bag
- 6 Belt & Bag
- 7 Helmet
- 8 Other
- 9 Not Applicable

Factors Affecting EMS

- 01 Adverse weather
- 02 Adverse road conditions
- 03 Vehicle problems
- 04 Unsafe scene
- 05 Language barrier
- 06 Extrication >20 minutes
- 07 Hazardous materials
- 08 Crowd control
- 09 Med. control failure
- 10 Other ________
- 11 Not Applicable

Treatment Authorization

- 1 On-line (radio/telephone)
- 2 On-scene
- 3 Protocol
- 4 Written orders (patient specific)
- 5 Orders refused
- 6 Unknown
- 7 Not Applicable

Trauma Assessment

	Amputation	Burn	Crush	Dislocation/FX	Blunt	Gunshot	Laceration	Puncture/Stab	Pain	Soft Tissue
Head	00	10	20	30	40	50	60	70	80	90
Face/Eye/Ear	01	11	21	31	41	51	61	71	81	91
Neck	02	12	22	32	42	52	62	72	82	92
Spine	03	13	23	33	43	53	63	73	83	93
Thorax	04	14	24	34	44	54	64	74	84	94
Abdomen/Pelvic Contents	05	15	25	35	45	55	65	75	85	95
Upper Arm/Shoulder	06	16	26	36	46	56	66	76	86	96
Lower Arm/Hand/Elbow	07	17	27	37	47	57	67	77	87	97
Upper Leg/Hip	08	18	28	38	48	58	68	78	88	98
Lower Leg/Foot/Knee	09	19	28	39	49	59	69	79	89	99

Cause of injury

Illness Assessment

- 01 Abdominal pain/problems
- 02 Airway obstruction
- 03 Allergic reaction
- 04 Altered level consciousness
- 05 Behavioral/psychiatric
- 06 Cardiac arrest
- 07 Cardiac rhythm disturbance
- 08 Chest pain/discomfort
- 09 Diabetic symptoms
- 10 Hyperthermia
- 11 Hypothermia
- 12 Hypovolemia/shock
- 13 Inhalation injury (toxic gas)
- 14 Poisoning/drug ingestions
- 15 Pregnancy/O.B. delivery
- 16 Respiratory arrest
- 17 Respiratory distress
- 18 Seizure
- 19 Smoke inhalation
- 20 Stroke/CVA
- 21 Synope/fainting
- 22 Vaginal hemorrhage
- 23 Other ____________
- 24 Unknown
- 25 Not applicable

Destination Determination

- 01 Closest facility (none below)
- 02 Patient/family choice
- 03 Patient physician choice
- 04 Managed care
- 05 Law enforcement choice
- 06 Protocol
- 07 Specialty resource center
- 08 On-line medical direction
- 09 Diversion ____________ (name of hospital diverted from)
- 10 Other
- 11 Unknown
- 12 Not applicable

Treatment

D	Att.		D	Att.		D	Att.		D	Att.	
01	02	Bag mask/Demand valve	19	20	Drug administered	39	40	I.V. administered # _____	59	60	Oxygen by mask ____ lpm
03	04	Bleeding controlled	21	22	Endotracheal intubation	41	42	I.V. failed # _____	61	62	P.C.P.D. applied
05	06	Blood specimen drawn	25	26	Other airway	43	44	I.V. maintained	63	64	Pulse oximetry
07	08	C.P.R.	27	28	EKG monitor	47	48	Intraosseous infusion # _____	65	66	Spinal immobilization
09	10	Cardiac pacing	29	30	Extremity splint	53	54	N.G. tube	69	70	Suction airway
13	14	Cricothyrotomy	31	32	Extrication ____ time	55	56	O.B. delivery	71	72	Thoracentesis
15	16	Defibrillation ___ watts/sec.# __ attempts	35	36	Glucose test _____ mg/dl	57	58	Oxygen by cannula ____ lpm	75	76	Other ____________

MO 580-0597 (R1-99) Missouri Ambulance Reporting System

FIGURE 36.6 EMTs play a critical role in data collection. Efforts to collect accurate and concise data assist in continuous quality improvement.

Primary Survey

Airway
- ☐ Clear
- ☐ Noisy
- ☐ Obstructed
- ☐ ETT/NTT
- ☐ OPA/NPA
- ☐ Chin Lift/Jaw Thrust
- ☐ C-Spine Precautions

Breathing
- ☐ Normal
- ☐ Labored
- ☐ Shallow
- ☐ Absent
- ☐ BVM
- ☐ Lung Sounds: _____

Circulation
Pulse:
- ☐ Normal
- ☐ Weak
- ☐ Absent
- ☐ Regular
- ☐ Irregular
- ☐ CPR

Skin:
- ☐ Warm
- ☐ Cool
- ☐ Dry
- ☐ Moist
- ☐ Pink
- ☐ Pale
- ☐ Cyanotic

Neuro
- ☐ Alert
- ☐ Verbal
- ☐ Pain
- ☐ Unresponsive

Intubation Record

Time	Tube Size	BBS/Time	ETCO2/Time	BBS/Time	ETCO2/Time	CM @ Teeth

Vital Signs/Fluids/Drugs

Time	BP	Pulse	Resp	SaO2	Time	Fluid/Drug	Site/Rt.	Vol/Dose
	/							
	/							
	/							
	/							
	/							
	/							
	/							
	/							

Pre-existing Conditions:
- ☐ Behavioral/Psych
- ☐ Blood Disorder
- ☐ Cardiac
- ☐ Cancer
- ☐ Communicable Disease
- ☐ Diabetes
- ☐ Dialysis/Renal Failure
- ☐ Hypertension
- ☐ Neuro/Seizure
- ☐ Respiratory
- ☐ Other: _____
- ☐ Unknown
- ☐ None

Pediatric Trauma Score
- Weight _____
- Airway _____
- Systolic BP _____
- CNS _____
- Wounds _____
- Fractures _____
- Total PTS _____

Revised Trauma Score
- Systolic BP _____
- Resp. Rate _____
- Glasgow CS _____
- Eye Opening _____
- Best Verbal _____
- Best Motor _____
- Total RTS _____

Allergies: _____

Medications: _____

Chief Complaint: _____

FIGURE 36.6, cont'd For legend see opposite page.

The Emergency Medical Technician's Role in Quality Assurance

A good continuous quality improvement program can assist the EMT in providing excellent patient care. The EMT can expect to participate in such a program in various ways. Many of these methods require the EMT to work together with the medical director in assessing and improving quality. A successful continuous quality improvement program provides the EMT with the skills and confidence to constantly improve the care he or she provides, as well as the ability to appropriately document that care. The EMT can expect to participate in the following methods of continuous quality improvement: data collection, case reviews, continuing education, and remediation.

Data Collection

Data collection and evaluation of data have become increasingly important as EMS system managers and researchers have come under pressure to become more efficient and demonstrate quality of care. EMTs are the most important tools in data collection because they must make every effort to accurately document the care being delivered by the system (Figure 36.6). All EMTs are required to complete a patient care report to document an EMS call. These forms are used to collect data on such items as response times, treatment given, and other data that can measure the quality of care delivered by the EMS system. These data can provide the medical director and other EMS system personnel with the information necessary to make changes in how the system responds to patient needs. Chapter 35 discusses this issue in greater detail.

Case Reviews

Many continuous quality improvement programs review cases with EMTs to learn from situations that have already occurred. Case reviews may be offered by the medical director or his or her staff so all of the EMTs can learn from interesting or challenging calls. The **case review** provides an opportunity for the EMT to receive positive feedback and constructive criticism from the medical director on actual cases handled by the system. The emphasis here is on "positive" and "constructive." These sessions are not intended and should not be conducted to achieve public humiliation or discipline. As mentioned previously, the quality process (and its components) are not designed to punish—they must be designed to inform, educate, and correct when necessary. Case reviews also help the EMT identify the aspects of patient care that are important to the medical director.

Continuing Education

Continuing education plays a critical role in any continuous quality improvement program. Medical directors provide feedback to the training staff on the particular skills that must be reviewed or new skills that must be taught. A good continuing education program gives EMTs a chance to keep their skills sharp and provides a method of staying current on trends in the profession.

Remediation

From time to time the continuous quality improvement process identifies a single EMT who needs additional training or coaching. **Remediation** is a process that uses individual performance information gathered in the quality assessment process to help an EMT improve his or her performance. Additional training classes, one-on-one skills practice, or other educational methods may be used. Remediation is not designed to reprimand the EMT, but it is used to give a specific EMT additional help to improve his or her skills and the care delivered to patients.

> ✓ The EMT's role in continuous quality improvement is very important. EMTs will be involved in many aspects of a quality assurance plan, including data collection, case reviews, continuing education, and remediation.

Summary

- Quality assurance includes measuring the quality of care delivered by an EMS system and comparing that performance with standards of care.
- Continuous quality improvement has replaced traditional quality assurance methods with a method of constantly improving all aspects of an EMS system.
- The three types of quality assessment are retrospective evaluation, concurrent evaluation, and prospective evaluation.
- The quality improvement loop ensures continuous improvement of patient care in the system.

Summary (cont'd)

- EMTs are able to improve the care they deliver to patients by actively participating in various continuous quality improvement methods. These methods include data collection, case reviews, continuing education, and remediation.

Scenario Solution

In the scenario, the type of quality evaluation that is used is concurrent. Evaluating an EMT's skills as they are being performed is termed *concurrent quality evaluation.* Concurrent evaluation is the most useful kind of evaluation to the medical director. In this scenario the medical director, Dr. Quentin, benefits tremendously from this concurrent evaluation. He has the opportunity to see firsthand how the EMTs perform in the field and can provide them with positive feedback immediately. Patient care is improved by this method as the medical director provides immediate and valuable feedback to the EMTs on their skills and how to improve or enhance their patient care abilities.

Key Terms

Case review A method of quality assurance that involves reviewing actual cases with EMTs in order to review the quality of care delivered by the EMS system.

Concurrent evaluation Evaluating the quality of care as it is being given (e.g., physician ride-along with the EMT).

Continuing education Ongoing educational experiences provided to EMS personnel; an essential part of any quality assurance program in which the EMTs can maintain and improve their skills.

Continuous quality improvement A method of continuously evaluating and improving the care delivered in the EMS system.

Data collection Collection of data through various means, such as EMS patient care reports completed by EMTs responding to calls.

Prospective evaluation The quality evaluation method used before an EMS response (e.g., skills check-off).

Quality assurance Evaluating the performance of an emergency medical system's response to a given standard.

Remediation A method of improving a certain aspect or skill of an EMT by providing one-on-one training or coaching.

Retrospective evaluation The quality evaluation tool used after an EMS response has occurred (e.g., run sheet review).

Review Questions

1. Which of the following would be considered a prospective form of quality evaluation?
   a. Patient care report review
   b. Physician ride-along
   c. Skills check-off
   d. On-line medical direction
2. What are the three types of evaluation used to measure quality? Give an example of each.
3. Name four methods of continuous quality improvement with which the EMT may become involved.
4. Why is a quality process in EMS so important?
5. What is the difference between quality assurance and continuous quality improvement?

Answers to these Review Questions can be found at the end of the book on page 869.

37

Ambulance Operation

Lesson Goal

The goal of this chapter is to review with the EMT the importance that the preparation of the ambulance plays in overall care of the patient. This chapter reviews the maintenance required for the ambulance and equipment. This chapter also presents an overview of local laws that govern the safe operation of an ambulance.

Scenario

As a newly certified emergency medical technician (EMT) eager to start your career, your first day on "the job" will be a special time. You meet your new partner, a veteran of many years, and ask her what you should do first. She replies that the last shift never does anything so the unit should be in pretty good shape. If you want to you can grab a cup of coffee and wait for the first call. You decide that you would like to familiarize yourself with your new unit. You climb in and start opening compartments, finding the location of equipment and materials. You spend the first hour restocking—the previous shift sure used a lot of expendables considering their easy tour. You get the unit in proper shape while your partner visits with the other crews. You feel good that your equipment is in order and you are reassured that your unit is ready.

 What are your responsibilities? What are the responsibilities of your partner, the emergency vehicle operator (EVO) on this shift?

Key Terms to Know

Emergency vehicle operator (EVO)

Type I ambulance

Type II ambulance

Type III ambulance

Learning Objectives

As an EMT-Basic, you should be able to do the following:

DOT

- Identify the medical and nonmedical equipment needed to respond to a call.
- List the phases of an ambulance call.
- Describe the general provisions of state laws relating to the operation of an emergency vehicle, including speed, warning lights, right-of-way, parking, and turning.
- List contributing factors to unsafe driving conditions.
- Describe the considerations that should be given to requests for escorts, following an escort vehicle, and intersections.
- Describe the concept of due regard for safety of others while operating an emergency vehicle.
- Identify the essential information for responding to a call.
- Identify factors that may affect response to a call.
- Summarize the importance of preparing the unit for the next response.
- Differentiate among the various methods of moving a patient in the unit based on injury or illness.
- Apply the components of the essential patient information in a written report.
- Identify what is essential for completion of a call.
- Distinguish among the terms *cleaning*, *disinfection*, *high-level disinfection*, and *sterilization*.
- Describe how to clean or disinfect items after patient care.

Supplemental

- Explain the rationale for preparing the unit to respond.

The emergency medical technician (EMT) and the ambulance are vital links in the chain of human and physical resources that are necessary to deliver emergency medical care in the prehospital environment. Preparation for this service cannot be overemphasized. EMTs must be prepared to respond and render care under a variety of conditions. The ambulance and the associated equipment must be maintained in a safe and usable condition. The EMT who arrives at a scene without functioning equipment is of no use to the patient. All components must be checked at the beginning of a shift for proper functioning.

The driver of the ambulance, also known as the **emergency vehicle operator (EVO)**, must have a thorough knowledge of the local laws governing the safe operation of an ambulance. The EVO and the unit must adhere to laws governing all motor vehicle traffic. Knowledge of these laws enables the EVO to operate the ambulance safely and accomplish the mission of emergency medical services (EMS).

Ambulance

The largest and most complex piece of EMS equipment is the vehicle itself—the ambulance. An ambulance is designed to get EMTs and equipment to the emergency scene safely and to transport patients to a medical facility. These units require a large amount of maintenance. The safety of EMTs, patients, and other members of the public depends on a safe, well-maintained ambulance. In addition, the operator of the ambulance must have the appropriate skills, training, attitude, and level of fitness necessary to operate the vehicle safely under varying conditions.

Ambulance Types

Type I

The **type I ambulance** has a conventional cab (which looks like the front end of a pickup truck) and chassis with a modular ambulance body (box) (Figure 37.1). No passageway is present between the patient's and EVO's compartment, other than a window. The modular part can be remounted on a new cab and chassis when the original is worn out.

Type II

The **type II ambulance** is essentially a converted van, usually with a raised roof (Figure 37.2). The EVO's and patient's areas form an integral unit.

Type III

The **type III ambulance** is similar to the type I, in that it is a cab-chassis unit with a modular box mounted on the frame (Figure 37.3). Most commonly, the type III is mounted on a van chassis and a walkway or passage connects the patient's compartment and the EVO's compartment. Like the type I, the modular patient compartment on a type III can be removed from a used chassis and remounted on a new chassis to prolong its useful life.

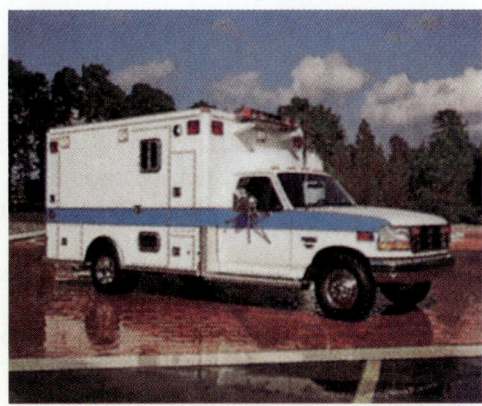

FIGURE 37.1 Type I ambulance.

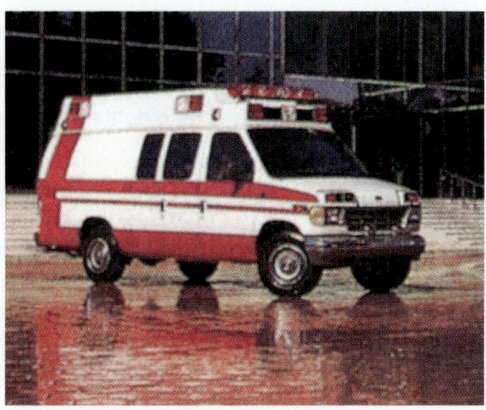

FIGURE 37.2 Type II ambulance.

KKK-A-1822C Federal Requirements for Ambulances

The federal government, through the General Services Administration (GSA), has established specifications for ambulances purchased by the federal government or those purchased with federal funds. Over time, these standards have also been adopted by many state and local jurisdictions as a minimum standard for all ambulances. Even in places where the KKK standards do not carry the weight of law, the ambulance industry has accepted these specifications as standard. These specifications help ensure that the equipment purchased performs as expected. Throughout this chapter, the specification applying to a piece of equipment is included in the discussion.

Occupational Safety and Health Administration Requirements for Contagious and Infectious Diseases

In addition to the federal specifications for ambulance construction, the Occupational Safety and Health Administration (OSHA) has developed a variety of requirements concerning ambulances and equipment as they relate to the prevention of transmission of infectious diseases. This subject is covered in more detail in Chapter 6. In this chapter, we discuss OSHA requirements only as they directly relate to design or operations of the ambulance.

✓ The largest and most complex piece of equipment in an EMS system is the ambulance. National standards for ambulance construction have been developed by the federal government. These standards, known as the KKK standards, have also been adopted by many state and local jurisdictions.

Medical Equipment

Basic supplies as listed in the next section should be carried by all ambulances. The quantities listed are suggested minimum quantities for basic service. The type of service normally delivered in your response area, the transport times, and the local statutes or regulations may dictate different quantities and kinds of equipment.

Basic Supplies

The following supplies are the basic items that should be stored on the ambulance to protect a patient from any environmental elements and to reduce the possibility of contamination:

- Pillows (disposable or nondisposable)
- Pillowcases (disposable or nondisposable)
- Sheets (disposable or nondisposable)
- Blankets (disposable or nondisposable)
- Emesis bags/basins (disposable)
- Bedpan (disposable)

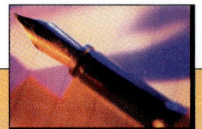 **Tips from the Pros**

- Keep a couple of older towels near the rear of the ambulance. They can be used for quick cleanups. Do not use these for other purposes.
- Location, location, location. Locate equipment and supplies near the areas they are used the most. Certain equipment is needed for every patient—keep it handy.
- Store spare sheets and pillowcases with the litter. Even if the hospital normally supplies the linens, they sometimes run out.

- Urinal (disposable)
- Toilet paper
- Boxes of tissue
- Paper drinking cups
- Towels
- Wet wipes
- Sterile water
- Soft restraints
- Biohazard disposal bags (OSHA compliant)
- Disinfectant
- Spray bottle (with bleach and water)

Patient Monitoring Equipment

The following items are necessary to monitor a patient's condition and should be stored on the ambulance for ready access:

- Sphygmomanometers (blood pressure cuff)—adult, obese, pediatric, infant
- Stethoscopes—adult, pediatric
- Thermometers (disposable)—regular fever, hypothermia
- Penlights

Patient Lifting and Moving Equipment

Lifting and moving patients is discussed in more detail in Chapter 33. This section simply lists suggested lifting and moving devices to be carried on the ambulance. The devices should be designed to safely carry the patient. Clearly label all equipment with permanent identification. Labeling will help in returning any equipment left at the hospital.

The following devices for lifting and moving patients should be stored in the ambulance:

- Wheeled ambulance stretcher
- Reeves stretcher
- Folding stair chair
- Scoop stretcher
- Stokes stretcher
- Child safety seat
- Backboards
- Other lifting and carrying devices as identified in local protocols or agency policies

> ✓ Label everything—not only so the items are easily retrieved but so the items can be seen readily when needed.

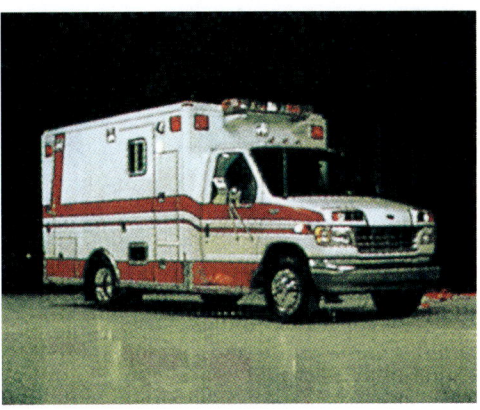

FIGURE 37.3 Type III ambulance.

Airway Supplies

Ambulances should carry the following devices for maintaining an open airway (local requirements may dictate the types and quantities of this equipment):

- Set of oropharyngeal airways
- Set of nasopharyngeal airways
- Esophageal obturator airway (if approved by jurisdiction having authority or the medical director, or both)
- Esophageal gastric tube airway (if approved by jurisdiction having authority or the medical director, or both)
- Pharyngotracheal lumen airway (if approved by jurisdiction having authority or the medical director, or both)
- Endotracheal tubes and laryngoscopes if the optional intubation skill is being used

Resuscitation Supplies

Resuscitation devices enable EMTs to maintain open airways, administer high levels of oxygen to patients, and avoid direct contact with the patient's body fluids. The following resuscitation supplies should be stored in the ambulance:

- Bag-valve-masks, in various sizes appropriate for use on adults and children and oxygen enriched with reservoir (disposable recommended)
- Various sized masks with standard 15 mm/22 mm fittings
- Disposable pocket masks with one-way valve and standard 15 mm/22 mm fittings
- Bite sticks/jaw block

Oxygen Equipment

Oxygen equipment (which must meet KKK-A-1822C specifications) is used to treat various patient conditions. Oxygen is a pressurized, combustible gas and must be used in accordance with strict policies and safety procedures. The regulatory requirements of federal, state, local, and gas industry agencies must be followed for safe and effective use of oxygen.

Fixed Oxygen System

A fixed oxygen system should have the following characteristics:

- Appropriate piping
- Connections
- Regulators
- Flowmeters
- Positive pressure/demand valve with standard 15 mm/22 mm fittings
- Various sized masks with standard 15 mm/22 mm fittings

Portable Oxygen System

The portable oxygen system is designed to deliver 300 L at 15 L/min and should have the following characteristics:

- Appropriate connecting tubing
- Connections
- Regulators
- Flowmeters
- Positive pressure/demand valve with standard 15 mm/22 mm fittings
- Various sized masks with standard 15 mm/22 mm fittings
- Spare portable cylinders

Other Oxygen Supplies

Clear masks afford a view of the patient's breathing and airway. All models are available in disposable versions; these are highly desirable. The following additional oxygen supplies should be stored in the ambulance:

- Adult nonrebreather masks
- Pediatric nonrebreather masks
- Adult nasal cannula
- Pediatric nasal cannula

Suction Equipment

Fixed Suction System

The fixed suction system should be designed to meet the KKK-A-1822C Federal Requirements for Ambulances and have the following characteristics and features:

- Accessible to patient compartment
- Sound and vibration insulated
- 20 L/min free air flow
- 300 mm Hg vacuum 4 seconds after suction tube is closed
- Rinsing water bottle
- Reservoir no less than 640 cubic inches
- Electric powered (can be engine powered if vehicle is gasoline powered and meets minimum requirements under all operating conditions)
- Gauge
- Tubing
- Catheters, hard and soft versions of various sizes with fingertip control
- Instructions for use, cleaning, and service

Portable Suction System

The portable suction system must be capable of operating from the ambulance's 12-volt electrical system. Additionally, the portable suction system must operate off rechargeable self-contained batteries for 20 minutes. The system should meet the following requirements:

- 20 L/min free air flow
- 300 mm Hg vacuum 4 seconds after suction tube is closed
- Rinsing water bottle
- Tubing
- Catheters, hard and soft versions of various sizes with fingertip control
- Instructions for use, cleaning, and service

Although the reservoir is not specified by standard, the suction unit cannot function without a reservoir. It is strongly recommended that a "universal" reservoir be used for both types of suction systems.

Automatic Resuscitators

Automatic resuscitators are designed to mechanically perform artificial ventilation and chest compression. In other words, they automatically perform cardiopulmonary resuscitation (CPR). All automatic resuscitators should meet the federal specifications for ambulances.

Additionally, all automatic resuscitators should meet current cardiac resuscitation standards of the American Heart Association. All connections should be compatible with the appropriate vehicle oxygen and electrical systems.

Fracture Management Equipment

Fracture management equipment is used to manage and care for fractures, dislocations, strains, and sprains as discussed in Chapter 28. The following equipment should be stored in the ambulance:

- Traction splints
- Padded board splints (amounts are minimums)—two 54-inch splints, two 36-inch splints, and two 15-inch splints
- Wire ladder splints, padded
- Air splint kit, various sizes and forms
- Cardboard splints
- Aluminum splints
- Vacuum splints
- Tongue depressors
- Triangular bandages with safety pins
- Tape
- Chemical cold packs
- Self-adhering roller gauze

Spinal Immobilization Equipment

Chapters 24 and 27 discusses the need for spinal immobilization and the various methods that may be used. Spinal immobilization devices should be readily recognizable. Ideally, equipment should be interchangeable with other units, because personnel from other organizations may help you in the application of these devices. All personnel should be educated about and familiar with these devices.

The following spinal immobilization devices should be stored in the ambulance:

- Full spine boards (72 × 16 inches minimum)—wood, aluminum, plastic, and disposable
- Short spine boards (autoextrication type)—wood and vest type (vinyl, plastic, or other material)
- Nine-foot straps or commercial straps as supplied by manufacturer of full and short devices
- Extrication collars
- Towels or large trauma dressings
- Head immobilizer or blanket roll
- Tape
- Triangular bandages with safety pins

Wound and Burn Care Supplies

Wound and burn care materials should be clean and preferably sterile. The following wound and burn care supplies should be stored in the ambulance:

- Sterile gauze
- Trauma dressings
- Triangular bandages with safety pins
- Tape
- Self-adhering roller gauze
- Occlusive dressings (sterile)
- Aluminum foil (sterile)
- Burn sheets (sterile)
- Water gel dressings (if approved locally)
- Adhesive bandages
- Scissors
- Disposable gloves (sterile)

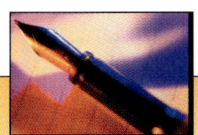

Tips from the Pros

Use a plastic irrigation bottle as a rubber glove dispenser. Cut out the bottom, mount on a vertical surface, and fill with gloves, and they will come out the opening one at a time.

Shock Equipment

Caring for a patient with the signs and symptoms of shock requires the EMT to treat the underlying causes and also the symptoms as discussed in Chapter 9. Total patient care will help the EMT in treating the signs and symptoms of shock, and the items listed below aid in treatment. There is much debate about the value of the pneumatic antishock garment (PASG) in the treatment of the signs and symptoms of shock. Use in the local system will be determined by system protocols. Even if the PASG is not used for the treatment of the signs and symptoms of shock, it is still a useful tool for management of lower-extremity fractures.

The following items used in the treatment of the signs and symptoms of shock should be stored in the ambulance:

- PASG
- Survival blankets
- Litter

Childbirth Supplies

Chapter 21 discusses the subject of childbirth in detail. The supplies necessary to accomplish an emergency childbirth are discussed here. Many emergency childbirth kits are available. The supplies can be obtained in commercially available "OB kits" or may be assembled and packaged locally. Kits should contain the items listed below as a minimum. Most of these items are available at little cost and can be put together very easily using the supplies normally carried in the ambulance.

The obstetrics kit should be stored on the ambulance and should contain the following items:

- Towels
- Bulb syringe

- Baby blankets
- Gown
- Masks
- Umbilical clamps
- Umbilical tape
- Scissors
- 4 × 4 sterile dressings
- Maternity dressings
- Disposable gloves (sterile)
- Infant swaddler (baby blanket and solar blanket)
- Plastic bags
- Skull cap

Poisoning Supplies

Toxicologic emergencies (poisonings) are discussed in Chapter 19. To effectively manage these patients, the following supplies are necessary:

- Drinking water (change daily)
- Syrup of ipecac (if approved locally)
- Activated charcoal (if approved locally)
- Paper cups
- Contact lens remover
- Irrigation equipment (for flushing eyes)
- Constriction bands (for snake bites)

Advanced Life-Support Equipment

In some areas, ambulances carry advanced life-support (ALS) equipment in addition to basic supplies. This equipment is used by advanced EMTs and EMT-Paramedics responding with the unit. Chapter 38 discusses the issues of EMTs and ALS in more detail. An EMT should be familiar with ALS equipment, where it is stored, and his or her role when the equipment is used. Local requirements may vary, and the EMT should learn about local system stipulations.

The following ALS equipment may be stored in the ambulance:

- Intravenous kit
- Fluids
- Administration sets
- Needles and catheters
- Preparation materials
- Tape
- 2 × 2 and intravenous dressings
- Adhesive bandages
- Endotracheal intubation kit—laryngoscope; adult and pediatric blades; endotracheal tubes, all sizes; endotracheal securing devices; tape
- Chest decompression kit
- Drugs and medications
- Esophageal obturator airway
- Esophageal gastric tube airway
- Pharyngotracheal lumen airway
- Tracheostomy/cricothyrotomy kit
- Cardiac monitor/defibrillator

Other Medical Equipment

Other equipment may be carried for use in special situations. This equipment may vary and be regulated by the jurisdiction having authority. The following additional medical equipment may be stored on the ambulance:

- Ring cutter
- Multiple casualty kit (used for large-scale incidents)
- Sharps disposal equipment (for the safe disposal of needles, etc.)
- EpiPens® (if approved locally for the administration of epinephrine during anaphylactic emergencies)
- Automatic defibrillator (if approved locally)
- Glucose paste (if approved locally for diabetic emergencies)

> ✓ Every ambulance should carry a basic set of supplies and equipment. The specific supplies and equipment are often identified in state or local laws and regulations.

Portable Kits

Portable kits (jump kits, aid boxes, backpacks, etc.) can greatly enhance patient care. By assembling the necessary supplies and equipment in a single carrying case or bag, the EMT can easily carry the necessary items to the patient in a single trip. Assembling equipment ahead of time prevents the EMT from returning to the unit for necessary items and reduces confusion at the scene. The items contained in each kit depend on local requirements and needs but should contain the items necessary to handle the task or tasks intended. The following are some examples of portable kits that can be preassembled:

- The airway kit contains those items used for airway management.
- The breathing/airway kit contains all of the items in an airway kit plus items needed to administer oxygen.
- The bleeding and bandaging kit contains items necessary for controlling bleeding.
- The spinal immobilization kit contains items necessary for spinal immobilization, not including backboards.

- The exposure kit contains items necessary to protect EMTs from exposure to contagious or infectious diseases.

> ✔ Prepackaging commonly used equipment and supplies into kits that are easily stored and carried makes the job of the EMT easier. Instead of having to manage an armload of loose supplies, a portable kit is a quick and efficient method of transporting supplies from the vehicle to the patient.

Nonmedical Equipment

Nonmedical equipment includes safety equipment and equipment that enables EMTs to gain access to or extricate victims. Much of this equipment requires training beyond an EMT course. *Use only the equipment you are trained and authorized to use.* Death or serious injury could result.

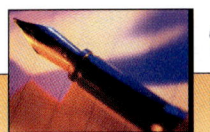

Tips from the Pros

Keep small "child-safe" items on your ambulance. During a time of crisis these can help calm a child. Be prepared to let the child keep them.

Safety Equipment

Safety equipment includes those items necessary to protect EMTs and patients. The following safety equipment (some equipment requires special education beyond the EMT course) may be stored in the ambulance:

- Heavy, fire-resistant coat (e.g., fire department "turnout" coat)
- Leather gloves
- Goggles or other shatter-resistant eye protection
- Helmet

Extrication and Rescue Tools and Equipment

Although many EMS systems have access to specialized rescue units to assist with patient extrication, the tools necessary for making uncomplicated rescues, particularly from automobiles, should be carried in the ambulance. This subject is discussed in greater detail in Chapter 39.

Personnel

The personnel available for emergency response can be a critical factor in patient outcomes. Not all areas can provide 24-hour staffs for EMS. Some departments may be staffed by personnel performing dual roles (e.g., fire, police, hospital staff). Volunteer units may have "on-call" personnel, who are alerted by radio, telephone, siren, or pager. Other units may be staffed by part-time employees during certain hours of the day and staffed by volunteers for the remainder.

Staffing should not be left to chance. Whatever the arrangements, it is important that all personnel understand the "who, what, where, when, and how" of staffing the EMS units in your area. Cooperative working relationships with all personnel enhance the operation and improve the delivery of EMS.

Qualifications

Ambulance staffing requirements are often established by state or local laws or regulations. In the absence of these regulations, the generally accepted national standard (as discussed in Chapter 1) is for at least one of the patient care personnel to be trained at the EMT-Basic level or higher.

Emergency Vehicle Operator

EVOs should be specially trained for the job. Ambulances are more than small trucks made to go fast. They are large, heavily loaded vehicles with complex systems, operating under adverse conditions. The training must be specific to ambulances. A variety of emergency vehicle driving courses are offered. These courses have been developed by the Department of Transportation, the National Safety Council, insurance companies, and state and local agencies. Specific courses or training may be required in some locations.

> ✔ Driving the ambulance requires special skills. These skills are often taught in specific emergency vehicle operator training courses developed by national, state, or local agencies. Some states require specific training and licensing to operate emergency vehicles.

Daily Inspections

One of the duties of an EMT is to be prepared to respond to emergency calls. This preparation includes making sure that the ambulance is prepared. A regular and systematic inspection ensures that a unit is in safe operating condition and contains the necessary supplies and equipment to respond to an emergency. These inspections also identify repairs and maintenance needed before a major breakdown occurs. While performing these inspections, EMTs become familiar with the ambulance equipment and where it is stored. After several inspections, the EMT will be able to restore the unit to a "ready" condition rapidly and efficiently.

EMTs must ask themselves at the beginning of every shift, "Am I sure that I have everything I need to care for my patients? Is my ambulance safe and ready to respond?"

Systematic Inspection of Vehicle Systems

A systematic approach helps the EMT perform a complete inspection. If all personnel involved use the same system, omissions, backtracking, and duplication will be reduced. Forms and "check-off" sheets help the EMT perform the inspections safely and completely. Seek advice from a qualified mechanic in creating a thorough system to inspect your EMS units.

Inspection of Exterior with Engine Off

Start the inspection on the exterior of the ambulance with the engine off (Figure 37.4). Visually check the following items:

- Regular lights
- Emergency lights
- Fuel cap
- Fluid leaks
- Oil leaks
- Cooling leaks

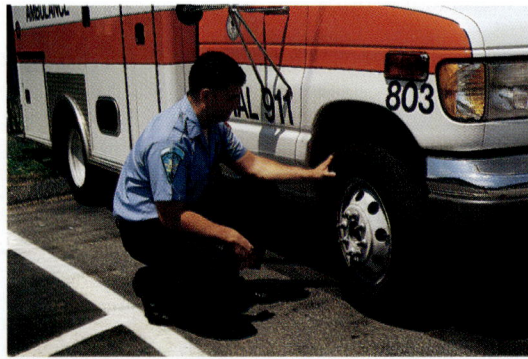

FIGURE 37.4 Start the inspection on the exterior, visually, and with the engine off.

- Condition of the wheels and lug nuts
- Lug nuts tightened to manufacturer's specifications
- Tires—condition, pressure, tread depth
- Wipers
- Doors and latches—passenger compartment, patient compartment, and storage compartments

Next, open the hood to the engine compartment and, with the engine off, check the following (Figure 37.5):

- Brake fluid
  - Level—should be near the top of the reservoir; check the manual.
  - Color—should be clear to amber; dark fluid could indicate the need for service.
  - Smell—should not smell burnt.
- Oil
  - Level—check the owner's manual for proper level.
  - Color—should be amber to light brown; dark and opaque oil could indicate the need for an oil change. Check the manual for proper oil change intervals. Use the schedule for "severe service." White film could indicate a major engine problem; in this case, have the unit checked by a qualified mechanic.
  - Feel—the oil should feel slippery and not gritty.
- Battery
  - Water level or charge indicator.
  - Connections should be tight and free of corrosion.
  - Mounting should be firm.
- The hood and latch should operate easily and smoothly.
- The hood should stay firmly latched when closed.
- Drive belts should be in good condition and firmly tensioned.
- Power steering fluid
  - Level—should be near the top of the reservoir; check the manual.
  - Color—should be clear or red (check the manual); dark fluid could show the need for service.
  - Smell—should not smell burnt.

Other items may be present that need regular maintenance. Check the manufacturer's manuals for further instructions.

Equipment Vehicle Operator's Seat with Engine Off

Continue the inspection in the EVO's seat with the engine off. Perform the following tasks:

- Adjust seat
- Adjust mirrors
- Check visors

- Check accessibility to all controls (vehicle, communications, and emergency warning devices)

Equipment Vehicle Operator's Seat with Engine Running

Set the parking brake, and ensure that the vehicle's transmission is in park or neutral. Start the engine according to the manufacturer's directions. (See owner's manual for procedures.) Check the dash indicators, lights, and gauges to ensure that they are operating correctly.

Stop the engine if any of the following occur, and seek repairs:

- Oil pressure low or nonexistent
- Temperature exceeding specifications
- Unusually loud noises
- Smoke or fire coming from any part of the vehicle (Exception—the exhaust system may produce some white smokelike vapor on startup. This smoke should dissipate when the engine warms.)

Pull the vehicle out of station or attach exhaust hoses to carry exhaust outside of the building. *Do not operate unit inside any building unless provisions are made to get rid of exhaust gases. Carbon monoxide can build up very quickly. Serious injury or death can occur.*

Check for correct operation of all the following lighting systems:

- Headlights
- Parking lights
- Turn signals
- Brake lights
- Marker lights (if equipped)
- Four-way flashers
- Emergency lights
- Passenger compartment lights
- Spotlights
- Other lighting systems

Check all audible warning devices. Wear hearing protection, and check in all modes.

Engine Compartment with Engine Running

Set the parking brake, and ensure vehicle transmission is in park or neutral. If not started previously, start the engine according to the manufacturer's procedures. With the vehicle running, the vehicle's transmission in park or neutral, and the parking brake set, open the hood.

Observe extreme caution when inspecting a running engine. Wear eye and hearing protection.

Check the following items:

- Observe for smooth running
- Observe belts operating smoothly
- Listen for excessive or unusual noise
- Operate air conditioning and observe belt
- Check automatic transmission according to manufacturer's recommendations
- Allow the engine to warm up to operating temperature before turning off

Inspection of Equipment and Supplies

Outside Compartments

Check that all equipment is present and is working properly (Figure 37.6). Make sure equipment is secured so that it does not move around the compartments. Check the water-resistant seals on or around the compartment doors to ensure that there will be no water leaks.

Patient Compartment

Check that the following equipment is present and working properly:

- Fixed and portable oxygen
- Fixed and portable suction
- Splinting supplies
- Dressings and bandages
- Other supplies as necessary

Using a regular check-off sheet reduces the chance of overlooking something. Check-off sheets assist in locating all necessary equipment. Additionally, check-off sheets provide a record of activities and help in the scheduling of routine and nonroutine maintenance, resulting in efficient inspections and a rapid return to service after a run.

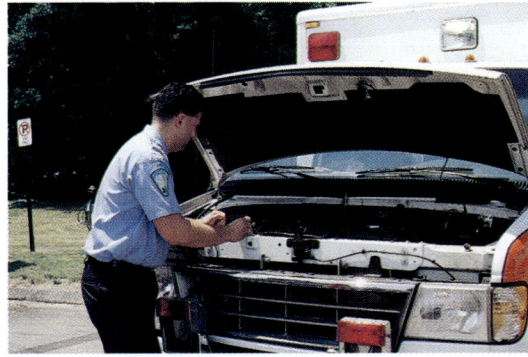

FIGURE 37.5 Open the hood to the engine compartment and, with the engine off, check the brake fluid, oil, battery, and power steering fluid.

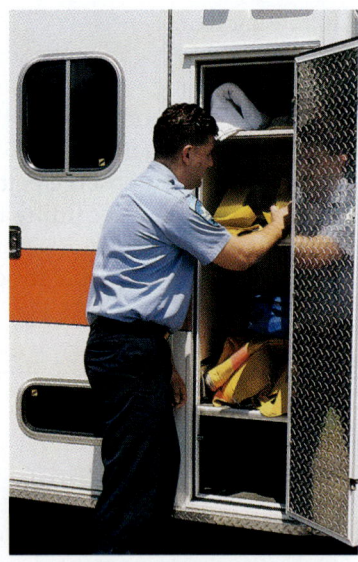

FIGURE 37.6 Check that all equipment in the outside compartments is present and working properly.

> ✓ A regular, systematic process for inspection of the ambulance will aid in the identification and resolution of mechanical problems before the emergency call arrives.

Dispatch (Communications Center)

Once the ambulance and equipment are inspected and made ready, the ambulance is ready to respond to the next call. The communications center receives calls for assistance and dispatches the appropriate EMS vehicle or vehicles. Chapter 34 discusses the systems and processes used for providing public access to EMS. Chapter 34 also describes the components of an EMS dispatch center and the activities that normally take place there.

> ✓ The communications center provides a connection between the public and the EMS system. It receives calls for assistance, dispatches the necessary equipment, and often provides initial verbal emergency care instructions over the phone.

En Route

With the dispatch information, safe and efficient travel to the scene is the next step. Seatbelts must be worn by the EMTs. Ideally, airbag protection should also be available; however, the bags are not yet universally available in ambulances. When seatbelts are secure, ensure that all mirrors, seats, and other items are adjusted. Start the engine, and scan the instruments for normal operation. Activate the emergency lights, headlights, and any other items necessary for emergency operation. Proceed out of quarters, and go into the traveled portion of the roadway only when safe.

Notify dispatch of your response, and verify the location of the emergency. This verification is often done as you respond to let dispatch know that you are not only responding but that you are also responding to the correct location. You should confirm all the essential information, such as the nature of the emergency, hazards, other agencies, and so on.

> **Tips from the Pros**
>
> Mount a vinyl-coated "basket" for storing the report clipboard in the patient compartment. This will keep it from being tossed about as the ambulance is moving.

Driving the Ambulance

Before driving any emergency vehicle, all operators should have specific training. This training should include both classroom and practical sessions. The training course should be approved by the jurisdiction having authority. Many courses are available to train the ambulance EVO. Check with the National Safety Council, the Department of Transportation (state and federal), and insurance companies for courses and guidance.

Characteristics of Good Ambulance Operators

Good EVOs should be physically fit to safely operate the ambulance in all environments. Their vision must meet state minimum requirements. Their hearing must be adequate to hear radio conversations, directions, and orders and to monitor other responding emergency vehicles. Additionally, the EVO must be physically able to perform any lifting and moving tasks normally expected of an EMT.

The EVO must be able to work under extreme stress. The EVO is expected to operate the vehicle during conditions that normally keep people at home, including ice, snow, rain, floods, and civil emergencies and other catastrophic events. The EVO is expected to perform effectively and safely and is often looked to for emotional stability by the public and others.

EVOs must be confident and positive yet realistic in their expectations of themselves, their crews, and the EMS system. Limitations exist for all members of EMS, and these factors should be known and understood. Red lights and sirens can lead one to a perception of invincibility. However, nothing could be farther from the truth. The EVO is just as vulnerable as anyone else.

The EVO must be tolerant of the driving of others. The other drivers on the road have different missions. They have no idea of the seriousness of the emergency to which the ambulance is responding. They may not even hear or see the ambulance. Many of their actions are unpredictable. Give the other vehicles on the road distance, allow for escape routes, allow for the lights and sirens to be heard, and allow the other drivers time to react. Observe the other drivers for their reactions and proceed with caution.

The EVO must avoid drugs, alcohol, and fatigue when operating the ambulance. These factors are killers. If an EVO is fatigued or under the influence of drugs or alcohol, he or she *must not* drive.

In some areas, the EVO must take specific tests and be licensed to operate ambulances. If glasses or contacts are needed for driving, EVOs should make sure that their prescriptions are up to date and that the glasses or contacts are in good condition. Good vision is essential for viewing the hazardous driving environment and for identification of the appropriate patient location.

> ✓ Emergency vehicle operation requires special skills, physical and mental preparedness, and common sense.

Safe Driving

Safe driving of the ambulance is a considerable responsibility. If the ambulance does not arrive safely at the scene, EMTs cannot deliver care.

Seatbelts are needed for all occupants. EVO training should include not only formal, generic driver training but also training aimed at safe operation of the specific vehicle that will be driven by the EVO. All vehicles have different operating characteristics. Driving to a scene is not the time to discover what those characteristics are. Learn the vehicle before you are dispatched to an emergency.

Planning Your Response Route

When the call is received, the EVO should first plan how and where to respond. Check the map and note any detours, road closings, bridges, railroad crossings, tunnels, schools, and heavy traffic areas. All of these factors can affect route selection and the speed of response. Plan the route and be prepared with a backup route should the first choice be blocked. Allow for environmental conditions such as ice, snow, or rain. Think about the time of day or day of the week—a busy thoroughfare during the day may be empty at night or may not be busy on the weekend. The key is to know the response area and plan the emergency response accordingly.

Situations Affecting Response to a Call

Ambulance calls often involve some sort of an encounter with an uncooperative motorist. The run is never as smooth as television and movies would lead us to believe. The motoring public can greatly influence the speed and safety of the response by their actions and inactions.

Day of the week. Weekdays are usually full of traffic, particularly on the main commuter routes, because people go to work and school. On weekends these routes are less crowded, but the areas surrounding city and suburban shopping areas may be full. Increased traffic increases the likelihood of accidents. Learn the traffic patterns for the response area and plan accordingly.

Time of day. Traffic into, out of, and around cities and suburbs increases during the morning and evening rush hours. Traffic jams can eliminate routes normally taken to get to hospitals. Plan an alternate route during rush hours.

Weather. Adverse weather creates conditions that reduce the speed of safe travel. In heavy snowfall, travel may be impossible.

Detours. Road construction can slow or stop traffic, making routes impassable. Unless the call is located in the detour area, detours usually do not affect an ambulance's ability to go from one point to another. However, when multilane highways are funneled down to one lane, the resulting backup can preclude responses on that route.

Railroads. At-grade crossings (railroad crossings on the same level as the roadway) can stop traffic for extended periods when a train is present. Plan an alternate route to avoid them.

Bridges and tunnels. Bridges and tunnels have very narrow shoulders, and many have none at all. Narrow or nonexistent shoulders will cause a very minor accident to back up traffic. Bridges have more accidents in the winter because they freeze much quicker than regular road surfaces.

Schools and school buses. Any encounter with schools or school buses should slow the response. Children are naturally curious about emergency vehicles and will rush to see them, often without regard to their safety. The ambulance operator must look out for them. Create strict guidelines for encounters with school zones and school buses. These procedures should be known not only by the EVO but by the school bus drivers as well.

Remember, it is the EVO's responsibility to operate the ambulance with due regard for the safety of others.

> ✓ Knowledge of the response area and careful planning of the response route to a call ensures a rapid and safe response to the scene of the emergency.

Emergency Warning Devices

Are warning lights and sirens friends or enemies? They are devices that only warn others of the emergency vehicle's presence, both visually and audibly. Neither device can physically move anything. They are not "shields" that protect the ambulance or its occupants. The warning devices are only a request for other drivers to yield. The laws in most states require the use of warning devices while responding to emergencies or while en route to the hospital with critical patients. Use all warning lights during a response. Also turn on headlights during an emergency response, because other motorists can see headlights for quite a distance during the day. The white light is more easily seen in the bright light of day.

Caution is the word here. Many drivers cannot see or hear these warning devices. Cars today have superior soundproofing and sophisticated stereo systems. Wait for the drivers to see or hear the ambulance and to react before taking the right of way. Always use caution. Some drivers have been known to make sudden changes in direction or come to a sudden stop when faced with responding emergency vehicles. The use of lights and sirens does not in any way exempt an EVO from the requirement to drive with due regard for the safety of others. The privilege granted to EVOs by emergency vehicle laws must be used with great caution.

> ✓ The visual and audible warning devices on an ambulance are *warnings* to other vehicles. They are not a shield around the responding ambulance, and they do not guarantee that other motorists will get out of the way.

Maintaining Safe Following Distance

Many guidelines and strategies exist to help maintain a safe following distance. All of them allow for reaction time and the time it takes the vehicle to slow or stop. However, many of these guidelines are designed for the family station wagon, operating under normal conditions, on clean dry roads, and with good visibility. An ambulance is not the family station wagon. Ambulances do not operate under these ideal conditions. An ambulance is a large, heavily loaded vehicle, expected to operate in adverse conditions. The standard guidelines for following distance are not enough.

Many organizations (such as the National Safety Council, the Department of Transportation, and the insurance industry) have made recommendations based on their experience and knowledge of emergency vehicles. They have recommended both the 3-second rule and the 4-second rule. Both rules have merit and, when used with a degree of caution, provide a reasonable margin of safety.

The 4-second rule requires that an EVO follow the vehicle ahead at a distance so that an object passed by the first vehicle is passed by the emergency vehicle 4 seconds later. Simply stated, count 4 seconds between the ambulance and the vehicle ahead when passing the same object.

Positioning the Unit

As you approach the scene, look for clues that may indicate hazards. The EVO's job is to position the ambulance in a safe area that is convenient to the patient. The emergency scene can be an extremely dangerous location. Chapters 5, 12, and 40 discuss in great detail scene dangers and steps to take to avoid problems.

Once a parking site is selected, park and secure the vehicle from moving. Place the transmission in park (automatic transmission) or neutral (manual transmission), and set the parking brake. Chock the wheels. Ensure that all the warning lights are on and operating. Additional warning devices such as highway flares may be used. Do not use flares where flammable liquids or vapors are suspected. Turn off the headlights unless they are needed for scene illumination. The white light of the headlights can overpower the warning lights and may lead other drivers to believe the vehicle is not an emergency vehicle. Position the ambulance so if it is hit by another vehicle, it is not driven into the emergency scene and the personnel working there. Consider how the vehicle will leave the scene once the patient is loaded. How will other emergency vehicles get to the scene? Will the vehicle block them? If so, select a better site.

Emergency Driving Privileges

The laws granting certain emergency driving privileges vary from state to state. However, some general legal principles of emergency vehicle operations are found in almost every instance.

These laws generally provide that emergency vehicles are exempt from following normal traffic laws in highly specific circumstances. However, the operator of the emergency vehicle must continuously exercise caution and safety when operating the vehicle. Strict conditions must be met to allow these exemptions. Specifically, emergency vehicle operators must

- Operate all visual and audible warning devices
- Drive with due regard for other occupants of the roadway

Under these conditions, emergency vehicles may generally

- Exceed posted speed limits
- Ignore red or stop signals
- Ignore parking or standing regulations
- Ignore flashing red lights
- Proceed through stop signs
- Proceed through yield or merge signs
- Cross solid double or single lines
- Disregard proper traffic lanes
- Proceed the wrong way on a divided highway or one-way street
- Proceed without regard to emergency or disaster routes
- Proceed when encountering a school bus while loading
- Pass on the right side of other moving vehicles
- Drive left of the center line
- Change direction
- Ignore "no turns" (right and left turns)
- Proceed against the right-of-way at uncontrolled intersections

No matter how many exemptions to traffic laws may be allowed, the EVO must *always* operate the ambulance with *due regard for the safety of others*. The exemptions do not give the EVO the right to injure or damage anything while exercising these exemptions. If due regard is not practiced, the protection provided by the traffic laws is no longer in effect.

When operating the ambulance under normal conditions (not responding in an emergency mode), all applicable laws, rules, and regulations must be obeyed.

> ✔ Laws concerning the operation of emergency vehicles generally allow the operator to disregard normal traffic laws and traffic control devices as long as all visual and audible warning devices are in use and as long as the emergency vehicle is operated with due regard for the safety of others.

Escorts and Multiple Unit Response

The concept of one emergency vehicle "escorting" another through traffic used to be popular but is rarely used today. The idea that two vehicles responding under emergency conditions can somehow travel faster to or from a scene is without merit. Escorts in themselves can add a level of danger that is both unnecessary and unacceptable. The most important consideration is the increased potential for collisions with other motorists. Many motorists do not expect a second emergency vehicle. Thinking the way is safe, they often pull into the path of the second emergency unit.

The need for or the use of escorts generally falls into two categories: lack of knowledge of the area and tradition. Training all EMTs in area familiarization reduces the need for escorts. Should escorts be needed, the ability to communicate with the escorting units increases the safety of the escort.

All ambulance operators should know the area in which they are responding, the best routes of travel, and the location of all local hospitals and must follow accepted safety precautions when operating an emergency vehicle. Should escorts still be necessary, all agencies involved should have clear and written procedures. These procedures should address how each unit will communicate with each other, what distance is to be placed between units (500 feet minimum), and who will proceed first. The procedures should also include how intersections are handled.

Multiple units will occasionally respond to the same call or to calls close to one another. This situation greatly increases the likelihood of two or more responding units encountering each other. The chances of collisions are increased dramatically, particularly at intersections. As with escorts, other motorists do not expect the second emergency vehicle and may pull into the path of responding units. Multiple audible warning devices coming from different directions can confuse motorists. Other emergency vehicles may block a motorist's view.

To make multiple responding units as safe as possible, the following guidelines are recommended:

- If following another emergency vehicle, maintain a distance of at least 500 feet.
- Use a different siren time or tone to help other motorists distinguish multiple units.
- Use radios to coordinate responses to reduce the likelihood of multiple units arriving at the same spot (intersection) simultaneously.
- Plan alternate routes to reduce conflict.

Training, clear procedures, and prearranged working relationships will help eliminate the need for escorts and make multiple responses safer.

> ✓ Two emergency vehicles traveling together creates a situation that is uniquely dangerous. Operators of the emergency vehicles in this situation must exercise extreme caution.

Intersection Collisions

Most crashes involving emergency vehicles occur at intersections. Motorists do not expect vehicles to go against their perceived right-of-way. Often they do not look to both sides and do not hear or see the responding unit. The EVO has the legal obligation to ensure that the way is clear before going through an intersection. This obligation is especially necessary when going against a traffic-control device. The same can be said for operating an emergency vehicle in the oncoming lane. Most often, collisions occurring in the oncoming lane are the fault of the EVO. The other motorists do not expect to encounter another vehicle and often cannot react quickly enough to avoid a collision. Therefore the emergency vehicle should never proceed in the oncoming lane when in areas of hills, curves, intersections, bridges, or any other areas of reduced visibility or reduced hearing.

Accidents and Accident Reports

If the unfortunate happens and a crash occurs while operating an emergency vehicle, follow these steps:

1. Pull off the road and stop the vehicle as safely as possible.
2. Turn off the ignition and turn on the vehicle's four-way flashers and other visual warning devices.
3. Check for injuries.
4. Check the other vehicles for injuries.
5. Notify dispatch and request additional resources.
6. If possible, start triage and management of any injured persons.
7. Start the documentation process as soon as possible, noting the position, direction, and condition of all vehicles and other physical items involved in the accident before and after the accident.
8. Follow any local procedures as necessary. Read and follow the instructions from the insurance carrier for your vehicle. If you are involved with a "self-insurance" situation, follow the procedures of your risk-management office (in this situation, it is the insurance company).
9. Complete all appropriate forms.

Accident reports *must* be completed completely and accurately. Do not take this responsibility lightly. These documents are used in courts. Juries and judges can and will make decisions based, in part, on the content of accident reports. Completing these reports is usually required by state or local laws. Every EVO should be familiar with local requirements for accident reporting.

When the report is complete, have someone not connected with the accident review it to ensure completeness and accuracy. Double-check everything. If accident reconstruction is done, get the names of the agency and personnel involved. Get the police report number.

Completeness and accuracy are the watchwords for accident reports. Avoid the accident with safe driving habits. However, if the unfortunate does occur, document it accurately.

Arrival at the Scene

Arrival at the scene can be a most important step in the successful delivery of EMS. The initial assessment and decisions set many actions by the crew and others into play.

Notify dispatch when arriving at the scene and, if first on the scene, give a brief initial report (BIR). This report creates a mental picture of the situation for dispatch and other EMTs. Initiate any incident command per local procedures.

Park safely, uphill and upwind, keeping a safe distance (100 feet minimum) from potentially hazardous scenes. Some EMS organizations specify a safe distance. Park so you have convenient and safe access to the patient. Consider the impact to traffic flow, the public, and other agencies. Avoid backing up if possible. Consider how immediate evacuation of the patient could be accomplished if necessary. If the scene is too dangerous to enter, can the patient self-evacuate? If the patient cannot, call for appropriate assistance and wait. Do not become part of the problem. Evaluate the situation on a risk-versus-benefit basis.

After the scene is found safe or made safe, assess the mechanism of injury or nature of the illness. Communicate this assessment as part of your BIR so other responding units can have the benefit of your assessment.

Arrival at the scene should be an orderly, safe, and efficient process. The approach should take in the big picture with the emphasis on safety. Do not let the scene become emotionally overwhelming. Clear thinking is the order of the moment.

Transferring the Patient to the Ambulance

When the patient is ready for transport, all critical interventions must be addressed. Begin basic life support immediately and completely. The airway must be opened, the patient must be breathing, or artificial respiration must be administered. Start CPR immediately on any patient without a pulse or respirations. Major severe bleeding should be controlled. Remember, in the case of unstable trauma, rapid transport to the receiving facility is going to be the most beneficial treatment. Splinting and backboarding of major fractures and back or neck injuries should be done while transport is being accomplished. These treatments and the equipment used must be appropriate for the type of transport. Remember the space constraints of the transporting unit. A 9-foot package will not fit in an 8.5-foot ambulance. Take vital signs regularly during treatment, after treatment, and during transport.

The patient should be secured to the moving device that is appropriate for the injury or illness. All lifting and moving should be accomplished using the guidelines in Chapter 33.

If the scene is unsafe or the patient is unstable, use the most appropriate emergency move to rapidly move the patient to the ambulance.

Gather any of the patient's effects (property) and transport to the receiving facility. Note these items on the patient care report. If available, place these in a bag designed for this purpose.

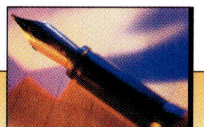

Tips from the Pros

Plastic, disposable blankets can be used as a rain cover for the patient. Be careful when using these around a patient's airway.

En Route to the Receiving Facility

Dispatch should be notified when the vehicle leaves the scene en route to the medical facility. This notification typically identifies the facility to which the patient will be transported.

The EVO must, again, plan the route and take appropriate steps to ensure a safe and efficient transport to the receiving facility. Observe all laws applicable to the local area. The patient's condition should dictate the use of emergency warning devices. If the patient is stable and the injury or illness is not life threatening, the transport should be at a speed and urgency that match that condition. Remember that the EMT with the patient must perform patient care en route. The manner in which the ambulance is driven can affect the patient's condition and care.

Notify the receiving facility of the patient's condition, treatments, and so on (see Chapter 34). Local requirements may dictate the procedure or the timing of medical communications.

Complete the prehospital care reports. These reports are notes of prehospital care that can be of assistance when transferring patient information at the hospital. Include the mechanism of injury or illness, injuries found, treatments, vital signs, and any changes en route. Some EMTs use carbon paper to make an immediate copy of these notes to hand to the medical staff at the receiving facility.

At the Receiving Facility

Notify the dispatch center on arrival at the receiving facility. Prepare the patient and the necessary equipment for transfer out of the unit and into the facility. If oxygen is in use, shift the source from the on-board supply to a portable unit and secure the unit on the litter. Do not place the oxygen cylinder between the patient's legs; place it in a carrier designed for this purpose or beside the patient. Disconnect any other items and connect portable units as necessary. Take any equipment needed for continuous patient care. Avoid the "mad rush" into the emergency department.

Make a verbal report to the medical staff. Point out any situations involving airway, breathing, circulation, or bleeding. Continue care until relieved. Report the mechanism of injury or the nature of the illness. Include all care given to this point and any changes in the patient's condition. Use the notes taken en route and, if possible, give a copy to the medical staff. Follow up with a written report of the notes when possible if a copy is not immediately available. The verbal report can be forgotten. A written report will not lose its memory and can be referred to later.

Transfer the patient's effects to the medical staff. Many emergency departments have specific containers or bags for this purpose. Make sure you know to whom you have given these items and note his or her name on the prehospital care report.

En Route to the Station

Restock any supplies used during the call from the ambulance inventory, or get them from the receiving facility if arrangements have been made previously. Many areas have prearranged agreements with the receiving facilities for restocking some supplies. Some have third-party billing, which places the cost of these items on the patient's hospital bill. Paperwork and forms should be properly completed and turned in. Do *not* take any supplies from the receiving facility without proper authorization. It is stealing and against the law.

Clean the ambulance, particularly the patient compartment. Most facilities have supplies available for this purpose. Dispose of any biohazardous material (body fluid–soaked dressings, etc.) properly. If the hospital does not accept them, your organization must dispose of them according to OSHA regulations. Do *not* dispose of these items with the regular trash. It is dangerous. Specific guidelines on cleaning the vehicle and disposing of hazardous waste are discussed in Chapter 6.

Inspect the unit for any "sharps" (e.g., needles, catheters) and dispose of them in an approved sharps container. Do *not* dispose of these items with the regular trash. It is dangerous and can be fatal.

Clean and disinfect any reusable supplies and equipment or store for transport to quarters for cleaning there.

Collect any equipment left from previous calls or left by other units that you will travel near and can drop off. Note any equipment you have had to leave at the hospital. Using this form can save thousands of dollars every year by rigorously tracking all reusable equipment left at hospitals.

Return and secure any equipment to its storage area. Replace any discharged batteries or reconnect to vehicle chargers. Replace empty oxygen cylinders.

Notify dispatch when leaving the receiving facility. If available for another call, the unit should be adequately restocked. All equipment and the ambulance should be ready for another call. All personnel should assess themselves and each other for their emotional states. If personnel are not ready for another call, return to quarters, unavailable.

If the ambulance cannot be restocked, or if necessary equipment has been left at the hospital, return to quarters unavailable. The ambulance should be stocked with extra supplies and equipment. Returning unavailable should be a rare occurrence.

Post-run

Notify dispatch when the vehicle is back at its station or post. Refuel the unit if necessary. Do not procrastinate about refueling, because it is easily overlooked. Inspect the unit as necessary. Check the oil, lights, tires, and anything unusual noticed during the run. Replenish or replace any supplies used. Complete any cleaning or disinfection of the ambulance or equipment. Complete and file all reports per local requirements.

Summary

- Successful ambulance operations start with preparation. Equipment must be prepared, maintained, and designed to meet the needs of patients and victims in a variety of situations. A failure at any level can make the difference between life and death. The EMS unit that cannot respond or responds without the resources needed is worse than no unit at all.
- Dispatch centers must be prepared to locate and dispatch calls accurately and in the most expeditious manner possible. Additionally, the dispatch center must have a well-trained staff, capable of giving telephone instructions for CPR, bleeding control, and so on.
- The ambulance operator must be trained specifically to operate the technically oriented equipment of the large modern ambulance. He or she must possess a working knowledge of traffic laws. The ambulance and its crew must survive travel to and from emergencies while sharing the road with other vehicles.
- The unit must be restocked and prepared for the next call. The EMT's job is not complete until the unit and its crew are ready to respond to another emergency.

Scenario Solution

With introductions complete, you and your new partner complete the ambulance inspection. The station radio blares out a call. The new EMT grabs the printout and checks the map. Both of you climb in the ambulance and buckle your seat belts. You start the engine and activate the emergency lights, confident that everything is working properly, and pull out of the station. The new EMT tells you about a detour and suggests an alternate route. You are impressed with his preparation.

Key Terms

Emergency vehicle operator (EVO) An appropriately trained and qualified ambulance driver.

Type I ambulance An ambulance with a conventional cab and chassis with a modular ambulance body (box).

Type II ambulance An ambulance that is essentially a converted van, usually with a raised roof; the EVO's area and the patient's area form an integral unit.

Type III ambulance An ambulance that is similar to the type I ambulance, in that it is a cab-chassis unit with a modular box mounted on the frame. Most commonly, the type III is mounted on a van chassis with a walkway or passage between the patient's compartment and the EVO's compartment.

Review Questions

1. True or False: An ambulance will handle just like any other pickup truck or van.
2. In general, motor vehicle laws grant special privileges to the operators of emergency vehicles. For example, they may ignore traffic control devices and speed restrictions. What does the EVO need to do to exercise these privileges?
3. Most collisions involving emergency vehicles occur at what type of location?
   a. The shoulder or breakdown lane on the freeway
   b. Intersections
   c. Backing into the station
   d. Parking lots
4. List at least four of the seven factors that must be considered by the EVO when planning a response.
5. True or False: If an EVO uses the visual and audible warning devices on the emergency vehicle, he or she can be assured that all traffic will get out of the way.
6. What are the phases of an ambulance call?
7. List three factors that contribute to unsafe driving conditions.
8. Identify two factors that may affect your response to an emergency call.
9. Why is it important to have your ambulance or emergency vehicle prepared for the next call?
10. Identify five medical and five nonmedical pieces of equipment required when responding to an emergency call.

Answers to these Review Questions can be found at the end of the book on page 869.

38

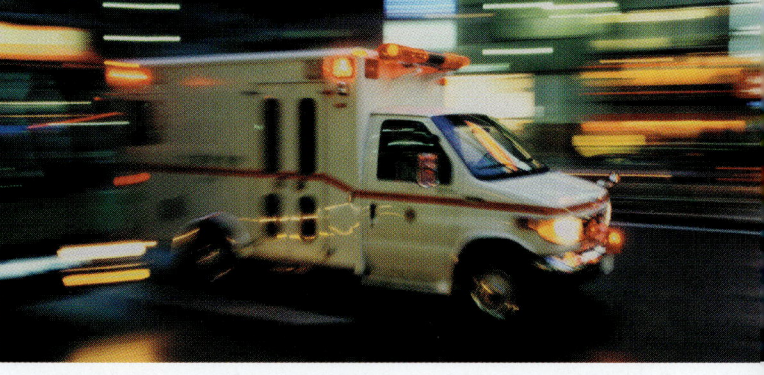

Interagency Interface

Lesson Goal

The goal of this chapter is to examine the decision-making process and support services available when the emergency medical technician has to interface with other emergency care providers.

Scenario

You and your partner, who are assigned to a basic life support (BLS) ambulance, respond to a local nursing home for a patient who needs to be transported to the hospital. On arrival you find that the patient, a 68-year-old man, is experiencing chest pain that radiates to his arms and jaw. The nurse tells you that Mr. Jones has had chest pain for the past 2 hours without relief from three nitroglycerine tablets. He has a past medical history of heart problems and diabetes. Your partner obtains the following vital signs: pulse 72 beats/min and irregular, respiratory rate 22 breaths/min, and blood pressure 142/78 mm Hg.

You begin to transport your patent to the hospital after beginning BLS care. The paramedic unit intercepts your ambulance on the way to the hospital. The paramedics board your unit and take a report from you. They begin to examine the patient and take a set of vital signs. They take a history from your patient, attach an electrocardiograph (ECG) monitor, and begin an intravenous (IV) line.

One of the paramedics leaves the ambulance, and you resume transport to the hospital. The remaining paramedic administers another nitroglycerin tablet. He then contacts medical control and reports on the patient. The medical control physician orders morphine to be given. Within a few minutes the patient is pain free and you arrive at the hospital. The paramedic gives his report to the nurse and doctor.

This is now a good time to discuss the call with the paramedics. Take the opportunity after the call to ask why they gave a certain medication or performed a certain procedure—or, just as important, why they did *not* give a medication. If you have a question, the time to ask it is after the call, away from the patient. If questions of patient care are asked in front of the patient, the patient may misconstrue it as disagreement regarding the care that the patient is going to receive. This may cause an increase in anxiety in the patient. On the other hand, you are still a member of the prehospital care team. You should not be afraid to offer observations or assist in the care of the patient.

 Why do you need to call for paramedics for this patient? What information would you relay to the paramedics while they are responding? Is there any other information that you need from the nurse before you leave? Why did the paramedic perform the same examination and history on the patient that you performed?

Key Terms to Know

Advanced life support (ALS)
Appropriate facility
Child protective services
Cold load
Fixed-wing aircraft
Fuselage
Hot load
Intercept

Landing zone
Landing zone coordinator
Landing zone hazards
Main rotor
Mandated reporter
Managed care organizations (MCOs)

Mechanism of injury
Neglect
Respond request
Rotor wash
Rotor-wing aircraft
Search and rescue (SAR)
Social service agency

Stand-by request
SWAT unit
Tactical unit
Tail rotor
Urban search and rescue (USAR)

Learning Objectives

As an EMT-Basic, you should be able to do the following:

Supplemental

- Discuss interactions with and how to access the following emergency care providers:
    - Dispatcher
    - First responder
    - Advanced life support (paramedic)
    - Aeromedical response
    - Crisis intervention team
    - Child protective services
    - Elder abuse services
    - Managed care organizations
    - Law enforcement agencies (street patrol, criminal investigation, tactical units, SWAT teams)
    - Rescue groups (wilderness search and rescue, urban search and rescue, hazardous materials, ski patrol)
- Identify safety precautions to consider when approaching and loading patients in an aeromedical helicopter.
- Describe the purpose and procedure for identifying a landing zone.

Since early childhood you have had to interact, relate, and resolve conflict with other people. These people may have been parents, teachers, or friends, but now that you have undertaken a career in emergency medical services (EMS) these interactions will become much more important. This is because patients will be placed in your care. The way you interact with other responders and hospital staff and resolve conflict with them is important to the outcome for the patient. The primary goal in EMS is to give the best patient care possible, and how you deal with other responders will directly affect your ability to accomplish this goal. This chapter provides an overview of other responders that you may encounter in your daily activity as an emergency medical technician (EMT). You must always use professionalism and respect when dealing with others.

As EMTs you will interact with many other prehospital providers in carrying out your job. Some providers, such as dispatchers and first responders, you deal with on almost every call. Other providers you may interact with only once or twice a year. Interaction with different levels of health care providers can be difficult, but it is important to remember that all the agencies involved have one thing in common—providing the best and most appropriate care for the patient.

Dispatcher

The old saying "dispatchers tell you where to go" still applies, but the days of just answering the phone, taking the address, and calling the ambulance on the radio are over. Modern dispatch centers multitask all aspects of emergency response, from call taking and triage to prearrival instructions. These centers employ dispatchers who are highly trained in extracting the needed information, determining the appropriate response to the situation, and providing simple medical instruction to the family or bystanders on the scene until the emergency personnel arrive.

When a call is received by a dispatch center, the call taker has to immediately determine what kind of emergency is involved. Some centers then send the call to a secondary dispatcher depending on whether the emergency is police, fire, or EMS. The dispatcher at this point has a set of predetermined questions to ask the caller. From the data gathered, the dispatcher then determines what kind of response is needed. Responses may vary according to system protocols, but the most serious (priority one) calls receive a full response. In a large urban system this may include an engine company with first responders, a basic life support (BLS) ambulance, and an **advanced life support (ALS)** unit with paramedics. In a more rural setting the response may be the local police or sheriff as first responder and the local volunteer ambulance. Protocols vary from area to area and are modified to take best advantage of the area's resources. You should get to know the protocols for dispatch in your area.

Most modern dispatch centers provide prearrival instructions to the bystanders on the scene of a serious medical or trauma situation. Once the appropriate units are dispatched, the dispatcher follows a written script, asking questions and providing instruction to bystanders. These may involve how to control bleeding, removal of airway obstruction, cardiopulmonary resuscitation (CPR), and childbirth. The dispatcher in less serious cases might not provide treatment instruction but gathers information that may be of value to the responding units, such as age, sex, chief complaint, past medical history, and medications. This information is then transmitted to the responding personnel so they can begin to develop a plan of treatment. The dispatchers will also try to determine any scene safety issues while on the phone (e.g., dispatchers may hear an argument in progress or a large dog barking, both of which can present problems for responders). In certain situations the dispatchers may have emergency personnel stage near the area until the scene can be secured by the police.

First Responders

First responders take many forms, from firefighters and police officers to organized first responder units. The commonality among all of them is that they are located closer to the sick or injured patient than the responding ambulance. In large urban areas, the job of first response usually, but not always, goes to the closest engine company from the fire department. In more rural areas, police officers or sheriff's deputies may be used. In some very rural areas, organized first response units are used. These units may be ski patrols located in resort areas or volunteer units in remote towns where response time for the ambulance may be up to an hour. The goal of the first responder is to find and treat any life-threatening conditions that the patient may have. In many systems, the first responders may accompany the EMTs in the ambulance if additional personnel are needed. These situations may include multiple patients, CPR, critical trauma patients, or whenever an "extra set of hands" is needed.

Before arrival of the ambulance, the first responders should be in contact with ambulance personnel. They should update the responding ambulance with patient status and, if needed, directions on how to find the patient's location. In some systems, the first responders may also downgrade or cancel the responding units based on what they find when they arrive. In preparation for the transfer of care from the first responder to the EMT, the first responder should introduce the EMT to the patient and provide a report that includes medical history, examination findings, and care rendered.

The first responders have developed a relationship with the patient in the few minutes that they have been providing care, so it may be appropriate to contact them after the call to let them know how the patient did during transport. This communication is important because it opens up the lines of communication, leading to the opportunity for discussion of any problems that may have arisen on the scene.

Advanced Life Support Paramedics

In the course of your practice as an EMT, you no doubt will interact with paramedics. In many systems, paramedic response is dictated by dispatch information. In others, the basic-level ambulance has to request a paramedic response. In either case, paramedics should be used when appropriate to patient care. It is important to have an understanding of the care that they can and cannot deliver to the patient and when it is appropriate to request a paramedic response. In some systems, the primary crew of an ALS ambulance is made up of an EMT-Basic (EMT-B) and an EMT-Paramedic (EMT-P). In this crew configuration, the EMT-B serves as assistant to the EMT-P and is usually the emergency vehicle operator. Some services provide additional training to EMT-Bs. This training may involve how to set up an IV bag or how to ventilate an endotracheal tube. You must become familiar with the names and locations of the paramedic's equipment on the ambulance. You can be of great help to the paramedic and the patient by anticipating and quickly getting the needed equipment.

Paramedics start their careers as EMT-Basics and then go on to further train as paramedics. Modern paramedic training consists of an average of 1300 hours of training. This includes classroom, laboratory, hospital, and clinical training and a comprehensive field internship. Training includes breathing tube placement, IV fluid replacement, defibrillation, ECG interpretation, and medication administration, to mention a few. More important, the paramedic is trained to gather and interpret data obtained from the physical examination and history. The paramedic must understand what disease or pathology is affecting the patient. Without this knowledge, paramedics cannot treat the patient appropriately.

Medical Control

Paramedics work under the control of a licensed physician. The paramedic may be in direct contact (on-line control) or working under a defined set of standing orders (protocols) that the physician has determined to be appropriate prehospital care for a patient with the presenting medical condition. Whether paramedics are in direct contact with medical control or not, they are working as an extension of the physician, and under his or her medical license.

Other Levels of Advanced Life Support

Many states have levels of prehospital care between EMT-B and EMT-P. The most common of these is the EMT-Intermediate (EMT-I). The basic and paramedic levels are essentially the same from state to state, but the intermediate program has over 40 different variations. Learn the levels of prehospital care personnel in your area.

Aeromedical Services

Transporting the sick and injured from the field to a hospital has been the role of EMS since its origination. The means of transport and the care given have progressed and developed through the years. Warfare has led to the development of innovative means of treating and transporting the injured. The value of aeromedical transport was realized many years ago. It was used during the Korean and Vietnam conflicts and saved many lives. These methods have been applied to the civilian population as well. Using aircraft such as fixed-wing airplanes and rotor-wing helicopters, patients can be airlifted over terrain and transported rapidly to an appropriate facility. Furthermore, highly trained and advanced medical teams can be transported by air to the patient on scene. It is important to know when to request aeromedical transport, how to find an appropriate place for the aircraft to land, how to work safely around an aircraft, and how to properly prepare the patient for the flight.

Types of Aeromedical Services and Their Purpose

A variety of aeromedical programs have been established. The types of services include the military and Coast Guard, state police and county sheriff services, park services and emergency medical programs, and hospital-based aeromedical services. Some services are solely for the transport of the ill or injured, whereas other services perform other duties such as search and rescue, patrol and observation, and other law enforcement activities. The types of aircraft also differ. Some are modified aircraft, and some are designed specifically for patient transport. The crew configuration may also vary. Different services fly different combinations of EMT-Ps, nurses, physician assistants, doctors, state troopers, and sheriff's deputies. There may be one or two pilots and one to three crewmembers. Depending on the terrain and distances involved, services may use helicopters or airplanes. Helicopters accomplish the majority of emergency air transports in the United States, and this section deals primarily with this type of aircraft.

> ✓ Aeromedical transportation is provided by a variety of types of services in a variety of types of aircraft. Helicopters are the most common means of transport.

Anatomy of a Helicopter

A variety of **rotor-wing aircraft** are available to fly patients. Some have one engine, and others have dual engines. The usual design consists of a **main rotor** system, which lifts the aircraft, and a **tail rotor,** which aids in the direction of the aircraft (Figure 38.1).

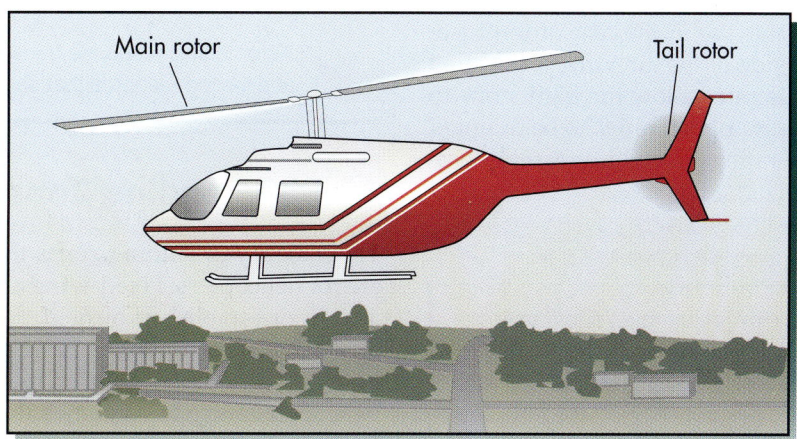

FIGURE 38.1 The main rotor system lifts the aircraft. The tail rotor helps control the aircraft.

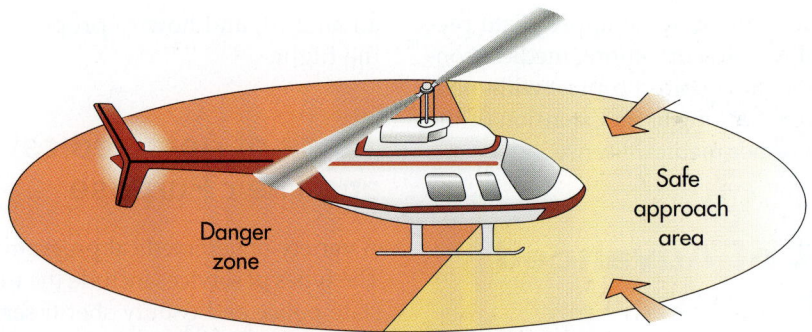

FIGURE 38.2 Extreme care must be taken whenever the rotor systems are turning.

All aircraft have danger areas of which the EMT must be aware (Figure 38.2). Extreme care must be taken whenever the rotor systems are turning. Depending on the aircraft, the rotor blades may be 3 to 15 feet off the ground. Whenever a person enters the perimeter of the main rotor system, that person is at risk. The prime rule to remember is never to approach the aircraft until directly instructed by the flight crew. When the aircraft is approached, the EMT should approach from a direction that will put him or her in the pilot's field of vision (i.e., from the front of the aircraft). The most dangerous area on most helicopters is the tail rotor area. *These blades may be low enough to the ground to cause decapitation.* Most aeromedical services provide outreach education to field providers on safety issues regarding the aircraft. You may want to contact the service in your area and attend one of these safety classes.

It is important for the EMT to know that a variety of sensitive equipment is mounted on the aircraft, and accidental damage by bumping, pulling, or grabbing may injure the EMT and may disable the aircraft. The aircraft has many doors and covers, or cowlings, as well as external antennas and equipment. Some aircraft have handles for routine use, and some handles are for emergency release. The loading doors may be in the rear of the **fuselage** or may open on the side of the aircraft. Never open or operate doors on the aircraft—allow the flight crew to do it. EMTs should seek out opportunities to be oriented or briefed on normal operating procedures by the local aeromedical service.

 Helicopters are complex, dangerous, and fragile vehicles. Extreme caution must be exercised at all times to avoid injury to the EMTs and patient, as well as damage to the aircraft.

Special Situations

Certain circumstances and patient medical conditions may warrant the use of aeromedical support. Transport time and the need for specialized care should be the determining factors. Examples include certain obstetric emergencies, unexpected or complicated premature deliveries, the need for smooth transport, and medical problems that require ALS with none available by ground.

Always remember to weigh the resources available, the need for advanced medical care on the scene, and the transport time to the nearest appropriate facility. In other words, situations in which the patient may not survive the ground transport time with the level of care available may require aeromedical support.

✓ The decision to use aeromedical transportation may be based on a number of criteria, including the **mechanism of injury,** physical findings, and other special circumstances.

✓ Aeromedical response transportation is an expensive and limited resource that should be used carefully.

Aircraft Landing Zone

The majority of landing zones that the EMT will prepare are for helicopters. **Fixed-wing aircraft** usually require an airport or established airfield. However, in some remote areas, makeshift airfields may be established or landings on water or ice may be an option. The **landing zone** for helicopters may vary somewhat, but the following is generally acceptable. During daylight hours, the minimum

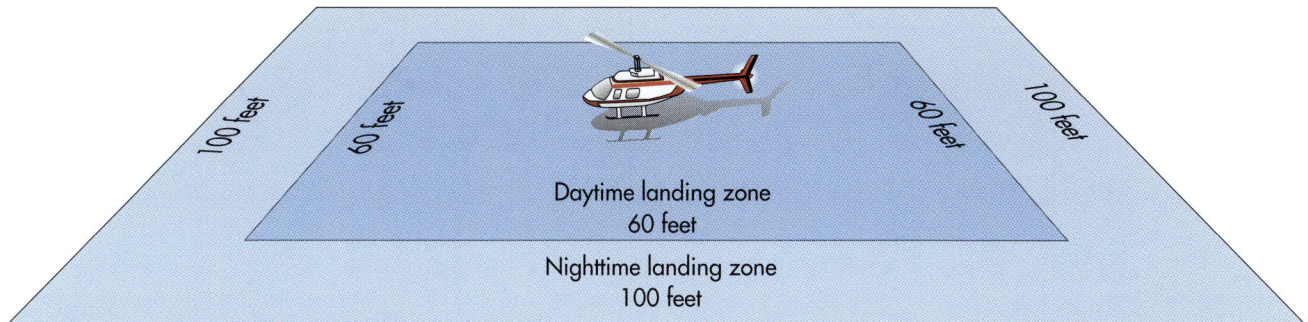

FIGURE 38.3 During daylight hours, the minimum dimensions for a helicopter landing zone are 60 feet by 60 feet. Nighttime operations require 100 feet by 100 feet.

dimensions are 60 feet by 60 feet, and nighttime operations require 100 feet by 100 feet (Figure 38.3). The area must be free of obstacles such as wires, debris, vehicles, personnel, trees, and high brush. Keep in mind that wires are difficult to see from the air and account for many of the incidents that occur with helicopters. Another consideration is the ground condition and slope. A slope greater than 8 degrees puts too great a stress on a helicopter's rotor system (Figure 38.4). The exact degree of slope is hard to determine at the accident scene. If the area has more than a gentle slope, it is probably too much; however, the final decision is the pilot's. The ground condition is also important to the landing and takeoff. Rocks and grooves in rocks that may wedge the skid system or wheels may prevent smooth takeoff and landing.

The ground must also be firm enough to support the aircraft, not boggy or soggy. On the other hand, dry and dusty landing zones can also be a hazard. As the helicopter hovers to land, dust, snow, or debris may obscure the vision of the pilot or may be thrown at EMTs or victims. Dry brush can also create a fire hazard if flares are used. Having your local fire department "water down" the landing zone may help with dust and fire hazards.

Once an acceptable landing zone has been found, it must be isolated from vehicle and pedestrian traffic. An evaluation of the landing zone must be conducted, looking for hazards such as wires, debris, and unmarked towers or poles. Appointing a **landing zone coordinator** is helpful. The coordinator should have a good idea of the **landing zone hazards,** ground conditions, and wind di-

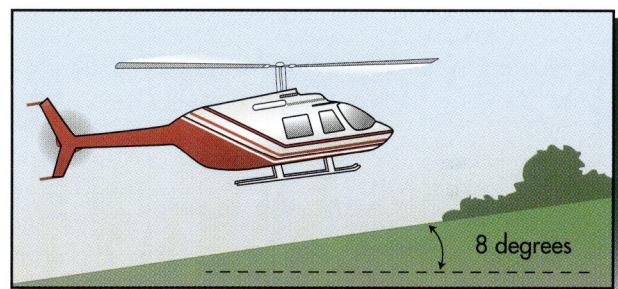

FIGURE 38.4 Landing zone considerations include ground condition and slope. A slope greater than 8 degrees puts too great a stress on a helicopter's rotor system.

rection. The coordinator should also have a means of direct communication with the helicopter personnel. This communication may be via radio or visual hand signals (Figure 38.5). Briefing the pilot of the landing zone hazards is important, and direct communication during touchdown and liftoff is helpful.

Setting up the Landing Zone

Mark the area for landing with objects that will not move with the downwash, or **rotor wash,** of the rotor blades. If flares are used, place them in a triangle or square (Figure 38.6). The aircraft will land in the middle of the triangle (i.e., do *not* place a flare in the middle). When flares are used, keep in mind the risk of fire. Mark all hazards that may interfere with the landing or takeoff. Vehicles can be used to mark the landing zone; however, use only the red flashers or beacons and avoid use of white light, especially at night. Never point bright lights, such as headlights or spotlights, into the landing area (Figure 38.7). These lights will interfere with the pilot's night vision at the critical point of landing or liftoff. No flash photography should be allowed at a landing zone. Remember, the

Tips from the Pros

Work with the aeromedical service in your area to establish predesignated landing zones in places commonly near accidents. Check all landing zones twice for wires and other hazards.

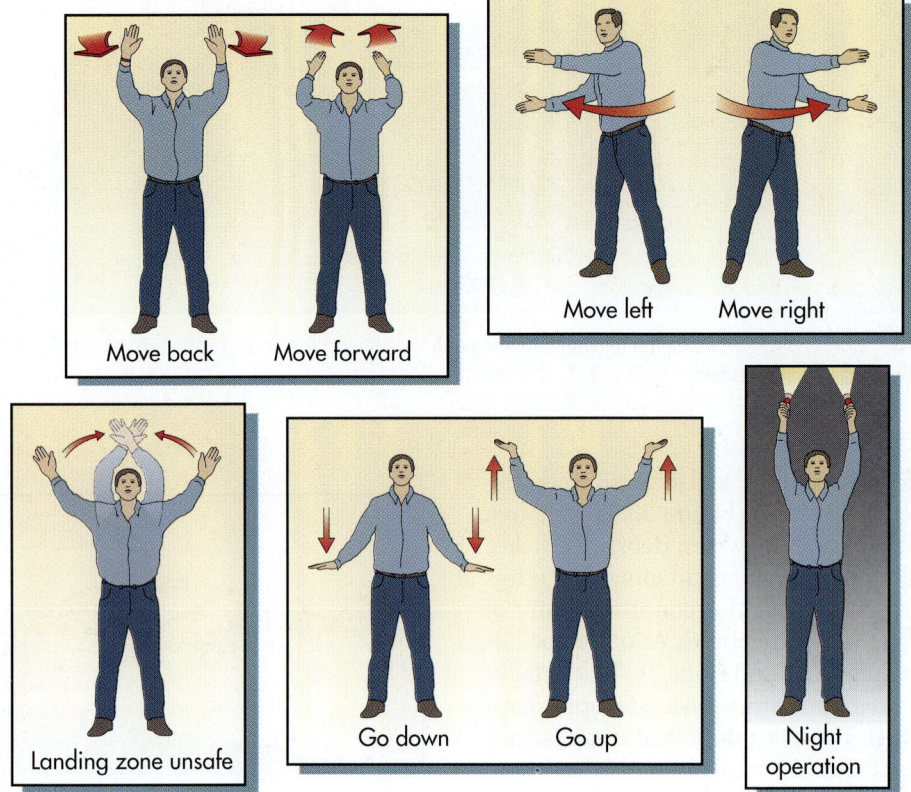

FIGURE 38.5 Landing zone hand signals. "Move back" and "move forward" have similar positioning, but with "move back" the thumbs are in and the signaler waves back to front, and with "move forward" the thumbs are out and the signaler waves front to back.

pilot has the absolute last say on the appropriateness of the landing zone and may at any point abort the landing or move the landing zone.

Directing an Aircraft

Always use references in relationship to the aircraft. In other words, if the landing zone is to the left of the aircraft as it is flying, inform the pilot that the landing zone is off to the left of the aircraft position. One can also use the positions of the clock. For instance, in the last example, one could say the landing zone is at 9 o'clock, remembering that the direction is related to the aircraft flying toward 12 o'clock. These directions are used because the pilot does not know the position of the landing zone coordinator, and any references using the landing zone are useless.

As the aircraft begins to hover to land, a gust of downward air will blow light objects around and can potentially be dangerous. All personnel near the landing zone should be shielded and should turn away from the aircraft as it lands. The landing zone coordinator may keep in direct visual contact with the pilot but must have adequate eye and body protection at all times.

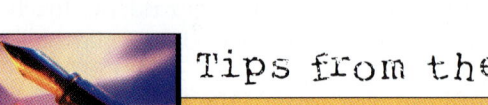 **Tips from the Pros**

Good direct communication during landings is essential; earphones or headsets may be helpful. Several devices are available to relay the accident scene location to the helicopter, such as a global positioning system and compasses. They all work well. If these devices are not available, relaying obvious landmarks such as churches, intersections, or playing fields will aid the pilot in locating the landing zone.

Safety Around an Aircraft

When an aircraft has arrived at the landing zone, safety of all personnel is essential. First, never approach a helicopter unless specifically requested to by the flight crew. Always approach from the front where the pilot can see you. Never approach from behind where the tail rotor is

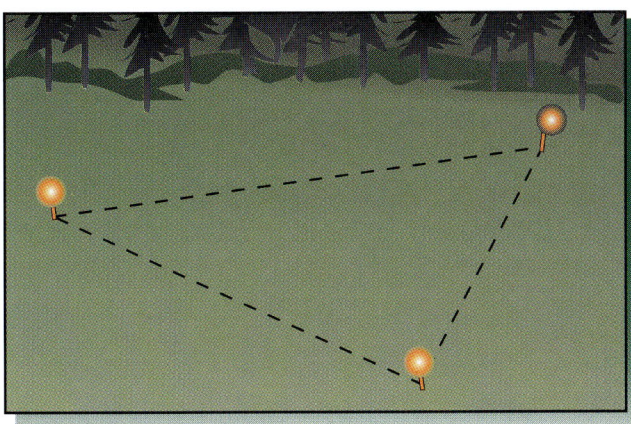 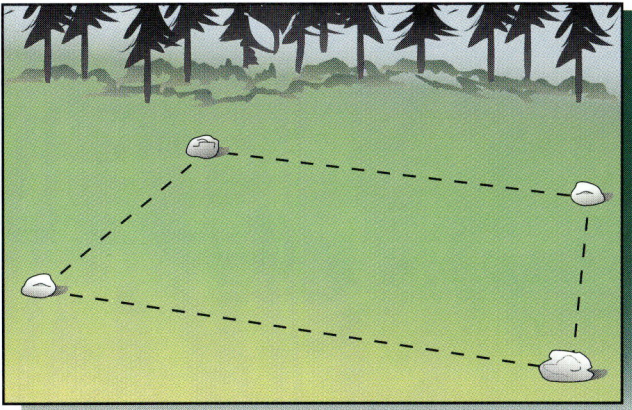

FIGURE 38.6 Mark the area for landing with objects that will not move in the downwash, or rotor wash, of the rotor blades. If flares are used, place them in a triangle or square. The aircraft will land in the middle of the triangle; therefore do not place a flare in the middle.

located. The tail rotor is usually 3 to 6 feet off the ground and spins so fast that you cannot see it. Accidentally walking into a tail rotor can be fatal. The loading or unloading of a helicopter with the rotor system running is called a **hot load**. It is usually safer to load or off-load when the rotor system has stopped, which is called a **cold load**. Extreme caution must be used while the rotor system is turning. Not only is there a danger to personnel, but if a vehicle or its radio antenna or piece of equipment such as a backboard or intravenous pole strikes the rotor system, the aircraft must be taken out of service (Figure 38.8). Therefore always approach the aircraft from the "downhill" side, and never carry objects above head level (Figure 38.9). Do not wear hats under the rotor system. Do not use loose sheets or cushions that may fly off and become entangled in the rotor system. Allow only the required number of personnel and equipment in the landing zone. Keep personnel and patients protected from rotor wash. Never park a vehicle less than 50 feet from the aircraft. Instead, carry the patient a few more feet for safety's sake. There should be absolutely *no* smoking near an aircraft.

A member of the aeromedical crew will direct all activity around the aircraft on the ground. This direction may come from the pilot or another crewmember. He or she may not allow personnel past a certain point while loading or unloading. Do not open or pull on any part of the aircraft. Several handles on the airframe are for door or cowling removal and can disable the aircraft if moved or opened. Move carefully around the aircraft, avoiding antennas and external equipment. It is difficult to hear around the aircraft, so move carefully and pay attention to the directions of the flight crew. Keep safety a priority.

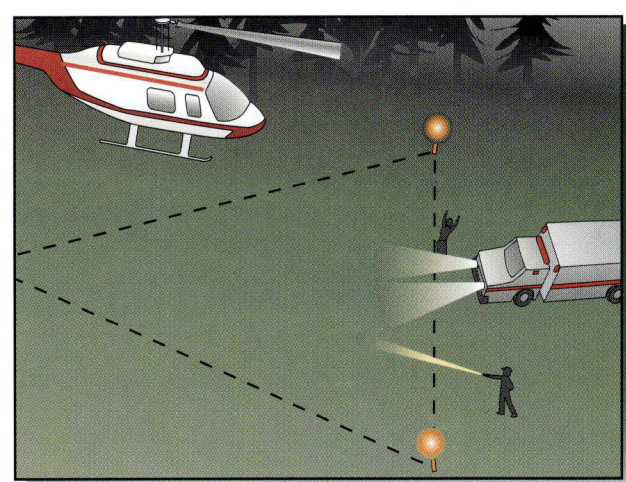

FIGURE 38.7 Never point bright lights, such as headlights or spotlights, at the landing area.

✓ The landing zone is a dangerous location for the patient, ground personnel, and the aircraft crew. A well-planned and well-coordinated effort is required to safely land the helicopter and transport the patient quickly.

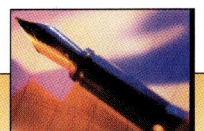 **Tips from the Pros**

Never run or rush around the aircraft; move deliberately as directed by the flight crew.

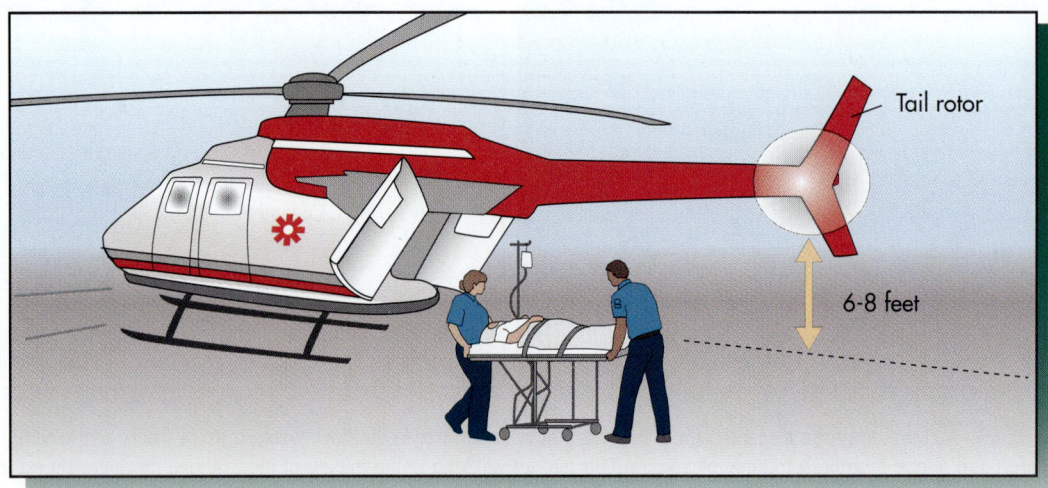

FIGURE 38.8 Extreme caution must be used while the rotor system is turning. Not only is there danger to personnel, but if a radio antenna, vehicle, or piece of equipment such as a backboard or intravenous pole strikes the rotor system, the aircraft must be taken out of service.

Patient Preparation

The success of an aeromedical mission depends on everyone involved. The ground personnel, including EMTs, are an integral part of the team. The ground crew should start the care and prepare the patient for transport. These preparations will reduce the on-scene time of the flight crew and improve care. Remember that the aircraft patient compartment space is limited, and several preflight preparations are important (Box 38.1).

Ensure adequate airway control, breathing, and circulation first, and treat life-threatening injuries. Place the patient on oxygen. If indicated, place the patient on a long backboard or equivalent device and completely immobilize the spine. The use of certain splints for long-bone fractures may be appropriate if time permits. Be careful not to extend splints to a length that prevents proper loading in the aircraft.

While caught up in the chaos of an accident scene, ground crews may overlook the basics of prehospital care. As a result, the aircraft medical team must perform basic packaging tasks that could have been completed before their arrival. Proper patient preparation and packaging are essential to the delivery of good aeromedical care.

Last, a concise but thorough assessment must be performed, and all pertinent information must be relayed directly to a member of the flight crew. Any bandaged or covered injury or any physical finding must be described to the flight medical crew, along with a brief but detailed history of the event.

> ✓ Space is limited in the helicopter; therefore it is important that as much treatment and stabilization as possible be accomplished on the ground before loading the patient into the helicopter.

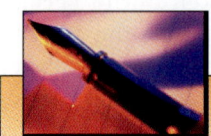 **Tips from the Pros**

Use the absolute minimum number of personnel in the landing zone to load the patient.

Aeromedical Services Review

1. Aircraft have become an important means of transporting injured people. The two types used are fixed-wing airplanes and rotor-wing helicopters.
2. The aircraft delivers highly trained, advanced medical care to the scene and rapidly transports patients over terrain to an appropriate facility.
3. Identification of patients needing aeromedical transport can be based on the mechanism of injury and physical findings.
4. The EMT may activate the aeromedical system according to local protocols. If time permits, request that the helicopter stand by when information indicates the potential need for aeromedical transport

> **Box 38.1   Preloading Steps**
>
> Because of space limitations in the helicopter, the following steps should be taken before loading the patient:
>
> - Control the patient's airway, breathing, and circulation.
> - Place the patient on oxygen.
> - Treat life-threatening injuries.
> - Completely immobilize the spine when appropriate.
> - Use splints carefully.

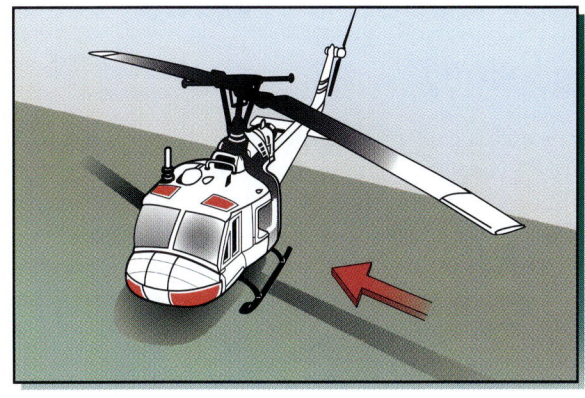

FIGURE 38.9 Always approach the aircraft from the "downhill" side, and never carry objects above head level.

(stand-by request). Once on scene, or when adequate information is obtained, request that the helicopter respond **(respond request).**

5. Safely guiding the helicopter to the landing zone and assisting the helicopter with landing is the responsibility of the landing zone coordinator, and direct radio communication is helpful.
6. Moving people and vehicles around an aircraft must be done with great care. Never park a vehicle less than 50 feet from the aircraft. Never approach the aircraft until directed to do so by the flight crew. Never approach the aircraft from the rear or from uphill. Keep clear of all of danger zones.
7. Have the patient ready for transport while optimally treating the patient's injuries.

Child Protective Services

Sometime in your EMS career you most likely will have to deal with the issue of child abuse or suspected abuse. Although the issues of child abuse may be troubling and images may stay with you long after the call, it is your ethical and in some cases your legal duty make sure these issues do not go uncorrected.

Physical injuries from abuse may be easily seen on examination; however, in many cases it may be extremely difficult to determine if these injuries happened due to accidental causes or from child abuse. Child abuse may also take forms other than physical injuries that may not be healthy for the child. Neglect and malnutrition may be present, as well as psychological factors. As an EMT you may be the only health care provider with the opportunity to see the child's home. Careful observation of the environment may help determine if the incident was an accident or child abuse.

Some states classify EMTs as mandated reporters, along with physicians and nurses. A **mandated reporter** is a person who is required by law to report any suspected child abuse. Whether you are a mandated reporter or not, it is still your moral and ethical duty to report your suspicions of child abuse. In states that require mandatory reporting, a toll-free number is usually available to report suspected incidents. You should also voice your concerns to the physician involved. **Child protective services** should be contacted. The police may also become involved in conducting the initial investigation. Child protective services may require you to provide a written statement and in some instances may interview you directly. After child protective services has received all the facts in the case, it makes a determination on whether to request placement of the child into "protective custody." In most cases this requires a court order.

Child abuse does not always take the form of physical abuse. Many times the situation may be that of **neglect.** Unlike abuse, neglect may be more difficult to detect or prove. For example, if you respond to a drug overdose and find a young child in the same household, you should have a high index of suspicion that this child may not be in a healthy environment. Although you may not have direct contact with the child, you may have some direct knowledge of a situation that should be further investigated by a child advocacy agency.

In any case of suspected child abuse, it is important to remember that you, the EMT, may be the voice for the child. Children from abusive families usually do not appear to be scared of those who hurt them; in fact, they may cling to their abusers. Your voice and that of the other members of the health care team may be the only chance a child from an abusive family has to have a normal childhood. Report anything that seems suspicious to the appropriate authorities.

Elder Abuse Services

Case Study

You receive a call from the police to check on the welfare of an 82-year-old man who has not been seen by his neighbors for the past 2 days. You and the police arrive on the scene at the same time. On your initial assessment of the scene, you see three newspapers on the front steps, a few meals that were left by meals-on-wheels, and a mailbox full of unopened mail. You hear a dog barking inside the house.

- Does anything raise your index of suspicion?
- Are there any personal safety issues?

The police officers break a small glass window in the door and unlock it. The dog appears to be a friendly, small dog that runs by the officers and out the door. You and the officers enter the house and find an elderly man lying on the floor at the bottom of a small landing. You assess the patient, treat him, and transport him to the local hospital.

- Is it important to convey the situation at the scene to the hospital staff?
- After recovery, can this gentleman return home?

There are certain common aspects between child abuse and elder abuse, but elder abuse has a tendency to take the form more of neglect than physical abuse. This neglect may not be anyone's fault, but rather the decreasing ability of an elderly person to care for himself or herself. Malnutrition and poor hygiene are signs that the patient can no longer meet self-care needs.

You may be called to care for an elderly person who has sustained an injury or a fall. There may have been multiple calls to the same address in the last few weeks, or you may notice that the patient cannot stand or walk without the risk of falling. Involvement of a **social service agency** at this point could prevent a fractured hip or other injuries from future falls.

Other issues that may impair self-care abilities among the elderly include inability to manage medication, recent death of a spouse, depression, and recent or multiple illnesses. In many of these situations the EMT may be the only person aware of the situation. To assume that someone else will deal with the problem is not the right course of action.

Depending on where you work, there may be different avenues to get the elderly person the needed help. In some states, the EMT is a mandated reporter and is required to report to a specific state agency. In other states, the social services department at the hospital may be able to assist the patient. In all cases, talking to the emergency department physician is a good place to start. Elder services and the social worker have many options to assist the patient.

The elderly patient may resist help at first for fear of being placed in a long-term nursing facility. This is a last resort, because everyone involved would like to see the patient remain at home. You may find that many elderly persons are afraid to admit that they need assistance; they may see this as the first step in losing their independence. Whatever the case, they should be referred to an appropriate support service.

Managed Care Organizations

Managed care organizations (MCOs) are becoming more involved in how the average American receives health care. It is not the intention of this section to debate the merits and shortfalls of such organizations, but rather to discuss how EMTs interact with these agencies.

The mission of MCOs is to provide quality health care at a reasonable cost. Toward this end, one of the goals of MCOs is to have the patient cared for in the **appropriate facility**. For example, if you are having a heart attack, you should call 911 and be transported to the closest emergency department; if you have had the flu for 3 days, you do not need to call 911 and go the emergency department. Most MCOs have a phone triage system in place so the patient can call and get advice on the appropriate care. This system is not without problems that EMTs have to deal with. One of the most common is that patients may be afraid to go to the emergency department or call 911 because they believe that their MCO will not pay the bill without prior approval. However, if the situation is a true emergency the patient does not have to call for prior approval. Most states require that ambulances transport emergency patients to approved emergency departments only.

Interacting with Law Enforcement Agencies

In the early days of modern EMS, the EMT had limited interaction with law enforcement. The primary time that EMTs dealt with the police was at the scene of automobile collisions. More recently, with increases in violent crime, EMTs are being called to many more crime scenes and asked to care for more patients with substance abuse problems. All of these require the involvement of the police. This section discusses some interactions that are commonly encountered.

It is important to understand the basic function and structure of a police department and how EMS providers will interact in each situation. Police officers are charged and empowered to "protect and serve" the citizens within their jurisdiction. To accomplish this, most departments have three major divisions: street patrol, detectives/criminal investigations, and tactical/SWAT units.

Street Patrol

Street patrol units are the police officers that EMS providers most commonly interact with. These are the officers who respond to most 911 calls. They are commonly assigned to a certain sector or area of the city and patrol this area when not answering calls. They are the officers in the marked patrol cars that are highly visible to the public. Although this high visibility has been shown to be a deterrent to crime, it also makes them targets for violent acts. EMS providers respond to calls for assistance with these officers. EMTs must always be cognizant of the fact that when in uniform and standing near these officers, they may be mistaken for police officers. Some EMS departments are now changing their uniforms so that they do not look like police uniforms.

EMTs respond to a variety of situations with the street patrol officer. One of the most common is automobile collisions. The police officer's responsibilities at the scene of an automobile collision are fluid and change over time. Officers may provide medical care until the arrival of EMS, direct traffic to provide a safe working area for EMS, and then investigate and reconstruct the crash scene. The EMS personnel interaction at automobile collisions is usually straightforward and uneventful. Interactions on the scene usually revolve around care for the patient, scene safety, and access to and egress from the crash site. Occasionally, investigation into motor vehicle crashes may involve drivers who were operating under the influence of alcohol or intoxicating drugs. In these situations you may be called on to testify in court. Testimony in court will be focused on what you observed and found during your examination. It is important to remember that the credibility of your testimony revolves around what you documented on your run report immediately after the call. If you did not put it down on the run report, your statement will carry less weight in the courtroom. Document what you see and what information the patient told you. In most states the patient-doctor privilege does not apply to EMTs, so whatever the patient tells you, you may be required testify to that in court. You should discuss this with you instructor to determine what laws exist in your area.

Response to violent and domestic crime is another common situation for EMS providers. The police officer has many tasks to perform when called to a crime scene. The first priority the officer has to deal with is safety. The officer is responsible for the safety of all on the scene. He or she must quickly assess the scene to determine overall safety and what steps must be taken to secure the situation. Until the scene is secured, EMS personnel will not be allowed to enter the area. This is for the protection of both the EMTs and the officers. Once the scene is deemed secure, the EMTs will be allowed in to care for the patient.

Although it is the primary job of the police officers to provide a secure, safe area for the EMTs to care for the patient, the EMTs should stay alert for any changes in the environment. Violence-related situations can change rapidly. If you notice a situation escalating, the prudent thing to do is to rapidly package your patient and continue care in the back of the ambulance. It may be necessary to drive a few blocks away and stop to continue care.

Police officers also must investigate the crime that has occurred. Although they are concerned with the patient receiving appropriate care, they are also responsible for preservation of the crime scene until a proper investigation can be completed. It is important that EMTs look for ways to provide good patient care with as little impact to the crime scene as possible. The following is a short list of things that EMTs should do at a crime scene:

- Try not to step in any pooled blood; extra bloody footprints on the scene will complicate the investigation.
- If the patient must be removed from a house, carry the patient from the house and then place the patient on the stretcher, if possible. Using a stretcher indoors will usually require moving furniture, which should be minimized or avoided.
- If it is necessary to cut off the patient's clothing, care should be taken not to cut though any bullet or stab holes. All clothing should be given to the police. If the clothing is removed on the way to the hospital, it should be placed in a bag and given to the police as soon as possible.
- If possible, do not set equipment down in the middle of the crime scene. Position it nearby but out of the immediate area.
- Make notes on what you see at the scene; if you move anything, report this to the officers immediately.
- Any statements the patient makes on the way to the hospital may be important to the investigation of the crime; report all statements to the police.

You may be called to transport a patient who is in police custody. This may be from the scene of a crime where the suspect was apprehended or from the jail or police station. If transporting the patient from the scene, care must be taken by both the EMTs and the police officers to ensure that the suspect has been searched and secured. Although the patient/perpetrator has the right to proper medical care, the EMT has the right to be safe while providing care. If the patient has been paced under arrest, a police officer should accompany the patient in the back of the ambulance.

You will often be called to attend to a jailed suspect requesting medical attention. In larger municipalities, the jail will have medical personnel available to assess the patient before a request for transport is made. However, in smaller cities these medical personnel may not be available; when a patient makes a complaint of any illness or injury, no matter how small, jail personnel must call EMS. If the patient requests transport to the hospital, the EMT usually has no choice but to comply, regardless of the nature of the complaint. Many habitual criminals know this, and they may use this ploy as a way to get some time out of the jail. It may also be used as a means of attempted escape. For this reason, you must have a police officer accompany the patient and, if possible, a second police officer following in a car.

When entering the jail, EMTs must realize that they are entering a secure area. They should not bring anything into this area that could be used as a weapon (e.g., pocketknife, bandage scissors).

Detectives

Most of the interactions that EMS providers have with detectives will take place a few hours after they have finished caring for the patient. The detective's job is to gather evidence and conduct interviews in preparation of a case against a criminal. You should make yourself available as soon as possible for this interview. The detectives may interview you and your partner separately, so that one person's statement will not influence the other's. You will be asked to read and sign this statement; it may be used in court at a later date. The detectives may ask for a copy of the run report. In most states, this information is considered to be part of the patient's medical record and cannot be obtained without permission of the patient or a court order. Contact your supervisor for assistance.

Tactical and SWAT Units

The **tactical unit,** or **SWAT unit,** consists of a small group of police officers who are highly trained in dealing with situations that have a high risk of violence. These situations include hostage situations, barricaded suspects, drug raids, and high-risk warrant service. Officers on these units are seasoned officers who undergo continuous training in the use of high-capacity weapons.

In recent years, these units have begun to realize that medical care can and should be available on the scene of tactical operations. Two different models are used: (1) The police agency trains a police officer to perform medical care at the tactical situation. This can work well if the police officer has prior emergency medical training. (2) Paramedics from the local EMS agency are trained to act within the tactical environment.

You may be called on to stand by for a tactical operation. When standing by, the police will have you stage in an area well outside the inner perimeter of the operation. In the event of an injury on the scene, the patient may be transported to you by the police, or, if the scene is deemed secure, you may be called into the area.

Transportation of an Injured Police Officer

One of the most difficult calls to deal with is the call for an injured police officer. Police officers can be injured in many ways—for example, they can be involved in a motor vehicle collision while responding to a call, or they can be injured while trying to subdue a violent person. In either case, tension will be high on the scene.

The EMT must remember that the officer is armed with a weapon. Whenever transporting an officer for anything other than a minor injury, the officer's firearm must be secured by another police officer. If possible, a police officer should accompany the injured officer to the hospital.

Search and Rescue

Rescue has become a highly technical and specialized practice in today's prehospital environment. It is beyond the scope of this text to explain the medical details specific to each of these areas, but an overview of the situations encountered by each of the specialties is provided. EMTs assigned to these teams are given special training required to deal with the specific working environments and patient injury patterns that they will encounter. It is important to remember that without specific training in technical rescue, EMTs are placing themselves and their team in danger. Never engage in rescue unless trained to do so.

Urban Search and Rescue

Urban search and rescue (USAR) teams are highly trained, multidisciplined teams designed to conduct search and rescue operations in the urban environment. Most of the missions these teams are deployed on involve some type of building collapse. The cause of such a collapse may be natural (e.g., earthquake, hurricane, tornado) or unnatural (e.g., construction accident, terrorist activity).

USAR team are made up of firefighters, engineers, and medical personnel. Firefighters specialize in gaining access to trapped victims within the collapsed structure. Engineers deal with building design and structural stability. The job of the firefighters and engineers is to gain access to trapped patients. Once access is gained, medical personnel (paramedics and physicians) treat patients until they can be removed from the structure. The removal process may take several hours or days. Medical personnel on USAR teams are also responsible for the condition of the team. USAR teams are under tremendous stress, both physical and emotional. The medical team constantly assesses this and determines when relief of the team is needed. USAR teams are located in major metropolitan areas throughout the United States. They are deployed within the United States and internationally when disasters strike. Major incidents may require the deployment of multiple teams or task forces.

Hazard Materials Teams

Hazardous materials are transported daily on the nation's highways and rail systems. Once these materials are transported, they must be stored before use. Although precautions are taken to ensure safe transportation of hazardous materials, unforeseen situations can arise causing the leakage of these materials. Hazardous materials teams are trained to enter these areas, retrieve and decontaminate patients, and then stop or isolate the leaking product. To allow entry into the area, the hazardous materials technicians wear special suits designed to insulate them from the particular chemical involved. Although these suits provide protection, they are heavy and hot. Medical personnel assigned to these teams monitor the condition of technicians to determine if they need to be withdrawn for rehabilitation. These medical personnel are also trained to treat and decontaminate chemicals that are beyond the scope of regular EMTs.

Search and Rescue and Wilderness Medicine

Traditional **search and rescue (SAR)** teams have been around for decades. These teams are used when a person is lost or injured in a wilderness area. The makeup of SAR teams varies. Some teams are made up of or supervised by law enforcement agencies. Others are made up of volunteer outdoor enthusiasts who receive special training in SAR techniques. This training may be available locally or on a national level from organizations such as the National Association for Search and Rescue (NASAR). Some SAR teams have members who are trained in wilderness medicine. There are many levels of wilderness medicine, ranging from wilderness first responders to physicians. These persons have special skills and experience in dealing with patients in remote areas that require extended transport time out of the wilderness. This increased transport time is further complicated by environmental factors such as rain, snow, and subfreezing temperatures. Medical care rendered in a backcountry rescue may take hours.

When interacting with SAR groups, EMTs must remember their abilities and limitations. Can EMTs trained and equipped to take care of patients in the urban setting safely travel into the wilderness to care for an injured party without putting their own lives in jeopardy? The answer to this question is *no*. If you are going to be involved in wilderness medicine, get the training that is necessary for good patient care and your own survival.

Ski Patrols

Ski patrols are standard at ski areas in the United States. Ski patrollers receive basic medical training of about 80 hours. This training concentrates on injuries and illnesses commonly seen on the ski slopes. Many patrols have ALS available, and paramedics and physicians commonly work on or volunteer for patrol duty.

Your interactions with the ski patrol will usually take place in the ski patrol first aid room. This is the area at the base of the hill where the injured skier is brought to after evacuation off the mountain. You should expect to get a report from the patroller who is caring for the patient; it is your job to constantly reassess the patient. Perform a comprehensive examination if patient condition allows. Remember that while on the hill, the patroller could not effectively remove clothing or inspect certain areas because of heavy clothing. Remove clothing as much as possible. Ski boots should be removed (you may want to ask the ski patroller for help doing this).

Conflict Resolution

There may be times when conflict arises between EMTs and paramedics. Conflicts can also develop between any level of providers. It should be noted that regardless of tact (or lack thereof), the highest-trained provider assumes medical supervision and responsibility for the patient. Arguments regarding patient care in the presence of the patient undermine the patient's confidence in your ability and may generate a request to "just take me to the hospital." Such behaviors do not serve the best interests of patient care.

Disagreements must be settled after the patient is safely delivered to the hospital and when an opportunity for private discussion is available. Should conflict occur, the following guidelines are offered to help facilitate resolution:

- If the situation is "too hot to handle," allow for a cooldown period.
- Do not escalate the conflict (feed off each other's anger).
- Remain open and objective throughout the discussion.
- Identify the issue or problem, and focus on it to the exclusion of extraneous concerns.
- Compromise—there may be more than one appropriate solution.
- Display mutual respect.
- Forgive, forget, and move on.

Case Study

The EMT has called for an ALS **intercept** for a patient complaining of severe difficulty breathing. On arrival, the ALS provider asks where the patient is and sweeps past the EMT, who is trying to explain the patient's situation. The EMT, after persisting in her presentation of the patient's present condition, asks if there is anything that she can do to assist in caring for the patient. The ALS provider says, "Sure, go direct traffic and leave the real care to someone who can make a difference." The EMT continues to prepare the patient for transport and discusses the process with the family members present.

Transport is accomplished. At the conclusion of the call and in the privacy of the EMS room, the EMT asks the ALS provider what caused him to act in such an inappropriate manner. The ALS provider relates the story of a patient call in which the EMT was clueless as to how to interact with other providers or the patient's family. After a long conversation, the EMT and ALS provider have garnered a better understanding of each other.

The ALS provider in this scenario arrived on the scene of this call with a preconceived view of the EMT. The EMT remained calm and acted in a professional manner in continuing to care for the patient. She worked with the ALS provider to the best of her ability, and the call went smoothly. The EMT further demonstrated her professionalism by working to resolve the situation through open communication without anger. It is important to realize that had the EMT taken a different stance, resentment and lack of team effort could have resulted. The resentment could have grown over time and damaged the overall team effort to provide quality care.

> ✓ Conflicts between EMTs and ALS providers should be resolved in a calm, professional manner outside of the scene.

After reading this chapter, it is easy to see that several different groups are involved in patient care. As an EMT you have a job to do, but it is important to realize that other responders have jobs to do also. These tasks vary, and conflicts may occur. Deal with these conflicts, but remember that the care the patient receives comes first and foremost.

Summary

- To achieve positive patient outcomes, it is imperative that EMTs at all levels work together as a team.
- The strength of the team effort depends on the clinical, rescue, and interpersonal skills of all participants on the scene.
- As clinicians, EMTs must be able to determine when it is in the best interest of the patient to request assistance.

Scenario Solution

You need to call for paramedics for this patient because the patient can benefit from advanced life support. Medication may be administered to relieve pain and to prevent progression to cardiac arrest.

You would relay the following information to the paramedics while they are responding: age, sex, presenting complaint, level of consciousness, and vital signs. The paramedics may also ask for any examination and history findings. You may

Scenario Solution (cont'd)

also need to communicate directions and instructions for an intercept point.

Before you leave, you will need to get a copy of the patient's chart, medication sheet, and transfer orders; the hospital staff will need these. You may also need forms filled out by the nursing home that are necessary for submitting bills for insurance reimbursement.

The paramedic repeats the examination and history to make absolutely sure that the information you provided is correct and has not changed. The paramedic should listen to what you have to report on your patient, but will do his or her own examination.

Key Terms

Advanced life support (ALS) Level of emergency care that is higher than the EMT-Basic level of emergency care. In the prehospital care environment, EMTs who are educated and credentialed at the EMT-Intermediate and EMT-Paramedic levels perform ALS. ALS personnel perform more complex procedures, such as administering medications and inserting intravenous lines.

Appropriate facility A hospital staffed and equipped to immediately handle the patient's specific injuries.

Child protective services A branch of the state or local government that is charged with caring for lost, displaced, or neglected children. Children removed from the parents by the court will be placed in their custody.

Cold load Loading a patient onto an aircraft after the rotor systems have completely stopped turning.

Fixed-wing aircraft An aircraft with wings that are solidly attached to the main fuselage; as the entire aircraft moves through the air, lift is created as air passes over the wings; commonly called an *airplane*.

Fuselage The main body of an aircraft.

Hot load Loading a patient onto an aircraft while the rotor systems are still turning.

Intercept An established location where two units (emergency vehicles) rendezvous.

Landing zone Area where an aircraft lands. Must be of sufficient size for the craft and flat, firm, and free of hazards.

Landing zone coordinator The person in charge of the landing zone. Responsible for identifying and controlling all hazards, directing the aircraft to the landing zone, guiding the aircraft during landing and takeoff, and ensuring safe operations around the aircraft.

Landing zone hazards Anything that interferes with the safe landing or takeoff of an aircraft, including debris, tall brush, pedestrians, poles, towers, and especially wires.

Main rotor The main set of rotor blades on a helicopter, usually located over the center of the fuselage, that creates the lift for flight.

Mandated reporter A health care professional who is required by law to report abuse.

Managed care organizations (MCOs) A form of health care insurance. Managed care plans control costs by monitoring how medical professionals treat patients, limiting referrals to specialists, and requiring authorization before care is rendered. Managed care usually includes negotiated payment rates with providers that are discounted below the normal fee-for-service rates.

Mechanism of injury The manner in which an injury occurs; important in determining whether aeromedical support is required.

Neglect Failure to exercise the degree of care that a reasonable person would exercise under the same circumstances.

Respond request The second phase of activating aeromedical support; requests aeromedical service launch the aircraft because appropriate guidelines have been met. Stand-by request may or may not precede the respond request.

Rotor wash Downward gust of air created by the main rotor system as an aircraft lands or takes off; can blow dust and rocks, cause injuries, and obscure vision.

Rotor-wing aircraft An aircraft with multiple blades that rotate at high speed and create lift as they turn; commonly called a *helicopter*.

Search and rescue (SAR) Specially trained members or groups that respond to lost or injured persons in the wilderness or urban environment.

Social service agency Specially trained health care professionals who deal with patients' continuing medical needs.

Stand-by request The first phase of activating aeromedical support; requests aeromedical service prepare to respond; allows time to prepare the aircraft and find the location, as well as check local weather conditions.

SWAT unit Specially trained law enforcement group that deals with high-risk situations and criminal activity.

Key Terms (cont'd)

Tactical unit Specially trained unit that deals with tactical situations such as armed hostage situations and sniper situations.

Tail rotor Set of rotor blades located at the rear of the fuselage and perpendicular to the main rotor; counters the inherent spin of the aircraft created by the rotation of the main rotor.

Urban search and rescue (USAR) Specially trained unit that responds to lost or injured persons in an urban setting.

Review Questions

1. List five of the guidelines used to help resolve conflicts.
2. True or False: At a crime scene, when removing a patient's clothing it is important to cut though bullet holes.
3. Which of the following might be considered advantages of air transportation as compared with ground transportation?
   a. Rapid transportation.
   b. Transportation not affected by roads, traffic, or terrain.
   c. Air transport vehicle often comes with personnel with more advanced training and equipment than is available on ground units.
   d. All of the above.
4. What is a mandated reporter? Are you one in your state?
5. All of the following statements are true about search and rescue *except*:
   a. You should not engage in rescue unless trained to do so.
   b. USAR primarily deals with building collapses and confined-space rescue.
   c. SAR may involve treatment and transport times of several hours or even days.
   d. You are adequately protected in the hazardous materials situation by wearing fire department turnout gear.

Answers to these Review Questions can be found at the end of the book on page 869.

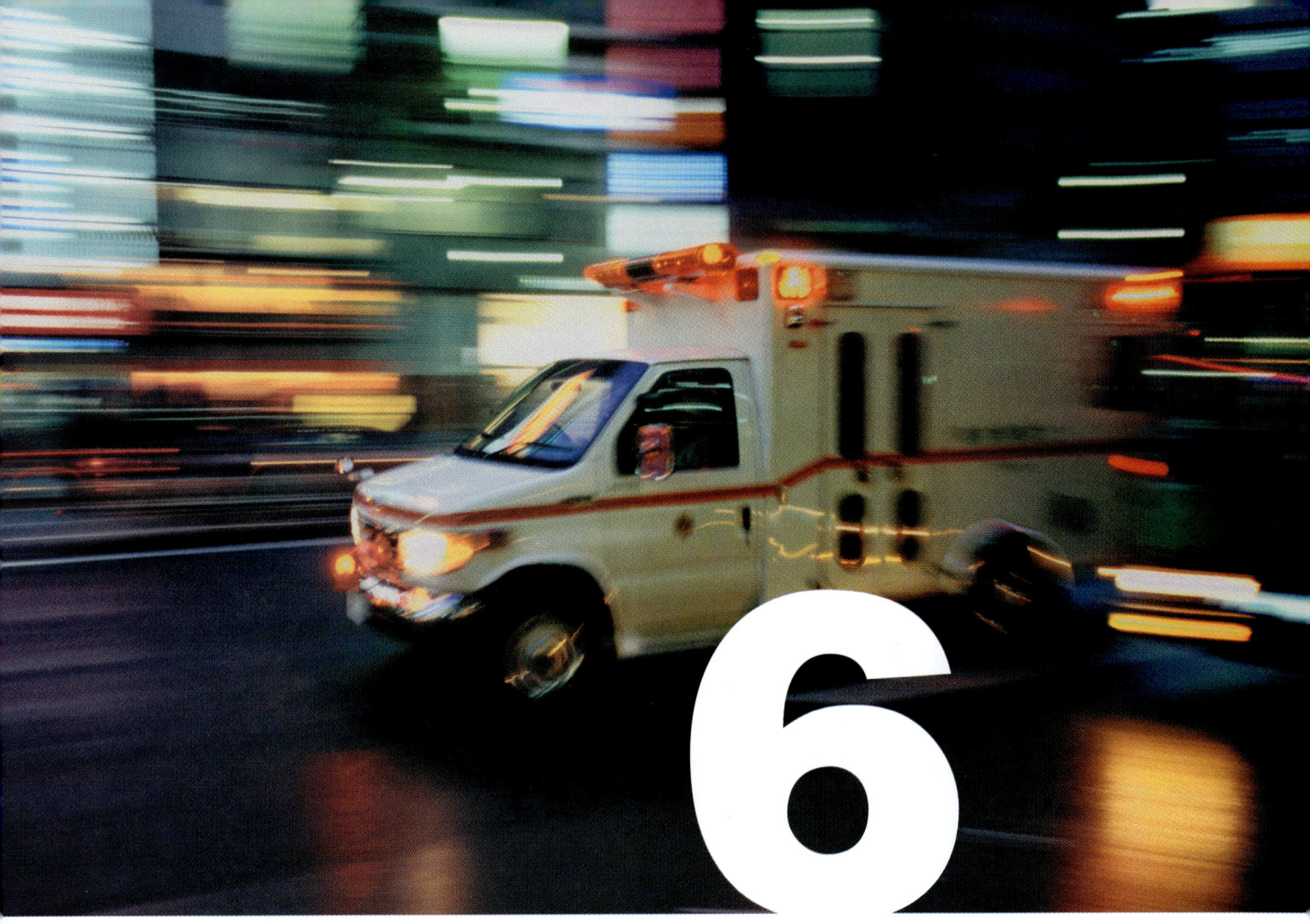

section six

Special Topics

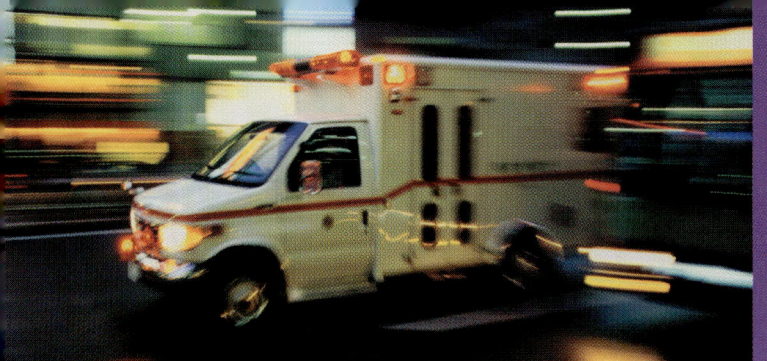

Gaining Access

Lesson Goal

The goal of this chapter is to review the various types of rescue operations, types of vehicles and equipment, personal safety, the emergency medical technician's role, and priorities at the rescue scene.

Scenario

As you are returning to quarters from the hospital, your unit is dispatched to a single-car collision on a high-speed, two-lane road. It is 01:30 on a Saturday morning, and the traffic is light. The weather is clear and cool. As you approach the scene, it appears that the car has contacted a wooden power pole before winding up in the middle of the road. The pole is heavily damaged and leaning away from the street, and the wires are still intact. It is a 1999-model car equipped with both front and side air bags. The front bags have deployed, but both side bags have not. The driver is the only person visible in the car; he appears to be unconscious and possibly trapped in the wreckage.

 What are the first actions you take when you arrive on the scene? How would you gain simple access? How would you handle this incident?

Key Terms to Know

Air restraint bag
Circle survey
Cribbing
Disentanglement
Entrapment
Extrication

Fend-off position
Full protective clothing
Golden hour
Hand tools
Hazardous materials
   (HAZMAT)

Initial patient access
Kendrick Extrication Device®
Laminated plate glass
Pedi-Immobilizer®
Rescue action plan
Size-up

Stabilization
Step chocks
Sustained access
Tempered safety glass
Wedge cribbing

Learning Objectives

As an EMT-Basic, you should be able to do the following:

DOT

- Describe the purpose of extrication.
- Describe the role of the EMT-Basic in extrication.
- Identify the personal safety equipment that is required for the EMT-Basic.
- Define fundamental components of extrication.
- State the steps that should be taken to protect the patient during extrication.
- Evaluate various methods of gaining access.
- Distinguish between simple and complex access.

Supplemental

- Differentiate among the various types of rescue operations.
- List 10 steps in a rescue plan of action.
- Describe four categories of vehicle rescue situations.

Emergency medical technicians (EMTs) are often called on to provide emergency care to one or more patients who are trapped. In these cases, the EMT-Basic (EMT-B) becomes an integral part of the overall rescue effort by providing patient stabilization and critical intervention as the rescue team frees the patient.

Rescue situations can range from something as simple as a child with a finger caught in a candy machine, to an incident as complex as a trench or building collapse. Environmental hazards from severe weather, electricity, fires, and even earthquakes can all present danger to everyone involved. Although it appears at first glance that each type of rescue is very different, most can be handled by following the same sequence of steps to organize the scene. This is called the **rescue action plan**. Though the skills required for each step in the plan differ, it is important that the EMT-B know the concepts of each step to be a safe, productive part of the rescue effort.

Your first duty on any scene, regardless of the complexity, is to maintain a high level of attention to your personal safety. If you are injured, the patient will suffer from the lack of care you would have provided and from the lack of attention of other EMTs who must now provide medical care to you. Your personal safety concerns on a given event start the minute the call comes in and continue until you arrive safely in quarters and begin preparations for the next call.

Because the vast majority of rescue situations you respond to will involve motor vehicle collisions, we will use these situations to illustrate the overall rescue action plan. However, being a member of a rescue team requires extensive training in general rescue practices, as well as specific types of rescue operations. This will vary with your agency's response capabilities.

Types of Rescue Operations

As an EMT-B you will respond to many different types of rescue situations. It is important to remember that a good rescuer will be able to use a systematic approach to organize every scene regardless of the circumstances. A good rescuer should also be able to apply basic rescue disciplines, following a rescue action plan, to obtain a successful rescue outcome for both patient and rescuer.

EMTs may be a part of the rescue team, being further trained in technical rescue operations, or they may be with an outside agency that provides emergency prehospital care. In this capacity, they may be required to wait for the rescue team to deliver the patient to a safe area for evaluation and treatment by the EMT.

It is important to keep in mind that in all situations, EMTs must stay within their scope of training and job requirements when working at these scenes. They must also be trained in and able to use proper personal protective equipment if they are to enter the danger zone that surrounds the scene and the trapped victim. Additional injuries or even death of untrained or unprotected rescue personnel cannot be allowed. This is unsafe not only for the EMT-B but also for the rest of the rescue team.

Rescue situations may include, but are not limited to, the following:

- Building collapse
- Trench/excavation collapse
- Confined spaces
- Low angle/high angle
- Wilderness
- Water
- Machinery/industrial
- Vehicles

Building Collapse

These are rescue situations in which a structure has collapsed, trapping victims inside the debris. They may be caused by tornadoes, hurricanes, earthquakes, fires, or structural failure. In lightweight, wood-frame buildings, it is possible for properly protected EMTs to assist in surface checks. In many cases, however, a specially trained rescue team will properly crib and shore the structure and use specialized tools to reach trapped patients. They will then free the patients and bring them to a safe location for the EMTs to assess and treat.

Trench/Excavation Collapse

A trench or excavation collapse occurs when an opening in the earth collapses on people inside it. These cave-in situations are extremely dangerous to rescue personnel. In fact, more rescuers than entrapped victims are killed and injured in these circumstances. A highly trained rescue team, with training in the disciplines of trench and excavation rescue, is needed to properly handle these situations. They require special sheeting and shoring equipment and specialized tools to safely rescue trapped victims.

Confined Spaces

A *confined space* is generally defined as any space large enough for a person to enter and perform work and that has a limited entry and egress. It is not designed for continuous human occupancy and has one or more of the following characteristics:

- It has a potential for a hazardous atmosphere.
- There is material inside that may engulf a person.
- It has inwardly converging walls, or a floor that slopes downward and tapers to a smaller opening.
- It contains any serious health hazards such as fall, equipment, or environmental.

Rescue teams trained and equipped for confined space rescue operations will be required to access and remove the victims.

Low Angle/High Angle

Low-angle rescue situations occur whenever the victim is located below or above grade level and within reach of ground ladders. This means one or two stories above or below ground level, where rescue systems can be assembled with ropes, pulleys, rope appliances, and ladders to safely access, disentangle, and remove the patient.

High-angle rescue situations occur when the victim is located beyond the reach of ground ladders. This can be on the outside of a high-rise building or other structure, on a cliff, down a cave, or on a tower. In these situations rescuers, specially trained in rope anchoring, rescue harness utilization, rappelling, proper patient removal practices, and safety operations will be needed.

Wilderness

Wilderness is considered any natural area that is uncultivated and uninhabited. It can be remote from populated areas, but not necessarily in all cases. Locating victims in these situations takes rescue teams trained in proper wilderness search techniques. They will use safe patient access and removal techniques for victims located in remote locations. EMTs may be a part of the rescue team, or they may accompany the team to the patient in order to provide initial care.

Water

Water rescue scenes can include surf, swift water, ice, and standing water. Rescuers trained in special water rescue skills and techniques are used to access the victim and bring the victim to a safe area for initial patient care and evaluation. Water rescue personnel will also have access to rescue boats and equipment designed for the job. It is dangerous for an EMT-B untrained in water rescue techniques to attempt to perform this type of rescue operation.

Machinery/Industrial

Incidents involving elevators, escalators, machinery, and industrial machinery present unique rescue challenges. Rescuers trained in working with special tools, as well as the general operating processes of the machinery involved, will operate at these scenes. In these instances, if it is safe enough, EMTs may be able to get close to the victim and begin patient care while the rescue is being performed. It is important to work closely with rescuers who are working to free the patient. You may need to move to a safe area during the operation, and then return to continue your care.

Vehicles

Vehicles include planes, trains, buses, trucks, and passenger cars. The rescue of persons trapped in planes and trains is less common for EMTs. These situations are usually large operations involving many agencies. They also require rescue personnel specially trained and equipped to safely access and remove trapped and injured patients.

Collisions involving buses, trucks, and passenger cars are common in all areas and are a major contributor to trauma injuries and death. Of all the rescue situations discussed so far, EMTs will respond to these types of incidents most frequently. Motor vehicle collisions may or may not involve patients who are trapped in the vehicle. If the patient is trapped, the operation to free and remove the patient is referred to as **extrication.** EMT-Bs should be aware of techniques to approach the scene, stabilize the vehicles, recognize hazards, gain initial access, and properly remove the injured patient. A simple action such as opening an obstructed airway until the patient is freed from the wreckage can save a life.

Many areas have agencies responsible for the utilization of special rescue tools and techniques to free patients trapped in vehicles. It is important that EMTs work closely with these agencies and their personnel to prepare for the vehicle rescue incident.

Tips from the Pros

An extrication situation automatically means that scene time is going to be longer than normal. While this extra time is ticking away, the patient may be exposed to the elements for an extended period of time. If the weather is cool or cold, hypothermia may result and may cause a further decline in the patient's condition. If the weather is hot, heatstroke or shock may result, adding further complications to the patient's medical condition. Always be aware of the environmental conditions, particularly during a lengthy extrication process. In cold weather, consider arranging blankets or tarps to block wind. Portable lights generate a great deal of heat and may be used (cautiously) inside a vehicle to provide warmth. If intravenous (IV) fluids are being administered by advanced life support, remember to keep them out of the cold and out of the wind. IV bags can be placed inside of coats of EMTs, where body heat will help maintain temperature.

Rescue Action Plan

Using a rescue action plan builds good habits. By standardizing your approach, a natural order of tasks becomes automatic. Having a basic rescue plan will help make even the most severe incidents less intimidating. Establishing and following a natural order results in less wasted time and confusion with safer conditions for everyone involved.

The following is a sample rescue action plan for most rescue situations.

Step 1: Preparation

- Train as a team, addressing the hazards and safety procedures associated with each type of rescue you may encounter.
- Check all tools, equipment, and response vehicles periodically and after each use. Maintain them in a "ready-to-respond" condition.

Step 2: Response

- The call taker should gather the appropriate information to help the responders begin their size-up and be prepared to give qualified advice to the caller regarding his or her safety and clear direction for patient care.
- Always respond in a safe manner, using preplanned routes when possible.

Step 3: Arrival and Size-up

- On arrival at the emergency, park in a manner that will protect the scene from traffic. It is imperative that you and your team members not become victims of speeding traffic. Wear reflective and brightly colored clothing, even during daylight hours.
- Perform a **circle survey,** looking at the entire scene. This is where you will check for hazards and locate patients. Address all hazards as you encounter them.
- Establish command. There must be one incident commander. Even if only two EMTs arrive initially on the scene, someone must be in charge.

Step 4: Stabilization

- Call for additional resources as soon as it is apparent that they are needed. Additional help will be needed at most incidents involving persons trapped in vehicles.
- Stabilize the situation (vehicle, machinery, or area) and establish a tool staging area.

Step 5: Access the Patient

- Once the situation is stabilized, make **initial patient access** and begin critical intervention.
- Establish **sustained access** to the patient. This usually involves opening a larger area around the patient, such as a door or roof of a vehicle, moving obstructions out of the way, or providing additional ladders to a person above or below ground level.
- Prioritize patients by their medical condition and degree of entrapment.

Step 6: Disentanglement

- Now that the scene, area, and patient are stabilized, prepare the patient for **disentanglement** and move anything that blocks the patient's egress.

Step 7: Removal

- Protect the patient as you remove him or her from the hazardous area.

Step 8: Transport

- Remove the patient and transport immediately to the appropriate medical facility.

Step 9: Secure Scene; Prepare for Next Call

- Secure your tools and prepare for the next call.

Step 10: Postincident Analysis

- There is no such thing as a perfect rescue. Every significant event should be discussed in a highly organized way, so everyone involved can learn from what went right and what went wrong.

Vehicle Rescue Incidents

The rescue action plan will work on almost every rescue scene, but the EMT-B will most often employ the plan at the scene of a motor vehicle collision. By following the plan, the EMT-B will be able to function as a vital member of the rescue team.

Categorizing Vehicle Rescue Situations

Vehicle rescue situations can be categorized by severity (degree of **entrapment**), with each category describing the patient's situation:

- *No entrapment,* in which the occupants of the vehicle can be readily removed without the use of tools
- *Light entrapment,* in which minimal use of tools is necessary to remove the patient (e.g., it is necessary to free a jammed door, but the patient is otherwise free)
- *Moderate entrapment,* in which one or more occupants are trapped in a way that requires roof and door removal, but no displacement of the dash or other parts of the car
- *Heavy entrapment,* in which extrication goes beyond removing the roof and doors

Preparation

Preparation begins with being equipped with the proper personal protective gear (**full protective clothing**). For all rescue personnel this must include approved head, hand, foot, and body protective clothing. Shatter-resistant safety glasses or goggles are mandatory. If the rescue requires exposure to a potential for fire, a fire-protective garment such as firefighter's bunker gear or a jumpsuit made of Nomex® or fire-resistive cotton is mandatory. Wear brightly colored and reflective clothing, such as a traffic safety vest, for additional safety while working near traffic.

Keep in mind that because of the potential for body fluids to be present at any vehicle collision, body substance isolation must be in place, particularly when working near or handling the patient (Figure 39.1).

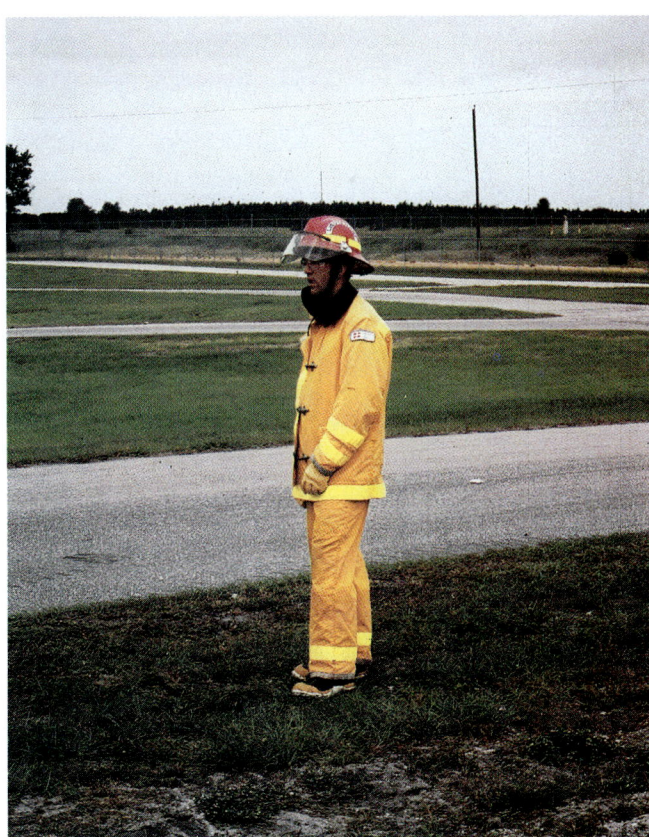

FIGURE 39.1 Preparation begins with being equipped with the proper personal protective gear.

Response

When the call taker is gathering information from the caller, it is essential to gather the correct information so the appropriate information is dispatched. When gathering information on a vehicle collision, for example, ask the caller, "Does it look like we will have to cut the car apart to get the patient out?" This will help you dispatch the appropriate level of response to the incident.

Most agencies dispatch an emergency medical services (EMS) unit and a fire engine to any report of a significant vehicle collision. This level of response should escalate if the initial call indicates that a person is trapped. If information is received that indicates the potential for **hazardous materials (HAZMAT)** on the scene, a HAZMAT team should be dispatched to assist. If HAZMAT are indicated, approach the scene with extreme caution, usually from the upwind, uphill side.

Arrival and Size-up

On arrival at the emergency, park in a manner that will protect the scene from traffic. It is imperative that you and your team members not become victims of speeding traffic. This is called the **fend-off position** (Figure 39.2).

Perform a circle survey, looking at the entire scene. This is where you will check for hazards and locate patients. The outer circle survey allows you to assess for ejected patients, area hazards, and patients who may have wondered off from the scene.

Address all hazards as you encounter them. Be ready to secure any hazards that may occur at a vehicle collision. Hazards can include electrical shock from the vehicle battery and electrical system.

Make certain the vehicle is not being charged from a domestic power source such as downed lines or underground feeds. Look above and beneath the car for a pos-

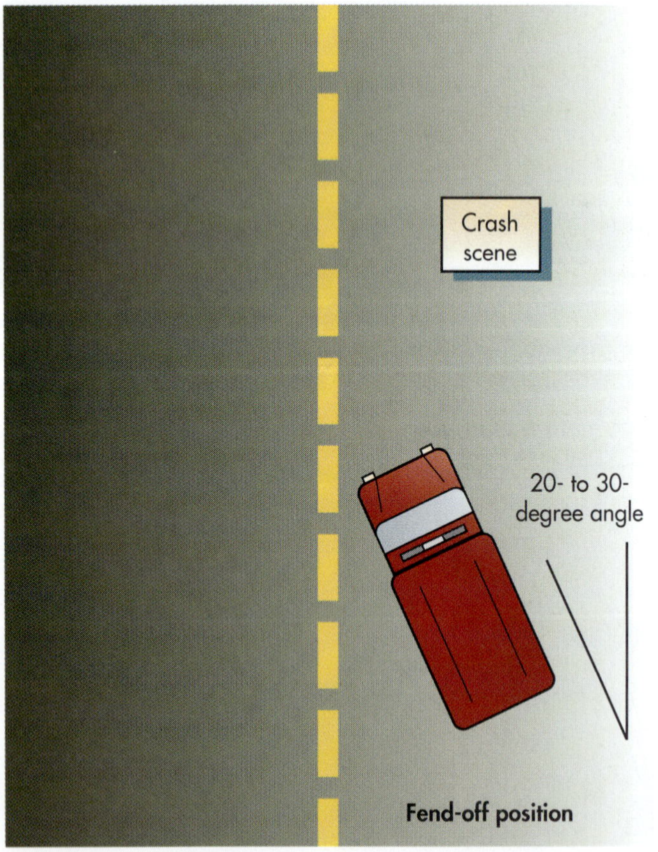

FIGURE 39.2 On arrival at the emergency, park in a manner that will protect the scene from traffic.

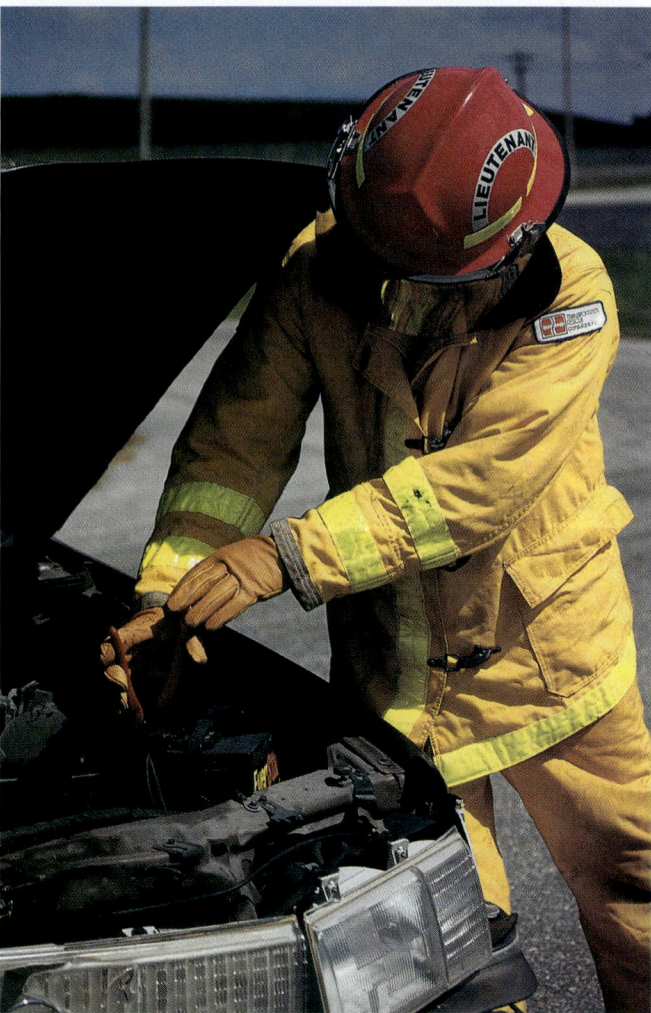

FIGURE 39.3 If possible, disconnect the battery by removing the ground wire first to reduce the chance of sparks, and finish by removing the other cable and isolating the cables from the battery.

sible electrical source. Many progressive agencies use an electrical detection device to ensure that energized electrical power is not present.

If possible, disconnect the battery by removing the ground wire first to reduce the chance of sparks, and finish by removing the other cable and isolating the cables from the battery. A damaged battery can release flammable, caustic fluids and gases into the area. This increases the risk of respiratory system irritation, eye injury, or burns to the skin of anyone exposed. Fire is also a possibility if fuel spills are present (Figure 39.3).

There are many laceration hazards on a vehicle collision scene. Sharp metal edges and broken glass must be covered. Tarps, blankets, and duct tape are good for this. Cover the hazards as you encounter them and as the extrication process creates them.

Air restraint bags will be present in newer-model cars. Once deployed, air restraint bags present little hazard. If undeployed, these restraints do not usually present a critical danger to rescue personnel as long as rescuers stay out of the path of possible air bag inflation. However, new systems are being developed, and there is a need to stay updated on advanced air bag restraint system technology. Maintain a safe zone of 5 inches from side bags, 10 inches from driver's-side front bags, and 15 inches from passenger-side front bags. Do not place anything, including yourself, within the strike zones of each type of air bag (Figure 39.4).

Remember to secure any hazards that can endanger the patient or the rescue team *before beginning extrication efforts*. Additional injuries to the patient should not occur at well-managed extrication scenes.

Stabilization

Cars usually wind up in one of three positions following a collision: upright, on the side, or on the roof. To avoid further harm to the patient and for your own safety, it is necessary to secure the car in place before beginning extrication efforts. This is called **stabilization.**

Box 39.1 Equipment List for Primary Access Duties

- Spring-loaded center punch
- Long screwdriver
- Flat pry bar
- Four step chocks
- Large pliers
- Windshield saw
- Flat axe

The tools most often used for stabilization include **cribbing** and jacks. The types of cribbing most agencies use include step chocks, 4 × 4 inch cribbing blocks, and wooden **wedge cribbing**. Although space is limited on many EMS units, a limited amount of cribbing can go a long way toward making the scene safe and is well worth the space it takes up on your unit (Box 39.1).

If the car is upright, it is best to isolate the body from its springs and tires. This will keep the car from moving in a way that might compromise the patient's cervical spine. A majority of agencies use step chocks to accomplish this type of stabilization. Start by checking underneath the car to make sure there is no one trapped beneath the vehicle or other reason not to lower the car. Now, simply place four **step chocks** under the patient area, two behind the front tires and two just in front of the rear tires. If there is not enough room for a step chock, use a wedge. Deflate the tires by pulling the valve stems with pliers, allowing the car to settle on the step chocks.

If the car has come to rest on its side, it is in a highly unstable position. Because of space limitations, most EMS units do not carry sufficient cribbing to safely stabilize a car on its side. Use extreme caution when working around a vehicle in this position. Do not climb on top of the vehicle or open a door, which can throw the car off balance. Whenever possible, wait for help to arrive and stabilize the vehicle before entering it.

When you encounter a car on its side or roof, you should be prepared to handle any fuel leaks. Contain the fuel, oil, and other fluids with absorbent material. Next, insert wedges under any voids you may find and secure them in place. If the car is on its roof and on a slope, it will be susceptible to sliding downhill. Keep clear of the downhill side (Figures 39.5 and 39.6).

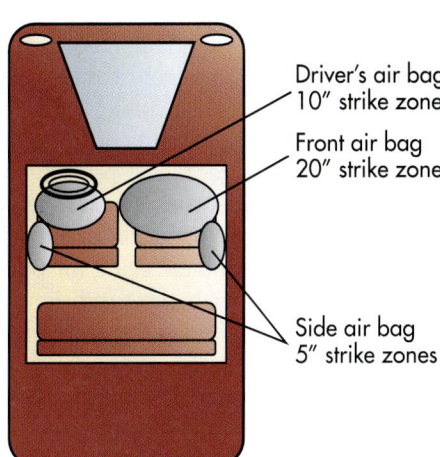

FIGURE 39.4 Do not place anything, including yourself, within the strike zones of each type of air bag.

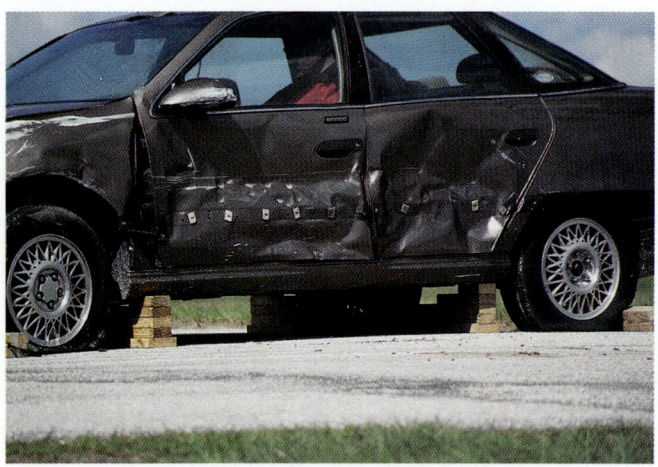

FIGURE 39.5 Step chocks are used to stabilize a car in its upright position before rescue personnel enter the vehicle.

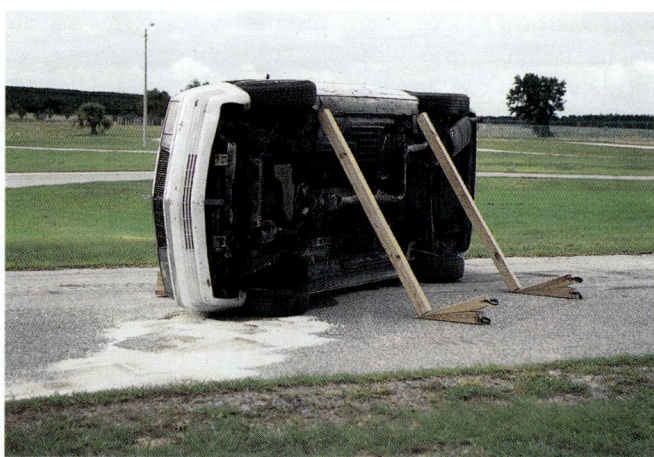

FIGURE 39.6 A vehicle on its side is in a highly dangerous, unstable position.

Access the Patient

Once the hazards are controlled and the vehicle is stabilized, establish initial access to the patient. This usually involves reaching into an open window or door (simple access) or breaking a remote window and crawling in (complex access). Remember to avoid placing yourself in the inflation path of an undeployed air bag.

There are two types of glass on an automobile: **laminated plate glass** used for windshields, which holds together when it breaks, and **tempered safety glass** used for rear and side windows, which breaks into small pieces. A number of **hand tools** can be used for glass removal. These include the spring-loaded center punch, a long screwdriver, a pry bar, various axes, and glass-cutting tools designed specifically for extrication.

Cover the patient with soft protection to protect him or her from broken glass. Respiratory protection from a dust mask may be necessary if the windshield is being cut with a reciprocating saw. If a facemask is used to deliver oxygen, it should be a non-rebreather type to help protect the patient from fine glass dust.

It is important to give the patient continuous psychological support during the rescue, especially when the patient is covered with soft protection. It is likely that the patient is already experiencing claustrophobia from the tight confines of the car, and covering the patient with a heavy tarp will only exacerbate the condition. It is often helpful to position yourself under the tarp with the patient to give calming support.

Tempered safety glass breaks when the most force is applied to the smallest area. The spring-loaded center punch is highly effective for this. By pressing it against a corner of a side or rear window, the point of the punch makes a hole and the glass shatters. Make sure to use the corner, because this will keep your hand from following through the glass when it breaks. Using the point of a screwdriver blade in a snapping motion accomplishes the same thing by concentrating force on a small area.

A safe and efficient way to remove a windshield is to cut around the edges. This can be done with an axe or a specialized windshield-cutting tool. A windshield-cutting tool will not take up much room on a smaller EMS vehicle.

Start at the top center of the windshield. If you are using an axe, grip the handle near the head for best control. Take small chops, just cutting through the glass. Support the windshield as soon as one rescuer can get his or her hand behind it. After a few hits on the bottom, it can be folded downward and pulled out.

If you are using a windshield-cutting tool, saw away the circumference of the windshield. Most of these specialized saws have a point at one end for making a hole in the windshield, which is where you begin cutting with the blade. The blade is designed to cut on the outward stroke to help minimize glass particles inside the vehicle.

> ✓ When breaking glass, always wear proper safety attire, including eye, head, foot, and hand protection, and keep your mouth closed.

Disentanglement

The EMT's role in the disentanglement phase of the rescue is to maintain patient contact, in-line spinal stabilization, and continued critical intervention. A more focused assessment should be conducted as the patient is freed from the wreckage.

It is helpful for the EMT-B to know the order in which the disentanglement will take place. The first step toward disentangling a patient is to provide a more sustained access route so additional patient care can be delivered. This usually involves cutting or flapping the roof out of the way. This will make some noise that may startle the patient, so continue with strong psychological support by preparing the patient for each noise. With the roof out of the way, a patient who is not pinned by the wreckage can be removed along his or her long axis by sliding the patient up a long spine board. This is especially helpful if the patient's condition is critical or takes a sudden turn for the worse (Figure 39.7).

Before moving the patient, more sustained immobilization efforts must be completed. This usually involves the application of a short spinal immobilization device such as the **Kendrick Extrication Device®**.

To remove a patient through the roof, tilt the seat back if possible. Next, insert a long spine board between the patient and the seat. The rescuer at the patient's head is in command of the action. Lift under the patient's legs, on each side, and use the two side lift handles on the immobilization device. After the rescuer at the head gives the command, lift together and move the long board to a level position. Immediately secure the patient to the board before carrying him or her away from the vehicle.

Because children are anatomically different from adults, pediatric immobilization devices such as the **Pedi-Immobilizer®** have been designed to address their special needs. Follow the instructions on the device your agency uses, and practice applying it often.

As long as the patient's condition remains stable, it is usually best to continue with conventional extrication efforts and remove the patient through openings in the side of the vehicle. This will require the interior rescuer's utmost attention to any negative effects during metal movement operations. Monitor the patient's condition and relay updates to the extrication team periodically.

Once the roof is out of the way, the rescue team will probably focus on removing one or both sides of the vehicle. Specialized hydraulic tools are often used to pry the doors off the vehicle. In some cases, the entire side of the vehicle will be pried out of the way. Prepare the patient for sudden noises, loud "pops," and increased vibrations.

Now that there is more room for rescuers, make yet another survey of the patient's situation. Relay any changes to the extrication team so they can continue developing their rescue plan. Look closely at trapped extremities to see if they are truly trapped. For example, you may be able to simply manipulate a person's foot from behind a pedal to free the person from the wreckage.

If the dash assembly traps the patient, the front of the car will be pushed out of the way. This may involve using long hydraulic rams or lifting the dash with a hydraulic spreader. Be prepared to control the patient's movements at this point. Most traumatized patients are also experiencing claustrophobia and will try to "self-extricate" at this point. Explain each step as you go.

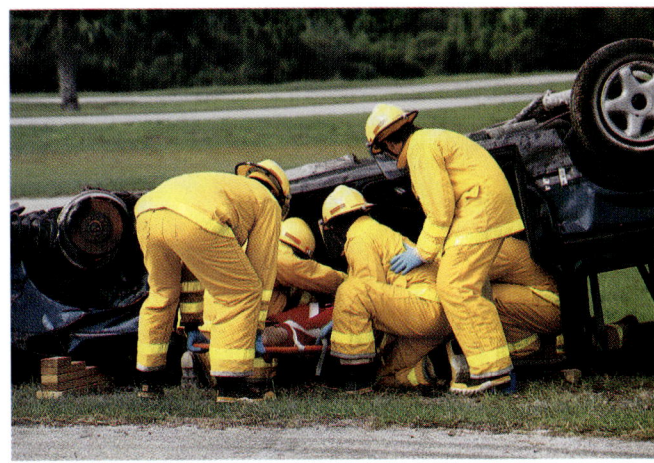

FIGURE 39.7 It is important that the EMT-B understand the order of extrication so that he or she can be prepared for what will be done next.

Removal

Once the side of the car is out of the way and steps have been taken to ensure that the patient is no longer trapped by the wreckage, it is time to transfer the patient from the car to the long spine board for further immobilization and continued care. This is perhaps the most difficult time to maintain spinal immobilization.

Even though the patient is in a short spine immobilization device, the spine is not totally immobilized. Total immobilization is achieved only after the patient is secured to a long spine board and a cervical immobilization device is in place.

How the patient is removed from the car usually depends on the path of egress provided by the extrication team. If possible, it is usually best to remove the patient feet first, directly onto a long spine board, especially if there is trauma to the lower extremities. The short spinal immobilization device will help achieve this because it has handles in place to help move the patient. Always try to have plenty of help moving the patient, and remember to use proper lifting techniques to avoid back injury to the rescuers. Lift the patient at the hips so the immobilization device does not catch on the long backboard as the rescuers slide the patient out.

Removing the patient head first is also an option and can be accomplished in much the same way. While doing this, make sure to provide ample support to the lower

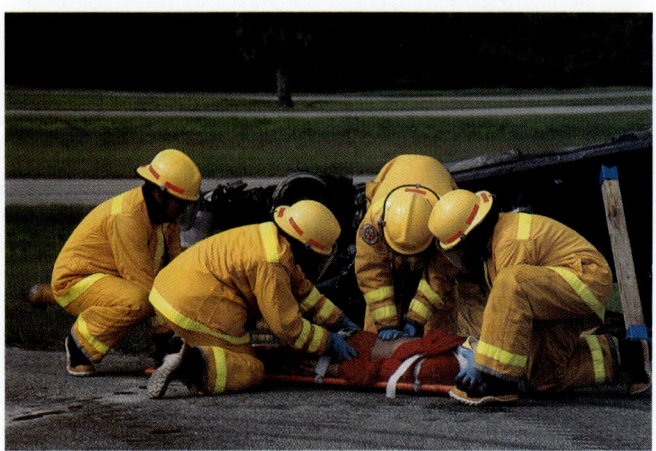

FIGURE 39.8 If time allows, place the patient on a short backboard to immobilize the victim's head, neck, and spine. The patient must be secured and then transferred to a long spine board and then to the wheeled ambulance stretcher.

extremities, because moving the hips and legs has a direct effect on the lower spine.

Once the patient has been extricated and secured to a long spine board, the care team has better access to all sides of the patient. Continue monitoring the patient's condition (Figure 39.8).

Transport

An average extrication time is about 30 minutes from the time of call to the point where the patient is ready for transport to the hospital. This means that much of the **golden hour** has elapsed. If air transport is available in your area and the patient's condition meets the criteria for using this service, it may be necessary to transfer the patient to a special spine board that will fit in the helicopter. Preplan for this event and try to follow the air transport agency's recommendations when purchasing spine boards, if possible.

Most health care systems require a radio report to be called in while transporting the patient to the emergency department. This allows the trauma team time to prepare for uninterrupted patient treatment. Your early observations of the patient's condition will serve as a benchmark for further comparison, so it is essential to efficiently communicate this information to the hospital.

Secure the Scene/Prepare for the Next Call

After the incident, prepare your equipment for the next rescue. Take a good look around the scene for anything you may have missed, such as a clue that there may have been other patients in the collision. Remember to continue with universal precautions during the cleanup. If possible, take pictures of the collision site for your use later.

Postincident Analysis

Once the equipment is back in service, prepare yourself for the next call by conducting a critique of your actions. View this critique as an opportunity to improve the next patient's chance for survival. Look at each step of the rescue action plan and review your procedures, analyzing each component for deficiencies that should be corrected. Share what you have learned with others.

> ### Tips from the Pros
>
> All EMTs must recognize that rescue operations are inherently dangerous scenes, particularly where wreckage, unstable building debris, collapsed soil, water, HAZMAT, or hazardous atmospheres are potentially present. They must be properly protected with personal protective equipment when entering these areas. If EMTs are not trained in technical rescue operations, they may need to stay at a designated safe area until the patient has been freed and brought to them. They must be familiar with and understand the steps of the rescue action plan and how it is used to organize all types of rescue scenes. They should be thoroughly familiar with the procedures required at motor vehicle collisions, because those will probably be the most common trauma incidents to which they will be called.

Summary

- EMTs respond to a wide variety of rescue situations. They must recognize the specialized training, personal protective equipment, and specialized rescue tools required to free patients.
- The rescue action plan provides a systematic method to organize any rescue scene.
- There are eight major types of rescue situations, all of which require specialized training and equip-

Summary (cont'd)

ment: building collapse, trench/excavation collapse, confined spaces, low angle/high angle, wilderness, water, machinery/industrial, and vehicles.
- The rescue action plan has 10 steps: preparation, response, arrival and size-up, stabilization, access the patient, disentanglement, removal, transport, secure the scene/prepare for the next call, and postincident analysis.

- Vehicle collision incidents can be placed into four categories: no entrapment, light entrapment, moderate entrapment, and heavy entrapment.
- A vehicle collision scene can be managed by dividing the incident into the basic elements of the rescue action plan.

Scenario Solution

Your first concern should be for your own safety, as well as the safety of your partner. Park your unit in a fend-off position that will protect the scene from traffic. Check the overhead power lines once again, before leaving your vehicle. Your partner transmits a short radio report: "Unit Ten on the scene of a single-vehicle collision, appears to be moderate entrapment, request fire department to respond for extrication. We have a power pole involved, but power lines appear to be intact; notify the power company to respond. Unit Ten will be establishing Elm Street Command, assessing scene at this time."

Your partner turns on the side flood lights of your vehicle and quickly lights up the scene. Both of you put on your safety coat, helmet, goggles, and gloves as you exit the unit. You walk cautiously around the car, being careful not to touch it. The patient's window is open and he appears to have an open airway and is breathing. When you get completely around the car you check the air bag status and see that the front ones have deployed and the side ones have not. You did not see or smell any fuel leaks as you circled the car.

Your partner completes an outer circle survey, clearing loose debris and looking for other hazards and patients. He then returns to the unit and begins taking out a small tarp for tools staging and cribbing. He also removes a small hand tool pouch.

You look again at the patient and the interior of the car. You check to see how the patient is trapped. The dash is not down on him at all. You help you partner stabilize the car with cribbing. Then you try the doors; they are jammed and will not open. During all procedures, you and your partner tell each other what you find and what you are doing.

Now you take control of the patient's C-spine, maintaining the head in an eyes-front, neutral position. Your partner breaks out the rear glass and enters the rear seat area with the medical trauma kit. He conducts an initial survey of the patient while you maintain C-spine care. The patient has a cut on his head, and pulse and blood pressure are normal. The patient's level of consciousness is unresponsive. Your partner now applies a cervical collar on the patient, places a quick bandage on the head laceration, and then takes control of C-spine.

You get the patient soft protection cover from your unit and place it over the front seat area and the patient. You now take the windshield cutting tool and begin to cut out the broken windshield. At this time, the fire department arrives with the extrication tools.

The fire department supervisor comes to you for a situation report. You report type of entrapment, number of patients, location, condition, and what steps you have taken so far. The supervisor states that he will take over and assigns you and your partner to take care of the patient while they attempt to remove the roof and force open the door with powered hydraulic tools. The fire department can reach the battery terminals through the bend in the hood and disconnect the battery. You get your long backboard, straps, KED®, and cervical immobilization device ready at the tool staging area. An additional EMT-B unit arrives and wheels up a stretcher to the tool staging area.

Fire department personnel remove the remaining side glass and cut the roof off. They then open the door next to the driver, closely monitoring how their work affects the patient. The door is opened and the cover removed from the patient. The fire department supervisor now tells you that the patient is free and they are ready to remove him. You and the firefighters place the KED® on the patient. Then all of you work together to move the patient onto the long backboard. He is quickly strapped onto the board, and a cervical immobilization device is placed at the head and neck and then secured. The patient is then lifted from the side of the car and placed on the waiting stretcher. After the patient is placed on the transporting unit, you do a quick reevaluation of vital signs and condition. There is no change. You pass on everything to the transport unit personnel; they leave immediately for the emergency department.

You check with your partner; she is fine. Then both of you check with the fire department supervisor to see if it is all right to retrieve your equipment. All equipment is retrieved and checked while placing it back on the unit.

At the station, you and your partner go over the call as you do a check of your tools and restock your supplies. You talk about what went well and what did not go so well. This helps you prepare for the next incident.

Key Terms

Air restraint bag A part of the passive passenger restraint system of a passenger car; consists of a deflated air bag that fills quickly with a gas, either electrically or mechanically activated on impact of the vehicle; provides extra protection for the front-seat occupants during a vehicle collision.

Circle survey A method for rescue personnel to conduct a thorough survey of the accident scene; includes walking in a 360-degree circle around the entire scene.

Cribbing Specially cut or assembled pieces of wood used to support raised objects; used as ground pads or bases on which to place tools, and as blocks over which chains and cables pass while moving objects.

Disentanglement The process of freeing a trapped patient on the rescue scene.

Entrapment State of a patient trapped in a vehicle. The four degrees of entrapment are no entrapment, light entrapment, moderate entrapment, and heavy entrapment.

Extrication Procedures used by rescue personnel to remove trapped patients (trapped by the wreckage or by their injuries) from vehicles involved in collisions.

Fend-off position A method of positioning emergency apparatus at a vehicle collision scene that provides added protection to the scene from traffic.

Full protective clothing Specially designed protective clothing that is worn by rescue personnel while performing vehicle rescue procedures in and around the vehicle. Specifications depend on local requirements; however, they should include head, hand, foot, and body protection. See also *personal protective gear*.

Golden hour The first hour after an incident; period in which a trauma patient has the best chance for recovery if safely delivered to an emergency medical facility.

Hand tools For extrication work, these include cutting, prying, and lifting tools. They may be electrically driven, such as a reciprocating saw; pneumatically powered, such as an air chisel; or manually operated, such as a hacksaw.

Hazardous materials (HAZMAT) Any materials exposed on an emergency scene that are hazardous by being poisonous, flammable, explosive, carcinogenic, or environmentally pollutant; abbreviated *HAZMAT* in emergency services.

Initial patient access Usually considered the first contact of a collision victim by rescuers. This is done before stabilization to provide immediate C-spine and airway care.

Kendrick Extrication Device® A specially designed device used in removing automobile collision patients; composed of the body sling with straps and handles, chin and head straps, and a space filler pad; also referred to as a KED.

Laminated plate glass Specially designed glass used in automobile windshields that is comprised of layered plate glass separated by clear plastic.

Pedi-Immobilizer® A spinal immobilization device designed for use on small children.

Rescue action plan A system that helps rescuers organize the actions and procedures at the scene of an emergency.

Size-up The act of gathering information about the emergency in order to formulate an action plan.

Stabilization In vehicle rescue this usually refers to securing the wrecked vehicle in which an injured patient is trapped; can also refer to gaining control of and handling a chaotic emergency scene or hazardous condition.

Step chocks Specialized cribbing assemblies made out of wood blocks assembled in a stair-step configuration; used to stabilize vehicles.

Sustained access For rescue situations, this refers to a path of access to the patient that is secure and readily useable by rescuers during the rescue operation.

Tempered safety glass Specially designed glass used in automobile side and rear windows that is resistant to breakage.

Wedge cribbing Cribbing shaped in the form of a wedge; used to tighten and secure cribbing assemblies supporting weight; usually used as a gap filler.

Review Questions

1. What is the most common type of rescue performed by EMTs?
   a. Trench rescue
   b. High-angle rescue
   c. Vehicle extrication
   d. Water rescue
2. True or False: Disentanglement on the rescue scene occurs before scene stabilization.

Review Questions (cont'd)

3. A vehicle collision that requires roof and door removal to extricate trapped occupants is considered a _____ entrapment situation.
   a. No
   b. Light
   c. Moderate
   d. Heavy
4. Laminated safety glass is generally used on the _____.
5. The first step in disentangling a patient is to provide a more sustained _____.
6. True or False: Total immobilization is only achieved after the patient is secured to a long spine board and a cervical immobilization device is in place.

Answers to these Review Questions can be found at the end of the book on page 869.

40

Emergency Preparedness

Lesson Goal

The goal of this chapter is to provide the basic information necessary for the emergency medical technician to function effectively in disaster or multiple-casualty situations and hazardous materials incidents. This chapter also reviews the role that the EMT plays when responding to a situation in which hazardous materials are involved and may have contaminated the area.

Scenario

Your day starts off routinely enough for you and the "new guy," your partner. The ambulance checks out, and you have enough supplies to carry you through your shift. The morning passes quickly with two calls: an elderly woman who fell and possibly dislocated her hip, and a transport from the police lockup to the hospital for a psychologic evaluation of a young man the police found swimming naked in the town's fountain.

Just after lunch, you and your partner receive a radio call to respond to a trucking company in town for a sick patient. You acknowledge and respond to the call, and begin your size-up in your mind: "This is a large trucking company that handles a variety of cargoes from around the country. They receive, then ship, everything from single boxes to large barrels and containers of anything from dry goods to chemicals. I hope it's just a bad case of the flu."

The security guard at the gate tells you the problem is in the bulk receiving dock area, and now there are three persons who have gotten sick since the 911 call was originally made. He also informs you that the suspected cause is a leaking barrel inside one of the transport trucks. Plant security has evacuated the dock area and has kept everyone from that area confined in another warehouse, a safe distance from the contaminated area. Security placed another call to 911 asking for the fire department and hazardous materials team to respond also.

In the distance you hear sirens approaching. You move through the gate so as not to block the entrance, pull over to the side of the road, and wait for the fire department. The little voice in your head says, "This is *not* just a bad case of the flu."

 How do you think you need to handle this situation?

Key Terms to Know

Decontamination
Disaster
Hazardous materials (HAZMAT)
Incident command system (ICS)
Infrastructure
Mass (multiple) casualty incident (MCI)
Risk assessment
Triage

Learning Objectives

As an EMT-Basic, you should be able to do the following:

DOT

- Explain the roles and responsibilities of the emergency medical technician (EMT) in a disaster or multiple-casualty situation.
- Describe the EMT's roles and responsibilities at a hazardous materials incident.
- Describe what the EMT-Basic (EMT-B) should do if there is reason to believe that there is a hazard at the scene.
- Describe the actions that an EMT-B should take to ensure bystander safety.
- State the role the EMT-B should perform until appropriately trained personnel arrive at the scene of a hazardous materials situation.
- Break down the steps to approaching a hazardous situation.
- Discuss the various environmental hazards that affect emergency medical services (EMS).
- Describe the criteria for a multiple-casualty situation.
- Summarize the components of basic triage.
- Define the role of the EMT-B in a disaster operation.
- Describe basic concepts of incident management.
- Explain the methods for preventing contamination of self, equipment, and facilities.
- Review the local multiple-casualty incident plan.
- Given a scenario of a multiple-casualty incident, perform triage.

Supplemental

- Describe the characteristics of a disaster, and differentiate these characteristics from normal operational conditions.
- Identify the importance of disaster planning in disaster preparedness.
- Demonstrate the ability to use the principles of triage in a multiple-casualty situation.
- Define *hazardous materials* and explain their significance for EMS operations.
- Explain the federal regulations concerning hazardous materials training for emergency responders.
- Review the rules for scene safety, and identify the tools that are available to the EMT for managing a hazardous material situation.

The day-to-day routine of emergency medical services (EMS) system operations can become familiar and comfortable to the personnel in the system. Requests for emergency response or nonemergency transportation are received, units dispatched, emergency care provided, and transportation accomplished in an organized and efficient manner. Occasionally, however, specific types of incidents occur that are anything but routine. They stretch (and sometimes exceed) the capacity of the system. Providers' lives are endangered, and normal operations are no longer sufficient to deal with the situation.

This chapter deals with two of the most common types of these "uncommon" incidents: disaster or multiple-casualty situations (Figure 40.1) and hazardous materials (HAZMAT) incidents (Figure 40.2). These incidents occur often enough that EMS systems and providers need to be specifically trained to deal with them but infrequently enough that providers and systems never quite feel comfortable with handling them. These situations often result in unusual types or numbers of injuries and require different methods of sorting, treating, and transporting patients. Disaster and hazardous materials responses also present unique dangers to EMS providers.

The goal of this chapter is to provide the basic information necessary for the emergency medical technician (EMT) to function effectively in these situations. However, complete mastery of these topics requires specialized training and experience that far exceed the boundaries of an EMT course and this text. EMTs who will be

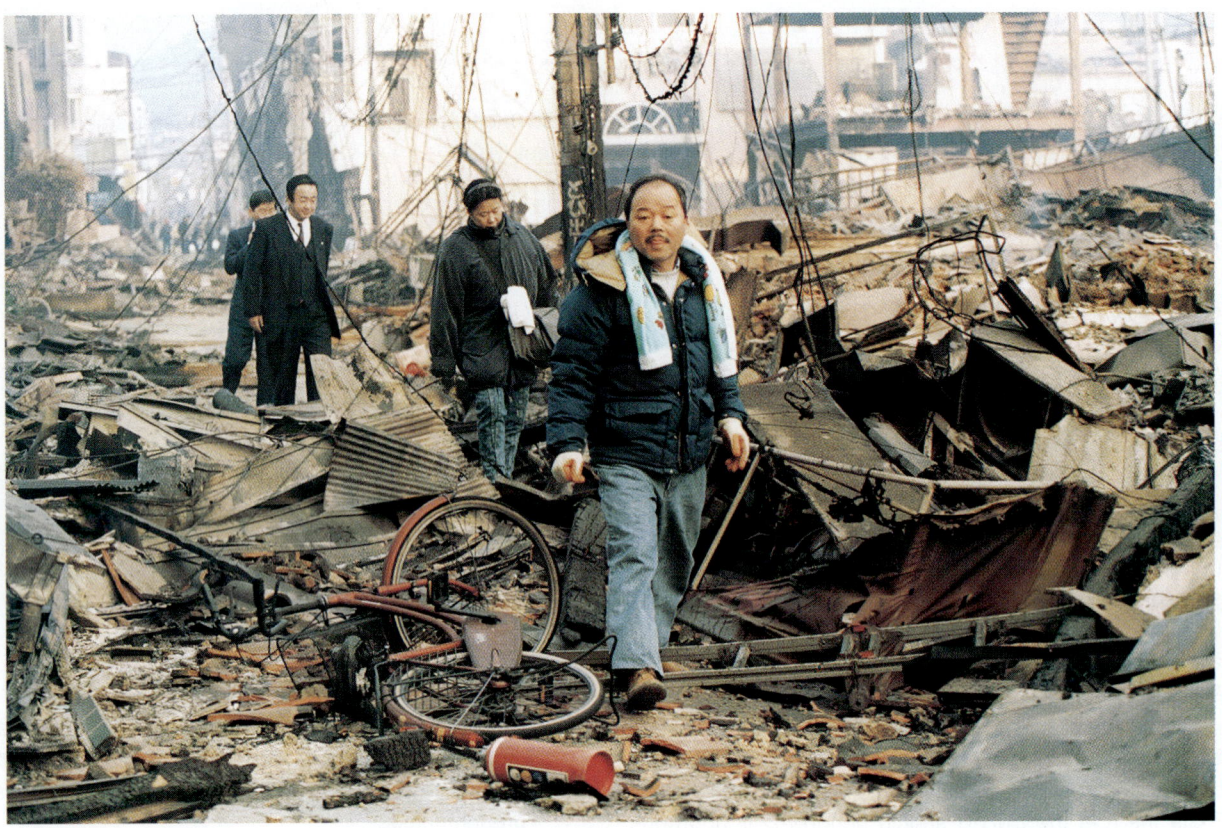

FIGURE 40.1 Natural disasters, such as earthquakes, provide a challenge to EMS systems because of the infrastructure damage that occurs, as well as the possibility of injuries.

involved in routine response to these specialized situations should complete additional specialized training.

Disaster and Multiple-Casualty Response

The nightly news brings dramatic images from disaster scenes throughout the world. A large, crippled jet almost makes a successful landing but falters at the last minute, spewing fire and bodies over an area the size of several football fields. Deep below a major city, two subway trains collide in a fiery crash, which not only causes injuries but also threatens victims and EMTs alike with the prospect of escape or rescue through miles of tunnels. Office buildings, freeways, and private homes are reduced to rubble by an earthquake that strikes in the predawn hours. People are injured by debris or trapped in collapsed buildings.

Each of these situations has dramatic implications for EMS systems and for the EMTs who work within them. Experts agree that the keys to successful handling of these types of situations are preplanning, practice, and careful management. The EMT may play a number of roles in the disaster situation. However, a good place to start is with a basic understanding of the elements of a disaster situation.

Definitions and Classifications

The vast majority of EMS responses involve a single patient and a single EMS response vehicle. Usually, the number of EMTs exceeds the number of patients, and the EMS system focuses a large amount of personnel and equipment resources on managing the problem experienced by that single patient. A lot of help is available, and plenty of equipment is on hand (Figure 40.3).

In general, a disaster exists when a large incident has occurred that changes this normal ratio of EMTs and equipment to patients. Simply put, EMTs are outnumbered by those needing assistance (at least in the short term), and not enough equipment or vehicles are available to take care of everyone. In practice, a valuable distinction should be made between different types of disasters.

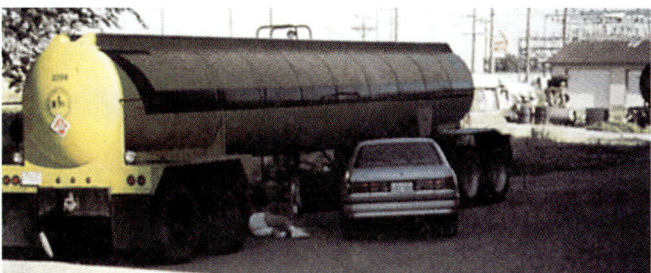

FIGURE 40.2 Hazardous materials incidents are a challenge to EMS systems because of the danger to EMTs and other emergency responders.

> ✔ Disasters create situations that are significantly different from the normal EMS response situation. Successfully managing a disaster situation requires a different approach or mind-set.

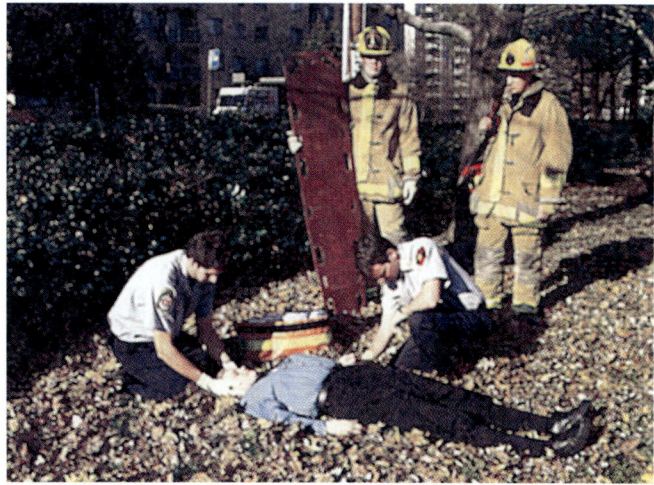

FIGURE 40.3 In the normal EMS response, there are more EMTs than patients.

Disaster

The term **disaster** is generally associated with a manmade or natural event that involves tremendous damage across a large geographic area. For example, earthquakes, hurricanes, and floods are considered disasters. Disasters typically involve a lot of damage to community **infrastructure**—roads, power, communications, housing. However, disasters may or may not involve large numbers of injuries or fatalities. Hurricane Hugo was clearly a major disaster, but it did not cause many injuries or fatalities. The other extreme is illustrated by the earthquake in Turkey in 1999, which resulted in thousands of deaths and tens of thousands of injuries. Disasters also frequently result in significant public health challenges due to the disruption of public sanitary systems. In addition, refugees are often crowded together in cramped quarters, providing an excellent environment for disease transmission.

Multiple-Casualty Incident

Another type of disaster that EMS providers may face is more appropriately called a **mass (multiple) casualty incident (MCI)**. An MCI is an event that overburdens the EMS response team but usually does not cover a large geographic area. For example, an airplane or bus crash creates large numbers of victims but is a highly localized event.

Whereas the chief challenge of a disaster is the infrastructure destruction that accompanies the event, the primary challenge in an MCI is the ratio of responders to victims. The number of patients exceeds the capacity of the normal emergency response system, at least for a short period of time. Because systems have varying amounts of personnel and equipment available, the definition of an MCI may change from one system to another depending on local resources and conditions. A two-car collision with four serious injuries in a remote rural community may quickly exceed the capacity of a small local ambulance service, whereas such an event is easily handled in a routine manner by a large, urban EMS system (Figure 40.4).

> ✔ Disasters and MCIs are large, challenging incidents that exceed the capacity of local emergency response agencies to handle them, at least in the short term.

Preplanning

Experts uniformly agree that the principal factors in successful management of disasters are preplanning and practice. Because disasters force emergency response agencies to depart from normal operational methods, systems and people are automatically challenged by trying to operate in a new way. Because disasters also exceed local system capacity, successful management forces multiple agencies to work together in ways in which they do not normally operate. Although response to disasters involves the same people and equipment as everyday operations, it is a far different environment. Careful thought must go into planning for these extraordinary events, and frequent practice is essential so that participants become comfortable with the plans and operations (Box 40.1).

Preplanning Activities

Disaster planning activities involve several common components that can be found in most EMS systems. First, the system typically carries out a risk assessment.

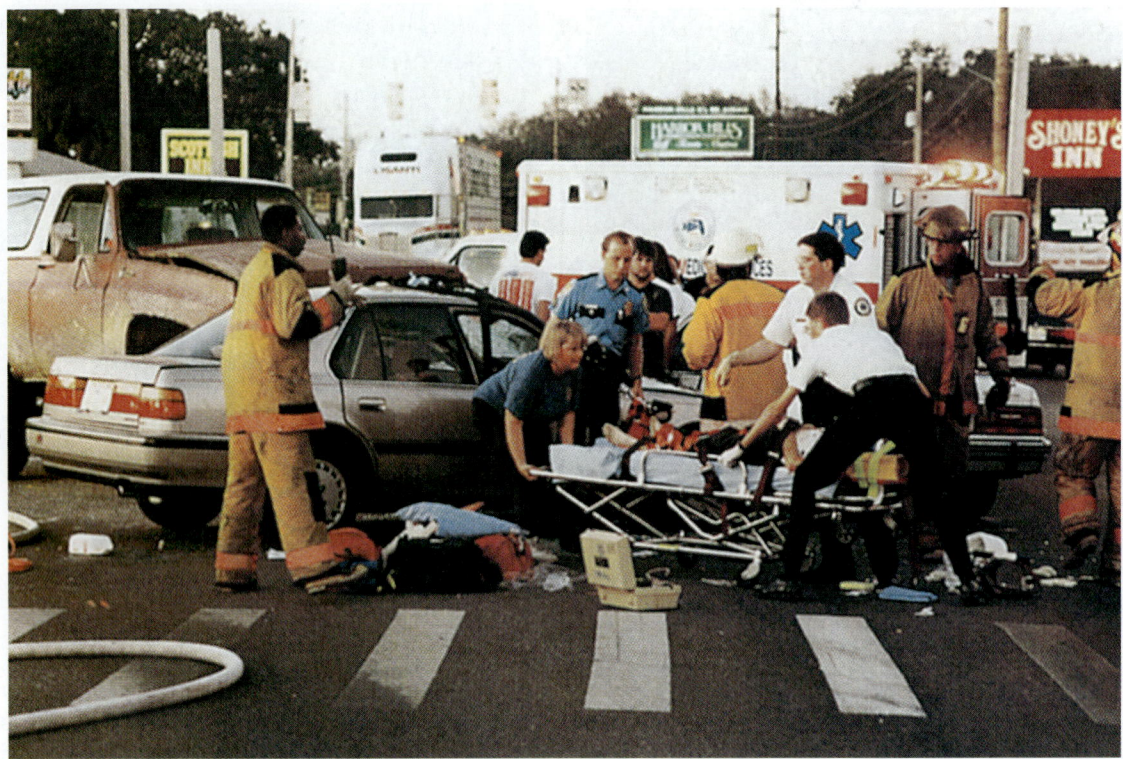

FIGURE 40.4 This accident might be handled routinely by a major urban EMS system but would be a major multiple-casualty incident for a rural, isolated ambulance service.

Risk assessment is a process of analyzing the kinds of disaster or MCI incidents that are likely to happen in a given community. For example, Omaha probably does not need to worry about hurricane preparedness, but Miami clearly does. Los Angeles needs to address a significant risk for a major earthquake, whereas Baltimore has significantly less risk for an earthquake. A community with a major interstate highway has a much higher risk for a major transportation incident than does a small rural community without major roads or rail lines. Risk assessment identifies the types of incidents for which a community should plan.

A second major activity in disaster planning is resource identification. Because a disaster, by definition, exceeds the capacity of the local emergency response system, it is critical that planners have a firm grasp of the actual resources (people, equipment, and vehicles) available in the community, as well as the sources of additional resources. For example, a train derailment calls for immediate access to extrication equipment not usually available within an EMS system, such as cranes and heavy cutting tools. An airplane crash on a snowy runway in subzero weather requires access to portable heaters for victims and EMTs. A comprehensive resource inventory identifies the resources available inside and outside of the local EMS system.

With potential community risks identified and local resources inventoried, planners can proceed with development of the disaster plans that will guide system activities. These plans include specific procedures and activities for each of the phases of a disaster response. Because every community faces different combinations of risks and resources, it is impossible to discuss specifics of disaster plans in this chapter. However, all EMTs should make it an early priority to study disaster plans for their own system.

Exercises

Disaster plans are useless if they are placed in loose-leaf binders and kept on the shelf. Practice is essential if the plans have any hope of working. Agencies and providers must clearly understand their roles in the disaster response. Because the types of action and interaction required in a disaster response are not the same as normal operations, participants must be given the opportunity to work through the plans. The disaster exercise has several goals:

- Allow participants to practice the activities that they will be required to perform.
- Allow planners to test the assumptions and guesswork that went into plan development.

- Provide an opportunity to review the positive and negative aspects of the implementation of the plan.

Exercises can be accomplished in a number of ways, ranging from the "tabletop," or "paper," exercise, in which participants meet and talk through a plan without actually carrying out each activity, to a full-scale disaster simulation that includes simulated patients and complete treatment and transportation. How often disaster plans are exercised varies by EMS system. However, most EMTs can expect to participate in disaster exercises frequently throughout their careers.

> ✓ Effective management of disaster situations requires careful planning and frequent practice. Planning involves risk assessment, resource identification, and careful thought. Practice may be accomplished by a variety of exercises ranging from tabletop to full-scale simulations.

Incident Command System

Because disaster response involves a large number of resources (people, equipment, vehicles) and the interaction of a large number of different agencies that do not work together on a routine basis, effective coordination or management of the disaster response is an essential factor leading to successful resolution of the incident. The need for good incident management systems has been a tremendous challenge for emergency response organizations, and it has only been in the past 10 years or so that significant progress has been made. Today, the standard for coordination of significant events is called the **incident command system (ICS)**. The origins of the ICS can be traced to the military and to the United States Forest Service's systems for managing wildfires. However, the ICS has been adapted for use in almost every situation that requires the management of complex responses to major incidents. A detailed discussion of ICS theory is beyond the scope of this chapter and is more than the EMT needs to know initially. However, excellent resources are available that discuss the ICS.

The basic concept of ICS involves a chain of command and organizational structure. The management function is divided and subdivided into specific areas of responsibility that allow managers to focus their attention on small pieces of the overall response. For example, an EMS sector, rescue sector, or transportation sector may be set up on the scene of an MCI (Figure 40.5). The commander of each sector is responsible for the activities described in the sector title. Personnel within a given sector carry out specific duties assigned by the sector commander. Sector commanders coordinate with each other and report to the next level in the organizational structure. This segmentation of management responsibility has proved to be an extremely effective tool for complex incident management. The EMT will most likely be involved in doing detailed assignments within a sector (e.g., triage), although EMTs may also find themselves in the role of sector commanders if they have specific additional training or experience that prepares them for this more advanced role.

> ✓ Disaster response requires the effective management of a complex incident with many individual providers and agencies. Most EMS systems use the ICS, or a variation of the ICS, as the preferred management method.

Triage

By definition, a disaster or MCI results in a number of patients that exceeds the normal capacity of the EMS system. Patients outnumber rescuers in an MCI, particularly in the early stages of the incident. **Triage** is the generic term used

---

Box 40.1 Chronologic Sequence of Events in Response to a Disaster or Multiple-Casualty Incident

Activation Phase
Phase 1: Notification and initial response
Phase 2: Organization of command and scene assessment

Implementation Phase
Phase 3: Search and rescue
Phase 4: Victim extrication, triage, stabilization, and transport
Phase 5: Definitive scene management

Recovery Phase
Phase 6: Scene withdrawal
Phase 7: Return to normal operations
Phase 8: Debriefing

From Roush WR, editor: *Principles of EMS systems*, ed 2, Dallas, 1994, American College of Emergency Physicians.

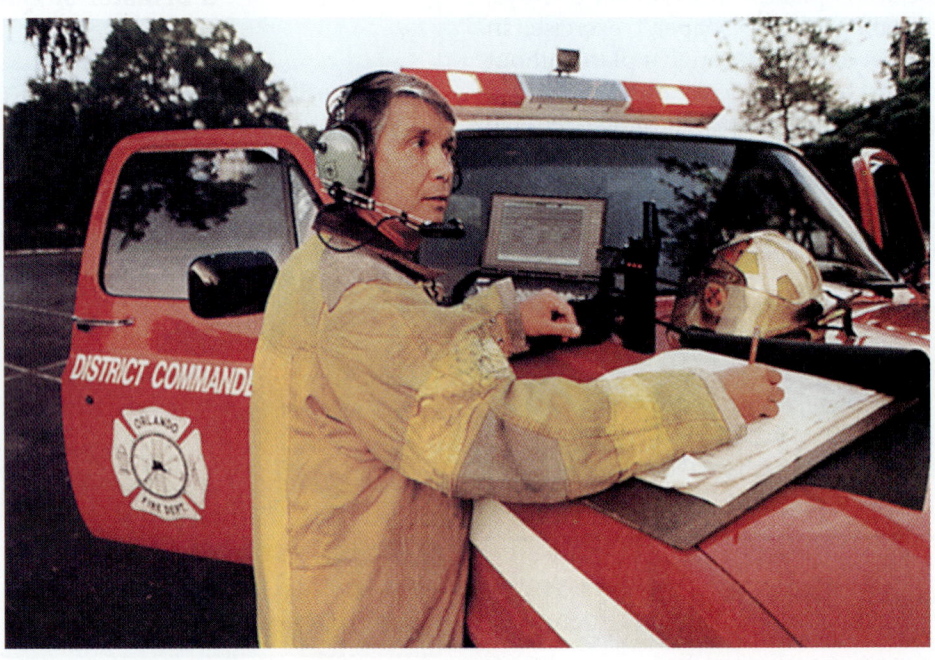

FIGURE 40.5 An incident command system breaks the management function down to small pieces that function independently but with good communication.

to describe the system of sorting or prioritizing patients so that the most effective use is made of limited resources.

A number of different schemes or methods of triage have been developed and used all over the world. The EMT must study and become familiar with the triage method used in his or her local system. Although the specific systems vary, the general principles of triage remain the same.

Triage is initiated by the first-arriving EMS personnel at the disaster scene. As soon as scene safety has been ensured and the necessary notifications accomplished to implement the disaster plan, the EMTs begin the process of sorting and prioritizing patients. Triage is often difficult for EMTs, because the normal mode of operation for EMTs is to find a patient and stay with that patient. In triage, it is absolutely critical that the EMT not become committed to a single patient until the overall sorting and prioritizing are accomplished.

Triage involves rapid movement from patient to patient to gain a quick, overall view of the situation. For each patient, a quick examination is performed to determine the severity of the injury. The only interventions provided are those that are lifesaving. The highest-priority patients are those with the most serious injuries. However, an important exception is a patient who is still alive but has wounds that are obviously fatal. This patient is placed in the lowest category immediately ahead of the dead. The principle here is that valuable, scarce resources should not be used on patients who will die anyway. An additional point is that triage is a dynamic process and patient status or priority can change. For example, a patient can suddenly deteriorate and go from a lower level of priority to a higher one.

The basic priority levels in most triage systems are as follows:

1. Highest priority
   a. Airway and breathing difficulties
   b. Uncontrolled or severe bleeding
   c. Decreased mental status
   d. Severe medical problems (heart attack, stroke, etc.)
   e. Shock (hypoperfusion)
   f. Severe burns
2. Second priority
   a. Burns without airway problems
   b. Major or multiple bone or joint injuries
   c. Back injuries with or without spinal cord damage
3. Lowest priority
   a. Minor painful, swollen, deformed extremities
   b. Minor soft-tissue injuries
4. No priority*
   a. Injuries incompatible with life
   b. Death

---

*The NHTSA (DOT-NSC) only lists three classifications in triage—highest, second, and lowest. They have combined "no priority" with lowest.

As each patient is triaged, his or her status or priority is marked in a way that is easily identified by other EMTs as they arrive (Figure 40.6). There is a tremendous amount of variation between systems in how this identification is accomplished. Some EMS systems use colored tags, some use colored ribbons, some mark directly on the patient with colored markers, and some systems use plain paper. As mentioned earlier, it is important for EMTs to learn and become familiar with the triage marking system used in their EMS system. Once the triage process is complete, incoming EMTs can then be assigned to the highest-priority patients.

> ✔ Because patients outnumber EMTs and other resources in a disaster situation, triage is used to sort and prioritize the patients. Many EMTs find it difficult to change gears and function in a triage mode rather than the normal ratio of multiple EMTs to a single patient.

One other aspect of the management of an MCI does not match the normal or intuitive process of EMS response. When transportation begins, the highest-priority patients are not always transported first. The goal of transportation is to get all of the patients to the appropriate medical facility as soon as possible. However, destination decisions must be governed by knowledge about the individual capacities of hospitals. In general, most medical facilities can easily handle a steady stream of seriously injured people. The hospital's capacity to provide care, however, begins to deteriorate if multiple seriously ill or injured patients arrive at the same time. Therefore the typical disaster plan calls for mixing the patient loads to each hospital, so that no single institution is completely overwhelmed. For example, an ambulance may transport one critical patient, another patient with less severe injuries on a stretcher, and two "walking wounded" to a hospital. This type of mix allows the hospital to integrate the patients into normal operations in an efficient manner.

Roles and Responsibilities of the Emergency Medical Technician

EMTs may find themselves in a variety of situations related to disaster response or an MCI. If EMTs are on the first-arriving EMS vehicle, they will be involved in initial notifications and activations of the system disaster plan. They will also be involved in initial patient triage. EMTs on units arriving later may find themselves assigned to care for individual patients or assigned to manage a part of the activity through assignment as a sector commander. Later-arriving providers will most often be involved in transportation activities. In addition to these major

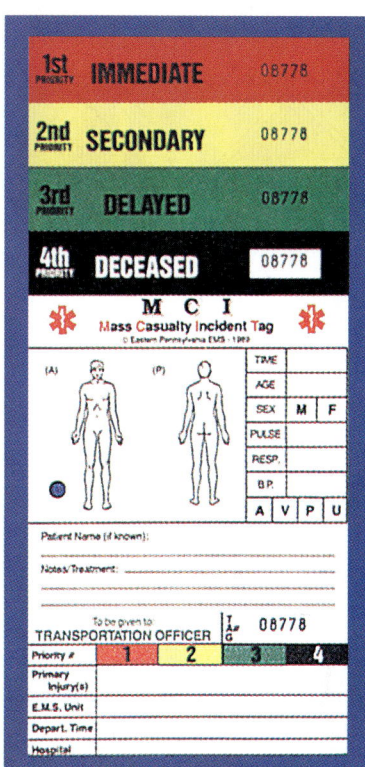

FIGURE 40.6 A triage tag used to sort and prioritize patients at a multiple-casualty incident.

roles and responsibilities, many other jobs must be carried out at a disaster. The bottom line is that EMTs could find themselves involved in almost any aspect of the disaster response. Therefore it is critical that EMTs study and understand disaster plans for their own system.

An important point about disaster response that is often ignored or neglected is the emotional well-being of the EMTs themselves. Disasters and MCIs place extraordinary psychologic pressure on emergency responders. Feelings of being overwhelmed by the sheer magnitude of the disaster and the wrenching emotions involved in having to bypass patients who need help to focus efforts on triage or the more seriously injured can combine with a number of other feelings to cause tremendous emotional stress. The emotional well-being of the EMTs must be considered, both in the planning phase and in the actual disaster management

> ✔ EMTs will find themselves highly stressed in disaster response. In addition, they will be called on to be extremely flexible and innovative in meeting the many challenges of a disaster situation. The EMT needs to be aware of the emotional challenges of disaster response, and the EMS system must provide for CISD for disaster responders.

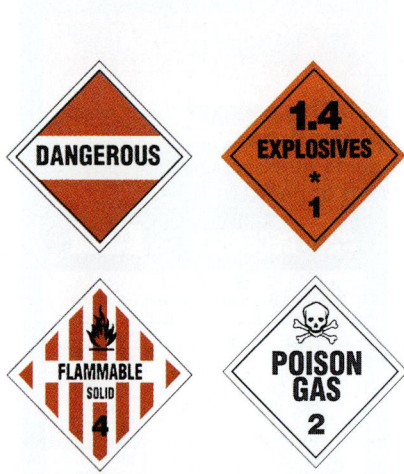

FIGURE 40.7 Examples of domestic placards used on trucks and rail cars.

phase. Chapter 5 discusses the concept of critical incident stress debriefing (CISD) in detail. CISD must be included in system disaster planning activities.

Hazardous Materials (HAZMAT) Response

Many substances in the environment are hazardous to humans. Modern technology, modern manufacturing processes, and modern transportation methods have put **hazardous materials (HAZMAT)** in our lives more often than at any time in the past. Dangerous substances are handled routinely in many industrial processes, and dangerous chemicals are routinely transported through cities and towns by rail and highway. The mere presence of a toxic chemical does not mean that a hazardous situation exists. Instead, a hazardous materials incident involves the possibility of unprotected human exposure to toxic chemicals as a result of an unplanned event such as a highway collision, train derailment, industrial spill, or other accidental incident.

Hazardous Materials Incidents and the Emergency Medical System

HAZMAT incidents are of particular concern to EMS providers because of the nature of EMS work. EMS providers are often the first emergency responders to arrive at the scene of an incident involving HAZMAT. However, EMS providers rarely carry all of the sophisticated protective equipment necessary to operate safely in a HAZMAT environment. Also, many EMS providers have no specific training in the management of HAZMAT incidents. Finally, the first impulse of any EMS provider anywhere, when faced with a situation in which people are obviously ill or injured, is to run in as quickly as possible to help. In a HAZMAT incident, these factors can combine to create a dangerous—even deadly—situation for EMS providers. Dead EMTs are of no help to anyone.

> ✓ HAZMAT incidents are particularly dangerous for EMS providers because they require such a radically different thought process and approach than do traditional EMS responses. Failure to recognize this need and adjust conditioned responses can lead to dead or seriously injured EMTs.

Laws, Regulations, and Training Requirements

Because of the extremely dangerous characteristics of HAZMAT responses and the tremendous value of education and experience, the Occupational Safety and Health Administration, the Environmental Protection Agency, and the National Fire Protection Association have developed regulations and training guidelines to ensure that emergency responders are appropriately prepared to respond to HAZMAT incidents. The most basic level of training is a brief class (approximately 8 to 12 hours) focused on recognition and initial management of HAZMAT incidents. This course focuses on giving emergency responders enough information to recognize a HAZMAT incident and to know what to do to keep themselves and others safe. A number of other training levels are also identified, and the most sophisticated level, for individuals and teams that specialize in HAZMAT response, involves hundreds of hours of training and experience.

Emergency Medical Technician Roles and Responsibilities

As mentioned earlier, the EMT plays a vital role in a number of aspects of HAZMAT response. The EMT is often the first emergency responder to arrive at a HAZMAT incident. The EMT's choice of initial actions can make a major difference in lives saved.

Recognition

The first key step in successfully managing a HAZMAT response is recognition. Someone has to recognize that the incident involves a potentially dangerous environment.

To recognize a HAZMAT incident, the EMT first needs a heightened sense of awareness about HAZMAT. Whenever EMS is dispatched to a transportation incident, whether on the highway, on the rails, or in the air, the EMT must think about HAZMAT. Any response to a fire or accident at an industrial facility should prompt the EMT to consider HAZMAT as a possibility. Similarly, a response to an incident in which multiple patients are experiencing similar complaints (e.g., everyone is having trouble breathing) should send warning signals to the EMT.

The government, the chemical industry, and the transportation industry have developed several uniform methods for identifying HAZMAT. For transportation vehicles (truck or train), a system of placards (signs) is used to identify HAZMAT (Figure 40.7). The presence of these placards is required by law. Vehicles carrying these placards have shipping papers that identify the substance contained in the vehicle. The placards also contain a four-digit number in the center that corresponds to the United States Department of Transportation's *Emergency Response Handbook: Guidebook for Hazardous Materials Incidents.* This guidebook provides basic emergency information for known HAZMAT and should be carried by every emergency response vehicle. Although the presence of a placard is a good indication that hazardous substances may be present, the absence of a placard does not mean that the incident is perfectly safe. For many hazardous substances, a placard is not required until the weight of the substance exceeds a minimum limit, most often 1000 lb. Therefore it is possible for a significant amount of hazardous materials to be present without a placard to serve as a warning.

Department of Transportation (DOT) placarding is not the only means of recognizing hazardous materials available to the EMT:

- The National Fire Protection Association (NFPA) 704 placard (Figures 40.8 and 40.9) is used to indicate the properties of bulk storage in the industrial setting.
- Specific information on hazardous materials (chemical composition, effects on the body, recommended treatments, etc.) is available in the Materials Safety Data Sheet (MSDS) (Figure 40.10). Commercial and industrial environments are required to maintain MSDSs on all chemicals used or stored in their operations. EMTs should demand to see the MSDS when there has been an exposure even to a single patient *before patient contact.*
- Another source of information on hazardous materials is CHEMTREC® (1-800-424-9300; www.chemtrec.org). CHEMTREC® is an emergency information center offering assistance 24 hours a day, 365 days a year. CHEMTREC® is run by the Chemical Manufacturers Association in close association with the DOT.

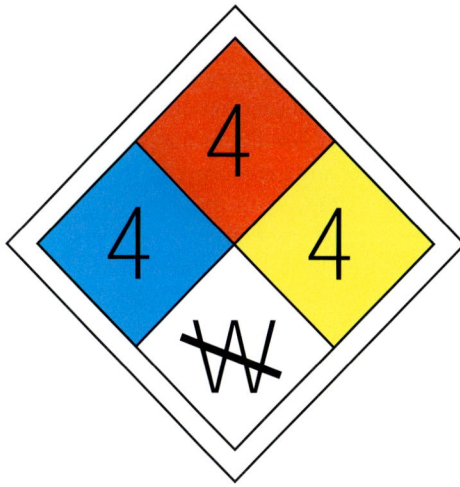

FIGURE 40.8 A National Fire Protection Association 704 placard that is placed in or on a building to indicate the presence of hazardous materials.

CHEMTREC® has information on over 1 million chemicals on file, and it can serve as a resource for EMS and HAZMAT operations.

> ✓ EMS units are frequently the first to respond and the first on the scene of incidents such as highway or rail accidents that may involve HAZMAT. Therefore EMTs play a particularly important role in the early stages of the recognition of and response to HAZMAT incidents.

Scene Safety

As mentioned earlier, an EMT must have a heightened sense of awareness when responding to incidents or locations where HAZMAT might be involved. As soon as the scene is in sight, particularly if it is obvious that a truck or train car is involved, the EMS vehicle should stop and look for HAZMAT placards or markings from a distance. Because placards may be difficult to see, emergency response vehicles should carry binoculars so that observation can be conducted from a safe distance. If placards or other markings indicative of HAZMAT are detected, the EMT has several immediate responsibilities.

First, resist the urge to drive right up to the scene and rush in to help the victims. If hazardous materials are actually involved, this approach may lead to injury or death for the EMT. Instead, attempt to identify the substance by using any of the recognition methods discussed earlier. Request assistance from personnel or units familiar with HAZMAT response, and take the necessary steps to establish response zones around the

NFPA 704 System

Health (Blue)

In general, health hazard in fire fighting is that of a single exposure which may vary from a few seconds up to an hour. The physical exertion demanded in fire fighting or other emergency conditions may be expected to intensify the effects of any exposure. Only hazards arising out of an inherent property of the material are considered. The following explanation is based upon protective equipment normally used by fire fighters.

4 Materials too dangerous to health to expose fire fighters. A few whiffs of the vapor could cause death or the vapor or liquid could be fatal on penetrating the fire fighter's normal full protective clothing. The normal full protective clothing and breathing apparatus available to the average fire department will not provide adequate protection against inhalation or skin contact with these materials.

3 Materials extremely hazardous to health but areas may be entered with extreme care. Full protective clothing, including self-contained breathing apparatus, coat, pants, gloves, boots, and bands around legs, arms and waist should be provided. No skin surface should be exposed.

2 Materials hazardous to health, but areas may be entered freely with full-faced mask self-contained breathing apparatus, which provides eye protection.

1 Materials only slightly hazardous to health. It may be desirable to wear self-contained breathing apparatus.

0 Materials which on exposure under fire conditions, would offer no hazard beyond that of ordinary combustible material.

Flammability (Red)

Susceptibility to burning is the basis for assigning degrees within this category. The method of attacking the fire is influenced by this susceptibility factor.

4 Very flammable gases or very volatile flammable liquids. Shut off flow and keep cooling water streams on exposed tanks or containers.

3 Materials which can be ignited under almost all normal temperature conditions. Water may be ineffective because of the low flash point.

2 Materials which must be moderately heated before ignition will occur. Water spray may be used to extinguish the fire because the material can be cooled below its flash point.

1 Materials that must be preheated before ignition can occur. Water may cause frothing if it gets below the surface of the liquid and turns to steam. However, water fog gently applied to the surface will cause a frothing which will extinguish the fire.

0 Materials that will not burn.

Reactivity (Stability) (Yellow)

The assignment of degrees in the reactivity category is based upon the susceptibility of materials to release energy either by themselves or in combination with water. Fire exposure was one of the factors considered along with conditions of shock and pressure.

4 Materials which (in themselves) are readily capable of detonation or of explosive decomposition or explosive reaction at normal temperatures and pressures. Includes materials which are sensitive to mechanical or localized thermal shock. If a chemical with this hazard rating is in an advanced or massive fire, the area should be evacuated.

3 Materials which (in themselves) are capable of detonation or of explosive decomposition or of explosive reaction which require a strong initiating source or which must be heated under confinement before initiation. Includes materials which are sensitive to thermal or mechanical shock at elevated temperatures and pressures or which react explosively with water without requiring heat or confinement. Fire fighting should be done from an explosive-resistant location.

2 Materials which (in themselves) are normally unstable and readily undergo violent chemical change but do not detonate. Includes materials which can undergo chemical change with rapid release of energy at normal temperatures and pressure or which can undergo violent chemical change at elevated temperatures and pressures. Also includes those materials which may react violently with water or which may form potentially explosive mixtures with water. In advance or massive fires, fire fighting should be done from a safe distance or from a protected location.

1 Materials which (in themselves) are normally stable but which may become unstable at elevated temperatures and pressures or which may react with water with some release of energy, but not violently. Caution must be used in approaching the fire and applying water.

0 Materials which (in themselves) are normally stable even under fire exposure conditions and which are not reactive with water. Normal fire fighting procedures may be used.

From *Hazardous Material Awareness for Minnesota First Responders*—Minnesota State Board of Technical Colleges.

FIGURE 40.9 The numbers on a 704 placard correspond to health, flammability, and reactivity hazards described in NFPA standard 704.

MATERIAL SAFETY DATA SHEET

SUPPLIER: UPRIGHT INCORPORATED ADDRESS: 10715 KAHLMEYER DRIVE ST. LOUIS, MO 63132	EMERGENCY NO.: (800) 248-7007 PHONE NO.: (314) 426-3336 FAX NO.: (314) 426-0145

SECTION I - MATERIAL IDENTIFICATION

CHEMICAL NAME & SYNONYMS: AMORPHOUS MINERAL SILICATE
All ingredients are Non-Hazardous, Inert, Non-Toxic and Non-Biodegradable

CHEMICAL FAMILY: Alumino-Silicate

TRADE NAME & SYNONYMS: WYK SAFETY SORBENT
All 500 Series Stock No's
MIRACLE SWEEP   SU-40
UPRIGHT ANTI-SLIP UP-40

SECTION II - INGREDIENTS AND HAZARDS

This product is NOT hazardous as defined by CFR 1910.1200. All elements are chemically and physically bound.

Typical Chemical Analysis:
SiO_2 (66-72%) Al_2O_3 (11-17%) Fe_2O_3 (2-4%)
CaO (1-4%) K_2O (1.5-4.7%) Na_2O (3-5%)

SECTION III - PHYSICAL DATA

Boiling point at 1 atm, deg. F:	N/A	Specific gravity (H2O = 1):	2.2 - 2.4
Vapor pressure at (mm HG.):	N/A	Evap. Rate:	N/A
Vapor density (Air = 1):	N/A	Volatiles, % by Volume:	N/A
Water Solubility:	Negligible	Melting Point:	N/A
Appearance and Odor:	Gray Powder/Odorless		

SECTION IV - FIRE AND EXPLOSION DATA

Flash Point: Non-Flammable   **Autoignition Temp:** N/A

Flammability Limits In Air: Lower = N/A / Upper = N/A

Extinguishing media: N/A

Special fire fighting procedures: N/A

Unusual fire and explosion hazards: N/A

N.F.P.A HAZARD INFORMATION LABEL

Hazard Code
4 = Extreme
3 = High
2 = Moderate
1 = Slight
0 = Negligible

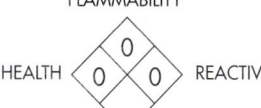

SECTION V - HEALTH HAZARD INFORMATION   TLV: N/A

<u>This product is not considered a carcinogen. It is certified *free of respirable silica* using NIOSH Method #7500 and X-ray Defraction Testing.</u>

Summary of risks: Under windy conditions or in enclosed areas, sorbent can be a nuisance dust.
Medical conditions which may be aggravated by contact: N/A
Target organs: N/A
Primary entry route (s): N/A
Acute effects: N/A
Chronic effect (s): N/A

FIGURE 40.10 Materials Safety Data Sheet.

Continued

Page 2	UPRIGHT, INC.	STK # 500 Series

SECTION V: - HEALTH HAZARD INFORMATION - Continued

EFFECTS OF OVEREXPOSURE

FIRST AID:

- **Eye Contact:** Flush eyes with water. Seek medical attention if necessary.
- **Skin Contact:** Remove with soap and water.
- **Inhalation:** Remove to fresh air. If needed, seek medical help.
- **Ingestion:** Under normal conditions, material is non-toxic.

SECTION VI - REACTIVITY DATA

Material is stable. Hazardous polymerization will not occur.

Chemical Incompatibility (Materials to Avoid): HYDROFLUORIC ACID and HF Compounds.

Hazardous Decomposition Products: N/A

SECTION VII - SPILL LEAK, AND DISPOSAL PROCEDURE

Spills, leaks: (steps to be taken): Vacuum or sweep up. Maintain good housekeeping procedures.

Waste Disposal Method: Observe all Federal, State, and Local laws concerning health and environment.

SECTION VIII - SPECIAL PROTECTION INFORMATION

Personal protective equipment:
- **Goggles:** Normally not required
- **Gloves:** Normally not required
- **Respirator:** Normally not required
- **Other:** Special considerations may be required given the nature of the liquids to be absorbed.

Work Place Consideration:
- **Ventilation:** Under certain conditions.
- **Safety Station:** N/A
- **Contaminated Equipment:** N/A

SECTION IX - SPECIAL PRECAUTIONS AND COMMENTS

- **Storage and Handling Information:** No special requirements. Keep dry.
- **Engineering Controls:** N/A
- **Other Precautions:** N/A

Judgments as to the suitability of information herein for purchaser's purposes are necessarily purchaser's responsibility. Therefore, although reasonable care has been taken in the preparation of such information, UPRIGHT, INC. extends no warranties, makes no representations and assumes no responsibility as to accuracy or suitability of such information for application to purchaser's intended purposes or for the consequences of its use.

Signed: *GC Katzenburger*

Title: President

Date: 08/01/00   MSDS No.: 500

FIGURE 40.10 cont'd   Materials Safety Data Sheet.

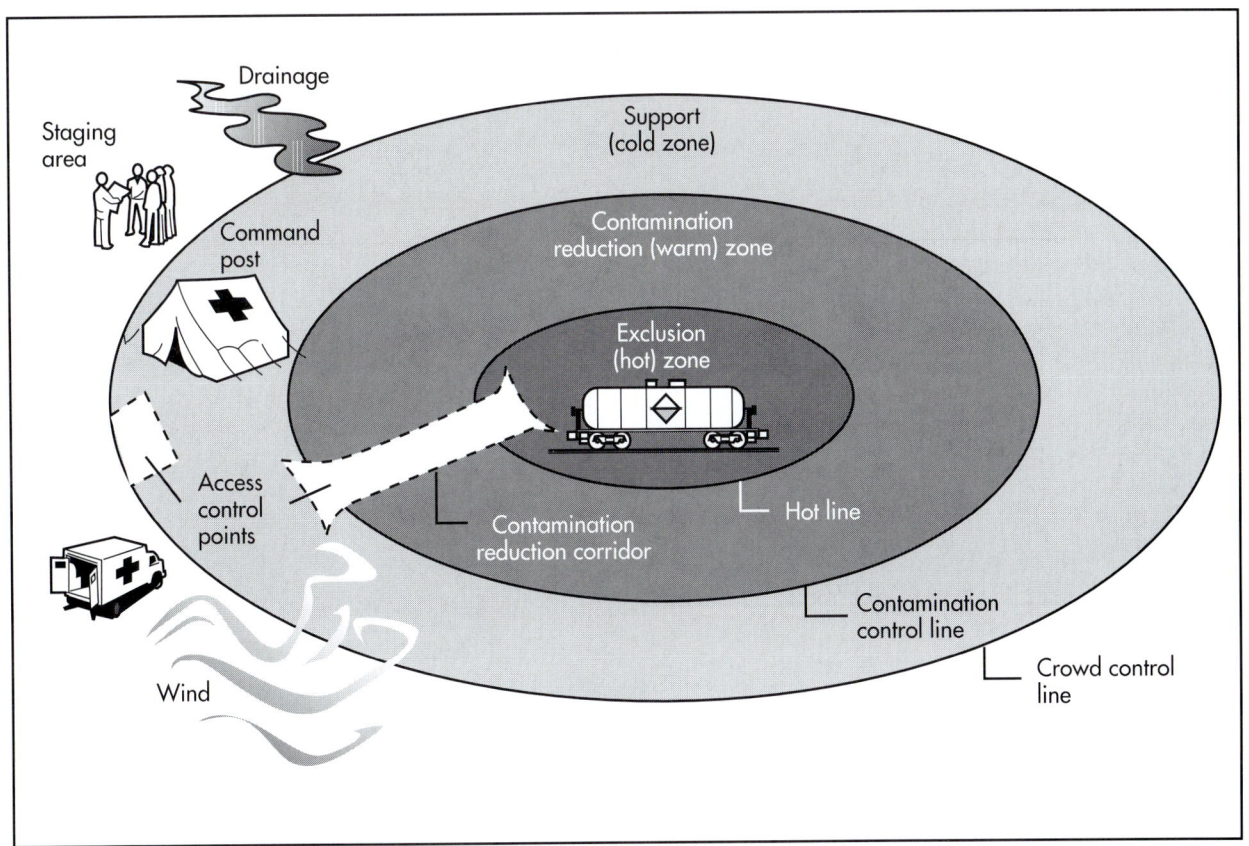

FIGURE 40.11 Response zones around an incident. The red zone is in the middle, yellow is the second zone, and green is the outermost zone.

incident (Figure 40.11). Communicate any relevant information about the identity of the chemical or specifics of the incident to the dispatch center, and notify the hospital that a HAZMAT incident is under way. Consider notifying the local poison control center so that they can be prepared to provide necessary advice.

At this point, the EMS provider will usually have to wait until victims are extricated and decontaminated by the HAZMAT specialists before starting any medical treatment. Local HAZMAT management teams will likely have specific procedures for establishing safety zones and decontamination processes. The EMT should learn the procedures used in his or her local system before responding to a HAZMAT incident.

> ✓ The EMT must resist the urge to rush in and help if the incident involves hazardous materials. Instead, the EMT needs to identify the hazardous substance and establish the necessary safety zone around the location.

Decontamination and Management

Management for victims of HAZMAT incidents must be accomplished with a number of priorities in mind. The first priority is safety for the EMTs and other rescuers. The second priority is the safety of other bystanders, and the third priority is safety of the patient. Although it may seem strange to consider the patient third in this priority list, the simple fact remains that the patient has already been exposed, whereas EMTs and bystanders have not.

Decontamination. Before any management can occur, the patient should be decontaminated by the HAZMAT professionals before being turned over to the EMTs. **Decontamination** is the process of removing as much of the hazardous substance as possible from the patient. Decontamination often involves the removal of clothing and hosing down the patient with large amounts of water. However, it is rare that a patient is completely decontaminated, so EMTs should take the necessary steps to protect themselves while treating the patient. In addition, EMTs must protect the transport vehicle from contamination. A

> **Box 40.2 Equipment Items on Ambulance to Deal with HAZMAT Incident**
>
> - Plastic trash bags (3 to 4 mm thick)
> - Plastic sheeting (6 mm thick) to cover doors, benches, windows, and essential portable equipment and perhaps to wrap the patient
> - Plastic body bag (alternative to wrap the patient)
> - Duct tape to seal cabinets
> - Rubber boots
> - Rubber gloves (neoprene is more resistant to chemicals than latex)
> - Rubber aprons
> - Disposable gowns or coveralls
> - Face masks, eye shields
> - Reference books

few basic supplies give the EMT the necessary equipment to deal with a contaminated patient (Box 40.2).

Management. Once the patient is decontaminated and the EMTs are dressed in appropriate protective equipment, medical management can begin. The management itself is most likely unremarkable, and the same techniques learned elsewhere in this text are used for the appropriate injuries or illnesses. For example, a fractured leg will be splinted in the same way using the same devices. In rare instances, there may be subtle differences in management that are dictated by the nature of the contamination. In this case, specific instructions usually will be available from on-line medical direction or from a HAZMAT guidebook.

Transportation. The receiving facility must be given plenty of advance warning that a patient exposed to hazardous materials is being transported. The hospital must take steps to prevent the entire emergency department or the hospital itself from being contaminated. The hospital may request that the patient be transported to an area other than the normal ambulance entrance. Medical personnel may see and treat the victim in the ambulance rather than move the patient into the building.

Postincident Activities. After the patient is delivered to the medical facility, the EMTs will need to proceed with decontamination of themselves and the vehicle. The specific procedures that will be involved will be dictated by the hazardous substance that was encountered, but at a minimum, the EMTs will need to remove and clean (and perhaps discard) the clothing worn during the response. A complete and vigorous hand washing, followed by a shower as soon as possible, will also be required. If the EMTs are actually exposed to a hazardous substance, medical testing and follow-up also may be required. The EMS agency should have specific policies and processes in place for personnel decontamination and medical follow-up. The EMTs should become familiar with local requirements or guidelines.

For the vehicle, any contaminated equipment must be cleaned or disposed of. As with the decontamination of personnel, the specific processes used for the vehicle will vary depending on the hazardous substance that was encountered. EMTs should follow local guidelines to prepare the vehicle for the next call.

Disposal of clothing and other contaminated equipment must be handled appropriately. The important point is that anything that is contaminated with a hazardous substance cannot be discarded in the station or hospital trash can. The EMS agency should have specific policies in place for dealing with disposal of contaminated items, and EMTs must become familiar with and follow these policies.

Summary

- Disasters and MCIs are complex events involving many different providers and agencies. Management is a particular challenge. The ICS is used by most emergency services as a model for organization and function.
- Triage is a process for sorting and prioritizing patients in an MCI. The priority of patients is determined by the severity of their illness or injury combined with their likelihood of survival. A wide variety of different marking or identification systems are in use around the country, so EMTs must familiarize themselves with the methods used locally.
- HAZMAT response requires a heightened awareness and a change in normal response methods to avoid serious injury to EMTs. The emphasis must be placed on early recognition of the HAZMAT incident and rapid mobilization of trained HAZMAT response personnel.

Summary (cont'd)

- Once the patient is decontaminated, medical management is accomplished using routine methods. The receiving facility must be given as much warning as possible if a contaminated patient is being transported. The hospital must make advance preparations that might include treating the patient somewhere other than the emergency department.

Scenario Solution

You *know* you have a hazardous materials accident. You *know* you already have more patients than you can effectively manage. You radio for more EMS help. Your partner grabs the triage kit, and you report to the fire department officer, who has established the incident command. You inform him that you are the first-arriving medical unit and will assume the role of medical sector command. He is advised that there are additional ambulances and EMS crews responding to handle the patients. You know you must establish triage and treatment areas after those who were exposed are decontaminated. You direct your partner to the triage area you have chosen in the safe zone. As the additional ambulances and EMS crews arrive, you direct them to their treatment areas and appoint a treatment sector officer for each of the three treatment sectors. The incident commander has received information on the chemical causing the exposure, relays that to you, and informs you there are three patients with direct exposure to the chemical complaining of nausea, vomiting, and difficulty breathing, and there are another six who were exposed to the fumes but are not showing signs yet. The decontamination crew starts bringing out patients to your partner in the triage area. You contact medical control and inform them that you have instituted a multiple-casualty operation. You relay the information given to you by the incident commander, and notify medical control that you will be selecting a communications officer to assume the responsibility of maintaining contact with them.

After the last of your patients has been stabilized and transported by EMS and the fire department and HAZMAT team have controlled the spill, the incident commander strikes the call and declares the area safe. During your cleanup, the incident commander thanks you and your partner for a job well done, and congratulates you for your key role in avoiding what could have been a fatal situation.

Key Terms

Decontamination The process of removing hazardous substances from the patient, rescuers, and equipment.

Disaster Human-caused or natural event that involves tremendous damage across a large geographic area; may or may not involve large numbers of injuries.

Hazardous materials (HAZMAT) Any materials exposed on an emergency scene that are hazardous by being poisonous, flammable, explosive, carcinogenic, or environmentally pollutant; abbreviated *HAZMAT* in emergency services.

Incident command system (ICS) A system or method of management of complex events involving large amounts of resources (people, equipment, vehicles). The origins of ICS can be traced to the fire service, but it has now been adapted for use in almost every situation requiring management of complex events.

Infrastructure Physical components of a community that are necessary for normal, everyday operations, such as roads, bridges, electrical power, and telephone communications.

Mass (multiple) casualty incident (MCI) Commonly accepted definition is any incident involving one or more patients that cannot be handled by the first-responding units to a scene.

Risk assessment A process of analyzing disasters or multiple-casualty incidents that are most likely to occur in a given community.

Triage A process used to sort patients and determine which will be treated or transported first; often used to describe the sorting process used in a disaster situation but also can apply to any situation in which sorting of patients is necessary.

Review Questions

1. A *multiple casualty incident* is best defined as:
   a. Any incident involving five or more patients
   b. Any incident involving a moving vehicle
   c. Any incident that overburdens the response unit's ability to handle
   d. None of the above
2. The primary consideration for the EMT when responding to a hazardous materials incident is:
   a. Identifying the hazard
   b. Controlling the hazard
   c. Safety of the EMS crew
   d. Safety of the patients
3. The phone number for CHEMTREC® is:
   a. 1-800-424-9300
   b. 1-800-424-3939
   c. 1-800-424-3900
   d. CHEMTREC® could be contacted by any of these numbers
4. You and your partner respond to a two-car motor vehicle collision. Which of the following patients requires the *highest* priority of treatment?
   a. 24-year-old man, ejected from the vehicle, pulseless and not breathing
   b. 22-year-old woman with bilateral tibia/fibula open fractures
   c. 45-year-old man, restrained passenger, complaining of neck pain, moving all extremities, denies numbness
   d. 65-year-old man, restrained driver, complaining of crushing chest pain that started before impact; patient states it is the worst pain he has ever felt
5. Referring to review question 4, which patient has the *lowest* priority of care?
   a. a
   b. b
   c. c
   d. d

Answers to these Review Questions can be found at the end of the book on page 869.

Diving Emergencies

Lesson Goal

Presently the Department of Transportation does not list learning objectives for this presentation. Information presented is for enrichment of the student. The emergency medical technician (EMT) who is in a position where management of these types of injuries can occur needs to obtain more complete training in the management of these patients and their specific injuries. Information presented is designed as an overview of the types of injuries that can occur to these individuals and how these patients may be transferred. Although the EMT-Basic may not initially treat these patients, he or she may be intimately involved in their transfer to the hospital and therefore must understand the processed involved.

Scenario

At 10:43 A.M. on a mild and sunny day in late December, you and your partner are dispatched to the local marina in reference to a reported call for medical assistance from a charter dive boat operator. Initial reports indicate that a male subject, 47 years old, was found floating on the surface, shortly after beginning a dive on a submerged wreck at a popular dive site, using scuba equipment.

The boat captain further advises that the subject was pulled from the water, unconscious, and is presently receiving oxygen. His vital signs are pulse 122 and regular, respiration rate 28 and shallow; his skin is cool and pale. His diving gear has been removed and he is covered with a blanket. The dive master advises that the subject is unresponsive with frothy sputum in his airway, which they are attempting to clear. The weather is sunny with an air temperature of 70 degrees Fahrenheit.

Because you are located in a resort community where scuba diving is a popular tourist sport, you have been trained in management of scuba diving emergencies. However, you have not responded to this type of call in over a year.

? As you respond to the marina you mentally process the following questions. What type of diving accident is this—ascent or descent? What are the particular types of barotrauma that could have occurred in each incidence? How will you initially manage these types of injuries? What other information would you like to obtain, either en route or once you have arrived on the scene? Are there any support services that you would like to notify to assist in the management or transport of this patient?

Key Terms to Know

Ascent injury
Barotrauma
Decompression sickness
Descent injury
Recompression chamber
Scuba

Learning Objectives

As an EMT-Basic, you should be able to do the following:

- Explain the mechanics of water, air, and oxygen pressure and how these effects are measured in relationship to the human body.
- Define *Boyle's law* as it relates to pressure and volume relationships for scuba diving accidents.
- Define *Dalton's law of partial pressure* and the effect this has on a scuba diver who is using compressed air.
- Define *barotrauma* as it relates to the human body and how this can affect a scuba diver.
- Describe the pathophysiology and field management of the following barotrauma descent injuries that can be found in a scuba diver: ear, sinus, dental, pulmonary, and mask.
- Describe the pathophysiology and field management of the following barotrauma ascent injuries that can be found in a scuba diver: pneumothorax, hemothorax, pneumomediastinum, air embolism, subcutaneous emphysema.
- Define *decompression sickness,* and describe how it occurs in a scuba diver and its emergency management.
- Understand the different methods of transfer of patients with barotrauma and other diving injuries.

The opportunities for an emergency medical technician (EMT) to encounter a medical or trauma-related emergency secondary to a **scuba** diving accident is related to the location of the emergency medical service (EMS). With the current advances in both the science of scuba diving and modern equipment used by the recreational diver, the incidence of injury or medical emergencies is small. However, many U.S. communities have a great exposure to diving because of close access to the ocean, the Gulf of Mexico, or inland lakes (Figure 41.1).

For the EMT it is not necessary to possess a complete understanding of the underlying physiologic process. Rather it is important to understand the stabilization priorities and urgency of seeking a functional recompression facility. The National Association of Underwater Instructors (NAUI), the Professional Association of Diving

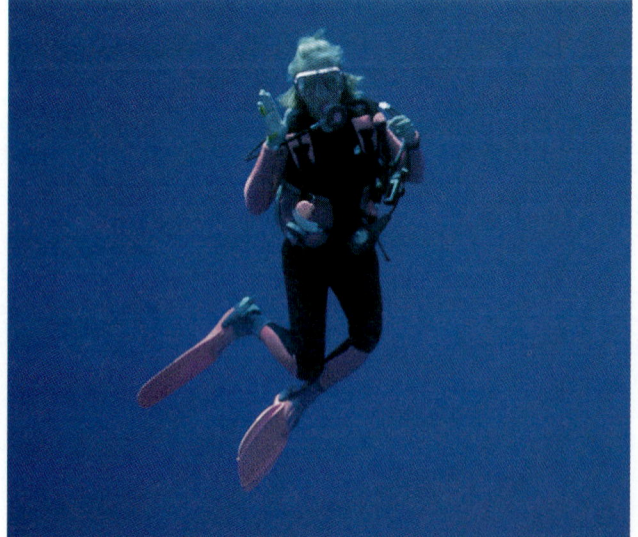 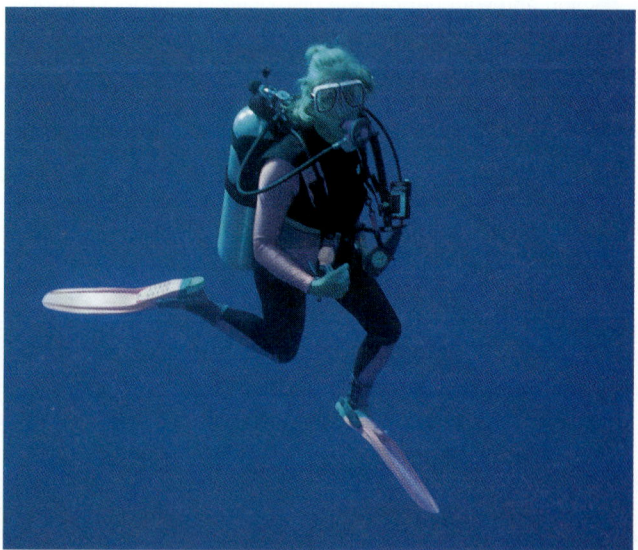

FIGURE 41.1 Scuba diver.

Instructors (PADI), and the Young Men's Christian Association (YMCA) teach the complete basic and advanced diving course, as well as the specialized information that is required to teach diving, to run a diving operation as a dive master, and to work as a search and rescue diver. This chapter in no way is constructed to teach diving, its complications, or their medical management. Rather it is meant to assist the EMT in the understanding of how to assist in the management during the time of transfer to the hospital by the scuba rescue team. EMTs interested in becoming certified divers should consult one of the aforementioned organizations.

Traumatic injuries that can occur as a result of scuba diving accidents will not be discussed, because they are treated the same as any other trauma event.

The Physics of Air

Air is a mixture of gases. These gases are odorless, colorless, and tasteless in their natural forms. Breathing is a natural event in our lives, and most of the time we are not conscious of it happening. The most important gas related to life on this planet is oxygen. Making up approximately 21% of the air we breathe, it is essential to survival. The other major gas in air is nitrogen, which makes up approximately 78% of the air we breathe at sea level. Considered an inert gas because it does not react inside our bodies under normal conditions, it can have serious consequences for scuba divers when it is not eliminated properly and completely (Figure 41.2).

Air can be easily compressed into a cylinder by the use of force. A good example is filling the EMS unit tire to its recommended pressure. This same principle applies to the cylinder of air the scuba diver uses. Because of the atmosphere's own weight, the air at sea level is denser than air in the stratosphere, and air in mountainous and other high-elevation regions is less dense than that at sea level.

All three forms of a substance (gas, liquid, and solid) are compressible. Gas, however, is much more easily compressed than is liquid, which, in turn, is more compressible than are solids. Enough pressure applied to a cylinder of air or water will exceed the tensile strength of the walls of the container, resulting in rupture of the container.

An example to better understand the issue of density as applied to water and air is two containers, one filled with water, the other with air. The container filled with water is much heavier because water molecules are more compact (dense). One cubic foot of air weighs only 0.08 pounds. One cubic foot of seawater weighs approximately 64 pounds (63 pounds for freshwater), approximately 800 times the same volume of air. The difference is caused by the greater density of the water.

The effects of pressure on divers and on the patient in a hyperbaric compression chamber are the same. During descent, while at the maximum depth of their dive, and on ascent back to the surface, pressure of the surrounding environment (either air or water) compresses the air being breathed and the solution of gases in the blood (Figure 41.3).

A 1 inch by 1 inch column of air that extends up into the earth's atmosphere exerts a pressure of 14.7 pounds per square inch at sea level. In technical terms this is referred to as *1 atmosphere of pressure.* This pressure is exerted continuously on the human body, but it generally goes unnoticed for two reasons. First, the body is primarily composed of fluids (approximately 60% to 70% water). The response of water to pressure is small enough to be unnoticeable. Second, the air spaces in the body, such as the lungs and sinuses, are open to the surrounding atmospheric pressure, which allows the pressure within and outside of these air-containing spaces to equilibrate.

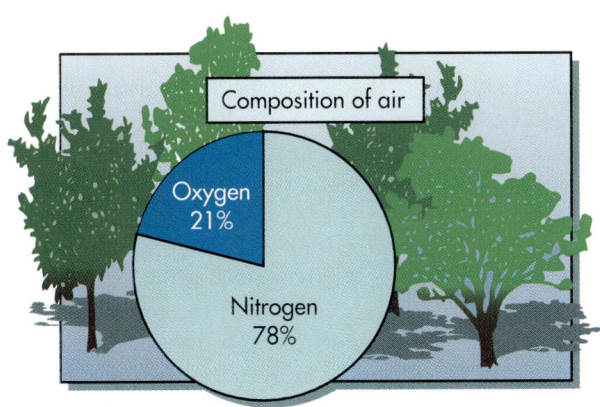

FIGURE 41.2 Air and its components.

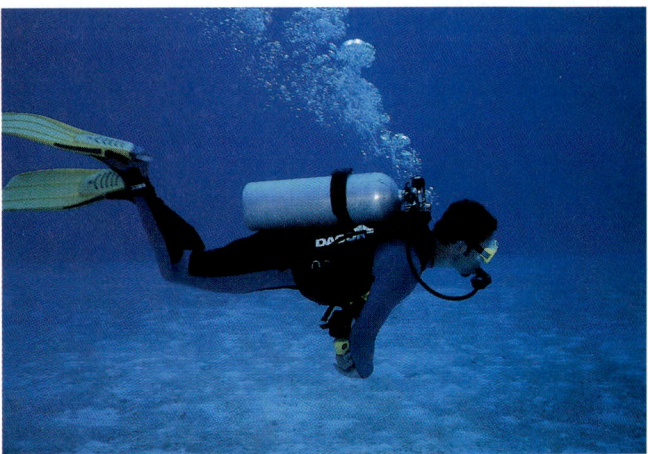

FIGURE 41.3 The pressure of water on the body must be overcome by pressure of air from the tank if the diver is to breathe under water.

A 1 inch by 1 inch column of air that extends up into the atmosphere exerts a pressure of 14.7 pounds per square inch. A 1 inch by 1 inch column of seawater that is only 33 feet tall (34 feet for freshwater) exerts the same pressure of 14.7 pounds per square inch. This is because of the difference in density. Water is only minimally compressed and transmits its pressure freely, and its effects increase at a constant rate. A 1 inch column of water that is 33 feet tall would, if doubled to a height of 66 feet, exert twice as much pressure. At 99 feet the pressure increases by another 14.7 pounds (or 1 atmosphere [atm]). At any depth in water, the weight of the column of air (atmospheric pressure) at the surface must be added to the weight of the column of water to describe the correct pressure being applied to the body.

> ✓ A 1 inch by 1 inch column of air that extends up into the stratosphere exerts 14.7 psi on the human body. A 1 inch by 1 inch column of seawater that has a height of 33 feet (34 feet for freshwater) exerts the same amount of pressure, 14.7 psi, on the body.

Pressure, Volume, and Density

Several *gas laws* apply to scuba diving. The two that most directly affect patients likely to be managed by EMTs are the focus of this discussion. More detail can be found in any good physics book or scuba text. The first of these laws is called *Boyle's law* and refers to the relationship between pressure and volume. A closed container that is filled with atmospheric air at sea level would, when taken under water, respond to the pressure of the increasing depth. The pressure would begin to compress the volume of air into a smaller and smaller space, collapsing the walls of the container, while not affecting the amount of air that is in the container. This results in increased density. When the container is returned to the surface and the pressure is reduced, the volume would expand back to its original density.

The same container is returned to the same depth under water, is filled with an air hose to the same volume, and is maintained at the depth that we had at the surface. Upon returning the container to the surface without releasing any air, the volume expands as the pressure decreases. If this volume expansion exceeded the capacity of the container, it would rupture.

> ✓ Boyle's law states that as pressure increases, volume decreases, and as pressure decreases, volume increases.

The second important gas law is *Dalton's law of partial pressure*. This gas law states that, in a mixture of gases, the pressure exerted by each gas is the same as it would exert if it alone occupied the same volume. It further states that the total pressure equals the sum of all the partial pressures in a component gas.

Although this law applies to all gases that are found in air, the gas that most affects the scuba diver is nitrogen. Nitrogen is an inert gas, or a gas that in normal concentrations and under normal conditions has no effect on the human body. However, in the scuba diver, the effects of increasing depth and pressure begin to affect the physiology of nitrogen in the body.

Nitrogen is constantly being exchanged within the tissues on a one-to-one basis, as are other gases. The system is said to be in a state of equilibrium. This equilibrium is lost when the pressure on the air one breathes begins to increase. Because air density increases as the diver descends, the amount of nitrogen absorbed by the body increases at a faster rate than it is breathed off. The result is an increase in blood nitrogen levels. Different tissues absorb nitrogen at different rates and, likewise, off-load the gas at different rates. As more nitrogen is absorbed, the diver becomes at increased risk if the nitrogen is not eliminated from the body as fast as the pressure decreases. If the nitrogen is not eliminated as the pressure decreases, the bubbles enlarge, producing pain, blocking blood flow, and tearing tissue in the lungs. This condition is termed *the bends*.

> ✓ Dalton's law of partial pressure relates to the percentage of any single gas occurring in air. In the case of scuba diving, it is most directly related to the inert gas nitrogen.

Barotrauma Injuries Occurring During Descent

As previously stated, the human body is mostly fluid, but it does have some air spaces. Included are the lungs, middle ear, and sinuses. As a scuba diver makes his or her descent into the water, the density, and thus the pressure, of the water begins to compress existing air in these spaces.

Lungs are like large paper sacks that fill with air during inspiration and expel that air during expiration. In between these two mechanical acts, the process of diffusion occurs, which transfers oxygen into the hemoglobin of the red blood cells and removes the waste products of cell metabolism in the form of carbon dioxide. As the diver descends and pressure increases, the air spaces are compressed, and eventually the diver's lungs would no longer function **(descent injury)**. To offset this problem,

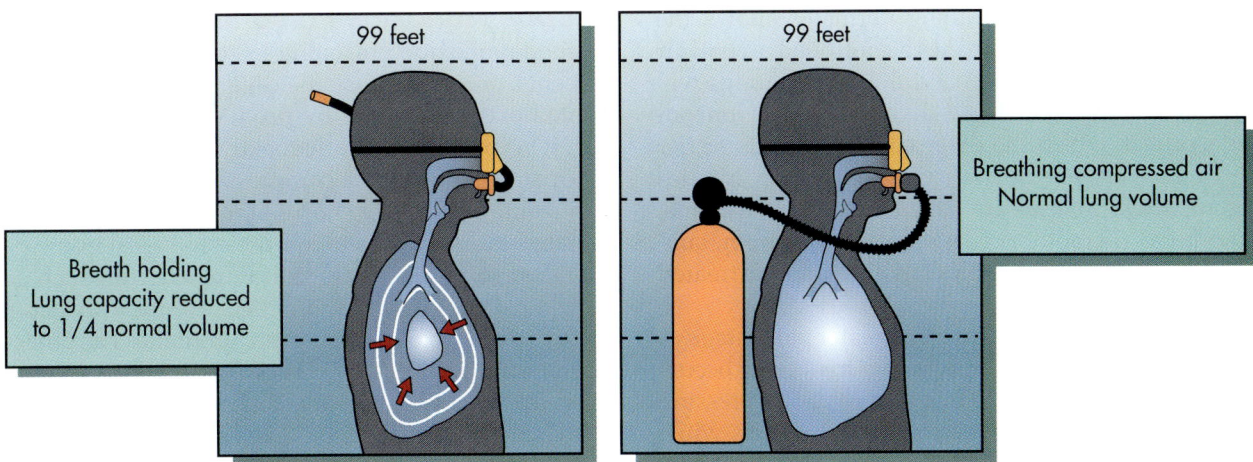

FIGURE 41.4 Effects of pressure on free diver's lungs and effects of breathing compressed air on scuba diver's lungs.

the pressurized air from the scuba tank allows for the lungs to compensate and remain fully inflated with each breath (Figure 41.4).

Sinuses are cavities within the head that are lined with mucous membranes and normally contain only air. Each sinus is connected to the nasal passage by way of a tube. These passageways are normally open and allow for the free movement of air, but when one has a cold or allergies, they become inflamed and can easily clog. Once clogged, the sinuses can trap air. The pathway into the sinuses will frequently allow the ingress of air under pressure, but when the pressure decreases, egress will not occur. To the scuba diver this means that the sinus will respond as will a container with additional air added under pressure. This can case severe pain as the diver returns to the surface.

Another important air space in the diver's body is the middle ear. As the scuba diver descends, the pressure on either side of the tympanic membrane (eardrum) equalizes through the eustachian tube in the throat and the external canal of the ear that opens to the outside. The problem that occurred in the sinuses can occur with the middle ear. If the diver has a cold or allergies, he or she may have blocked eustachian tubes and thus be unable to move air into the middle ear space as the pressure increases. The difference in the two pressures is most apparent on the tympanic membrane. The eardrum has a limited ability to stretch and can easily be ruptured. If this happens, water will rush into the middle ear, causing a disruption in the equilibrium or balance of the individual. To the scuba diver this can be painful and, at worst, deadly.

These same types of "squeeze injuries" can occur to the diver who does not equalize the pressure inside the mask. As the diver descends, the increased pressure from the water will increase the pressure on the outside of the mask and can, if enough pressure is exerted, cause rupture of small vessels on the diver's face. If the diver has a filling in a tooth that has air trapped in it, the increased pressure from the descent can create pain in that tooth.

Emergency care for these types of injuries generally consists of supportive care and, in the case of a sinus squeeze with hemorrhage, protecting the airway.

> ✓ A scuba diver who has a cold or allergies resulting in congestion of the sinuses or eustachian tubes is at increased risk for a squeeze injury, resulting in significant pain or hemorrhage.

Barotrauma Injuries Occurring During Ascent

The opposite force occurs during ascent as pressure is reduced on the body and air expands. Under normal circumstances, it is harder to get air into a space, such as a sinus, than it is to get it to release, provided the connecting passageways are open. Therefore most divers experience few, if any, problems with air spaces during ascents.

The two main areas that may be involved in an **ascent injury** are the sinuses and the lungs. The problem with a sinus, as described previously, is with expanding air or fluids that are trapped and cause pressure and pain. The EMT would be called as a result of the pain and bleeding that can occur. Treatment for this patient is primarily supportive in nature and referral to a physician.

The biggest issue for the scuba diver is a lung expansion injury during ascent. While a diver is descending, the increasing pressure will cause the air to become compressed (more dense) and occupy less space. During ascent, air in the lungs will expand as pressure is decreased.

As long as the diver is breathing normally, allows the glottis to remain open, and makes a controlled ascent, air will escape during expiration and the diver's lungs will be protected. However, if the diver makes an uncontrolled ascent in which the diver either holds his or her breath or ascends too quickly, lung expansion injuries will occur. These injuries are similar to thoracic trauma, pneumothorax, hemothorax, pneumomediastinum, subcutaneous emphysema, and air embolism and are treated the same way (Figure 41.5).

Because pressure increases by a greater percentage as the diver nears the surface, barotrauma frequently occurs near the surface. From 0 to 33 feet of water the pressure has doubled (1 atm to 2 atm). The reverse occurs while descending; the bubble size doubles between 33 and 0 feet. This is the same change that has occurred from 99 to 33 feet (4 atm to 2 atm)

Emergency care for these individuals is the same as would be delivered if the injury were from a traumatic incident, such as a motor vehicle collision. Attention is directed toward maintaining an open airway, supporting ventilation, and treating for shock. The major difference is that these injuries have occurred while the patient was using scuba equipment; therefore the patient should be transported to a facility that is prepared to treat diving-related injuries.

Secondary Effects of Pressure on Scuba Divers

Two more subtle effects that can occur to divers are carbon monoxide poisoning and decompression sickness, more commonly known as the bends.

Carbon Monoxide Poisoning

Carbon monoxide poisoning in scuba divers, as in other patients, occurs because the diver is breathing air that is contaminated with the by-products of fossil fuel burning. It becomes worse in scuba divers because the air that he or she breathes in is compressed. This contamination is a result of the dive shop filling the diving tanks with exhaust gases from their compressor. Precautions should be taken so that clean air is not mixed with such gases. This most commonly occurs because the exhaust gases are vented too close to the fresh air intake. The other way contamination occurs is because the compressor has been improperly maintained, as could occur if the oil is not changed on a scheduled basis and becomes too hot, or the air filtration system becomes contaminated, resulting in carbon monoxide being pumped into the scuba diver's tanks.

Carbon monoxide, in and of itself, is dangerous and life threatening to any individual, but particularly so to scuba divers because they are underwater, may not recognize the effects early enough to return to the surface, and may drown. Although carbon monoxide itself is tasteless and odorless, the air that is contaminated with it tends to taste and smell oily or foul. If a diver's signs and symptoms appear to be related to carbon monoxide poisoning, ask if the air in the tank tasted or smelled different. Also, if possible, take the tank so the air can be tested.

Good diving shops do not have this problem very often. The diving industry is very sensitive to providing "good air"; however, there are unlicensed operations that will fill tanks cheaply and sell to those who are not certified divers. It is for this reason that the EMT must keep the carbon monoxide problem in mind.

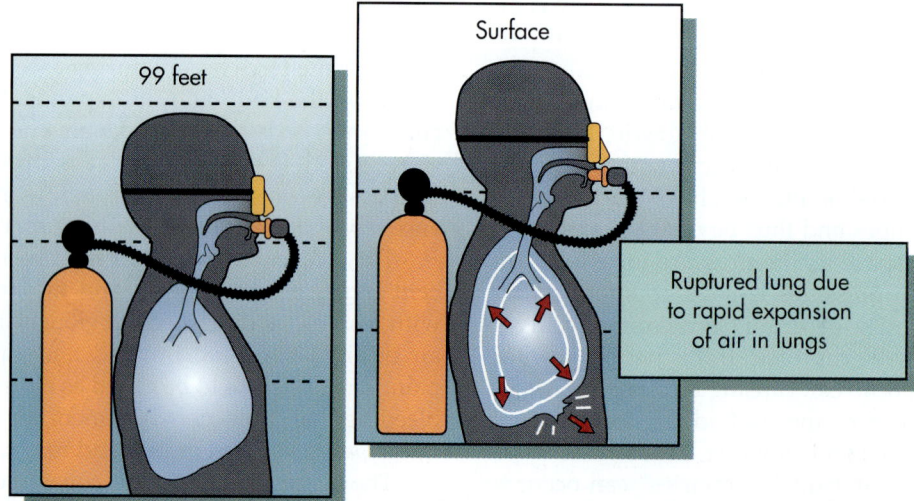

FIGURE 41.5 The diver who holds his or her breath after pressurization at depth will experience expansion of the gas contained in the lungs, which can cause the lungs to rupture.

> ✓ Carbon monoxide poisoning and decompression sickness are both secondary effects of using compressed air for scuba divers. However, they must not be considered less serious than primary effects of pressure on divers, because they can both be life threatening if not recognized and properly treated.

Decompression Sickness

Another major threat to scuba divers is that of **decompression sickness,** or *the bends* as it is commonly known. Nitrogen is an inert gas, moving freely into and out of our bodies at a one-to-one ratio. Imbalance in nitrogen concentration occurs when pressure is increased and more of the gas is driven into the tissues. The deeper a scuba diver descends, the greater the amount of nitrogen absorbed by various tissues of the body. If a diver remains at depth too long, his or her body tissues will become saturated with nitrogen and will not be able to off-load the gas during ascent at a fast enough rate. As a result, the nitrogen, which is in solution in the bloodstream, will begin to form bubbles as the pressure is reduced. These nitrogen bubbles are what cause decompression sickness. The bubbles will travel through the body, in the bloodstream, until they become lodged in a smaller vessel and stop blood flow.

Signs and symptoms of decompression sickness include skin rash, fatigue, and joint pain, particularly the shoulders and hips in the early stages. Paralysis and unconsciousness can occur in more serious cases (Box 41.1).

The depth and time of the dive is important to obtain in the history of the event to arrange transport to an appropriate facility with a hyperbaric compression chamber. Recompression of the diver is the only treatment for decompression sickness. It is not correct to attempt to treat a diver with decompression sickness by placing the diver back into the water and returning him or her to depth. The diver will not have enough air to remain in the water for the several hours that it would take to off-load the nitrogen, and it would place the diver at risk for other serious injury, such as hypothermia. Treatment should consist of maintaining an open airway, administering high-flow oxygen, and putting the patient in the left lateral recumbent position, if possible. This will help prevent a nitrogen bubble from being pumped though the heart and possibly causing a stroke.

Pathophysiology

If the patient has been breathing underwater at any time, it is possible that he or she could suffer from diving **barotrauma.** Gas embolism can occur in depths as shallow as 2 to 4 feet of sea water (fsw) (70 mm Hg). Even an experienced diver can suffer injury because of inherent respiratory medical problems. Asthma, broncholithiasis, congenital or acquired cysts, emphysema, fibrosis, tuberculosis, and infection (especially fungal or obstructive lung diseases) may result in trapped air that will expand on ascent to surface pressure. This expansion of trapped air may be sufficient to rupture air spaces. The escaping air may cause air to be trapped in the skin or mediastinum; a pneumothorax; or an arterial gas embolism.

Decompression sickness, in most presentations, is less serious with regard to immediate life-threatening consequences of the injury. Decompression sickness is caused by improper or incomplete decompression following exposure to depths usually deeper than 30 fsw. Do not rule out decompression sickness because a diver was within the safe limits of the dive tables or diving computer. Some studies of diving data have shown that as many as 70% of decompression sickness presentations were in divers who were well within "safe" limits.

In 1986, Rutkowski originally coined the catch-all phrase "bubble trouble" to denote the unspecified variances of pressure-related injuries. These can happen to anyone exposed to the hyperbaric environment far out to sea, as well as in home swimming pools, lakes, harbors, canals, water drainage pipes, and submerged cars. To ensure a successful treatment, dive instructors and dive masters, EMTs, rescue personnel, physicians, and emergency department staff must be able to recognize the problem, begin diving accident treatment procedures, and move the victim into the hyperbaric recompression system as soon as possible.

In the presence of a medical emergency exhibiting signs resembling those of a diving accident, there is one primary question: "Did the subject breathe underwater?" If the answer is "Yes," the subject is a diving accident victim, especially in the case of unconsciousness, until proven otherwise.

Box 41.1 Decompression Sickness

1. Types
    a. Type I—pain only
    b. Type II—neurologic symptoms
2. Decompression sickness may take several hours to manifest signs and symptoms that the diver will recognize or accept are present.
3. Decompression sickness is related to effect of nitrogen on the tissues.

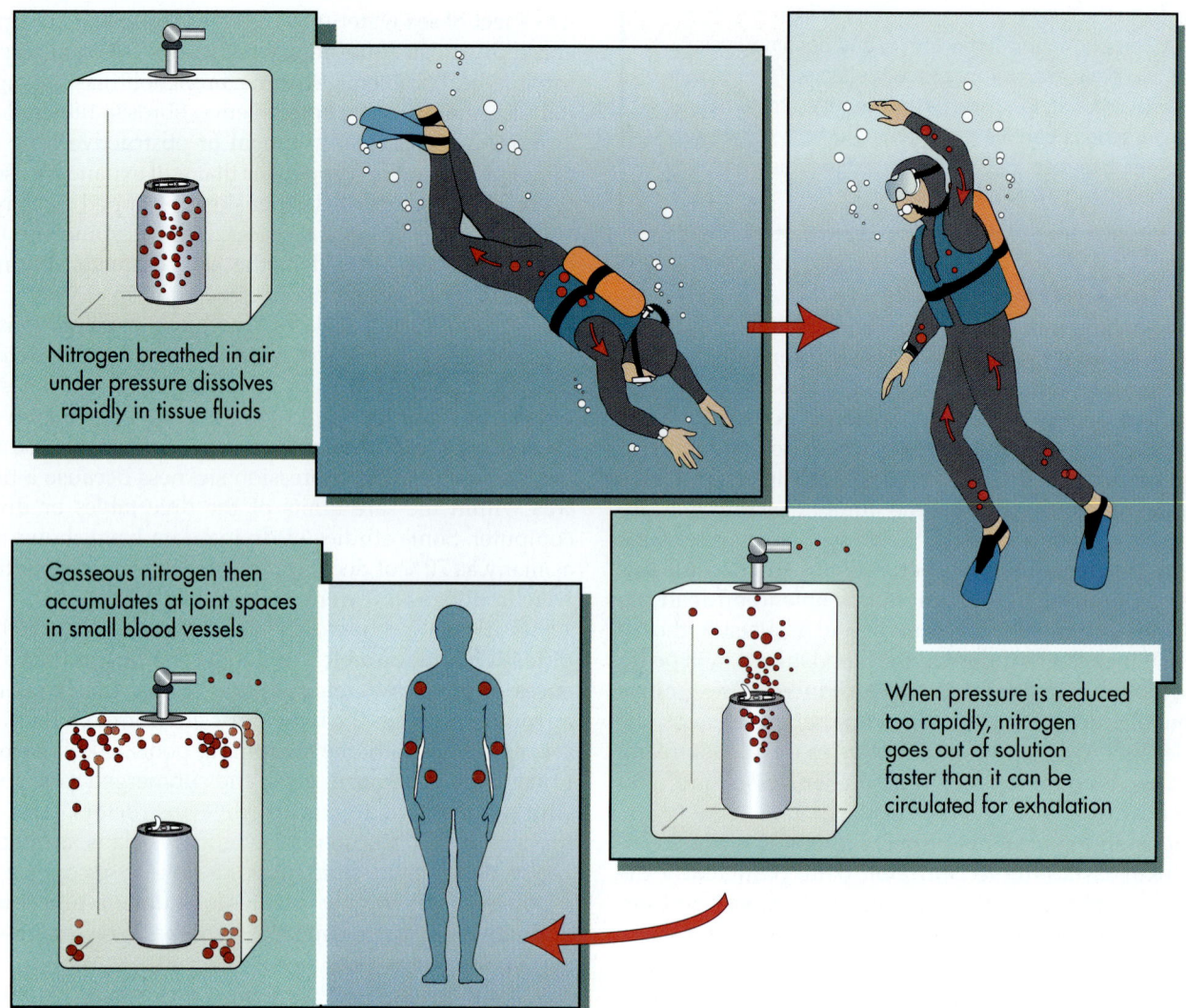

FIGURE 41.6 Air is forced into the tissue under pressure, oxygen comes out rapidly, and nitrogen comes out much more slowly. If ascent is too rapid, the nitrogen comes out of solution into the tissue space and blocks small blood vessels or expands into bones or joints producing pain.

Gas Embolism

As the diver surfaces, the gas trapped in the lungs expands, rupturing the alveoli. Bubbles of gas are forced into the circulatory system, travel to the heart, and are distributed to the body tissues. Because the ascending diver is normally in a vertical position, these bubbles tend to travel upward to the brain. As the bubbles enlarge and pass into smaller arteries, they reach a point where they can move no further, and cut off circulation (Figure 41.6). The effects of halting circulation, especially to the brain, are serious and require immediate treatment. Symptoms of embolism occur within 3 to 5 minutes of surfacing in most cases (Box 41.2).

Decompression Sickness

In a nutshell, improper decompression resulting in occlusive inert gas bubble formation is probably the major culprit in decompression sickness. Although some would argue to the contrary, most experts generally agree that *all* dives are decompression dives. Even those without stage decompression obligations have ascent rates factored into their model as a means of decompression. Divers should routinely practice slow ascents in the last 2 atm, 66 fsw (20 m), to the surface in conjunction with a recommended 5-minute "safety stop" around the 10 to 15 fsw (3.03 to 4.5 m) level.

A detailed treatment of the pathophysiology of decompression sickness is available in most standard diving texts, so only a brief review is offered in this section. The primary concern is with divers and EMTs being able to recognize symptomatology effectively and react accordingly. Those with a desire to delve deeper into the mechanisms of decompression sickness are encouraged to access these separate materials.

At the surface, the body is basically saturated with nitrogen at 1 atm. As the diver descends, pressure increases and nitrogen is dissolved and absorbed by the body's tissues and blood. The deeper the dive, the more nitrogen is "loaded." Theoretically, after a period of time (based on the longest half-time used in the model) at any given depth, be it 60 fsw (18.2 m) or 600 fsw (181.8 m), the body is saturated with all the nitrogen it can hold, and no further decompression obligation would be incurred no matter how long a diver stayed down. This is the basis of "saturation diving" theory in which aquanauts are placed underwater in a bell or habitat to work for as much as a week or more and then decompressed when the project is finished.

Untethered free-swimming divers do not have the luxury of saturation support equipment and must come back to the surface. Herein lies the problem with the nitrogen being absorbed during the brief, by comparison, sojourn into the deep.

It was originally thought that dive tables would serve the purpose of preventing bubble formation in the blood as pressure was decreased on ascent. Haldane and other pioneers in decompression sickness originally thought that no bubbles would form if their decompression models were followed. Through the use of modern Doppler devices, it is now known that bubbles may exist on every dive. Such scanning is frequently employed to monitor divers during test criteria for new table development and as a benchmark of decompression stress. Concern with inert gas bubbles, not air bubbles, is the problem in lung overexpansion accidents typical of breath-holding ascents. The size and location of these bubbles dictates the presentation of decompression sickness symptoms.

Assessment

Other texts divide decompression sickness symptomatology into type I (pain only) or type II (serious symptoms, central nervous system involvement) (Box 41.3). To the diver in the field or the EMT, this distinction is not of great importance and requires special training in many instances to classify presentations. More important is the ability to be able to recognize any symptoms or signs of decompression sickness and leave diagnosis and treatment selection to trained chamber staff or medical consultants. All observations recorded by the EMT will be of significant aid to and ultimate hope of recovery.

> **Box 41.2 Signs and Symptoms of Gas Embolism**
>
> **Symptoms**
> Fatigue
> Weakness
> Dizziness
> Paralysis of extremities or face
> Visual disturbances such as blurring
> Feeling of blow on chest, progressively worsening
> Cough or shortness of breath
>
> **Signs**
> Sudden unconsciousness (usually immediately before or after surfacing)
> Bloody, frothy sputum
> Staggering
> Confusion or difficulty in seeing (e.g., moving in wrong direction, bumping into objects, uneven gait)
> Paralysis or weakness
> Collapse or unconsciousness
> Convulsions
> Cessation of breathing

One of the most frustrating aspects of sport divers and decompression sickness is sport divers' stubborn denial of symptoms and failure to accept early treatment. This denial has historically led to the majority of sport diver incidents being unnecessarily delayed for treatment. Even divers who knew beyond a doubt that they were at risk from their profile, and even divers with early onset of symptoms, have refused oxygen that was readily available. This denial is often due to some perceived ego threat or for fear that fellow divers would think less of them. Others refuse to accept the possibility that decompression sickness could be involved, thinking, "I can't be bent, I was within the limits of the tables."

Early recognition, reporting, and treatment of decompression sickness dramatically improves patient outcome.

> ✓ Barotrauma events such as decompression sickness and embolism are of first priority. Although both can be treated in part by aggressive administration of 100% oxygen, the need for recompression is vital. The speed with which the patient can be pressurized will often determine prognosis for full resolution and recovery.

Box 41.3 Decompression Sickness Symptomatology

Type I (pain only, mild symptoms)
"Skin bends"—skin blotching or mottling of the skin producing a red or purplish-blue tinge

Itching similar to fiberglass irritation

Fatigue

Indifference, personality or mood swings, irritable behavior, diver unaware of surroundings

Pain usually in or near a joint such as shoulder or knee; onset may be gradual and pain transient

Type II (CNS involvement)
CNS spinal and cranial abnormalities, usually gradual in onset with initial subtle symptoms often masked by pain distractions

Cardiopulmonary symptoms typically manifested by "chokes," a dry, persistent nonproductive cough; cerebral symptoms may follow; all effects in this group should be considered life threatening

Unusual fatigue

Dizziness or "staggers," vertigo

Numbness, paralysis, progressive loss of feeling in skin patches

Shortness of breath

Unconsciousness, collapse, syncope

Loss of bladder and bowel control, inability to urinate

Muscular weakness, poor grip, poor resistance to restraint of motion

Visual disturbances, inability to hear fingers rubbed close to ears

Headache

Abdominal pain or lower back pain precursor of overt spinal symptoms (may be misdiagnosed as less serious type I)

Convulsions

Any symptoms developing while still underwatrer

The prudent diver and his or her dive group should encourage prompt relation of any ailment that even remotely resembles a symptom of decompression syndrome. Divers may mistake unrelated symptoms, such as muscle strains or limb numbness due to sitting on a leg, for decompression sickness. *Always err on the side of caution.*

Five-Minute Neurologic Examination

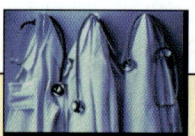

Physician Notes

Most of the time, the ambulance crew that interfaces with the patient will have a nearby hospital where the 5-minute neurologic examination can be more efficiently performed while treating the patient's condition. This examination is included in this book for those rare instances when such information must be relayed to the physician when the patient and the EMT are *not* close to the medical facility. Do NOT DELAY patient transportation to perform this examination in the field.

Examination of a victim's central nervous system soon after an accident may provide valuable information to the EMT or chamber supervisor responsible for treatment. The 5-minute neurologic examination is easily learned and performed.

The examination can be done step-by-step while reading from this text. Perform the steps in order, and record the time and results.

1. Orientation
Does the diver know name and age?
Does the diver know present location?
Does the diver know what time, day, or year it is?

Even though a diver appears alert, the answers to these questions may reveal confusion. Do *not* omit them.

2. Eyes
Have the diver count the number of fingers displayed using two or three different numbers. Check each eye separately and then together. Have the diver identify a distant object.

Tell the diver to hold his or her head still, or the EMT should gently hold the diver's head still, while placing the other hand about 18 inches in front of the face. Ask the diver to follow the EMT's hand with his or her eyes. Move the hand up and down and then side to side. The diver's eyes should smoothly follow the EMT's hand and should not jerk to one side and return. Check that pupils are equal in size.

3. Face

Ask the diver to whistle. Look carefully to see that both sides of the face have the same expression while whistling. Ask the diver to grit the teeth. Feel the jaw muscles to confirm that they are contracted equally.

Instruct the diver to close the eyes while you lightly touch your fingertips across the forehead and face to be sure sensation is present and the same everywhere.

4. Hearing

Hearing can be evaluated by holding your hand about 2 feet from the diver's ear and rubbing your thumb and finger together. Check both ears, moving your hand closer until the diver hears it. Check several times and confirm with your own hearing. If the surroundings are noisy, the test is difficult to evaluate. Ask bystanders to be quiet and turn off unneeded machinery.

5. Swallowing Reflex

Instruct the diver to swallow while you watch the Adam's apple to be sure that it moves up and down.

6. Tongue

Instruct the diver to stick out the tongue. It should come out straight in the middle of the mouth without deviating to either side.

7. Muscle Strength

Instruct the diver to shrug the shoulders while you bear down on them to observe for equal muscle strength. Check the diver's arms by bringing the elbows up level with the shoulders, hands level with the arms and touching the chest. Instruct the diver to resist while you pull the arms away, push them back, and push them up and down. The strength should be approximately equal in both arms in each direction. Check leg strength by having the diver lie flat and raise and lower the legs while you gently resist the movement.

8. Sensory Perception

Check on both sides by touching as done on the face. Start at the top of the body and compare sides while moving downward to cover the entire body. The diver's eyes should be closed during this procedure. The diver should confirm the sensation in each area before you move to another area.

9. Balance and Coordination

Be prepared to protect the diver from injury when performing this test. Have the diver stand up with feet together, close eyes, and stretch out arms. The diver should be able to maintain balance if the platform is stable. Your arms should be around but not touching the diver. Be prepared to catch the diver who starts to fall.

Check coordination by having the diver move his or her index finger back and forth rapidly between the diver's nose and your finger held approximately 18 inches from the diver's face. Instruct the diver to slide the heel of one foot down the shin of the other leg. The diver should be lying down when attempting this test. Perform these tests on both right and left sides, and observe carefully for unusual clumsiness on either side.

Although this test is important for documenting the patient's neurologic status, it should not delay transport and should not be performed if the mechanism of injury suggests a possible spinal injury. The diver's condition may prevent the performance of one or more of these tests. Record any omitted test and the reason. If any of the tests are not normal, injury to the nervous system should be suspected. The tests should be repeated at frequent intervals while awaiting assistance to determine if any change occurs. Report the results to the emergency department personnel or chamber personnel responding to your call.

Management

1. *Airway.* Check for obstruction, air exchange, dentures, foreign bodies, vomitus, and orofacial burns or trauma. Check ear canals for otitis or obstruction. Palpate the neck for subcutaneous emphysema due to pulmonary barotrauma.
2. *Breathing.* Check for stridor, retraction of accessory muscles, wheezing, or localized decreased breath sounds.
3. *Cardiac status.* Check for pulse quality, deficits, and baseline blood pressure. Palpate pulse for irregularity. Assess electrocardiogram monitoring quality.
4. *Neurologic.* Check pupils for asymmetry and reactivity. Check deep tendon reflexes and Babinski's reflex. Assess sensorium.

Stabilization checklist:

1. Stabilize the patient, including treating for shock, hydration, thermal protection, and cardiopulmonary resuscitation if necessary.
2. Immediately give the patient oxygen for surface breathing. This may be delivered via hood, nonrebreather reservoir mask, bag-valve-mask with reservoir, scuba cylinder and regulator (if properly cleaned), or standard demand/valve mask system, or by assisted ventilations. The seal should be tight to ensure the maximum level of O_2 delivered to the patient. Air leaks around the mask will dilute the percentage of O_2 inspired. Care must be taken to ensure

> **Box 41.4 Helicopter Procedures**
>
> 1. Post lookout to watch for helicopter's arrival on scene.
> 2. Attempt to establish radio communication via VHF channel 16 or 9.
> 3. Maintain vessel speed at 10 to 15 knots if possible. Pilot will count on constant speed for approach. Do not slow down or stop.
> 4. Assume a course that places vessel with the prevailing wind approximately 40 degrees on port bow. If wind is calm or insignificant, maintain course to shore.
> 5. Lower antennas, masts, flagstaffs, etc. that could interfere with helicopter's deployment of uplifting device.
> 6. Secure all loose objects and equipment on decks. Prop wash from rotor blades can be severe.
> 7. Do not touch the lift device or cable until it has touched the deck of the vessel and grounded. Electric shock can result otherwise.
> 8. Have patient and EMT wear life jackets. If available, also give patient smoke flare for day or night flare if dark. This will help find the patient if he or she falls out of the basket or if the basket is dropped. Have lookout watch patient until secure inside chopper. If patient goes into sea, follow man-overboard drill immediately. Have crew member ready to go overboard to rescue patient and establish buoyancy. Swift action and anticipation of contingencies are vital to ensure patient's survival.
> 9. Secure patient in basket (stretcher) via provided harness or tie in with sizing line, ideally with quick-release knots that patient can access if necessary.
> 10. If patient cannot communicate or is unconscious, fasten (duct tape, safety pin, etc.) as much information about his or her condition, dive profile, name, age, address, next of kin, emergency phone numbers, etc. as possible. If patient was using a computer, send it with the patient. Make note of tables used to acquire profile.
> 11. Advise or reconfirm that patient is diving victim and requires evacuation to recompression facility.
> 12. If patient goes into cardiac arrest while helicopter is en route, inform flight crew or Coast Guard operator. This may prevent a needless heroic effort at rescue by the flight crew if bad weather is a factor.

the integrity of the mask seal, especially in patients with facial hair or any patient with pronounced facial wrinkles. As a rule of thumb, the mask seal should be good enough for the patient to breathe on his or her back underwater. If a scuba regulator is used, sealing the nose with a dive mask or clip is recommended. Free-flow oxygen systems, although still widely in use, are not advisable because they do not deliver 100% O_2 and are extremely wasteful of the gas. Do not discontinue oxygen breathing even if symptoms disappear.

3. There should be sufficient oxygen available to keep the patient on this therapy during all phases of transit. A single small cylinder as provided in most emergency kits will not meet this criterion. If oxygen supplies are exhausted, consideration can be given to use of hyperoxic nitrogen-oxygen mixtures if available.

4. Until recently, patient management included positioning the diver in either Trendelenburg (head down, legs bent at knees, left side tilted down) or Scultetus (head down, legs straight) position. Beginning in 1990, this advice has been modified to suggest use of simple supine positioning (patient lies flat on back). Trendelenburg position proved to be of little efficacy except in the first 10 to 15 minutes of surfacing, primarily in arterial gas embolism cases, and the difficulty of maintaining this posture was not thought to be significantly beneficial.

5. Depending on site conditions, it may be desirable to remove the patient's wet suit or dry suit to maintain thermal core stability. In any event, see that the patient is kept warm and comfortable. Cover with blankets, towels, or dry clothing.

6. Observe and record all signs and symptoms of injury, including results of the 5-minute neurologic examination, if performed. These observations should be repeated for comparison if transit is prolonged.

7. Oral fluids should be given if the patient is conscious. Regular drinking water or unsweetened apple juice in amounts of 12 to 16 ounces every 30 minutes will keep the patient properly hydrated. This amount may (and should) require urination if transit is prolonged. Urination is a good sign and should be accommodated in the supine position. Inability to urinate may indicate more serious type II decompression sickness. Such retention will ultimately become painful. If the patient is unable to pass water within a reasonable time period, catheterization will be needed. Urine should be checked for volume and specific gravity.

If an IV has been started in the field, continue IV of normal saline or lactated Ringer's, and run at 250 ml/hr. If no IV was established, do so and administer normal saline or lactated Ringer's bolus 500 ml and run at 250 ml/hr until the patient is hydrated.

8. As a general rule, pain medications are not appropriate in the field because they may mask symptoms or progressive development of same.
9. Record dive profiles, decompression schedules, and all relevant aspects of the dive plan for transmittal to treatment professionals.
10. Confirm that the local hyperbaric facility or **recompression chamber** is functional and staffed. If in doubt, call the Divers Alert Network (DAN) at 919-648-8111 for advice and directions to the closest facility.

If at sea, call the Coast Guard via radio or cellular phone. It may be necessary to relay messages through another vessel if sufficiently offshore that the radio cannot reach the mainland. Make certain that the Coast Guard knows that this emergency is a diving accident victim and requires transportation to a recompression facility. At this point, the Coast Guard may direct the EMTs to proceed to a designated port. An evacuation helicopter to intercept and extract the diver for faster transport may be dispatched (Box 41.4).

Portable Chambers

Recent advances in lightweight, low-pressure designs have resulted in a practical portable field chamber (sometimes referred to as a "hyperbaric stretcher") that can actually be transported in two hand-carried cases easily stowed in a van or dive vessel. Weighing approximately 160 pounds for the pressure tube and control panel, this unique package allows for a patient to be placed under pressure immediately in the field, blown down to 60 fsw with a patient O₂ BIBS mask including overboard dump, and then the entire unit evacuated to a full-size field chamber or hospital-based unit. Procedure for patient transfer without decompression is simple: put the portable chamber inside the treatment chamber and remove the patient after pressures are equalized.

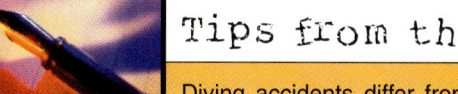

Tips from the Pros

Diving accidents differ from other aspects of emergency medicine because of the compelling need for recompression in the hyperbaric environment. Be certain that the plan for transportation includes confirmation of status and location of such facility. The patient's prognosis for recovery depends on such treatment. Needless delay would be incurred by transporting a victim to a standard hospital facility when recompression is dictated. The administration of 100% oxygen and proper hydration methods cannot be overemphasized. When in doubt, seek the medical advice of DAN's trained staff, who are on call 24 hours.

✓ Signs and symptoms of decompression sickness include skin rash, fatigue, and joint pain, particularly the shoulders and hips in the early stages. Paralysis and unconsciousness can occur in more serious cases. Transport to a facility that has a recompression chamber is critical for these patients.

Summary

- Barotrauma in scuba diving accidents is a result of changes in pressure exerted on the body. It is sometimes termed *squeeze injury*.
- Air consists of 21% oxygen, 78% nitrogen, and traces of other gases.
- Air is compressible (becomes denser and heavier); water is not.
- Increasing the external pressure on a given volume of air will result in it being compressed and becoming heavier and denser.
- Saltwater is heavier than freshwater, 34 pounds per gallon vs. 33 pounds per gallon.
- Any given volume of water, at sea level, is 800 times heavier than the same volume of air.
- A 1 inch by 1 inch column of air extending up into the earth's atmosphere exerts 14.7 psi at sea level.
- A 1 inch by 1 inch column of water that is 33 feet tall will exert 14.7 psi at sea level.
- Boyle's law states that as pressure increases, volume decreases, and as pressure decreases, volume increases.
- Dalton's law of partial pressure states that each gas produces a pressure as if it were in the container alone.
- Nitrogen under pressure is absorbed at different rates for different tissues within the body.
- Barotrauma descent injuries are most commonly associated with pressure on air spaces such as the lungs, sinuses, ears, mask, and teeth.
- Barotrauma ascent injuries are most commonly associated with expansion of air in the lungs and include pneumothorax, hemothorax, air embolism, and subcutaneous emphysema.

Summary (cont'd)

- The secondary effects of scuba diving while on compressed air include carbon monoxide poisoning and decompression sickness.
- Decompression sickness (the bends) is caused by nitrogen forming bubbles in the circulatory system and becoming lodged in smaller vessels, disrupting blood flow.
- Decompression sickness is caused by diving too deep for too long and becoming saturated with nitrogen.
- The majority of barotrauma injuries associated with scuba diving accidents can be treated as any other trauma injury similar in pathophysiology.
- The only safe treatment for a scuba diver with decompression sickness is transport to and treatment in a recompression chamber.

Scenario Solution

Because this a scuba diving–related call, you will want the communications center to immediately notify the regional trauma center that maintains a hyperbaric chamber. This is important in the event that the chamber operator must be called in or there are other patients within the facility that are treated in the chamber. Additionally, you will want to request additional assistance, if available, if you and your partner are the only medical personnel responding, due to the serious condition of the patient. If you will be using a helicopter to transport the patient to the trauma center, the trauma center will need to be given an immediate call to determine availability and warm-up time.

If you are able to obtain a direct link with the boat captain, obtain an update on the patient's condition and offer suggestions to the crew to support initial care. Additionally, you will need to have the diver's profile, how long he was in the water, and at what depth, to facilitate treatment decisions. If you do not have direct communications with the boat captain, this information will have to be obtained at the dock.

When the boat arrives you find a male subject, age 46, lying on the deck supine with oxygen being applied by mask at 10 L/min. He is unconscious and responds only to deep pain reflex, in a nonpurposeful manner. He is cool to the touch, pale in color, and covered with a blanket. The dive master states that he has been in this condition since he was pulled from the water. His brother states that he has no known medical history and that they dive twice a year. Each diver has approximately 25 dives.

The captain states that the diver was last seen at a depth of 90 feet, shortly after beginning the dive with a group of six. He had been in the water for approximately 10 minutes when his partner could not find him. The diver was observed floating on the surface, face down, by the dive master, who pulled him onto the boat. The captain states that the diver had been acting very nervous at the dock and bragging about his diving experiences. At the same time, he appeared anxious and had to be helped with the assembly of his equipment.

While you have been obtaining this information, your partner has assessed the patient and found that his airway is clear, his respiratory rate is 20 and shallow, he has diminished breath sounds on the right side, his pulse is 128 and weak, his blood pressure is 90/64, and his skin is pale. Based on the history and physical findings, you treat this patient as though he has an ascent injury, probably an air expansion. Oxygen is maintained at high flow, the patient is strapped to a backboard, confirmation of dive profile is made, and the patient is loaded into your vehicle for transport to the trauma center, which is 10 minutes away.

Key Terms

Ascent injury Injury that can occur to scuba divers as they ascend to the water surface.

Barotrauma Trauma to hollow organs or spaces in the body as a result of significant pressure difference. Sometimes called *squeeze injury.*

Decompression sickness A medical condition that can occur to scuba divers as a result of body tissues becoming saturated with nitrogen during a dive on compressed air; results in the formation of small inert gas bubbles that can block blood flow.

Descent injury Injury that can occur to a scuba diver while descending from the water surface.

Recompression chamber A specialized chamber in which a diver who is suffering from decompression sickness is placed and artificially returned to a diving depth that will force nitrogen bubbles back into solution and then be slowly removed from the bloodstream.

Scuba Self-contained underwater breathing apparatus.

Review Questions

1. One of the keys to understanding scuba diving accidents and their management is Boyle's law. This law revolves around the relationship of pressure, either air or water, and volume. Boyle's law in simple terms states that:
   a. As pressure increases, the volume of a given gas will increase.
   b. As pressure decreases, the volume of a given gas will decrease.
   c. The sum of a total pressure is equal to that of partial pressures combined.
   d. As pressure increases, the given volume of a gas will decrease.

2. Much of the discussion concerning scuba diving accidents centers around the physics of air and water pressure. In the discussion concerning this topic, the chapter identified that:
   a. Both air and water can be put under pressure and compressed to greater density.
   b. Air can be compressed and its density increased, but water cannot.
   c. Water can be compressed and its density increased, but air cannot.
   d. When compressed, the density of water and air will always be equal.

3. Scuba divers are subject to a variety of potential injuries due to the changes in pressure that are exerted on their bodies while using compressed air. Generally, injury patterns are described as either ascent or descent in nature. Divers who are descending into water are most at risk for:
   a. Decompression sickness.
   b. Expansion injuries.
   c. Compression injuries.
   d. CO_2 poisoning.

4. Scuba divers are subject to several types of expansion injuries that can occur while they are ascending to the surface. Which of the following has the greatest potential for a life-threatening injury during the ascent?
   a. Decompression sickness.
   b. Pneumothorax.
   c. Sinus squeeze.
   d. Rupture of the eardrum.

5. A scuba diver who dives to and remains at any given depth beyond a predetermined time limit is at risk for development of decompression sickness (the bends). This diving malady is a result of absorption of too much:
   a. Oxygen.
   b. Carbon monoxide.
   c. Carbon dioxide.
   d. Nitrogen.

6. The correct management of a scuba diver with signs and symptoms of decompression sickness would include:
   a. Returning the diver to the water immediately, and remaining at a depth of 60 feet for 2 hours.
   b. Placing the patient in the left lateral recumbent position, if possible; administering high-flow oxygen; and transporting to a facility that has a recompression chamber.
   c. Having the diver vigorously exercise to force the gas from the tissues in order to off-load the residual effects.
   d. Having the diver rest for a period of 6 hours while breathing oxygen and receiving IV fluid therapy.

Answers to these Review Questions can be found at the end of the book on page 869.

42

Military EMS

Lesson Goal

The first goal of this chapter is to define patient care during combat situations. Protection, speed, hazards of transportation, and delay in transportation produce a different set of variables than most civilian situations. The corpsman must take these conditions into consideration as priorities are established and the types of patient care are defined. The second goal of this chapter is to describe the differences between civilian and military medicine so that the student who works in both areas can understand the two philosophies and adapt easily to both. The third goal of this chapter is to provide an understanding of biologic warfare agents and their effects in military and civilian situations.

Scenario

A 24-person special operations forces (SOF) team is ordered to raid a cocaine laboratory in South America. The cocaine lab is located in a dense jungle area protected by an estimated hostile strength of 15 men with automatic weapons. Insertion will be accomplished by a riverine craft approximately 6 kilometers from the target. As the patrol reaches the target area, a booby trap is tripped, injuring the point man (no pulse or respiration) and the patrol leader (massive trauma to the leg with femoral arterial bleeding). There is heavy incoming direct and indirect fire as the lab security force responds to the explosive blast. The planned extraction of the SOF team is by boat, 1 kilometer from the target area.

? As the medic accompanying the SOF team, how would you triage the patients identified in this scenario with regard to treatment and order of evacuation? What additional information would be helpful in making medical management decisions at this point? Are there any barriers to proper patient management at the scene? How can you work around these barriers? Outline the steps you would take to manage these patients.

Key Terms to Know

Biologic warfare agents	Combat lifesaver program	SWIMS	Weapons of mass destruction
Casevac	Medevac	Triage	

Learning Objectives

As an EMT-Basic, you should be able to do the following:

Supplemental

- Define and describe military echelons of care.
- Identify potential threats in a tactical combat situation.
- Identify the stages of care associated with battlefield assessment.
- Describe the threats from biologic and chemical weapons.
- Compare and contrast military and civilian mass casualty situations and the conduct of patient triage in these two scenarios.

Editor's Note

This chapter was originally titled "Unconventional Prehospital Care." The title has been changed to "Military EMS," which more accurately describes the intent of the chapter. It provides the basis for the military medic taking the first EMT-B course to understand the differences between the two systems in which he or she must function.

This chapter describes the care given in a very specialized condition—combat. The methods by which care is provided in combat are different. There are patients in conditions that require special access and a different type of care by the EMTs who are there to serve them.

The information contained in this chapter is not a substitute for the National Standard Curriculum objectives. It is in addition to that material to meet the needs of those who are or may be in combat situations.

Why not just refer the civilian EMT or the military corpsman to the published works on the subject of combat care? The reasons for that and the objectives for the inclusion in this book are as follows:

1. The type of EMS practiced in the military is different for several reasons:
   a. It is highly regimented, as the military must be to function in a dangerous, stressful environment.
   b. The situations that exist in combat do not usually exist in the civilian environment in the United States.
   c. There are needs for patient care that are different under combat situations.

2. As much as we do not want to think about it, there may come a day when a situation will arise in any of our communities that combat conditions will exist and civilian and military medics will have to function side by side. We each need to know how the other thinks.

3. Many of the military medics will practice in a civilian environment working with a civilian EMS. Therefore they must be trained first to function as a conventional EMT. Many will use this textbook for that knowledge. Most if not all are certified by the National Registry of EMTs in these skills and knowledge.

4. In addition to the basic EMT knowledge and skills these military medics will need to know, there are different skills and knowledge that are required in combat. This chapter provides some of that information. It also explains why two different skill sets are needed and why the civilian skill set may not work in combat.

For those who will read this chapter and never use it, it makes for interesting and thought-provoking reading. For those who may enter situations in which the information is required, the authors of this chapter and the editors of this textbook hope that the information is both useful and important.

James Paturas, NREMT-P
Norman McSwain, MD, Capt, MC, USNR (Ret)

Military and civilian health care agencies are increasingly involved in cooperative efforts to provide relief operations in natural or man-made disasters such as hurricanes, floods, earthquakes, chemical spills, and terrorist incidents. Civil-military interoperability has become critical, and the two communities can learn from and complement each other as we continue to fine-tune our emergency response skills. Both need to know how the other operates and thinks.

Military medicine differs from routine civilian care in several areas and poses unique challenges to the health care provider, from first responder to definitive care. This is particularly true in a tactical situation where significant differences exist between civilian emergency response and military requirements on a battlefield (Table 42.1). The gap between battlefield trauma management and civilian responders is diminishing, however, as the threat of a terrorist attack grows worldwide. Conventional explosive devices and weapons of mass destruction (chemical, biologic, and nuclear) make the civilian population vulnerable to mass casualty situations traditionally faced only by those in combat. Tactical-type situations are becoming more common as well, and civilian emergency medical service (EMS) personnel may be responding to such emergencies at the local level. One of the main priorities will be to respond in a manner that maintains EMS safety and minimizes injury to others, just as in any other EMS response. If faced with a mass casualty triage situation and limited resources, recognize those limitations and work to save the maximum number of victims. Understanding tactical concepts will prove valuable to military and civilian providers alike. Civilian emergency medical technicians (EMTs) may never have to use what is presented here, but if such a situation happens these basic concepts make the difference for the survival of both the EMS personnel and the patients.

The majority of combat-related deaths occur near the site of injury before the casualty reaches an established medical treatment facility (MTF). Highly trained nonphysicians provide health care at or near the front lines, and patients are transported to various levels of facilities for further care. Combat medics have a scope of practice beyond that of their civilian counterparts. Basic first aid is the starting point, but modifications and ingenuity are expected and acceptable when applying basic protocols in a hostile situation. The restrictive environment of the battlefield significantly influences patient care decisions.

Mission accomplishment may have a higher priority than immediate evacuation, an apparent conflict with generally accepted patient care standards. Immediate evacuation may not even be an option, and long-term supportive care may be required. Lessons learned in combat can be extended into civilian practice.

Military Echelons (Levels) of Care

Medical assets of the U.S. military are organized into five increasingly sophisticated levels of care. Each echelon builds on the capabilities of the previous level and adds additional services. Echelons extend from the point of wounding, illness, or injury (usually at the lowest level) and provide a continuum of care. Military medical doctrine is evolving from a fixed-facility concept to a more fluid system in order to improve survivability of wounded soldiers. Advanced capabilities are being moved further forward with the idea of balancing maximal care and required mobility.

Echelon of Care I

Echelon I is care at the unit level, accomplished by individual soldiers or a trained medic or corpsman. Military personnel are taught basic first aid on entry into the service. The United States Army augments this capability with the **combat lifesaver program,** which instructs nonmedical personnel in skills beyond basic first aid. Echelon I also includes mobile aid stations, staffed by medical technicians and a physician or a physician assistant, that move with the units they support. These stations function out of small tents or vehicles (such as armored personnel carriers, when in a mechanized unit). Care at this level includes basic airway management, including intubation, restoration of an airway by surgical procedure, administration of intravenous fluids and antibiotics, and stabilization of wounds and fractures. The goal of medical management at echelon I is to return the patient to duty or to stabilize the patient for evacuation to the next appropriate level.

Echelon of Care II

Echelon II involves a team of physicians, physician assistants, nurses, and medical technicians capable of basic resuscitation, stabilization, and surgery along with x-ray, pharmacy, and temporary holding facilities. Many eche-

TABLE 42.1 Differences Between Civilian and Military First Response

Civilian	Military
Patients are usually limited in number, and medical resources are not overwhelmed.	Large number of injuries can quickly overwhelm available resources.
Patients are located in secure areas.	Patients are located in nonsecure areas.
EMT access to supplies and advice is available.	There are limited supplies and an isolated provider.
The prehospital phase is short.	The prehospital phase may be extended.
Evacuation times to definitive care are generally short.	Evacuations may be delayed.

lon II facilities have limited laboratories, and this is the first level of care that has transfusion capabilities (group O liquid packed red blood cells). Surgical procedures are limited to emergency procedures to prevent death, loss of limb, or loss of bodily function. Echelon II may be augmented by specialized surgical support teams capable of more extensive procedures, but this varies among the services.

Like echelon I facilities, echelon II units must be small and mobile. Size is determined by the predicted number and type of casualties during an operation based on previous experience and an analysis of the enemy threat. One example of an echelon II unit is the United States Air Force 10-bed facility. It has 51 personnel assigned in support of 10 holding beds and one operating room, with enough supplies to perform 50 major surgical cases. Ground or air evacuation is available to transfer patients to more capable treatment facilities as required.

Echelon of Care III

Echelon III facilities have capabilities normally found in fixed MTFs and are located in lower-threat environments. The goal at echelon III is restoration of functional health and includes resuscitation, initial or delayed wound surgery, and postoperative management. More extensive services such as laboratory, x-ray, and pharmacy are available, along with a full range of blood products. Care proceeds with greater preparation and deliberation.

Echelon of Care IV

Echelon IV further expands on the capabilities of the echelon III facility by providing definitive therapy within a theater of operations for patients who can be returned to duty within a set time. Theater evacuation policy (the amount of time a casualty can remain in theater) is dependent on the enemy threat, type of mission, size of the force, airframe availability, and bed occupancy and availability. If the patient cannot be returned to duty within the specified time, evacuation is required, usually to the continental United States. Definitive care in an echelon IV facility is normally provided by a fleet hospital ship, a general hospital, or an overseas MTF.

Echelon of Care V

Convalescent, restorative, and rehabilitative care is provided at echelon V. This care is provided by military hospitals, Department of Veteran Affairs (VA) hospitals, or civilian hospitals located in the United States.

Comparison of Military and Civilian Systems of Care

The military system of echeloned medical care may be compared to the civilian trauma system. The integrated trauma system, when examined in parts, closely matches the military system. Echelon I is comparable to care rendered by paramedics and civilian critical care helicopter units. Echelon II facilities are comparable to the resuscitation areas in level I trauma centers. Echelons III and IV provide the restorative surgery and medical care provided in acute and intermediate trauma center wards. Echelon V units provide the rehabilitative and support services that are offered in the follow-up phase of care in truly integrated trauma systems.

Echelon Coordination

Military medical units tend to be small and geographically separated; close coordination is required to make the system work. Central control of patient movement within and out of the theater is critical and relies on good communications, visibility of casualty flow through all facilities in theater (to minimize overload of any one facility), and the availability and control of evacuation assets. Proper triage is aimed at minimizing stress at any one level by ensuring that workloads are appropriate for the level of care, degree of specialization, and resources. Stable patients, even with serious wounds, may bypass intermediate echelons and be sent directly to definitive care if the transport time is short or if the intermediate echelon is overloaded.

Emergent Care in the Tactical Environment

Tactical Combat Casualty Care— General Considerations

Ninety percent of those who die from wounds sustained in combat do so on the battlefield before ever reaching an MTF.[1] Trauma management training for military corpsmen and medics is critical. Recognized principles taught in such courses as Advanced Trauma Life Support (ATLS), Prehospital Trauma Life Support (PHTLS), and Basic Trauma Life Support (BTLS) provide well-thought-out, standardized approaches to the management of trauma that have proven successful at various stages of trauma care. The same principles are used in a tactical setting but must be applied differently because of differences between combat and noncombat situations.[2-13]

The combat setting is complicated by such factors as darkness, hostile fire, medical equipment limitations, prolonged evacuation times, limited provider experience levels, mission-related command decisions, hostile environments (aquatic, mountain, desert, and jungle settings), and the unique problems entailed in transporting casualties on the battlefield. Casualty care guidelines for combat medics will therefore differ from those of their civilian counterparts. Military as well as civilian organizations have developed recommendations for the care of trauma patients and other medical emergencies that take into account the special conditions encountered by their membership.[13,14]

Stages of Care

It is useful to consider the management of casualties that occur during combat missions as being divided into several distinct phases of care.[13] This approach is essential for combat trauma, because guidelines for combat medics and corpsmen must consider not only the appropriate elements of treatment but the appropriate time in the continuum of care from battlefield to hospital facility to render that care.

1. *Care under fire* is the care rendered by the medic or corpsman at the scene of the injury while both the caregiver and the casualty are still under effective hostile fire. The risk of additional injuries being sustained at any moment is extremely high for both casualty and rescuer. Available medical equipment is limited to that carried by each operator on the mission or by the medical personnel in their medical packs.
2. *Tactical field care* is the care rendered by the medic or corpsman once he and the casualty are no longer under effective hostile fire. It also applies to situations in which an injury has occurred on a mission, but there has been no hostile fire. Medical equipment is still limited to that carried into the field by mission personnel. Time before evacuation may range from a few minutes to many hours.
3. *Combat casualty evacuation care* is rendered once the casualty has been picked up by an aircraft, vehicle, or boat for transportation to a higher echelon. Additional personnel and medical equipment that have been prestaged in these assets should be available during this phase of casualty management. The term **casevac** should be used to describe this phase instead of the commonly encountered term **medevac**

because the Air Force reserves the term *medevac* to describe a noncombat medical transport.

Basic Tactical Combat Casualty Care Plan

Having defined these three phases of casualty management in the tactical setting, the next step is to outline care that is appropriate to each phase. A basic tactical casualty management plan is presented in Boxes 42.1 through 42.3.[13] This management plan is a generic sequence of steps that often requires modification for specific casualty scenarios. The basic plan is important, however, as a starting point from which development of individualized scenario-based management plans may begin. A detailed rationale for the steps outlined in the basic management plan for each of these stages of care has been presented.[13] In general, basic EMT principles and treatment methods may be followed unless specific combat considerations are believed to justify a departure. A few of the major differences between this recommended combat casualty care plan and EMT standards will be reviewed here and the reasons for these differences discussed.

Care Under Fire

A minimum of medical care should be attempted while the casualty and provider are actually under effective hostile fire. This is reflected in the recommended care shown in Box 42.1. Suppression of hostile fire and moving the casualty to a position where adequate cover allows more complete evaluation and treatment are major considerations. Significant delays for detailed examination or in-depth treatment of the patient's wounds are ill-advised while under effective hostile fire. It may be criti-

---

Box 42.1 Basic Tactical Combat Casualty Management Plan—Phase One: Care Under Fire

1. Return fire as directed or required.
2. Try to keep yourself from getting shot.
3. Try to keep the casualty from sustaining additional wounds.
4. Airway management is generally best deferred until the tactical field care phase.
5. Stop any life-threatening external hemorrhage using necessary means.
6. Take the casualty with you when you leave.

cal for the combat medic or corpsman to help suppress the hostile fire before attempting to provide care at all, especially in small-unit operations where friendly firepower is limited and each person is essential to the successful outcome of an engagement. If hostile fire is not effectively suppressed, there is a need to move the casualty to cover. Management of the airway is temporarily deferred because this movement will entail the rescuer carrying or dragging the casualty for some distance, during which time airway management will be difficult or impossible.

The temporary use of a tourniquet to manage life-threatening extremity hemorrhage in this phase may be required. Hemorrhage from extremity wounds is the number one cause of preventable death on the battlefield and was responsible for the deaths of more than 2500 casualties in Vietnam who had no other major injuries.[15] Use of direct pressure or compression dressings may result in delays in getting the casualty to cover, exposing both casualty and rescuer to increased hazard and additional injury. They are less effective than a tourniquet at stopping the bleeding during the initial combat rescue in which the casualty may have to be dragged or carried to cover by the rescuer. Treatment of non–life-threatening bleeding should be deferred until the patient is moved to cover or effective hostile fire is suppressed.

The usual requirement of immobilizing the cervical spine before moving a casualty with a penetrating neck or head wound does not apply when moving the casualty out of a firefight. In less than 2% of patients with penetrating neck injuries in Vietnam would immobilization of the cervical spine have been of possible benefit.[10] The risk of additional injuries to both casualty and rescuer during attempted immobilization poses a much greater threat in this setting than that of damage to the spinal cord from failure to immobilize the cervical spine.[10]

Tactical Field Care

Recommended guidelines for this phase of care are shown in Box 42.2. Attempts at cardiopulmonary resuscitation are not appropriate for most blast or penetrating trauma patients found in arrest on the battlefield.[13] Prehospital resuscitation of trauma patients in cardiac arrest has been found to be futile even in the urban setting where the victim is in close proximity to trauma centers. Resuscitation of trauma victims in cardiopulmonary arrest should not be attempted unless the arrest is secondary to an immediately manageable airway injury. In the tactical combat setting, the cost of attempting to resuscitate patients in full arrest will be measured in additional lives lost. Combat medical personnel will be exposed to hostile fire during resuscitation efforts and care is withheld from casualties with potentially survivable wounds. Successful completion of the unit's mission

---

Box 42.2 Basic Tactical Combat Casualty Management Plan—Phase Two: Tactical Field Care

1. Airway management:
   - Chin-lift or jaw-thrust.
   - Unconscious casualty without airway obstruction: nasopharyngeal airway.
   - Unconscious casualty with airway obstruction: cricothyroidotomy.
   - Cervical spine immobilization is not efficient for casualties with penetrating head or neck trauma.
2. Breathing:
   - Consider tension pneumothorax and decompress if a casualty has unilateral penetrating chest trauma and progressive respiratory distress.
3. Bleeding:
   - Control any remaining bleeding using necessary means.
4. IV:
   - Start an 18-gauge IV or saline lock.
5. Fluid resuscitation:
   - Controlled hemorrhage without shock: no fluids necessary.
   - Controlled hemorrhage with shock: Hespan 1000 ml if available; otherwise lactated Ringer's 2000 ml.
   - Uncontrolled (intraabdominal or thoracic) hemorrhage: no IV fluid resuscitation.
6. Inspect and dress wound.
7. Check for additional wounds.
8. Analgesia as necessary:
   - 5 mg IV of morphine.
   - Wait 10 minutes.
   - Repeat as necessary.
9. Splint fractures and recheck pulse.
10. Antibiotics:
    - 2 g slow IV push (over 3 to 5 minutes) of cefoxitin for penetrating abdominal trauma, massive soft tissue damage, open fractures, grossly contaminated wounds, or long delays before casualty evacuation.
11. Cardiopulmonary resuscitation:
    - Resuscitation on the battlefield for victims of blast or penetrating trauma who have no pulse, no respirations, and no other signs of life will not be successful and should not be attempted.

> **Box 42.3** Basic Tactical Combat Casualty Management Plan—Phase Three: Combat Casualty Evacuation (Casevac) Care
>
> 1. Airway management:
>   - Chin-lift or jaw-thrust.
>   - Unconscious casualty without airway obstruction: nasopharyngeal airway, endotracheal intubation, combitube, or laryngeal mask airway.
>   - Unconscious casualty with airway obstruction: cricothyroidotomy if endotracheal intubation or other airway devices are unsuccessful.
> 2. Breathing:
>   - Consider tension pneumothorax and decompress with needle thoracostomy if a casualty has unilateral penetrating chest trauma and progressive respiratory distress.
>   - Consider chest tube insertion for all penetrating chest trauma.
>   - Oxygen.
> 3. Bleeding:
>   - Consider removing tourniquets and using direct pressure to control bleeding if possible.
> 4. IV:
>   - Start an 18-gauge IV or heparin lock if not already done.
> 5. Fluid resuscitation:
>   - No hemorrhage or controlled hemorrhage without shock: lactated Ringer's at 250 ml/hr.
>   - Controlled hemorrhage with shock: Hespan 1000 ml initially if available; otherwise lactated Ringer's 2000 ml.
>   - Uncontrolled (intraabdominal or thoracic) hemorrhage: no IV fluid resuscitation.
>   - Head wound patient: Hespan at minimal flow to maintain infusion unless there is concurrent controlled hemorrhagic shock.
> 6. Monitoring:
>   - Institute electronic monitoring of heart rate, blood pressure, and hemoglobin oxygen saturation.
> 7. Inspect and dress wound if not already done.
> 8. Check for additional wounds.
> 9. Analgesia as necessary:
>   - 5 mg IV of morphine.
>   - Wait 10 minutes.
>   - Repeat as necessary.
> 10. Splint fractures and recheck pulse if not already done.
> 11. Antibiotics (if not already given).
>   - 2 g slow IV push (over 3 to 5 minutes) of cefoxitin for penetrating abdominal trauma, massive soft tissue damage, open fractures, grossly contaminated wounds, or long delays before casualty evacuation.

may also be jeopardized by these efforts. Only in cases of nontraumatic disorders such as hypothermia, near-drowning, or electrocution should cardiopulmonary resuscitation be considered in the tactical setting.

Unconscious casualties should have their airways opened with the chin-lift or jaw-thrust maneuvers. If spontaneous respirations are present and there is no respiratory distress, a nasopharyngeal airway is the airway of choice. The two main advantages of this device over an oropharyngeal airway are that it is better tolerated should the patient suddenly regain consciousness and it is less likely to be dislodged during transport.

Should an airway obstruction develop or persist despite the use of a nasopharyngeal airway, a more definitive airway is required. Experienced paramedical personnel can quickly insert an endotracheal tube in the field. This technique may be more problematic in the tactical environment, however, for a number of reasons:[13]

1. No studies were found that documented the ability of well-trained but relatively inexperienced paramedical military intubationists to accomplish endotracheal intubation on the battlefield.
2. Many corpsmen and medics have never performed an intubation on a live patient or even a cadaver.
3. Standard endotracheal intubation techniques entail the use of the white light in the laryngoscope, which is tactically compromising on the battlefield, primarily at night.
4. Maxillofacial injuries that cause blood and other obstructions in the airway could make endotracheal intubation more difficult.
5. Esophageal intubations would be much less likely to be recognized on the battlefield and may result in fatalities.

Endotracheal intubation has been shown to be a difficult task, even in the hands of more experienced paramedical personnel under much better conditions. First-time intubationists, trained with mannequin intubations alone, were noted to have an initial success rate of only 42% in the ideal confines of the operating room with paralyzed patients.[16] Most of the previously cited studies documenting the success of paramedical personnel in performing endotracheal intubation noted that they used cadaver training, operating room intubations, supervised initial intubations, or a combination of these methods in training their paramedics. They also stress the importance of continued practice of this skill in maintaining proficiency.

Significant airway obstruction in the combat setting is likely to result from penetrating wounds of the face or neck in which blood or disrupted anatomy precludes visualization of the vocal cords. Although not proven under combat conditions, cricothyroidotomy has been reported to be safe and effective in trauma victims, and it might be a better choice than intubation if the corpsman or medic has been trained in this procedure.[17] This procedure is not without complications,[18,19] but a prepackaged cricothyroidotomy kit for combat medical use has recently been developed at the Walter Reed Army Institute of Research and approved by the Food and Drug Administration (FDA). The kit contains additional equipment for an over-the-wire technique. Combat medical personnel should be trained to use this technique in the case of airway obstruction where intubation is not possible. These techniques work well in an urgent environment, but in an emergent setting the time required to achieve oxygenation using over-the-wire techniques can be excessive.

A presumptive diagnosis of tension pneumothorax should be made when progressive, severe respiratory distress develops in the case of unilateral penetrating chest trauma. Diagnosis in the tactical situation should not rely on typical clinical signs such as decreased breath sounds, tracheal shift, distended neck veins, and hyperresonance on percussion. These signs may not always be present and, if they are, they may be exceedingly difficult to appreciate on the battlefield. A patient with penetrating chest trauma will generally have some degree of hemothorax or pneumothorax as a result of the primary wound. The additional trauma caused by a needle thoracostomy would not significantly worsen the patient's condition in the absence of a tension pneumothorax. Combat corpsmen and medics should be trained in this technique and perform it in this setting. Paramedics are authorized to perform needle thoracostomy in some civilian emergency medical services. Tube thoracostomy is generally not part of the paramedic's scope of care in civilian EMS settings, nor were any studies found that address the use of this procedure by corpsmen and medics on the battlefield. Chest tubes are not recommended in this phase of care for the following reasons:

1. They are not needed to provide initial treatment for a tension pneumothorax.
2. They are more difficult and time consuming for relatively inexperienced medical personnel to perform, especially in the austere battlefield environment.
3. Chest tube insertion would be more likely to cause additional tissue damage and subsequent infection than a less traumatic needle thoracostomy.
4. No documentation was found in the literature that demonstrated a benefit from tube thoracostomy performed by paramedical personnel on the battlefield.[13]

Tourniquets applied during the care under fire phase should be replaced with direct pressure or compression dressings when the tactical situation allows, as long as these measures are equally effective at controlling the hemorrhage.

Although standard trauma care involves starting two large-bore (14- or 16-gauge) intravenous catheters, the use of an 18-gauge catheter is preferred in the field setting because of the increased ease of starting. The larger catheters are necessary to administer large volumes of blood products rapidly, but this is not a factor in the tactical setting because blood products will not be available. Crystalloid solutions can be administered rapidly through an 18-gauge catheter. Larger-bore catheters may subsequently be started at an MTF. IVs placed in the field may be discontinued or changed because of concerns about contamination at the IV site.

Fluid Resuscitation

Despite its frequent use, the benefit of prehospital fluid resuscitation in trauma patients has not been established. The beneficial effect from crystalloid and colloid fluid resuscitation in hemorrhagic shock has been demonstrated largely on animal models where the volume of hemorrhage is controlled experimentally and resuscitation is initiated after the hemorrhage has been stopped. In uncontrolled hemorrhagic shock models, multiple studies have found that aggressive fluid resuscitation in the setting of an unrepaired vascular injury is associated with either no improvement in survival or an increased mortality rate when compared with no fluid resuscitation or hypotensive resuscitation. This lack of benefit is presumably due to interference with vasoconstriction as the body attempts to adjust to the loss of blood volume and establish hemostasis at the bleeding site.

A large prospective trial examining this issue in 598 victims of penetrating torso trauma was published by Bickell and colleagues.[3,7] They found that aggressive prehospital fluid resuscitation of hypotensive patients with penetrating wounds of the heart was associated with a higher mortality rate than seen in those for whom aggressive volume replacement was withheld until the time of surgical repair. This difference was most significant in those patients with wounds of the heart; patients with abdominal wounds showed little difference in survival between early and delayed fluid resuscitation. Although confirmation of these findings in other randomized, prospective studies has not yet been obtained, no human studies were found that demonstrated any benefit from fluid replacement in patients with ongoing hemorrhage. Battlefield casualties with penetrating abdominal or thoracic trauma must be presumed to have ongoing hemorrhage before surgical repair of their injuries.

If fluid resuscitation is required for controlled hemorrhagic shock in the tactical field care phase, Hespan (6% hetastarch) is recommended as an alternative to lactated Ringer's (LR) solution.[13] Lactated Ringer's solution is a crystalloid, which means that the primary osmotically active particle is sodium. Because the sodium ion distributes throughout the entire extracellular fluid compartment, LR moves rapidly from the intravascular space to the extravascular space. This shift has significant implications for fluid resuscitation. If one infuses 1000 ml of LR into a trauma patient, 1 hour later only 200 ml of that volume remains in the intravascular space to replace lost blood volume. This is not a problem in the civilian setting, because the average time for transport of the patient to the hospital in an ambulance is less than 15 minutes.[7,8] Once the patient has arrived at the hospital, infusion of blood products and surgical repair of the patient's injuries can be rapidly initiated. In the military setting, several hours or more may elapse before a casualty arrives at an MTF, and effective volume resuscitation may be difficult to achieve with LR.

Hespan offers an alternative. The large hetastarch molecule in Hespan is retained in the intravascular space with little or no loss of fluid to the interstitium. Hespan actually draws fluid into the vascular space from the interstitium such that an infusion of 500 ml of Hespan results in an intravascular volume expansion of almost 800 ml, and this effect is sustained for 8 hours or longer. In addition to providing more effective expansion of the intravascular volume, a significant reduction in medical equipment weight is achieved by carrying Hespan instead of LR into the field. Four liters of LR weigh almost 9 pounds, whereas the 500 ml of Hespan needed to achieve a similar sustained intravascular volume expansion weighs just over 1 pound.[13] Hespan in volumes greater than 500 ml may produce increased hemorrhage from small vessels. It is used widely in Europe for trauma management but is not used in the United States for this purpose.

Another theoretical complication with the use of any volume expander is the increased blood loss associated with increased blood pressure in uncontrolled hemorrhage (see Chapter 9).

If the casualty is conscious and requires analgesia, it should be achieved with morphine, preferably administered intravenously. This mode of administration allows for much more rapid onset of analgesia and for more effective titration of dosage than intramuscular administration. An initial dose of 5 mg is given with 2 to 5 mg boluses repeated at 10-minute intervals until adequate analgesia is achieved.

Infection is an important late cause of morbidity and mortality in wounds sustained on the battlefield. Cefoxitin (2 g IV) is an accepted monotherapeutic agent for empiric treatment of abdominal sepsis and should be given without delay to all casualties with penetrating abdominal trauma. Cefoxitin is effective against gram-positive aerobes (except some enterococcus species) and gram-negative aerobes (except for some *Pseudomonas* species). It also has good activity against anaerobes (including *Bacteroides* and *Clostridium* species). Because it is effective against the clostridial species that cause myonecrosis, cefoxitin is also recommended for casualties who sustain wounds with massive soft tissue damage,[20] grossly contaminated wounds, open fractures, or patients for whom a long delay until casevac is anticipated.[21]

Casevac Care

The use of a casevac asset to evacuate the wounded from the battlefield presents the opportunity to bring in additional medical equipment and personnel to treat the casualties. This opportunity led to the recommendation to establish designated combat casualty transportation teams for special operations forces (SOF).[13] This concept, when implemented, will serve to provide a physician skilled in trauma or critical care management as far forward as possible in the SOF combat environment. This additional medical expertise and equipment will allow for the expanded diagnostic and therapeutic measures outlined in Box 42.3 for the casevac phase of care. The concept of combat casualty transportation teams and the additional care that they provide must be evaluated by the combat units of the conventional forces to determine whether this concept might have applicability for their forces as well.

The tactical combat casualty care guidelines described previously have now been implemented in the Naval Special Warfare community[22] and incorporated into the undersea medical officer course conducted by the Navy's Bureau of Medicine and Surgery. They are currently scheduled for inclusion in the *Textbook of Military Medicine* being sponsored by the Office of the Surgeon General of the Army[23] and are being considered for use by units in the Marine Corps and the Air Force. Like all medical management strategies, these guidelines will require periodic review and updating, and the establishment of a standing Department of Defense (DOD) committee on the tactical management of combat trauma has been called for by the commander of the Naval Special Warfare Command.[24] Such guidelines will never be able to anticipate all of the difficulties that may confront the combat medic or corpsman, however, and the need for well-trained combat medical personnel to further modify treatment methods for trauma patients on the battlefield based on the specifics of a given casualty scenario must be recognized. Several scenarios that dramatically illustrate this fact are provided in Boxes 42.4 through 42.7. Scenarios such as these are useful in the planning phase of combat operations to help medical personnel develop customized management plans. Specialized workshops that combine the expertise of both physicians and combat medical personnel to review treatment strategies for specific types of casualty scenarios help provide insights that may be of use to combat medical personnel as they develop these management plans.

Weapons of Mass Destruction

Weapons of mass destruction (WMD) include nuclear devices, biologic agents, and chemical substances. Historically, WMD have been considered as a single class of weapons, but they differ significantly in their use, presentation, and concepts of casualty management. Nuclear weapons may be encountered in the civilian sector as radiation accidents or spills. The technology required to use a nuclear weapon is still substantial in comparison with that required for chemical or biologic agents. A significant threat exists that terrorist groups or hostile nations may use chemical or biologic weapons against the United States. These weapons are readily available to determined parties. Each type of weapon is discussed, along with its general management principles.

Nuclear Weapons

Thermal burns and a variety of traumas complicated by differing degrees of radiologic contamination are the most likely injuries to be encountered in survivors of a nuclear blast. Multiple delayed effects may be anticipated, but early treatment will deal with relatively standard trauma management. Decontamination should be conducted as soon as possible but should not delay lifesaving treatment. A radiologic spill or incident may occur with or without associated trauma. The acronym **SWIMS** describes the procedure that should be followed in most incidents:

Stop the spill
Warn others
Isolate the area
Minimize contamination
Secure ventilation if in an enclosed building

Many civil defense agencies are well versed in the management of nuclear events, and further information can be obtained through these sources.

Biologic Warfare Agents

Biologic weapons are among the most insidious and dangerous ever devised by humankind. They have been

---

Box 42.4 Parachute Insertion Casualty Scenario

- Twelve-person patrol
- Interdiction operation for weapons convoy
- Night static line jump from C-130
- Four-mile patrol over rocky terrain to objective
- Planned helicopter extraction near target
- One jumper has canopy collapse at 40 feet
- Open facial fractures with teeth and blood in oropharynx
- Bilateral ankle fractures
- Open, angulated fracture of the left femur

Box 42.5 Delayed Evacuation Land Warfare Scenario

- Eight-person special operations team
- Dropped into unfriendly Middle Eastern country
- Four-day scud hunt
- Planned helicopter extraction at end of operation
- Lost communications—no casevac or extraction plan changes possible
- Chance encounter on second day
- One soldier shot in abdomen—unconscious
- One soldier shot in leg—external hemorrhage
- One soldier with fragment in eye—light perception vision
- Hostiles all dead

> **Box 42.6 Combat Swimmer Casualty Scenario**
>
> - Limpet mine attack on hostile ship
> - Launch from coastal patrol craft 12 miles out
> - One-hour transit in small boats
> - Seven swim pairs using closed-circuit oxygen rigs
> - Launch craft approach to approximately 2 miles from the harbor
> - Divers wearing wet suits—78° F (26° C) water
> - Surface swim for a mile, then begin dives
> - One man shot in chest by patrol boat during peek in harbor
> - Casualty conscious

> **Box 42.7 Combined Land Warfare–Diving Scenario**
>
> - Two open submersible SEAL delivery vehicles (SDVs)
> - Eight-person SEAL element
> - Insertion from a submarine with 2-hour transit to beach
> - Target is heavily defended harbor in a bay
> - Divers wearing dry suits in 43° F (6° C) water
> - Air temperature 35° F (1° C)
> - Boats bottomed for across-the-beach operation
> - One man shot in chest at the objective
> - Mission plan calls for SEALs to extract by SDV

characterized as the poor person's atomic bomb, a cheaper and less sophisticated alternative to chemical, nuclear, or conventional weapons. Biologic agents may be produced at low cost, in a covert manner, and may be spread easily using readily available equipment. They are capable of producing large numbers of casualties, and the first sign of an attack may be days after the actual event when symptoms of a disease begin to appear. **Biologic warfare agents** (BWAs) fall into four broad categories: true biologic agents, biologic vectors, toxins, and bioregulators.

True biologic agents are living microorganisms (pathogens) that have the ability to cause disease in humans or animals and can cause plant destruction. These include viruses, bacteria, fungi, and rickettsiae.

Biologic vectors are insect vectors that have been purposefully infected with a pathogen in an attempt to propagate the spread of a disease. A variety of insect vectors exist within nature, usually endemic to a specific region, and often act as intermediate breeding grounds for local pathogens. Mosquitoes act in this way for the spread of malaria, and infected fleas do the same for plague.

Toxins of biologic origin constitute the third broad category of BWA. Strictly speaking, these agents are chemicals, but they are generally classified as BWA due to their production within living things. Examples include botulinum and cholera toxins.

The final category of BWA is chemicals that act on the human system as bioregulators. These are chemicals that occur naturally, in small amounts within the body, to regulate such functions as heart rate and blood pressure; they may be synthetically derived to achieve the same purposes. In altered concentrations, these agents may lead to a wide variety of adverse actions such as paralysis, loss of consciousness, or death. Given their specificity for use against the human system, they are included as BWA.

The primary means of exposure to most of these agents is via the respiratory tract. The gastrointestinal tract is the second major route of exposure for many infectious agents and toxins, normally through the ingestion of contaminated food or water supplies. Weight for weight, BWAs are inherently more toxic than either chemical or conventional weapons, have a much higher specificity for their intended targets than chemical weapons, and, effectively disseminated, provide the largest area coverage of any type of weapon. Once disseminated, however, BWAs tend to degrade quickly.

There are two primary methods of dissemination of BWAs, both of which depend on weather conditions for maximum effectiveness. The first is from a point-source weapon such as a bomb or stationary aerosol generator, which disseminates the agent from a single location. The second is a line-source weapon that disseminates the agent from a moving platform such as a spray tank mounted on a vehicle (truck or aircraft). Line-source weapons can disperse large amounts of agent over much wider areas than point-source weapons and are significantly more effective.

Factors Affecting Dissemination and Spread of Biologic Warfare Agents

Atmospheric conditions can dramatically alter the dispersal and subsequent effectiveness of BWA. High winds tend to disperse BWA over a wider area and dilute concentrations. Unstable winds, especially those with gusty, unpredictable patterns, will provide less uniform spread. Sunlight, particularly the ultraviolet portion, tends to break down toxic agents and kill pathogens through rapid drying. Rain tends to wash an agent out of the air and clear surfaces.

Terrain is equally important in the dispersal patterns and subsequent effectiveness of BWA. Flat, unobstructed territory or an open expanse of water allows for maximum potential distribution. Urban settings or hilly, rugged terrain prevents even distribution, increases vertical dilution, and tends to reduce effective concentrations over distance.

Early detection allows personnel to take protective cover in time to prevent exposure. Limitations in technology, however, make this extremely difficult to achieve. Biologic warfare agent detectors are in development but of questionable reliability at the present time.

Personnel entering a targeted area may lack effective protection, become casualties themselves, and spread the disease further. Delayed effects make it difficult even to discern when and where the attack was conducted. An outbreak of disease may cause significant death or illness yet mimic a naturally occurring epidemic.

Should biologic agents be of concern, three points should be remembered:

1. Avoid contamination, if possible.
2. Decontamination should be conducted, if possible, to eliminate or reduce the hazard from exposed personnel and equipment. Decontamination often involves caustic materials and bleaches to neutralize the agent and thus may damage equipment. The secondary infectious hazard is minimal and treatment may proceed even in the absence of full decontamination.
3. Maintain a high index of suspicion. Look for unusual diseases or patterns of disease if a biologic incident was possible. Seek treatment early if symptoms develop after responding to a call. Prompt and effective medical treatment is necessary to counteract the effects of the agents and minimize casualties. Treatment is effective in the majority of commonly used agents, but, in some cases, by the time symptoms appear, it may be too late to treat effectively; in others, no effective treatment exists.

Characteristics of Biologic Warfare Agents

General characteristics that determine the usefulness of BWAs include the following:

1. *Infectivity.* This involves the ability of an agent to reliably infect a person or animal exposed to it.
2. *Virulence.* This characteristic relates the agent's ability to incapacitate or kill an intended target once exposure and infection have occurred.
3. *Incubation period.* The incubation period is the lag between the time when infection occurs and the time when symptoms of the disease become apparent. Biologic agents rarely cause instant casualties. With the exception of certain toxins, BWA tend to have effect only after their incubation period.
4. *Stability.* Most biologic agents are unstable when compared with chemical agents. Stability is the ability to maintain virulence and other characteristics over time and under varying ecologic conditions.
5. *Environmental persistence.* Persistence is closely related to stability and is the ability of an organism to survive in the environment long enough to have the desired effect.
6. *Resistance.* Resistance is the ability of an agent to withstand normal medical countermeasures.
7. *Protection.* Protection is the ability of an attacker to protect his or her troops with a vaccine or other protective measure not available to the opponent.
8. *Controllability.* This is the ability to predict, with some measure of assuredness, the extent and nature of the BWA effects given a specific set of employment parameters.
9. *Producibility.* The most likely agents used by developing countries will be those that are cheap, are easy to produce, and can be readily obtained on the global market. Only about 30 pathogens have been considered as likely BWA out of the several hundred known to affect humans and animals.

Anthrax. Anthrax is often discussed as the prototypical biologic warfare agent. *Bacillus anthracis,* the causative organism for anthrax, occurs naturally in horses, cattle, and sheep. Anthrax is highly toxic and stable in an aerosolized form. Once released, exposure can occur through inhalation, ingestion, or wounds in the skin. An inhalational dose of less than 1 μg can be fatal in days. The normal incubation period is 3 to 5 days but may be as little as 24 hours with a larger exposure. Cutaneous anthrax has a mortality rate approaching 20% if left untreated, but less than 1% following treatment. Inhalational anthrax, however, approaches 100% mortality rate. Treatment of suspected cases must begin before the onset of symptoms or it is likely to be ineffective. Even with treatment, survivors may be incapacitated for months and require retreatment due to relapses.

Protection against an anthrax attack currently includes the use of personal protective gear and a mask if the attack is detected in time. Current detection methods may be unreliable, however, in warning of an attack early enough to prevent exposure, and detectors are not routinely deployed with at-risk units. A well-tested, safe, and reliable anthrax vaccine is available.

Chemical Warfare Agents

Chemical agents fall into five main categories: nerve agents, vesicants, cyanide, lung agents, and riot control agents. In addition to the potential for terrorist activity, these agents may be encountered during cleanup of lands where old chemical munitions were stored or during hazardous material accidents involving spills of organophosphate insecticides or other industrial chemicals such as phosgene or cyanide. Chemical agents are primarily

> **Box 42.8 Nerve Agents—Summary**
>
> **Signs and Symptoms**
> - Small vapor exposure—miosis, runny nose, shortness of breath
> - Large vapor exposure—loss of consciousness, convulsions, apnea, flaccid paralysis
> - Small to moderate liquid exposure—localized sweating, fasciculations; nausea, vomiting, diarrhea, feeling of weakness (may start hours later)
> - Large liquid exposure—loss of consciousness, convulsions, apnea, flaccid paralysis
>
> **Decontamination**
> - Thoroughly flush with hypochlorite and water
>
> **Emergency Medical Care**
> - Atropine (2–6 mg); 2 PAMCl; diazepam (depending on severity); ventilation; suction of airways if secretions are copious; supportive care

> **Box 42.9 Vesicants—Summary**
>
> **Signs and Symptoms**
> - Normally a latent period of hours followed by the onset of erythema and blisters, conjunctivitis, and upper respiratory signs. All may worsen over the following hours. Mustard does not cause pain on contact; lewisite and phosgene oxime cause pain on exposure to liquid or vapor.
>
> **Decontamination**
> - Hypochlorite or large amounts of water to flush agent away. Must be within seconds to be maximally effective.
>
> **Emergency Medical Care**
> - Immediate decontamination. None otherwise (no early effects). Suspected casualty should be observed for at least 8 hours. Later, symptomatic management of lesions.

liquids that produce contact hazards but are even more dangerous as they vaporize. They may be "persistent" (staying on the ground for more than 24 hours) or nonpersistent if they evaporate within 24 hours. In liquid form, these agents are heavier than water and may be covered by puddles. In vapor form, they are heavier than air and tend to collect in low spots. Like biologic agents, the primary considerations are contamination avoidance, decontamination, and movement of decontaminated patients from a contaminated to a clean area. In many circumstances, it is best to treat patients on site and move them after appropriate decontamination is achieved. Failure to do this may result in widespread contamination and increased casualties. Responders to a chemical incident must themselves be protected by appropriate suits and masks, or they risk becoming casualties as well.

Nerve Agents

Nerve agents cause involuntary skeletal muscle activity and excessive secretion from lachrymal, nasal, salivary, and sweat glands into the airways and gastrointestinal tract (Box 42.8). Constriction of muscles within the airway produces bronchoconstriction similar to that seen in asthma. In the gastrointestinal tract it leads to cramps, vomiting, and diarrhea. The single most effective treatment for exposure to nerve agents is atropine. Atropine will reduce secretions and reduce activity in smooth muscle but has little effect on excess activity of skeletal muscles. Nerve agents penetrate normal clothing and skin to be absorbed into the body. Clinical effects depend on the route and amount of agent exposure.

Vesicants

Vesicants are substances that cause burning of the skin with redness and blistering (Box 42.9). These agents are liquids but produce damage in the vapor form as well. Damage begins to occur almost immediately on contact with the skin, and the best management is early and thorough decontamination of the affected areas. Clinical effects may be delayed for several hours and increase in severity over several days; death usually occurs from damage to the respiratory tract. Early responders may not see significant lesions because the effects are often delayed.

Cyanide

Cyanide is a common industrial chemical that has been used as a poison for centuries (Box 42.10). It is found in cigarette smoke and in some types of foods. Cyanide inhibits the ability of cells to use oxygen and causes death by cellular hypoxemia. Although large doses produce rapid death, smaller doses may be effectively treated with rapid administration of the antidotes, support of circulation as necessary, and oxygen.

Lung Agents

Lung agents are a class of compounds that cause pulmonary edema (Box 42.11). The most important of these is phosgene, a common industrial compound. Teflon, when it burns, may give off perfluoroisobutylene, another agent in this class. Generally, these agents produce damage to the alveolar-capillary membrane with onset of symptoms between 2 and 24 hours depending on the level of exposure. Patients should be observed for a 24-hour period and triaged based on the severity of symptoms that develop.

> **Box 42.10** Cyanide—Summary
>
> **Signs and Symptoms**
> - Few. After inhalation of a large amount: loss of consciousness, convulsions, apnea, and cardiac arrest.
>
> **Decontamination**
> - Not usually necessary in vapor. Wet clothing should be removed, and underlying skin decontaminated (hypochlorite or water).
>
> **Emergency Medical Care**
> - Amyl nitrite in bag-valve-mask followed by IV sodium nitrite and sodium thiosulfate; ventilation with oxygen.

> **Box 42.11** Lung Agents—Summary
>
> **Signs and Symptoms**
> - Eye and airway irritation early on in some cases. Later development of pulmonary edema with shortness of breath, cough, and clear sputum.
>
> **Decontamination**
> - None usually necessary. Remove wet clothing, decontaminate underlying skin with hypochlorite or water. Fresh air.
>
> **Emergency Medical Care**
> - Termination of exposure. Oxygen with positive pressure for respiratory distress. No physical activity.

Riot Control Agents

Riot control agents (RCAs) are in common use by law enforcement agencies but are not usually of great concern to first responders (Box 42.12). Medical treatment is not generally indicated following exposure because the effects are self-limiting. There are, however, some rare complications worthy of note. Persons with reactive airway disease may develop prolonged bronchospasm following exposure to RCAs. Standard treatment for a severe asthmatic attack may be required. Moderate to severe conjunctivitis has been reported following exposure that occasionally requires treatment by an ophthalmologist. Finally, a delayed-onset contact dermatitis may develop that may require follow-up medical care.

Decontamination

Decontamination is vital in any chemical incident and has two main goals. The first is to minimize injury to the casualty. This must be done within minutes after exposure in order to be effective. The best and most effective decontamination is that performed within the first minute after exposure to a liquid chemical agent. If decontamination is delayed 15 to 60 minutes, it may do little to assist the casualty. If the agent was a nerve agent, the casualty may be dead. The best and often quickest decontamination is physical removal of the agent. Remove any clothing that has been contaminated and clean the skin of any residual. Large amounts of water under pressure or a scraper-type object may be effective. Substances that chemically destroy or detoxify the agent are commonly used for decontamination. Sodium hypochlorite is a primary agent. Undiluted bleach followed by washing may be effective, and specially prepared decontamination kits are available. The second goal is to prevent contamination of rescue personnel, EMS personnel, transport units, and the receiving medical facility.

Before a casualty is decontaminated, all personnel in contact with the casualty must wear appropriate protective equipment. There is a significant risk of contaminating vehicles and medical facilities from a chemical casualty. A strict decontamination area must be established with a clean area on one side and the contaminated area on the other. Any person (symptomatic or asymptomatic), casualty, or medical care provider who goes from a contaminated area to a clean uncontaminated area, such as a medical treatment area, must be decontaminated. Casualties or medical personnel who have not undergone decontamination procedures may contaminate the entire air system of a hospital by spreading a vapor agent.

Specific protective equipment includes the following:

> **Box 42.12** Riot Control Agents—Summary
>
> **Signs and Symptoms**
> - Burning and pain on exposed mucous membranes and skin, causing eye pain and tearing, respiratory discomfort, and stinging on the exposed skin.
>
> **Decontamination**
> - Fresh air. Flush eyes with water or saline. Flush skin with alkaline soap and water or weak bicarbonate solution (not hypochlorite).
>
> **Emergency Medical Care**
> - Usually none needed; effects are self-limiting.

1. Personal equipment
   - Masks, the M40 or older M17A2, and suits
   - Self-contained breathing apparatus (SCBA) approved for civilian use
   - Standard chemical clothing available to civilian emergency agencies through the Defense Logistics Agency
   - Responder suit (civilian responders)

2. Detection equipment
   - Chemical detection kits
3. Medical items
   - Mark I nerve agent antidote kit
   - Litter made of monofilament polypropylene fabric, which allows drainage of liquids, does not absorb chemical agents, and is easily decontaminated for reuse
   - Fiberglass long spine boards—nonpermeable and easily decontaminated

Triage

The most important concept in successful management of mass casualties is triage. **Triage** is the sorting of casualties into treatment categories by a designated officer. Categories are determined based on the severity of injury, likelihood of recovery, and availability of treatment resources. Resources consist of time, personnel, and equipment. The objective is to provide survival for as many as possible. The triage officer's responsibility is to sort the casualties; he or she does not treat patients and is often alone and without equipment. In an ideal situation, a senior experienced trauma or general surgeon should conduct triage because these individuals are most qualified to make the necessary life-and-death decisions. In practice, many other personnel may be forced to do triage based on circumstances. Patients are triaged and retriaged at each level of care, and treatment categories may change based on availability of resources or a change in condition. Two categories deserve special mention: field triage and hospital triage.

Field Triage

Field triage occurs at or near the site of injury. This is the battlefield in wartime or the site of a disaster in peacetime. The triage officer may be a physician but will more likely be a corpsman or nurse. There are three broad categories of patients in the field: agonal (those who are about to die); those who are more scared than wounded; and all others. Little can be done for the agonal, and the minimally injured should be removed from the scene and returned to duty as soon as possible. Those with more serious injuries need to be treated initially and moved to an MTF as quickly as possible. Two categories are designated based on injury severity and threat to integrity of airway, breathing, and circulation (the ABCs). These include the traditional "immediate" and "urgent" categories. After initial intervention, little can be accomplished at the scene in terms of reversing instability, and eventual outcome will likely be determined at the MTF.

Hospital Triage

Hospital triage is considerably more precise. The triage officer is the surgeon most experienced in trauma care. He or she only sorts patients and rarely treats them. Three categories constitute the simplest, most-used method of triage. "The walking wounded" are those patients whose injuries would heal with little or no therapy. They constitute approximately 65% of the patients seen. They are moved to a separate area of the MTF where their injuries are treated by a physician and a nurse if staffing permits. "The expectant" are those patients who will probably die no matter what treatment is performed and would tie up significant resources in the process. They are moved to a separate area of the MTF and made as comfortable as possible. They number less than 10% of the casualties and are attended by only a single nurse. "The priority" are those patients where a meaningful survival can be achieved by immediate or prompt intervention and treatment. They number about 25% of the patient load. Despite obvious differences, military (battlefield) triage and civilian (disaster) triage adhere to those basic levels of casualty sorting.

Extenuating Factors Related to Battlefield Triage

Triage in the combat zone is stressed by obvious extenuating circumstances. The ongoing conflict poses risks to the integrity of the MTF and those components integral to patient transport and evacuation. Casualty care is problematic but may be remarkably efficient despite the difficulties.

Resource limitations are present in both battlefield and domestic occurrences. Contingency planning can minimize shortfalls in both scenarios, and protocols should be established for each. A major treatment facility, whether it be a combat casualty support hospital or a level I trauma center, must have a disaster plan. It should be published, updated routinely, and periodically rehearsed.

Environmental Concerns with Triage

Environmental concerns in disaster management include casualty and medical personnel protection against heat, cold, wind, rain, dust, flood, and storm. Sources of water and electricity may be jeopardized, communications disrupted, and transportation rendered impossible. Contingency planning is essential, and these issues should be addressed in standard disaster plans. Exposure to nuclear, biologic, or chemical agents has become of increased concern in recent years.

Triage is best done at a distance from the actual scene of a terrorist act. An initial blast may be followed by a second, larger detonation designed to maim and kill those responding to the first.

Comparison of Civilian versus Military Casualty Management

This section provides a comparison of casualty management following the terrorist bombing of the U.S. Marine Corps facility in Beirut, Lebanon, in 1983 and the terrorist bombing of the A. P. Murrah Federal Building in Oklahoma City in 1995.

The Beirut bomb resulted in 346 casualties, among whom 234 (68%) died immediately. The battalion aid station, located on the fourth floor of the building, was destroyed; the medical officer and numerous corpsmen were killed, resulting in a lack of initial medical capability at the scene. Of the 112 survivors, 7 subsequently died (6%). Six of these succumbed in association with a delay in treatment secondary to entrapment within the building. Most of the survivors (64%) were flown by helicopter off shore to the USS Iwo Jima, where they were triaged. Twenty-four casualties were flown from the scene to Europe and Cypress after the arrival of U.S. and British Air Ambulance Units. Fifteen survivors with minor injuries remained on shore; all survived. Eight casualties were taken to local Lebanese hospitals, where one died.

The Oklahoma City bomb caused 759 casualties, among whom 167 (22%) died immediately. Of the 83 (11%) survivors who were hospitalized, 1 died. The remaining 509 casualties were treated as outpatients. The field triage officer in this disaster was an emergency medicine resident from the nearby University Hospital.

Summary

- Levels (echelons) of care improve the survivability of wounded soldiers by moving more advanced capabilities further forward in the echelon system. The military-derived system of levels of care is the civilian counterpart spread across a theater of operation.
- Prehospital care in the tactical environment requires specialized training for physicians, corpsmen, and medics. Because of the complicating effects of battlefield conditions (e.g., darkness, enemy fire, and equipment limitations), scene safety is not always feasible. Care under fire calls for an occasional variance from normal protocol due to these unique circumstances. Before any combat operation or mission can be undertaken, special attention must be directed at a basic medical care plan.
- Weapons of mass destruction are the most insidious and dangerous threat devised by humankind. Early detection and decontamination are the most important priorities in countering biologic or chemical warfare agents. Treat concurrent injuries as in a conventional setting.
- The most important concept in successful management of mass casualties, whether in the battlefield or on the home front during peacetime, is triage. Understand that triage in the combat zone is stressed by extenuating circumstances.

Scenario Solution

The point man who sustained the injuries resulting in no pulse or respirations would be placed in the "expectant" category. No time or equipment would be used in a resuscitation attempt. The point man will be extracted with the team. The patrol leader with the femoral hemorrhage would be placed in the "immediate" category.

Can the patient be stabilized well enough to be extracted with the team as planned? If not, what is the medical evacuation (medevac) plan? How soon can medevac arrive at the patrol's present location? Does the medevac aircraft have the necessary equipment to extract the patients from the patrol's present location (i.e., jungle penetrator, Stokes litter)?

Incoming direct and indirect fire make it necessary for the patrol to either suppress hostile fire using fire support (artillery, naval gunfire, close air support) or break contact and move out of their present position immediately. Transport of the patient is a priority, and more definitive care may be delayed until the patrol is in a suitable location.

The patrol leader will receive a pressure dressing or a tourniquet placement until the medic or corpsman can remove

Scenario Solution (cont'd)

him from hostile fire. Later, during movement or at the extraction site, the patient will receive a more definitive dressing and advanced lifesaving procedures, including 3:1 volume replacement with lactated Ringer's and a full primary and secondary survey to identify any other conditions that may have previously gone unrecognized.

Key Terms

Biologic warfare agents True biologic agents, biologic vectors, toxins, and bioregulators.
Casevac Combat casualty evacuation care.
Combat lifesaver program U.S. military program that provides nonmedical personnel education beyond basic first aid.
Medevac Noncombat medical transport.
SWIMS *S*top the spill, *W*arn others, *I*solate the area, *M*inimize contamination, and *S*ecure ventilation.
Triage Sorting of casualties into treatment categories.
Weapons of mass destruction Nuclear devices, biologic agents, and chemical substances.

Review Questions

1. Which echelon of care is characterized by its mobility and staffing of medical technicians, one physician, and one physician assistant?
   a. Echelon I.
   b. Echelon II.
   c. Echelon III.
   d. Echelon IV.
2. Which stage of care applies to a situation in which care of an injury is provided while on a mission with no hostile fire?
   a. Combat casualty evacuation care.
   b. Care under fire.
   c. Tactical field care.
   d. Battlefield care.
3. Which nerve agent causes loss of consciousness, convulsions, apnea, and cardiac arrest?
   a. Lung agents.
   b. Cyanide.
   c. Riot control agents.
   d. Anthrax.
4. Field triage will most likely be performed by whom?
   a. Surgeon.
   b. Corpsman or nurse.
   c. Physician assistant.
   d. Physician.

Answers to these Review Questions can be found at the end of the book on page 869.

References

1. Bellamy RF: The causes of death in conventional land warfare: implications for combat casualty care research, *Milit Med* 149:55, 1984.
2. Alexander RH, Proctor HJ: *Advanced trauma life support 1993 student manual*, Chicago, 1993, American College of Surgeons.
3. Bickell WH, Wall MJ, Pepe PE, et al: Immediate versus delayed fluid resuscitation for hypotensive patients with penetrating torso injuries, *N Engl J Med* 331:1105, 1994.
4. Honigman B, Rohwder K, Moore EE, et al: Prehospital advanced trauma life support for penetrating cardiac wounds, *Ann Emerg Med* 19:145, 1990.
5. Smith JP, Bodai BI: The urban paramedic's scope of practice, *JAMA* 253:544, 1985.
6. Stern SA, Dronen SC, Birrer P, et al: Effect of blood pressure on hemorrhage volume and survival in a near-fatal hemorrhage model incorporating a vascular injury, *Ann Emerg Med* 22:155, 1993.

References (cont'd)

7. Martin RR, Bickell WH, Pepe PE, et al: Prospective evaluation of preoperative fluid resuscitation in hypotensive patients with penetrating truncal injury: a preliminary report, *J Trauma* 33:354, 1992.
8. Kaweski SM, Sise MJ, Virgilio RW: The effect of prehospital fluids on survival in trauma patients, *J Trauma* 30:1215, 1990.
9. Krausz MM, Bar-Ziv M, Rabinovici R, et al: "Scoop and run" or stabilize hemorrhagic shock with normal saline or small-volume hypertonic saline? *J Trauma* 33:6, 1992.
10. Arishita GI, Vayer JS, Bellamy RF: Cervical spine immobilization of penetrating neck wounds in a hostile environment, *J Trauma* 29:332, 1989.
11. Zajtchuk R, Jenkins DP, Bellamy RF, et al, editors: *Combat casualty care guidelines for Operation Desert Storm,* Washington, DC, 1991, Office of the Army Surgeon General Publication.
12. Ekblad GS: Training medics for the combat environment of tomorrow, *Milit Med* 155:232, 1990.
13. Butler FK, Hagmann J, Butler EG: Tactical combat casualty care in special operations, *Milit Med* 161(suppl):1, 1996.
14. Wilderness Medical Society: *Practice guidelines for wilderness medical emergencies,* Indianapolis, 1995, Wilderness Medical Society.
15. Maughon JS: An inquiry into the nature of wounds resulting in killed in action in Vietnam, *Milit Med* 135:8, 1970.
16. Trooskin SZ, Rabinowitz S, Eldridge C, et al: Teaching endotracheal intubation using animals and cadavers, *Prehosp Disaster Med* 7:179, 1992.
17. Salvino CK, Dries D, Gamelli R, et al: Emergency cricothyroidotomy in trauma victims, *J Trauma* 34:503, 1993.
18. McGill J, Clinton JE, Ruiz E: Cricothyrotomy in the emergency department, *Ann Emerg Med* 11:361, 1982.
19. Erlandson MJ, Clinton JE, Ruiz E, et al: Cricothyrotomy in the emergency department revisited, *J Emerg Med* 7:115, 1989.
20. Bowen TE, Bellamy RF, editors: *Emergency war surgery: second United States revision of the Emergency War Surgery NATO Handbook,* Washington, DC, 1988, United States Government Printing Office, p 175.
21. Ordog GJ, Sheppard GF, Wasserberger JS, et al: Infection in minor gunshot wounds, *J Trauma* 34:358, 1993.
22. Commander, Naval Special Warfare Command letter of 9 April 1997.
23. Butler FK: Medical support of special operations. In Burr RE, Bellamy RF, editors: *Medical operations in harsh environments. Textbook of military medicine,* Washington, DC, Office of the Surgeon General of the Army Publication (in press).
24. Commander, Naval Special Warfare Command letter of 29 May 1997.

Appendix A

CPR Review*

Introduction

Cardiopulmonary resuscitation (CPR) and its ability to save lives is one of the cornerstones of prehospital care. Laypersons and trained professionals have been using CPR to save lives for decades. CPR training to hospital personnel was recommended 30 years ago; now it is mandatory in most states for physicians, nurses, laboratory technicians, and environmental services—anyone who might come into contact with a patient. Dr. B.B. Milstein published in 1963 that one of the greatest hindrances to reviving cardiac arrest patients was the delay in starting open heart chest massage. He also points out that the closed-chest cardiac massage "represents a brilliant advance, for it is now possible to perform effective cardiac massage without opening the chest, and thus the greatest hindrance to successful resuscitation has been removed." Imagine how he would feel knowing how many people practice CPR today. His biggest hindrance to this philosophy was trying to convince physicians the same thing.

The use of defibrillators were first described in 1956, and they have been used in hospitals and advanced life support (ALS) ambulances ever since. In the past few years, automated external defibrillators (AED) have been in use by laypersons to save lives in the public. Chicago's O'Hare International Airport boast that it has an AED within 1 minute and 30 seconds of any person in need.

History

Vesalius recorded the first attempts to resuscitate a cardiac arrest patient. His idea was that the heart would restart if air was used to inflate the lungs artificially by "insufflating air into the trachea." John Hunter was also successful in his studies of patients who had drowned. He showed that if artificial respirations were initiated in the first 10 minutes, the heart would often recover. In 1776, 224 years ago, Hunter proposed that "anything salutary to life applied to the lungs would restore the heart's action after it had been at rest some time" (Milstein, 1963†).

In November of 1848 a new introduction was made in the world of medicine—chloroform. It was an important introduction for the obvious reason of anesthesia but also for another important reason. Patients were dying with its use. This was an unfortunate adverse effect of chloroform, but it brought about the thought process of what to do to revive the patient and why the patients were dying. Was it a question of respiratory failure that stopped the heart, or was it that the heart stopped and caused respiratory failure?

A great physiologist and innovator, Moritz Schiff, started studying cardiac arrest in patients who received chloroform versus ether in 1874. He concluded that cardiac arrest occurred before respiratory failure in patients anesthetized with chloroform. His attempts with chest compression, breathing of air into the lungs, and the use of electrical currents were unsuccessful, "but if one opens the thorax while air is slowly blown into the lungs and compresses the heart rhythmically with the hand to squeeze out the blood . . . one can restore the heart as long as eleven and a half minutes after it has been arrested." Through his continuous studies "he understood that the heart revived because oxygenated blood was supplied to the myocardium by the artificial coronary circulation produced by cardiac massage. These experiments demonstrated for the first time the salutary effect of thoracotomy for cardiac massage in the resuscitation of the heart. This work [and the work of Wiggers in 1940] remains the basis for the current treatment of cardiac arrest, which differs little today from the methods which Schiff used in animals" (Milstein, 1963†). This was what is now termed as *open-cardiac massage*; it was not until later that closed-chest cardiac massage was documented.

Milstein (1963†) continues his discussion of *"great advances"* in cardiac arrest and resuscitation by stating the following: "The greatest advance which has been made since the time of Schiff is the demonstration by Kouwenhoven that cardiac massage can be carried out effectively by external compression of the thorax (1960). In his original report Kouwenhoven was able to show a 70 per cent survival rate in twenty patients. The heart beat returned in every case. Because this method can be applied anywhere and by anybody and because thoracotomy can be avoided, it is to be hoped that the high mortality of cardiac arrest can now be diminished."

In 1974, the American Heart Association (AHA) published *The Standards and Guidelines of the American Heart Association*. This publication defined with relative precision the algorithms for intervention of the cardiac arrest victim.

Cardiac compression was described initially in the Bible but was not used medically until the nineteenth century. In 1858, documentation describes an 18-year-old female with a history of severe asphyxia attacks caused by tuberculosis who was found pulseless and apneic. Janos Balassa of Hungary performed a laryngotomy, after which he began compressing the patient's anterior chest wall with one hand, he felt a pulse after 6 minutes, and later the patient achieved consciousness. In 1878, studies were conducted on cats that had been placed in cardiac arrest, and external chest compressions were performed. With these studies it was found that the blood pressure was maintained, and with visualization of the carotid artery a pulse could be found with each chest compression. Further case studies on chest compressions were described in 1892 when a 9-year-old boy under chloroform anesthesia went into cardiac arrest and Friedrich Maass initiated chest compressions at a rate of 30 to 40 compressions a minute. Some improvement in the boy was made; however, he did not regain a

---
* Written by Merry J. McSwain and Catherine A. Parvensky Barwell.
† Milstein BB: *Cardiac arrest and resuscitation*, London, 1963, Lloyd-Luke.

pulse until a tracheostomy was performed, and after 30 minutes a pulse was detected. The boy recovered with some mental confusion.

Maass described another case in which compressions were continued at a rate of 120 compression a minute. He concluded the following (Tang and Weil, 1999*) : "So long as compression is applied at the speed of the patient's breathing, there is slow deterioration. When compression is speeded up, gradual improvement follows . . . At this point it becomes clear that, first of all, forceful pressure on the heart region with its relatively small effect on respiration has accomplished more than the very extensive artificial respiration according to Silvester; second, that compressions at the speed of a fast pulse were more effective than those that were executed at the speed of respirations."

Almost a century later, when the *Journal of the American Medical Association* published the article "Closed-Cardiac Chest Massage," what is now termed *CPR* came into use.

Importance and Statistics

CPR has come under scrutiny of late for various reasons. CPR saves lives; that is not under dispute. What is under dispute is at what cost does it save lives? It is very expensive and time consuming to run a "full code." Is it judicious to send time, energy, and resources to try and "save a dead person," or would the time, energy, and resources be better used on the living if the choice can between the two? The family members of the patient certainly want "everything possible done," and if that patient walks out of the hospital with a good quality of life, then surely the effort was well worth the cost. However, what about the hundreds of patients for whom this is not true? Some of these patients are saved to be a vegetable or cannot recover enough to be removed from the ventilator, not to mention the cost of the code or the further cost of the patient. It is not within the scope of this chapter to debate this ethical issue; this is only meant to inform the reader of some of the ethical dilemmas that modern medicine produces. In some aspects of medicine these decisions are an everyday occurrence, and prehospital care is one of those pathways.

Much of medicine and many medical decisions are based on statistics. Unfortunately, the statistics concerning CPR or sudden death are difficult to define. The difficulty is in determining which patients to place within these statistics. Does one place all of cardiac arrest patients in that category or just the sudden death cases? In the world of prehospital medicine, this would seem a fairly easy question to answer. All patients who receive CPR should be considered, but then there are so many variables, such as trauma deaths, congestive heart failure (CHF), cancer, and other previous medical conditions. Do you account for the patients who were in cardiac arrest upon arrival and/or all patients who received CPR? Should sudden infant death syndrome (SIDS) patients be included in that statistic? It is not uncommon to code an infant for the sake of the parents knowing that the baby is not viable. If one were to include those numbers, the statistics could be skewed. There is a considerable amount of difficulty in differentiating these numbers, hence the problem of accurately describing the statistics involving the survival rate of patients who receive CPR.

---
* Tang W, Weil MH: *CPR: resuscitation of the arrested heart,* Philadelphia, 1999, W.B. Saunders

The survival rate of patients who receive CPR is not known. Who do you include in the survival rate? Surely it cannot be just the patients who walk out of the hospital? Experts estimate that the overall survival rate in the United States is 3% to 5%. The statistics are broken down by state and city, and the results vary. One city estimates its survival rate at 18% and another at 1.4%, thus it is difficult to be sure.

What is known is that the use of the AED, bystander CPR, basic life support (BLS) and ALS prehospital providers, and short arrival time are of the essence to increase the survival rate. CPR saves lives; this is an undisputed fact. The difficulty lies in knowledge of when to start, response times, and when to stop.

Who Writes the CPR Guidelines and Why?

The AHA writes the guidelines for hospital personnel and laypersons. They started training hospital personnel in 1961 and in 1973 recommended that CPR training programs be available to the general public. The AHA established guidelines for resuscitation and has continued to improve and update with developing changes, studies, and discoveries in modern medicine. At the writing of this text new guidelines have been published and are discussed later in this appendix. These changes are a new global standard for the treatment of cardiovascular emergencies such as sudden death, myocardial infarction, and stroke. Experts from Australia, Europe, Canada, Japan, New Zealand, Latin America, Saudi Arabia, Southern Africa, and Thailand have contributed to the process. They are the first truly international guidelines. The *Guidelines 2000* are designed for laypersons and health care providers. As stated previously, everyone working in most hospitals must be BLS certified, from physicians to housekeepers. This measure is to ensure the quick response of "bystander CPR," which as been shown to increase the survival rate.

Advanced Cardiac Life Support

Advanced cardiac life support (ACLS) also comes under the umbrella of the AHA and is taught to physicians, nurses, and paramedics. The use of ACLS includes BLS, definitive airway management, defibrillation, and drug therapy. With the advent of ALS in the prehospital setting, it allows the paramedic to perform or "run a code" (in effect, the same as a physician would in an emergency department), thus enabling the patient to have access to a mobile emergency department. The paramedic is able to insert a definitive airway (i.e., an endotracheal tube) and deliver oxygen and drug therapy much like in the hospital. ACLS ensures that the most that can possibly be done for a patient in cardiac arrest will be done as soon as possible. ACLS provides an algorithm for all of the major cardiac arrhythmias and the treatment for each of them. They are the same algorithms that are used in any setting in the hospital.

Guidelines 2000 for Cardiopulmonary Resuscitation and Emergency Cardiovascular Care

Upon the writing of this text, the AHA just published new guidelines on CPR and emergency cardiovascular care (ECC). The following are recommendations and changes for both health care providers and laypersons. These guidelines were published on August 22, 2000 in *Circulation: Journal of the American Heart Association.*

Chain of Survival

The *chain of survival* is the term used to explain the necessary steps that must occur to ensure that CPR has the highest benefit possible. When a patient is found unresponsive, complaining of chest pain, or exhibiting signs and symptoms of cardiac arrest, the "links" in the chain must be activated for the system to work at its best. Each link has its own importance, but if not connected, the chance for survival is greatly reduced.

The links in the chain of survival are as follows:

1. Recognition of early warning signs
2. Activation of the emergency medical system (EMS)
3. Basic CPR
4. Early defibrillation
5. Management of the airway
6. Intravenous administration of medications

The EMT-B is involved in each of these links. With the help of AEDs supplied on the ambulance and the IV administration of medications provided by paramedics or physicians in the emergency department, the EMT-B is a vital link in the chain of survival. Early detection and treatment of patients before the patient arrives at the hospital is the goal of EMS, and sudden death ranks is one of the primary focuses of prehospital providers. Many lives are saved because EMTs are on the streets. If any of these links is missing or weak, the chance of survival is lessened and the EMS and its patients are condemned to poor results.

The AHA has also developed the adult chain of survival, which includes the following links:

1. Early access
2. Early CPR
3. Early defibrillation
4. Early ACLS

The importance of the first three links in the adult chain of survival cannot be overstated. Time is of the essence when sudden death is an issue and should not be prolonged. The United States is pushing hard for AEDs that are easy to use and readily accessible because time is the enemy. Prolonged access to defibrillation and CPR could literally mean the difference between life and death. It could be the difference between walking to the ambulance or the scene and running with proper equipment in hand.

The reason that time is of the essence is because the brain is the most susceptible organ to hypoxia and is irreversibly damaged. The reason behind CPR is to provide the brain with oxygen, which is only accomplished by getting oxygen into the blood (breathing) and pumping it to the brain (compressions). The AHA is using the term *cardiopulmonary-cerebral resuscitation* to further emphasize the need to preserve cerebral viability.

CPR was originally used to maintain viability long enough to transport the patient to a defibrillator machine. BLS is most often successful if defibrillation occurs sooner than 6 to 10 minutes after collapse. Brain damage is not as likely from 0 to 4 minutes after collapse. After 6 to 10 minutes, brain damage is likely and the hope of regaining a pulse is doubtful. Therefore response times and early access are critical aspects of EMS and saving lives.

Criteria for Initiating and Terminating CPR

When to start and stop CPR can be a complex decision in the prehospital setting. Neither the AHA nor medical control desire for the EMT to make a judgment call on when to start or stop CPR, so criteria are set as a guideline. Not every scene is the same, and not every patient or family is the same. People act differently, and not every situation can be documented; therefore these are only guidelines and are not hard and fast rules. One must make his or her own decision.

No clear criteria will help the EMT predict the futility of CPR accurately; therefore it is recommended that all patients receive CPR except in the following situations:

- Attempts to perform CPR would place the EMT at risk of physical injury.
- The patient has a valid do not attempt resuscitation (DNAR) order (to be discussed in the next section).
- The patient has signs of irreversible death (e.g., rigor mortis, decapitation, or dependent lividity).
- No physiological benefit can be expected because the vital functions have deteriorated despite maximal therapy of such conditions as progressive shock or cardiogenic shock.

Do Not Resuscitate (DNR) and Do Not Attempt Resuscitation (DNAR) Orders

The do not resuscitate (DNR) order has been the common lingo to state that the patient does not want any form of CPR initiated on them for any reason. In recent years DNR has come to mean various forms of resuscitation, such as the following:

1. Do not intubate, but perform other efforts of resuscitation.
2. Do not perform chest compressions, but perform other efforts of resuscitation
3. Perform CPR, but do not use any drugs or intubation.

All of these orders get confusing to health care providers, patients, and family members, not to mention EMTs who do not acknowledge anything but "all or nothing." The EMT performs either all resuscitative efforts or none of them with proof of a written DNR order from the family or significant other, preferably before resuscitative measures have begun. Once resuscitation has begun, legal problems can occur.

The general rule for DNR or DNAR is that the family must produce written documentation of the DNAR order before resuscitation begins. If they do not and the EMT does not perform CPR, the EMT is considered to have abandoned the patient, which leads to serious consequences to the EMT-B who left the patient regardless of what the family said. Protocols regarding this issue should be adhered to and medical control should be contacted in all situations.

The existence of a living will or advance directives is not the same as a DNR. The living will may or may not include the patient's willingness to forego CPR. The document must be read well before forgoing CPR. With time being of the essence, the EMT faces a predicament at that exact moment and must make decisions quickly and legally. The EMT may need to look over such documents and familiarize himself or herself with the different documents and what they mean.

Another tricky document is the power of attorney. A power of attorney is a document that allows another person to make decisions for the patient if required. The EMT should be careful because this document should spell out what the indicated person or persons can handle and will not include situations that the person or persons cannot handle. Therefore the indicated person may be able to handle the patient's financial responsibilities or some medical decisions if the patient is not able to do so but not necessarily be able to dictate whether the patient can receive CPR. If the decision to resuscitate or not resuscitate is included in the power of attorney, it will be stated specifically and should be spelled out for easy interpretation. If not, the EMT should initiate CPR. Asking for identification and documentation of the person with the power of attorney is also helpful. The EMT should always contact medical control for advisement.

The EMT should always initiate CPR if he or she has a reason to believe that the DNAR order is invalid, the patient may have changed his or her mind, or there is reasonable doubt not to initiate CPR. Resuscitative measures can be discontinued at the hospital once all information is obtained. It is not the responsibility of the EMT to decipher the ifs and maybes. The EMT should follow the rule of "all or nothing" until he or she has no doubt about the wishes of the patient.

The AHA and other medical communities are shying away from the term *DNR* because it might be misleading. It might suggest that resuscitation would be successful if initiated, which is not always the case; therefore new nomenclature of the AHA is *DNAR*, with no implementation of CPR.

When to terminate CPR by an EMT is usually not the decision of the provider or the family. Most EMS systems are not allowed by law to terminate CPR efforts once they have been initiated. The patient should be transferred to the emergency department with all efforts being maintained, and it is up to the physician to make the decision to discontinue CPR. Some services have strict protocols written, medical control must be contacted and advised of the situation, and the EMT must wait to received further orders. The EMTs must know under what protocols he or she is functioning. The only two unquestionable reasons to terminate CPR are (1) the rescuers are exhausted with no help in sight or (2) the patient starts breathing and has a pulse. If the patient has a pulse with no spontaneous respirations, then rescue breathing should be maintained.

Dispatch-Assisted CPR

Dispatch is the first link of the public to the 911 or emergency response. These trained professionals are the first people with whom a patient, family member, or bystander can speak to gain access in the chain of survival. This link in the chain is one of the most important for one reason—dispatch-assisted CPR. In the situation of sudden death, when a bystander calls 911 the dispatcher can send a unit to the call while keeping the bystander on the phone. Because time is of the essence in these situations, CPR can be initiated over the phone with the help of the dispatcher. The dispatcher should also be trained in CPR so that the instructions are easy to follow. The dispatcher must be able to calm the bystander down and instill the confidence in the person to initiate CPR in a probable panic condition. If the bystander is already trained in CPR, he or she may only need to be prompted in the steps or the dispatcher can "teach" the bystander step-by-step on what to do. In layperson CPR the new guidelines have eliminated assessment of the pulse, so the bystander is responsible for assessing the rise and fall of the chest and, if none is present, for beginning CPR.

CPR can save lives, but the time constraint is critical. With dispatch-assisted CPR, the bystander can initiate and continue CPR until the ambulance arrives and has support and help from the person on the other end of the phone. Dispatch-assisted CPR can only be effective if the dispatcher takes the initiative to assist the bystander and is knowledgeable about CPR. Dispatch-assisted CPR is a critical step in increasing the survival rate.

Compression-Only CPR

One concern of bystanders to initiate CPR is a fear of contracting a contagious disease. Despite studies that have shown the safety of CPR, this is a real fear for the layperson that cannot be ignored. Surveys have been administered and have published that because of this concern laypersons are reluctant to administer CPR. Because of this apprehension, other attempts have been made to overcome the problem and try to save lives. Evidence has shown that chest compression only with no mouth-to-mouth contact is significantly better than no CPR at all because some oxygen remains in the body that can be circulated to the brain. Animal studies have suggested that positive-pressure ventilation is not essential during the initial 6 to 12 minutes of adult CPR. Evidence has suggested that spontaneous gasping helps in maintaining oxygenation levels in the body. Chest compressions only generate 25% of normal output, so there is a reduced requirement for ventilations during this time.

Compression-only CPR is *not* to take the place of the AHA's CPR guidelines; it is not the ideal method to increase survival rates. Compression only CPR is recommended only (1) when a rescuer is unwilling or unable to perform mouth-to-mouth rescue breathing or (2) for use in dispatch-assisted CPR instructions in which the simplicity of this modified technique allows untrained bystanders to rapidly intervene.

Complications

CPR is not without complications even when performed properly. Nevertheless, the complications are not a contraindication to performing CPR. It should still be performed because it saves lives.

The most common complication of CPR is gastric distention caused by overinflation of the lungs. Air that is pushed into the body from the mouth can only go into two places—the lungs via the trachea or the stomach via the esophagus. With a properly positioned airway, the majority of the air goes into the lungs; however, any excess goes into the stomach. For these reasons it is important to properly open and maintain the airway and to limit breath volume enough to see a rise and fall in the chest. Once the chest has risen sufficiently, the breath should be terminated to prevent excess air from entering the stomach. For this reason it is important to watch for the rise and fall of the chest and pay attention. Allowing 2 seconds per breath also can decrease the chance of gastric distention. If possible, having another rescuer apply pressure on the cricoid (Adam's apple) can also diminish gastric distention. This provides for a more direct route of the air into the lungs. Other factors that can lead to gastric distention are forceful breaths, rapid breaths, and short inspiratory breaths. These factors should be avoided and stopped if they are present.

If the stomach becomes distended during CPR, the EMT should not attempt to place pressure on the external portion of the patient's stomach to try to expel its contents. One of the complications of gastric distention is regurgitation and aspiration of its contents into the lungs. The air and pressure in the stomach can increase so much as to cause regurgitation. If this happens, the EMT should roll the patient to one side, wipe out the contents of his or her mouth and nose as much as possible, and continue CPR.

When performed properly, CPR can cause rib fractures. This can cause other rare complications or injuries to the child or infant patient. Rib fractures from CPR are usually seen in elderly patients who have fragile bones. These fractures can be minimized with proper hand placement and correct compression depths.

Current Changes in the International Guidelines for CPR

One of the major changes in the new international guidelines for CPR is in the teaching and simplification of the skills for the layperson. The emphasis is placed only on CPR and not on obstructed airway. Obstructed airway education will no longer be taught in the layperson CPR class for simplification of the course. Studies indicate that the layperson can get bogged down with the details of CPR and obstructed airway and come away from the class without a clear knowledge of the most important aspects. Another change is in teaching the layperson how to detect a pulse. The layperson may not be able to remember where the pulse can be found, may get confused, and may not initiate CPR. Therefore this step has been removed from the skills. These changes are for the layperson only, not the health care provider. The goal of the changes is to give the layperson more confidence and desire to want to initiate CPR. This is because CPR saves lives—the sooner it is initiated, the better the chance of survival.

The following skill sheets are to be used as a refresher tool:

Appendix A

Student Name: _____ Date: _____
Examiner: _____

RELIEF OF FOREIGN BODY AIRWAY OBSTRUCTION (FBAO)
Responsive Adult or Child Victim Standing or Sitting

	POINTS POSSIBLE	POINTS AWARDED
Take or verbalize body substance isolation precautions	1	
Determine if the victim is choking and obtain consent to intervene	1	
Stand behind the victim, wrap arms around the victims waist and make a fist with one hand	1	
Place the thumb side of your fist against the victim's abdomen, in the midline slightly above the navel and well below the tip of the xiphoid process	1	
Grasp the fist with the other hand and press the fist into the victim's abdomen with a quick inward and upward thrust	1	
Repeat the thrusts until the object is expelled from the airway or the victim becomes unresponsive	1	
Each new thrust should be a separate and distinct movement administered with the intent of relieving the obstruction	1	
Repeat the sequence of attempts (and reattempts) to ventilate, Heimlich maneuver, and tongue-jaw lift and finger sweep until the obstruction is cleared or advanced procedures are available to establish a patent airway	1	
If the FBAO is not removed, follow the procedures for FBAO in an unconscious victim	1	
If the FBAO is removed and the airway is cleared, check breathing	1	
If the victim is not breathing, provide rescue breaths. Then check for signs of circulation (pulse check and evidence of breathing, coughing, or movement). If there are no signs of circulation, begin chest compression.	1	
If the victim is breathing or resumes effective breathing, place in recovery position.	1	
TOTAL:	12	

Critical Criteria

_____ Failure to take or verbalize body substance isolation precautions
_____ Did not determine if victim was choking and obtain consent
_____ Incorrect hand placement
_____ Did not follow the correct sequence
_____ Did not perform the Heimlich maneuver until FBAO was relieved or the victim became unresponsive
_____ Did not assess breathing or circulation after relieving the FBAO
_____ Did not provide rescue breathing or CPR as necessary after relieving the FBAO

Student Name: _____   Date: _____

Examiner: _____

RELIEF OF FOREIGN BODY AIRWAY OBSTRUCTION (FBAO)
Adult Victim Found Unresponsive

	POINTS POSSIBLE	POINTS AWARDED
Take or verbalize body substance isolation precautions	1	
Establish unresponsiveness	1	
Open the airway and attempt to provide rescue breaths	1	
If unable to make the chest rise, reposition the victim's head (reopen the airway) and try to ventilate again	1	
If the victim cannot be ventilated even after attempt to reposition the airway, straddle the victim's knees and perform the Heimlich maneuver (up to 5 times)	1	
After 5 abdominal thrusts, open the victim's airway using a tongue-jaw lift and perform a finger sweep to remove the object	1	
Repeat the sequence of attempts (and reattempts) to ventilate, Heimlich maneuver, and tongue-jaw lift and finger sweep until the obstruction is cleared or advanced procedures are available to establish a patent airway	1	
If the FBAO is removed and the airway is cleared, check breathing	1	
If the victim is not breathing, provide rescue breaths. Then check for signs of circulation (pulse check and evidence of breathing, coughing, or movement). If there are no signs of circulation, begin chest compression.	1	
If the victim is breathing or resumes effective breathing, place in recovery position.	1	
TOTAL:	10	

Critical Criteria

_____ Failure to take or verbalize body substance isolation precautions
_____ Failure to establish unresponsiveness
_____ Did not open the victim's airway
_____ Did not establish that the victim was not breathing
_____ Did not attempt to provide rescue breaths
_____ Did not reposition the victims airway and re-attempt to provide rescue breaths
_____ Did not perform the Heimlich maneuver (up to 5 times)
_____ Did not follow the correct sequence
_____ Did not repeat the sequence of attempts (and re-attempts) to ventilate, Heimlich maneuver, and tongue-jaw lift and finger sweep until the obstruction is cleared
_____ Did not assess breathing or circulation after relieving the FBAO
_____ Did not provide rescue breathing or CPR as necessary after relieving the FBAO

Appendix A

Student Name: _____   Date: _____
Examiner: _____

RELIEF OF FOREIGN BODY AIRWAY OBSTRUCTION (FBAO)
Adult Victim Who Becomes Unresponsive

	POINTS POSSIBLE	POINTS AWARDED
Take or verbalize body substance isolation precautions	1	
Establish unresponsiveness	1	
Perform a tongue-jaw lift, followed by a finger sweep to remove the object	1	
Open the airway and attempt to ventilate	1	
If unable to make the victim's chest rise, reposition the head and try to ventilate again	1	
If the chest does not rise with attempted breaths, even after repositioning the airway, straddle the victim's thighs and perform the Heimlich maneuver (up to 5 times)	1	
After 5 abdominal thrusts, open the victim's airway using a tongue-jaw lift and perform a finger sweep to remove the object	1	
Repeat the sequence of attempts (and reattempts) to ventilate, Heimlich maneuver, and tongue-jaw lift and finger sweep until the obstruction is cleared or advanced procedures are available to establish a patent airway	1	
If the FBAO is removed and the airway is cleared, check breathing	1	
If the victim is not breathing, provide rescue breaths. Then check for signs of circulation (pulse check and evidence of breathing, coughing, or movement). If there are no signs of circulation, begin chest compression.	1	
If the victim is breathing or resumes effective breathing, place in recovery position.	1	
TOTAL:	11	

Critical Criteria

_____ Failure to take or verbalize body substance isolation precautions
_____ Failure to establish unresponsiveness
_____ Did not open the victim's airway
_____ Did not establish that the victim was not breathing
_____ Did not attempt to provide rescue breaths
_____ Did not reposition the victims airway and re-attempt to provide rescue breaths
_____ Did not perform the Heimlich maneuver (up to 5 times)
_____ Did not repeat the sequence of attempts (and re-attempts) to ventilate, Heimlich maneuver, and tongue-jaw lift and finger sweep until the obstruction is cleared
_____ Did not assess breathing or circulation after relieving the FBAO
_____ Did not provide rescue breathing or CPR as necessary after relieving the FBAO

Student Name: _____   Date: _____

Examiner: _____

RELIEF OF FOREIGN BODY AIRWAY OBSTRUCTION (FBAO)
Child Victim Found Unresponsive

	POINTS POSSIBLE	POINTS AWARDED
Take or verbalize body substance isolation precautions	1	
Establish unresponsiveness	1	
Open the airway and attempt to provide rescue breaths	1	
If unable to make the chest rise, reposition the victim's head (reopen the airway) and try to ventilate again	1	
If the victim cannot be ventilated even after attempt to reposition the airway, straddle the victim's knees and perform the Heimlich maneuver (up to 5 times)	1	
After 5 abdominal thrusts, open the victim's airway using a tongue-jaw lift and look for an object in the pharynx. If an object is visible, perform a finger sweep to remove the object. *DO NOT* perform a blind finger sweep.	1	
Repeat the sequence of attempts (and reattempts) to ventilate, Heimlich maneuver, and tongue-jaw lift, visualize, and finger sweep if appropriate, until the obstruction is cleared or advanced procedures are available to establish a patent airway	1	
If the FBAO is removed and the airway is cleared, check breathing	1	
If the victim is not breathing, provide rescue breaths. Then check for signs of circulation (pulse check and evidence of breathing, coughing, or movement). If there are no signs of circulation, begin chest compression.	1	
If the victim is breathing or resumes effective breathing, place in recovery position.	1	
TOTAL:	10	

Critical Criteria

_____ Failure to take or verbalize body substance isolation precautions
_____ Failure to establish unresponsiveness
_____ Failure to open the victim's airway
_____ Failure to establish that the victim was not breathing
_____ Failure to attempt to provide rescue breaths
_____ Failure to reposition the victims airway and re-attempt to provide rescue breaths
_____ Failure to perform the Heimlich maneuver
_____ Performed a blind finger sweep
_____ Failure to look for an object in the pharynx after abdominal thrusts but before attempting ventilation
_____ Failure to follow the correct sequence
_____ Failure to assess breathing or circulation after relieving the FBAO
_____ Failure to provide rescue breathing or CPR as necessary after relieving the FBAO

Student Name: _____ Date: _____
Examiner: _____

RELIEF OF FOREIGN BODY AIRWAY OBSTRUCTION (FBAO)
Child Victim Who Becomes Unresponsive

	POINTS POSSIBLE	POINTS AWARDED
Take or verbalize body substance isolation precautions	1	
Perform a tongue-jaw lift and look for an object in the pharynx. If an object is visible, remove it using a finger sweep. DO NOT perform a blind finger sweep.	1	
Open the airway and attempt to ventilate	1	
If unable to make the victim's chest rise, reposition the head and try to ventilate again	1	
If the chest does not rise with attempted breaths, even after repositioning the airway, straddle the victim's hips and perform the Heimlich maneuver (up to 5 times)	1	
After 5 abdominal thrusts, open the victim's airway using a tongue-jaw lift and look for an object in the pharynx. If visible, remove it with a finger sweep.	1	
Repeat the sequence of attempts (and reattempts) to ventilate, Heimlich maneuver, and tongue-jaw lift, visualize, and finger sweep if appropriate until the obstruction is cleared or advanced procedures are available to establish a patent airway	1	
If the FBAO is removed and the airway is cleared, check breathing	1	
If the victim is not breathing, provide rescue breaths. Then check for signs of circulation (pulse check and evidence of breathing, coughing, or movement). If there are no signs of circulation, begin chest compression.	1	
If the victim is breathing or resumes effective breathing, place in recovery position.	1	
TOTAL:	10	

Critical Criteria

_____ Failure to take or verbalize body substance isolation precautions
_____ Failure to open victim's airway
_____ Failure to visualize for an object before attempting ventilation
_____ Incorrect hand placement
_____ Failure to follow the correct sequence
_____ Performed a blind finger sweep
_____ Failure to assess breathing or circulation after relieving the FBAO
_____ Failure to provide rescue breathing or CPR as necessary after relieving the FBAO

Student Name: _____ Date: _____

Examiner: _____

RELIEF OF FOREIGN BODY AIRWAY OBSTRUCTION (FBAO)
Infant Victim Who Becomes Unresponsive

	POINTS POSSIBLE	POINTS AWARDED
Take or verbalize body substance isolation precautions	1	
Perform a tongue-jaw lift and look for an object in the pharynx. If an object is visible, remove it using a finger sweep. DO NOT perform a blind finger sweep.	1	
Open the airway and attempt to ventilate	1	
If unable to make the victim's chest rise, reposition the head and try to ventilate again	1	
If the chest does not rise with attempted breaths, even after repositioning the airway, perform the sequence of up to 5 back blows and up to 5 chest thrusts.	1	
Open the victim's airway using a tongue-jaw lift and look for an object in the pharynx. If visible, remove it.	1	
Attempt to ventilate	1	
Repeat the sequence of attempts (and reattempts) to ventilate, up to 5 back blows, up to 5 chest thrusts, open the airway, visualize for an object and finger sweep if appropriate, and attempt to ventilate until the obstruction is cleared or advanced procedures are available to establish a patent airway	1	
If the FBAO is removed and the airway is cleared, check breathing	1	
If the victim is not breathing, provide rescue breaths. Then check for signs of circulation (pulse check and evidence of breathing, coughing, or movement). If there are no signs of circulation, begin chest compression.	1	
If the victim is breathing or resumes effective breathing, place in recovery position.	1	
TOTAL:	11	

Critical Criteria

_____ Failure to take or verbalize body substance isolation precautions

_____ Incorrect hand placement

_____ Performed a blind finger sweep

_____ Failure to open the victim's airway

_____ Failure to perform a tongue-jaw lift and visualize for an object before attempting to ventilate

_____ Failure to follow the correct sequence

_____ Failure to perform the Heimlich maneuver until FBAO was relieved or the victim became unresponsive

_____ Failure to assess breathing or circulation after relieving the FBAO

_____ Failure to provide rescue breathing or CPR as necessary after relieving the FBAO

Student Name: _____ Date: _____
Examiner: _____

RELIEF OF FOREIGN BODY AIRWAY OBSTRUCTION (FBAO)
Infant Victim Found Unresponsive

	POINTS POSSIBLE	POINTS AWARDED
Take or verbalize body substance isolation precautions	1	
Establish unresponsiveness	1	
Open the airway and attempt to ventilate	1	
If unable to make the victim's chest rise, reposition the head and try to ventilate again	1	
If the chest does not rise with attempted breaths, even after repositioning the airway, perform the sequence of up to 5 back blows and up to 5 chest thrusts.	1	
Open the victim's airway using a tongue-jaw lift and look for an object in the pharynx. If visible, remove it.	1	
Repeat the sequence of attempts (and reattempts) to ventilate, up to 5 back blows, up to 5 chest thrusts, open the airway, visualize for an object and finger sweep if appropriate, and attempt to ventilate until the obstruction is cleared or advanced procedures are available to establish a patent airway	1	
If the FBAO is removed and the airway is cleared, check breathing	1	
If the victim is breathing, check for signs of circulation (pulse check and evidence of breathing, coughing, or movement). If there are no signs of circulation, begin chest compression.	1	
If the victim is not breathing, provide rescue breaths.	1	
If the victim is breathing and has a pulse place in recovery position.	1	
TOTAL:	11	

Critical Criteria

_____ Failure to take or verbalize body substance isolation precautions
_____ Incorrect hand placement
_____ Performed a blind finger sweep
_____ Failure to open the victim's airway
_____ Failure to assess for breathing
_____ Failure to follow the correct sequence
_____ Failure to perform a tongue-jaw lift and visualize for an object before attempting to ventilate
_____ Did not assess breathing or circulation after relieving the FBAO
_____ Did not provide rescue breathing or CPR as necessary after relieving the FBAO

Student Name: _____ Date: _____

Examiner: _____

CARDIOPULMONARY RESUSCITATION
Adult One-Rescuer - EMS Responder

	POINTS POSSIBLE	POINTS AWARDED
Take or verbalize body substance isolation precautions	1	
Establish unresponsiveness	1	
Open the airway (head tilt - chin lift or jaw thrust maneuver)	1	
Assess breathing (look, listen and feel) to identify absent or inadequate breathing taking no more than 10 seconds	1	
If victim is breathing or resumes effective breathing, place in recovery position	1	
If victim is not breathing, give 2 slow breaths (without O_2 supplement over 2 seconds each; with O_2 supplement over 1 to 2 seconds)	1	
If unable to give initial breaths, reposition the head and re-attempt ventilation. If still unsuccessful, follow unresponsive FBAO sequence	1	
Assess for signs of circulation by feeling for a carotid pulse - taking no more than 10 seconds	1	
If there are no signs of circulation, begin chest compressions by locating proper hand position - Consider AED use if available and appropriate	1	
Perform 15 chest compressions at a rate of approximately 100 per minute, depressing the chest 1½ to 2 inches with each compression	1	
Open the airway and deliver 2 slow rescue breaths (2 seconds each)	1	
Find the proper hand position and begin 15 more compressions at a rate of 100 per minute	1	
Perform 4 complete cycles of 15 compressions and 2 ventilations	1	
Re-assess for signs of circulation (10 seconds)	1	
If there are still no signs of circulation, resume CPR, beginning with chest compressions, checking for signs of circulation and spontaneous breathing every few minutes	1	
If signs of circulation are present, check for breathing	1	
If breathing is present, place the victim in a recovery position and monitor breathing and circulation	1	
If breathing is absent but signs of circulation are present, provide rescue breathing at 10 to 12 times per minute (1 breath every 4 to 5 seconds) and monitor for signs of circulation every few minutes	1	
TOTAL:	18	

Critical Criteria

_____ Failure to take or verbalize body substance isolation precautions
_____ Failure to establish unresponsiveness
_____ Did not open the victim's airway
_____ Did not establish that the victim was not breathing
_____ Did not deliver two adequate rescue breaths
_____ Took longer than 10 seconds to establish that the patient was not breathing
_____ Did not assess for a pulse
_____ Took longer than 10 seconds to establish that the patient had no pulse
_____ Did not consider AED use
_____ Did not deliver compressions at an appropriate depth, location, or rate
_____ Did not re-assess the patient's circulatory or respiratory status
_____ Did not assess breathing status after the return of a pulse
_____ Did not provide rescue breathing as necessary after the return of a pulse

Appendix A

Student Name: _____ Date: _____

Examiner: _____

CARDIOPULMONARY RESUSCITATION
Adult Two-Rescuer - EMS Responder

	POINTS POSSIBLE	POINTS AWARDED
Take or verbalize body substance isolation precautions	1	
Establish unresponsiveness	1	
RESCUER #1 Remains at the victim's head		
Open the airway (head tilt - chin lift or jaw thrust maneuver)	1	
Assess breathing (look, listen and feel) to identify absent or inadequate breathing taking no more than 10 seconds	1	
If victim is breathing or resumes effective breathing, place in recovery position	1	
If victim is not breathing, give 2 slow breaths (without O_2 supplement over 2 seconds each; with O_2 supplement over 1 to 2 seconds)	1	
If unable to give initial breaths, reposition the head and re-attempt ventilation. If still unsuccessful, follow unresponsive FBAO sequence	1	
Assess for signs of circulation by feeling for a carotid pulse - taking no more than 10 seconds	1	
RESCUER #2 Positioned at the victim's side		
If there are no signs of circulation, begin chest compressions by locating proper hand position - consider AED use if available and appropriate	1	
Perform 15 chest compressions at a rate of approximately 100 per minute, depressing the chest 1½ to 2 inches with each compression	1	
RESCUERS #1 and #2		
Continue CPR with a compression to ventilation ratio of 15:2, with a pause for ventilation of 2 seconds each until the airway is secured by a cuffed endotracheal tube	1	
When the person performing chest compressions becomes fatigued, the rescuers should change positions with minimal interruption of chest compressions	1	
RESCUER #1		
Assess the effectiveness of the partner's chest compressions by checking the pulse during compressions	1	
Determine whether the victims has resumed spontaneous breathing and circulation by stopping compressions for 10 seconds at approximately the end of the first minute of CPR and every few minutes thereafter	1	
If signs of circulation are present, check for breathing	1	
If breathing is present, place the victim in a recovery position and monitor breathing and circulation	1	
If breathing is absent but signs of circulation are present, provide rescue breathing at 10 to 12 times per minute (1 breath every 4 to 5 seconds) and monitor for signs of circulation every few minutes	1	
TOTAL:	17	

Critical Criteria

_____ Failure to take or verbalize body substance isolation precautions

_____ Failure to establish unresponsiveness

_____ Did not open the victim's airway

_____ Did not establish that the victim was not breathing

_____ Took longer than 10 seconds to establish that the patient was not breathing

_____ Did not assess for a pulse

_____ Took longer than 10 seconds to establish that the patient had no pulse

_____ Did not consider AED use

_____ Did not deliver two adequate rescue breaths

_____ Did not deliver compressions at an appropriate depth, location, or rate

_____ Did not re-assess the patient's circulatory or respiratory status

_____ Did not assess breathing status after the return of a pulse

_____ Did not provide rescue breathing as necessary after the return of a pulse

Student Name: _____   Date: _____

Examiner: _____

CARDIOPULMONARY RESUSCITATION
Child Victim - EMS Responder

	POINTS POSSIBLE	POINTS AWARDED
Take or verbalize body substance isolation precautions	1	
Establish unresponsiveness	1	
Open the airway (head tilt - chin lift or jaw thrust maneuver)	1	
Assess breathing (look, listen and feel) to identify absent or inadequate breathing taking no more than 10 seconds	1	
If victim is breathing or resumes effective breathing, place in recovery position	1	
If victim is not breathing, give 2 slow breaths (mouth-to-mouth, with enough volume to make the chest rise, taking 1 - 1½ seconds per breath)	1	
If unable to give initial breaths, reposition the head and re-attempt ventilation. If still unsuccessful, follow unresponsive FBAO sequence	1	
Assess for signs of circulation by feeling for a carotid pulse - taking no more than 10 seconds	1	
If there are no signs of circulation, begin chest compressions by locating proper hand position	1	
Perform 5 chest compressions at a rate of approximately 100 per minute	1	
Open the airway and deliver one ventilation (1-1½ seconds per breath; use bag-mask ventilation if readily available)	1	
Perform 10 complete cycles of 5 compressions and 1 ventilation (5:1 ratio)	1	
Re-assess for signs of circulation (10 seconds)	1	
If there are still no signs of circulation, resume CPR, beginning with chest compressions, checking for signs of circulation and spontaneous breathing every few minutes	1	
If signs of circulation are present, check for breathing	1	
If breathing is present, place the victim in a recovery position and monitor breathing and circulation	1	
If breathing is absent but signs of circulation are present, provide rescue breathing at 20 breaths per minute (1 breath every 3 seconds) and monitor for signs of circulation every few minutes	1	
TOTAL:	17	

Critical Criteria

_____ Failure to take or verbalize body substance isolation precautions
_____ Failure to establish unresponsiveness
_____ Did not open the victim's airway
_____ Did not establish that the victim was not breathing
_____ Took longer than 10 seconds to establish that the patient was not breathing
_____ Did not assess for a pulse
_____ Took longer than 10 seconds to establish that the patient had no pulse
_____ Did not deliver two adequate rescue breaths
_____ Did not deliver compressions at an appropriate depth, location, or rate
_____ Did not re-assess the patient's circulatory or respiratory status
_____ Did not assess breathing status after the return of a pulse
_____ Did not provide rescue breathing as necessary after the return of a pulse

Student Name: _____ Date: _____

Examiner: _____

CARDIOPULMONARY RESUSCITATION
Infant Victim - EMS Responder

	POINTS POSSIBLE	POINTS AWARDED
Take or verbalize body substance isolation precautions	1	
Establish unresponsiveness - attempt to stimulate	1	
Open the airway (head tilt - chin lift or jaw thrust maneuver)	1	
Assess breathing (look, listen and feel) to identify absent or inadequate breathing taking no more than 10 seconds	1	
If victim is breathing or resumes effective breathing, place in recovery position	1	
If victim is not breathing, give 2 slow breaths (mouth-to-mouth-and-nose, with enough volume to make the chest rise, taking 1 - 1½ seconds per breath)	1	
If unable to give initial breaths, reposition the head and re-attempt ventilation. If still unsuccessful, follow unresponsive FBAO sequence	1	
Assess for signs of circulation by feeling for a brachial pulse - taking no more than 10 seconds	1	
If there are no signs of circulation or if the pulse rate is <60 bpm with signs of poor perfusion, begin chest compressions by locating proper hand position	1	
Perform 5 chest compressions at a rate of approximately 100 per minute at a depth of ½ to 1 inch, using the 2 finger technique for 1 rescuer and 2 thumb technique for 2 rescuers	1	
Open the airway and deliver 1 slow rescue breath (1 - 1½ seconds, using a bag-mask ventilation for 2 rescuers, if readily available)	1	
Find the proper hand position and continue with a series of 5 compressions and 1 breath at a rate of 100 per minute	1	
Perform 10 complete cycles of 5 compressions and 1 ventilation each	1	
Re-assess for signs of circulation (taking no more than 10 seconds)	1	
If there are still no signs of adequate circulation, resume CPR, beginning with chest compressions at a ratio of 5 compressions to 1 ventilation, checking for signs of circulation and spontaneous breathing every few minutes	1	
If signs of adequate circulation are present, check for breathing	1	
If breathing is present, place the victim in a recovery position and monitor breathing and circulation	1	
If breathing is absent but signs of adequate circulation are present, provide rescue breathing at a rate of 20 per minute (1 breath every 3 seconds) until breathing resumes, and monitor for signs of circulation every few minutes	1	
TOTAL:	18	

Critical Criteria

_____ Failure to take or verbalize body substance isolation precautions
_____ Did not open the victim's airway
_____ Did not establish that the victim was not breathing
_____ Took longer than 10 seconds to establish that the patient was not breathing
_____ Did not assess for a pulse
_____ Took longer than 10 seconds to establish that the patient had no pulse
_____ Did not begin chest compressions with heart rate of 60 bpm or less with signs of poor perfusion
_____ Did not deliver two adequate rescue breaths
_____ Did not deliver compressions at an appropriate depth, location, or rate
_____ Did not re-assess the patient's circulatory or respiratory status
_____ Did not assess breathing status after the return of a pulse
_____ Did not provide rescue breathing as necessary after the return of a pulse

Student Name: _____   Date: _____

Examiner: _____

CARDIOPULMONARY RESUSCITATION
Newborn Infant Victim - EMS Responder

	POINTS POSSIBLE	POINTS AWARDED
Take or verbalize body substance isolation precautions	1	
Establish unresponsiveness - attempt to stimulate	1	
Prevent heat loss - keep newborn as warm as possible	1	
Open the airway (head tilt - chin lift or jaw thrust maneuver to a neutral position)	1	
Assess breathing (look, listen and feel) to identify absent or inadequate breathing - taking no more than 10 seconds	1	
If victim is not breathing, give 2 slow breaths (mouth-to-mouth-and-nose, with enough volume to make the chest rise, taking ½ to 1 second per breath)	1	
Assess for signs of circulation by feeling for a brachial pulse - taking no more than 10 seconds	1	
If heart rate is 60 to 80 bpm and not rising, ventilation should be the priority in resuscitation. If there are no signs of circulation or if heart rate is <60 bpm, begin chest compressions by locating proper hand position.	1	
Perform 3 chest compressions at a rate of approximately 120 per minute at a depth of ½ to 1 inch, using the 2 finger technique for 1 rescuer and 2 thumb technique for 2 rescuers [unless local protocols require a 5:1 ratio]	1	
Open the airway and deliver 1 slow rescue breath (½ second, using a bag-mask ventilation for 2 rescuers, if readily available)	1	
Find the proper hand position and continue with a series of 3 compressions and 1 breath at a rate of 120 per minute [unless local protocols require a 5:1 ratio]	1	
After approximately 1 minute, re-assess for signs of circulation (taking no more than 10 seconds)	1	
If there are still no signs of circulation, resume CPR, beginning with chest compressions, checking for signs of circulation and spontaneous breathing every few minutes	1	
If signs of circulation are present, check for breathing	1	
If breathing is present, place the victim in a recovery position and monitor breathing and circulation	1	
If breathing is absent but signs of adequate circulation are present or if heart rate continues at a rate <100 bpm, provide rescue breathing at 40 to 60 per minute using a neonatal BVM and monitor for signs of circulation every few minutes	1	
TOTAL:	16	

Critical Criteria

_____ Failure to take or verbalize body substance isolation precautions
_____ Did not take steps to prevent heat loss
_____ Did not open the victim's airway
_____ Did not establish that the victim was not breathing or that breathing was inadequate
_____ Took longer than 10 seconds to establish that the patient was not breathing
_____ Did not assess for a pulse
_____ Took longer than 10 seconds to establish that the patient had no pulse
_____ Did not begin assisted ventilations with heart rate of 100 bpm or less
_____ Did not begin chest compressions with heart rate of 60 bpm or less
_____ Did not deliver adequate rescue breaths
_____ Did not deliver compressions at an appropriate depth, location, or rate
_____ Did not re-assess the patient's circulatory or respiratory status
_____ Did not assess breathing status after the return of a pulse
_____ Did not provide appropriate rescue breaths as necessary after the return of a pulse

Appendix B

National Registry of Emergency Medical Technicians (NREMT) Skill Sheets

Since its inception in 1970 the primary goal of the National Registry of Emergency Medical Technicians (NREMT) has been to promulgate the standardization of certification and licensure standards. At this time 40 states use the NREMT.

Although the skill sheets are used for testing, they are in reality the way that patient care should flow and therefore are good teaching guides and patient care guides. Included with the skill sheets are the "Instructions to the Candidate" for each of the skill stations. These instructions are used for each EMT student being tested. They have been written so that each candidate has a clear understanding of the requirements of the station and to ensure consistency when the candidate is given instructions from the evaluator.

Instructions to the Candidate

Patient Assessment and Management—Trauma

This station is designed to test your ability to perform a patient assessment of a victim of multisystem trauma and voice treat all conditions and injuries discovered. You must conduct your assessment as you would in the field, including communicating with your patient. You may remove the patient's clothing down to shorts or swimsuit if you feel it is necessary. As you conduct your assessment, you should state everything that you are assessing. Clinical information not obtainable by visual or physical inspection, such as blood pressure, will be given to you after you demonstrate how you would normally gain that information. You may assume that you have two EMTs working with you and that they are correctly carrying out the verbal treatments that you indicate. You have 10 minutes to complete this skill station. Do you have any questions?

Instructions to the Candidate

Patient Assessment and Management—Medical

This station is designed to test your ability to perform a patient assessment of a victim with a chief complaint of a medical nature and voice treat all conditions and injuries discovered. You must conduct your assessment as you would in the field, including communicating with your patient. As you conduct your assessment, you should state everything that you are assessing. Clinical information not obtainable by visual or physical inspection, such as blood pressure, will be given to you after you demonstrate how you would normally gain that information. You may assume that you have two EMTs working with you and that they are correctly carrying out the verbal treatments that you indicate. You have 10 minutes to complete this skill station. Do you have any questions?

Instructions to the Candidate

Cardiac Arrest Management

This station is designed to test your ability to manage a prehospital cardiac arrest by integrating CPR skills, defibrillation, airway adjuncts, and patient and scene management skills. There will be an EMT assistant in this station. The EMT assistant will only do as you instruct. As you arrive on the scene, you will encounter a patient in cardiac arrest. A first responder will be present performing single rescuer CPR. You must immediately establish control of the scene and begin resuscitation of the patient with an automated external defibrillator. At the appropriate time, you must control the airway and ventilate the victim using adjunctive equipment. You may not delegate this action to the EMT assistant. You may use any of the supplies available in this room. You have 15 minutes to complete this skill station. Do you have any questions?

Instructions to the Candidate

Airway, Oxygen, and Ventilation Skills—Bag-Valve-Mask for Apneic Patient with Pulse

This station is designed to test your ability to ventilate a patient using a bag-valve-mask (BVM). As you enter the station, you will find an apneic patient with a palpable central pulse. There are no bystanders, and artificial ventilation has not been initiated. The only patient intervention required is airway management and ventilatory support using a BVM. You must initially ventilate the patient for a minimum of 30 seconds. You will be evaluated on the appropriateness of ventilator volumes. I will inform you that a second rescuer has arrived and will instruct you that you must control the airway and the mask seal while the second rescuer provides ventilation. You may use only the equipment available in this room. Do you have any questions?

Instructions to the Candidate

Spinal Immobilization—Supine Patient

This station is designed to test your ability to provide spinal immobilization on a patient using a long spine immobilization device. You arrive on the scene with an EMT assistant. The assistant has completed the scene size-up and the initial and focused assessments. As you begin the station, the patient has no airway, breathing, or circulatory problems. You are required to treat the specific isolated problem of an unstable spine using a long spine immobilization device. When moving the patient to the device, you should use the help of the EMT assistant and the evaluator. The EMT assistant should control the head and cervical spine of the patient while you and the evaluator move the patient to the immobilization device. You are responsible for the direction and subsequent action of the EMT assistant. You may use any equipment available in this room. You have 10 minutes to complete this procedure. Do you have any questions?

Instructions to the Candidate

Spinal Immobilization—Seated Patient

This station is designed to test your ability to provide spinal immobilization on a patient using a half-spinal immobilization device. You arrive on the scene with an EMT assistant. The EMT assistant has completed the scene size-up and initial and focused assessments. As you begin the station, the patient has no airway, breathing, or circulatory problems. You are required to treat the specific isolated problem of an unstable spine using a half-spinal immobilization device. Continued assessment of airway, breathing, and central circulation is not necessary. You are responsible for the direction and subsequent actions of the EMT assistant. Transferring the patient to the long spine board should be accomplished verbally. You may use any equipment available in this room. You have 10 minutes to complete this procedure. Do you have any questions?

Instructions to the Candidate

Immobilization Skills—Long Bone

This station is designed to test your ability to properly immobilize a closed, nonangulated long bone injury. You are required to treat only the specific, isolated injury. The scene size-up and initial assessment have been completed, and during the focused assessment a closed, nonangulated injury of the _____ (radius, ulna, tibia, fibula) was detected. Ongoing assessment of the patient's airway, breathing, and central circulation is not necessary. You may use any equipment available in this room. You have 5 minutes to complete this procedure. Do you have any questions?

Instructions to the Candidate

Immobilization Skills—Joint Injury

This station is designed to test your ability to properly immobilize a noncomplicated shoulder injury. You are required to treat only the specific, isolated injury. The scene size-up and initial assessment have been accomplished on the victim, and during the focused assessment a shoulder injury was detected. Ongoing assessment of the patient's airway, breathing, and central circulation is not necessary. You may use any equipment available in this room. You have 5 minutes to complete this procedure. Do you have any questions?

Instructions to the Candidate

Immobilization Skills—Traction Splinting

This station is designed to test your ability to properly immobilize a midshaft femur injury with a traction splint. You will have an EMT assistant to help you in the application of the device by applying manual traction when directed to do so. You are required to treat only the specific, isolated injury. The scene size-up and initial assessment have been accomplished on the victim, and during the focused assessment a midshaft femur deformity was detected. Ongoing assessment of the patient's airway, breathing, and central circulation is not necessary. You may use any equipment available in this room. You have 10 minutes to complete this procedure. Do you have any questions?

Instructions to the Candidate

Bleeding Control and Shock Management

This station is designed to test your ability to control hemorrhage. This is a scenario-based testing station. As you progress through the scenario, you will be offered various signs and symptoms appropriate for the patient's condition. You will be required to manage the patient based on these signs and symptoms. A scenario will be read aloud to you, and you will be given an opportunity to ask clarifying questions about the scenario; however, you will not receive answers to any questions about the actual steps of the procedures to be performed. You may use any of the supplies and equipment available in this room. You have 10 minutes to complete this skill station. Do you have any questions?

Instructions to the Candidate

Airway, Oxygen, and Ventilation Skills—Upper Airway Adjuncts and Suction

This station is designed to test your ability to properly measure, insert, and remove an oropharyngeal and a nasopharyngeal airway and suction a patient's upper airway. This is an isolated skill test comprised of three separate skills. You may use any equipment available in this room. Do you have any questions?

Instructions to the Candidate

Airway, Oxygen, and Ventilation Skills—Mouth-to-Mask with Supplemental Oxygen

This station is designed to test your ability to ventilate a patient with supplemental oxygen using a mouth-to-mask technique. This is an isolated skill test. You may assume that mouth-to-mouth ventilation is in progress and that the patient has a central pulse. The only patient management required is ventilator support using a mouth-to-mask technique with supplemental oxygen. You must ventilate the patient for at least 30 seconds. You will be evaluated on the appropriateness of ventilatory volumes. You may use any equipment available in this room. Do you have any questions?

Instructions to the Candidate

Airway, Oxygen, and Ventilation Skills—Supplemental Oxygen Administration

This station is designed to test your ability to correctly assemble the equipment needed to administer supplemental oxygen in the prehospital setting. This is an isolated skill test. You will be required to assemble an oxygen tank and regulator and administer oxygen to a patient using a nonrebreather mask. Because the patient cannot tolerate the mask at this point, you will be instructed to discontinue oxygen administration by the nonrebreather mask and start oxygen administration using a nasal cannula. Once you have initiated oxygen administration using a nasal cannula, you will be instructed to discontinue oxygen administration completely. You may use only the equipment available in this room. Do you have any questions?

Patient Assessment/Management - Trauma

Start Time: _____
Stop Time: _____   Date: _____
Candidate's Name: _____
Evaluator's Name: _____

		POINTS POSSIBLE	POINTS AWARDED
Takes, or verbalizes, body substance isolation precautions		1	
SCENE SIZE-UP			
Determines the scene is safe		1	
Determines the mechanism of injury		1	
Determines the number of patients		1	
Requests additional help if necessary		1	
Considers stabilization of spine		1	
INITIAL ASSESSMENT			
Verbalizes general impression of the patient		1	
Determines responsiveness/level of consciousness		1	
Determines chief complaint/apparent life threats		1	
Assesses airway and breathing	Assessment Initiates appropriate oxygen therapy Assures adequate ventilation Injury management	1 1 1 1	
Assesses circulation	Assesses/controls major bleeding Assesses pulse Assesses skin (color, temperature and condition)	1 1 1	
Identifies priority patients/makes transport decision		1	
FOCUSED HISTORY AND PHYSICAL EXAMINATION/RAPID TRAUMA ASSESSMENT			
Selects appropriate assessment *(focused or rapid assessment)*		1	
Obtains, or directs assistance to obtain, baseline vital signs		1	
Obtains S.A.M.P.L.E. history		1	
DETAILED PHYSICAL EXAMINATION			
Assesses the head	Inspects and palpates the scalp and ears Assesses the eyes Assesses the facial areas including oral and nasal areas	1 1 1	
Assesses the neck	Inspects and palpates the neck Assesses for JVD Assesses for tracheal deviation	1 1 1	
Assesses the chest	Inspects Palpates Auscultates	1 1 1	
Assesses the abdomen/pelvis	Assesses the abdomen Assesses the pelvis Verbalizes assessment of genitalia/perineum as needed	1 1 1	
Assesses the extremities	1 point for each extremity includes inspection, palpation, and assessment of motor, sensory and circulatory function	4	
Assesses the posterior	Assesses thorax Assesses lumbar	1 1	
Manages secondary injuries and wounds appropriately **1 point for appropriate management of the secondary injury/wound**		1	
Verbalizes re-assessment of the vital signs		1	
	TOTAL:	40	

Critical Criteria

_____ Did not take, or verbalize, body substance isolation precautions
_____ Did not determine scene safety
_____ Did not assess for spinal protection
_____ Did not provide for spinal protection when indicated
_____ Did not provide high concentration of oxygen
_____ Did not find, or manage, problems associated with airway, breathing, hemorrhage or shock (hypoperfusion)
_____ Did not differentiate patient's need for transportation versus continued assessment at the scene
_____ Did other detailed physical examination before assessing the airway, breathing and circulation
_____ Did not transport patient within (10) minute time limit

Appendix B

Patient Assessment/Management - Medical

Start Time: _____
Stop Time: _____ Date: _____
Candidate's Name: _____
Evaluator's Name: _____

	POINTS POSSIBLE	POINTS AWARDED
Takes, or verbalizes, body substance isolation precautions	1	
SCENE SIZE-UP		
Determines the scene is safe	1	
Determines the mechanism of injury/nature of illness	1	
Determines the number of patients	1	
Requests additional help if necessary	1	
Considers stabilization of spine	1	
INITIAL ASSESSMENT		
Verbalizes general impression of the patient	1	
Determines responsiveness/level of consciousness	1	
Determines chief complaint/apparent life threats	1	
Assesses airway and breathing — Assessment	1	
Assesses airway and breathing — Initiates appropriate oxygen therapy	1	
Assesses airway and breathing — Assures adequate ventilation	1	
Assesses circulation — Assesses/controls major bleeding	1	
Assesses circulation — Assesses pulse	1	
Assesses circulation — Assesses skin (color, temperature and condition)	1	
Identifies priority patients/makes transport decision	1	
FOCUSED HISTORY AND PHYSICAL EXAMINATION/RAPID ASSESSMENT		
Signs and symptoms *(Assess history of present illness)*	1	

Respiratory	Cardiac	Altered Mental Status	Allergic Reaction	Poisoning/ Overdose	Environmental Emergency	Obstetrics	Behavioral
*Onset? *Provokes? *Quality? *Radiates? *Severity? *Time? *Interventions?	*Onset? *Provokes? *Quality? *Radiates? *Severity? *Time? *Interventions?	*Description of the episode. *Onset? *Duration? *Associated Symptoms? *Evidence of Trauma? *Interventions? *Seizures? *Fever?	*History of allergies? *What were you exposed to? *How were you exposed? *Effects? *Progression? *Interventions?	*Substance? *When did you ingest/become exposed? *How much did you ingest? *Over what time period? *Interventions? *Estimated weight?	*Source? *Environment? *Duration? *Loss of consciousness? *Effects - general or local?	*Are you pregnant? *How long have you been pregnant? *Pain or contractions? *Bleeding or discharge? *Do you feel the need to push? *Last menstrual period?	*How do you feel? *Determine suicidal tendencies. *Is the patient a threat to self or others? *Is there a medical problem? *Interventions?

	POINTS POSSIBLE	POINTS AWARDED
Allergies	1	
Medications	1	
Past pertinent history	1	
Last oral intake	1	
Event leading to present illness (rule out trauma)	1	
Performs focused physical examination *(assesses affected body part/system or, if indicated, completes rapid assessment)*	1	
Vitals *(obtains baseline vital signs)*	1	
Interventions *(obtains medical direction or verbalizes standing order for medication interventions and verbalizes proper additional intervention/treatment)*	1	
Transport (re-evaluates the transport decision)	1	
Verbalizes the consideration for completing a detailed physical examination	1	
ONGOING ASSESSMENT (verbalized)		
Repeats initial assessment	1	
Repeats vital signs	1	
Repeats focused assessment regarding patient complaint or injuries	1	
TOTAL:	**30**	

Critical Criteria

_____ Did not take, or verbalize, body substance isolation precautions when necessary
_____ Did not determine scene safety
_____ Did not obtain medical direction or verbalize standing orders for medical interventions
_____ Did not provide high concentration of oxygen
_____ Did not find or manage problems associated with airway, breathing, hemorrhage or shock (hypoperfusion)
_____ Did not differentiate patient's need for transportation versus continued assessment at the scene
_____ Did detailed or focused history/physical examination before assessing the airway, breathing and circulation
_____ Did not ask questions about the present illness
_____ Administered a dangerous or inappropriate intervention

Appendix B

Cardiac Arrest Management/AED

Start Time: _____
Stop Time: _____   Date: _____
Candidate's Name: _____
Evaluator's Name: _____

	POINTS POSSIBLE	POINTS AWARDED
ASSESSMENT		
Takes, or verbalizes, body substance isolation precautions	1	
Briefly questions the rescuer about arrest events	1	
Directs rescuer to stop CPR	1	
Verifies absence of spontaneous pulse (**skill station examiner states "no pulse"**)	1	
Directs resumption of CPR	1	
Turns on defibrillator power	1	
Attaches automated defibrillator to the patient	1	
Directs rescuer to stop CPR and ensures all individuals are clear of the patient	1	
Initiates analysis of the rhythm	1	
Delivers shock (up to three successive shocks)	1	
Verifies absence of spontaneous pulse (**skill station examiner states "no pulse"**)	1	
TRANSITION		
Directs resumption of CPR	1	
Gathers additional information about arrest event	1	
Confirms effectiveness of CPR (ventilation and compressions)	1	
INTEGRATION		
Verbalizes or directs insertion of a simple airway adjunct (oral/nasal airway)	1	
Ventilates, or directs ventilation of, the patient	1	
Assures high concentration of oxygen is delivered to the patient	1	
Assures CPR continues without unnecessary/prolonged interruption	1	
Re-evaluates patient/CPR in approximately one minute	1	
Repeats defibrillator sequence	1	
TRANSPORTATION		
Verbalizes transportation of patient	1	
TOTAL:	21	

Critical Criteria

_____ Did not take, or verbalize, body substance isolation precautions
_____ Did not evaluate the need for immediate use of the AED
_____ Did not direct initiation/resumption of ventilation/compressions at appropriate times.
_____ Did not assure all individuals were clear of patient before delivering each shock
_____ Did not operate the AED properly (inability to deliver shock)
_____ Prevented the defibrillator from delivering indicated stacked shocks

Appendix B

BAG-VALVE-MASK
APNEIC PATIENT

Start Time: _____
Stop Time: _____   Date: _____
Candidate's Name: _____
Evaluator's Name: _____

	POINTS POSSIBLE	POINTS AWARDED
Takes, or verbalizes, body substance isolation precautions	1	
Voices opening the airway	1	
Voices inserting an airway adjunct	1	
Selects appropriately sized mask	1	
Creates a proper mask-to-face seal	1	
Ventilates patient at no less than 800 ml volume *(The examiner must witness for at least 30 seconds)*	1	
Connects reservoir and oxygen	1	
Adjusts liter flow to 15 liters/minute or greater	1	
The examiner indicates arrival of a second EMT. The second EMT is instructed to ventilate the patient while the candidate controls the mask and the airway		
Voices re-opening the airway	1	
Creates a proper mask-to-face seal	1	
Instructs assistant to resume ventilation at proper volume per breath *(The examiner must witness for at least 30 seconds)*	1	
TOTAL:	11	

Critical Criteria

_____ Did not take, or verbalize, body substance isolation precautions
_____ Did not immediately ventilate the patient
_____ Interrupted ventilations for more than 20 seconds
_____ Did not provide high concentration of oxygen
_____ Did not provide, or direct assistant to provide, proper volume/breath *(more than two (2) ventilations per minute are below 800 ml)*
_____ Did not allow adequate exhalation

SPINAL IMMOBILIZATION
SUPINE PATIENT

Start Time: _____

Stop Time: _____   Date: _____

Candidate's Name: _____

Evaluator's Name: _____

	POINTS POSSIBLE	POINTS AWARDED
Takes, or verbalizes, body substance isolation precautions	1	
Directs assistant to place/maintain head in the neutral in-line position	1	
Directs assistant to maintain manual immobilization of the head	1	
Reassesses motor, sensory and circulatory function in each extremity	1	
Applies appropriately sized extrication collar	1	
Positions the immobilization device appropriately	1	
Directs movement of the patient onto the device without compromising the integrity of the spine	1	
Applies padding to voids between the torso and the board as necessary	1	
Immobilizes the patient's torso to the device	1	
Evaluates and pads behind the patient's head as necessary	1	
Immobilizes the patient's head to the device	1	
Secures the patient's legs to the device	1	
Secures the patient's arms to the device	1	
Reassesses motor, sensory and circulatory function in each extremity	1	
TOTAL:	14	

Critical Criteria

_____ Did not immediately direct, or take, manual immobilization of the head

_____ Released, or ordered release of, manual immobilization before it was maintained mechanically

_____ Patient manipulated, or moved excessively, causing potential spinal compromise

_____ Patient moves excessively up, down, left or right on the patient's torso

_____ Head immobilization allows for excessive movement

_____ Upon completion of immobilization, head is not in the neutral position

_____ Did not assess motor, sensory and circulatory function in each extremity after immobilization to the device

_____ Immobilized head to the board before securing the torso

SPINAL IMMOBILIZATION
SEATED PATIENT

Start Time: _____
Stop Time: _____   Date: _____
Candidate's Name: _____
Evaluator's Name: _____

	POINTS POSSIBLE	POINTS AWARDED
Takes, or verbalizes, body substance isolation precautions	1	
Directs assistant to place/maintain head in the neutral in-line position	1	
Directs assistant to maintain manual immobilization of the head	1	
Reassesses motor, sensory and circulatory function in each extremity	1	
Applies appropriately sized extrication collar	1	
Positions the immobilization device behind the patient	1	
Secures the device to the patient's torso	1	
Evaluates torso fixation and adjusts as necessary	1	
Evaluates and pads behind the patient's head as necessary	1	
Secures the patient's head to the device	1	
Verbalizes moving the patient to a long board	1	
Reassesses motor, sensory and circulatory function in each extremity	1	
TOTAL:	12	

Critical Criteria

_____ Did not immediately direct, or take, manual immobilization of the head
_____ Released, or ordered release of, manual immobilization before it was maintained mechanically
_____ Patient manipulated, or moved excessively, causing potential spinal compromise
_____ Device moved excessively up, down, left or right on the patient's torso
_____ Head immobilization allows for excessive movement
_____ Torso fixation inhibits chest rise, resulting in respiratory compromise
_____ Upon completion of immobilization, head is not in the neutral position
_____ Did not assess motor, sensory and circulatory function in each extremity after voicing immobilization to the long board
_____ Immobilized head to the board before securing the torso

IMMOBILIZATION SKILLS
LONG BONE INJURY

Start Time: _____

Stop Time: _____   Date: _____

Candidate's Name: _____

Evaluator's Name: _____

	POINTS POSSIBLE	POINTS AWARDED
Takes, or verbalizes, body substance isolation precautions	1	
Directs application of manual stabilization of the injury	1	
Assesses motor, sensory and circulatory function in the injured extremity	1	
Note: The examiner acknowledges "motor, sensory and circulatory function are present and normal"		
Measures the splint	1	
Applies the splint	1	
Immobilizes the joint above the injury site	1	
Immobilizes the joint below the injury site	1	
Secures the entire injured extremity	1	
Immobilizes the hand/foot in the position of function	1	
Reassesses motor, sensory and circulatory function in the injured extremity	1	
Note: The examiner acknowledges "motor, sensory and circulatory function are present and normal"		
TOTAL:	10	

Critical Criteria

_____   Grossly moves the injured extremity

_____   Did not immobilize the joint above and the joint below the injury site

_____   Did not reassess motor, sensory and circulatory function in the injured extremity before and after splinting

IMMOBILIZATION SKILLS
JOINT INJURY

Start Time: _____

Stop Time: _____   Date: _____

Candidate's Name: _____

Evaluator's Name: _____

	POINTS POSSIBLE	POINTS AWARDED
Takes, or verbalizes, body substance isolation precautions	1	
Directs application of manual stabilization of the shoulder injury	1	
Assesses motor, sensory and circulatory function in the injured extremity	1	
Note: The examiner acknowledges "motor, sensory and circulatory function are present and normal."		
Selects the proper splinting material	1	
Immobilizes the site of the injury	1	
Immobilizes the bone above the injured joint	1	
Immobilizes the bone below the injured joint	1	
Reassesses motor, sensory and circulatory function in the injured extremity	1	
Note: The examiner acknowledges "motor, sensory and circulatory function are present and normal."		
TOTAL:	8	

Critical Criteria

_____ Did not support the joint so that the joint did not bear distal weight

_____ Did not immobilize the bone above and below the injured site

_____ Did not reassess motor, sensory and circulatory function in the injured extremity before and after splinting

IMMOBILIZATION SKILLS
TRACTION SPLINTING

Start Time: _____

Stop Time: _____   Date: _____

Candidate's Name: _____

Evaluator's Name: _____

	POINTS POSSIBLE	POINTS AWARDED
Takes, or verbalizes, body substance isolation precautions	1	
Directs application of manual stabilization of the injured leg	1	
Directs the application of manual traction	1	
Assesses motor, sensory and circulatory function in the injured extremity	1	
Note: The examiner acknowledges "motor, sensory and circulatory function are present and normal"		
Prepares/adjusts splint to the proper length	1	
Positions the splint next to the injured leg	1	
Applies the proximal securing device (e.g. . . . ischial strap)	1	
Applies the distal securing device (e.g. . . . ankle hitch)	1	
Applies mechanical traction	1	
Positions/secures the support straps	1	
Re-evaluates the proximal/distal securing devices	1	
Reassesses motor, sensory and circulatory function in the injured extremity	1	
Note: The examiner acknowledges "motor, sensory and circulatory function are present and normal"		
Note: The examiner must ask the candidate how he/she would prepare the patient for transportation		
Verbalizes securing the torso to the long board to immobilize the hip	1	
Vearbalizes securing the splint to the long board to prevent movement of the splint	1	
TOTAL:	14	

Critical Criteria

_____ Loss of traction at any point after it was applied

_____ Did not reassess motor, sensory and circulatory function in the injured extremity before and after splinting

_____ The foot was excessively rotated or extended after splint was applied

_____ Did not secure the ischial strap before taking traction

_____ Final Immobilization failed to support the femur or prevent rotation of the injured leg

_____ Secured the leg to the splint before applying mechanical traction

Note: If the Sagar splint or the Kendricks Traction Device is used without elevating the patient's leg, application of manual traction is not necessary. The candidate should be awarded one (1) point as if manual traction were applied.

Note: If the leg is elevated at all, manual traction must be applied before elevating the leg. The ankle hitch may be applied before elevating the leg and used to provide manual traction.

BLEEDING CONTROL/SHOCK MANAGEMENT

Start Time: _____
Stop Time: _____ Date: _____
Candidate's Name: _____
Evaluator's Name: _____

	POINTS POSSIBLE	POINTS AWARDED
Takes, or verbalizes, body substance isolation precautions	1	
Applies direct pressure to the wound	1	
Elevates the extremity	1	
Note: The examiner must now inform the candidate that the wound continues to bleed.		
Applies an additional dressing to the wound	1	
Note: The examiner must now inform the candidate that the wound still continues to bleed. The second dressing does not control the bleeding.		
Locates and applies pressure to appropriate arterial pressure point	1	
Note: The examiner must now inform the candidate that the bleeding is controlled		
Bandages the wound	1	
Note: The examiner must now inform the candidate the patient is now showing signs and symptoms indicative of hypoperfusion		
Properly positions the patient	1	
Applies high concentration oxygen	1	
Initiates steps to prevent heat loss from the patient	1	
Indicates the need for immediate transportation	1	
TOTAL:	10	

Critical Criteria

_____ Did not take, or verbalize, body substance isolation precautions
_____ Did not apply high concentration of oxygen
_____ Applied a tourniquet before attempting other methods of bleeding control
_____ Did not control hemorrhage in a timely manner
_____ Did not indicate a need for immediate transportation

AIRWAY, OXYGEN AND VENTILATION SKILLS
UPPER AIRWAY ADJUNCTS AND SUCTION

Start Time: _____

Stop Time: _____   Date: _____

Candidate's Name: _____

Evaluator's Name: _____

	POINTS POSSIBLE	POINTS AWARDED
OROPHARYNGEAL AIRWAY		
Takes, or verbalizes, body substance isolation precautions	1	
Selects appropriately sized airway	1	
Measures airway	1	
Inserts airway without pushing the tongue posteriorly	1	
Note: The examiner must advise the candidate that the patient is gagging and becoming conscious		
Removes the oropharyngeal airway	1	
SUCTION		
Note: The examiner must advise the candidate to suction the patient's airway		
Turns on/prepares suction device	1	
Assures presence of mechanical suction	1	
Inserts the suction tip without suction	1	
Applies suction to the oropharynx/nasopharynx	1	
NASOPHARYNGEAL AIRWAY		
Note: The examiner must advise the candidate to insert a nasopharyngeal airway		
Selects appropriately sized airway	1	
Measures airway	1	
Verbalizes lubrication of the nasal airway	1	
Fully inserts the airway with the bevel facing toward the septum	1	
TOTAL:	13	

Critical Criteria

_____ Did not take, or verbalize, body substance isolation precautions

_____ Did not obtain a patent airway with the oropharyngeal airway

_____ Did not obtain a patent airway with the nasopharyngeal airway

_____ Did not demonstrate an acceptable suction technique

_____ Inserted any adjunct in a manner dangerous to the patient

MOUTH TO MASK WITH SUPPLEMENTAL OXYGEN

Start Time: _____

Stop Time: _____   Date: _____

Candidate's Name: _____

Evaluator's Name: _____

	POINTS POSSIBLE	POINTS AWARDED
Takes, or verbalizes, body substance isolation precautions	1	
Connects one-way valve to mask	1	
Opens patient's airway or confirms patient's airway is open (manually or with adjunct)	1	
Establishes and maintains a proper mask to face seal	1	
Ventilates the patient at the proper volume and rate *(800-1200 ml per breath/10-20 breaths per minute)*	1	
Connects the mask to high concentration of oxygen	1	
Adjusts flow rate to at least 15 liters per minute	1	
Continues ventilation of the patient at the proper volume and rate *(800-1200 ml per breath/10-20 breaths per minute)*	1	
Note: The examiner must witness ventilations for at least 30 seconds		
TOTAL:	8	

Critical Criteria

_____ Did not take, or verbalize, body substance isolation precautions

_____ Did not adjust liter flow to at least 15 liters per minute

_____ Did not provide proper volume per breath *(more than 2 ventilations per minute were below 800 ml)*

_____ Did not ventilate the patient at a rate a 10-20 breaths per minute

_____ Did not allow for complete exhalation

OXYGEN ADMINISTRATION

Start Time: _____

Stop Time: _____   Date: _____

Candidate's Name: _____

Evaluator's Name: _____

	POINTS POSSIBLE	POINTS AWARDED
Takes, or verbalizes, body substance isolation precautions	1	
Assembles the regulator to the tank	1	
Opens the tank	1	
Checks for leaks	1	
Checks tank pressure	1	
Attaches non-rebreather mask to oxygen	1	
Prefills reservoir	1	
Adjusts liter flow to 12 liters per minute or greater	1	
Applies and adjusts the mask to the patient's face	1	
Note: *The examiner must advise the candidate that the patient is not tolerating the non-rebreather mask. The medical director has ordered you to apply a nasal cannula to the patient.*		
Attaches nasal cannula to oxygen	1	
Adjusts liter flow to six (6) liters per minute or less	1	
Applies nasal cannula to the patient	1	
Note: *The examiner must advise the candidate to discontinue oxygen therapy*		
Removes the nasal cannula from the patient	1	
Shuts off the regulator	1	
Relieves the pressure within the regulator	1	
TOTAL:	15	

Critical Criteria

_____ Did not take, or verbalize, body substance isolation precautions

_____ Did not assemble the tank and regulator without leaks

_____ Did not prefill the reservoir bag

_____ Did not adjust the device to the correct liter flow for the non-rebreather mask *(12 liters per minute or greater)*

_____ Did not adjust the device to the correct liter flow for the nasal cannula *(6 liters per minute or less)*

VENTILATORY MANAGEMENT
ENDOTRACHEAL INTUBATION

Start Time: _____

Stop Time: _____   Date: _____

Candidate's Name: _____

Evaluator's Name: _____

Note: *If a candidate elects to intially ventilate the patient with a BVM attached to a reservoir and oxygen, full credit must be awarded for steps denoted by "**" provided the first ventilation is delivered within the initial 30 seconds*

		POINTS POSSIBLE	POINTS AWARDED
Takes, or verbalizes, body substance isolation precautions		1	
Opens the airway manually		1	
Elevates the patient's tongue and inserts a simple airway adjunct (oropharyngeal/nasopharyngeal airway)		1	
Note: *The examiner must now inform the candidate "no gag reflex is present and the patient accepts the airway adjunct."*			
**Ventilates the patient immediately using a BVM device unattached to oxygen		1	
**Hyperventilates the patient with room air		1	
Note: *The examiner must now inform the candidate that ventilation is being properly performed without difficulty*			
Attaches the oxygen reservoir to the BVM		1	
Attaches the BVM to high flow oxygen (15 liter per minute)		1	
Ventilates the patient at the proper volume and rate *(800-1200 ml/breath and 10-20 breaths/minute)*		1	
Note: *After 30 seconds, the examiner must auscultate the patient's chest and inform the candidate that breath sounds are present and equal bilaterally and medical direction has ordered endotracheal intubation. The examiner must now take over ventilation of the patient.*			
Directs assistant to hyper-oxygenate the patient		1	
Identifies/selects the proper equipment for endotracheal intubation		1	
Checks equipment	Checks for cuff leaks	1	
	Checks laryngoscope operation and bulb tightness	1	
Note: *The examiner must remove the OPA and move out of the way when the candidate is prepared to intubate the patient.*			
Positions the patient's head properly		1	
Inserts the laryngoscope blade into the patient's mouth while displacing the patient's tongue laterally		1	
Elevates the patient's mandible with the laryngoscope		1	
Introduces the endotracheal tube and advances the tube to the proper depth		1	
Inflates the cuff to the proper pressure		1	
Disconnects the syringe from the cuff inlet port		1	
Directs assistant to ventilate the patient		1	
Confirms proper placement of the endotracheal tube by auscultation bilaterally and over the epigastrium		1	
Note: *The examiner must ask, "If you had proper placement, what would you expect to hear?"*			
Secures the endotracheal tube *(may be verbalized)*		1	
	TOTAL:	21	

Critical Criteria

_____ Did not take or verbalize body substance isolation precautions when necessary
_____ Did not initiate ventilation within 30 seconds after applying gloves or interrupts ventilations for greater than 30 seconds at any time
_____ Did not voice or provide high oxygen concentrations (15 liter/minute or greater)
_____ Did not ventilate the patient at a rate of at least 10 breaths per minute
_____ Did not provide adequate volume per breath (maximum of 2 errors per minute permissible)
_____ Did not hyper-oxygenate the patient prior to intubation
_____ Did not successfully intubate the patient within 3 attempts
_____ Used the patient's teeth as a fulcrum
_____ Did not assure proper tube placement by auscultation bilaterally over each lung **and** over the epigastrium
_____ The stylette (if used) extended beyond the end of the endotracheal tube
_____ Inserted any adjunct in a manner that was dangerous to the patient
_____ Did not immediately disconnect the syringe from the inlet port after inflating the cuff

VENTILATORY MANAGEMENT
DUAL LUMEN DEVICE INSERTION FOLLOWING
AN UNSUCCESSFUL ENDOTRACHEAL INTUBATION ATTEMPT

Start Time: _____

Stop Time: _____   Date: _____

Candidate's Name: _____

Evaluator's Name: _____

	POINTS POSSIBLE	POINTS AWARDED
Continues body substance isolation precautions	1	
Confirms the patient is being properly ventilated with high percentage oxygen	1	
Directs the assistant to hyper-oxygenate the patient	1	
Checks/prepares the airway device	1	
Lubricates the distal tip of the device *(may be verbalized)*	1	
Note: *The examiner should remove the OPA and move out of the way when the candidate is prepared to insert the device*		
Positions the patient's head properly	1	
Performs a tongue-jaw lift	1	
❏ USES COMBITUBE	❏ USES THE PTL		
Inserts device in the mid-line and to the depth so that the printed ring is at the level of the teeth	Inserts the device in the mid-line until the bite block flange is at the level of the teeth	1	
Inflates the pharyngeal cuff with the proper volume and removes the syringe	Secures the strap	1	
Inflates the distal cuff with the proper volume and removes the syringe	Blows into tube #1 to adequately inflate both cuffs	1	
Attaches/directs attachment of BVM to the first (esophageal placement) lumen and ventilates	1	
Confirms placement and ventilation through the correct lumen by observing chest rise, ausculation over the epigastrium and bilaterally over each lung	1	
Note: *The examiner states, "You do not see rise and fall of the chest and hear sounds only over the epigastrium."*		
Attaches/directs attachment of BVM to the second (endotracheal placement) lumen and ventilates	1	
Confirms placement and ventilation through the correct lumen by observing chest rise, auscultation over the epigastrium and bilaterally over each lung	1	
Note: *The examiner states, "You see rise and fall of the chest, there are no sounds over the epigastrium and breath sounds are equal over each lung."*		
Secures device or confirms that the device remains properly secured	1	
TOTAL:	15	

Critical Criteria

_____ Did not take or verbalize body substance isolation precautions

_____ Did not initiate ventilations within 30 seconds

_____ Interrupted ventilations for more than 30 seconds at any time

_____ Did not hyper-oxygenate the patient prior to placement of the dual lumen airway device

_____ Did not provide adequate volume per breath (maximum 2 errors/minute permissible)

_____ Did not ventilate the patient at a rate of at least 10 breaths per minute

_____ Did not insert the dual lumen airway device at a proper depth or at the proper place within 3 attempts

_____ Did not inflate both cuffs properly

_____ **Combitube** - Did not remove the syringe immediately following the inflation of each cuff

_____ **PTL** - Did not secure the strap prior to cuff inflation

_____ Did not confirm, by observing chest rise and auscultation over the epigastrium and bilaterally over each lung, that the proper lumen of the device was being used to ventilate the patient

_____ Inserted any adjunct in a manner that was dangerous to the patient

VENTILATORY MANAGEMENT
ESOPHAGEAL OBTURATOR AIRWAY INSERTION FOLLOWING AN UNSUCCESSFUL ENDOTRACHEAL INTUBATION ATTEMPT

Start Time: _____

Stop Time: _____   Date: _____

Candidate's Name: _____

Evaluator's Name: _____

	POINTS POSSIBLE	POINTS AWARDED
Continues body substance isolation precautions	1	
Confirms the patient is being properly ventilated high percentage oxygen	1	
Directs the assistant to hyper-oxygenate the patient	1	
Identifies/selects the proper equipment for insertion of EOA	1	
Assembles the EOA	1	
Tests the cuff for leaks	1	
Inflates the mask	1	
Lubricates the tube *(may be verbalized)*	1	
Note: The examiner should remove the OPA and move out of the way when the candidate is prepared to insert the device		
Positions the head properly with the neck in the neutral or slightly flexed position	1	
Grasps and elevates the patient's tongue and mandible	1	
Inserts the tube in the same direction as the curvature of the pharynx	1	
Advances the tube until the mask is sealed against the patient's face	1	
Ventilates the patient while maintaining a tight mask-to-face seal	1	
Directs confirmation of placement of EOA by observing for chest rise and auscultation over the epigastrium and bilaterally over each lung	1	
Note: The examiner must acknowledge adequate chest rise, bilateral breath sounds and absent sounds over the epigastrium		
Inflates the cuff to the proper pressure	1	
Disconnects the syringe from the inlet port	1	
Continues ventilation of the patient	1	
TOTAL:	17	

Critical Criteria

_____ Did not take or verbalize body substance isolation precautions
_____ Did not initiate ventilations within 30 seconds
_____ Interrupted ventilations for more than 30 seconds at any time
_____ Did not direct hyper-oxygenation of the patient prior to placement of the EOA
_____ Did not successfully place the EOA within 3 attempts
_____ Did not ventilate at a rate of at least 10 breaths per minute
_____ Did not provide adequate volume per breath (maximum 2 errors/minute permissible)
_____ Did not assure proper tube placement by auscultation bilaterally and over the epigastrium
_____ Did not remove the syringe after inflating the cuff
_____ Did not successfully ventilate the patient
_____ Did not provide high flow oxygen (15 liters per minute or greater)
_____ Inserted any adjunct in a manner that was dangerous to the patient

Appendix C

National Highway Traffic Safety Administration (NHTSA) Technical Advisory Panel (TAP) Standards

Each of the NHTSA TAP standards (commonly accepted criteria) are reviewed briefly with the goal to provide an overview of the EMS system. The actual NHTSA standards are quoted with any necessary explanation or clarification. Although these standards are worded so as to apply formally to statewide systems, the standards have equal applicability at the regional and local levels.

Regulation and Policy

Standard: To provide a quality, effective system of emergency medical care, each EMS system must have in place comprehensive enabling legislation with provision for a lead EMS agency as well as a funding mechanism, regulations, and operational policies and procedures.

Resource Management

Standard: The provision of centralized coordination to identify and categorize the resources necessary for overall system implementation and operation is essential to an effective EMS system. This provision is required to maintain a coordinated response and appropriate resource utilization throughout the state. It is essential that victims of medical or traumatic emergencies have equal access to basic emergency care, including triage (sorting or prioritizing) and transport of all victims by appropriately certified personnel in a licensed (approved for use by a government agency) and equipped ambulance to a facility that is appropriately equipped, staffed, and ready to administer to the needs of the patient.

Human Resources and Training

Standard: EMS personnel can perform their mission only if adequately trained and available in sufficient numbers throughout the state. Each prehospital training program should use a standardized curriculum for each level of EMT personnel. In an effective EMS system, training programs are routinely monitored, instructors must meet certain requirements, and the curriculum is standardized throughout the state. In addition, the state EMS lead agency must provide a comprehensive plan for stable and consistent EMS training programs with effective local and regional support.

Transportation

Standard: Safe, reliable ambulance transportation is a critical component of an effective EMS system. Most patients can be effectively transported in a ground ambulance staffed by qualified emergency medical personnel. Other patients with more serious injuries or illnesses, particularly in remote areas, require rapid transportation provided by rotor craft (helicopter) or fixed wing (airplane) air medical services. Routine, standardized methods for inspection and licensing of all emergency medical transport vehicles are essential to maintain a constant state of readiness throughout the state.

Facilities

Standard: It is imperative that the seriously ill patient be delivered in a timely manner to the closest appropriate facility. This determination needs to consider both stabilization and definitive care. This determination should be free of political considerations and requires that the capabilities of the facilities be known in advance so that appropriate primary and secondary transport decisions can be made.

Standard: An effective communications subsystem is an essential component of an overall EMS system. Beginning with a universal access number, such as 911, the communications network should provide for prioritized dispatch, dispatch to ambulance communication, ambulance to ambulance, ambulance to hospital, and hospital to hospital communications to ensure the receiving facility is ready and able to accept the patient.

Standard: EMS is a medical care system that includes medical practice as delegated by physicians to nonphysician providers who manage patient care outside the traditional confines of the office or hospital. As befits this delegation of authority, it is the physician's obligation to be involved in all aspects of the patient care system. Specific areas of involvement include planning and protocols, on-line medical direction and consultation, and audit and evaluation of patient care.

Standard: To provide a quality, effective system of trauma care, each state must have in place a fully functional EMS system. Enabling legislation should exist for the development of the trauma component of the EMS system. This should include trauma center designation (using national standards as guidelines), triage and transfer guidelines for trauma patients, data collection and trauma registry definitions and mechanisms, mandatory autopsies, system management, and quality assurance of any statewide system.

Standard: A comprehensive evaluation program is needed to effectively plan and implement a statewide EMS system. Each EMS system must be responsible for evaluating the effectiveness of services provided to victims of medical- or trauma-related emergencies. The statewide EMS system should be able to state definitively what influence has been made on the patients serviced by the system. EMS system managers must be able to evaluate resource use, scope of service, patient outcome, and the effectiveness of operational policies, procedures, and protocols. An effective EMS system evaluates itself against preestablished standards and objectives so that improvements in service, particularly direct patient care, can occur. These requirements are a part of an ongoing quality assurance system to review system performance. The evaluation process should be educational and ongoing. Quality assurance reviews should occur at all phases of EMS system management so that needed policy changes or treatment protocol revisions can be made.

Answers to Review Questions

Chapter 1
1. National Highway Traffic Safety Administration (NHTSA)
2. The role of the EMT is to be the eyes and ears of the physician in the field and perform initial care and stabilization until the patient reaches the emergency department.
3. Assessment-based
4. Hospital based, fire service, industrial, military, private ambulance company
5. *Fee-for-service* is a charge based on the level of care that is provided, and *managed care* is a set fee based on a preexisting contract no matter what level of care is provided.
6. Basic and advanced life support care and specialty rescue in a unified manner

Chapter 2
1. In 1948, the World Medical Association adopted the Oath of Geneva. In 1978, the National Association of Emergency Medical Technicians adopted the EMT Oath and a Code of Ethics. These three documents detail the guiding principles for professional EMT service, and all EMTs should be familiar with them.
2. An EMT is an individual who has completed the educational process according to a national standard curriculum and who possesses the knowledge to provide initial assessment and emergency care for the ill and injured. Any one of a group of trained professionals may provide treatment of the ill or injured patient at the scene of an emergency. These trained professionals have various knowledge bases received from formal training. All have a responsibility to provide care for the patient. In most states, someone trained to provide care at the level of standard first aid provider, first responder, EMT, or paramedic is recognized as a prehospital care provider. Training and responsibilities vary accordingly.
3. EMTs may encounter many other job-related functions depending on the setting in which they find themselves. Not all EMTs work on ambulances. For example, some EMTs work as community educators, some in industry, and others in sports medicine. The EMT's ability to perform the various functions and tasks required by the job provides stimulation and rewards. The EMT should be a well-rounded individual willing to accept challenge.
4. You will need to portray a professional appearance and exhibit a professional attitude. Most of your time as an EMT will not be spent in emergency situations, but when the time arrives you must be prepared to respond. You will most likely have the opportunity at some point to make a monumental difference in someone's life.
5. For an EMS system to be its best it must have a means to continuously monitor and measure the quality of care delivered. A quality assurance program evaluates data such as response times, scene times, adherence to protocols, and other indicators of quality to identify trends. This helps a system know what it does well and what it needs to work on based on a uniform set of data. After a system has identified a weakness, it can improve through education.
   EMS systems may also use a quality improvement program for evaluating system performance. It is usually based on the perceptions of the customer. It is also an ongoing effort to refine and enhance the system. Its focus may be on clinical issues or different aspects such as billing, unit maintenance, or other support functions. Quality improvement relies on the customer as the ultimate indicator of quality.

Chapter 3
1. a
2. b
3. a
4. c
5. b

Chapter 4
1. b
2. a
3. b
4. a
5. a

Chapter 5
1. b
2. d
3. a
4. a
5. b
6. d
7. b

Chapter 6
1. b
2. c
3. b
4. a
5. c
6. d
7. a
8. c

Chapter 7
1. c
2. b
3. c
4. b
5. b
6. b
7. d
8. d
9. b
10. c
11. c
12. d

Chapter 8
1. b
2. c
3. b
4. c
5. a
6. b

7. a
8. d
9. d

Chapter 9
1. Vein
2. b
3. b
4. c
5. d
6. True
7. b

Chapter 10
1. b
2. c
3. b
4. d
5. b
6. a
7. b
8. b

Chapter 11
1. b
2. a
3. b
4. d
5. d

Chapter 12
1. c
2. b
3. b
4. b
5. c, f, d, h, g, a, b
6. True
7. True
8. e
9. False
10. c
11. b
12. b

Chapter 13
1. a
2. b
3. b
4. c
5. b
6. b
7. b

Chapter 14
1. a
2. c
3. c
4. b

5. b
6. c

Chapter 15
1. c
2. b
3. d
4. a
5. d
6. c

Chapter 16
1. b
2. d
3. c
4. b
5. d
6. b

Chapter 17
1. c
2. b
3. d
4. a
5. c
6. c
7. d, b, c
8. d
9. b
10. c

Chapter 18
1. Antigen
2. Immune
3. False
4. True
5. d

Chapter 19
1. False
2. False
3. c
4. Respiratory depression or arrest
5. Poison control center
6. b
7. b
8. f
9. a
10. d

Chapter 20
1. Acute anxiety, phobias, depression, suicide, paranoia, disorientation, and disorganization
2. Depression; male over 55 years of age; recent loss of spouse, significant other, or family member; chronic debilitating illness; financial setback or job loss, previous suicide attempt; family history of suicide; substance abuse; children of alcoholic parent; mental disorder
3. b
4. d
5. a

Chapter 21
1. False
2. b
3. a
4. c
5. False

Chapter 22
1. a
2. a
3. a
4. c
5. b

Chapter 23
1. c
2. a
3. a
4. c
5. c

Chapter 24
1. a
2. a
3. a, d
4. a, c
5. b
6. d
7. b
8. a

Chapter 25
1. d
2. d
3. a
4. a
5. b

Chapter 26
1. a
2. c
3. b
4. e
5. b
6. c
7. d

Chapter 27
1. c
2. a

3. c
4. a
5. b

Chapter 28
1. d
2. c
3. b
4. b
5. b
6. d
7. b

Chapter 29
1. Breathing, conduction, convection, evaporation, and radiation
2. Age and medical condition
3. 70
4. 18% front and 18% back; 36% total BSA
5. 10
6. Anaphylactic

Chapter 30
1. b
2. e
3. False
4. d
5. b
6. The period of old age is characterized, in general, by frailty, slower mental processes, impairment of psychologic functions, diminished energy, the appearance of chronic and degenerative diseases, and decline in sensory acuity. Functional abilities are lessened and the well-known superficial signs and symptoms of older age appear, such as skin wrinkling, changes in hair color and quantity, osteoarthritis, and slowness in reaction time. Organ systems have reached maturation, and a turning point in physiologic growth has been reached. The body gradually loses its ability to maintain homeostasis (state of relative constancy of the internal environment of the body), and viability declines over a period of years until death occurs. The fundamental process of aging occurs at the cellular level and is reflected in anatomic structure and physiologic function.
7. Many elderly persons are on some form of prescribed medication; in addition, the elderly take many over-the-counter drugs. Many patients take multiple medications, and drug interactions are common. Many hospital admissions are the result of drug-induced illness. Underdosing is usually more of a problem than overdosing.

    The following are some of the causes of underdosing:
    Confusion
    Forgetfulness
    Arthritis of the hands, resulting in inability to take the proper amount
    Economics (trying to save money)
    The following are some of the causes of overdosing:
    Confusion
    Vision impairment
    Arthritis of the hands, resulting in inability to take the proper amount
    Misselection of the medication
    Self-destruction (suicide)

    One factor that may be responsible for underdosing and overdosing is "bagging" the drugs (in plastic lunch sacs or brown lunch bags, hence "brown bagging"). In this activity, elderly patients either "save-up" the drugs and take them all at one time or take a few at a time. Elderly persons often do this to save money, because they think more of the drug at one time will be better for them, or because they are confused about the directions for taking the drug.

    The absorption and use of medications (drug pharmacokinetics) are altered in the elderly. These changes depend on the particular drug and patient. The following are some of the causes of these alterations:
    Decline in kidney function (decreased excretion)
    Poor nutritional state
    Decline in liver metabolic activities
    Changes in body composition, such as increased fat, decreased lean body mass
    Decline in plasma volume and total body water
8. Categories of abuse
    - Physical
    - Psychologic
    - Financial
    After comprehensive physical examination and appropriate documentation of findings, inform the physician in the emergency department of suspicions.
9. This patient fits the clinical picture of someone who has suffered a cerebrovascular accident (stroke). The dilated right pupil may indicate hemorrhage in the brain. Digoxin is an antiarrhythmic drug usually administered for supraventricular tachycardia; Coumadin (warfarin) is usually prescribed as an anticoagulant in patients with chronic atrial fibrillation or who have undergone valve replacement using a ceramic device and for other conditions. Long-term use of warfarin for patients 70 years of age and older has a risk of stroke. This patient's cardiovascular and cerebrovascular status is grave. Treatment requires maintenance of the airway, insertion of an airway, administration of oxygen at 15 L using a nonrebreather mask, and prompt transportation to the emergency department. EMTs should be prepared to administer basic life support if cardiac arrest occurs.
10. Dementia is the progressive, organic mental disorder that is marked by chronic personality disintegration, confusion, disorientation, stupor, and deterioration of intellectual capacity and function. Approximately 15% of persons over 65 years of age have some degree of dementia. Dementia is also characterized by impairment of control of memory, judgment, and impulsive behavior. Causes of dementia, many of which are treatable, include the following:
    Insulin shock
    Anemia
    Subdural hematoma
    Benign brain tumor
    Drug intoxication
    Hyperthyroidism
    Drug intoxication

    Some forms like traumatic brain injury, Alzheimer's disease, and Huntington's chorea are not responsive or very minimally amenable to treatment. In assessment of the elderly the EMT must take into consideration physical factors that may affect mental status.

    The essential feature of dementia is loss of intellectual abilities, especially those involved in higher cortical functions such as memory and reasoning. The presenting symptoms of dementia are usually multifaceted. The loss of higher mental functions can be severe enough to cause significant problems in social situations, job-related situations, and activities of daily living (ADLs). Clinical findings of dementia include the following:

- Memory impairment (forgetting the usual things involved in ADLs); as the impairment progresses to full memory loss, an inability to learn and adjust to new activities becomes apparent
- Inability to assemble items, copy dimensional objects, recognize objects, and execute motor functions
- Communications difficulties, including vague language, imprecise pronunciation, and signs of aphasia (defective or absent language function)
- Faulty judgment, including disregard of social conventions, inappropriate language and jokes, and neglect of personal hygiene
- Changes in personality, including paranoid or compulsive patterns, signs of irritability and uncooperativeness, and impulsive behavior
- Maladjustment, including heightened anxiety, depression, and overcompensation for mental deficits

Emergency medical evaluation of the mentally impaired elderly patient must be an essential part of the focused assessment. EMTs must note alterations of mental status so that definitive psychiatric assessment may be made.

Chapter 31
1. d
2. b
3. d
4. c
5. b
6. c
7. b
8. c

Chapter 32
1. False. "D" for disability still refers to the patient's neurological status.
2. d. Down syndrome is an inherited disorder and may include mental retardation.
3. The family should be respected and involved in the patient's care in whatever way possible. In most cases, they should be used as a resource and regarded as experts in their loved one's care.
4. True
5. b. With an Arnold-Chiari malformation, hyperextending the head can put pressure on the brain stem and cause apnea.
6. Developmental disability
7. False. Ideally, the ambulance service should be notified by hospital personnel when a patient with specialized equipment returns to the community. The EMT-B can visit the residence before an emergency to gain information about the type of equipment being used in the home.
8. False. Never assume that the patient cannot understand what you are saying. Communicate and explain procedures using language appropriate to the level of the person's understanding.
9. d
10. Latex. Latex-free equipment should be available in the ambulance to use in this instance or the person may have a life-threatening allergic reaction.
11. Ketogenic. This diet is high in fat and causes the body to metabolize fat instead of glucose, thus producing ketosis. The state of ketosis is thought to control some seizure activity.
12. Central venous access device
13. c
14. American Academy of Pediatrics and American College of Emergency Physicians
15. False. An individual should be identified at the scene to take responsibility for the wheelchair. If no one is available or interested, ask the police for assistance.

Chapter 33
1. Know or find out the weight to be carried.
   Know the limitations of the crew's abilities.
   Work in a coordinated manner and communicate with partners.
   Keep the weight as close to your body as possible.
   Keep your back in a locked-in position and refrain from twisting.
   Flex at the hips, not the waist, and bend at the knees.
   Do not hyperextend your back (do not lean back from the waist).
2. Stair chair
    Advantages
      Provides easy access in tight spots
      Fits into elevators
      Fits on aircraft
    Disadvantages
      Patient has to be conscious
      Patient has to sit upright
      Patient's spine cannot be immobilized
   Scoop (orthopedia) stretcher
    Advantages
      Can be used on unconscious patients
      Has good hand straps
    Disadvantages:
      Not good for spinal immobilization
      Difficult to move in very tight spaces
   Flexible stretcher
    Advantages
      Has good hand straps
    Disadvantages
      Not good for spinal immobilization
      Difficult to move in very tight spaces
3. The one-person stretcher has special loading wheels at the head end, allowing it to be rolled in and out of the ambulance by one person if needed. The advantage of the one-person stretcher is that it does not have to be lifted into the ambulance, only rolled. The two-person stretcher requires two EMTs to lift the stretcher from each side when loading and unloading from the ambulance.
4. These include any medical emergencies that place the patient at immediate risk of dying or sustaining irreversible damage. The following are examples:
   Cardiac arrest
   Heart attack
   Airway compromise
   Anaphylactic reaction
   Stroke
   Severe respiratory distress
   Decreased level of consciousness

Chest pain, difficulty breathing, or any condition that causes severely abnormal vital signs
5. Presence of life-threatening injury
Location of nearest trauma center
Availability of advanced life support
Availability of aeromedical support
Number of patients

Chapter 34
1. b
2. c
3. d
4. a
5. a
6. c

Chapter 35
1. d
2. SAMPLE is a quick and easy abbreviation for items you check or ask about in obtaining a patient history after completing your rapid assessment. SAMPLE stands for S (signs and symptoms of the episode), A (allergies), M (medications), P (past medical history), L (last meal or oral intake), E (events leading up to emergency).

    OPQRST is an abbreviation for the circumstances or details about the patient's chief complaint that you will want to explore when obtaining the history of the present problem. OPQRST stands for O (onset of problem [When did the pain start?]), P (provoke [Does anything provoke or make the pain worse?]), Q (quality [Describe the pain for me—aching, crushing, tingling.]), R (radiation [Is the pain in one specific area or does it move to another area?]), S (severity [Rate the pain on a scale from 1 to 10 for me with 1 being normal and 10 being the worst pain you've ever felt]), T (time and treatment [Is this similar to previous episodes of the same problem? Have you done anything for the pain? Did that help?]).

    SAMPLE and OPQRST assist the EMT in obtaining good patient information about their chief complaint and history and also serve as valuable tools when documenting the current problem.
3. c
4. False
5. c

Chapter 36
1. c
2. *Retrospective.* Patient care report review, complaint investigation, other data collection methods
Concurrent. Physician ride-alongs, EMTs working with physician in clinic or emergency department, on-line medical direction
Prospective. Skills check off, continuing education, testing
3. Data collection
Case reviews
Continuing education
Remediation

Chapter 37
1. False
2. Maintain control of the vehicle and proceed with due regard for the safety of others.
3. b
4. Time of day, traffic, weather, route, construction, bridges and tunnels, and detours
5. False
6. Dispatch, en route to the scene, at the scene, en route to the hospital, transfer of patient at the hospital, return to station, preparation for the next call
7. Weather, speed, traffic, detours, time of day, school zones, hospital zones, detours, construction, railroads
8. Detours, school zones, construction, weather, time of day, traffic
9. The next call may come at any time.
10. Medical-stethoscope, sphygmomanometer, thermometer, oropharyngeal airway, bag-valve-mask, non-medical pillows, sheets, blankets, towels, aluminum foil

Chapter 38
1. • If the situation is too hot to handle, allow for a "cool-down" period.
   • Do not escalate the conflict (feed off each other's anger).
   • Remain open and objective throughout the discussion.
   • Identify the issue or problem, and focus on it to the exclusion of extraneous concerns.
   • Compromise because there may be more than one appropriate solution.
2. The hole created by the bullet or penetrating object can be useful in the investigation of the crime scene. Avoid cutting through holes.
3. d
4. A mandated reporter is a health care professional who is required by law to report abuse.
5. d

Chapter 39
1. c
2. b
3. c
4. Windshield
5. Access route
6. a

Chapter 40
1. c
2. c
3. a
4. d
5. a

Chapter 41
1. d
2. b
3. c
4. b
5. d
6. b

Chapter 42
1. a
2. c
3. b
4. b

Glossary

A

Abandonment Failure to provide continuing care for the patient once it has been initiated.

Abdominal quadrants Sections of the abdomen: right upper, left upper, right lower, left lower.

Abortion Expulsion of an embryo or fetus from the uterus before the twentieth week; can occur spontaneously or through a medical procedure.

Abrasion Damage to the epidermis and dermis from shearing forces; commonly referred to as a *scrape*.

Abruptio placentae Sudden separation of the placenta from the wall of the uterus; signs and symptoms include sudden severe low abdominal pain with or without vaginal bleeding.

Abscess Localized collection of pus (white cells, bacteria, and debris) usually contained within a fibrous sac.

Absence Seizure characterized by a sudden, momentary loss of consciousness; also known as a *petit mal seizure*.

Absorption Uptake of medications into tissues.

Accessory muscles Muscles located primarily in the neck that contract to increase tidal volume during respiratory distress.

Acidosis Abnormal increase in hydrogen ion concentration in the body; blood pH below 7.40 (normal blood pH is 7.5).

Acromion Lateral edge of the shoulder.

Action Desirable effect of a drug (e.g., the action of oral glucose is to raise the blood sugar level).

Action circle "Clear zone" established early on an extrication scene, 10 to 15 feet in all directions from the vehicles involved in an accident.

Activated charcoal Form of charcoal with a high surface area that is specially formulated to bind to substances; used to prevent absorption of swallowed substances from the intestine.

Active rewarming Process of rapidly rewarming the body.

Activities of daily living (ADLs) Activities usually accomplished during a normal day (e.g., eating, dressing, washing).

Acute Injury or disease characterized by rapid onset, severe symptoms, and a short course.

Acute care Short-term medical treatment for an injury or disease with rapid onset, severe symptoms, and short duration, such as injuries resulting from an automobile collision.

Advance directives Legally binding document prepared and signed by an individual that clearly states his or her personal wishes regarding implementation of lifesaving techniques in the event that the individual is severely injured or terminally ill and cannot make decisions at that time.

Advanced life support (ALS) Care provided to patients with use of drugs, advanced invasive airway procedures using cardiac monitor defibrillators, and advanced knowledge and judgment. these skills are generally reserved for prehospital care providers trained above the EMT-Basic level.

Advanced life support intercept Arranged rendezvous with paramedics while en route to the hospital when the patient is in need of an advanced level of care not available at the scene.

Advocate Person who assists another person in carrying out desired wishes; an EMT should function as a patient's advocate in all aspects of prehospital care.

Aerobic In the presence of oxygen.

Aging Set of expected, inevitable changes in biologic and psychologic function, some of which are detrimental, that occur with the passage of time.

Agonal ventilations Occasional, gasping breaths that occur just before death.

Airborne pathogens Microorganisms, present in the air, that cause disease.

Air chisel Metal-cutting hand tool adapted from industry for use on the extrication scene. It is a system comprised of an air chisel gun, compressed air hose, regulator, and compressed air supply.

Air rescue bags Extrication tool, consisting of air sacs or bags, filler hoses, air regulator, control valves, and a supply of compressed air. Also referred to as *air lifting bags*.

Air restraint bag Part of the passive passenger restraint system of a passenger car. It consists of a deflated air bag, which fills quickly with a gas when either electrically or mechanically activated on impact of the vehicle. This bag system affords extra protection of the front seat occupants during a vehicle accident.

Airway adjuncts Devices such as oropharyngeal and nasopharyngeal airways that are designed to prevent airway obstruction by the tongue.

Allergen Substance that can produce a hypersensitive reaction in the body; not always harmful (e.g., pollen, dust, animal dander, feathers, and various foods).

Allergic reaction Response of the body's immune system when challenged by a foreign substance either on the surface or into the body.

Alveolar/capillary exchange Gas exchange that occurs in the lungs; oxygen enters the capillaries and is transported by the blood, and carbon dioxide enters the alveoli and is exhaled.

Alveoli Small air sacs in the lungs where the exchange of gas takes place.

Ambient temperature Outside or environmental air temperature that surrounds the body.

Amniotic fluid Clear to straw-colored fluid in the amniotic sac that acts as a shock absorber and maintains a uniform pressure and temperature for the fetus.

Amniotic sac Fibrous sac filled with a clear to straw-colored fluid called *amniotic fluid*; protects the fetus; also called *bag of waters*.

Amputation Injury or surgical procedure in which a limb or other body part is removed completely from the body.

Amylase Class of enzymes that split or hydrolyze starch.

Anaerobic In the absence of oxygen.
Anaphylactic reaction Extreme allergic reaction that is caused by the release of histamine from the cells.
Anaphylaxis Exaggerated, life-threatening hypersensitivity reaction to a previously encountered antigen.
Anatomic position Patient facing forward, arms at the sides, with the palms facing forward.
Anatomic splinting Splinting the body by completely immobilizing it on and fully securing the patient to a long spine board.
Anatomy Structure of the body and relationship of the parts to one another.
Aneurysm Ballooned-out area of a blood vessel.
Angina pectoris Chest pain or pressure frequently brought on by exercise and relieved by rest; caused by ischemia in the heart and often treated with nitroglycerin.
Angular-impact collision Off-center impact.
Anoxia Deficiency of oxygen.
Anterior Toward the front.
Anterior axillary line Line that extends directly caudad from the pectoralis major skin fold and the skin of the arm to the anterior superior iliac spine.
Anterior flail chest Two or more adjacent ribs fractured in two or more places, resulting in an unstable or potentially unstable segment of the chest wall.
Antibodies Complex system of circulating protective proteins used to fight off foreign material in the body.
Antidote Agent that directly blocks or reverses the effect of a poison.
Antigen Substance, usually a protein, that causes the formation of an antibody and reacts specifically with that antibody; antigens are usually found on the surfaces of microorganisms.
Aorta Largest artery in the body, extending from the left ventricle through the thorax and abdomen to the navel, where it divides into the iliac arteries; carries blood from the heart to the body.
Aortic insufficiency Incompetent aortic valve.
Apex Rounded tip of an organ (e.g., bottom of the heart, top of the lung).
APGAR score Scoring system used to evaluate the condition of the infant after 1 and 5 minutes of life; scores of 0, 1, or 2 are given for **A**ppearance, **P**ulse, **G**rimace, **A**ctivity, and **R**espiration. Most newborns have a calculated APGAR score of 8 to 10 1 minute after birth.
Apical pulse Pulse that is heard over the apex of the heart using a stethoscope; beats heard per minute at this location.
Apnea Complete lack of respirations.
Apnea monitor Technological aid used to warn of cessation of breathing in a premature infant; also may warn of bradycardia and tachycardia.
Appendicitis Inflammation of the appendix usually seen in young patients between 15 and 25 years of age. In adults, it is more common in males than in females. It can be acute, subacute, or chronic and usually requires surgical removal.
Appropriate facility Hospital equipped and staffed to immediately handle the patient's specific injuries.
Arachnoid membrane Second membrane of the meninges; a transparent, spiderlike membrane interlaced with fibers.

Arnold-Chiara malformation Complication of spina bifida in which the brainstem and cerebellum extend down through the foramen magnum into the cervical portion of the vertebrae.
Arrhythmia Abnormality in the conduction system of the heart (e.g., ventricular fibrillation).
Arteries Vessels that carry blood away from the heart to the body under pressure.
Arteriole Smallest branch of an artery; supplies capillaries with oxygenated blood.
Arytenoid cartilage Small structures that serve as the posterior attachments for the vocal cords; located behind the glottic opening on each side of the larynx.
Ascent injury Injury that can occur to a scuba diver upon ascent to the water surface at the end of the dive.
Aspiration Accidental inhalation of fluid or other particles into the lower airway.
Assault Creation of immediate fear of harm in another individual.
Assessment Process that includes an oral interview and a physical examination. Assessment allows the EMT to gather information or clues that are useful in deciding which emergency medical interventions will be used. The results of the assessment are communicated to the medical personnel at the receiving hospital.
Asthma Respiratory disorder characterized by recurring episodes of sudden onset of breathing difficulty, wheezing on expiration and inspiration as a result of constriction of the bronchi, coughing, and thick mucous bronchial secretions; also known as *reactive airways disease*.
Atelectasis Collapsed alveoli in the lung. These sections are not ventilated and contribute to lack of oxygenation of the red blood cells and can lead to pneumonia.
Atherosclerosis Disease in which arteries are narrowed by collections of cholesterol and cellular debris; increases the risk for angina pectoris and myocardial infarction.
Atonic Weak; lacking normal tone, as in the case of a flaccid muscle.
Atria Upper chambers of the heart; the right atrium receives blood from the superior and inferior venae cavae; the left atrium receives blood from the pulmonary veins.
Aura Period immediately preceding a seizure.
Auscultate Listen through a stethoscope.
Auscultation Listening to sounds of the body with a stethoscope or blood pressure cuff; listening to the blood pressure.
Automated external defibrillator (AED) Device used in cardiac arrest to perform a computer analysis of the patient's cardiac rhythm and deliver defibrillatory shocks when indicated.
Automated transport ventilator (ATV) Oxygen-powered device with settings for tidal volume and respiratory frequency designed to provide artificial ventilation for intubated patients.
Automaticity Ability of an organ, such as the heart, to generate an electrical impulse.
Autonomic Having the ability to perform independently without outside influence; pertaining to the autonomic nervous system.
Autonomic nervous system Part of the nervous system that regulates involuntary vital functions, including the activity

of the cardiac muscle, smooth muscles, and glands; divided into the sympathetic nervous system and the parasympathetic nervous system.

Availability Amount of drug that is absorbed from the site of administration.

AVPU Acronym for **A**lert, **V**erbal, **P**ainful, and **U**nresponsive; used to describe patient's responsiveness.

Avulsion Injury in which flaps of skin or tissue are torn either partially or completely off the body.

Axial skeleton Division of the skeletal system comprised of the head and trunk of the body.

Axillary region "Armpit" region of the body.

B

Ball-and-socket joint Joint that moves freely in all directions, such as the shoulder.

Bandage Material that holds a dressing in place over a wound.

Barotrauma Term used to identify injury occurring as a result of greater pressure on the external body than within body cavities. Often referred to as a *squeeze*.

Base Flat end of an organ (e.g., top of the heart, bottom of the lung).

Base plate Metal support provided in some powered hydraulic rescue tool systems. It is used to strengthen the push-off point of a powered hydraulic ram.

Base station Radio that is operated at a fixed site such as a dispatch center, hospital, or some other location that does not move; usually runs off of community electrical power (as opposed to battery power) and transmits at a much higher power than do smaller portable radios.

Battery Touching another person without his or her consent.

Battle's sign Discoloration behind the ears found in basilar or occipital skull fractures.

Behavior How a person functions or acts.

Bent-arm drag Type of inline drag using the patient's arms in a bent position to provide leverage for dragging the patient away from immediate danger.

Bicuspid valve Two-flap valve that covers the opening between the left atrium and the left ventricle.

Bilateral Pertaining to both sides.

Bioethical considerations Term that relates to living tissue and the moral principles or values concerning the life and/or death of that living tissue; the principles of conduct governing an individual or professional group.

Biological warfare agents (BWAs) True biological agents, biological vectors, toxins, and bioregulators.

Birth canal Structure located between the anus and the urethral orifice; also known as the *vagina*.

Blanch (blanching) Skin's ability to change from a lighter color to a normal color after slight pressure is applied to the area; indication of adequate circulation.

Blanket drag Type of inline drag using a blanket placed under the patient to pull him or her away from immediate danger.

Blood Fluid consisting of blood cells and plasma that carries nutrients to the tissues and removes waste.

Bloodborne pathogens Microrganisms present in the blood that cause disease.

Blood pressure Pressure that blood exerts on the walls of arteries; measured with a sphygmomanometer.

Blood vessels Vessels that carry blood throughout the body.

Blunt trauma Injury that is not immediately evident to the human eye.

Body fluids/substances Any matter excreted or emitted by the body that may contain infectious microorganisms.

Body position General term applied to the positioning of the rescuer's body away from dangerous areas near rescue tools while they are in operation under force.

Body substance isolation (BSI) Isolation of substances that are excreted from the body to prevent the spread of communicable diseases.

Body surface area (BSA) Measured area of the body involved, usually dealing with thermal injuries.

Bolt cutter Hand tool that is used to cut steel on chains, locks, or other items.

Bounding pulse Strong pulse that is easily palpated.

Box crib This is an arrangement of 4" by 4" or 2" by 4" wood cribbing where it is stacked in parallel pairs at right angles to the parallel pair immediately below.

Brachial artery Artery located on the inside of the elbow on the same side as the small finger; extends from the elbow to the armpit.

Brachial pulse Pulse palpated at the brachial artery of the arm, found on the inner aspect of the upper arm.

Bradycardia Heart rate less than 60 beats per minute; a patient with bradycardia may or may not have symptoms.

Brain edema Swelling in the brain.

Brain stem Part of the brain responsible for consciousness; contains the medulla oblongata, pons, and mesencephalon.

Brain stem herniation Occurs when the portion of the brain that contains the medulla oblongata, pons, and mesencephalon is forced down through the foramen magnum when pressure inside the cranium is increased.

Braxton Hicks contractions Contractions that occur at irregular intervals but do not increase in pain intensity; also known as *false contractions*.

Breech birth Birth in which the presenting part of the fetus is either the buttocks, foot, or leg.

Bronchi Two branches of the trachea. Also known as *bronchial tubes*.

Bronchiole Small airway of the respiratory system extending from the bronchi into the lobes of the lungs.

Bronchiolitis Acute viral infection of the lower respiratory tract that occurs primarily in infants under 18 months of age; characterized by expiratory wheezing, respiratory distress, inflammation, and obstruction at the level of the bronchioles.

Bronchodilators Medications that relax constricted airways, making airflow easier; commonly used in patients with chronic obstructive pulmonary disease and asthma.

Bronchospasm Condition seen in patients with asthma in which airways constrict tightly in response to irritants, cold air, exercise, or unknown factors.

Bronchus (Plural, *bronchi*) One of several large air passages in the lungs through which inspired air and exhaled waste gases pass.

Bruit Sound made ("whoosh") when blood flows through a narrowed blood vessel or through a ballooned-out area in a blood vessel.

C

Capillaries Smallest blood vessels in the body; in the tissues, capillaries surround the cells, allowing gas and nutrient exchange to take place.

Capillary refill Time it takes for a patient's skin color to return to normal after the skin or nailbed has been pressed or blanched; normal time is less than 2 seconds; assesses perfusion.

Capitation Payment scheme within the managed care industry in which payments are made to health care providers for a specified menu of services to a specified patient population. Payments are made on a cost per member per month basis. This method shifts the insurance risk from the payer to the provider.

Cardiac arrest Condition in which the heart no longer generates blood flow, causing pulselessness and apnea; two of the many causes are arrhythmias and myocardial infarction.

Cardiac contusion Bruise to the heart.

Cardiac muscle Made up of three layers—epicardium (external layer), myocardium (middle layer), and endocardium (internal layer).

Cardiac muscle cell Specialized muscle cell that is present only in the heart. Its internal makeup and function are different from those of other muscle cells in the body.

Cardiac output Total amount of blood pumped by the heart in 1 minute; usually 5 liters.

Cardinal Key, critical, common sign.

Cardiogenic shock Condition in which the heart's output is not strong enough to meet the body's needs, causing widespread hypoperfusion.

Cardioversion Restoration of normal cardiac function and rhythm to the heart using electrical energy.

Cargo compartment Rear (or front area on vehicles with a rear engine) compartment area of a passenger vehicle that is used to store or carry items.

Cargo strap Tool used to secure objects together. It consists of a strap and a wratcheting device to tighten the strap.

Carina Division of the lower end of the trachea into the two mainstem bronchi.

Carotid arteries Major arteries of the neck, supplying the face, head, and brain with oxygenated blood.

Carotid pulse Pulse palpated at the carotid artery of the neck, on either side of the neck beside the larynx.

Carpals Wrist bones.

Carryout Removing a patient from the scene to the transport vehicle.

Cartilage Form of connective tissue that is more elastic than bone and is considered part of the skeleton.

Case review Method of quality assurance that involves reviewing actual cases with EMTs to review the quality of care delivered by the EMS system.

CASEVAC Combat casualty evacuation care.

Cavitation Open area in an organ or tissue.

Cellular/capillary exchange Exchange of oxygen that occurs in the body tissues; oxygen enters the cells to be metabolized, and carbon dioxide enters the capillaries to be carried to the lungs.

Centers for Disease Control and Prevention (CDC) Division of the United States Public Health Service that is responsible for activities related to control and prevention of disease processes.

Central nervous system Part of the nervous system comprising the brain and spinal cord.

Cerebellum Portion of the brain located beneath the cerebrum and surrounding the brain stem; coordinates movement.

Cerebral edema Accumulation of fluid in the brain tissues. Because the skull cannot expand to accommodate the increase in pressure, the brain is compressed; early symptoms are changes in level of consciousness, sluggish to dilated pupils, and a gradual loss of consciousness; can be fatal.

Cerebral palsy Neuromuscular condition in which the patient has difficulty controlling the voluntary muscles because of damage to a portion of the brain.

Cerebrospinal fluid (CSF) Fluid that circulates around the brain and spinal cord; acts as a cushion to protect the brain, allowing the brain to literally float; also helps remove byproducts of brain metabolism.

Cerebrovascular accident (CVA) Medical term for stroke.

Cerebrum Portion of the brain divided into left and right hemispheres and further divided into several lobes, each of which has a unique responsibility in the control of specific intellectual, sensory, and/or motor functions.

Certification Act of certifying or state of being certified. In the legal sense, certification is analogous to licensure.

Cervical collar Device used to provide partial C-spine immobilization; only 50% in the three major motions of anterior/posterior, lateral bending, and rotation. It is applied to the neck area of an injured patient suspected of having a cervical spine injury.

Cervical immobilization Reduction of motion of the spine by immobilization of the bones above and below the cervical spine (head and thoracic spine).

Cervical spinal immobilization Important procedure of initial patient care where the cervical area of the spine is controlled by the rescuer with a little movement as possible of this area to prevent further injury to the cervical spine.

Cervical vertebrae First seven vertebrae.

Cervix Opening to the uterus.

Chain of survival Critical interventions needed to improve survival from prehospital cardiac arrest, including early access, early cardiopulmonary resuscitation, early defibrillation, and early advanced cardiac life support.

Cheyne-Stokes breathing Specific breathing pattern characterized by a period of slow and shallow breathing, a period of deep ventilation, a period of slow shallow breathing, and a period of apnea.

Chief complaint Description of the patient's reason for seeking medical attention; should be stated in the patient's words if possible; abbreviated CC or C/C.

Cholecystitis Inflammation of the gallbladder, which may be acute or chronic. Pain is increased by ingestion of fatty foods.

Chronic Long, drawn out; applied to a disease that is not acute.

Chronic bronchitis Form of chronic obstructive pulmonary disease commonly seen in smokers, characterized by a chronic productive cough and obstructive airway symptoms.

Chronic care Health care provided for a persistent injury or disease with little change or slow progression, such as

Alzheimer's disease; typically this care is provided in an extended-care facility.

Chronic obstructive pulmonary disease (COPD) Condition characterized by diminished inspiratory and expiratory capacity of the lungs.

Circle survey Method for rescue personnel to conduct a thorough survey of the accident scene, which includes walking in a 360 degree circle of the entire scene.

Civil (tort) law Part of the law that deals with noncriminal matters such as contract disputes, divorce, and medical malpractice.

Clavicle Bone running from the manubrium to the shoulder.

Closed fracture Fracture in which the skin integrity has not been compromised.

Closed head injury Injury to the brain or skull that does not penetrate the skin.

Closed injury Blunt trauma that has no break in the integrity of the skin.

Closed soft-tissue injury Damage to the skin and underlying tissue layers in which the skin remains intact (see *Contusion*, *Hematoma*, and *Crush injury*).

Clothing drag Type of inline drag using the patient's clothing to pull him or her away from immediate danger.

Coccyx vertebrae Last four vertebrae after the cervical, thoracic, lumbar, and sacral vertebrae.

Cold load Loading a patient on an aircraft after the rotor systems have completely stopped turning.

Collision bar Reinforced part of the interior of a modern automobile door. It is designed to add strength to the vehicle and provide some protection to the occupants from side impacts.

Colon Portion of the large intestine that is divided into three parts—ascending colon, transverse colon, and descending colon.

Colostomy Incision in the colon for the purpose of making a more or less permanent opening between the bowel and the abdominal wall.

Combat Lifesaver Program U.S. military program that provides nonmedical personal education beyond basic first aid.

Combination tool Powered hydraulic tool that consists of spreader arms with cutting edges on the inside of the arms. They can spread metal and cut it.

Come along Lifting or pulling tool. This is a portable hand-operated winch. It includes an operating handle, cable spindle and casing, cables, and hooks. It is designed to be used with rescue chains or rescue chain sling devices.

Command Term used to describe the person in control of an emergency scene or to denote the action of controlling an emergency scene.

Common duct Duct that carries bile to the duodenum and receives it from the cystic duct of the gallbladder and the hepatic ducts. The distal portion runs through the head of the pancreas. Also known as the *common bile duct*.

Communicable disease Disease that can be transmitted from one person to another through body fluids, air ingestion, or skin contact.

Communication Ability to send and receive information.

Compartment syndrome Condition commonly caused by crush injuries or prolonged lack of blood flow to an extremity. Muscle tissue dies, causing swelling, which increases pressure in the muscle compartment, which decreases blood flow, which kills more muscle, leading to more swelling, etc. It can result in complete death of the extremity if not stopped by surgical intervention.

Complete fracture Fracture in which the bone ends separate.

Compliance When used to describe the lungs, this term refers to the relative stiffness of the lungs. As compliance decreases, the lungs become more stiff and difficult to artificially ventilate.

Compression Squeezed together.

Compression fracture Fracture of a bone resulting from a force from above and below the bone.

Computer-aided dispatch (CAD) Computerized dispatch communications program.

Computer-based report One format for a patient care report. A computer-based report is completed using an electronic clipboard or mobile data terminal in which the information is entered by a special instrument or keyboard. The information then can be downloaded or printed at the hospital or ambulance base.

Concurrent evaluation Evaluating the quality of care as it is being given (e.g., physician ride-along with the EMT).

Conduction Direct heat exchange that occurs when two or more surfaces come into contact with one another; movement of heat will be from the surface of higher temperature to the surface of lower temperature. A patient will lose body heat when lying on the cold ground as a result of conduction.

Confidentiality Privacy that is afforded to patient-related information.

Confusion Inability to understand the situation.

Congestive heart failure Condition in which the heart is an inadequate pump, causing fluid to build up in the lungs (pulmonary edema) and venous system (distended neck veins).

Consent Doctrine that states that before a health care provider may render medical treatment, the patient must express consent.

Constrict Make smaller or narrower, as in pupils reacting to light.

Continuing education Ongoing educational experiences provided to EMS personnel; an essential part of any quality assurance program in which EMTs can maintain and improve their skills.

Continuous quality improvement (CQI) Method of continuously evaluating and improving the care delivered in the EMS system.

Contraction Tightening and hardening of the uterus, which expels the fetus.

Contraindications Conditions or situations in which a drug should not be given (e.g., lack of consciousness is a contraindication to giving oral medications).

Controlled glass removal Dislodging of vehicle glass that is obstructing tool application or patient access in a vehicle crash entrapment situation. Glass is removed in a safe and controlled action.

Contusion Minor damage in the dermal layer of the skin, causing discoloration from blood leaking into surrounding tissue; a bruise.

Convection Heat exchange that occurs when air currents move across an exposed surface.
Convulsive Producing motor activity, as in a seizure.
Core Central part; the heart and lungs of the human body.
Core area Area of the body containing the major organs (head, thorax, and abdomen).
Core temperature Temperature in the center, or core, of the body.
Coronary arteries First branches off the aorta, which supply the heart with blood. If occluded, a myocardial infarction often occurs.
Costovertebral angle Angle of the junction of the lower ribs and the spine. The kidneys lie just beneath this area. Pain produced by percussion of this area is usually associated with kidney conditions.
Countershock Electrerical termination of atrial fibrillation.
Court system State or federal forum in which legal issues and disputes are resolved.
Crackles Low-pitched bubbling sounds produced by fluid in the lower airways; often described as either fine or coarse.
Cranial cavity Cavity that houses the brain.
Cranium Portion of the skull that encloses the brain, consisting of the frontal, occipital, sphenoid, and ethmoid bones.
Crash Impact between vehicles or people.
Crepitus Crackling sensation that can be felt when air escapes from the lungs and gets into surrounding tissue. Similar in feel to pressing on "bubble packs." The sound and the feeling bones can make when they are fractured, caused by the rubbing together of loose bone ends.
Cribbing Generally refers to the specially cut and/or assembled pieces of wood used to support raised objects (e.g., a car).
Cricoid cartilage Complete ring of cartilage at the lower end of the larynx that marks the beginning of the lower airway; compressed during the Sellick maneuver.
Crime scene Location where the crime occurred. Everything present in and around the scene is a potential clue or evidence and should not be disturbed.
Criminal law Part of the law that deals with crime and punishment.
Criteria-based dispatch (CBD) Type of dispatch based on the recognition that the level of care at either the EMT-Basic or EMT-Paramedic level required for patients and the urgency of that prehospital care can be identified by established medical criteria.
Critical incident Event or circumstance that overwhelms one or more of the people present.
Critical incident stress debriefing (CISD) Confidential meeting in which a team consisting of mental health professionals and police, fire, and EMS disaster management personnel meet with prehospital providers to discuss a critical incident for the purpose of debriefing and alleviating stress.
Critiquing Discussion of the rescue effort during the postincident phase in order to learn from the rescue effort.
Croup Viral infection seen in children, characterized by a "barking" cough and moderate to severe ventilatory distress.
Crowd control Safe and efficient removal of unnecessary people from in and around the vehicles involved in an accident. This can be accomplished by initially arriving rescuers and law enforcement personnel.
Crowning Bulging of the perineum when birth is imminent.
Crush injury Damage that results from a body part being compressed between two surfaces; deep damage to muscle and compartment syndrome may result.
C-spine Neck area; common term in vehicle extrication trauma patient care; short for *cervical spine*.
Curriculum Description of an education program; usually includes learning objectives for the students and guidelines or rules for conducting the program (e.g., number of hours, number of lessons, etc.).
Cushing's triad Phenomenon seen with increased cranial pressure, distinguished by a rise in blood pressure, change in respirations, and decrease in pulse.
Cutter Powered hydraulic tool that is used for cutting metal and other wreckage on the extrication scene.
Cyanosis Slightly bluish, grayish, slatelike, or dark purple discoloration of the skin caused by a deficiency of oxygen and excess of carbon dioxide in the blood.
Cyanotic Bluish color of the skin associated with unoxygenated hemoglobin.

D

Dash lift Lifting maneuver on the front dash of an automobile used to lift the dash assembly up and off of trapped patients. This is usually done with heavy hydraulic spreaders, cutters, and/or rams.
Data collection Collection of data through various means, such as EMS patient care reports (PCRs) completed by EMTs responding to calls.
Dead space Space in the lungs that contains air that is inhaled but does not reach the alveoli for exchange; includes the upper and lower airways and is usually about 150 ml in volume.
Debriefing Activity in which rescuers, patient, and patient's family discuss the rescue effort to relieve emotions and anxiety
Deceleration sensor Type of sensing device used on air bag restraint systems that, when activated by a sudden collision, activates the deployment of the air bag.
Decerebrate posturing Extension of the upper extremities with the lower extremities rigid and extended.
Decompression sickness Medical condition that can occur in scuba divers as a result of body tissues becoming saturated with nitrogen during a dive with compressed air and results in the formation of small inert gas bubbles that can block blood flow.
Decontamination Process of removing hazardous substances from the patient, rescuers, and equipment.
Decorticate posturing Flexion of the upper extremities with the lower extremities rigid and extended.
Defibrillation Delivery of an electrical shock to the myocardium in an attempt to convert ventricular fibrillation or ventricular tachycardia to a normal rhythm.
Definitive care Treatment provided to cure or resolve a patient's current illness or injury (e.g., surgery to repair a badly fractured bone or reattach an amputated limb).
Dehydration Excessive loss of water from the body tissues; signs include poor skin turgor, flushed and dry skin, coated tongue, low urine output, irritability, and confusion.
Demarcation Clear, visible line of color change.

Dementia General mental deterioration caused by organic or psychologic factors.

Dermis Middle layer of the skin that contains the blood vessels, glands, hair follicles, and nerve endings.

Descending aorta Part of the aorta between the arch and the iliac bifurcation.

Descent injury Injury that can occur to a scuba diver while descending from the water surface to the dive depth.

Detailed physical examination Follows the focused history and physical examination; this portion of patient assessment comprises a region-by-region evaluation of the entire body to check for hidden problems.

Developmental disability Disability that involves some degree of impaired adaptation in learning, social adjustment, and/or maturation.

Diabetes A metabolic disorder that results from inadequate insulin secretion.

Diagnosis Identification of a disease or condition. The results of the assessment are compared with known injury or illness patterns to identify a disease or condition.

Diagnostic reserve airbag module (DRAM) Device that stores electricity for the deployment of air bag restraint systems in vehicles. They provide a back up capacity in the event of electrical failure.

Diagonal slide Movement used to place a patient on a long spine board.

Diaphoresis Secretion of sweat.

Diaphoretic State of sweating (e.g., patients with cardiac chest pain are often diaphoretic).

Diaphragm Dome-shaped muscle that separates the thoracic cavity from the abdominal cavity. When it contracts, the thoracic cavity enlarges, allowing air to enter the lungs.

Diastolic pressure Pressure in the heart when the heart muscle is relaxing; lower reading of a blood pressure measurement.

Digital radio equipment Computer-controlled radio equipment that is used in a sophisticated communication system, usually in the 800 MHz range.

Dilate Get larger, as in the pupils reacting to darkness.

Direct ground lift Lift used for patients who are not suspected of having a spinal injury; allows the movement of the patient from the ground to a piece of equipment.

Direct medical direction Clinical type of medical direction that involves real-time direction of prehospital providers in the delivery of emergency care; also known as *on-line medical direction*.

Direct pressure Controlled pressure applied over a wound with the hands or with bandages; first-resort measure to control bleeding.

Disaster Human-made or natural event that involves tremendous damage across a large geographic area; may or may not involve large number of injuries (e.g., earthquakes, hurricanes, or floods).

Disentanglement Process of freeing a trapped patient on the rescue scene, usually by removal of the vehicle from around the victim.

Dislocation Separation of two bones from their normal relationship within a joint.

Displacement Describes the moving of a part of a vehicle beyond its normal operating range, making space for the access and removal of trapped patients.

Distal Located away from the center of the body; situated away from the point of attachment or origin or a central point.

Distraction injury Injury in which the spine is pulled apart.

Do-not-resuscitate (DNR) orders Instructions to withhold resuscitation efforts. These can be issued by a physician after consultation with the patient or surrogate decision maker or by the medical command authority via radio communication.

Door latch assembly Device that keeps the door of a vehicle closed. It is generally made up of a pin in the door jamb upon which a clasping device in the door itself hooks when the door is closed.

Dorsal Toward the back

Dorsalis pedis artery Artery located on the upper surface of the foot; usually palpable and can be used to assess blood supply distal to a leg injury.

Down syndrome Genetic syndrome characterized by varying degrees of mental retardation and multiple physical defects.

Dressing Sterile material that is placed directly on a wound.

Drowning Death resulting from asphyxiation after submersion in a liquid.

Duodenum First portion of the small bowel. It is approximately 12 inches long (hence the name) and has a combined blood supply with the pancreas.

Dura mater Outermost layer of the meninges.

Durable power of attorney Legally binding document signed by a party that designates an individual to make health care decisions for the person executing the document.

Duration of action Length of time a drug is effective after one dose.

Duty to act Responsibility to provide appropriate medical care.

Dyspnea Symptom of having difficulty breathing or shortness of breath.

Dysrhythmia Abnormal rhythm.

E

Ecchymosis Discoloration or bluing of the skin.

Eclampsia In the pregnant patient, predelivery increase in blood pressure with resultant seizure activity.

Edema Abnormal accumulation of fluid in tissues in response to injury.

Elder abuse Physical, psychologic, and financial mistreatment of the elderly.

Elderly Traditional term given to those persons 65 years of age or older.

Electrical detection device Specialized tool that is used to detect the presence of alternating current electrical charge on the emergency scene.

Electrocardiogram (ECG) Tracing of the electrical conduction system in the heart; normally occurs in predictable patterns.

Elevation To raise an extremity or injured part above the level of the heart; measure used to control severe bleeding.

Emancipated minor Minor whose parent or guardian has relinquished authority and control over him or her; minor surrenders the right to maintenance and support by the parent or guardian.

Emancipation Legal doctrine that allows a person to make legal decisions regarding his or her health.

Embryo Fertilized egg to the first 8 weeks of pregnancy.

Emergency medical dispatch (EMD) Approach to the dispatch function of an EMS system that involves the dispatcher in making decisions about the type and priority of EMS response that is necessary, providing critical information to responding units while they are en route, and providing prearrival instructions to callers until the EMS units are on the scene.

Emergency medical services (EMS) system Complex organization composed of people, equipment, and facilities designed to respond to the emergency health care needs of the community.

Emergency medical technician (EMT) Person trained in and responsible for the administration of specialized emergency care and transportation to a medical facility of victims of acute illness or injury. The U.S. Department of Transportation training guidelines for EMTs include a 110-hour course of instruction and clinical time.

Emergency move Any move that is initiated because of immediate danger to the patient and rescuer.

Emergency vehicle operator (EVO) Term used to describe an appropriately trained and qualified ambulance driver.

Emphysema Form of chronic obstructive pulmonary disease characterized by destruction of alveoli and obstructive airway symptoms; commonly seen in smokers.

EMS do not resuscitate (DNR) legislation Legislation providing for a legally binding order signed by a physicians and by the person that precludes life-saving techniques being started on a patient who has a terminal illness and who arrests.

EMT-Basic (EMT-B) Basic level of emergency medical technician education identified by the U.S. Department of Transportation; provides basic emergency medical care.

EMT-Intermediate (EMT-I) Level of emergency medical technician between the level of EMT-Basic and EMT-Paramedic. The EMT-I generally has additional education in assessment over the EMT-B level. In addition, the EMT-I generally will be educated to use intravenous therapy and a limited selection of medications.

EMT-Paramedic (EMT-P) Most advanced level of prehospital emergency care provider identified by the U.S. Department of Transportation. The EMT-P has advanced assessment skills and is trained in a wide variety of invasive interventions. The EMT-P can use a variety of medications, intravenous solutions, and other advanced treatment techniques.

Endocardium Inner layer of the heart.

Endocrine Enzymes secreted by various glands in the body.

Endotracheal tube Specialized tube designed to definitively control the airway. The tube has a cuff that is inflated in the trachea to prevent aspiration and improve oxygenation.

Endotracheal tube cuff Small balloon that is inflated with 5 to 10 ml of air to prevent aspiration around the endotracheal tube; it should be checked for leaks before insertion.

End-tidal carbon dioxide Carbon dioxide that is exhaled with each breath. After endotracheal intubation, documenting the presence of end-tidal carbon dioxide helps confirm tube position.

Energy Molecular activity.

Engine compartment Area of the vehicle in which the engine is located. It is generally separated from the vehicle passenger area by a heavily constructed fire wall.

Enhanced 911 (E-911) Fully integrated, computerized 911-access telephone system.

Environmental stressors Strains and pressures from factors in the environment that can affect the EMT (e.g., weather conditions, noise levels, and shift work).

Epicardium Outer layer of the heart.

Epidermis Outermost layer of the skin; consists of cells only.

Epidural hematoma Condition in which blood leaks into the epidural space.

Epidural space Potential space located between the skull and the dura mater.

Epigastrium Area between the umbilicus and the xiphoid process. The EMT auscultates in this area after endotracheal intubation to ensure that an esophageal intubation has not occurred.

Epiglottis Leaf-shaped structure just above the larynx that prevents food and liquids from entering the trachea during swallowing.

Epiglottitis Inflammation of the epiglottis; a bacterial infection seen most often in children. The epiglottis becomes swollen and may cause airway obstruction; patients often have excessive drooling.

Epilepsy Group of neurologic disorders characterized by recurrent episodes of convulsive seizures, sensory disturbances, unusual behavior, loss of consciousness, or all of these; uncontrolled electric discharge from the nerve cells of the cerebral cortex.

Epinephrine Hormone secreted by the adrenal gland; causes tachycardia, vasoconstriction, and release of insulin.

Epi-Pen® Autoinjector that contains epinephrine used subcutaneously to counteract the effects of histamine.

Erythrocytes Blood cells that contain hemoglobin; primary function is to carry oxygen back to the tissues; also called *red blood cells*.

Esophageal intubation detection device Specially designed syringe or a self-inflating bulb used to determine whether air can be aspirated freely; used to help confirm correct endotracheal tube placement.

Esophagus Muscular canal extending from the back of the mouth to the stomach.

Evaporation Heat exchange that occurs when a liquid is changed into a gas. When perspiration evaporates, it uses body heat as the energy source and results in a reduction of body heat.

Evisceration Injury in which organs protrude from the abdominal cavity through a wound in the abdominal wall.

Exhalation Breathing air out of the lungs.

Expert witness Witness who has special knowledge of the subject about which he or she is called to testify.

Exposure control plan Plan that an employer is required to develop to comply with the Occupational Safety and Health Administration standard; to minimize the risk that employees will become exposed to a communicable disease.

Expressed consent Patient states consent either in writing or orally for EMTs to provide treatment.

Extended-care facility Facility providing inpatient chronic or restorative patient care; often referred to as a *nursing home*.

Extremity lift Lift used for patients who are not suspected of having a spinal injury that uses the patient's arms and legs to move him or her a short distance.

Extrication Common vehicle rescue term that is used in this text to describe procedures used by rescue personnel to remove trapped patients, trapped by the wreckage or by their injuries, from vehicles involved in accidents.

Extrication officer Designation of a subcommand level of control on the scene that is generally responsible for supervising the actual rescue efforts of moving wreckage and freeing the patient for removal.

Extubation Process of removing an endotracheal tube. If a patient becomes more responsive after endotracheal intubation, he or she may attempt self-extubation because of discomfort.

F

Face Bones of the anterior section of the skull.

Fallopian tube Paired canals approximately 4 inches long connecting the ovary to the uterus; also called *oviducts*.

False contractions Contractions that occur at irregular intervals but do not increase in pain intensity; also known as *Braxton Hicks contractions*.

False imprisonment Intentional and unjustifiable detainment of a person.

Febrile Pertaining to elevated body temperature; a body temperature of over 100° F commonly is considered febrile.

Fee-for-service In a fee-for-service model, the patient accesses a health service and pays a fee for such care. In this approach, no limits are placed on the patient in selection of medical providers or access to the health care system.

Femoral arteries Major vessels supplying the legs with oxygenated blood; can be palpated in the groin area.

Femoral pulse Pulse palpated at the femoral artery of the groin on either side of the pelvis.

Femur Bone of the thigh.

Fend-off position Method of positioning emergency apparatus at a vehicle accident that provides added protection to the scene from traffic.

Fetus The developing unborn offspring from 8 weeks after conception until birth.

Fibula Posterior bone of the lower leg.

Field assessment card Form used for making notes during the assessment and history-taking process; serves as a way for the EMT to organize information informally before entering it on the patient care report.

FiO$_2$ Percentage of inspired oxygen.

Firewall Area that separates the engine compartment from the passenger compartment in a vehicle. For vehicle extrication it is considered one of the strongest points in a vehicle.

Fistula Abnormal tubelike passage from a normal cavity or tube to a free surface or another cavity, which can be due to congenital incomplete closure of parts or a result of abscesses, injuries, or inflammatory processes.

Fixed-wing aircraft Aircraft with wings solidly attached to the main fuselage. As the entire aircraft moves through the air, lift is created as air passes over the wings; commonly called an *airplane*.

Flexible stretcher Piece of equipment, also known as a *pole stretcher*, designed for use when space is limited.

Flexion Movement allowed by certain joints of the skeleton that decreases the angle between two adjoining bones, such as bending the elbow.

Focused history and physical examination Follows the initial assessment; this portion of patient assessment focuses on regions of the body that the EMT-Basic suspects may have sustained illness or injury. History may be assessed using the SAMPLE mnemonic.

Foramen magnum Opening at the base of the skull.

Fowler's position Sitting up.

Fracture surrounding a joint Fracture around a true joint that makes that joint more freely movable and creates a greater tendency for the joint to impinge on surrounding structures such as arteries, veins, and nerves.

Fragmentation Breaking apart.

Freeze International term used when a rescuer wants other rescuers to make an emergency stop to their activities on the scene.

Frontal Anterior section of the skull.

Frostbite Injury to the skin caused by prolonged exposure to cold. The liquid content of the skin cells freezes and ruptures the cell membranes; may be superficial (frostnip) or deep.

Frostnip Frostbite that is superficial in nature; affects only the topmost layers of the skin.

Fuel systems Systems within a vehicle that provide fuel for the engine. The components include the fuel tank, fuel lines which carry the fuel to the engine, fuel pumping device, and fuel distributing device at the engine itself.

Full frame Type of vehicle construction in the undercarriage that is used in some station-wagon–type automobiles and light trucks.

Full protective clothing Specially designed protective clothing that is worn by rescue personnel while performing vehicle rescue procedures in and around the vehicle. Specifications depend on local requirements; however, they should include head, hand, foot, and body protection. See also *personal protective gear*.

Full pulse Strong, normal pulse.

Full-thickness burn Burn involving all skin layers and, in some cases, the underlying bone and muscle; characterized by charring of the skin and complete absence of feeling as a result of destruction of nerve endings; also called *third-degree burn*.

Functional disorder Disorder in which the performance or operation of an organ or organ system is abnormal but not as a result of known changes in structure.

Fuselage Main body of the aircraft.

G

Gallbladder Pear-shaped sac on the undersurface of the right lobe of the liver holding bile from the liver. The bile is stored and, while in the gallbladder, is concentrated by removing water.

Gastric lavage Use of a tube passed through the nose or mouth into the stomach to remove material from the stomach.

Gastroenteritis Inflammation of the stomach and intestines that accompanies numerous gastrointestinal disorders; symptoms are lack of appetite, nausea, vomiting, abdominal discomfort, and diarrhea.

Gastrointestinal Of or pertaining to the organs of the gastrointestinal tract, from mouth to anus.

Gastrointestinal tract Area that includes the stomach and intestines.

Gastronomy tube Tube placed in a patient's stomach that allows continuous feeding for an extended period of time.

Gatekeeper Health care provider, often a primary care physician, who is used in many managed care systems to direct or control the flow of patients within the system. Patients and other health care providers must contact the gatekeeper and receive authorization before initiating treatment.

General impression EMT's overall "gut feeling" about the scene and patient based on knowledge and tempered by experience.

General injury Involvement of one or more of the body's major systems.

Generic name Simple form of the chemical name of the drug; each drug has only one generic name.

Gerontologists Specialists who treat the elderly.

Glasgow coma scale Standardized rating system used to evaluate the degree of consciousness impairment based on eye opening, motor response, and verbal response. Points are scored for the patient's best response in each of the three categories.

Glottic opening Opening between the vocal cords through which an endotracheal tube is passed.

Glottis Slitlike opening between the vocal cords.

Glucagon Hormone secreted by the pancreas that stimulates the breakdown of glycogen and the release of glucose by the liver.

Glucose Simple sugar used by the cell for energy; derived from the digestion of complex carbohydrates that are eaten, from the breakdown of glycogen in the liver, or by conversion of protein in the liver.

Glycogen Starch that is the major storage form of glucose; stored in the liver and can be broken down to glucose when needed.

Golden hour Special first hour after the incident in which a traumatized patient has the best chance for recovery from the trauma if he or she can be safely delivered to an emergency medical facility and a surgeon.

GPM Fire service abbreviation term for gallons per minute flow of a liquid.

Grand mal Generalized full tonic-clonic seizure.

Gravida Pregnant or the number of times that a person has been pregnant.

Great vessels Major vessels in the chest.

Gynecologic Pertaining to the study of the diseases of women's reproductive organs.

Gynecology Study of the diseases of women's reproductive organs.

H

Hack saw Hand operated metal cutting tool consisting of a frame and removable blade. It uses a sawing action to cut metal.

Halligan bar Hand tool originally designed for forcible entry in the fire service. For vehicle rescue it is used as a prying and glass-breaking tool. It is usually used with a flat-head axe.

Hand tools For extrication work, these include cutting, prying, and lifting tools. They may be electrically driven like a reciprocating saw; pneumatically powered like an air chisel, or manually operated like a hack saw.

Hard protection In vehicle rescue, a type of patient protection that consists of a hard barrier between the patient and tool action.

Hatch back Common description of a vehicle that has a rear access door to the passenger compartment area or rear storage area.

Hazard control Handling of hazards on the extrication scene. It can also denote a command sector or subdivision of command on the scene that is concerned with hazards.

Hazardous materials (HAZMAT) Chemical substances (solid, gas, or liquid) that are toxic to humans; unprotected exposure to these chemicals may result in severe illness or death. They may be poisonous, flammable, explosive, carcinogenic, or environmentally pollutant. HAZMAT is the part of emergency services that handles these field situations.

Hazardous materials team Group of emergency workers trained in all aspects of safely handling emergency incidents that involve hazardous materials.

Head injury Damage to the brain.

Head-on collision Frontal impact.

Head-tilt chin-lift Maneuver that opens the airway of unconscious patients; the neck is extended with one hand on the forehead and one hand under the chin.

Health care delivery system Large and complex network of people, equipment, and facilities designed to meet the general health care needs of the population.

Health maintenance organization (HMO) Type of health care provider, most often associated with "managed care," which offers a specified menu of health services to an enrolled population for a fixed payment, usually an annual fee.

Heart Four-chambered organ that pumps blood through the blood vessels to distribute oxygen to the cells of the body.

Heart rate Number of heart beats that occur in 1 minute.

Heat cramps First and mildest form of heat exposure; muscle cramping caused by excessive loss of body fluids and salts.

Heat exhaustion Form of heat exposure that occurs when the body's circulatory system fails to maintain its normal functions as a result of excessive loss of body fluids and salts; patient presents with shocklike symptoms.

Heat index Measurement of the combined effect of temperature and humidity on the apparent temperature.

Heat stroke Life-threatening condition that results from the failure of the body's normal temperature regulatory processes; body temperature rises out of control, and critical body functions deteriorate.

Hematoma Damage similar to a contusion but more extensive with larger blood vessels torn and more blood collected in deep tissues.

Hemiparesis Partial paralysis that affects only one side of the body.

Hemiplegia Total paralysis that affects only one side of the body.

Hemoglobin Specialized protein that binds to oxygen in red blood cells; gives red blood cells their color.

Hemopneumothorax Collection of both blood and air in the pleural space; always abnormal and may cause collapse of the underlying lung.

Hemorrhage Severe loss of blood.

Hemothorax Accumulation of blood and fluid in the pleural cavity usually caused by trauma.

High-efficiency particulate air (HEPA) respirator Mask worn over the mouth and nose that decreases the spread of infection of airborne pathogens such as tuberculosis.

High-energy weapons Weapons with a muzzle velocity less than 2000 feet per second.

High-lift jack Lifting device that is designed to mechanically lift a vehicle that sits high off the ground level. Used in vehicle extrication for metal moving and stabilization.

Hinged joint Joint that moves freely in only one direction.

Hinged-side-first method Type of vehicle door removal technique that starts at the hinges of the door and ends on the latch side of the door.

Hip joint Joint formed by the head of the femur and the acetabulum.

Histamine Specific substance produced by the body responsible for the attack.

History of present illness or injury (HPI) Events or complaints associated with the patient's current health problem; should correspond to the reason the patient is now seeking medical attention.

Hives Raised, blanched, irregularly shaped lesions with surrounding redness. Hives cause severe itching.

Home care Health care provided to the patient outside of a licensed health care facility, such as in the patient's home or home of a relative.

Homeostasis State of relative constancy of the internal environment of the body.

Hormones Chemicals that regulate body activities and functions.

Hose line Fire services term that denotes water hose lines that carry water to the emergency scene from the fire engine.

Hot load Loading a patient on the aircraft when the rotor systems are still turning.

Humerus Bone of the upper arm.

Humidity Measurement, usually expressed in percentage, of the amount of water or moisture in the air.

Hydraulic jack Lifting tool that comes in a kit with several attachments. It is a piston operated by a manual hydraulic pump.

Hydrocephalus "Water on the brain"; can cause increased intracranial pressure if allowed to accumulate.

Hypercarbia High concentration of carbon dioxide in the blood.

Hyperextension Position of a joint in maximum extension.

Hyperglycemia Elevated blood glucose level.

Hypersensitivity Abnormal condition characterized by an excessive reaction to a particular stimulus.

Hypertension Abnormally high blood pressure; a risk factor for atherosclerosis, stroke, and other vascular events.

Hyperthermia Condition in which the core temperature of the body exceeds normal limits and starts to malfunction.

Hyperventilation Process in which minute ventilation is increased above normal; purposely done for patients with head injuries or prolonged apnea.

Hypoglycemia Low blood glucose level.

Hypoperfusion State of inadequate supply of oxygen and nutrients to the tissues, most commonly caused by decreased blood flow. If widespread hypoperfusion exists, the patient is in shock.

Hypopharynx Lower third of the pharynx.

Hypotension Abnormally low blood pressure; may be a sign of shock.

Hypothermia Abnormal and dangerous condition in which the core body temperature falls below 35° C (95° F) and the body's normal functions are impaired; usually caused by prolonged exposure to cold.

Hypoventilation Process of lowering minute ventilation below normal. Patients who are hypoventilating have higher carbon dioxide and lower oxygen levels than normal.

Hypovolemia Abnormally low circulating blood volume.

Hypovolemic shock State of physical collapse caused by massive blood loss, circulatory dysfunction, and inadequate tissue perfusion.

Hypoxemia Abnormal deficiency of oxygen in the arterial blood.

Hypoxia Condition in which the patient has a shortage of oxygen at the cellular level. Signs and symptoms of hypoxia include dyspnea, restlessness, confusion, lethargy, and poor skin color.

I

Ileostomy Creation of a surgical passage through the abdominal wall into the ileum.

Iliac crest Superior, lateral bones of the hip.

Immediate medical control Range of activities that a medical director provides while the emergency is actually taking place (e.g., giving instructions to EMTs via radio or telephone).

Immersion To be completely soaked in a wet substance (e.g., to be caught in the rain or to be drenched in sweat).

Immune Protected from a disease; protected from a disease by vaccination or inoculation.

Immune system Recognizes foreign invaders and eliminates them from the body.

Immunosuppression (or immunity suppression) Prevention of formation of immune responses.

Impact wrench Heavy bolt-driving tool that may be pneumatically or electrically powered. It comes in a kit with several sizes of specially designed sockets.

Implied consent Consent implied when a patient is unable to give expressed consent; the law assumes that such a patient would want to have life-saving treatment administered.

Incident command system (ICS) System of control of the emergency scene that is set up by predetermined procedures for effective control of complex emergency operations, such as extrication operations. The origins of ICS can be traced to the fire service, but it has now been adapted for use in almost any situation requiring management of complex events.

Incident commander Person in charge of the incident command system.

Incompetent patient Patient who is unable to make legal decisions. Usually an act of the court may be judged to be in such a state because of a medical or mental condition.

Increased intracranial pressure (ICP) Increased pressure in the cranium caused by insult.

Indications Conditions under which a drug is given (e.g., chest pain is an indication for giving nitroglycerin).

Indirect medical control Administrative duties carried out by the EMS medical director (e.g., writing of protocols, negotiation of destination policies, and retrospective review of EMT performance); also known as *off-line medical direction*.

Inertia Basic law of physics that states that an object at rest will tend to remain at rest and an object in motion will tend to remain in motion until acted upon by an outside force.

Infectious disease Disease that can be transmitted from one organism to another; an active state of infection.

Inferior Below.

Inferior vena cava Major vein of the abdominal cavity; returns blood from the lower extremities, pelvis, and abdomen to the right atrium.

Inflammation Tissue reaction to injury in which the inflamed tissue undergoes continuous change as the body's repair processes start to heal and replace the injured tissue.

Inflatable curtain Type of air restraint system primarily designed to give side-impact protection to occupants of a vehicle.

Inflatable tubular structure Woven fabric tube that is inflated on impact. It is a type of air restraint system designed to protect occupants of a vehicle in side-impact crashes.

Informed consent Doctrine that allows a patient to accept or refuse treatment based on disclosure of information about the medical condition and the risks, benefits, complications, potential outcome, and alternatives of the suggested treatment.

Infrastructure Physical components of a community that are necessary for normal, everyday operations, such as roads, bridges, electrical power, and telephone communications.

Inhalation Breathing air into the lungs.

Initial assessment Assessment that is completed by the EMT-Basic after scene size-up. Includes assessment of major body systems (airway, breathing, circulation, and level of consciousness) to identify life-threatening problems and initiation of interventions, including transportation.

Initial patient access Usually considered the first contact of a crash victim by rescuers. This is done before stabilization to provide immediate C-spine and airway care.

Injury location chart Anterior and posterior anatomic figure diagram located on the prehospital care report; used to diagram the patient's injuries.

Inline drag Move used to drag a patient to safety when immediate danger is present.

Inline stabilization Immobilization of a bone or bones in the axis of the bones.

Inner circle survey Term that describes the procedure of assessing a vehicle that has been involved in an accident. This involves the full circling of the vehicle and assessment of the area in, around, and under the vehicle.

Inner skin Part of the vehicle door anatomy that is the inside sheet metal of the door. This holds support for the outer skin, collision bar, window operating hardware, locks, and inside door handles.

Insulin Hormone produced in the pancreas needed for the proper metabolism of blood sugar.

Insulin-dependent diabetes mellitus Condition characterized by an inability to metabolize carbohydrates (sugar) because of a lack of insulin.

Integumentary system Made up of the skin, sebaceous glands, and sweat glands. Its function is to protect the body and help with temperature and water regulation.

Intercept Established location where two units (emergency vehicles) come together.

Intercostal muscles Muscles located between the ribs that lift the ribs upward and outward during inhalation, increasing tidal volume.

Internal fixation Use of wires, pins, and screws to place bones in proper position.

Interthoracic pressure Pressure inside the thorax that changes with ventilation.

Intervention Action or skill performed by the EMT in response to a finding in the initial assessment or focused history and examination.

Intervertebral disc Padding between vertebrae.

Intoxication Above the legal limit of alcohol or drugs.

Intracranial Within the cranium or skull.

Intracranial pressure (ICP) Pressure that builds up inside the cranial cavity.

Involuntary muscles Muscles that carry out the automatic functions of the body.

Ischemia Inadequate blood flow to a tissue; can cause anginal pain or a myocardial infarction.

Ischium Inferior, posterior bones of the hip.

Islets of Langerhans Cluster of cells in the pancreas that produce insulin.

J

Jaw thrust Maneuver for opening the airway in unconscious patients; enables cervical spine stabilization and is often used with trauma patients.

Joints Area where two bones connect.

K

Kendrick extrication device® (KED) Specially designed device used in removing automobile accident patients. It is composed of the body sling with straps and handles, chin and head straps, and a space filler pad.

Ketogenic diet Special diet high in fats and low in carbohydrates and protein; produces a state of ketosis in which fat is used for energy instead of glucose; used for children with ongoing seizures that do not respond to customary medication and other therapies.

Ketone bodies Group of chemicals formed by the metabolism of fat.

Kidney Organ located behind the peritoneum on each side of the vertebral column; form urine by the process of filtration, reabsorption, and secretion.

Kinematics Branch of biomechanics concerned with movement of the body, especially with respect to time.

Kinetic energy Law of physics that defines the amount of energy present in a moving object.

Kussmaul's respirations (air hunger) A deep, rapid breathing rate directly attributed to diabetic ketoacidosis.

Kyphosis Curvature of the thoracic spine.

L

Labor Regular uterine contractions that increase in frequency and intensity and propel the fetus from the uterus.

Laceration Break in the skin of varying depths resulting from a forceful impact with a sharp object; deeper injury than is seen with abrasions, with larger blood vessels involved and more bleeding.

Laminated glass Safety glass used for automotive windshields; a layer of plastic sandwiched (laminated) between two layers of glass to reduce shattering on impact.

Landing zone (LZ) Area established for the aircraft to land; for helicopters during the day, LZ is 60 ft × 60 ft and at night 100 ft × 100 ft; must be flat, firm, and free of hazards.

Landing zone (LZ) coordinator Person in charge of the LZ; responsible for identifying and controlling all hazards, directing the aircraft to the LZ, guiding the aircraft to landing and take-off, and ensuring safe operations around the aircraft.

Landing zone (LZ) hazards Anything that interferes with the safe landing or take-off of the aircraft, including debris, tall brush, pedestrians, poles, towers, and especially wires.

Large intestine Extends from the end of the small intestine to the anus. It is divided into the cecum, colon, sigmoid colon, rectum, and anus.

Laryngoscope Instrument used to visualize the vocal cords for endotracheal tube insertion; it has two parts: a handle and a blade.

Laryngotracheobronchitis Inflammation of the major respiratory passages, usually causing hoarseness, nonproductive cough, and difficulty breathing; also known as *croup*.

Larynx Structure consisting of cartilage, muscle, and soft tissues; located between the pharynx and the trachea; often called the *voice box*.

Latch assembly Part of a vehicle's door that closes around the striker bolt and holds the door shut. It releases when the door handle is operated.

Latch-side-first method Type of vehicle door removal technique that starts at the latch of the door and ends on the hinge side of the door.

Lateral Away from the midline.

Lateral bending Injury caused by the head bending too far in one direction.

Lawsuit Legal action filed by one party against another.

Lethargy State or quality of being indifferent, apathetic, or sluggish; stupor or coma resulting from disease or hypnosis.

Leukocytes White blood cells; function in the body's immune system.

Level of consciousness (LOC) Indirect measurement of cerebral oxygenation.

License Document issued by the government that grants permission to perform certain activities, such as operating a car. Often a license also attests to compliance with standards. An ambulance license implies that the ambulance has complied with government licensing criteria and is granted permission to operate as an ambulance in the state or community.

Licensure Process by which the EMT-B is issued a license or certification by the state government agent. The licensure process implies compliance with federal and state guidelines.

Ligaments Connective tissue that holds bones together at a joint.

Lipase Lipolytic or fat-splitting enzyme found in the blood, pancreatic secretions, and tissues.

Liver Largest organ in the body; situated on the right side beneath the diaphragm; has four lobes. The liver receives blood from the portal vein and this is the first organ to receive blood from the intestines, where the blood has absorbed the final products of digestion and decomposition.

Living will Legal document, signed and witnessed, outlining the types of medical interventions that may or may not be implemented on the signer, who may or may not have been diagnosed with a terminal or permanently disabling injury or medical condition.

Local injury Injury limited to a small area.

Locally acting medication Drug that is applied directly to an affected area; usually has very low absorption into the bloodstream.

Long spine board Device to immobilize the entire body as a single unit.

Loss of skeletal integrity Condition in which skin, bones, arteries, nerves, and veins are in a state of impairment, usually related to trauma.

Low-energy weapons Handheld weapons with a cutting edge.

Lumbar vertebrae Next five vertebrae after the cervical and thoracic vertebrae.

Lungs Two large air sacs that are made up of lobes. The right lung has three lobes, and the left lung has two.

M

Main rotor Main set of rotor blades on a helicopter, usually located over the center of the fuselage, that creates the lift for flight.

Mainstem bronchi Two primary divisions of the trachea that supply the lungs with oxygen.

Malnutrition Any disorder of nutrition; may result from an unbalanced, insufficient, or excessive diet or from the impaired absorption or metabolism of foods.

Managed care Form of health care insurance. Managed care plans control costs by monitoring how medical professionals treat patients, limiting referrals to specialists, and requiring preauthorization before care is rendered. Managed care also usually includes negotiated payment rates with providers that are discounted below the normal fee-for-service rates.

Managed care organization (MCO) The organization that runs managed care.

Mandated reporter Health care professional who is required by law to report abuse.

Mandible Bone of the lower jaw.

Manual cervical immobilization Type of spinal immobilization in which the cervical spine is immobilized by hand until further devices can be applied.

Manubrium Superior section of the sternum.
Mass (multiple) casualty incident (MCI) Commonly accepted definition of any incident involving one or more patients that cannot be handled by the first responding units to a scene.
Material safety data sheet (MSDS) Government-prescribed form describing the actions and toxicities of substances used in the workplace.
Maxilla Two bones that form the upper jaw.
Mechanical sensor Type of air bag restraint sensor that operates by mechanical means to activate the air bag system.
Mechanism of injury Manner in which injuries occur; actions or objects that cause trauma injury to a patient during a vehicle accident.
Meconium Fetal intestinal contents that stain the amniotic fluid green or black; fetus may expel contents of bowels before birth as a result of stress; indicates a birth complication.
MEDEVAC Noncombat medical transport.
Medial Toward the midline.
Medical command authority Base station physician to which the EMT can communicate by telephone or radio for directions in delivery of patient care.
Medical control See *medical direction*.
Medical control emergency physician (MCEP) See *medical director*.
Medical direction Various duties that a physician provides in support of an EMS system; includes protocols, case reviews, educational programming, etc.
Medical director Physician who provides medical direction to an EMS system.
Medical terminology Specialized language of the medical profession that allows concise and effective communication.
Medications Chemicals that change the way the body functions; used to treat a variety of diseases and symptoms.
Medium-energy weapons Weapons with a muzzle velocity greater than 1500 feet per second.
Meninge One of three highly vascular membranes that separate the cranium from the brain; includes the dura mater, pia mater, and arachnoid.
Meningitis Any infection or inflammation of the meninges.
Menopause Permanent absence of menstruation (menses or period).
Menstrual period See *menstruation*.
Menstruation Periodic sloughing of the uterine lining, which is composed of blood, tissue, and cells.
Mental disorder Illness with psychologic or behavioral manifestations and/or impairment in functioning as a result of social, psychologic, genetic, physical and chemical, or biologic disturbance.
Mental retardation Developmental disability characterized by a lower-than-normal intelligence quotient (IQ).
Metabolism Chemical reactions that take place within an organism to maintain life; the work of the cells.
Metacarpals Hand bones.
Metatarsals Foot bones.
Metered dose inhaler Device designed to give a fixed dose of inhaled medication with each puff; most inhalers are used by patients with chronic obstructive pulmonary disease or asthma.

Microorganism Microscopic organism (plant or animal).
Midaxillary Imaginary line running vertically from the middle of the armpit to the ankle.
Midclavicular line Vertical line on a standing patient that runs caudad from the center of the clavicle on either side.
Midline Imaginary line running vertically from the nose through the umbilicus (belly button).
Minor Below the age to make a legal decision.
Minute ventilation Amount of air inhaled in 1 minute; calculated by multiplying the tidal volume by the respiratory rate.
Miscarriage Natural or spontaneous abortion.
Mobile radio Vehicular-mounted radio that operates off of the vehicle's electrical supply; has a range of approximately 20 miles and a broadcast strength less than a base station.
Motor nerve Nerve that carries responses from the central nervous system to an organ or muscle.
Mottling Condition seen in patients with severe hypoxia; skin has diffuse patches of red and white discoloration.
Mucous plug Accumulation of mucus that forms and interlocks with the capillaries of the cervix during pregnancy; acts as a protective barrier between the cervix and the vagina for the length of pregnancy.
Muscles Contractile tissue that works with the skeleton to provide movement and protection for the body.
Musculoskeletal system Includes the muscles and skeletal system and provides a framework for movement and protection for internal organs. The bones are also important in the production of red blood cells.
Myelomeningocele Developmental anomaly of the central nervous system in which a hernial sac containing a portion of the spinal cord, its meninges, and cerebrospinal fluid protrudes through a congenital cleft in the vertebral column; occurs in approximately 2 out of every 1000 live births, is readily apparent, and is easily diagnosed at birth.
Myocardial infarction (MI) Condition in which part of the heart muscle (myocardium) dies because of inadequate supply of oxygen and nutrients; may be caused by a thrombosis, coronary artery spasm, or emboli; also called *heart attack*.
Myocardium Muscle tissue that makes up the inner layer of the heart.

N

Nasal bone Bone of the nose.
Nasal flaring Widening of the nostrils that occurs during inhalation in patients with respiratory distress.
Nasal prongs Device used to deliver low concentrations of oxygen to patients who need supplemental oxygen but who are not in acute respiratory distress.
Nasogastric (NG) tube Tube that is placed through the nose and esophagus into the stomach; can be used for gastric decompression, medication administration, nutrition, or gastric lavage.
Nasopharyngeal (nasal) airway Airway adjunct inserted into a nostril and designed to prevent airway obstruction by the tongue.
Nasotracheal intubation Type of endotracheal intubation in which the tube is passed through the nose and into the trachea; performed only by advanced life support personnel in patients who are breathing.

Nature of illness Generally describes the medical condition that prompts an individual to be sick and to subsequently request EMS.

Near drowning Asphyxia after submersion with at least temporary survival.

Needle cricothyrotomy Insertion of a needle into the cricothyroid membrane to create a temporary airway opening.

Negligence Failure to exercise the degree of care that a reasonable person would exercise under the same circumstances.

Newton's first law of motion Physical law that states that an object in motion will stay in motion until acted on by an outside force.

Nitroglycerin Medication that dilates blood vessels and decreases the workload on the heart; often used to treat angina pectoris.

Non–insulin-dependent diabetes mellitus A diabetic condition that usually occurs in individuals over 40 years of age and usually can be controlled by diet and oral insulin.

Nonurgent move Type of move designed to provide the best care based on the patient's status in a safe, controlled environment.

Nonrebreather mask Device used to deliver high concentrations of oxygen to patients in acute respiratory distress; has a reservoir bag and one-way valve to prevent rebreathing.

O

Obstetrics Branch of medicine that deals with the management of women during pregnancy, childbirth, and 42 days after the expulsion of all contents of pregnancy.

Occipital Pertaining to the posterior section of the skull.

Occiput Posterior part of the skull that rests on the ground when a patient is supine; a towel is placed under the occiput to put the patient in the sniffing position.

Occupational Safety and Health Administration (OSHA) Division of the United States Department of Labor that is responsible for establishing and enforcing safety and health standards in the workplace.

Off-line medical direction Administrative duties carried out by the EMS medical director (e.g., writing of protocols, negotiation of destination policies, retrospective review of EMT performance); also known as *indirect medical direction*.

Olecranon Elbow joint.

Ongoing assessment Follows the detailed physical examination; this portion of the patient assessment checks for problems that arise after the initial assessment and evaluates whether the interventions initiated are working.

On-line medical direction Clinical type of medical direction that involves real-time direction of prehospital providers in the delivery of emergency care; also known as *direct medical direction*.

One-person stretcher Piece of equipment designed to allow one person to load the stretcher into the ambulance, if necessary.

Open fracture Fracture in which the integrity of the skin has been interrupted.

Open head injury Injury to the skull or brain in which the skin has been broken.

Open injury Blunt or penetrating trauma in which the skin has been penetrated; potentially associated with a bony injury.

Open pneumothorax Injury that penetrates the skin, subcutaneous tissue, and intracostal muscles and into the thoracic cavity.

Open reduction Use of surgery to place bones in proper position.

Open soft-tissue injury Damage to the skin and underlying tissue layers in which the skin integrity is lost (see *abrasion, laceration, avulsion, penetrating/puncture wounds, amputations,* and *evisceration*).

Operating parameters Guideline for emergency medical personnel that provides approved procedures for patient care under certain circumstance.

Operator's shift checklist Daily checklist used to assess automated external defibrillator function, including the ability to recognize ventricular fibrillation and an assessment of battery function.

Oral hypoglycemics Medication taken orally that stimulates the pancreas to produce insulin.

Orbit Eye socket.

Organic brain syndrome Transient or permanent dysfunction of the brain caused by disturbance of physiologic functioning of brain tissue.

Oriented Describes a patient who can state name, current location, date, etc.

Orogastric tube Same tube used for nasogastric insertion, only placed through the mouth instead of the nose; orogastric route is required in patients with suspected facial or skull fractures.

Oropharyngeal (oral) airway Airway adjunct designed to prevent airway obstruction by the tongue in unconscious patients; inserted upside down and rotated 180 degrees.

Oropharynx Portion of the pharynx that is inside the mouth.

Osteoporosis Increased porosity of bone, occurring most frequently in postmenopausal women and sedentary or immobilized persons.

Ostomy Surgical procedure in which an opening is made to allow the passage of urine from the bladder or intestinal contents from the bowel to an incision or stoma surgically created in the wall of the abdomen.

Outer circle survey Method of surveying the scene of a vehicle crash that is used in combination with an inner circle survey. It is used to gather information by the rescue team when they first arrive on the scene.

Ovaries Paired, almond-shaped organs suspended by ligaments in the left and right lower quadrants of the abdomen that release a mature egg once a month in females from the approximate ages of 9 to 50 years.

Overall scene safety Terminology describing the safety concerns of rescuers for the entire scene of a vehicle accident. It is subdivided into personal safety, patient safety, hazard control, traffic control, crowd control, and agency control.

Over ride Term in vehicle rescue that describes a crash in which one vehicle has driven over the top of another vehicle.

Oviducts Paired canals approximately 4 inches long connecting the ovary to the uterus; also called *fallopian tubes*.

Ovulation Release of a mature egg from an ovary once a month.

Oxygenation Onloading of oxygen to the red blood cells or the tissue cells.

P

Pacing Regulation of the rate of contraction of the heart muscle by use of an artificial cardiac pacemaker; can be external or internal.

Packaging Preparing the victim for transfer from the vehicle to the ambulance.

Palmar Relating to the palm.

Palm rule Size of the palm is equal to 1% of the total body skin surface area.

Palpation To use the sphygmomanometer and locate the radial pulse with the fingers to obtain a blood pressure.

Pancaked vehicle Vehicle rescue term used to describe an accident situation in which the vehicle has come to rest on its roof, with the roof crushed in upon the passenger compartment.

Pancreas Gland located in the abdomen that makes digestive enzymes and insulin.

Para Woman who has produced a viable infant regardless of whether the infant is alive at birth.

Paradoxical motion Describes a movement of the chest during respiration when one section of the bony rib cage moves in an opposite direction from the rest of the rib cage, indicating that a section of the rib cage has broken loose.

Paralysis Loss of muscle function and/or sensation.

Paraplegia Paralysis of the lower limbs and trunk.

Paraspinal muscles Muscles along the spine that provide support and motion.

Parasympathetic nervous system Segment of the autonomic nervous system that works to slow down the functions of the body.

Paresthesia Any subjective sensation experienced as numbness, tingling, or a "pins and needles"; may be a symptom of hyperventilation or a spinal cord injury.

Parietal Pertaining to the top of the skull.

Parietal pleura Interior lining of the chest wall.

Partial fracture Fracture in which bone ends remain together.

Partial spinal immobilization Immobilization of the spine using manual stabilization of the head (or using a head block), placement on the backboard, and use of gurney straps to stabilize the torso; avoids cumbersome strapping techniques and is used only when the patient is unstable.

Partial-thickness burns Burns involving the topmost and middle layers of the skin; often associated with blisters and intense pain; also referred to as *second degree burns*.

Passenger compartment Portion of a vehicle that is designed to carry the occupants.

Passive rewarming Controlled, slow process of rewarming.

Patella Kneecap.

Patient advocacy Process by which the patient places responsibility for his or her care and well-being in the hands of others.

Patient care report (PCR) Official or formal documentation of the physical assessment and care provided to a particular patient; may either be in a written or computer-based format.

Patient care team On the vehicle crash scene, this is the group of rescuers that will deliver care and assist in removing the injured victim.

Patient data Specific information about a patient that is documented on the patient care report. This information may include, but is not limited to, patient name, address, date of birth, age, and sex; nature of call; mechanism of injury; location of patient; level of consciousness; sensation; pupillary response; skin color, moisture, and temperature; vital signs; history; trauma or medical assessment (as appropriate); care administered to the patient; and any medical care provided prior to the arrival of EMS.

Patient safety Term describing the well-being and protection that is necessary for patients involved or entrapped in vehicle accidents.

Pediatric trauma score (PTS) Standardized injury severity index used in pediatric patients; see also *revised trauma score* and *Glasgow coma scale*.

Pedicle Supporting part of the bone.

Pedi-immobilizer® Spinal immobilization device designed for use on small children.

Penetrating/puncture wounds Injuries that result when the skin is pierced by a sharp object (e.g., knife stabs, gunshots).

Penetrating trauma Injury that is evident immediately to the human eye; usually involves a sharp object or high-velocity weapon.

Perfusion State of adequate supply of oxygen and nutrients to the tissues; ability of the circulatory system to distribute blood containing nutrients and oxygen to the tissues.

Pericardium Thin sac surrounding the heart.

Perineum Space located between the vaginal opening and the anal opening.

Peripheral nervous system Part of the nervous system consisting of all the nerves that extend from the brain and spinal cord.

Periphery Outside part; the legs, arms, abdomen, and brain of the human body.

Peritoneum Serous membrane covering the organs and lining the abdominal cavity.

Peritonitis Inflammation of the peritoneum, the membranous coat lining the abdominal cavity and investing the viscera.

Permanent cavity Cavity that remains in the tissue after the complete dissipation of energy.

Permanent vegetative state Condition in which the human body no longer exists in a conscious state. This condition is caused by massive trauma to the brain or by extended periods of anoxia to brain tissue, resulting in no conscious activity within the nervous system.

Personal protection Steps taken to decrease the risk that the rescuer will become exposed to a communicable disease.

Personal safety This term describes the well-being and protection of rescue personnel during extrication operations.

Personal stressors Strains and pressures caused by the stress a person places on himself or herself from factors such as expectations, anxiety, and guilt.

Pertinent negative Absence of a sign or symptom that helps substantiate or identify a patient's condition (e.g., in a patient complaining of abdominal pain, finding that the abdomen is soft and nontender is a pertinent negative and should be documented).

Pertinent past medical history Any prior or current medical conditions, surgeries, hospitalizations, illnesses, or injuries suffered by the patient; specific attention is focused on major problems that might be related to the patient's current medical condition.

Pertinent positive Presence of a sign or symptom that helps substantiate or identify a patient's condition (e.g., if patient falls and complains of wrist pain, the positive sign is deformity of the wrist).

Petit mal Usually refers to a partial seizure that is seen in children.

Phalanges Bones of the fingers and toes.

Pharmacology Study of how chemicals work in the human body.

Pharynx Hollow space behind the nose and mouth and above the larynx and esophagus; divided into the nasopharynx, oropharynx, and hypopharynx.

Physical assessment Head-to-toe, hands-on examination.

Physical disability Disability that involves limitation of mobility.

Physician extenders Specially trained individuals who are prepared to act as the physician's eyes, ears, and hands in the prehospital evaluation and management of the emergency patient.

Pia mater Innermost layer of the meninges.

Pillars Vehicle design term used for the posts that connect the roof of a vehicle to the rest of the body.

Pilot balloon Small balloon near the adapter end of the endotracheal tube that verifies inflation of the endotracheal tube cuff.

Placenta Highly vascular dishlike structure that links the tissue of the mother with that of the fetus. The placenta exchanges oxygen and carbon dioxide between fetus and mother, transports nutrients and waste byproducts, and serves as a temporary source for hormone production necessary to sustain pregnancy.

Placenta previa Condition in which the placenta implants itself either on or near the opening of the cervix; severe bleeding in late pregnancy occurs when the cervix begins to dilate in early labor.

Plantar Relating to the sole of the foot.

Plasma Liquid component of blood that contains proteins such as blood clotting factors.

Platelets Cellular fragments in the blood that form plugs at the site of bleeding, starting the clotting process.

Pleura Thin membrane that covers the lungs and lines the thoracic cavity.

Pleural space Potential space between the two layers of pleura surrounding the lungs.

Pneumatic antishock garment (PASG) Device used to externally vasoconstrict blood vessels for the purpose of moving blood from the periphery to the core of the body.

Pneumatic struts Specially designed shoring tools that are normally operated by air pressure. They are pistonlike metal shafts with inserts and an assortment of tips and bases. They are locked in place with screw adjusters and pins.

Pneumonia Infection of the lungs that may be caused by bacteria, viruses, or fungi; patients often have fever, dyspnea, and a cough.

Pneumothorax Collection of air in the pleural space; always abnormal and may cause collapse of the underlying lung.

Poison Food, plant, chemical, or drug that has an adverse effect on the body.

Poison control center Regional center that provides telephone poison information and advice to patients and health care providers.

Poisoning Method by which a food, plant, chemical, or drug has a toxic effect on the patient's body.

Portable stretcher Piece of equipment designed to easily carry patients down stairs or over rough terrain; sometimes referred to as *shippers* or *folding stretchers*.

Postcrash After the impact.

Posterior Toward the rear.

Posterior tibial artery Artery located on the inside of the ankle.

Postictal state Period of time immediately after a seizure.

Postincident phase Time frame after a rescue.

Posts Vehicle anatomy term meaning the rolled sheet metal assemblies on vehicles that attach the roof to the main body of the vehicle (e.g., A-Post, B-Post, etc.).

Powered hydraulics Hydraulically powered rescue tools in which the hydraulic operation is powered by a gasoline engine, electric motor, or PTO off the rescue unit.

Power unit In a powered hydraulic rescue tool system, this generates the hydraulic pressure to operate the various tools on the system. It consists of a motor-driven pump and reservoir with a distributing manifold.

Prearrival assessment Assessment of anticipated medical problems based on initial dispatch information.

Prearrival planning Discussing the role of each provider and anticipating equipment and personnel needs.

Precrash Before the impact.

Prefix Word element placed before the root word that changes the meaning of the word.

Prehospital advanced life support interface (PHALSI) Cooperative interaction of basic and advanced life support skills for the betterment of patient outcome.

Prehospital care Health-related services provided to the patient outside of the hospital, generally at home, work, or in the field.

Prehospital provider Generic term for an individual who provides clinical prehospital care (e.g., EMT-B, EMT-I, EMT-P).

Prehospital system Component of the emergency medical services (EMS) system that includes care rendered before arrival at a medical facility.

Prehospital Trauma Life Support (PHTLS) Continuing education for trauma education developed by the National Association of EMTs (NAEMT) in cooperation with the American College of Surgeons Committee on Trauma.

Preincident planning Planning that takes place before a rescue in which equipment needs are assessed and roles and responsibilities are assigned.

Preoxygenation Process of hyperventilating a patient with 100% oxygen before attempting endotracheal intubation; should occur before each attempt.

Presenting part Part of the fetus that protrudes initially during the birthing process.

Preventive care Programs that give individuals information and skills that help prevent illness and injury.

Primary care Type of health care that focuses on prevention of illness and continuity of care; includes health screening, physical examinations, immunizations, and other routine medical care.

Primary care provider Physician who oversees the medical care for a patient in the managed care system; also called a *gatekeeper*.

Primary injuries Injuries that result from the blast wave.

Primary survey In vehicle rescue, this is the initial patient check done by rescuers of trapped patients.

Professional Someone who practices a particular profession; a person who conforms to technical and ethical standards of his or her profession.

Professionalism Actions and attitudes that reflect responsible and consistent performance of the duties of one's chosen profession.

Prolapsed cord Premature expulsion of the umbilical cord.

Prone Lying face down.

Prospective evaluation Quality evaluation method used before an EMS response (e.g., skills check-off).

Prospective medical direction Range of activities with which a medical director may be involved that occur before the emergency occurs (e.g., training of EMTs).

Protective equipment Equipment that is used to decrease the risk that the rescuer will become infected with a communicable disease.

Protocols Written or printed instructions or plans for carrying out an activity. In EMS, a protocol is a document that describes, usually in a step-by-step manner, the method that is used to deal with a particular set of symptoms or conditions.

Proximal Located toward the center of the body; situated next to or near the point of attachment or origin or a central point.

Psychogenic Causation of a symptom or illness by mental or psychic factors as opposed to organic ones.

Psychosocial stressors Stressors that are initiated by contact with other people.

Pubis Inferior, anterior bone of the hip.

Pulmonary arteries Vessels that carry oxygen-poor blood from the right side of the heart to the lungs; the only arteries in the body that carry oxygen-poor blood.

Pulmonary contusion Bruise of the lung.

Pulmonary edema Condition in which fluid builds up in the alveoli and small airways causing hypoxia and dyspnea; most commonly caused by congestive heart failure.

Pulmonary embolism Obstruction of blood flow to the lungs caused by a clot that has traveled from a deep leg vein to a branch of the pulmonary arteries; can cause acute dyspnea, hypoxia, and/or sudden death.

Pulmonary veins Vessels that carry oxygen-rich blood from the lungs back to the left side of the heart; the only veins in the body that carry oxygen-rich blood.

Pulse Wave of blood produced by the contraction of the left ventricle; can be felt wherever an artery passes over a bone close to the skin surface.

Pulse character Force of the wave of blood created by the pumping of the heart.

Pulse point pressure Method of bleeding control in which pressure is applied to the strongest pulse point above an injury for 5 minutes and then released.

Pulse pressure Difference between the systolic and diastolic pressures.

Pulse rate Number of heart beats per minute.

Pulse rhythm Intervals between the beats of the heart.

Purchase point A small opening made in wreckage that makes room for the insertion of rescue tools to move that wreckage.

Q

Quadriplegia Paralysis affecting all four extremities.

Quality In patient assessment, strength, depth, and completeness of assessment. In patient care, accuracy, completeness, and correctness of care.

Quality assurance (QA) Evaluating the performance of an EMS system's response to a given standard.

Quality improvement Term used interchangeably with *quality assurance*. However, in quality improvement the emphasis is placed on improving performance at individual and system levels.

R

Raccoon's eyes Raccoonlike appearance caused by blood accumulated in the tissue around the eyes.

Radial artery Artery located on the thumb side of the wrist of each arm; extends from the wrist to the elbow.

Radial pulse Pulse palpated at the radial artery of the arm at the wrist, on the outer aspect of the inner arm.

Radiation Form of heat exchange that occurs when heat is transmitted through air or water (e.g., the heat that can be felt when sitting in front of a fireplace).

Radius Bone on the lateral side of the lower arm.

Rales Fine breath sounds that represent opening of collapsed alveoli or fluid in the small airways near the alveoli; simulated by rubbing hair between the fingers.

Rams In a powered hydraulic rescue tool system, these are hydraulic driven pistons that extend and retract, providing a lifting capability.

Rapid patient removal Procedure of quick removal of a patient caused by the patient's condition or exposure to hazards present on a vehicle accident scene.

Rapid trauma or medical focused history and physical examination Complete evaluation of the patient limited to the area of most concern based on the kinematics of the trauma or the presentation of the medical condition.

Rate Number of occurrences in a period of time, such as ventilations per minute.

Reactive airways disease See *asthma*.

Reciprocating saw Rescue tool designed for cutting metal and wreckage. It consists of an electrically powered saw unit that moves the blade in and in-and-out motion.

Recompression chamber Specialized chamber in which a diver who is suffering from decompression sickness is placed and artificially returned to a diving depth that will force nitrogen bubbles back into solution and then slowly removed from the blood stream.

Recovery position Position in which an unconscious patient is placed on his or her side and balanced by the positioning of the arms and legs.

Rectus abdominus Large muscle in the center of the anterior abdominal wall.

Red blood cells Blood cells that contain hemoglobin; primary function is to carry oxygen to the tissues.

Refusal of care Declined treatment based on an informed consent.

Regulation Rule; regulations are used to implement laws and provide more detail than is provided in the actual statutory language. Regulations are developed by government agencies and implemented only after a formal process designed to provide the opportunity for public comments and input. They can be modified at any time by simply repeating the announcement and public comment process used initially.

Relative humidity Ratio of the amount of water vapor in the air at a specific temperature to the maximum capacity of the air at that temperature.

Remediation Method of improving a certain aspect or skill of an EMT by providing one-on-one training or coaching.

Renal failure Inability of the kidneys to excrete wastes, concentrate urine, and conserve electrolytes.

Renal (kidney) stones Calculus or crystalline mass present in the pelvis of the kidney, composed principally of urates, oxalates, phosphates, and carbonates and varying in size from small granular masses to 1 inch or more in diameter.

Repeater Radio unit that receives a signal from another radio unit and rebroadcasts it, boosting the signal strength in the process; used to overcome distance or geographic obstacles, such as mountains.

Reportable incident Any incident that is to be reported to the appropriate authority under local, state, and/or federal regulation or law (e.g., in some states, health care providers are required to report suspected child or elder abuse).

Rescue Removal of a person from a dangerous scene.

Rescue action plan System that helps rescuers organize the actions and procedures at the scene of an emergency..

Rescue chain assemblies Chain assemblies that are used as anchor devices to which pulling tools are attached to move metal. These are made in the configuration of chain, hooks, and identification tag.

Rescue chain sling assembly Chain assemblies, usually provided in pairs, that are used as anchor devices to which pulling tools are attached to move metal. These are made in the configuration of a sling and include hooks, connectors, chain, round or oblong link, chain shorteners, and an identification tag.

Respiration Physiologic process of moving oxygen into the red blood cells and tissue cells and metabolizing the oxygen to make energy (ATP).

Respiratory alkalosis Caused by excessive elimination of carbon dioxide produced by an excessive ventilatory rate.

Respiratory arrest Lack of breathing; a patient in respiratory arrest may have agonal respirations, however, these are not effective breaths.

Respiratory depth (tidal volume) Volume of air inhaled with each breath; normally about 500 ml of air in an adult.

Respiratory quality Assessment of breath sounds, chest expansion, and effort.

Respiratory rate Breaths per minute.

Respiratory rhythm Measure of the regularity of breathing.

Respond request Second phase of activating aeromedical support; requests aeromedical service to launch the aircraft because appropriate guidelines have been met. "Stand-by" request may or may not precede this request.

Restorative care Health care provided to a patient, generally after acute care, designed to return the patient to normal form or function.

Restraint Physical "restraints" to prevent a patient from injuring himself, herself, or others.

Resuscitation not indicated (RNI) Term applied in the prehospital setting to those patients who, because of their medical condition or injuries, have no chance of survival and in which resuscitative efforts would be futile; sometimes referred to as *futile intervention*.

Retraction Sign of respiratory distress often seen in infants and children marked by inward pulling of the skin above the clavicles and below the rib cage with inspiration.

Retroperitoneal space Space posterior to the abdominal cavity that contains the kidneys.

Retrospective evaluation Quality evaluation tool used after an EMS response has occurred (e.g., run sheet review).

Retrospective medical direction Activities conducted by the medical director after the call is complete (e.g., review of the patient care report).

Revised trauma score (RTS) Standardized injury severity index that incorporates the Glasgow coma scale and measurements for the systolic blood pressure and respiratory rate.

Rhythm Cadence or equality in repetition.

Ribs Twelve pairs of bones that line the wall of the thorax.

Rights Liberties, allowed for by law, to which each individual is entitled.

Right to refusal Court-granted right of a competent person to refuse medical care.

Risk assessment Process of analyzing disasters or mass casualty incidents that are most likely to occur in a given community.

Risk-benefit ratio Estimation of the risk of a medical intervention versus the benefit to the patient.

Roof flap Displacement procedure on an extrication scene that involves the cutting and folding up and away the roof of the vehicle.

Roof rails Part of vehicle roof anatomy that provides support to the edge of the roof; located along the outer edge of the roof assembly.

Roof ribs Part of vehicle roof anatomy that provides support to the sheet metal of the roof; located along the bottom of the roof sheet metal straddling the middle of the roof.

Root word Basic stem word used as a building block with the addition of prefixes and suffixes.

Rotor wash Downward blast of air created by the main rotor system as the aircraft lands or takes off; can blow dust and rocks, cause injuries, and obscure vision.

Rotor wing aircraft Aircraft with multiple blades that turn at a high speed and create lift as they turn through the air; commonly called a *helicopter*.

Route of administration Way a drug is put into the body.

Rule of Nines System for measuring the percentage of body surface area (BSA) involved in a burn.

Run data Specific information about an ambulance call that is documented on the patient care report. Run data may include, but is not limited to, ambulance service name and unit number, crew license numbers and/or names, location of the ambulance call, response times, and mileage.

S

Sacral vertebrae Next five vertebrae after the cervical, thoracic, and lumbar vertebrae.

SAMPLE history Mnemonic to help EMT-Basics assess history. *S*—Signs and symptoms; *A*—Allergies; *M*—Medications; *P*—Past pertinent medical history; *L*—Last oral intake; *E*—Event.

Scapula Flat bone located bilaterally in the posterior, superior thorax.

Scene size-up Quick, broad overview of the scene that the EMT-Basic performs upon arrival at the scene. During scene size-up, the EMT-Basic checks for scene safety, looks for the mechanism of injury or nature of illness, counts the number of patients, and calls for additional help if needed.

Scope of practice Knowledge and skills that an EMT is permitted to use in caring for patients as defined by the pertinent state laws and regulation governing medical practice; usually based on the knowledge and skills in the Department of Transportation EMT curriculum.

Search and rescue (SAR) Specially trained members or groups that respond to lost or injured persons in the wilderness or urban environment.

Seat-mounted air bags Air bag restraint system components that are located in the seat assembly of a vehicle. They are primarily designed to provide side-impact protection to the person sitting in that seat.

Secondary drowning Loss of the protective lining within the lungs caused by aspirated water, causing the alveoli to collapse and allowing additional fluids to accumulate in the lungs.

Secondary injuries Injuries that result from flying debris.

Seizure Sudden, abnormal electrical activity in the brain.

Sellick maneuver Maneuver designed to prevent passive aspiration during artificial ventilation; performed by applying posterior pressure to the cricoid cartilage.

Semilunar valve Two moon-shaped, pocketlike valves; one is located between the right ventricle and the pulmonary artery, and the other is located between the left ventricle and the aorta.

Senescence Aging; growing old.

Sensory nerve Nerve that carries impulses from the sensory receptors to the central nervous system.

Separation of power Doctrine that prohibits one branch of government from exercising the powers that belong to another.

Sepsis Infection; contamination.

Septic shock Form of shock that occurs from an infection when toxic products are released from pathogenic bacteria into the bloodstream.

Shape Configuration.

Shear Tearing apart.

Shear capsule Part of the dash and steering column assembly of a vehicle. It provides a way for the steering mechanism to collapse on impact of the occupant during a frontal collision.

Sheet drag Type of inline drag using a sheet placed under the patient to pull him or her away from immediate danger.

Shock Failure of the circulatory system to perfuse tissues; hypoperfusion of the circulatory system.

Shoring A vehicle rescue tool that supports a load by using shafts of wood or other devices.

Short spine board Device that will immobilize the entire spine using the pelvis and the head as the bone above and the board below.

Side effects Unwanted or harmful effects of a drug. Almost all medicines have some side effects, the severity of which often depend on the dose of the drug.

Signs Any observable indication of illness or injury.

Six-way communications model (1) Sender formulates the idea that he or she wishes to convey to another member, (2) Sender transmits the message, (3) Message is transferred through the medium, (4) Receiver obtains the message, (5) Receiver interprets the message, (6) Receiver confirms the message.

Size-up Act of gathering information about the emergency to formulate an action plan.

Skeleton Major component of the musculoskeletal system; framework for the body.

Skull Bones that house and protect the brain.

Small intestine First portion of the intestine with three parts—duodenum, jejunum, and ileum. Also known as the *small bowel*.

Sniffing position Desired patient position for endotracheal intubation; the patient's neck is flexed slightly (C_5 and C_6) and the head is extended at the base of the skull (C_1 and C_2).

SOAP Specific format used in completing the narrative section of the patient care report. SOAP is the acronym for the components of the narrative: *S*—Subjective findings; *O*—Objective findings; *A*—Assessment; *P*—Plan of action for caring for the patient.

Social service Specially trained health care professionals who deal with patients' continuing medical needs.

Soft protection Type of patient protection that is used when working with tools near the trapped patient.

Somatic nervous system Part of the nervous system that is voluntary; used in activities such as kicking a ball or reading this text.

Source of the exposure Event that caused exposure to heat or cold, such as cold weather, fire, overdressing, etc.

Spaceframe Type of vehicle construction that uses a "bird cage" type of frame assembly to which body panels and parts are attached.

Special needs Any condition with the potential to interfere with usual growth and development; may involve physical disabilities, mental disabilities, chronic illnesses, or forms of technological support.

Special needs patient Patient who has any condition with the potential to interfere with usual growth and development; may involve physical disabilities, mental disabilities, chronic illnesses, or forms of technological support.

Specialty care Type of health care provided outside the scope of primary care; requires specific expertise in a defined area such as emergency medicine, surgery, or cardiology.

Sphygmomanometer Pressure cuff device used on a peripheral extremity to determine the pressure in the heart on relaxation and contraction; blood pressure cuff.

Spina bifida Birth defect in which the back portion of the vertebrae fails to close, usually in the area of the lower back.

Spinal column Column of bones that encloses the spinal cord.

Spinal immobilization Critical trauma patient care that involves the maintenance of the spinal column, in-line, in place so that further injury to that area will be prevented during patient removal or handling.

Spinal trauma Physical injury to the spinal cord.

Sprain Injury in which ligaments are stretched or partially torn.

Spreader Part of a hydraulic rescue tool system that is used to spread apart wreckage. It can be manually powered or powered by mechanically driven power units.

Spring-loaded center punch Tool adapted to the vehicle extrication scene that is used to break tempered glass for controlled removal. It is a small spring-loaded cylinder with a pointed tip that loads into the handle as it is being pressed down and fires out rapidly as pressure is applied, thus breaking tempered glass.

Stabilization Process of bringing a patient's emergency medical condition under control.

Stack crib Configuration of 2" × 4" or 4" × 4" wood cribs that are placed in a stack as an object is being lifted by tools. Also known as a *box crib*.

Staging area Designated area away from the extrication scene where additional apparatus and manpower are placed in reserve until needed at the scene.

Standard Commonly accepted description or set of criteria and characteristics. For example, the fact that red traffic signals mean stop and green signals mean go is a standard that is accepted around the world. The EMT-Basic training course is a national standard description of how EMTs are trained. Standards may be developed by government, industry, or other interested groups. Standards often are enforced or implemented through laws or regulations.

Standard cardiac care Management of a patient with cardiac complaints; includes maintaining patient comfort and administering oxygen.

Standard of practice The level of care that a reasonable EMT would provide for the patient in a similar situation.

Standard operating procedures Formal guidelines developed by emergency organizations to assist in preplanning emergency operations and procedures before the incident.

Stand-by request First phase of activating aeromedical support; requests aeromedical service to get ready to respond; allows time to prepare the aircraft, find the location, and check local weather conditions.

Standing orders Patient care instructions in writing that authorize specific steps in patient assessment and intervention without the requirement of direct medical direction contact by radio or telephone; usually very specific in what can be done and contained within the patient care protocols.

Status asthmaticus Acute, severe, and prolonged asthma attack; hypoxia, cyanosis, and unconsciousness may follow.

Status epilepticus Continuous seizure lasting more than 30 minutes or a seizure in which the patient does not regain consciousness.

Statute Law that is introduced, debated, and passed by a legislative body at the state or federal level. Once passed, the law may only be changed by the same legislative body that passed it. Statutes create programs and government agencies, control actions of people or industry, and enforce behavior. Some statutes have penalties associated with a failure to comply.

Steering column Part of the vehicle that controls its direction of travel. It consists of the shaft and connectors that extend from the steering wheel to the steering gear box.

Steering displacement Moving or forcing of a steering assembly out of its normal operating range to provide room for patient access and removal.

Step chocks Specialized cribbing assemblies made out of wood blocks assembled in a stair-step configuration. These are usually used to stabilize vehicles.

Sternum Flat bone lying in the anterior center of the thorax.

Stethoscope Device used to listen to the sounds of the body; consists of a bell and a diaphragm, which pick up the sounds, and rubber or vinyl tubing connected to ear pieces.

Stoma Artificially created opening between two passages or body cavities or between a cavity or passage and the body's surface.

Stomach Dilated, saclike, distensible portion of the alimentary canal below the esophagus and partly under the liver. The stomach secretes gastric juice and converts proteins into peptones.

Stopping distance Distance for something to stop.

Strain "Muscle pull"; a soft-tissue injury or muscle spasm that occurs around a joint or anywhere in the musculature.

Stress Internal response to an external factor such as work, family responsibilities, or lifestyle changes.

Striations Microscopic lines that differentiate voluntary muscle and give it its name of *striated muscle*.

Stridor Abnormal, high-pitched, musical sound caused by an obstruction in the trachea or larynx; usually heard during inspiration.

Striker bolt Pin located in a vehicle door jam on which the latch closes when the door is closed.

Stylet Malleable metal rod that is inserted into the endotracheal tube to provide stiffness for intubation; it should not extend beyond the tracheal end of the tube during insertion.

Subcutaneous tissue Deepest layer of the skin; made up of fatty and connective tissue.

Subdural hematoma Accumulation of blood between the arachnoid and the pia mater.

Sublingually Literally, "under the tongue" (e.g., nitroglycerin is often administered sublingually).

Submersion To enter a body of liquid (e.g., to dive or fall into a lake or pool).

Subpoena Command issued by a court to appear for a legal proceeding.

Suffix Word element placed at the end of a root word that changes the meaning of the word.

Sun roof Part of a roof assembly provided on some vehicles that contains an opening and a window. This may or may not be retractable into the roof.

Superficial Nearer the surface of the body.

Superficial burn Most minor of thermal injuries; involves the epidermis layer of skin and includes reddening of the skin without blistering.

Superior Above.

Superior vena cava Large vein that returns blood to the right atrium from the thorax, arms, head, and neck.

Supine Lying face up.

Supplemental restraint system Vehicle anatomical term that refers to any additional passenger restraints in a vehicle (e.g., air bag restraint systems).

Surrogate consent Informed consent provided by another.

Suspension system Anatomy of a vehicle that uses springs, torsion bars, or other mechanical means to further isolate the passengers from the road.

Sustained access For rescue situations, a path of access to the patient that is secure and readily usable by rescuers during the rescue operation.

Sutures Immobile interlocking joints that connect the cranial bones.

SWAT tactical unit Specially trained law enforcement group that deals with high-risk situations and criminal activity.

SWIMS *S*—Stop the spill; *W*—Warn others; *I*—Isolate the area; *M*—Minimize contamination; *S*—Secure ventilation.

Sympathetic nervous system Segment of the autonomic nervous system that works to "speed up" functions of the body.

Symptoms Indication of illness or injury that is not observable and must be related by the patient.

Syncope Brief lapse in consciousness.

Syrup of ipecac Medication used to induce vomiting in some cases of poisoning.

Systemically acting medication Drug that enters the blood and is carried to the whole body.

Systems status management (SSM) Approach to deployment of EMS resources (people and vehicles) that seeks to achieve maximum efficiency with minimal sacrifice in quality of care. SSM uses computer modeling techniques to predict EMS call volume and location, thereby allowing systems to preposition vehicles in most efficient locations.

Systolic pressure Pressure in the heart when the heart muscle is contracting; upper reading of a blood pressure measurement.

T

Table fracture Fracture in which the bone ends are separate.

Tachycardia Condition in which the heart contracts at a rate greater than 100 beats per minute.

Tachypnea Rapid respiratory rate.

Tail rotor Set of rotor blades located at the rear of the fuselage and perpendicular to the main rotor; counters the inherent spin of the aircraft created by the turning main rotor.

Targeting Procedure performed to determine if cerebral spinal fluid is mixed with blood.

Tarsals Ankle bones.

T-bone Descriptive term that denotes the type of vehicle accident in which one vehicle collides into the side of another vehicle.

Team approach Idea behind modern vehicle extrication procedures in which one person is placed in charge of a rescue team and coordinates the teams efforts into successful and efficient results.

Team effort Group of people working in cohesion to achieve a mutual goal.

Technical rescue First phase of a rescue effort, in which rescuers attempt to reach the patient and assess the estimated length of the rescue effort.

Telemetry Transmission of electronic signals over the radio. In EMS, the most frequent telemetry transmission is the electrocardiogram. To be useful, telemetry requires a very "quiet," or interference-free, frequency.

Tempered glass Glass used for automobile windows except for the windshield. When struck, tempered glass shatters into many tiny fragments instead of the large, pointed shards that result from breakage of plate glass.

Temporal Pertaining to the sides of the skull.

Temporary cavity Cavity that is present as a result of the maximum energy exchange. This cavity is present for only microseconds and depleted rapidly.

Tendons Straps of tissue that attach voluntary muscles to bone.

Tensioning devices Part of a seat belt system provided in some vehicles that automatically tightens the seat belt harness to the occupant during a vehicle crash.

Tension pneumothorax Pneumothorax that has increased pressure in one hemothorax that has collapsed the lung on the affected side and pushed the organs of the mediastinum into the opposite chest, restricting the ventilation of that lung as well.

Tertiary injuries Injuries produced by the victim being knocked down or into an object.

Testes Two egg-shaped glands that produce spermatozoa (sperm).

Third door Term that describes a displacement evolution used to open the rear side panel of a two-door automobile, creating a "third door" or access opening to the trapped patient.

Thoracic cavity Bony structure made of ribs, muscle, and cartilage that protects the lungs and vital organs.

Thoracic vertebrae Twelve vertebrae that are caudad to the cervical vertebrae.

Thorax Superior two thirds of the trunk.

Thready pulse Weak, thin, rapid pulse or heart rate.

Thyroid cartilage Most prominent part of the larynx; often referred to as the *Adam's apple*.

Tibia Anterior bone of the lower leg.

Tidal volume Volume of air inhaled with each breath; normally about 500 ml in an adult.

Tiered response system Level of service at which multiple response of first responders, EMT-Basics, and EMT-Paramedics work together at the scene of an emergency. The type of care will determine the level of care to be provided.

Time dependent Relationship of the effectiveness of many medical interventions to the time at which they are implemented.

Tinnitus Ringing in the ears.

Tire-deflating device Tool that allows air to escape when placed on a vehicle's valve stem, thus deflating the tire.

Tonic-clonic Rhythmic motion of the body and extremities that occurs with a seizure.

Tool reaction Describes the movement of rescue tools while force is being applied by them on wreckage. This reaction can be the turning of the tool, slipping off of the tool, or sudden release of the tool under force.

Tool staging General vehicle rescue scene operation in which tools and equipment are placed in a central designated area for potential use at the damaged vehicles.

Torso Trunk of the body.

Tourniquet Band of cloth placed around an extremity and twisted to increase pressure so that blood flow below the band is interrupted or stopped; last resort measure used to control severe bleeding.

Toxin Noxious or poisonous substance.

Trachea Cylinder-shaped tube in the neck composed of cartilage and membrane that extends from the vocal cords to about the level of the fifth thoracic vertebra where it divides into two bronchi; also called the *windpipe*.

Tracheostomy Surgical opening through the neck into the trachea through which an indwelling tube may be inserted.

Tracheotomy Incision made into the trachea through the neck below the vocal cords to gain access to the airway below a blockage with a foreign body, tumor, or edema of the glottis.

Trade name Drug name created by the company that sells the drug; one drug may have many trade names.

Traffic control Term used to describe the safe rerouting or halting of vehicle traffic on a roadway to provide for the safety of the rescue effort.

Training evolution Learning operations, generally practical in nature, that develop hands-on skills for fire and rescue personnel.

Transcultural Crossing cultural lines.

Transient ischemic attack (TIA) Temporary disruption in blood flow to the brain, which results in dizziness, imbalance, and generalized weakness.

Trauma General term that describes injuries to a person resulting from being struck by, hit against, or penetrated by an outside object or force.

Trauma center Hospital equipped and staffed to handle trauma patients. Trauma centers are divided into three levels based on response capability: *Level I*—A hospital staffed and equipped to place the patient in the operating room within minutes of arrival. All staff members are available in the hospital 24 hours a day. *Level II*—A hospital staffed and equipped to place the patient immediately in the operating room if necessary. Some of the staff members may not sleep in the hospital but are available in the emergency department when the patients arrive. *Level III*—A hospital with emergency department staff members who are available in the hospital 24 hours a day, but the operating room, surgical, and anesthesia staff may be at home and on call for rapid response when the need exists.

Trauma score Measurement of the physiologic response of the patient to the injury; includes assessment of respiratory rate, respiratory expansion, systolic blood pressure, and capillary refill.

Trendelenburg position Position of stretcher or cot in which the foot of the bed is raised and the head of the bed is lowered; sometimes used to treat shock.

Triage Process used to sort patients and determine which will be treated or transported first; often used to describe the sorting process used in a disaster situation but also can apply to any situation in which sorting of patients or sorting of casualties into treatment categories is necessary. Usually used in context with patient handling and treatment of injuries.

Tricuspid valve Three-flap valve that covers the opening between the right atrium and the right ventricle.

Trimester Three-month period; there are three 3-month periods, or trimesters, during a pregnancy.

True contractions Labor contractions; cramplike pain that may radiate to the lower back, generally regular, with intervals lasting between 5 and 15 minutes and increasing in pain intensity as labor progresses.

Tubal pregnancy Pregnancy in which the fertilized egg implants in a fallopian tube.

Tumble Over-and-over motion.

Turgor Normal resiliency of the skin caused by the outward pressure of cells and interstitial fluid; when grasped and raised between two fingers, the skin slowly returns to a position level with the surrounding tissue; decreased skin turgor results in dehydration.

Two-person stretcher Piece of equipment designed for two people to carry, move, and load the patient.

Type I ambulance Ambulance with a conventional cab and chassis with a modular ambulance body (box).

Type II ambulance Ambulance that is essentially a converted van, usually with a raised roof; the driver and patient areas form an integral unit.

Type III ambulance Ambulance that is similar to the type I ambulance in that it is a cab/chassis with a modular box mounted on the frame. Most commonly, the type III will be mounted on a van chassis with a passage between the patient compartment and the driver compartment.

U

UHF band Set of radio frequencies between 450 and 470 MHz; almost interference free but limited to line of sight and travel only short distances.

Ulcer Open sore or lesion of the skin or mucous membrane accompanied by sloughing of inflamed necrotic tissue.

Ulna Bone on the medial side of the lower arm.

Umbilical arteries Arteries that carry deoxygenated blood from the fetus to the placenta.

Umbilical cord Fibrous, whitish tube that connects the fetus to the placenta.

Umbilical vein Vein that carries oxygenated blood from the placenta to the fetus.

Umbilicus Navel.

Unit body Type of vehicle construction that uses the floor panels and undercarriage as a structural element of the vehicle, eliminating the need for a full chassis for vehicle body support; also known as *unibody*.

Under ride Type of vehicle crash in which a vehicle drives underneath another vehicle.

Urban search and rescue (USAR) Finding and removing patients in the city.

Ureter Narrow tube, about 12 cm in length, that carries urine from the kidney to the urinary bladder.

Urethra Tube that extends from the bladder to the outside of the body at the urethral meatus.

Urgent move Move performed when any factor at the rescue scene may contribute to the patient's decline or the rescuer's safety; requires that the patient be moved more quickly than usual.

Urticaria Another name for hives.

Uterine rupture Rupture of the uterus caused by trauma or previous cesarean scarring.

Uterus Single, pear-shaped, muscular organ located between the rectum and the bladder that houses the fetus during fetal development.

Uvula Small grapelike structure made of soft tissue that hangs from the roof of the mouth just in front of the oropharynx.

V

Vaccination Introduction of a vaccine, a mixture of weakened or dead microorganisms, into the body to produce immunity to a specific disease.

Vagina Fibromuscular sheath that leads from the uterus and extends to the vaginal opening.

Vaginal opening Opening to the vagina located between the anus and the urethral orifice.

Vallecula Valley formed between the base of the tongue and the pharyngeal surface of the epiglottis; the curved laryngoscope blade is inserted into the vallecula during endotracheal intubation.

Vasoconstriction Contraction of blood vessels.

Vasodilation Expansion of blood vessels.

Vehicle rescue Term denoting the rescue of injured victims of a vehicle crash incident.

Veins Vessels that carry blood back to the heart.

Velocity Speed.

Venae cavae (Singular, *vena cava*) Two major veins of the body, the inferior vena cava and superior vena cava, that return blood to the heart.

Ventilation Mechanical process of moving air into and out of the lungs.

Ventilatory arrest Lack of breathing. A patient in ventilatory arrest may have agonal respiration; however, these are not effective breaths.

Ventilatory character Strength of the ventilations.

Ventilatory depth Depth of each ventilation effort.

Ventilatory rate Number of ventilations per minute.

Ventilatory rhythm Regularity of the ventilations.

Ventral Toward the front.

Ventricles Lower chambers of the heart that pump blood; the right ventricle supplies blood to the lungs and the left supplies the body.

Ventricular fibrillation (VF) Arrhythmia in which the heart is in a state of disorganized electrical and mechanical activity, resulting in a lack of blood flow; treated with defibrillation.

Ventricular tachycardia (VT) Arrhythmia in which the ventricles are driven by an electrical impulse separate from the normal conduction system; pulses may or may not be present; if there are no pulses, defibrillation is necessary.

Venules Smallest veins in the body; carry blood from the capillaries to the veins.

Vertebrae Circular bones that make up the vertebral column.

Vertebral column The stack of vertebrae.

VHF high band Set of radio frequencies between 150 and 174 Mhz; less prone to interference than VHF low band but limited to line of sight communication because they cannot bend around obstacles or the curve of the earth.

VHF low band Set of radio frequencies between 32 and 50 MHz; can travel great distances but are subject to interference.

Visceral pleura Exterior lining of the lungs.

Vocal cords Thin membranes within the larynx that produce sound.

Volume Amount of fluid; may be measured in metric or apothecary units.

Voluntary muscles Muscles attached to bone that provide for movement.

W

Weapons of mass destruction Nuclear devices, biological agents, and chemical substances.

Wedge cribbing Cribbing shaped in the form of a wedge that is used to tighten and secure cribbing assemblies supporting weight. Usually used as a gap filler.

Wheezes High-pitched sounds heard when air moves through constricted airways; commonly occurs in patients with asthma.

White blood cells Blood cells that function in the body's immune system.

Wind chill Measurement of the combined effect of ambient temperature plus wind velocity on exposed surfaces; in general, the higher the wind, the lower the temperature will seem.

Windshield saw Specialized hand tool used for the removal of laminated plate glass found in most vehicle front windshields. Some windshield tools also have capability of breaking tempered glass.

Working load limit (WLL) Recommended limit of force, measured in pounds of weight, with which rope, chain, or cable can be safely operated. It denotes how much weight the rope, chain, or cable can lift safely.

Wrecker Towing vehicle that can be used to hoist heavy loads on the vehicle rescue scenes. They come in different classifications (A, B, and C) for different load-lifting capacities.

Written report One format for a patient care report; typically consists of a specific form that includes check boxes and a section for writing a narrative of the patient scenario, assessment, and interventions provided or attempted.

X

Xiphoid process Small bony structure located between the costal margins at the lower end of the sternum; used as a landmark for chest compressions and nasogastric tube insertion.

Z

Zygomatic bones Cheek bones.

Illustration Credits

All photos (unless otherwise noted) by Richard Brady
All drawings (unless otherwise noted) by Jeanne Robertson
Dedication photo: Courtesy National Registry of EMTs, Columbus, Ohio

Chapter 1
1.1, 1.2, 1.3, 1.4, 1.5, 1.6, 1.7, 1.8, 1.9, 1.10, 1.11, 1.12, 1.13, 1.14, 1.15, and **1.16** Kristen Burke

Chapter 2
2.3A, 2.4, 2.6, 2.7 Kristin Burke

Chapter 4
4.2, 4.3, 4.4 Kristin Burke

Chapter 5
5.1, 5.3, 5.4, 5.6, 5.10A, 5.11, 5.12 Craig Jackson; **5.2, 5.5, 5.7, 5.8, 5.9, 5.11, 5.14, 5.15, 5.16, 5.18, 5.19, 5.20, 5.22, 5.25** Krinstin Burke; **5.10B** Vincent Knauss; **5.21** Swindoll CR: *Strengthening your grip*, Dallas, 1994, Word I.C.

Chapter 6
6.2, 6.4A and B, 6.5 Kristen Burke; **6.3** Patrick Watson. From Grimes D: *Infectious diseases*, St Louis, 1994, Mosby.

Chapter 7
7.1, 7.26, 7.27A, 7.27B From Shade: *Mosby's EMT-Inermediate textbook*, St Louis, 1997, Mosby; **7.4** Sanders M: *Mosby's paramedic textbook*, St Louis, 1994, Mosby; **7.5, 7.13, 7.17, 7.20** From Pre-Hospital Trauma Life Support Committee of the National Association of Emergency Medical Technicians in Cooperation with the Committee on Traumaof the American College of Surgeons: *Pre-hospital trauma life support*, ed 3, St Louis, 1994, Mosby; **7.29** From Hafen BQ, Karren KJ, Mistovich JJ: *Prehospital emergency care*, Upper Saddle River, NJ, 1996, Prentice Hall.

Chapter 8
8.1, 8.3, 8.5A and B, 8.7, 8.15A to D, 8.17, 8.20, 8.21, 8.22, 8.23, 8.24A and B, 8.27 Kristen Burke; **8.2** Craig Jackson; **8.8** Sanders M: *Mosby's paramedic textbook*, St Louis, 1994, Mosby.

Chapter 9
9.11A to D Kristen Burke.

Chapter 10
10.1, 10.2, 10.16 From Pre-Hospital Trauma Life Support Committee of the National Association of Emergency Medical Technicians in Cooperation with the Committee on Trauma of the American College of Surgeons: *Pre-hospital trauma life support*, ed 3, St Louis, 1994, Mosby; **10.14, 10.17** Courtesy Life Support Products, Inc. From Sanders M: *Mosby's paramedic textbook*, St Louis, 1994, Mosby; **10.9A and B, 10.10, 10.15, 10.16, 10.19, 10.21A to D** Kristen Burke; **10.20** Vincent Knauss.

Chapter 11
11.3B Custom Medical stock photo. From Thibodeau GA: *Structure and function*, ed 9, St Louis, 1992, Mosby; **11.4** From Pre-Hospital Trauma Life Support Committee of the National Association of Emergency Medical Technicians in Cooperation with the Committee on Trauma of the American College of Surgeons: *Pre-hospital trauma life support*, ed 3, St Louis, 1994, Mosby; **11.5, 11.8B, 11.18, 11.19, 11.20, 11.21A to C** Kristen Burke; **11.16** Vincent Knauss. From Aehlert B: *Pediatric advanced life support study guide*, St Louis, 1994, Mosby; **11.17** Robert D. White, MD.

Chapter 12
12.1, 12.3, 12.4, 12.5, 12.6, 12.8, 12.12, 12.13 Kristen Burke; **12.2** Bendix King Radio, Inc., Lawrence, Kansas; **12.4, 12.7, 12.9, 12.10, 12.14** Craig Jackson; **12.11** U.S. Department of Transportation.

Chapter 13
13.1, 13.2C and E Vincent Knause; **13.2A, B, and D** Kristen Burke.

Chapter 14
14.1 From Pre-Hospital Trauma Life Support Committee of the National Association of Emergency Medical Technicians in Cooperation with the Committee on Trauma of the American College of Surgeons: *Pre-hospital trauma life support*, ed 3, St Louis, 1994, Mosby; **14.5A** Vincent Knauss; **14.5B** Kristen Burke.

Chapter 15
15.2 From LeFleur Brooks: *Exploring medical language*, St Louis, 1998, Mosby; **15.4** From Pre-Hospital Trauma Life Support Committee of the National Association of Emergency Medical Technicians in Cooperation with the Committee on Trauma of the American College of Surgeons: *Pre-hospital trauma life support*, ed 3, St Louis, 1994, Mosby; **15.6, 15.7, 15.8** From Wilson: *Respiratory disorders*, St Louis, 1990, Mosby; **15.10, 15.11** Kristen Burke.

Chapter 16
Box 16.1 From Eiberberg MS: Cardiac resuscitation in the community: importance of rapid provision and implication for program planning, *JAMA* 241:1905, 1979; **16.3, 16.4A and B, 16.6** From Aehlert B: *ECGs made easy*, St Louis, YEAR, Mosby; **16.7** Stoy: *Mosby's EMT-Basic textbook*, St Louis, 1996, Mosby.

Chapter 17
Table 17.1 From Pre-Hospital Trauma Life Support Committee of the National Association of Emergency Medical Technicians in Cooperation with the Committee on Trauma of the American College of Surgeons: *Pre-hospital trauma life support*, ed 3, St Louis, 1994, Mosby; **17.2A to E** Kristen Burke.

Chapter 18
18.3 Courtesy Gary Quick. From Sanders M: *Mosby's paramedic textbook*, St Louis, 1994, Mosby; **18.5A, B, D, E, F, G**, Kristen Burke; **18.5C** From Epi-Pen®, a registered trademark of Center, Division of EM Industries, Port Washing, New York.

Chapter 19
19.4, 19.5 Kristen Burke.

Chapter 20
20.1, 20.2, 20.3, 20.4, 20.5, 20.6, 20.7, 20.8 Kristen Burke.

Chapter 21
Table 21.3 From Aehlert B: *Pediatric advanced life support study guide*, St Louis, 1994, Mosby; **21.1; 21.1A and B, 21.3** From LeFleur Brooks: *Exploring medical language*, ed 4, St Louis, 1998, Mosby; **21.2, 21.20** Kristen Burke; **21.4** Lennart Nilsson; **21.9** From Al-Azzawi F: *Color atlas of childbirth and obstetrics*, London, 1995, Wolfe; **21.10, 21.12** Bobak, Lowddermilk, Jensen: *Maternity nursing*, ed 4, St Louis, 1995, Mosby; **21.11** Sanders: *Mosby's paramedic textbook*, St Louis, 1994, Mosby; **21.15** From Aehlert B: *Textbook of pediatric advanced life support*, St Louis, 1994, Mosby. Copyright American Heart Association; **21.19** From Mosby: *Mosby's medical nursing and allied health dictionary*, ed 4, St Louis, 1994, Mosby.

Chapter 22
22.1, 22.2, 22.6, 22.8, 22.9B, 22.10, 22.11, 22.12, 22.15, 22.16A, 22.16B, 22.17, 22.19, 22.21, 22.23, 22.27, 22.28, 22.29, 22.29, 22.30, 22.32, 22.36, 22.38, 22.40, 22.42, 22.44, 22.45A, 22.46A and B, 22.48, 22.50, 22.51, 22.57, 22.61, 22.65, 22.66, 22.68, 22.70 From Pre-Hospital Trauma Life Support Committee of the National Association of Emergency Medical Technicians in Cooperation with the Committee on Trauma of the American College of Surgeons: *Pre-hospital trauma life support*, ed 3, St Louis, 1994, Mosby; **22.58** Courtesy H. Tschan. From Vallotton, Dubas, editors: *Color atlas of mountain medicine*, St Louis, 1991, Mosby; **22.62, 22.80** From McSwain NE Jr: Pulmonary chest trauma. In Moylan JA, editor: *Principles of trauma surgery*, New York, 1992, Gower; **22.59** From Vallottan, Dubas, editors. *Color atlas of mountain medicine*, St Louis, 1991, Mosby; **22.64F** From London PS: *A colour atlas of diagnosis after recent injury*, London, 1990, Wolfe; **22.62, 22.80** From McSwain NE Jr: Pulmonary chest trauma. In Moylan JA, editor: *Principles of trauma surgery*, New York, 1992, Gower.

Chapter 23
23.2, 23.5, 23.15 From Pre-Hospital Trauma Life Support Committee of the National Association of Emergency Medical Technicians in Cooperation with the Committee on Trauma of the American College of Surgeons: *Pre-hospital trauma life support*, ed 3, St Louis, 1994, Mosby; **23.3, 23.4, 23.6A and B, 23.7, 23.8A and B, 23.9, 23.10, 23.11, 23.12A and B** From London PS: *A colour atlas of diagnosis after recent injury*, London, 1990, Wolfe; **23.13, 23.14, 23.17A and B, 23.19A to D** Kristen Burke.

Chapter 24
Table 24.1, Fig 24.2, 24.3, 24.4A, 24.5A, 24.16, 24.17, 24.18 From Pre-Hospital Trauma Life Support Committee of the National Association of Emergency Medical Technicians in Cooperation with the Committee on Trauma of the American College of Surgeons: *Pre-hospital trauma life support*, ed 3, St Louis, 1994, Mosby; **24.6** From ATLS, American College of Surgeons. Adapted with permission from Naryan RK: Head injury. In Grossman RG, Hamilton WJ, editors: *Principles of neurosurgery*, Philadelphia, 1999, Raven Press; **24.14, 24.15** From London PS: *A colour atlas of diagnosis after recent injury*, London, 1990, Wolfe.

Chapter 25
25.1, 25.2, 25.3, 25.4, 25.5, 25.6, 25.7, 25.8, 25.9, 25.10, 25.11 From Pre-Hospital Trauma Life Support Committee of the National Association of Emergency Medical Technicians in Cooperation with the Committee on Trauma of the American College of Surgeons: *Pre-hospital trauma life support*, ed 3, St Louis, 1994, Mosby.

Chapter 26
26.3, 26.4A From Pre-Hospital Trauma Life Support Committee of the National Association of Emergency Medical Technicians in Cooperation with the Committee on Trauma of the American College of Surgeons: *Pre-hospital trauma life support*, ed 3, St Louis, 1994, Mosby; **26.4B** From Thibodeau GA: *Anatomy and physiology*, ed 3, St Louis, 1997, Mosby.

Chapter 27
27.4, 27.5, 27.8A to 8D, 27.9, 27.10, 27.11, 27.12A to E From Pre-Hospital Trauma Life Support Committee of the National Association of Emergency Medical Technicians in Cooperation with the Committee on Trauma of the American College of Surgeons: *Pre-hospital trauma life support*, ed 3, St Louis, 1994, Mosby; **27.6A and B, 27.13A to C** Kristen Burke.

Chapter 28
28.1, 28.2 From Pre-Hospital Trauma Life Support Committee of the National Association of Emergency Medical Technicians in Cooperation with the Committee on Trauma of the American College of Surgeons: *Pre-hospital trauma life support*, ed 3, St Louis, 1994, Mosby; **28.9, 28.14, 28.15A to G, 28.16, 28.17A to H, 28.18, 28.20** Kristen Burke; **28.11B** From London PS: *A colour atlas of diagnosis after recent injury*, London, 1990, Wolfe.

Chapter 29
29.3, 29.5A and B, 29.8 Kristen Burke; **29.4A, 29.4B** Courtesy Cameron Bangs, MD; **29.8** From Mosby: *Mosby's medical, nursing and allied health dictionary*, ed 4, St Louis, 1994, Mosby; **29.9, 29.10** Courtesy St. John's Mercy Medical Center, St. Louis, Missouri. From Sanders M: *Mosby's paramedic textbook*, St Louis, 1994, Mosby; **29.11** From Pre-Hospital Trauma Life Support Committee of the National Association of Emergency Medical Technicians in Cooperation with the Committee on Trauma of the American College of Surgeons: *Pre-hospital trauma life support*, ed 3, St Louis, 1994, Mosby; **Table 29-1** Sanders MA: *Mosby's paramedic textbook*, St Louis, 1994, Mosby; **29.12A to C** Courtesy Paul Auerbach, MD; **29.13** Courtesy Cameron Smith. From Auerbach PS: *Wilderness medicine*, ed 3, St Louis, 1995, Mosby.

Chapter 30
30.1, 30.2 From Mosby: *Mosby's medical, nursing and allied health dictionary*, ed 4, St Louis, 1994, Mosby; **30.3, 30.4** Vincent Knauss; **30.5** From Pre-Hospital Trauma Life Support Committee of the National Association of Emergency Medical Technicians in Cooperation with the Committee on Trauma of the American College of Surgeons: *Pre-hospital trauma life support*, ed 3, St Louis, 1994, Mosby.

Chapter 31
Table 31.1 From American College of Emergency Physicians; **Table 31.5, 31.6** From Eichelberger M: *Pediatric emergencies: a manual for prehospital care providers*, Englewood Cliffs, NJ, 1992, Prentice-Hall; **Table 31.7** From Emergency Nursing Pediatric Course: Emergency Nurses Association, 1993, Mosby; **Fig 31.1** From Maternal and Child Health Bureau, 1994; **31.5** Vincent Knauss; **31.9, 31.10, 31.11A**

and B, **31.14, 31.15, 31.16, 31.17, 31.18** Kristen Burke; **31.19A to F** Craig Jackson; **31.20** From Sanders M: *Mosby's paramedic textbook*, St Louis, 1994, Mosby

Chapter 32

32.1 Courtesy of Assocaition for Retarded Citizens of the United States, Arlington, Texas; **32.2** Craig Jackson; **32.3** Courtesy of Beltimore Association for Retarded Citizens, Baltimore, Maryland; **32.4, 32.13, 32.16A** From Mosby: *Mosby's medical, nursing, and allied health dictionary*, ed 4, St Louis, 1994, Mosby; **32.5** From LeFleur Brooks: *Exploring medical language*, ed 4, St Louis, 1998, Mosby; **32.6** From Seidel, Ball, Dains et al: *Mosby's guide to physical examination*, ed 2, St Louis, 1991, Mosby; **32.7, 32.12, 32.13, 32.16C, 32.17** Kristen Burke; **32.9, 32.10, 32.11** From Whaley, Wong: *Nursing care of infants and children*, St Louis, 1999, Mosby; **32.14** From ACEP website.

Chapter 33

33.2 From Stoy WA, Center for Emergency Medicine: *Mosby's EMT-Basic textbook*, St Louis, 1996, Mosby; **33.3, 33.4, 33.5, 33.6, 33.7, 33.8, 33.9, 33.10, 33.11, 33.12, 33.13, 33.14A and B, 33.15A to D, 33.16, 33.17A to C, 33.18, 33.19, 33.20, 33.21, 33.25, 33.26, 33.27, 33.28** Kristen Burke; **33.22, 33.23** Vincent Knauss; **33.24** Courtesy Moore Medical.

Chapter 34

34.1, 34.2, 34.3, 34.4, 34.5, 34.6, 34.7, 34.8, 34.9, 34.10 Kristen Burke; **34.11** Craig Jackson.

Chapter 35

35.1, 35.5 Kristen Burke; **35.2** From Siren-Pro®, Courtesy of Digital Objectives, Inc.; **35.3** EMS Data Systems, Inc.; **35.4** Vincent Knauss.

Chapter 36

36.1 Craig Jackson; **36.2, 36.3, 36.4** Kristen Burke.

Chapter 37

37.1A, B, and C Courtesy Wheeled Coach, Orlando, Florida. From Sanders M: *Mosby's paramedic textbook*, St Louis, 1994, Mosby; **37.2, 37.3, 37.4** Kristen Burke.

Chapter 40

40.2, 40.3, 40.4, 40.5 Craig Jackson; **40.6** Courtesy Eastern Pennsylvania EMS; **40.7** From US Department of Transportation, Research and Special Programs Administration, 1993, Emergency Response Guidebook; **40.9** Hazardous Material Awaeness for Minnesota First Responders: Minnesota State Board of Technical Colleges. From Keuhl AE: *Prehospital systems and medical oversight*, ed 2, St Louis, 1994, Mosby; **40.10** From Upright Inc.; **40.11** From Currace, Bronstein: *EMS/hazardous materials response: practice and scene management*, St Louis, 1999, Mosby.

Index

A

Abandonment
 defined, 40
 examples of, 38
Abbreviations, 88, 89t
ABC mnemonic, 330–331
ABCs in head-injured patient, 473
Abdomen
 compartment syndrome of, 541
 compression injuries of, 417, *417*, *418*, *419*
 muscles of, *418*
 organs of, *132*
 physical examination of
  detailed, 136
  rapid focused, with medical conditions, 135
 quadrants of, *106*, 106–107, *107*, 108, *499*
Abdominal trauma, 493–503
 anatomic considerations, 494, *496*, 496–497
 appendix, 499
 assessment of, 500–501
  algorithm for, 495
 in children, 628
 female reproductive organs, 500
 gallbladder, 498–499
 gastrointestinal, 494, 497–498, *498*
 hemorrhage from, 494, 497
 kidneys, 499–500
 management of, 501
 pancreas, 499
 penetrating, 434–435
 physiology of, 497–500
 shear force, 417, *417*, *419*
Abortion
 defined, 394
 pathophysiology of, 379
 symptoms and care, 379t
Abrasions
 characteristics of, 444, *444*
 defined, 127, 146, 454
Abruptio placentae
 bleeding due to, 380
 defined, 394
 symptoms and care, 379t
Abscess
 as complication of abdominal trauma, 497
 defined, 502
Absence seizure, defined, 635
Absorption
 defined, 267
 drug, 263
Abuse; *see also* specific types
 categories of, 601
 defined, 600

Access, 761–773; *see also* Rescue operations; Vehicle rescue incidents
 sustained, defined, 772
Accessory muscles, 185
 defined, 209, 286
 in respiratory emergencies, 281
Accident reports, emergency vehicles in, 738
Accident scene, assessing for hazards, 54
Accidents, emergency vehicles in, 738
Acetone, 327
Acidosis
 defined, 635
 metabolic, 163
 in pediatric patient, 613
Acquired immunodeficiency syndrome (AIDS) in prehospital setting, 78t
Acromion, 93, *95*
 defined, 108
Action, drug, defined, 267
Activated charcoal, 269
 action, effects, contraindications, administration, 265t
 defined, 353
 for ingested poisons, 348–349
Activities of daily living, defined, 357, 371, 586, 602
Acute care
 characteristics of, 8
 defined, 18
Acute respiratory distress syndrome, 165
Adjustment, defined, 357
Adrenalin; *see* Epinephrine
Advance directives, 231, 247–248
 defined, 233, 251
Advanced cardiac life support, 289, 299, 300
 early, 300–301
Advanced life support
 with AED, 320
 in airway management, 213
 with altered mental status, 327
 characteristics of, 9
 defined, 757
 dispatching and, 48
 levels of, 745
 for patient in shock, 169
 pediatric, 617
 sudden cardiac death and, 307
Advanced life support-Paramedic, interagency interface and, 744–745
Advanced Trauma Life Support, 809
Advocacy, patient, 26
 defined, 30
Advocate
 defined, 657
 role of, 653

AED; *see* Automated external defibrillation
Aerobic, defined, 174
Aerobic metabolism, 151
Aeromedical services
 aircraft direction and, 748, *748*
 interface with, 745–751
 landing zone for, 746–747, *747*
 landing zone setup and, 747–748
 patient preparation for, 750
 review of, 750–751
 safety and, 748–749, *749*, *750*
 types of, 745
Affect, assessment of, 361
Age, classification of, 586
Agencies, interface with; *see* Interagency interface
Aging
 anatomy and physiology of, 587–591
 changes during, 586–587
 defined, 602
Agonal ventilation, 186, 279–280
 defined, 209, 286
Agonist muscles, 536
Air, physics of, 793–794
Air bags, 420–421
Air hunger, defined, 333
Air restraint bag
 defined, 772
 hazard from, 767, *767*
Air splint, 551–552, *552*
Aircraft
 directing, 748, *748*
 fixed-wing, 746
  defined, 757
 rotor-wing, 745
  defined, 757
 safety around, 748–749, *749*, *750*
Airway adjuncts, *188*, 188–189, *189*
 defined, 209
Airway management, 177–211, 186–208, 217–231
 advanced life support in, 213
 advanced skills in, 212–234
 airway-opening techniques in, 186–187, *187*
 algorithm for, 179
 in allergic reactions, 339–340
 ambulance supplies for, 727
 assisted ventilation in, *188*, 188–194
  with airway adjuncts, *188*, 188–189, *189*
  in infants and child, 189–191, *190*, *191*, *192*, *193*
  with supplemental oxygen, 194–196
  techniques for, 189–191, *190*, *191*, *192*, *193*
 with automated transport ventilators, 229–230

899

Airway management—cont'd
  basic life support in, 213
  basic techniques, 218
  with endotracheal intubation, 218–229
  with endotracheal suctioning, 229
  with nasogastric tube placement, 230–231
  practice opportunities, 218
  step-by-step procedures for, 196–208
    applying oxygen nasal prongs, 207
    applying oxygen regulator to tank, 201
    bag-valve-mask, 205–206
    jaw thrust, 196
    mouth-to-mask ventilation, 203–204
    nasopharyngeal airway insertion, 200
    nonrebreather mask, 208
    oropharyngeal airway insertion, 198–199
    suctioning, 187–188, 197
    turning on tank, 202
Airway obstruction, *180*
  causes of, 181
  in combat, 813
  in infants/children, 182–183
  pathophysiology of, 216
Airways, *97*
  assessment of, 121–122, 122*t*, 180
    algorithm for, 214, 478–479
    during shock, 167
  establishing, during shock, 168–169
  interventions for, 121–122, 122*t*
  lower, 181–182
  multilumen, 227
  pediatric, adjuncts to, 615–617
  in pediatric patient, 614, *614*
  upper, 181
    anatomy and physiology of, 215–216
Albuterol
  action, effects, contraindications, administration, 265*t*
  trade names for, 283*t*
Alcohol
  abuse of, 352
  altered mental status and, 330
  hypothermia and, 567
Alert, defined, 469
Alkalosis, respiratory
  defined, 287
  hyperventilation and, 277
Allergens
  defined, 635
  hypersensitivity reaction to, 619
Allergic reaction
  causes and types, 336
  defined, 342
  incidence of, 336
Allergies, 335–342
  anatomic and physiologic considerations, 336–337
  antigen-antibody response in, 336, *337*
  assessment of, 338–339
  drug, 279

Allergies—cont'd
  management of, 339–340
    airway management in, 339–340
    drug therapy in, 340–341
  pathophysiology of, 337–338
ALS; *see* Advanced life support
Altered mental status, 323–334
  assessment of, 330–332
    with ABC, 330–331
    algorithm for, 325
    with AVPU, 330
    focused history/physical exam in, 331–332
    with Glasgow Coma Scale, 331–332, 331*t*
    with SAMPLE, 332
  causes of, 324–325, 324–330
    diabetes, 324–327
    neurologic, 327–329
    toxicologic, 330
    traumatic, 330
  in organic brain syndrome, 329
  from seizures, 329
  in stroke, 327–329
Alveolar capillary relationship, *164,* 164–165
Alveolar/capillary exchange, 182, 184
  defined, 209, 286
  physiology of, 275
Alveolar/capillary membrane, 479, *481*
  defined, 491
Alveoli, 96, 181–182
  aging and, 588
  defined, 108, 209, 491
  lung injuries and, 484–485
Alzheimer's disease, 329
  characteristics and management, 367
  in elderly, 591–592
  screening for, 592
Ambient temperature, 565
  defined, 580
Ambulance
  accident procedures for, 738
  collisions involving, 738
  daily inspections of, 731–734
  dispatch and, 734
  driver characteristics, 734–735
  driving, 734
  emergency driving privileges and, 736–737
  en route to receiving facility, 739
  en route to station, 739–740
  equipment guidelines, 609*t*–611*t*
  escorts for, 737
  federal requirements for, 726
  HAZMAT equipment on, 788
  medical director's responsibilities and, 48
  medical equipment for, 726–730
  nonmedical equipment for, 731
  operation of, 724–741
  OSHA requirements for, 726
  personnel and, 731
  portable kits for, 730–731

Ambulance—cont'd
  positioning, 736
  postrun, 740
  at receiving facility, 739
  safety and, 735–736
  at scene, 738
  transferring patient to, 738–739
  types of, 725, *726*
    defined, 741
Ambulance driver; *see* Emergency vehicle operator
Ambulance services, EMS and, 9–10
American Association of Poison Control Centers, 345
American College of Emergency Physicians, ambulance equipment guidelines, 609*t*–611*t*
Amniotic fluid
  anatomy/physiology of, 376
  defined, 394
Amniotic sac
  anatomy/physiology of, 376
  defined, 394
Amphetamines, abuse of, 351
Amplitude, determining, 312–313, *313*
Amputation, *447*
  assessment of, 448
  defined, 454
  management of, 451–452
  tissue death and, 446
Amylase, defined, 502
Anaerobic, defined, 174
Anaerobic metabolism, 151
  prevention of, 307
Analgesia in tactical field care, 814
Anaphylactic reaction
  to bites/stings, 578
  defined, 342, 580
Anaphylactic shock, 162
Anaphylaxis
  defined, 342, 635
  in pediatric patient, 613
  signs and symptoms of, 338, *339*
Anatomic positioning, 530
  defined, 559
Anatomy, defined, 436
Angina pectoris
  defined, 303
  pathophysiology of, 296
Ankle, sprained, *537*
Antagonist muscles, 536
Anthrax, management of, 817
Antibodies
  antigens and, 336
  defined, 342
Antidepressants, indications and trade names for, 363*t*
Antidotes, 344
  defined, 353
Antigen/antibody response, 336
Antigens
  common types of, 338
  defined, 342
Antipsychotic agents, indications and trade names for, 363*t*

Anxiety
    acute, characteristics and management, 361–362
    in phobic patient, 362
Aorta, 99, *100*
    anatomy of, 291, 479, 481, *481, 482*
    defined, 108, 303
    descending, defined, 437
    trauma to, 409
Aortic dissection in elderly, 596
Aortic insufficiency
    abdominal trauma and, 417, *419*
    defined, 436
Aortic tear, 416, *416, 417*
APGAR score, defined, 394
Apnea
    after head injuries, 471, *471*
    in COPD patient, 283
    defined, 186, 209, 286
    intubation and, 217
    ventilation *versus* intubation in, 219
Apnea monitor, 647–648, *648*
    defined, 657
Appendicitis, 499
    defined, 502
Appendix, pain associated with, 499
Appropriate facilities, defined, 757
Arachnoid membrane, 459, 460, *461*
    defined, 474
Arborization, 157
ARDS; *see* Acute respiratory distress syndrome
Arm-a-Char; *see* Charcoal, activated
Arnold-Chiari malformation
    defined, 657
    in spina bifida, 642
Arterial pressure, 296
Arteries, 99, *99*
    aging and, 590
    anatomy of, 291–292, *293*
    defined, 109, 174, 303
    pulmonary, 157
    structure and function of, 157
Arterioles
    anatomy of, 292
    defined, 174, 303
    structure and function of, 157
Arteriosclerosis, cause of, 590
Arytenoid cartilage, 215
    defined, 233
Ascent injuries, 795–797
    defined, 804
Aspiration, defined, 181, 210
Assault
    defined, 40
    liability for, 35
Assessment, 24, 113–149; *see also* Evaluation
    algorithm for, 115
    of baseline vital signs, 137
    of blood pressure, 141–142
    defined, 4, 18, 116, 146–147
    detailed physical exam in, 135–137
    as EMS base, 14
    EMT's role in, 273–274
    formats for, 116

Assessment—cont'd
    general impression, 117–118
    initial, 120–125
        of airway patency, 121–122
        of breathing, 122–123, 123t
        calming patient during, 121
        of circulation, 123–124
        of disability, 124–125
        of general impression, 121
        of priority patient, 125
    of level of consciousness, 142–144
    ongoing, 137
    plan of action, 117–118
    of pulse, *138*, 138–140, *139, 140, 141*
    of pupils, 144
    rapid focused history in, 126
    rapid focused physical exam in, 126–127
        with medical problems, 133–135
        in trauma, 127–133
    SAMPLE history in, 126, 144–145
    scene survey, 118–120
        body substance isolation in, 119
        for determining need for additional help, 120
        for mechanism of injury, 120
        for nature of illness, 120
        for number of patients, 120
        for safety, 118–119
        triage in, 120
    signs *versus* symptoms in, 137–138
    of skin color and temperature, 142
    stages of, 116–117
    of ventilations, 140
    vital signs review in, 145
Asthma
    versus bronchiolitis, 619t
    characteristics of, 644
    in children, 618–619
    defined, 635, 657
    pathophysiology of, 276–277
    riot control agents and, 819
Atelectasis
    defined, 491
    preventing, 488
Atherosclerosis
    characteristics of, 590
    defined, 303, 320
    myocardial infarction due to, 307
    pathophysiology of, 296
Atmosphere of pressure, 793
Atria, 99, 155, 291, *292*
    defined, 109, 174, 303
Attitudes, stress and, 70
Aura, defined, 620, 635
Auscultation
    for assessing blood pressure, 142
    defined, 147, 174
    of lungs, during shock, 168
Automated external defibrillation, 300–302
    in cardiac arrest, 300
    continuing education for, 301–302
    public access to, 310, *311*
Automated external defibrillator, 123, 289, 309–315
    computerized, 311–312, *312*

Automated external defibrillator—cont'd
    defined, 303, 320
    design advances in, 310
    functions of, 310–313
    maintaining skills with, 315, *316, 317*
    maintenance of, 315
    postresuscitation care and, 315
    safety issues, 314
    step-by-step procedures for, 318–319
    treatment protocols for, 314
    use of, 313–314
    voice commands and prompts of, 314
Automated transport ventilators, 229–230, *230*
    defined, 233
Automatic crash notification, 691
Automatic resuscitators, 728
Automatic vehicle location, 690
Automaticity, defined, 95, 109
Automobile
    disentangling patient from, 768–769
    glass hazards in, 768
    removing patient from, 769–770
Autonomic, defined, 635
Autonomic nervous system
    defined, 109, 527, 635
    function of, 507
    in pediatric asthma, 619
    structure and function of, 101, *101*
AVPU mnemonic, 330
AVPU scale, 125, 469
    defined, 147
Avulsions
    assessment of, 448
    characteristics of, 444–445, *445*
    defined, 454
    tissue death and, 446

B
Back
    detailed physical exam of, 137
    in rapid focused physical exam, with medical conditions, 135
    rapid focused physical exam of, in trauma, 132
Backboards
    long, 676, *676*
    for pediatric patient, *627*, 627–628
    short, 677, *677*
Bag-valve-mask ventilation, *190*, 191, *191*
    administration of, 196
    versus intubation, 215
    pediatric, *616*, 616–617
    step-by-step procedure for, 205–206
    two-person, 218, *218*
Ball-and-socket joint
    defined, 109
    structure and function of, 90
Balloon, pilot, 220, 233
Bandages
    characteristics and uses, 448–449, *449*
    defined, 454
    triangular, *548*, 548–549
Barbiturates, abuse of, 350
Baroreceptors, 163

Barotrauma, 794–797
  during ascent, 795–797
  defined, 804
  during descent, 794–795
  pathophysiology of, 797
  as priority conditions, 799
Barrel chest deformity, 276
Base station
  characteristics of, 688, *688*
  defined, 699
Basic life support
  in airway management, 213
  in cardiovascular emergencies, 299
  characteristics of, 9
  dispatching and, 48
  pediatric, 614, 617
Basic trauma life support, 809
Battery
  defined, 40
  liability for, 35
Battle's sign, 127, 468, *469*
  defined, 474
Behavior, defined, 356, 357, 371
Behavioral emergencies, 355–371
  assessment of, 358–361
  causative factors, 358–359
  defined, 357
  management of, 369–370
  medicolegal considerations, 368–369
    consent, 368
    legal authority, 368
    potential violence, 369
    restraint, 368–369
    standard of care, 368
Benadryl; *see* Diphenhydramine
Bending, lateral, 510
  defined, 527
Bends, 794; *see also* Decompression sickness; Diving emergencies
  signs and symptoms of, 797
Benner, Ludwig, 243
Bent-arm drag, 670, *670*
  defined, 684
Benzisoxazole, indications and trade names for, 363*t*
Benzodiazepines
  abuse of, 350
  indications and trade names for, 363*t*
Bicuspid valve, 156
  defined, 174
Bioethical considerations, 247–249
Biologic warfare agents, 816–819
  anthrax, 817
  characteristics of, 816–817
  defined, 822
  dissemination of, 816–817
Biomechanics, 401
Birth canal, 375
  defined, 394
Births, multiple, 390
Bites, 578–579
  assessment of, 578–579
  disease transmission by, 77
  examples of, *578*, *579*
  management of, 579

Black eye, 468
Blanch, defined, 569, 580
Blanket drag, 669–670
  defined, 684
Blast injuries, 427–428, *428*
Bleeding
  control of, 446–447
  during first trimester, 379
  intracranial, in pediatric patient, 613
  during shock, 169
  during third trimester, 380
  trauma-related, 452–453
  uterine, after delivery, 385, *386*
  vaginal, 379–380, 379*t*
    during pregnancy, 391
Blood
  components of, 100, 295
  composition of, 158
  defined, 109
Blood flow, *154*, 158–159; *see also* Circulation
  to brain, 465
  interruption of, with musculoskeletal injuries, 546
  maintenance of, 159–160
  periphery to core shunting of, 160–161, 166
  in shock, 163
Blood loss; *see also* Bleeding; Hemorrhage
  shock and, 165
Blood pressure, 158–159; *see also* Diastolic pressure; Hypertension; Hypotension; Systolic pressure
  assessing, 141–142
    during initial assessment, 124
    methods of, 141–142
  characteristics and assessment, 295–296
  components of, 100
  defined, 109, 303
  estimating, 166
  maintenance of, 159–160
  measurement of, 159
  during pregnancy, 391
  during shock, 166
  in trauma patient, 486
Blood supply, reduced, from musculoskeletal injuries, 543–544
Blood transfusions, 158
  disease transmission by, 77
Blood vessels, 100, *100*, 156–157; *see also* specific blood vessels
  defined, 109
Blood volume during shock, 167
Bloodborne pathogens, 76, 77
  defined, 84
  protection guidelines, 78–80
BLS; *see* Basic life support
Blunt trauma, 406–421
  abdominal injuries from, 417, *417*, *418*, *419*
  blood loss after, 167
  defined, 174, 436
  and effects of restraints, 418–421, *420*
  head injuries from, *413*, 413–415, *414*, *415*

Blunt trauma—cont'd
  from motor vehicle collisions; *see* Motor vehicle collisions
  organ injuries from, 412–413, *413*
  pelvic injuries from, 418
  versus penetrating, 404–406
  versus penetrating trauma, 413
  thoracic injuries from, *415*, 415–416, *416*, *417*
Body, 86–112
  abbreviations pertaining to, 89*t*
  anatomic position of, *89*
  cardiovascular system of, 99, 99–101, *100*, *101*
  cavities of, 105–107, *106*, *107*
  cooling, 562–564
  digestive system of, 103, *103*
  endocrine system of, 103–104, *104*
  integumentary system of, 102–103
  muscular system of, 93–95, *96*, *97*
  nervous system of, *101*, 101–102, *102*
  renal system of, 104, *104*
  reproductive system of, 104–105, *106*
  respiratory system of, 95–99, *97*, *98*
  skeletal system of, 88–93, *91*, *92*, *93*, *94*, *95*
  terminology for, 87–88, 88*t*, 89*t*, *90*
Body fluids, 157–158
  compartments of, *157*, 157–158
  contact with, 83
  defined, 84
  risks of exposure to, 246
  spillage of, 79–80
Body substance isolation, 55
  during assisted ventilation, 188
  defined, 72, 84
  guidelines for, 76–77
  personal protection and, 80–83
  during scene survey, 119–120
  during suctioning, 187
Body surface area
  calculating, 574, *575*
  defined, 454
  determining, 443
Body temperature
  control of, 446
  core, 562
    defined, 580
  environmental factors affecting, 564–565
  increasing, 564
  lowering, 562–563
  normal, 561
  regulation of, 561–564
Bones
  anatomy of, 531–532
  classification of, 532
  cranial, anatomy of, 459
  facial, 91
  fractures of, 536–537, 540–541
  mineral loss in, 587
  movement and, 532, 536
  and point of insertion, 532
  as point of muscular origin, 532
Bounding pulse, defined, 147
Boyle's law, 794

Brachial artery, 100, *100*
 anatomy of, 291
 defined, 109, 174, 303
 in pediatric patient, 612, *613*
Brachial pulse
 assessing, 159
 defined, 174
Bradycardia, defined, 147, 293, 303
Brain
 aging and, 590
 anatomy of, 459, 460, 462
 blood flow to, 465
 components of, 103
 divisions of, 460, *463*
 edema of, *464*, 464–465
 herniation of, 467, *467*
 increased intracranial pressure in, *464*, 464–465
 infection of, 467
 pathophysiology of, *464*, 464–467, *465*, *467*
 shear force injuries to, 414, *414*
 space-occupying lesions of, 464
 trauma to, *413*, 413–414
Brain attacks, 327
Brainstem, 101
 anatomy of, 460, 462, *463*
 defined, 109, 474
 functions of, 103
 herniation of, defined, 635
Braxton Hicks contractions, 376
 defined, 394
Breastfeeding, uterine bleeding and, 385
Breath, shortness of, 273; see also Dyspnea
Breath sounds
 absent, 184–185
 assessing, 129, *131*, 184–185, 279
 in chest trauma, 487
 in pediatric patient, 612
 in respiratory emergencies, 281
Breathing; see also Respiration
 altered, with altered mental status, 331
 assessment and intervention, 122–123
 assessment of, 184–186
 defined, 580
 difficulty with, 121
 disorders of, in elderly, 596–597
 effort of, in respiratory emergencies, 281
 as heat loss mechanism, 563
 inadequate, 185–186
 versus respiration, 122
 seesaw, 186, 281, *282*
Breech birth, *389*, 389–390
 defined, 394
Bridges, response route and, 735
Bronchi, 96
 defined, 109
 mainstem, 181, *182*
  defined, 210
Bronchioles, defined, 635
Bronchiolitis
 versus asthma, 619t
 defined, 635
 management of, 619
Bronchitis, chronic, defined, 286

Bronchodilators, 271, 283–284, 283t, *284*
 defined, 286
Bronchospasm, defined, 286
Broselow tape, 611, *612*
Bruises; see also Contusions
 assessing, 131
 characteristics of, 443–444, *444*
Bubble trouble, 797
Building collapse, 762–763
Bullet wounds, 428–435, *429*, *431*, *432*, *433*, *434*, *435*
Burnout, characteristics of, 67–68
Burns, 573–576
 ambulance equipment for, 729
 assessing extent of, 443
 body surface area of, 574, *575*
 chemical, 574–575
 classification of, 573–574, 576
 critical, 574
 electrical, 575–576
 facial, 576
 full-thickness, 574
  defined, 580
 management of, 576
 partial-thickness, 574, *574*
  defined, 581
 in pediatric patient, 613
 skin damage from, *572*
 superficial, 573, *573*
  defined, 581
Butyrophenone, indications and trade names for, 363t

C

Calcium, bone integrity and, 532
Calming techniques, 121
Cannabis, abuse of, 351
Cannula, nasal, *versus* nasal prongs, 195
Capillaries, *99*, 100
 anatomy of, 292, *293*
 defined, 109, 174, 303
 structure and function of, 157
Capillary refill
 defined, 147, 174
 during shock, 166–167
Capillary refilling time
 assessing, 124, *125*
 increased, from musculoskeletal injuries, 544
Capillary/cellular exchange
 defined, 286
 physiology of, 275
Carbon dioxide
 end-tidal
  defined, 233
  measurement during intubation, *226*, 226–227
 exhalation of, 181
Carbon monoxide poisoning in scuba divers, 796
Cardiac arrest
 in children, 301
 deaths due to, 309
 defined, 303
 definitive care in, 310

Cardiac arrest—cont'd
 management of, 289, 299–300
 versus myocardial infarction, 296–297
 in pediatric patient, 613
 survival rates between CPR/defibrillation and, 308t
Cardiac care, standard, defined, 304
Cardiac compromise, signs and symptoms of, 298
Cardiac contusions, 415–416, *416*
 defined, 436
Cardiac death, sudden; see Sudden cardiac death
Cardiac emergencies
 in elderly, 589
 incidence of, 307
Cardiac failure, shock due to, 168
Cardiac muscle, 536
 defined, 109, 559
Cardiac output
 characteristics and assessment, 156
 defined, 174
 during shock, 163, 164, 166
Cardiac valves, 156–157, 291, *292*
 damage to, 157
Cardinal, defined, 174
Cardiogenic shock, 162
 defined, 303
 pathophysiology of, 297
Cardiopulmonary resuscitation, 123, 289
 AED and, 311
 during combat, 812
 early, 300–301
 limitations of, 310–311
 in pediatric patient, 614
 and survival of cardiac arrest, 308t
Cardiovascular conditions in special needs patient, characteristics and treatment issues, 654t
Cardiovascular emergencies, 288–305
 assessment of, 297–298
  algorithm for, 441
 automated external defibrillation in, 300–302
 management of, 298–300
  cardiac arrest management in, 299–300, *300*
  nitroglycerin in, 298–299
  standard cardiac care in, 298
 postresuscitation care in, 301
Cardiovascular system, *99*, 99–101, *100*, *101*; see also Circulatory system
 aging changes in, 589–590
 anatomy of, *291*, 291–292, *292*
 components of, 100–101, *101*
 physiology of, 292–296
Cardioversion, 310
 defined, 320
Carina, 96, 181, *182*
 defined, 109, 210
Carotid arteries, 99
 anatomy of, 291
 defined, 109, 147, 174, 303
 in pediatric patient, 612, *613*
Carotid pulse, assessing, 139, *139*, 159

Carpals, 93, *95*
  defined, 109
Carries
  direct, in supine patient transfer, 671, *672*
  end-to-end, *666*
  guidelines for, 666
  side-to-side, *666*
  on stairs, 666–668, *667*
Cartilage
  arytenoid, 215
    defined, 233
  cricoid, *97*, 181
    defined, 210
    in infants and children, 228
  growth of, 587, *587*
  structure and function of, 90
  thyroid, *97*, 181
    defined, 211
Case review
  defined, 303, 723
  quality assurance and, 722
Casevac care
  characteristics of, 815
  defined, 822
  versus medevac, 811
Casualties, military, 812–813
Cataracts, characteristics of, 591
Catheters for airway suctioning, 187–188
Cavitation, 404
  defined, 436
  energy exchange and, 404–406, *405*
Cavities
  permanent, defined, 437
  temporary, defined, 437
  types of, 404
CDC; *see* Centers for Disease Control and Prevention
Cellular telephones, 690
Cellular/capillary exchange, 184
  defined, 210
Centers for Disease Control and Prevention
  body substance isolation recommendations of, 55
  communicable disease guidelines, 76
  defined, 84
  infection control guidelines of, 78–80
Central nervous system
  components of, 507, *508*
  defined, 109, 527
  in elderly, 597
  structure and function of, 101, *101*
Central venous access devices, 646–647, 647*t*
Cephalad, *versus* proximal, 483
Cerebellum, 101
  anatomy of, 460, 462, *463*
  defined, 109, 474
  functions of, 103
Cerebral edema, defined, 635
Cerebral palsy
  characteristics of, 641, *641*
  defined, 657

Cerebrospinal fluid
  defined, 474
  epidural hematoma and, 460
  functions of, 462
  leakage of, 465, 467
Cerebrovascular accident
  altered mental status in, 327–329
  defined, 251
Cerebrum, 102
  anatomy of, 460, 462, *463*
  defined, 109, 474
  functions of, 103
Certification, 14, 27–28
  defined, 30
Cervical collar
  characteristics of, 514
  defined, 527
Cervical spine
  in children
    flexion of, 626
    immobilization of, 627
  compression injuries of, 414, *414*
  in elderly, 597
  fracture of, 483
  trauma to, 410–411
Cervical vertebrae, structure and function of, 92, *94*
Cervix
  anatomy of, 375
  defined, 394
Chain of survival, 289, 300–301
  defined, 303
Chair, stair, 675, *676*
Charcoaide; *see* Charcoal, activated
Charcoal, activated, 269
  action, effects, contraindications, administration, 265*t*
  defined, 353
  for ingested poisons, 348–349
Charcola; *see* Charcoal, activated
Chemical burns, 574–575
Chemical warfare agents, 817–819
  affecting lungs, 818
  cyanide, 818
  nerve agents, 818
  for riot control, 818–819
  vesicants, 818
CHEMTREC
  for burn information, 575
  HAZMAT information from, 783
Chest
  detailed physical exam of, 136
  flail; *see* Flail chest
  percussion of, 487
  rapid focused physical exam of
    with medical conditions, 135
    in trauma, 128–131
Chest pain
  assessment of, 297–298
  algorithm for, 290
  in elderly, 595, 596
Chest trauma, 128–129, 409, 410, *411*, 476–492
  anatomic considerations in, 477, 479, *480*, 481, *481*

Chest trauma—cont'd
  assessment of, 486–487
    algorithm for, 478–479
  in children, 628
  deaths due to, 477
  heart involvement in, 486
  management of, 487–490
    flail chest, 488
    open pneumothorax, 489
    pneumothorax, 488–489
    rib fractures, 487–488
    tension pneumothorax, 489–490
  pathophysiology of, 483–486
  physiological considerations in, 481–483
Chest wall
  aging and, 589
  expansion of, 483
  penetrating injuries of, 484
Chest wounds
  open, management of, 450, *450*
  penetrating, 448
Cheyne-Stokes breathing, *470*, 471
  defined, 474
Chickenpox in prehospital setting, 78*t*
Child abuse, 630–632
  indicators of, 632, *632*, 633
  reporting, 37
  risk factors for, 630*t*
  types of, 631–632
Child protective services
  defined, 757
  interface with, 751
Childbirth, ambulance supplies for, 729–730
Children; *see also* Pediatric patients
  assisted ventilation in, 193
  cardiac arrest in, 301
  communication with, 698
Cholecystitis
  defined, 502
  with and without infection, 499
Chronic, defined, 657
Chronic brain syndrome, 592
Chronic bronchitis, defined, 286
Chronic care
  characteristics of, 8
  defined, 18
Chronic illnesses, 644–645
  reactive airways disease, 644
  seizures/epilepsy, 644–645, 645*t*
  transplant recipients, 645
Chronic obstructive pulmonary disease
  in elderly, 596
  exacerbations of, 283
  kyphosis and, 587
  management of, 283
  pathophysiology of, 275–276, *276*
Circle survey, defined, 772
Circulation; *see also* Blood flow
  altered, with altered mental status, 331
  assessment of, 123–124, *124*
    algorithm for, 152
  cardiopulmonary, 483
  in elderly, 597
  interventions for, 123–124, *124*

Circulation—cont'd
  pulmonary, 155, *156*
  systemic, 155, *156*
Circulatory status in pediatric patients, 612
Circulatory system; *see also* Cardiovascular system
  algorithm for assessing, 308
  anatomy and physiology of, 153–159, *154*
  failure of, 153
  as pump system, 154, *155*
  vessels of, 156–157
Clavicle, 93, *95*
  defined, 109
Clinical experience, 13
Closed injuries
  characteristics of, 443
  defined, 454
Clothing, full protective, 765, *765*
  defined, 772
Clothing drag, 669
  defined, 684
Cocaine, abuse of, 351
Cold exposure
  generalized, 566–569
    management of, 568–569
    vital sign changes and, 568
  localized, 569–571
    assessment of, 569–570
    management of, 570–571, *571*
Cold load, 749
  defined, 757
Cold water submersion, 577–578
Cold weather, dressing for, 566
Colles' fractures, 425
Collisions
  angular-impact, defined, 436
  of emergency vehicles, 738
  factors affecting, 402–403
  head-on, defined, 437
  motor vehicle; *see* Motor vehicle collisions
  motorcycle, 421–423
Colon, 103
  defined, 109, 502
  infection of, 497
Colostomy, 649
  defined, 657
Combat, EMS care in; *see* Military EMS
Combat casualty evacuation care, 811
Combat lifesaver program
  characteristics of, 808
  defined, 822
Combat swimmer casualty scenario, 815
Combitube, indications for, 227
Common duct, 498
  defined, 502
Communicable (infectious) disease, 75–76
  classification of, 75–76
  defined, 84
  in prehospital setting, 78t
  transmission of, 77–78

Communication, 22–24, 686–700; *see also* Interagency interface
  with elderly, 594
  emergency medical dispatch and, 692–693
  EMS system for, 687–691
    personnel of, 691
    public access to, 691–692
  en route, 693, 695–696
  in-person, with facility staff, 696–697
  legal issues in, 698
  with medical control, 32–33, 35–36
  with medical direction/destination facility, 694–695
  with patient, 23–24
  personal, 22–23
  principles of, 697
  radio, 23, 693–694
  at scene, 245
  with special needs patient, 652, 697–698
  with team, 24
Compartment syndrome, 460, *463*
  abdominal, 466, 541
  characteristics of, 446, 466
  defined, 455, 559
  fracture-associated, 540–541
  of skull, 540
Compassion, role of, 246
Compliance
  defined, 233
  poor, development during intubation, 229
Compression, defined, 436
Compression force, 412–413
Compression fracture
  defined, 527
  spinal, 510–511
Compression injuries, 415–416
  abdominal, 417, *417, 418, 419*
  cardiac, 415–416, *416*
  of head, *413*, 413–414
  of neck, 414, *414*
  pulmonary, 416, *416*
  thoracic, 415, *415*
  of thorax, *415*, 415–416, *416*
Computer-aided dispatch, defined, 251
Computer-based reports, 703, *704*
  defined, 713
Conception, products of, 379
Concurrent evaluation, defined, 723
Conduction
  defined, 580
  as heat loss mechanism, 563
Confidentiality
  defined, 40
  duty of, 37
Confined spaces, 763
Conflict resolution, applications of, 755–756
Confusion
  causes of, 36–37
  defined, 40
Congestive heart failure, 165
  defined, 303
  pathophysiology of, *296*, 297

Consciousness, level of; *see* Level of consciousness
Consent
  with behavioral emergencies, 368
  defined, 40
  emergency doctrine for, 34
  expressed, 34
    defined, 40
  implied, defined, 40
  in incompetent patient, 35–36
  informed, 33–34
    defined, 40
  for medical care/transportation, 33–35
  by minors, 34–35
  surrogate, 36–37
    defined, 40
  treatment without, 36
Constrict, defined, 147
Continuing education, 14, 22, 28; *see also* Education; Training
  defined, 723
  quality assurance and, 722
Continuous quality improvement, defined, 723
Contractions
  defined, 376, 394
  false
    defined, 394
    versus true, 376
  true, defined, 395
Contraindications, 258
  defined, 267
Contusions
  cardiac, 415–416, *416*
  defined, 436
  characteristics of, 443–444, *444*
  defined, 127, 147, 455, 491
  pulmonary, 410, 485, 488
    defined, 437
Convection
  defined, 580
  as heat loss mechanism, 563
Convulsive, defined, 635
Core, defined, 174
Coronary arteries, 99, 291
  defined, 109, 303
Coronary heart disease, deaths due to, 289
Costovertebral angle, 496
  defined, 503
Cots, lifting, 665, *665, 666*
Counseling, EMT, 50
CPR; *see* Cardiopulmonary resuscitation
Crackles
  characteristics of, 184
  defined, 210, 286
  in respiratory emergencies, 282
Cramps, heat, 572
  defined, 581
Cranial cavity, 460
  defined, 474
Crash, defined, 437
Crash notification, automatic, 691
Crash phase, 401–402

Crepitus
  assessing, 543
  characteristics and significance, 129
  defined, 147, 559
Cribbing, 767
  defined, 772
Cricoid cartilage, *97*, 181
  defined, 210
  in infants and children, 228
Cricothyrotomy, needle
  for children, 618
  defined, 636
Crime scene, 59–60
  defined, 40
  treatment at, 37
Criteria-based dispatch, defined, 251
Critical incident, defined, 67, 72
Critical incident stress debriefing, 68–69
  defined, 72–73
Croup
  assessment and management of, 618
  defined, 286
  versus epiglottitis, 618*t*
  pathophysiology of, 278
Crowning, 382, *383*
  defined, 394
Crush injuries
  characteristics of, 444, *444*
  defined, 455
Curriculum
  defined, 18
  EMT, 11–13
Cushing's triad
  characteristics and significance, 466
  clinical significance of, 332
  defined, 333, 474
Cyanide, characteristics of, 818
Cyanosis, 186
  characteristics of, 280
  in chest trauma, 487
  defined, 210, 286, 635
  in pediatric patient, 612
  during shock, 166

D

Dalton's law of partial pressure, 794
Data
  patient, defined, 714
  types of, 703
Data collection, 26
  defined, 723
  for quality assurance, 722
DCAP-BTLS mnemonic, 126, 545
Dead space, defined, 185, 210
Death and dying, 60–62
  and family of patient, 60–62
  stages of, 60, 152
Decerebrate posturing, 471
  defined, 474
Decompression sickness
  assessment of, 799–801
  defined, 804
  pathophysiology of, 798–799
  scuba diving and, 797

Decompression sickness—cont'd
  signs and symptoms of, 797, 800, 803
  types of, 797
Decontamination
  with chemical warfare agents, 819
  defined, 789
Decorticate posturing, 471
  defined, 474
Defibrillation
  automated external; *see* Automated external defibrillation
  defined, 303, 320
  early, 306–322
  by EMT-Bs, 310
  history of, 310
  by lay rescuers, 310
  for life-threatening dysrhythmias, 307
  mechanism of, 310–311
  for patient in ventricular fibrillation, 308
  and survival of cardiac arrest, 308*t*
Defibrillators, automated external, 289
Definitive care, defined, 4, 18
Deformities
  of extremities, 537
  from musculoskeletal injuries, 542
Dehydration
  aging and, 591
  in children, 621–622, 622*t*
  defined, 635
  in pediatric patient, 612–613
  shock due to, 168
Delayed evacuation land warfare scenario, 814
Delirium *versus* dementia, 592
Delivery
  abnormal, 387–390
    with breech presentation, *389*, 389–390
    with meconium, 390, *390*
    multiple births, 390
    with prolapsed cord, 387–388, *388*
  EMT protection during, 382
  multiple, 390
  procedure for, 382, *383*, *384*, 384–385, *385*
  signs of readiness for, 381–382
Delivery kit, 382, *382*
Demand valve ventilators, 196
Dementia
  altered mental status and, 329
  characteristics of, 592
  in elderly, 591–592
Density, energy exchange and, 406
Dentures, handling of, 596
Department of Transportation, HAZMAT guidelines of, 783
Depression
  characteristics and management, 363–364
  in elderly, 599
Dermis
  characteristics of, 441
  defined, 109, 455
  structure and function of, 103
Descent injuries, 794–795
  defined, 804

Detailed physical examination, 135–137
  of abdomen, 136
  of back, 137
  of chest, 136
  defined, 147
  of ears, 135
  of extremities, 137
  of eyes, 135–136
  of face, 135
  of head, 135
  of mouth, 136
  of neck, 136
  of nose, 136
  of pelvis, 137
  of vital signs, 137
Detectives, interface with, 754
Developmental disabilities, 640
  assessment of, 649
  defined, 657
Diabetes
  altered mental status due to, 324–327
  classification of, 326
  defined, 333
  emergencies due to, 326–327
  incidence of, 324
  management of, 327
  metabolic effects of, 326
  pathophysiology of, 326
Diabetic ketoacidosis, 326–327
Diagnosis
  defined, 18
  as EMS base, 14
  EMT's role in, 273
  working, 273
Diagonal slide, 515–516
  defined, 527
Diaphoresis
  in children, 621
  defined, 635
Diaphoretic, defined, 303
Diaphoretic skin, 166, 186
  in cardiovascular emergencies, 298
  defined, 210
Diaphragm
  anatomy of, 183, 477, *480*
  defined, 109, 210, 491
Diastole, 154
  during shock, 164
Diastolic pressure, 100, 159
  assessment of, 141, 295
  characteristics of, 295
  defined, 109, 147, 174, 303
  during shock, 164
Dibenzoxazepine, indications and trade names for, 363*t*
Dietary guidelines, 70
Digestive system, structure and function of, 103, *103*
Digital radio equipment, 690
  defined, 699
Dihydroindolone, indications and trade names for, 363*t*
Dilate, defined, 147

Diphenhydramine (Benadryl) for allergic reactions, 340
Diphtheria-pertussis-tetanus vaccine, 83
Direct force, example of, 536
Direct ground lift, 670–671, 681
  defined, 684
Directives, advance, 231, 247–248
  defined, 233, 251
Disabilities; *see also* Special needs; Special needs patient
  assessment of, 124–125
    algorithm for, 639
  awareness about, 655, 656
  children with, 632–633
  developmental, 640
    assessment of, 649
    defined, 657
  myths about, 640
  permanent, in special needs patient, characteristics and treatment issues, 654t
  physical, 640–644
    assessment of, 649
    defined, 657
Disasters, 776–782
  definitions and classifications, 776–777, 789
  EMT roles in, 781–782
  incident command system in, 779
  natural, 776, 777
  preplanning for, 777–779
  response sequence in, 779
  triage in, 779–781
Discoloration; *see also* Bruises
  from musculoskeletal injuries, 542
Disease, communicable (infectious); *see* Communicable (infectious) disease
Disentanglement
  defined, 772
  process for, 768–769
  in rescue operations, 765
Dislocations
  characteristics of, 541
  defined, 559
  fracture with, 537, *539*
Disorganization, characteristics and management, 366–367
Disorientation, characteristics and management, 366–367
Dispatch; *see also* Emergency medical dispatch
  ambulance, 734
  BLS *versus* ALS, 48
Dispatcher
  interagency interface and, 743–744
  responsibilities of, 249
Distraction injuries
  defined, 527
  spinal, 511
Distress
  defined, 65
  preventing, 69–71
Divers Alert Network, 803

Diving emergencies, 791–805
  assessment of, 799–801
  barotrauma injuries, 794–797
  five-minute neurologic exam in, 800–801
  helicopter procedures in, 802
  management of, 801–803
  and physics of air, 793–794
  portable chambers for, 803
Diving reflex, 160
DKA; *see* Diabetic ketoacidosis
Documentation, 701–714; *see also* Patient care report
  by call type, 708–709
  by chronologic method, 710
  of multiple casualty incidents, 712
  of nonconsenting cases, 36
  of patient refusal of care, 711
  prehospital, 33
  by SOAP method, 706, 709–710
  of special situations, 712
Do-not-resuscitate legislation, 247–248
Do-not-resuscitate orders, 247
  defined, 252
  procedures pertaining to, 248
Dorsalis pedis artery
  anatomy of, 292
  defined, 303
Down syndrome, 640
  defined, 657
Draw sheet method, 671–672
Dressings
  characteristics and uses, 448, *449, 450*
  for controlling bleeding, 452
  defined, 455
  for evisceration, 450, *451*
  for open chest wounds, 450, *450*
Driving
  emergency privileges for, 736–737
  safe, 735–736
Drowning; *see also* Near-drowning
  defined, 577, 580
  secondary, 577
    defined, 581
Drug use, hypothermia and, 567
Drugs; *see also* Medications; specific drugs
  absorption of, 263
  actions of, 258
  administration of
    inhaled, 262–263, 262t
    intramuscular, 262, 262t
    intravenous, 262, 262t
    oral, 262, 262t
    rectal, 262
    subcutaneous, 262, 262t
    sublingual, 262, 262t
    topical, 263
  altered mental status and, 330
  assessment and management of, 264–266
  available for EMT use, 258, 258t, 264
  chemical composition of, 260
  contraindications to, 258
  duration of action of, 261

Drugs—cont'd
  dynamics of, 261–263
    absorption, 263
    elimination, 263
    and route of administration, 261–263
  elimination of, 263
  forms of, 259–261, *260*
    gases, 261
    gels, *260*, 260–261
    injectable, 261
    for nebulizers, 261
    powders, 261
    sublingual, 261
    suspensions, 261
    tablets, 260, *260*
  indications for, 258
  labels and prescriptions for, 263–264
  locally acting, defined, 267
  names for, 259
  overview of EMT use of, 258–259
  prescribed, 259
  route of administration of, 258
  side effects of, 258
  systemically acting
    defined, 267
    versus locally acting, 261
  terminology for, 258
Duodenum, 498
  defined, 503
Dura mater, 459, *461*
  defined, 474
Durable power of attorney, 247
  defined, 40, 252
  procedures pertaining to, 248–249
Duration of action, defined, 267
Duty to act, defined, 40
Dying; *see* Death and dying
Dyspnea
  defined, 85, 275, 286, 602
  in myocardial infarction, 595
Dysrhythmias
  cardiac arrest due to, 308
  deaths due to, 309
  defined, 303
  pathophysiology of, 293–294, *295*

E

Ears, detailed physical exam of, 135
Ecchymosis, periorbital, 468
Eclampsia
  defined, 394
  symptoms of, 380
Edema; *see also* Swelling
  assessing, 135
  of brain, defined, 474
  causes and effects of, 446
  cerebral, defined, 635
  defined, 147, 164, 455
  intracranial, 466–467
  pulmonary
    in congestive heart failure, 297
    defined, 287, 304
    pathophysiology of, 278
    during shock, 164–165

Edentulism, 587
Education; *see also* Continuing education; Training
   diagnosis- *versus* assessment-based, 14
   initial *versus* continuing, 14
   medical director's role in, 50
   philosophies of, 45
Effort of breathing in respiratory emergencies, 281
Elasticity, tissue, 404
Elder abuse, 599–601
   assessment of, 600–601
   categories of, 601
   defined, 600, 602
   profile of, 600
   reporting, 37
Elder abuse services, interface with, 752
Elderly; *see also* Geriatric patients
   definitions of, 584, 602
   leading cause of death in, 587
Electrical burns, 575–576
Electrocardiogram, 293, *294*
   defined, 303
   interpretation of, 313
Elevation, defined, 455
Emancipation
   defined, 40
   minors' rights and, 35
Embolism
   gas, 797–799
   pulmonary
      defined, 287
      pathophysiology of, 278
Embryo, defined, 375, 394
Emergencies; *see also* Behavioral emergencies; Cardiac emergencies; Cardiovascular emergencies; Diving emergencies; Environmental emergencies; Obstetric/gynecologic emergencies; Psychologic emergencies; Respiratory emergencies; Toxic emergencies; Water-related emergencies
   EMT's reaction to, 63–64
      disciplining, 64
      physiologic, 63–64
Emergency consent doctrine, 34
Emergency department
   EMT's interactions with, 249–250
   in in-hospital care continuum, 251
Emergency medical dispatch
   components of, 241
   computer-aided, 241
      defined, 251
   criteria-based, 241
      defined, 251
   defined, 252, 699
   hazardous materials and, 243
   information provided for, 241–243
   patient access and, 241
Emergency medical services
   access to, 22
   ambulance dispatch and, 241; *see also* Emergency medical dispatch

Emergency medical services—cont'd
   assessment- *versus* diagnosis-based, 14
   calls to, anatomy of, *250*
   challenges of, 15–17
   citizen access/communication and, 240
   components of, 4, 7, 21–22
   defined, 18, 30
   delivery models for, 9–10
   design of, 46
   do-not-resuscitate legislation for, 247–248, 252
   financing of, 10–11
   funding of, 7
   future of, 15
   in health care delivery, 7–9
   history of, 6–7
   introduction to, 3–19
   legislation for, 5
   level of, 9
   military; *see* Military EMS
   protocols for, 46–47
   quality assurance/improvement of, 22
   training for, 11–13
   types of calls received by, 238–240
      cardiovascular, 238
      geriatric, 239–240
      medical, 238–239
      pediatric, 239
      special needs, 240
      trauma, 239
   variables in, 9–14
Emergency Medical Services for Children, 606
Emergency Medical Services Systems Act of 1973, 6
Emergency medical technician
   certification/licensure of, 27–28
   communication and, 22–24
      patient, 23–24
      personal, 22–23
      radio, 23
      team, 24
   counseling of, 50
   defined, 30
   future of, 15
   history of, 5–6
   legal regulations and, 27
   levels of, 5
   medical director's relationship with, 43–44
   patient advocacy and, 26
   patient transportation/transfer and, 24, 26
   professional attributes of, 26
   professional ethics of, 27
   professional organizations for, 28–29
   record keeping and, 26
   responsible patient care and, 24
   roles and responsibilities of, 20–30
   safety and, 24
   scope of practice of, 37–38
   well-being of, 53–73
Emergency medical technician-Basic
   curriculum for, 12–13
   defined, 18

Emergency medical technician-Basic—cont'd
   licensure and certification of, 14
   number of, 5
   prerequisites for, 12–13
   role of, 4
   training curriculum for, 11–13
   volunteer *versus* paid, 11
Emergency medical technician-Intermediate
   defined, 18
   supervision of, 43
   training of, 5
Emergency medical technician-Paramedic; *see also* Advanced life support-Paramedic
   defined, 18
   supervision of, 43
   training of, 5
Emergency move, defined, 684
Emergency preparedness, 774–790; *see also* Disasters
Emergency Response Guidebook, 56
Emergency vehicle operator
   characteristics of, 734–735
   defined, 741
   responsibilities of, 725
   training for, 731
Emergency warning devices, 736
Emotional abuse, defined, 631
Emphysema
   defined, 286
   pathophysiology of, 275, *276*
Employers, infection control and, 78–79
EMS; *see* Emergency medical services
EMT-B; *see* Emergency medical technician-Basic
EMT-defibrillation
   defined, 320
   programs in, 310
EMT-I; *see* Emergency medical technician-Intermediate
EMT-P; *see* Emergency medical technician-Paramedic
Endocardium, 99
   defined, 109
Endocrine, defined, 503
Endocrine system, 103–104, *104*
Endotracheal intubation, 218–229
   in adults, 221–223, *222, 223, 224, 225,* 225–228, *226*
   in airway management, 213–215
   anatomic and physiologic considerations, 215–216
   in infants/children, 216
   upper airway, 215–216
   versus bag-valve-mask ventilation, 215
   barriers to, 221–222
   in combat, 812–813
   complications of, 218–220
   confirming placement of, 219
   equipment for, *220,* 220–221, *221*
   indications for, 216–217
   in infants and children, 228–229

Endotracheal intubation—cont'd
  larynx during, 217
  positioning for, 222, 222–223, 223
  preparation for, 222
  procedure for, 223, 224, 225, 225
  RISE mnemonic for, 226
  risks of, 218–220
  training needs, 218
  versus ventilation, in apneic patient, 219
  ventilation *versus*, 215
Endotracheal suctioning, 229
Endotracheal tube
  confirming placement of, 225–227, 226, 228–229
  defined, 233
  formula for size selection in children, 228
  measuring insertion of, 220–221
  sizes of, 220
Endotracheal tube cuff, 220
  defined, 233
End-tidal carbon dioxide
  defined, 233
  measurement of, with intubation, 226, 226–227
Energy
  defined, 437
  production of, 151
Energy exchange
  cavitation and, 404–406
  defined, 401
  density and, 406
  physics of, 402–406
  in sports injuries, 427
  surface area and, 406
Entrapment
  defined, 772
  degree of, 765
Envenomation, 349
Environment, algorithm for assessing, 442
Environmental emergencies, 560–581
  assessment of, 565–566
  bites and stings, 578–579
  burns, 573–576
    body surface area of, 574
    chemical, 574–575
    classification of, 573–574
    critical, 574
    electrical, 575–576
    management of, 576
  cold exposure
    generalized, 566–569
    localized, 569–571
  in elderly, 597–598
  heat exposure, 571–573
  management of, 566
  water-related, 577–578
Environmental stressors, 66
  defined, 73
Epicardium, 99
Epidermis
  characteristics of, 441
  defined, 109, 455
  structure and function of, 103

Epidural hematoma, 459–460, 462
  defined, 474
Epidural space, 459, 461
  defined, 474
Epigastrium
  breath sounds over, during intubation, 226
  defined, 233
Epiglottis, 96, 181
  defined, 109, 635
Epiglottitis
  assessment and management of, 618
  causes and symptoms, 278
  versus croup, 618t
  defined, 210, 286, 635
  pathophysiology of, 278
Epilepsy
  characteristics of, 644–645, 645t
  in children, 619–620
  control of, 329
  defined, 333, 620, 636, 657
Epinephrine, 269–270
  action, effects, contraindications, administration, 265t
  for allergic reactions, 340–341
  defined, 342
Epi-Pen, 340
  defined, 342
Epithelial cells, 441
Equipment; *see also* Supplies
  ambulance, 726–730
  for assessing blood pressure, 141
  carrying guidelines, 666
  HAZMAT, 788
  inspection of, 733–734
  nonmedical, for ambulance, 731
  oxygen, 728
  protective, 75t, 80–83, 81
    defined, 84
  resuscitation, infection control and, 82
Erythrocytes, 100, 295
  defined, 109
  production and function of, 158
Escorts, 737–738
Esophageal intubation detection device, 227
  defined, 233
Esophagus, 103, 103
  defined, 109, 636
  inadvertent intubation of, 215–216, 216, 218–219
    detecting, 227
  during pediatric ventilation, 617
Ethics
  EMT code of, 28
  professional, 27
Eustress, defined, 65
Evaluation; *see also* Assessment
  concurrent, defined, 723
  prospective, defined, 723
  retrospective, defined, 723
Evaporation
  defined, 580
  as heat loss mechanism, 563

Evisceration, *448*
  assessment of, 448
  defined, 455
  management of, *450*, 451
Excavation collapse, 763
Exercise, body temperature and, 571
Exhalation, defined, 140, 147
Exposure control plan
  components of, 78–79
  defined, 84
Expressed consent, 34
  defined, 40
Extended care facility, 8
  defined, 18
Extension injuries, spinal, 510–511
Extremities
  detailed physical exam of, 137
  passive motion of, 544
  penetrating trauma to, 435, *435*
  rapid focused physical exam of
    with medical conditions, 135
    in trauma, 132
  upper/lower, 93, *95*, *96*
Extremity lift, 667, *667*, 670, *671*
  defined, 684
Extrication
  defined, 772
  process for, 768–769
  rapid, 519–520
Extrication tools, 731
Extubation
  defined, 233
  preventing, 219
Eyes
  detailed physical exam of, 135–136, *136*
  exposure to poisons, 346, 348, 349
  protection of, 81

F
Face
  bones of, 91
  burns of, 576
  defined, 109
  detailed physical exam of, 135
Face masks; *see also* Nonrebreather masks
  infection control and, 82
Facilities, appropriate, 752
  defined, 757
Fainting, 162
Fallopian tubes
  anatomy/physiology of, 375
  defined, 394
Falls, *425*, 425–426, *426*
Family
  of dying patient, 60–62
  of EMT, 64–65
  of special needs patient, 655
Febrile, defined, 602
Febrile illness in elderly, 598
Febrile seizures, 329
Feeding, aging and, 591
Fee-for-service model, 9, 11
  defined, 18

Femoral arteries, 99–100, *100*
  anatomy of, 292
  defined, 109, 147, 174, 303
Femoral pulse
  assessing, 140, *140*, 159
  defined, 174
Femur, 93, *96*
  defined, 109
  injuries to, 408, *408*
  trauma to, 410–411, *411*
Fend-off position, 766, *766*
  defined, 772
Fetus, *377*
  defined, 375, 394
Fever in elderly, 598
Fibrillation, ventricular, cardiac arrest due to, 308
Fibula, 93, *96*
  defined, 109
Fick principle, 153, 177, 310
  statement of, 307
Field assessment card, 703
  defined, 713
Fight or flight syndrome, 508
Financing
  challenges of, 15–16
  EMS, 10–11
  fee-for-service, 9
FiO₂; *see* Inspired oxygen concentration
Fire department
  EMS and, 9
  hazardous materials units of, 243
Firearms, wounds from, 428–435, *429*, *431*, *432*, *433*, *434*, *435*
First responders
  interagency interface and, 744
  training of, 5
First response, civilian *versus* military, 808
Fistula
  as complication of abdominal trauma, 497
  defined, 503
Fixation, internal, 530
  defined, 559
Fixed-wing aircraft, 746
  defined, 757
Flail chest, 415, *415*, 485
  anterior, 409
  defined, 436
  management of, 488
Flexible stretcher, defined, 685
Flexion
  of child's cervical spine, 626
  defined, 636
Flexion injuries, spinal, 510–511
Flow-restricted oxygen-powered ventilators, 191–192, *192*, 196
Fluid resuscitation in military EMS, 813–815
Fluids; *see* Body fluids
Foramen magnum, 459, *460*
  defined, 474
Force, types of, 536

Fractures
  ambulance equipment for, 728–729
  closed, 540–541, *541*
    defined, 559
  Colles', 425
  compression, 510–511
    defined, 527
  descriptions of, 537
  with dislocation, 537, *539*
  in elderly, 598
  impacted, 537, *538*
  open, 537, *539*, 540, *540*
    defined, 559
  pathophysiology of, 536–537, 540–541
  reduction of, 540
  unstable, 537, *538*
Fragmentation, 406
  defined, 437
Frontal, defined, 109
Frostbite
  characteristics of, 570
  classification of, 569
  defined, 580
  management of, 570, *571*
Frostnip
  characteristics of, 569
  defined, 580
  management of, 570, *571*
Funding; *see* Financing
Fuselage, defined, 757

G
Gag reflex, intubation and, 217
Gallbladder
  defined, 503
  pain associated with, 498–499
Gallstones, 498–499
Gas embolism, 797
  pathophysiology of, 798
  signs and symptoms of, 799
Gas laws, 794
Gases, poisonous, 346
Gastric lavage
  defined, 353
  procedure for, 230–231
Gastroenteritis
  defined, 636
  in pediatric patient, 612
Gastrointestinal, defined, 636
Gastrointestinal disorders in children, 621
Gastrointestinal tract
  defined, 503
  thoracic part of, 481
Gastrostomy tube, defined, 657
Gastrostomy tube/button, 648, *649*
General impression
  defined, 147
  of patient, 121
  of scene, 117–118
General Services Administration, ambulance requirements of, 726
Generic names, 259
  defined, 267
Geneva, Oath of, 27

Genital herpes in prehospital setting, 78*t*
Geriatric patients, 585–603; *see also* Elderly
  abuse of, 599–601
  anatomic and physiologic changes in, 587–591
    cardiovascular, 589–590
    dermatologic, 588
    muscular, 588
    neural, 590
    nutritional, 591
    respiratory, 588–589
    sensory, 590–591
    skeletal, 587
    in thermoregulation, 591
    in thirst response, 591
  assessment of, 592–594
    for acute illness, 595–596
    case histories, 598–599
    for environmental problems, 597–598
    for trauma, 596–597
  communication with, 594, 698
  dementia and Alzheimer's disease in, 591–592
  medications and, 594–595
  suicide of, 599
German measles in prehospital setting, 78*t*
Gerontologists, defined, 586, 602
Glands, 103–104, *104*
Glasgow Coma Scale, 217, 331–332, 331*t*, 469, 472
  defined, 333, 474, 713
  in patient care report, 704, *705*
  use of, 470, 471*t*
Glass, auto, hazards from, 768
Glottic opening, 215
  defined, 233
  in infants and children, 228
Glottis, defined, 636
Gloves, infection control and, 81–82
Glucagon
  defined, 333
  in protein metabolism, 326
Glucose
  defined, 333
  in diabetes, 326
  metabolism of, 324
  oral, 269
    action, effects, contraindications, administration, 265*t*
Glutose; *see* Glucose, oral
Glycogen
  breakdown of, 325–326
  defined, 333
Goggles, protective, 81
Golden hour, 770
  defined, 772
Gonorrhea in prehospital setting, 78*t*
Gowns, infection control and, 82
Grand mal seizure, defined, 333
Grand mal seizures, 329
Gravida, defined, 381, 394
Great vessels
  defined, 437
  trauma to, 409

Gross, Samuel, 152
Ground lift, direct, defined, 684
Growth and development, approach strategies and, *607–608*
Gunshot wounds, 428–435, *429, 431, 432, 433, 434, 435,* 483
   to chest wall/lung, 485
Gynecologic, defined, 503
Gynecologic emergencies; *see* Obstetric/gynecologic emergencies
Gynecologic organs, *500*
   pain associated with, 500
Gynecology, defined, 373, 394

H

Haemophilus influenzae B vaccine, 83
Halo sign, 465, *465*
Hand tools, defined, 772
Hazardous materials
   assessing potential for, 766
   defined, 73, 243, 772, 789
   scene size-up and, 243
Hazardous materials incidents
   EMS and, 782
   laws, regulations, training requirements, 782
Hazardous materials response; *see* HAZMAT response
Hazardous materials scene, 55–57
Hazardous materials team, interface with, 755
Hazards
   assessing for, 54
   size-up and handling, 766–767
HAZMAT, defined, 772
HAZMAT incidents, *775, 776, 777*; *see also* Emergency preparedness
HAZMAT response, 782–788
   ambulance equipment for, 788
   decontamination and management in, 787–788
   EMS and, 782
   EMT roles in, 782, 787
   legal issues, 782
HAZMAT team, 55–56, 766
Head
   anatomy of, *458,* 458–463
   compression injuries of, *413,* 413–414
   detailed physical exam of, 135
   penetrating trauma to, 433–434, *434*
   in rapid focused physical exam, with medical conditions, 135
   rapid focused physical exam of, in trauma, 127
Head injuries
   in children, 623–624
   closed, 467
      defined, 474
   defined, 40
   open, 467
      defined, 475
   in pediatric patient, 613
   symptoms of, 35, 458

Head trauma, 456–475
   anatomic considerations, 458–462
   assessment of, 467–473
      Glasgow Coma Scale in, 470
      for level of consciousness, 468–470
      for miscellaneous signs, 470–471
      in open *versus* closed injuries, 471–472
      for pupillary changes, 470
      for related medical conditions, 472
      for scalp injuries, 467–468
      for skull injuries, 468
   brain involvement in, 470–471
   deaths due to, 467, 472
   head elevation after, 468
   pathophysiologic considerations, 463–467
Headrests, positioning of, *409,* 409–410, *410*
Head-tilt chin-lift maneuver, 186–187, *187*
   defined, 210
Healing, aging changes in, 591
Health care
   definitive, defined, 4
   managed, 9
   power of attorney for, 36
   prehospital, 5
Health care delivery system
   acute care in, 8
   changes in, 8–9
   chronic care in, 8
   components of, 7–9
   defined, 18
   home care in, 8
   restorative care in, 8
Hearing, aging and, 590
Hearing loss
   characteristics of, 643–644
   classifications of, 643*t*
Heart
   aging and, 590
   anatomy and physiology of, *99, 99,* 153–156, 479, 481
   blunt trauma to, 486
   chambers of, 158
   circulation through, 483
   contusions of, 415–416, *416*
   defined, 109, 174
   penetrating trauma to, 486
Heart attack; *see also* Myocardial infarction
   risk factors for, 590
Heart failure, congestive, 165
   pathophysiology of, *296,* 297
Heart rate
   in assessment of shock, 152
   defined, 174
   during intubation, 219
   pediatric, 612
   physiology of, 293
   during pregnancy, 391
Heart valves, 156–157
   damage to, 157
Heat cramps
   assessment of, 572
   defined, 581

Heat exhaustion
   assessment of, 572
   defined, 581
Heat exposure, 571–573
   assessment of, 572
      for heat cramps, 572
      for heat exhaustion, 572
      for heatstroke, 572
   management of, 573
   signs and symptoms of, 572, *572*
Heat illness in elderly, 597–598
Heat index
   calculation of, 565*t*
   defined, 581
   effects of, 565
Heat loss
   mechanisms of, 563, *563*
   preventing, 566
Heat-related emergencies, 573, 573*t*
Heatstroke
   assessment of, 572
   defined, 581
   in elderly, 591, 597–598
Helicopters
   anatomy of, *745,* 745–746, *746*
   procedures for diving emergencies, 802
Helmets
   immobilization and, *628, 628*
   on spinal trauma patients, 520–521, *521*
Hematoma
   of brain, 471
   characteristics of, 444
   in children, 624
   defined, 455, 636
   epidural, 459–460, *462*
      defined, 474
   intracranial, 465–466
   subdural, 460, *462*
      defined, 475
Hemiparesis
   defined, 333
   stroke-associated, 327
Hemiplegia
   defined, 333
   stroke-associated, 327
Hemoglobin, 100, 295
   defined, 109, 174, 303
   oxygen binding with, 182
Hemopneumothorax
   complications of, 487
   defined, 182, *183,* 210
Hemorrhage
   from abdominal trauma, 494, 497
   from amputation, 452
   assessment of, 124, 447
   cerebral, 328
   into chest cavity, 485
   defined, 174, 455
   epidural/subarachnoid, 414
   as fracture complication, 540
   fracture-associated, 545–546
   internal, 447, *448*
   intracranial, *464,* 465
      in pediatric patient, 613

Hemorrhage—cont'd
  from intracranial hematoma, 465–466
  management of, 447
  from scalp, 463–464, 466, 467–468, *468*
  during shock, 169
  skull fractures and, 467
Hemorrhagic shock in tactical field care, 814
Hemothorax, 185, 485–486
  defined, 182, 210, 491, 636
  pathophysiology of, 278
  in pediatric patient, 613
Hepatitis A in prehospital setting, 78*t*
Hepatitis B in prehospital setting, 78*t*
Hepatitis B vaccine, 83
Herpes infection, genital, in prehospital setting, 78*t*
High-efficiency particulate air respirator, 82
  defined, 84
Hinged joint
  defined, 109
  structure and function of, 90
Hip joint, 93, *96*
  defined, 109
Histamine
  defined, 342
  effects of, 337
Hives
  cause and characteristics, 337, *339*
  defined, 342
Home care
  characteristics of, 8
  defined, 18
Homeostasis
  aging and, 586
  defined, 602
Hormones
  defined, 109
  function of, 103–104
Hospital
  communication en route to, 695–696
  EMS in, 10
Hot load, 749
  defined, 757
Huffing in respiratory emergencies, 281
Human body; *see* Body
Humerus, 93, *95*
  defined, 109
  fracture of, 549
Humidity
  body temperature and, 565, 571
  defined, 581
Hydrocephalus, *643*
  defined, 657
  in spina bifida, 642
Hymenoptera, anaphylactic reactions to, 338
Hypercarbia
  aging and, 589
  defined, 602
Hyperextension
  defined, 636
  during pediatric ventilation, 616

Hyperflexion, spinal, 425, *425*
Hyperglycemia
  defined, 325, 333
  in diabetes, 327
  signs and symptoms of, *326*
Hyperpyrexia in elderly, 597–598
Hypersensitivity, defined, 636
Hypersensitivity reaction
  allergens in, 619
  immediate, 337
Hypertension, defined, 295, 303
Hyperthermia
  defined, 562, 581
  in elderly, 591
Hyperventilation
  in acute anxiety, 361
  causes of, 277
  defined, 210, 286
  pathophysiology of, 277–278
Hypoglycemia
  defined, 325, 333
  in diabetes, 327
  signs and symptoms of, *326*
Hypoglycemics, oral, 327
  defined, 333
Hypoperfusion, defined, 160, 174
Hypopharynx
  anatomy of, 479, *480*
  defined, 491
Hypotension
  defined, 174, 296, 303
  during shock, 165, 166, 169–173
Hypothermia
  in children, 629–630, 629*t*
  defined, 562, 581, 636
  in elderly, 591, 598
  predisposing factors, 567, 569
Hypoventilation, defined, 185, 210
Hypovolemia
  defined, 636
  in pediatric patient, 612
Hypovolemic shock, 162
  defined, 636
  hypotension in, 170
  management of, 170
  in pediatric patient, 613
Hypoxia
  altered mental status due to, 330
  defined, 233, 286, 491
  signs of, 169
  supplemental oxygen in, 217
  symptoms of, 280

I

Identification bracelets, 653
Ileostomy, 649, *653*
  defined, 657
Iliac crest, 93, *95*
Illness
  assessing nature of, 120
  chronic; *see* Chronic illnesses
  nature of, defined, 147
Immediate hypersensitivity reaction, 337

Immersion
  defined, 581
  hypothermia and, 567
Immobilization
  cervical, defined, 527
  in-line, 513–514
    defined, 527
    for spinal trauma, 522–523
  of joints, 553
  for pediatric patient, *626*, 626–628, *627*
  spinal, 514–519
    ambulance equipment for, 728–729
    with long spine board, 515–517, *516*, *517*
    with short spine board, 518, *518*
    with standing patient, 518–519, *519*
Immune response in allergic reactions, 336
Immune system
  components of, 336
  defined, 342
Immunization
  mechanism of, 337
  recommendations for, 83
Immunologic conditions in special needs patient, characteristics and treatment issues, 654*t*
Immunosuppression, medication-induced, 645
Immunosuppressive, defined, 657
Impaled objects, management of, 451, *451*
Implied consent, defined, 40
Implied consent emergency doctrine, 368
Incident command system, 779
  defined, 789
Incompetent patient
  consent for, 35–36
  defined, 40
Increased intracranial pressure
  increased, 466
  in spina bifida, 643
Indications, 258
  defined, 267
Indirect force, example of, 536
Industrial incidents, rescue in, 763
Industry, EMS services in, 10
Infants; *see also* Pediatric patients
  assisted ventilation in, 193
Infection
  respiratory, 278–282
  skin as defense against, 442
  in tactical field care, 814
Infection control, 74–85
  bloodborne pathogen protection in, 78–80
  body substance isolation in, 76–77
  disease transmission and, 77, 77–78, 78*t*
  EMT protection in, 80–83
Infectious disease; *see* Communicable (infectious) disease
Inflammation
  as complication of abdominal trauma, 497
  defined, 503

Informed consent, 33–34
　defined, 40
Infrastructure, defined, 789
Inhalants, abuse of, 351–352
Inhalation, defined, 140, 147
Inhaler medications, 283–284, 283t, 284
　contraindications to, 284
　indications for, 283
　metered dose
　　defined, 286
　　indications and contraindications, 283–284
Injuries; see also Trauma
　closed
　　characteristics of, 443
　　defined, 454
　crush
　　characteristics of, 444, 444
　　defined, 455
　history of, 713
　location chart for, 706, 707
　　defined, 713
　mechanisms of, 401, 507
　open
　　characteristics of, 443
　　defined, 455
Inline drag, defined, 685
In-line immobilization, defined, 527
In-line stabilization, 513–514
Insects, anaphylactic reactions to, 338
Insertion, point of, 532
Inspiration
　diaphramatic movement during, 480
　muscles of, 183, 184
Inspired oxygen concentration, 273–274
　defined, 286
Instachar; see Charcoal, activated
Insta-Glucose; see Glucose, oral
Insulin
　defined, 333
　in diabetes, 324–325
　in glucose metabolism, 326
　secretion and function of, 324, 325–326
Insulin-dependent diabetes mellitus, 326
　defined, 333
Integumentary system
　defined, 109–110
　structure and function of, 102, 102–103
Interagency interface, 742–758; see also Communication
　aeromedical services in, 745–751
　ALS paramedics in, 744–745
　child protective services in, 751
　conflict resolution and, 755–756
　dispatcher's role in, 743–744
　elder abuse services in, 752
　first responders in, 744
　law enforcement agencies in, 752–754
　managed care organizations in, 752
　search and rescue in, 754–755
Intercept
　case study of, 756
　defined, 757

Intercostal muscles, 98, 98, 183, 184
　anatomy of, 477
　defined, 110, 210, 491
　in respiratory emergencies, 281
Internal fixation, 530
　defined, 559
Interventions
　assessment-driven, 116
　defined, 116, 147, 713
　documentation of, 702; see also Patient care report
Intervertebral disk
　defined, 527
　function of, 508, 510, 510
Intestines, 103, 103
Intoxication
　defined, 40
　informed decisions and, 34
Intracranial, defined, 636
Intracranial edema, 466–467
Intracranial hematoma, 465–466
Intracranial pressure
　defined, 474
　increased, 464, 464–465
　in spina bifida, 643
Intrathoracic pressure
　changes in, 481–482
　defined, 491
Intubation, endotracheal; see Endotracheal intubation
Ipecac, 346
Ischemia, 159–160, 163
　defined, 304, 333
　fracture-associated, 540–541
　stroke-associated, 327
　toleration of, 263
Ischium, 93, 95
　defined, 110
Islets of Langerhans, 326
　defined, 333
Isoetharine, trade names for, 283t
Isolation, body substance; see Body substance isolation

J

Jaw thrust maneuver, 187
　defined, 210
　step-by-step procedure for, 196
Joints
　anatomy of, 90, 92
　ball-and-socket, 90, 109
　defined, 110
　hinged, 90, 109
　hip, 93, 96, 109
　immobilization of, 553
　splinting, 549–550
Journals, professional, 29
Jump kit, 300, 300, 301

K

KED for spinal trauma, 523–526
Kendrick Extrication Device, 769
　defined, 772
Ketoacidosis, diabetic, 326–327

Ketogenic diet, 644–645
　defined, 657
Ketone bodies, 326
Kidney stones, 499–500
　defined, 503
Kidneys
　anatomy of, 496
　defined, 110
　pain associated with, 499–500
　structure and function of, 104, 104
　trauma to, 408–409, 411
Kinematics
　application of, 401
　defined, 437
Kinetic energy
　defined, 437
　factors affecting, 403
Kits, portable, for ambulance, 730–731
KKK ambulance standards, 726
Knee, injuries to, 408, 408, 409
Krebs cycle, 151, 159, 181
Kübler-Ross, Elisabeth, 60
Kussmaul's respirations, 331
　defined, 333
Kyphosis
　causes of, 586, 587
　defined, 602

L

Labels, drug, 263–264
Labor
　active, 381–382
　defined, 394
　stages of, 376, 376t, 378, 378–379
Lacerations
　characteristics of, 444, 445
　defined, 127, 147, 455
Laminated plate glass, defined, 772
Land warfare-diving scenario, 815
Landing zone
　defined, 757
　helicopter, 746–748, 747
Landing zone coordinator, defined, 757
Landing zone hazards, defined, 757
Langerhans, islets of, 326
　defined, 333
Large intestine, 103, 103
　defined, 110
Laryngoscope, 220, 220
　defined, 233
　for determining tube placement, 227–228
　inserting, 223, 224
Laryngoscopy during intubation, 219
Laryngotracheobronchitis
　assessment and management of, 618
　defined, 636
Larynx, 96, 181, 215, 216
　defined, 110, 210
　during intubation, 217
Latex
　allergy to, in spina bifida, 643
　items containing, 642

Law enforcement agencies
  detectives, 754
  interface with, 752–754
  officer injuries and, 754
  street patrol, 753–754
  tactical and SWAT units, 754
Leadership, defined, 245
Leaky capillary syndrome, 165
Learning, aging and, 590
Legal authority for behavioral emergencies, 368
Legal issues, 27, 31–41
  communication and, 698
  in HAZMAT response, 782
Legislation
  do-not-resuscitate, 247–248
  EMS, 5
  EMS do-not-resuscitate, defined, 252
  on hazardous materials, 243
Lethargy
  defined, 636
  in pediatric patient, 613
Leukocytes, 100, 295
  defined, 110
  types of, 158
Level of consciousness
  after head injuries, 470–471
  assessment of, 124–125, 142–144, 474
    with head injuries, 468
  cold exposure and, 566
  in diabetic patient, 327
  in elderly, 597
  with head injuries, 458
  during shock, 166, 167
Licensure, 14, 27–28
  defined, 30
Life support; see Advanced life support; Basic life support
Lifting and moving, 24, 26, 661–685
  ambulance equipment for, 727
  with direct ground lift, 681
  equipment for, 672–678
    flexible stretcher, 678, 678
    long backboard, 676, 676
    maintenance of, 678–679
    portable stretcher, 675
    scoop stretcher, 677–678
    short backboard, 677, 677
    stair chair, 675, 676
    wheeled stretcher, 672–675
  guidelines for, 664–672
    for carrying patients/equipment, 666
    for cots and stretchers, 665
    for emergency moves, 668–670
    general, 664–665
    for nonurgent moves, 670–672
    for pushing and pulling, 668
    for reaching, 668
    on stairs, 666–668
    for urgent moves, 670
  mechanics of, 664
  minimizing risk in, 663–664
  with one-person stretcher, 682
  patient positioning for, 679

Lifting and moving—cont'd
  with scoop stretcher, 683
  and time-dependent medical problems, 662–663
  transportation considerations, 680
Lifts
  direct ground, 670–671, 681
    defined, 684
  extremity, 670, 671
    defined, 684
Ligaments
  defined, 110, 437
  dislocated, 407, 407–408
  injuries to, 541–542
  structure and function of, 90, 92
Lime, burns from, 575
Lipase, defined, 503
Lithium, burns from, 575
Liver
  anatomy of, 496
  defined, 503
  laceration of, 417, 419
  trauma to, 408–409, 411
Living wills, 231, 247–248
  defined, 233, 252
Loads, aircraft, 749
LOC; see Level of consciousness
Lower extremities, bones of, 93, 96
LSD, abuse of, 351
Lumbar vertebrae, structure and function of, 92, 94
Lung volumes in elderly, 596
Lungs, 96, 98
  aging and, 589
  anatomy and physiology of, 182, 479
  circulation through, 483
  compression injuries of, 416, 416
  contusions of, 410, 485, 488
  defined, 110
  injuries to, 484–485
  overinflation of, in children, 229
  thoracic wall and, 483–484
Lysergic acid diethylamine, abuse of, 351

M

Machinery incidents, rescue in, 763
Main rotor, defined, 757
Mainstem bronchi, defined, 210
Malnutrition, defined, 636
Managed care organizations
  defined, 757
  interface with, 752
Managed health care, 9
  defined, 18–19
Mandated reports, defined, 757
Mandible, 91
  defined, 110, 527
  resorption of, 587
Manubrium, 93
  defined, 110
Marijuana, abuse of, 351
Masks
  infection control and, 82
  nonrebreather; see Nonrebreather masks

Mass casualty incident
  characteristics of, 246–247, 247
  defined, 252, 437
Mass destruction, weapons of; see Weapons of mass destruction
Materials safety data sheet, 347, 783, 785–786
  defined, 353
Maxilla, 91
  defined, 110
MCI; see Mass casualty incident
McSwain-Paturas musculoskeletal assessment system, 542
McSwain-Paturas respiratory assessment system, 280
McSwain-Paturas spinal assessment system, 513
Measles, mumps, and rubella vaccine, 83
Measles in prehospital setting, 78t
Mechanism of injury
  aeromedical transportation and, 746
  defined, 147, 757
  in musculoskeletal trauma, 536
  spinal precautions and, 507
  in spinal trauma, 510
Meconium
  defined, 394
  delivery with, 390, 390
Medevac
  versus casevac, 811
  defined, 822
Medical care
  appropriate, without interruption, 38–39
  consent for, 33–35
  refusal of, 34
Medical command authority
  with AED, 314
  defined, 321
Medical conditions, rapid focused history/ physical exam for, 133–137
Medical control
  communication with, 35–36
  contact with, 32–33
  paramedic interface and, 744–745
Medical direction
  communication with, 694–695
    six-way model, 693–694
  components of, 45–50
  defined, 52, 252, 267
  direct, 49
    defined, 51
  immediate, 48–49
    defined, 52
  off-line, 44–45, 52
  on-line, 45, 52
  for prescribed drugs, 259
  prospective, 45–48
    defined, 52
  retrospective, 49–50
Medical director, 42–52
  background of, 44
  EMT relationship with, 43–44
  involvement of, 44–45
  quality improvement and, 718

Medical history, pertinent past, 704
  defined, 714
Medical identification bracelets, 653
Medical practice acts, 43
Medical problems, time-dependent, 662–663
Medical records; *see also* Patient care report
  prehospital documentation in, 33
Medical terminology, 87–88, 88t, 89t
  defined, 110
Medications; *see also* Drugs; specific medications
  defined, 267
  elderly and, 594–595
Medicolegal issues; *see* Legal issues
Medulla, anatomy of, 462, *463*
Memory loss, 592
Meninges
  anatomy of, 459–460, *461*
  defined, 475, 621, 636
Meningitis
  in children, 621
  defined, 636
  in prehospital setting, 78t
Menopause
  characteristics of, 375
  defined, 394
Menstruation, 374–375
  defined, 394
Mental disorder, defined, 357, 371
Mental health problems
  in elderly, 593
  magnitude of, 357
Mental illness, misconceptions about, 357
Mental retardation
  characteristics and treatment issues, 654t
  defined, 657
  incidence of, 640
Mental status
  altered; *see* Altered mental status
  assessment of, 359–361
    affect in, 361
    algorithm for, 358
    interview behavior in, 359
    motor behavior in, 359
    orientation in, 360
    proficiency in, 361
    speech in, 360
    thought content in, 360
Metabolic acidosis, 163
Metabolism
  aerobic, 151
  anaerobic, 151, 153, 159, *159*, 160, 161; *see also* Shock
    body's response to, 162–165
    prevention of, 307
  chemical reactions in, 159
  defined, 95, 110, 151, 174, 275, 286, 581
  temperature regulation and, 561
Metacarpals, 93, *95*
  defined, 110

Metaproterenol
  action, effects, contraindications, administration, 265t
  trade names for, 283t
Metatarsals, 93, *96*
  defined, 110
Metered dose inhalers
  defined, 286
  indications and contraindications, 283–284
Methaqualone, abuse of, 351
Microorganisms
  defined, 84
  pathogenic, 77, 77–78
Midclavicular line
  defined, 491
  needle decompression and, 489–490, *490*
Military EMS, 806–823
  versus civilian EMS, 809, 821
  echelons of care in, 808–809
  first response in, 808
  in tactical environment, 809–815
    care plan for, 811
    casevac care in, 815
    field care in, 812–813
    under fire, 810–812
    fluid resuscitation in, 813–815
    general consideratons, 809–810
    stages of, 810–811
  triage in, 820–821
  and weapons of mass destruction, 815–820
    and biologic warfare, 816–819
    decontamination and, 819–820
    nuclear weapons, 816
Military medicine *versus* civilian medicine, 807–808
Minor
  defined, 34, 40
  rights of, 34–35
Minute ventilation, 185
Miscarriage
  defined, 394
  pathophysiology of, 379
  symptoms and care, 379t
Mnemonics
  ABC, 330–331
  ABCDE, 120–121
  AVPU, 330
  DCAP-BTLS, 126, 545
  OPQRST, 126, 298
  RISE, 226
  SAMPLE, 279, 332
  SHOCK, 167–168
  SPINE, 513
Mobile radios, defined, 699
Mobile two-way radios, 688, *689*
Monitoring, ambulance equipment for, 727
Monro-Kellie doctrine, 460, *463*
Motion
  Newton's first law of, 402, *402*, 428–429
    defined, 528
    spinal injuries and, 510
  Newton's second law of, 403–404

Motor behavior, assessment of, 359
Motor nerves, 507
  defined, 528
Motor vehicle collisions, 406–412
  head-on (frontal) impact, *406*, *407*, 407–409, *408*
  impacts caused by, 407
  lateral (side) impact, *410*, 410–412, *411*, *412*
  pedestrian injuries due to, 423–425, *424*
  rear impact, *409*, 409–410, *410*
  rollover, 412
  rotational impact, 412
  types of, 406–407
Motorcycle collisions, 421–423
  angular-impact, 421–423, *423*
  head-on, 421, *422*
Mottling
  characteristics of, 280
  defined, 286
Mouth, detailed physical exam of, 136
Mouth-to-mask ventilation, 189–190, *190*
  step-by-step procedure for, 203–204
Movement, muscle-bone interactions in, 532, 536
Moves; *see also* Lifting and moving
  emergency, 668–670
    with bent-arm drag, 670, *670*
    with blanket drag, 669–670
    with clothing drag, 669
    defined, 684
    with sheet drag, 669
  nonurgent, 670
    defined, 685
  urgent, 670
Mucous plug
  defined, 394
  function of, 376
Multiple-casualty incident, 776–782
  defined, 713, 777, 789
  documenting, 712
  response sequence in, 779
Multisystem trauma, 546
Multisystem trauma patient, defined, 559
Mumps in prehospital setting, 78t
Muscles
  agonist-antagonist pairs of, 536
  cardiac, 95, *96*
  classification of, 536
  defined, 110
  functions of, 532
  heart, 158
  injuries to, 541–542
  intercostal, 98, *98*
  involuntary, 95, *96*
    defined, 110
  movement and, 532, 536
  point of origin of, 532
  voluntary, 93, *96*, *97*
Muscular system, 93, *95*, *97*
  aging changes in, 588
  anatomy and physiology of, 532
  components of, *534–535*
Musculoskeletal system, defined, 110

Musculoskeletal trauma, 529–559
  anatomic and physiologic
      considerations, 531–532
  assessment of, 542–544
    feel component of, 543–544
    listen component of, 542–543
    look component of, 542
  EMT's responsibilities in, 530
  flow of care and, 531
  management of, 545–546
    air splint in, 551–552
    general principles, 545
    for hemorrhage, 545–546
    for interrupted blood supply,
        movement, sensation, 546
    joint immobilization in, 553
    joint splinting in, 549–550
    for life-threatening injuries, 546
    pillow splint in, 551, 557
    sling and swathe in, 548–549, 549–550
    splinting in, 545, 546, 547, 548
    traction splinting in, 550–551, 554–556
  mechanism of injury in, 536
  pathophysiology of, 536–542
  terminology pertaining to, 532, 533
Myelomeningocele
  characteristics of, 642, 642–643
  defined, 657
Myocardial infarction
  versus cardiac arrest, 296–297
  cause of, 291
  defined, 304, 321
  in elderly, 595–596
  incidence of, 307
  pathophysiology of, 296–297
  risk factors for, 590
Myocardium, 99
  contraction of, 293
  defined, 110, 304

N
Naloxone (Narcan) as poison antidote, 349
Narcotics
  abuse of, 350
  altered mental status and, 330
  overdose of, 349
Narratives, writing, 706
Nasal bone, 91
  defined, 110
Nasal cannula, pediatric, 615
Nasal flaring, 185–186
  defined, 210, 286
  in respiratory emergencies, 281, 282
Nasal prongs, 195, 195
  defined, 210
  versus nasal cannula, 195
  step-by-step procedure for, 207
Nasogastric tube
  defined, 233
  placement of, 230, 230–231, 231
Nasopharyngeal airway, 189, 189
  defined, 210
  pediatric, 615, 615, 617
  step-by-step procedure for inserting, 200

Nasotracheal intubation
  characteristics of, 218
  defined, 233
National Association of Emergency
    Medical Technicians, 29
  ambulance equipment guidelines,
      609t–611t
National Association of EMS Physicians,
    statement on pneumatic antishock
    garment, 171–172
National Fire Protection Association,
    HAZMAT guidelines of, 783, 783,
    784
National Maternal and Child Health
    Clearinghouse, 606
National Registry of Emergency Medical
    Technicians, 29
Natural disasters, 776, 777
Near-drowning
  defined, 581
  management of, 577
Nebulizers, 261
Neck
  compression injuries of, 414, 414
  detailed physical exam of, 136
  rapid focused physical exam of
    with medical conditions, 135
    in trauma, 127–128
  shear force injuries to, 415, 415
  trauma to, 409, 409–410, 410
Neck wounds, management of, 452, 452
Needle cricothyrotomy
  for children, 618
  defined, 636
Needles, contaminated, 77, 80
Neglect, defined, 631, 757
Negligence
  defined, 40
  proof of, 38
Nerve agents, characteristics of, 818
Nervous system
  aging changes in, 590
  anatomy of, 507–508
  structure and function of, 101, 101–102,
      102
Neurologic conditions in special needs
    patient, characteristics and
    treatment issues, 654t
Neuromuscular conditions in special
    needs patient, characteristics and
    treatment issues, 654t
Newborn
  APGAR scoring of, 386, 386t
  care of, 385–386
  resuscitation of, 386–387
Newton's first law of motion, 402, 402,
    428–429
  defined, 528
  spinal injuries and, 510
Newton's second law of motion, 403–404
911, 22
  enhanced, 241, 252
Ni-tro; see Nitroglycerin
Nitro-Bid; see Nitroglycerin

Nitrogard; see Nitroglycerin
Nitrogen, characteristics of, 794
Nitroglycerin, 270–271
  actions, effects, contraindications,
      administration, 258, 265t
  administration of, 298–299
  defined, 304
  indications and contraindications, 299
Nitrol; see Nitroglycerin
Nitrolingual; see Nitroglycerin
Nitrostat; see Nitroglycerin
Non-insulin-dependent diabetes mellitus,
    326
  defined, 333
Nonketotic hyperosmolar syndrome, 327
Nonrebreather masks, 195, 195–196
  defined, 210
  pediatric, 615
  during shock, 169
  step-by-step procedure for, 208
Nonurgent, defined, 685
Nonurgent moves, 670
  defined, 685
Nose, detailed physical exam of, 136
Nutrition, stress and, 70

O
Oath of Geneva, 27
Obstetric/gynecologic emergencies,
    372–396
  abnormal delivery, 387–391
    with breech presentation, 389, 389–390
    with meconium, 390
    with multiple births, 390
    with prolapsed cord, 387–388, 388
  alleged sexual assault, 391–393
  anatomic and physiologic
      considerations, 373–379
  assessment of, 381–382
  delivery, 382, 383, 384, 384–385
  management of, 382, 383, 384–391
  newborn care, 385–386
  newborn resuscitation, 386–387
  postpartum bleeding, 385, 385
  trauma during pregnancy, 390–391
Obstetrics, defined, 373, 394
Occipital, defined, 110
Occiput
  defined, 233
  during intubation, 221
Occupational Safety and Health
    Administration
  ambulance guidelines of, 726
  communicable disease guidelines of, 76
  defined, 84
  infection control guidelines of, 78–80
Off-line medical direction, 44–45
Olecranon, 93, 95
  defined, 110
One-person stretcher, defined, 685
On-line medical direction, 45
Open injuries
  characteristics of, 443
  defined, 455

Open reduction, 530
  defined, 559
OPQRST mnemonic, 126, 298
Oral hypoglycemics, 327
  defined, 333
Orbit, 91
  defined, 110
Organ death, 159
Organ donation, 39
Organic brain syndrome
  altered mental status in, 329
  cause of, 356
  defined, 371
Organizations, professional, 28–29
Organs, trauma to, 412–418
Orientation, assessment of, 125, 360
Oriented, defined, 147
Origin, point of, 532
Orogastric tube, defined, 233
Oropharyngeal airway, 188, 189
  defined, 210
  pediatric, 615, 617
  step-by-step procedure for inserting, 198–199
Oropharynx
  anatomy of, 479, 480
  defined, 491
OSHA; see Occupational Safety and Health Administration
Osmotic pressure, 157
Osteoarthritis, characteristics of, 587, 587
Osteoporosis
  characteristics of, 587
  defined, 603
Ostomy, 649, 653
  defined, 657
Ovaries, 104, 105
  anatomy/physiology of, 374
  defined, 110, 395
Overdose
  defined, 346
  narcotic, 349
  from substance abuse, 350
Oviducts
  anatomy/physiology of, 375
  defined, 395
Ovulation, defined, 374, 395
Oximeter, pulse, 186
Oxygen, 271
  action, effects, contraindications, administration, 265t
  administration of, 260, 261
    for shock, 168–169
  ambulance equipment for, 728
  hemoglobin binding with, 182
  metabolism of, 81
  supplemental, 194–196
    equipment for, 194, 194
    with nasal prongs, 195, 195
    with nonrebreather mask, 165, 195, 195–196, 208
Oxygen concentration, inspired, 273–274
Oxygen deprivation, effects on brain, 309

Oxygen regulator, step-by-step procedure for applying to tank, 201
Oxygen tank
  applying regulator to, 201
  turning on, 202
Oxygenation, 180–181
  defined, 491
  injuries affecting, 477
  optimal, 186
  during shock, 163–165, 169

P

Pacing, 310
  defined, 321
Pain
  abdominal, 497–498
  assessment of, 297
  chest; see Chest pain
  gynecologic, 500
  from musculoskeletal injuries, 544
  renal, 499–500
  in spinal assessment, 512
Pain control in pediatric patient, 633
Palm rule, 443
  defined, 455
Palpation, 127
  for assessing blood pressure, 141
  defined, 147
Pancreas
  anatomy of, 496, 496
  defined, 333, 503
  divisions of, 499
  insulin secretion by, 326
  pain associated with, 499
Para, defined, 381, 395
Parachute insertion casualty, 814
Paradoxical motion, 128–129, 483, 484
  defined, 147, 491
Paralysis
  defined, 333, 620, 636
  from musculoskeletal injuries, 543
  in spinal trauma, 512
  stroke-associated, 327
Paramedics; see also Emergency medical technician-Paramedic
  interagency interface and, 744–745
Paranoia, characteristics and management, 365–366
Paraplegia, defined, 511, 528, 657
Paraspinal muscles, 494
  defined, 503
Parasympathetic nervous system
  defined, 110
  function of, 507
  structure and function of, 101, 101
Paresthesia
  defined, 286, 333, 636
  in hyperventilation, 277
  from musculoskeletal injuries, 543
  stroke-associated, 327
Parietal, defined, 110
Parietal pleura, 98, 98
  defined, 110
PASG; see Pneumatic antishock garment

Patella, 93, 96
  defined, 110
  percussion of, 543
Pathogens
  airborne, defined, 84
  bloodborne, 76, 77
    defined, 84
  protection guidelines, 78–80
Patient
  accessing
    defined, 772
    in rescue operations, 764
    at rescue scene, 768
  advocacy for, 26
  assessment of, 24
  calming, 121
  communication with, 23–24
  general impression of, 121
  geriatric; see Geriatric patients
  incompetent
    consent and, 35–36
    defined, 40
  interactions with, 245–246
  lifting and moving; see Lifting and moving
  pediatric; see Pediatric patients
  priority, 121, 125
  safety of, 24
  special needs; see Special needs patient
  transfer of, 26
  transportation of, 24, 26
  unconscious, tongue in, 217
Patient advocacy, defined, 30
Patient care report, 702–711, 703
  completing, 703–711
    general guidelines for, 704, 706
    writing narrative for, 706, 709–710
  corrections to, 710
  defined, 714
  use of, 703
Patient data, defined, 714
Patient monitoring equipment, 727
Patient positioning, 679
Patient rights
  to appropriate care, 38–39
  to care without interruption, 38
  minor, 34–35
Pedestrians, injuries to, 423–425, 424
Pediatric patients, 604–637; see also Child abuse; Children
  abuse of, 630–632
  age classification for, 606
  approaching, 607
  assessment/management of emergencies in, 618–622
    asthma, 618–619
    bronchiolitis, 619
    croup, 618
    dehydration, 621–622, 622t
    epiglottitis, 618
    meningitis, 621
    seizures/epilepsy, 619–620
  basic airway and respiratory adjuncts for, 615–617

Pediatric patients—cont'd
  Basic Life Support for, 614
  developmental stages and approach strategies, 607t, 608
  EMS for, 606
  epidemiology of, 605–606
  general considerations, 633–634
  normal vital sign ranges for, 607, 611, 611t
  pain control in, 633
  pathophysiology in, 612–613
  poisoning in, 630
  resuscitation of, 617
  with special needs, 632–633
  sudden infant death syndrome and, 632
  trauma in, 622–630
    assessment of, 623
    of chest/abdomen, 628
    head, 623–624
    hypothermia, 629–630
    immobilization devices for, 626–628
    prevention of, 622
    spinal, 624–626
    unique characteristics of, 622–623
Pediatric trauma score, 706
  defined, 714
Pedicle
  defined, 437
  trauma to, 417, 419
Pedi-Immobilizer, 769
  defined, 772
Pelvis
  detailed physical exam of, 137
  injuries of, 418
  in rapid focused physical exam, with medical conditions, 135
  rapid focused physical exam of, in trauma, 131–132
  structure of, 93, 95
  trauma to, 410–411
Penetrating trauma, 428–437
  to abdomen, 434–435
  blood volume after, 167
  versus blunt trauma, 413
  of chest, 448
  to chest all, 484
  damage from, 429–430, 430, 431, 432
  defined, 175, 437
  effects of distance on, 431
  in entrance versus exit wounds, 431–433, 432, 433
  to extremities, 435, 435
  to frontal area, 429
  to head, 433–434, 434
  from high-energy weapons, 430–432, 432
  from low-energy weapons, 429–430
  from medium-energy weapons, 430, 431
  summary of, 435
  to thorax, 434, 435

Penetrating wounds
  characteristics of, 445, 446
  defined, 455
Perfusion
  assessment and intervention, 123
  decreased, in children, 624
  defined, 101, 110, 147, 160, 175, 297, 304, 636
  indicators of, 167
  preservation of, during shock, 168
Pericardial sac, 481
Pericardial tamponade, 541
Pericardium, 99
  defined, 110
Perineum
  anatomy of, 375, 376
  defined, 395
Peripheral nervous system
  components of, 507
  defined, 110, 528
  structure and function of, 101, 101
Periphery, defined, 175
Peristalsis during pregnancy, 391
Peritoneum, 107, 496, 496
  defined, 110, 503
Peritonitis
  after abdominal trauma, 497, 498
  defined, 503
Permanent vegetative state, defined, 309, 321
Personal protection, 80–83
  defined, 84
Personal protective equipment, 246
Personal stressors, 66
Personnel
  ambulance, 731
  in landing zone, 750
Pertinent negatives, 704
  defined, 714
Pertinent positives, 704
  defined, 714
Petit mal seizure, 329
  defined, 333
Phalanges, 93, 96
  defined, 110
Pharmacology, 257–271; see also Drugs; Medications; specific drugs
  defined, 258, 267
Pharyngeal-tracheal lumen, 227–228
Pharynx, 96
  anatomy and physiology of, 181, 181
  defined, 110, 210
  lateral view, 180
Phencyclidine, abuse of, 351
Phenol, burns from, 575
Phenothiazines, indications and trade names for, 363t
Phobia, characteristics and management, 362
Phosgene, characteristics of, 818
Physical abuse, defined, 631

Physical assessment, defined, 714
Physical disabilities, 640–644; see also Special needs
  assessment of, 649
  causes of, 640–641
  cerebral palsy, 641
  defined, 657
  hearing impairment, 643–644
  spina bifida, 642–643
  spinal cord injuries, 643
  visual impairment, 643
Physical examination; see also Detailed physical examination; Rapid focused physical examination
  during assessment, 117
Physician; see also Medical director
  on scene, 244
Physician extenders, 43
  defined, 52
Physician notes, 45
Pia mater, 459, 461
  defined, 475
Pillow splints, 551, 557
Pilot balloon, 220
  defined, 233
Placenta
  anatomy/physiology of, 375
  defined, 395
  delivery of, 385, 385
Placenta previa
  bleeding due to, 380
  defined, 395
  symptoms and care, 379t
Plan of action, 117–118
Plasma, 100, 158, 295
  defined, 110, 304
Plate glass, hazards from, 768
Platelets, 100, 295
  defined, 110, 304
  function of, 158
Pleurae, 98, 98, 182, 481
  defined, 210
Pleural space, 182, 481
  air accumulation in, 484
  defined, 210
Pneumatic antishock garment
  application of, 172
  for controlling bleeding, 452
  defined, 175, 455
  National Association of EMS Physicians on, 170–172
  recommendations for, 170–172
Pneumonia
  defined, 287
  in elderly, 598
  pathophysiology of, 278
Pneumothorax, 185
  characteristics of, 484
  collision-related, 410
  defined, 182, 210, 437, 491
  management of, 488–489
  open, 489
    defined, 491

Pneumothorax—cont'd
  pathophysiology of, 278
  tension; see Tension pneumothorax
Point of insertion, 532
Point of origin, 532
Poison control centers, 344–345
  for burn information, 575
  defined, 353
Poisoning; see also Toxic emergencies
  ambulance supplies for, 730
  anatomic and physiologic
      considerations, 345–346
  antidotes for, 344
  assessment of, 346–348
    with physical exam, 348
    with SAMPLE history, 347–348
    at scene, 347
  of children, 630
  defined, 344, 353
  incidence of, 344
  injury pyramid for, 344
  management of, 348–350
    for absorbed poisons, 349
    for ingested poisons, 348–349
    for inhaled poisons, 349
    for injected poisons, 349
Poisons
  absorption of, 346
    dermal, 346
    ocular, 346
  defined, 630
  information on, at scene, 346
  ingestion of, 345, 345–346
  inhalation of, 346
  injection of, 346
Police officers; see also Law enforcement
      agencies
  interface with, 754
Polio vaccine, 83
Polyuria
  defined, 333
  in diabetic patient, 326
Portable chambers for diving emergencies, 803
Positioning, anatomic, 530
  defined, 559
Postcrash phase, 401–402
  defined, 437
Postictal state, 329
  defined, 333, 620, 636
Posttraumatic stress disorder,
      characteristics of, 67
Posture, deviated, in respiratory
      emergencies, 281
Posturing
  decerebrate, 471
    defined, 474
  decorticate, 471
    defined, 474
Power of attorney, 36
  durable, 247
    defined, 40, 252
    procedures pertaining to, 248–249

Practice, scope of, 37–38
Precautions, universal, 55
Precrash phase, 401–402
  defined, 437
Prefixes, 88, 88t
  defined, 110
Pregnancy
  bleeding during, 379–380, 379t
  seizures during, 380
  structures of, 375–376
  trauma during, 390–391
  tubal, 375
    defined, 395
  vaginal bleeding during, 391
Prehospital care, 5
  defined, 19
Prehospital care report
  defined, 252
  function of, 250
Prehospital setting
  diseases encountered in, 78t
  protective equipment recommendations
      for, 76t
Prehospital Trauma Life Support, 809
Preoxygenation
  defined, 218, 218, 233
  for intubation, 222
  recommendations for, 219
Preplanning, 777–779
  activities in, 777–778
  exercises for, 778–779
Prescriptions, drug, 263–264
Presenting part, defined, 395
Pressure
  atmosphere of, 793
  effects on scuba divers, 796–797
Primary care provider, defined, 19
Priorities
  assessing, 121
  determining, 125
Products of conception, 379
Professional organizations, 28–29
Proficiency, assessment of, 361
Prolapsed cord, defined, 395
Prospective evaluation, defined, 723
Protective equipment, 80–83, 81
  defined, 84
Protocols, 21
  in cardiovascular emergencies, 301
  defined, 267
  drug, 265
  and family of injured patient, 61
  types of, 46–47
Proventil; see Albuterol
Proximal versus cephalad, 483
Pseudoaneurysm from shear force injury,
      416, 416, 417
Psychiatric disorders, medications for, 363t
Psychogenic, defined, 356, 371
Psychogenic shock, 162
Psychologic emergencies,
      primary/secondary, 361–367
  acute anxiety, 361–362

Psychologic emergencies, primary/
      secondary—cont'd
  Alzheimer's disease, 367
  depression, 363–364
  disorientation/disorganization, 366–367
  paranoia, 365–366
  phobia, 362
  suicide, 364–365
Psychosocial stressors, 66
PTSD; see Posttraumatic stress disorder
Pubis, 93, 95
  defined, 110
Public access, 691–692
  by enhanced 911, 692
  by 911, 691–692, 692
  by seven-digit access number, 691
Public third service, characteristics
      of, 10
Pulling, guidelines for, 668
Pulmonary arteries, 100, 100, 157,
      183, 183, 291, 292
  defined, 110, 175, 210, 304
Pulmonary circulation, 155, 156
Pulmonary contusions, 410
  defined, 437
Pulmonary edema
  chemical agents causing, 818
  in congestive heart failure, 297
  defined, 287, 304
  pathophysiology of, 278
Pulmonary embolism
  defined, 287
  pathophysiology of, 278
Pulmonary veins, 100, 100, 157, 183, 291, 292
  defined, 110, 175, 210, 304
Pulse
  absence of, with musculoskeletal
      injuries, 543–544
  assessment of, 123–124, 138–140, 159
  bounding, defined, 147
  brachial, defined, 174
  characteristics and assessment, 295
  defined, 147, 175, 304
  full, defined, 147
  identifying/locating, 138, 138
  interventions for, 123–124
  locations for assessing, 158
  marking site of, 545
  procedure for, 138, 138–139, 139
  rate, character, and rhythm of, 138
  during shock, 166
  thready, 166
    defined, 148
Pulse character, defined, 147
Pulse oximeter, 186
Pulse point pressure
  for controlling bleeding, 453
  defined, 175
Pulse pressure, 296
  assessing, 141
  characteristics and assessment, 295
  defined, 147, 304

Pulse rate, 156
  defined, 147
Pulse rhythm, defined, 147
Pulselessness from musculoskeletal injuries, 543–544, 550
Puncture wounds
  characteristics of, 445, *446*
  defined, 455
Pupils, assessment of, 144, *144*, 466
  with head injuries, 470
Pushing, guidelines for, 668

Q
QRS complex, height of, 312–313, *313*
Quadriplegia, defined, 511, 528, 657
Quality, defined, 210
Quality assurance, 22, 49, 717–718
  defined, 717, 723
  EMT's role in, *720–721*, 722
Quality improvement, 22, 715–723
  assessment of, 718–719
    with concurrent evaluation, 718–719
    with prospective evaluation tools, 718
    with retrospective evaluation, 719
  continuous, defined, 723
  defined, 30
  loop for, 719, *719*
  versus quality assurance, 717
  theories of, 715
  trackable, 717

R
Raccoon's eyes, 127
  after skull injuries, 468, *469*
  defined, 475
Radial artery, 100, *100*
  anatomy of, 291–292
  defined, 110, 147, 175, 304
Radial pulse
  assessing, 139, *139*, 159
  defined, 175
Radiation
  defined, 581
  as heat loss mechanism, 563
Radio
  digital equipment for, 690
  mobile, defined, 699
  mobile two-way, 688, *689*
Radio communication, 23
Radio equipment, digital, defined, 699
Radio frequencies, 689–690
Radius, 93, *95*
  defined, 110
Railroads, response route and, 735
Rales
  characteristics of, 184
  defined, 210, 287
  in respiratory emergencies, 282
Rape, alleged, 391–393
Rapid extrication, 519–520
Rapid focused history
  components of, 126
  defined, 147

Rapid focused history—cont'd
  with medical conditions, 133
  with trauma, 127–133
Rapid focused physical examination
  defined, 147
  indications for, 126–127
  with medical conditions, 133–135
  with trauma, 127–133
    back in, 132
    baseline vital signs in, 132–133
    chest in, 128–131
    extremities in, 132
    head in, 127
    neck in, 127–128
    pelvis in, 131–132
Rate, defined, 211
Reaching, guidelines for, 668
Reactive airway disease
  in children, 618–619
  riot control agents and, 819
Recompression chamber
  defined, 804
  for diving emergencies, 803
Record keeping, 26
Recovery position, defined, 685
Rectus abdominis muscle, 494
  defined, 503
Red blood cells, 100, 295
  defined, 304
  production and function of, 158
Reduction, open, 530
  defined, 559
Refilling time, 160
Refusal of care, 34
  defined, 40
  documenting, 711–712, *712*
  patient comptency and, 35
  right to, defined, 40
Remediation
  defined, 723
  quality assurance and, 722
Renal failure
  defined, 636
  from dehydration, 621
Renal stones, 499–500
  defined, 503
Renal system, structure and function of, 104, *104*
Repeaters, 688–689, *689*
  defined, 699
Reperfusion syndrome, 161
Reportable incidents, 712
Reports; *see also* Documentation; Patient care report
  accident, 738
  computer-based, 703, *704*
    defined, 713
  mandated, defined, 757
  written, 703, *703*
    defined, 714
Reproductive system, 104–105, *105*
  female, 373–379, *374*
    pain associated with, 500

Rescue action plan, defined, 772
Rescue operations
  action plan for, 764–765
  for building collapse, 762–763
  for confined spaces, 763
  for low angle/high angle situations, 763
  in machinery/industrial incidents, 763
  for trench/excavation collapse, 763
  types of, 762–764
  in vehicle incidents, 763–764
  for vehicle rescue incidents, 765–770; *see also* Vehicle rescue incidents
  in water, 577, 763
  in wilderness, 763
Rescue scene, 58–59
Rescue tools, 731
Research, EMS, 16–17
Respiration
  versus breathing, 122
  defined, 148, 273–274, 482
  versus ventilation, 273–274
Respirator, high-efficiency particulate air, 82
  defined, 84
Respiratory alkalosis
  defined, 287
  hyperventilation and, 277
Respiratory conditions in special needs patient, characteristics and treatment issues, 654t
Respiratory depth, 98
  defined, 110
Respiratory distress, 273
  assessment algorithm, 274
Respiratory distress syndrome, acute, 165
Respiratory emergencies, 272–287
  asthma, 276–277
  chronic obstructive pulmonary disease, 275–276, *276*
  color in, 280
  deaths due to, 273
  general care in, 282–283
  hyperventilation, 277–278
  in infants and children, 274, *282*, 284–285
  infections, 278
  McSwain-Paturas assessment of, 280
  pathophysiology of, 275–278
  pneumothorax/hemothorax, 278
  pulmonary edema, 278
  pulmonary embolism, 278
Respiratory infection, pathophysiology of, 278–282
Respiratory quality, defined, 110
Respiratory rate
  versus respiratory rate, 482
  versus ventilatory rate, 180
Respiratory rhythm, defined, 110
Respiratory status in pediatric patients, 612
Respiratory system, 95–96, *97*, *98*, 98–99
  aging changes in, 588–589
  anatomy and physiology of, 180–184, *181*, *182*, *183*, *184*

Respiratory system—cont'd
    functions of, 180–181
    physiology of, 275, *275*
Respond request, defined, 757
Response route, planning, 735
Restorative care, characteristics of, 8
Restraints
    automobile, 418–421, *420*
    with behavioral emergencies, 368–369
    defined, 40
    orders for, 35
Resuscitation
    after cold water submersion, 578
    ambulance supplies for, 727
    dilemmas in, 236–237
    equipment for, infection control and, 82
    fluid, in military EMS, 813–815
    Intiation/termination decisions, 247–248
    newborn, 386–387
    pediatric, 617
Resuscitation not indicated
    defined, 252
    legislation for, 248
Resuscitators, automatic, 728
Retractions
    assessing, 135
    characteristics of, 186
    defined, 148, 211, 287
    in respiratory emergencies, 281, *282*
Retroperitoneal space, 107, 496, *496*
    defined, 110, 503
Retrospective evaluation, defined, 723
Revenue; *see* Financing
Revised trauma score, 706
    defined, 714
Rhythm, defined, 211
Ribs, 92–93
    anatomy of, 477, 479
    cavitation phenomenon and, 405
    defined, 110, 437
    fractured, 487–488
Right to refusal, defined, 40
Riot control agents, 818–819
    summary of, 819
RISE mnemonic, 226
Risk, minimizing, 663–664
Risk assessment
    defined, 789
    process of, 778
Rollovers, 412, *412*
Root words, 87–88, 88*t*
    defined, 110
Rotor wash, 747
    defined, 757
Rotors, types of, 745, *745*
Rotor-wing aircraft, 745
    defined, 757
Route of administration, 258
    defined, 267
Rubella in prehospital setting, 78*t*
Rubeola in prehospital setting, 78*t*

Rule of nines, 443, *443*, 574, *575*
    defined, 455, 581
Run data, defined, 714

S

Safety
    with AED, 315
    aircraft, 748–749, *749*, *750*
    assessing, at scene, 118–119
    of crew, patient, bystanders, 24
    driving, 735–736
    following distance and, 736
    at HAZMAT scene, 783, 787
    personal, 24
    scene size-up and, 236
    substance abusing client and, 352
    transportation, 26
Safety glass, tempered, defined, 772
Safety seats, child, 626–627
SAMPLE history, 126, 144–145, 279
    for allergic reactions, 338–339
    for assessing altered mental status, 332
    defined, 148
    for poisoning, 347–348
    in rapid focused history, of medical conditions, 133
Scalp
    anatomy of, 459
    assessment of, 467–468
    pathophysiology of, 463–464
Scapula, 93, *95*
    defined, 111
Scene; *see also* Accident scene; Crime scene; Hazardous materials scene; Rescue scene; Trauma scene; Violent scene
    ambulance arrival at, 738
    assessment of, 116–117
        algorithm for, 75
    crime, 59–60
    hazardous materials, 55–57
    HAZMAT, 783, 787
    physician on, 244
    rescue, 58–59
    size-up of, defined, 148
    survey of, 118–120
        body substance isolation precautions and, 119
        and call for additional help, 120
        for mechanism of injury, 120
        for nature of illness, 120
        for number of patients, 120
        for safety, 118–119
        triage in, 120
    violent, 59
Scene size-up, 235–253
    algorithm for, 237
    bioethical considerations, 247–249
    compassion and, 246
    effective communication and, 245
    for environmental emergencies, 566
    information gathering and, 243
    with mass casualty incidents, 246–247

Scene size-up—cont'd
    patient interaction and, 245–246
    safety and, 236, 243
    scene control and, 244–245
    and taking command of scene, 245
    transportation considerations, 249
    at trauma scene, 244
School buses, response route and, 736
Scoop stretcher, 677–678, 682
Scope of practice, 37–38
    defined, 40
Scuba, defined, 804
Scuba diving
    courses in, 792–793
    gas laws and, 794
Scuba diving accidents, 792–793
    carbon monoxide poisoning and, 796
    decompression sickness and, 797
    and secondary effects of pressure, 796–797
Search and rescue
    defined, 757
    interface with, 754–755
    wilderness medicine and, 755
Seat belt sign, 496
Seat belts, 418–421, *420*
Seesaw breathing, 186, 281, *282*
Seizures
    absence, 620
    altered mental status from, 329
    characteristics of, 644–645, 645*t*
    in children, 619–620
    convulsive, 620
    defined, 619, 636
    febrile, 329
    generalized, 329
    management of, 329
    partial, 329
    postictal state after, 329
    during pregnancy, 380
Selective serotonin reuptake inhibitors, indications and trade names for, 363*t*
Sellick maneuver, 192
    defined, 211, 233
    during intubation, 225
Semiconscious, defining, 469
Semilunar valve, 156
    defined, 175
Senescence, 586; *see also* Aging
    defined, 603
Senile dementia, 592
Senility, altered mental status and, 329
Sensory nerves, 507
    defined, 528
Sensory system, aging changes in, 590–591
Sepsis
    defined, 636
    in pediatric patient, 613
Septic shock, 162
    defined, 636
    in pediatric patient, 613
Serosa, 481

Sexual abuse, defined, 631
Sexual assault, alleged, 391–393
Sexually transmitted diseases in prehospital setting, 78t
Shear, defined, 437
Shear force, 412–413
Shear force injuries
  abdominal, 417, *417*, 419
  of head, 414, *414*
  of neck, 415, *415*
  thoracic, 416, *416*
  of thorax, 416, *416*, 417
Sheet drag, 669
  defined, 685
Shock, 101, 150–176; *see also* Metabolism, anaerobic
  ambulance equipment for, 729
  anaphylactic, 162
  anatomic and physiologic considerations, 153–159
  assessment of, 165–167
  blood loss and, 165
  body fluid reaction in, 157
  cardiogenic, 162
  causes of, 151, 161
    determining, 168
  compensated, 160
  defined, 152, 175, 297, 304
  hemorrhagic, in tactical field care, 814
  hypothermia and, 567
  hypovolemic, 162
  irreversible, 161
  management of, 167–173
    mnemonic for, 167–168
    steps in, 168–173
  pathophysiology of, 159–165
  in pediatric patient, 612–613
  phases of, 161, *161*
  progression of, 160–161
  psychogenic, 162
  septic, 162
  signs of, 163, *165*, 165–167
  symptoms of, 167
  uncompensated, 160–161
SHOCK mnemonic, 167–168, *168*
Shortness of breath, 273; *see also* Dyspnea
Side effects, 258
  defined, 267
SIDS; *see* Sudden infant death syndrome
Signs
  defined, 148
  versus symptoms, 137–138
Sinus rhythm, normal, 293, *294*, *312*
Six-way communications model, defined, 700
Size-up, defined, 772
Skeletal integrity, loss of, 531
  defined, 559
Skeletal system
  aging changes in, 587
  anatomy and physiology of, 531–532
Skeleton
  components of, *533*
  defined, 111

Ski patrols, interface with, 755
Skin; *see also* Integumentary system
  aging changes in, 588
  anatomy and physiology of, 441–443, *443*
  in body temperature control, 446
  color and temperature of, 142
  diaphoretic, 166, 186
    in cardiovascular emergencies, 298
  exposure to poisons, 346
  fluid balance and, 446
  during shock, 166
Skull
  assessment of, 468
  bones of, 463
  compartment syndrome of, 540
  compression injuries of, *413*, 413–414
  defined, 111
  fractures of, 467, 468
  pathophysiology of, 467
  structure and function of, 91, *93*
  structure of, 106
Slide, diagonal, 515–516
Sling and swathe technique, 548–549, *549–550*
Small intestine, 103, *103*
  defined, 111, 503
  infection of, 497
Smooth muscle, 536
  defined, 559
Sniffing position, 222, *222*
  defined, 233
SOAP method, 706, 709–710
  defined, 714
Social service agency, defined, 757
Soda ash, burns from, 575
Soft tissue injuries, 438–455
  anatomic and physiologic considerations, 441–443
  assessment of, 447–448
    for hemorrhage, 447, *448*
    initial, 447
    by type, 447–448
  closed, 443–444, *444*
  hemorrhage from, 445–446
  management of, 448–452
    for amputations, 451
    with bandages and dressings, 448–449, *449*
    for closed injuries, 450
    for evisceration, *450*, 451
    for impaled objects, 451, *451*
    initial, 450
    for neck wounds, 452, *452*
    for open chest wounds, 450, *451*
    for open injuries, 450
  miscellaneous consequences of, 446–447
  open, *444*, 444–445, *445*, 446
  pathophysiology of, 443–447
  and underlying injuries, 440–441
Somatic nervous system
  defined, 528
  function of, 507
Spaces, confined, 763

Special needs; *see also* Disabilities
  assessment of, 648–652
  cerebral palsy, 641
  chronic illnesses, 644
  defined, 640, 657
  developmental disabilities, 640
  EMT-B considerations, 655
  family considerations, 655
  health conditions related to, 654t
  hearing impairment, 643–644
  information form for, 650–652
  management of, 652–655
  pathophysiology of, 640–648
  physical disabilities, 640–641
  reactive airways disease, 644
  seizures/epilepsy, 644–645, 645t
  spina bifida, 642–643
  spinal cord injuries, 643
  technologic aids for, 645–648, *646*, *647*, 647t, *648*
  transplant recipients, 645
Special needs patient, 638–658
  communication with, 697–698
    children, 698
    elderly, 698
    hearing- or speech-impaired, 697
    non-English-speaking, 697–698
  defined, 252
Speech, assessment of, 360
Sphygmomanometer, 158–159
  defined, 148, 175
  use of, 141
Spina bifida, characteristics of, *642*, 642–643
Spinal column
  bones of, 508
  defined, 528
  structure and function of, 92, *94*
Spinal cord trauma, 483
  characteristics of, 643
Spinal curvature, aging and, 589, *589*
Spinal immobilization, ambulance equipment for, 729
Spinal shock, 162
Spinal trauma, 504–528
  above clavicles, 511, *512*
  assessment of, 511–512
    algorithm for, 506
    with McSwain-Paturas system, 513
  in children, 624–626
    assessment of, 625
    causes of, 624
    immobilization devices for, *626*, 626–628, *627*
    management of, 625–626
  from compression fractures, 510–511
  from distraction injuries, 511
  from flexion and extension injuries, 510–511
  from lateral bending, 510
  management of, 513–514
    with cervical collar, 514
    in infants and children, 521
    with in-line immobilization, 522–523

Spinal trauma—cont'd
  management of—cont'd
    with in-line stabilization, 513–514
    with KED, 523–526
    with long spine board, 514, 515–517, *516, 517*
    for patients with helmets, 520–521, *521*
    with rapid extrication, 519–520
    with short spine board, 518, *518*
    skills for, 514–522
    with standing patient, 518–519, *519*
  mechanism of injury in, 510
  nervous system and, 507–508
  during pregnancy, 391, *391*
  signs and symptoms of, 512
Spine
  anatomy of, 508, *509*, 510
  pathophysiology of, 510–511
  trauma to, 408–409, *410*
Spine boards
  long, 515–517, *516*
    defined, 527
  short, 518, *518*
    defined, 528
SPINE mnemonic, 513
Spleen
  anatomy of, 496
  trauma to, 408–409, *411*
Splinting
  complications of, 545
  general guidelines for, 545, *546*
  of joints, 549–550
  with long bone splint, 546, *547*, *548*
  traction, 550–551, *551*, 554–556
Splints, *546*
  air, 551–552, *552*
  improvised, 548, *549*
  measuring for, 548
  pillow, 551, *557*
Sports injuries, 426–427, *427*
Sprain
  of ankle, *537*
  characteristics of, 542, *543*
  defined, 559
Squeeze injuries, 795
Stab wounds, *428*, 429–430, *434*
Stabilization
  defined, 4, 19, 772
  in-line, 513–514
    defined, 527
  open reduction and internal fixation and, 530
  at rescue scene, 767
Staff, communication with, 696–697
Stair chair, 675, *676*
Stairs, carrying on, 666–668, *667*
Standard of care for behavioral emergencies, 368
Standard of practice, defined, 40
Standard precautions; *see* Body substance isolation
Stand-by request, defined, 757

Standing orders, 265
  characteristics of, 47
  defined, 52, 267
Status asthmaticus
  in children, 619
  defined, 636
Status epilepticus, 329
  in children, 620
  defined, 333, 636
Step chocks, 767, *768*
  defined, 772
Sternum, 93, 477
  defined, 111, 491
Stethoscope, 141, *142*
  defined, 148
Stings
  assessment of, 578–579
  examples of, *579*
  management of, 579
Stoma, 192–193
  defined, 211
Stomach
  defined, 503
  leakage of contents of, 497
Stopping distance, 403
  defined, 437
Strain
  characteristics of, 541, *542*
  defined, 559
Stress, 65–71
  acute, 67
  alleviating, 69–71
  attitudes and, 70
  burnout and, 67–68
  categories of, 65
  chronic/cumulative, 66–67
  corrective action for, 68t
  debriefing and, 68–69
  defined, 65, 73
  dietary factors in, 70
  environmental, 66
  personal, 66
  posttraumatic, 67
  psychosocial, 66
  symptoms not requiring immediate action, 68t
  warning signals of, 67
Stressors, defined, 73
Stretchers
  defined, 685
  flexible, 678
    defined, 685
  lifting, 665, *665*, *666*
  one-person, 672, 682
    defined, 685
    loading from ambulance, 675
    loading into ambulance, 674
  portable, 675, *675*
    defined, 685
  scoop, 677–678, 682
  two-person, 672
    loading from ambulance, *674*, 674–675
    loading into ambulance, 673

Stretchers—cont'd
  wheeled, 672–673, *673*
    moving guidelines, 673
Striations
  defined, 559
  function of, 536
Stridor
  defined, 287, 342, 636
  in pediatric patient, 614
  in respiratory emergencies, 282
Stroke, altered mental status in, 327–329
Stroke volume, 156
Stuporous, defining, 469
Stylet, 221, *221*
  defined, 233
Subarachnoid space, 460
Subcutaneous tissue
  characteristics of, 441
  defined, 111, 455
  structure and function of, 103
Subdural hematoma, 460, *462*
  defined, 475
Sublingually, defined, 304
Submersion
  cold water, 577–578
  defined, 581
  hypothermia and, 567
Subscription systems, 11
Subsidies, EMS, 11
Substance abuse, 350–352
  with alcohol, 352
  with amphetamines, 351
  with barbiturates, 350
  with benzodiazepines, 350
  with cannabis, 351
  with cocaine, 351
  with inhalants, 351–352
  with lysergic acid diethylamine, 351
  management of, 352–353
  with methaqualone, 351
  with narcotics, 350
  with phencyclidine, 351
Suction equipment
  for ambulance, 728
  pediatric, 615–616
Suctioning
  for airway obstruction, 187–188
  endotracheal, 229
  step-by-step procedure for, 197
Sudden cardiac death, 307–310
  incidence of, 307
  risk factors for, 309
Sudden infant death syndrome, 632
Suffixes, 88, 88t
  defined, 111
Suicide
  assessing risk of, 364–365
  characteristics and management, 364–365
  depression and, 363, 364
  in elderly, 599
Supplies; *see also* Equipment
  airway, 727
  ambulance, 726–727
  resuscitation, 727

Surface area, energy exchange and, 406
Surrogate consent, 36–37
  defined, 40
Survival, chain of, 289, 300–301
  defined, 303
Sutures, 459
  defined, 475
SWAT unit
  defined, 757
  interface with, 754
Sweating, inadequate breathing and, 186
Swelling, 536–537, 537; see also Edema
  assessing, 131
  from musculoskeletal injuries, 542, 543
  reducing, 548
Swimmer casualties, combat, 815
SWIMS, defined, 822
Sympathetic nervous system
  defined, 111
  function of, 507–508
  structure and function of, 101, 101
Symptoms
  defined, 148
  versus signs, 137–138
Syncope
  defined, 603
  in elderly, 596
  in myocardial infarction, 595
Syphilis in prehospital setting, 78t
Systemic circulation, 155, 156
Systems status management
  characteristics of, 693
  defined, 699
Systole, 154
Systolic pressure, 100, 159
  assessing, 141
  characteristics and assessment, 295
  defined, 111, 148, 175, 304
  during shock, 164
  in trauma patient, 486

T
Tachycardia
  in children, 621
  defined, 148, 293, 304, 636
  ventricular
    defined, 304
    pathophysiology of, 294, 295
Tachypnea
  causes of, 277–278
  defined, 287
Tactical environment, emergent care in, 809–815
Tactical field care, 811, 812–813
Tactical unit
  defined, 758
  interface with, 754
Tail rotor, 745, 745
  defined, 758
TAP; *see* Technical Assistance Program
Tarsals, 93, 96
  defined, 111
Team building, 24
Technical Assistance Program, 7

Technology, challenges of, 17
Telemetry, 690, 690
  defined, 700
Telephones, cellular, 690
Temperature; *see also* Body temperature
  ambient, 565
    defined, 580
Temporal, defined, 111
Tendons, 93, 95, 97
  defined, 111, 437
  dislocated, 407, 407–408
  function of, 532
  injuries to, 541–542
Tension pneumothorax, 541
  in combat, 813
  defined, 491
  management of, 489–490
  signs of, 487
Terbutaline, action, effects, contraindications, administration, 265t
Terminology
  directional, 88, 89t, 90
  medical, 87–88
Testes, 105, 105
  defined, 111
Thermoregulation, aging changes in, 591
Thienbenzodiazepine, indications and trade names for, 363t
Thioxanthenes, indications and trade names for, 363t
Third service, public, characteristics of, 10
Thirst response in elderly, 591
Thoracic cage, bony stability of, 483
Thoracic cavity, 106, 182, 183
  defined, 211
  needle decompression of, 489–490, 490
Thoracic injuries; *see also* Chest trauma
  in children, 628
Thoracic pressure, increased, 487, 487
Thoracic vertebrae, structure and function of, 92, 94
Thoracic wall, lungs and, 483–484
Thorax
  anatomy of, 477, 480
  compression injuries of, 415, 415–416
  defined, 111
  penetrating trauma to, 434, 435
  shear force injuries to, 416, 416
  structure and function of, 92–93
Thought content, assessment of, 360
Thready, defined, 175
Thready pulse, 166
Thrombocytes, 100
Thyroid cartilage, 97, 181
  defined, 211
TIA; *see* Transient ischemic attack
Tibia, 93, 96
  defined, 111
Tibial artery
  anatomy of, 292
  defined, 304
Tidal volume, 98
  assessment of, 185
  defined, 110, 211

Tiered response system
  characteristics of, 9
  defined, 19
Time dependent medical problems, defined, 685
Tinnitus
  characteristics of, 591
  defined, 603
Tissue, subcutaneous
  defined, 111
  structure and function of, 103
Tongue
  intubation and, 215, 216
  in unconscious patient, 217
Tonic-clonic seizure, 329
  defined, 333
Tourniquet
  in care under fire, 812
  for controlling bleeding, 453
  defined, 455
  in field care, 813
Toxic emergencies, 343–354; *see also* Poisoning
Toxin
  from bites/stings, 578
  defined, 581
Trachea, 96, 181, 182
  assessing position of, 130
  defined, 111, 211, 636
  deviation of, 486
Tracheostomy, 192, 193
  for children, 618
  defined, 211, 636
  uses of, 646, 646
Traction splints, 550–551, 551, 554–556
Trade names, 259
  defined, 267
Training; *see also* Continuing education; Education
  about OSHA standards, 79
  diagnosis- *versus* assessment-based, 14
  EMS, 11–13
  medical director and, 47–48
  philosophies of, 45
Transfers
  to ambulance, 738–739
  bed to stretcher, of supine patient, 671–672, 672
  patient, 24, 26
Transfusions
  blood, 158
  disease transmission by, 77
Transient ischemic attack, 328–329
  defined, 333
Transplant recipients, risk of infection in, 645
Transport in rescue operations, 765
Transportation
  appropriate, 249
  issues in, 680
  patient, 24, 26
  of patient in shock, 169–173
  safety in, 26

Trauma; *see also* Abdominal trauma; Blunt
    trauma; Chest trauma; Head
    trauma; Musculoskeletal trauma;
    Penetrating trauma; Spinal trauma
  algorithm for assessing, 400, 440
  altered mental status due to, 330
  from blast injuries, 427–428, *428*
  deaths due to, 401
  definitions pertaining to, 401
  in elderly, 596–597
  from falls, *425*, 425–426, *426*
  kinematics of, 399–436
  mechanism of, 120
  multisystem, 546
  pediatric, 622–630
    assessment of, 623
    of chest/abdomen, 628
    of head, 623–624
    immobilization devices for, *626*,
        626–628, *627*
    prevention of, 622
    spinal, 624–626
    unique characteristics of, 622–623
  phases of, 401–402
  during pregnancy, 390–391
  rapid focused physical exam in, 127–133,
      128
  shock due to, 168
  from sports injuries, 426–427, *427*
  study of, 401
Trauma center
  defined, 252
  transportation to, 249
Trauma scene, evaluation of, 244
Trauma score
  pediatric, 706
    defined, 714
  revised, 706
Treatment
  consent for, 33–35
  at crime scene, 37
  without patient consent, 36
Trench collapse, 763
Trendelenburg position, 170, *170*
  defined, 175
Triage
  defined, 148, 246–247, 789, 822
  in disasters, 779–781
  in military EMS, 820–821
  during scene survey, 120
Tricuspid valve, 156
  defined, 175
Tricyclic antidepressants, indications and
    trade names for, 363*t*
Tridil; *see* Nitroglycerin
Trimester, defined, 375, 395
Tubal pregnancy, 375
  defined, 395
Tuberculosis
  in prehospital setting, 78*t*
  resistant strains of, 83
  testing for, 83
Tumble, 406
  defined, 437

Tunnels, response route and, 735
Twisting force, example of, 536
Two-person stretcher, defined, 685

U

UHF band, defined, 700
UHF band frequencies, 689–690
Ulcers
  as complication of abdominal trauma, 497
  defined, 503
Ulna, 93, *95*
  defined, 111
Umbilical arteries, 375
  defined, 395
Umbilical cord
  anatomy/physiology of, 375
  cutting, 384, *385*
  defined, 395
Umbilical vein, 375
  defined, 395
Umbilicus, 374
  defined, 395
U. S. Department of Transportation
  Emergency Response Guidebook of, 56
  first-responder training by, 5–6
  HAZMAT guidelines of, 783
Universal precautions, 55; *see also* Body
    substance isolation
Upper extremities, bones of, 93, *95*
Urban search and rescue
  defined, 758
  interface with, 754–755
Ureters, 104, *104*
  defined, 111
Urethra, 104, *104*
  defined, 111
Urgent moves, 670
  defined, 685
Urination, increased frequency of, 326
Urticaria
  cause and characteristics, 337, *339*
  defined, 342
Uterus
  anatomy/physiology of, 375
  defined, 395
  postpartum bleeding from, 385, *385*
  rupture of
    bleeding due to, 380
    defined, 395
    symptoms and care, 379*t*
Uvula
  anatomy of, 215, *215*
  defined, 233

V

Vaccination
  defined, 84
  mechanism of, 83
Vagal-vagal response, 162
Vagina
  anatomy of, 375
  defined, 395
Vaginal opening, 375
  defined, 395

Vagus nerve stimulator, 647
Vallecula, 215, *216*
  defined, 233
Valves, cardiac, 155–156
  damage to, 157
Vasoconstriction
  defined, 157, 175
  in shock, 163
Vasodilation, defined, 157, 175
Vasodilator
  defined, 342
  histamine as, 337
Vegetative state, permanent, defined, 309,
    321
Vehicle rescue incidents, 763–770
  accessing patient in, 768
  arrival and size-up, *766*, 766–767, *767*
  categories of, 765
  disentanglement process in, 768–769,
      769
  postaccident analysis, 770
  preparation for, 765
  removal process in, 769–770
  response to, 766
  securing scene, 770
  stabilization in, 767, *768*
  transport in, 770
Veins, 99, 100, *100*
  anatomy of, 292
  defined, 111, 175, 304
  pulmonary, 157
    defined, 304
  structure and function of, 157
Velocity, 403
  defined, 437
Venae cavae, 100, *100*, 291, *292*, *294*
  defined, 111, 304
Venom, injection of, 346
Ventilation
  agonal, 186, 279–280
    defined, 209, 286
  artificial *versus* assisted, 188
  assessing, 140, 190–191
  assisted, 188–194, 193–194
    with airway adjuncts, 188–189
  bag-valve-mask, pediatric, *616*, 616–617
  defined, 148, 274, 482, 491
  injuries affecting, 477
  versus intubation, 215
    in apneic patient, 219
  minute, 185
  versus respiration, 273–274
  structures involved in, 483–486
Ventilators
  automated transport, 229–230, *230*
    defined, 233
  demand valve, 196
  flow-restricted oxygen-powered,
      191–192, *192*, 196
Ventilatory arrest, 279
  defined, 287
Ventilatory character
  assessing, 140
  defined, 148

Ventilatory depth
  assessing, 140, 279
  defined, 148
Ventilatory quality, 98
  assessment of, 184
Ventilatory rate, 482
  assessment of, 122, 140, 184, 281
  defined, 111, 148
  management of, 281
  normal, 98, 99t
  physiology of, 279
  during pregnancy, 391
  versus respiratory rate, 180
  during shock, 165–166, 166, 169
Ventilatory rhythm, 98
  assessment of, 140, 184, 279
  defined, 148
Ventolin; *see* Albuterol
Ventricles, 99, 155, 291, *292*
  defined, 111, 175, 304
Ventricular fibrillation
  cardiac arrest due to, 308
  coarse *versus* fine, *312*
  defined, 304, 321
  management of, 300–301
  pathophysiology of, 293–294, *295*
Ventricular tachycardia
  defined, 304
  pathophysiology of, 294, *295*
Venules, 157
  anatomy of, *292*
  defined, 175, 304
Vertebrae, *509*
  defined, 111, 528
  function of, 508
  structure and function of, 92, *94*
Vertebral column
  defined, 437
  trauma to, 408–409
Vertebral disks, dehydration of, 587
Vesicants, characteristics of, 818
Vest devices for pediatric patient, 628

VHF high band, defined, 700
VHF high band frequencies, 689
VHF low band, defined, 700
VHF low band frequencies, 689
Violence, potential, with behavioral
  emergencies, 369
Violent scene, 59
Visceral pleura, 98, *98*
  defined, 111
Vision, aging and, 590, 591
Visual impairment, characteristics of, 643
Vital capacity, aging and, 588
Vital signs
  assessing, 144
  baseline, 137
  detailed physical exam of, 137
  normal pediatric values, 607, 611, 611t
  rapid focused physical exam of
    with medical conditions, 135
    in trauma, 132–133
  review of, 145
Vocal cords, 96, 215, *216*
  defined, 111
Volume, defined, 175
Voluntary muscles, defined, 111
Volvulus in elderly, 599

W

Water immersion, rescue from, 577
Water-related emergencies, 577–578
  rescue from, 763
Weapons
  high-energy, 430–432, *432*
    defined, 437
  low-energy, 429–430
    defined, 437
  of mass destruction, 815–820
    biologic warfare, 816–819
      anthrax, 817
      characteristics of, 816, 817
      dissemination of, 816–817
    chemical warfare, 817–819

Weapons—cont'd
  of mass destruction—cont'd
    decontamination procedures, 819–820
    defined, 822
    nuclear, 816
    types of, 815
  medium-energy, 430, *431*
    defined, 437
Wedge cribbing, 767
  defined, 772
Wheeled stretcher, 672–673, *673*
  moving guidelines, 673
Wheezing
  characteristics of, 184
  defined, 211, 287
  in respiratory emergencies, 282
White blood cells, 100, 295
  defined, 304
  types of, 158
Wilderness, rescue in, 763
Wilderness medicine, interface with, 755
Wind, body temperature and, 565
Windchill
  calculation of, 564t
  defined, 581
  effects of, 565
Working diagnosis, 273
Workplace, infection control in, 78–79
Wounds
  ambulance equipment for, 729
  penetrating/puncture
    characteristics of, 445, *446*
    defined, 455

X

Xiphoid process, 93
  defined, 111, 233

Z

Zygomatic bones, 91
  defined, 111

A Valuable Source of Information Delivered To You Each Month...

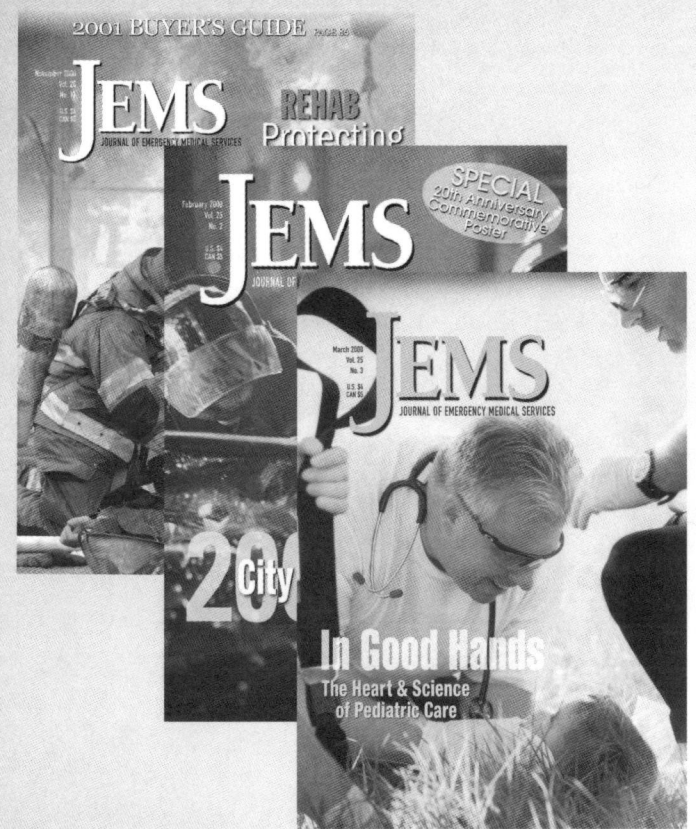

Vital Content Every Month:
Solid Clinical Features
Timely News Reporting
Continuing Education

Monthly Features:
Case of the Month
Hands On
Research Review
Tricks of the Trade

Annual Special Issues:
Resource Directory
Buyer's Guide
Salary Survey
Education/Careers

Special Student Subscription Offer!

Don't miss another month.
Subscribe Today!
(888) 456-5367

❏ **Yes!** Start my trial subscription to JEMS. If I like it, I'll pay just
❏ $15.77 for 9 months (only $1.75 per issue)
❏ $19.97 for 12 months (only $1.66 per issue)

JEMS

If I don't like it, I'll write "cancel" on the invoice and owe nothing. The first issue is mine to keep with no obligation.

Name _____
Title _____
Organization _____
Address _____
City _____ State _____ Zip _____
Phone ( ) _____
Fax ( ) _____
Email _____
We occasionally send promotions on products and services via email. If you do not wish to receive these messages, please check here ❏

❏ Bill me
❏ Payment enclosed
Charge my: ❏ VISA ❏ MasterCard ❏ Discover ❏ AMEX
Exp. Date ___ / ___ Card# _____
Signature _____

Occupation/Position
❏ A. Physician
❏ B. Nurse/Inst./Coord.
❏ C. Administrator/Supervisor
❏ D. Paramed./EMT-I/EMT-D
❏ E. EMT (Basic, 1st Resp.)
❏ F. Other _____ (Please Specify)

Employer/Affiliation
❏ 1. Hospital
❏ 2. Private Ambulance
❏ 3. Fire Dept./Rescue Squad
❏ 4. Third Serv./Mun. Agency
❏ 5. Industrial Commercial
❏ 6. Other _____ (Please Specify)

Canada please add $18 per year for postage. All other foreign please add $20 per year for surface mail postage; add $70 per year for air mail postage. Subscriptions must be paid in U.S. funds. Please allow 6-8 weeks for delivery of first issue.
*NEW SUBSCRIBERS ONLY

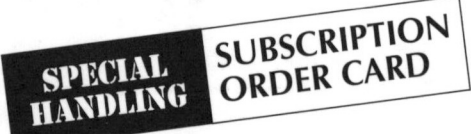

NO POSTAGE
NECESSARY
IF MAILED
IN THE
UNITED STATES

BUSINESS REPLY MAIL
FIRST-CLASS MAIL   PERMIT NO 806   CARLSBAD CA

POSTAGE WILL BE PAID BY ADDRESSEE

JEMS
PO BOX 469010
ESCONDIDO CA 92046-9976